A BIBLIOGRAPHY OF NURSING LITERATURE

THE HOLDINGS OF THE ROYAL COLLEGE OF NURSING
1976 — 1980

Edited and compiled by Frances Walsh

The Library Association

London

© The Royal College of Nursing 1986. Published by Library Association Publishing
Limited, 7 Ridgmount Street, London WC1E 7AE and printed and bound in Great
Britain at The University Press, Cambridge. Phototypeset by
Library Association Publishing Limited, London.

First published 1986

British Library Cataloguing in Publication Data

A Bibliography of nursing literature :
  holdings of the Royal College of Nursing,
  London 1976—80.
  Vol. 4
  1. Nursing——Bibliography
  I. Walsh, Frances II. Royal College of Nursing
  016.61073   Z6675.N7

ISBN 0-85365-746-7

A BIBLIOGRAPHY OF NURSING LITERATURE 1976—1980

8 7 0 13 4 1 / W 4 13

CONTENTS

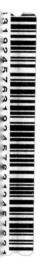

ACKNOWLEDGEMENTS

The work of producing the *Nursing Bibliography* on which this volume is based was carried out by members of staff of the Royal College of Nursing Library. Their efforts make this project possible and I am grateful to them for their hard work and commitment. Thanks are especially due to Patricia Bowen who was responsible for the initial work on the *Bibliography* and without whose contribution the work would not have been completed.

Frances M Walsh
Formerly Librarian
Royal College of Nursing

INTRODUCTION

Background
This volume is part of the programme of bibliographical work undertaken by the Library of the Royal College of Nursing as one of its most important functions.

It is a continuation of the *Bibliography of nursing literature 1859—1960* and *1961—1970*, compiled by Miss A M C Thompson, Librarian of the College from 1948 to 1968, and published in two volumes by the Library Association in 1968 and 1974.

This work is a revised cumulation of *Nursing Bibliography*, the monthly current awareness service issued since 1972 by the College Library, which presents a selection of English language material received in the Library.

Scope and content
The following are included:

(a) Books and monographs, including textbooks, both English and American and others published in the English-speaking world.

(b) Official publications, mainly United Kingdom government reports, but also publications of international organizations, such as the World Health Organization.

(c) Reports and pamphlets of various organizations, including nursing and medical organizations, health authorities and patients' groups. These include policy documents, research reports and other miscellaneous items.

(d) United Kingdom theses and dissertations, held in the Steinberg Collection of Nursing Research, a collection within the Royal College of Nursing Library.

Principles of selection
These follow the principles adopted by the *Nursing Bibliography* and take into account the existence of other sources such as *International Nursing Index*.

United Kingdom nursing literature. This has been extensively indexed except for very brief or ephemeral items. Even these have occasionally been included if they are significant or refer to a topic on which little has been written.

Overseas countries. The emphasis of the *Bibliography* is on nursing in the United Kingdom, but a selection of overseas material has been included, mostly from the United States and Commonwealth countries. If general in nature this has been placed in List 28, Nursing and health overseas, but items relating to specific subjects have been put within that subject. They have been listed in a separate sequence for convenience if the number of items has justified this.

Other subject fields. Items are included to show the development of nursing in the context of other trends and influences.

The three main areas are:

(a) Health service developments, mainly in the United Kingdom. These include the reorganization of the National Health Service, industrial relations in the health service and the development of community and occupational health services.

(b) The work of other professions, especially doctors, therapists and social workers, where it relates to the work of the nurse.

(c) Literature written from the patient's point of view, as this is of great concern to the nurse and is sometimes directed at both nurse and patient.

Arrangement
Because of the number of items, a broad classified arrangement has been used in preference to the alphabetical subject arrangement of the *Nursing*

Bibliography. Ninety-nine topics have been listed within fourteen broad subject groups. A comprehensive subject index is included.

As far as possible, the arrangement follows that of the previous volume, but in some cases, where new subjects have emerged or previous ones expanded, adjustments have been made to the numbering of individual subject lists.

SUBJECT LISTINGS

SUBJECT INDEX

THE
BIBLIOGRAPHY

NURSING AS A PROFESSION

1 BIBLIOGRAPHY AND REFERENCE BOOKS

a BIBLIOGRAPHIES

1 American Journal of Nursing Books of the year. Selected by nursing experts as significant reading for nurses. American Journal of Nursing, 76 (1), Jan 1976, 76-87.

2 Brandon, A.N. and Hill, D.R. Selected list of nursing books and journals. (Primarily of U.S. origin.) Nursing Outlook, 27 (10), Oct 1979, 672-680.

3 British Council British medical periodicals: a select and annotated list. 5th ed. British Council, 1977.

4 British Council Community health including community medicine, public health and social services: a select list of books, periodicals and non-book materials. British Council, 1977.

5 Georgetown University Medical Center Dahlgren Memorial Library Bibliography of nursing monographs, 1970-1978. Washington, D.C.: the Library, 1978.

6 Grosvenor, P. Nursing in theory 1972-1977. (Literature review reprinted from British Book News Feb 1978.) Nursing Times, 74, 27 Jul 1978, Occ. papers, 81-84; 3 Aug 1978, Occ. papers, 85-87.

7 Library Association Medical Section Books and periodicals for medical libraries in hospitals. 5th ed. Library Association, 1978.

b DICTIONARIES AND DIRECTORIES

1 Baillière's nurses' dictionary 19th ed. revised by Pamela M. Jeffries. Baillière Tindall, 1979.

2 Edwards, P. Know your nursing English. Hutchinson, 1979.

3 Lancaster, A. Nursing and midwifery sourcebook. Allen and Unwin; Beaconsfield: Beaconsfield Publishers, 1979.

4 McGraw-Hill nursing dictionary. New York: McGraw-Hill, 1979.

5 Miller, B.F. and Keane, C.B. Encyclopedia and dictionary of medicine, nursing and allied health. 2nd ed. Philadelphia: Saunders, 1978.

6 Morten, Honnor, compiler The nurse's dictionary; revised by Jean Cunningham. 28th ed. Faber, 1976. 29th ed. 1980.

7 Parkinson, J. English for doctors and nurses. 2nd ed. Evans, 1980.

8 Roper, N. compiler Nurses dictionary. 15th ed. Churchill Livingstone, 1978.

9 Roper, N. editor Pocket medical dictionary. 13th ed. Churchill Livingstone, 1978.

c INFORMATION NEEDS AND RESOURCES

1 American Nurses' Association Reference resources for research and continuing education in nursing. ANA, 1977.

2 Binger, J.L. and Huntsman, A.J. Keeping up: the staff development educator and the professional literature. (Survey of use of libraries, indexes and journals.) Nursing Education, 4 (3), May/Jun 1979, 19-22.

3 Clancy, H.G. The literature review: its structure and function. British Journal of Occupational Therapy, 43 (6), Jun 1980, 206-208.

4 Clark, J.M. and Stodulski, A.H. How to find out: a guide to searching the nursing literature. Nursing Times, 74, 23 Feb 1978. Occ. Papers, 21-23.

5 Crawford, M.L. Unique job eases retirement. (Author's work as indexer for Cumulative Index to Allied Health Literature, with description of it.) AORN Journal, 27 (4), Mar 1978, 754, 756, 758.

6 Davis, B. Information please! (Work of the Study Group on Information for Nurses.) Nursing Times, 76, 19 Jun 1980, 1109.

7 Ferguson, C.K. Reading skills versus success in nursing school. (Advice on helping students with poor reading ability.) Journal of Nursing Education, 18 (3), Mar 1979, 6-12.

8 Glatt, C.R. How your hospital library can help you keep up in nursing. (Reference sources including periodical indexes.) American Journal of Nursing, 78 (4), Apr 1978, 642-644.

9 Godbolt, S. Medical information services in Britain. British Medicine, 7 (3), Mar 1978, i-xi.

10 Going, M. Should community nurses be informed? (With list of basic information sources compiled by M. Going and K. Carter, p.160-161) Nursing Times, 75, 14 Jun 1979. Community Outlook, 157-158.

11 Interagency Council on Library Resources for Nursing Reference sources for nursing. Nursing Outlook, 24 (5), May 1976, 317-322; 26 (5), May 1978, 325-329.

12 Magrill, D. Information at the touch of a button. (Computerised retrieval systems, including Medline and BLAISE.) New Scientist, 77, 12 Jan 1978, 76-79.

13 Morton, L.T. editor Use of medical literature. 2nd ed. Butterworth, 1977. (Information sources for research and development series.)

14 Myco, F. Nursing research information: are nurse educators and practitioners seeking it out? (Survey of nurses' use of nursing journals and libraries and views on its inclusion in course curricula). Journal of Advanced Nursing, 5 (6), Nov 1980, 637-646.

15 Rajecki, A.A. and Muntz, M.L. An introduction to medical/nursing libraries and available resource tools. (Includes indexes and advice on literature searching.) Nursing Forum, 17 (1), 1978, 103-112.

16 Saba, V.K. and Skapik, K.A. Nursing Information Center. (New computerised centre which is part of the National Health Planning Information Center.) American Journal of Nursing, 79 (1), Jan 1979, 86-87.

17 Sparks, S.M. Avline for nursing education and research. (Computerised on-line data base of audio-visual material operated by National Library of Medicine.) Nursing Outlook, 27 (11), Nov 1979, 733-737.

18 Sparks, S.M. Letting the computer do the work. (Automated information retrieval systems including Medline.) American Journal of Nursing, 78 (4), Apr 1978, 645-647.

19 Strauch, K.P. and Brundage, D.J. Guide to library resources for nursing. New York: Appleton-Century-Crofts, 1980.

20 Tobiason, S.J. The indexes to nursing literature. (Advice on literature searching.) Supervisor Nurse, 9 (1), Jan 1978, 23, 25.

21 Tobiason, S.J. Making the library work for you. (Advice on American indexes including computerised indexes and recent nursing textbooks.) AORN Journal, 30 (3), Sep 1979, 466, 468, 470, 472, 474, 476, 478, 482, 487-488.

22 Tompkins, E.S. Get wise, organise. (Detailed advice on organising the collection of material for thesis writing.) Nursing Research, 26 (6), Nov/Dec 1977, 407.

23 Townsend, I. Information retrieval. (Letter describing the course held at the Newcastle upon Tyne Polytechnic.) Nursing Mirror, 143 (13), 23 Sep 1976, 43.

24 University of Sheffield Centre for Research on User Studies Pilot survey of the information needs of nursing staff within the central district of Sheffield. Sheffield: The Centre, 1978.

25 Welch, J. Computerised information retrieval services in a teaching hospital. (Wessex Medical Library of the University of Southampton.) British Medical Journal, 280, 14 Jun 1980, 1433-1434.

d NURSING LITERATURE

1 Ashton, K. To every nurse's aid. (150 years of Baillière Tindall.) Nursing Times, 72, 26 Feb 1976, 288-289.

2 Ball, D. We've been running on the spot for twenty-five glorious years. (Health and Social Service Journal since 1952.) Health and Social Service Journal, 87, 3 Jun 1977, 884-887.

3 Binger, J.L. Writing for publication: a survey of nursing journal editors. (Comments on nurses' writing skills and suggestions for improving writing.) Journal of Nursing Administration, 9 (1), Jan 1979, 50-52.

4 Binger, J.L. and Jensen, L.M. Lippincott's guide to nursing literature: a handbook for students, writers, and researchers. Philadelphia: Lippincott, 1980.

5 British Medical Journal Vancouver style. (And BMJ change in volume numbering.) British Medical Journal, 280, 5 Jan 1980, 3.

6 Brosnan, J. and Kovalesky, A. Perishing while publishing. (Views of authors and editors.) Nursing Outlook, 28 (11), Nov 1980, 688-690.

7 Burgett, G.L. Writing an article for a nursing journal. Journal of Practical Nursing, 30 (11), Nov/Dec 1980, 43, 44, 55.

8 Burkhalter, P. So you want to write! (The techniques of organising written work including literature surveys.) Supervisor Nurse, 7 (6), Jun 1976, 54-56.

9 Canadian Nurse A capsule history of your journal. (1905-1979). Canadian Nurse, 76 (3), Mar 1980, 20-21.

10 Carbary, L.J. Keep a nursing and medical reference library. (Advice to nurses on keeping personal file of literature and information.) Journal of Nursing Care, 12 (10), Oct 1979, 8-10.

11 Carnegie, M.E. The journal's contribution to research in nursing. (Contribution of the American Journal of Nursing from 1900-1952.) Nursing Research, 24 (6), Nov-Dec 1975, 403.

12 Chapman, C. Plagiarism — a form of stealing. (How to quote references when writing essays or articles.) Nursing Times, 76, 3 Jul 1980, 1160.

13 Claus, K.E. and Binger, J.L. How directors of nursing service use and share the nursing literature. (Survey.) Journal of Nursing Administration, 8 (11), Nov 1978, 17-21.

14 Community Outlook Fact sheet: getting through. (Advice on writing for newspapers and getting through to TV.) Nursing Times, 74, 12 Jan 1978. Community Outlook 12-13.

15 Crawford, C.O. On using words. (Hints on style in writing essays.) New Zealand Nursing Journal, 70 (4), Apr 1977, 8-10.

16 Creditor, H. Why don't nurses publish? Journal of Community Nursing, 1 (5), Nov 1977, 24.

17 Dopson, L. Celebrating 75 years. (Of the Nursing Times, including previous editors 933-936.) Nursing Times, 76, 22 May 1980, 923-936.

18 Driscoll, J. 1949-1957: AORN in retrospect. AORN Journal, 24 (1), Jul 1976, 140, 142, 146, 148.

19 Dunn, A. Confessions of an editor. Nursing Times, 76, 22 May 1980, 912-914.

20 Ellis, H. The art (or science) of book reviewing. British Medical Journal, 280, 19 Apr 1980, 1079-1080.

21 Ellis, R. Fallibilities, fragments, and frames. (Critique of articles on medical-surgical nursing in Nursing Research during the last 25 years.) Nursing Research, 26 (3), May/Jun 1977, 177-182.

22 Fitton, J.M. Why don't nurses read? Nursing Times, 76, 3 Jul 1980, 1159-1160.

23 Health Trends Health trends; readership survey (including senior nursing officers.) Health Trends, 1 (8), Feb 1976, 5.

24 Health Visitor Golden anniversary issue. (Three articles and editorial.) Health Visitor, 50 (10), Oct 1977, 323-330.

25 Henderson, V. Professional writing. (Encouragement to nurses to write for their professional journals.) Nursing Mirror, 146, 11 May 1978, 15-18.

26 Hodgman, E.C. On writing and writing workshops. Nursing Outlook, 28 (6), Jun 1980, 366-371.

27 Hospital and Health Services Review From gazette to review 1904-1979. (History of journal.) Hospital and Health Services Review, 76 (1), Jan 1980, 19-22. Editorial to mark 75th anniversary 1-2.

28 International Steering Committee of Medical Editors Uniform requirements for manuscripts submitted to biomedical journals. British Medical Journal, 1, 1979, 505-572.

29 James, P.D. With crime in mind. P.D. James. (Author of 'Shroud for a Nightingale'.) British Medical Journal, 281, 9 Aug 1980, 442-443.

30 Kaye (pseud) Tips for writers. Organising your papers and various formats. (Articles for nursing publications.) Journal of Continuing Education in Nursing, 8 (1), Mar-Apr 1977, 45-49.

31 Kolin, P.C. and Kolin, J.L. Professional writing for nurses in education, practice and research. St. Louis: Mosby, 1980.

32 LIPPINCOTT initiates award to mark 100 years of publishing for nurses. (Includes some information on early nursing textbooks.) American Journal of Nursing, 78 (6), Jun 1978, 982.

33 Longmore, J.M. Keeping up to date. (Describes system of constructing medical scrapbook of journal articles.) British Medical Journal, 1, 9 Jun 1979, 1547-1548.

34 Midwives Chronicle Ninety years of publication. (Outline of its history from 1887.) Midwives Chronicle, 90, Jun 1977, 136-141.

35 Nursing Mirror 90th anniversary issue. Nursing Mirror, 146, 13 Apr 1978, 6-68.

36 Nursing Research A quarter century of trial and editors; The people who made Nursing Research possible. (Outline of development of the Journal under five editors.) Nursing Research, 26 (3), May/Jun 1977, 228-229.

37 Nursing Times Celebrating 75 years. Nursing Times, 76, 22 May 1980, 903-936; Supplement 1-30.

38 Nursing Times How to write for publication. (Four articles on nursing care studies, research articles, style and grammar and the process of getting an article published.) Nursing Times, 74, 5 Oct 1978, 1632-1636.

39 Nuttall, P. A ride on the nursing roundabout. (Nursing Times, 1960-1980.) Nursing Times, 76, 22 May 1980, 918-919.

40 Olumide, F. Writing for scholarly journals — an editor's experience. Nigerian Nurse, 11 (2), Apr/Jun 1979, 13-15.

41 Perry, S.E. The trials and tribulations of a would-be author. (Advice on writing articles for journals.) Supervisor Nurse, 9 (1), Jan 1978, 13-16.

42 Powell, S.R. and others Writing for publication: a group approach. Nursing Outlook, 27 (11), Nov 1979, 729-732.

43 Schorr, T.M. On the subject of writing. (Editorial on writing style.) American Journal of Nursing, 77 (6), Jun 1977, 967.

44 Seager, C.P. Journal of Advanced Nursing. (Review of Vol.1, no.1, of Journal of Advanced Nursing.) Medical Education, 10 (4), Jul 1976, 330-331.

45 Stuart, G.W. and others Getting a book published. (Four nurses write a textbook.) Nursing Outlook, 25 (5), May 1977, 316-318.

46 Ward, M.J. Research Q and A. A. I'm preparing my first article for publication. Are there special suggestions that might be helpful? Nursing Research, 29 (4), Jul/Aug 1980, 263.

47 Watkin, B. Lord High Executioner. (Comments on book reviewing.) Nursing Mirror, 143, 5 Aug 1976, 42.

48 Williams, M. Writers' workshop for nurses. (Report on workshop at King's Fund Centre.) NATNews, 17 (9), Sep 1980, 16.

49 Young, P. History of Nursing Mirror. Nursing Mirror, 146, 13 Apr 1978, 11-14.

50 Young, Pat A valediction. Last editorial of Nursing Mirror Editor. Nursing Mirror, 147, 14 Sep 1978, 1.

e LIBRARIES

1 Bunch, Antonia J. Hospital and medical libraries in Scotland: an historical and sociological study. Glasgow: Scottish Library Association, 1975.

2 Caffarel, A. Classification of clinical nursing texts: a new approach. (Using a modification of NLM classification.) Bulletin of the Medical Library Association, 66 (1), Jan 1978, 52-55.

3 Cannon, G. Resource centre of distinction. (Work of the King's Fund Centre.) Nursing Focus, 1 (5), Jan 1980, 192-193.

4 Cumming, Eileen E. compiler Hospital and welfare library services: an international bibliography. Library Association, 1977.

5 Belleh, G.S. Libraries and nursing objectives. (Review of development of nursing libraries with special reference to Nigeria.) Nigerian Nurse, 9 (2), Apr/Jun 1977, 32-36.

6 Bond, S. Sources and resources. (New library services for nurses operated by Northern RHA and Newcastle Polytechnic.) Nursing Times, 76, 19 Jun 1980, 1106-1109. See also item in Health and Social Services Journal, 90, 1 Feb 1980, 144-145.

7 Fothergill, P. Library procedures in schools of nursing. Nursing Times, 73, 20 Jan 1977, 103-105; 27 Jan 1977, 140-141.

8 Gann, R. Displays in health service libraries. (With reference to Wessex Regional Library and Information Service.) Nursing Times, 75, 18 Jan 1979, 120-123.

9 Graves, K.J. and Dunavent, K.M. Hospital library consortia: a vital component of hospital-wide education. (Cooperative systems.) Journal of Continuing Education in Nursing, 9 (5), Sep/Oct 1978, 22-25.

10 Henderson, Virginia Awareness of library resources: a characteristic of professional workers, an essential in research and continuing education *in* American Nurses' Association Reference resources for research and continuing education in nursing... ANA, 1977.

11 Hodge, H.F. Service from the library. (Letter from librarian of Broadgreen Medical Library, Liverpool describing the service she gives to nurses.) Nursing Times, 75, 20/27 Dec 1979, 2210.

12 Library Association Guidelines for library provision in the health service: a consultative document. 2nd ed. The Association, 1980.

13 Library Association Medical Section Directory of medical libraries in the British Isles. 4th ed. The Association, 1976.

14 Library Association Medical Section Regional medical library systems: papers given at the annual conference... Liverpool, 10-13 Sep 1976. The Association, 1977.

15 Lindsay, M. Lack of library services for nurses. (Letter.) Nursing Times, 76, 24 Jan 1980, 160.

16 Lindsay, M. Shelving a learner's problem. (Library service for nurses at St. George's Hospital, London.) Nursing Mirror, 151, 10 Jul 1980, 30.

17 McNair, L. and Davis, S.M. Library facilities. (Letter about library in Nightingale School, St. Thomas's Hospital.) Nursing Times, 76, 7 Feb 1980, 250.

18 Matthews, D.A. The WILSH working party: an experiment in collaboration. (To examine the provision of NHS library service in Wales—Welsh Information and Library Services for Health.) Health and Social Service Journal, 86, 14 Feb 1976, 302.

19 Matthews, D.A. and Picken, F.M. Medical librarianship. Clive Bingley, 1979. (Outlines of modern librarianship, 12).

20 Morton, L.T. How to use a medical library. 6th ed. Heinemann, 1979.

21 National Health Service Regional Librarians Group Census of staff providing library services to NHS personnel, April 1978. The Author, 1978.

22 National Health Service Regional Librarians Group Make libraries an open book plead experts. (Evidence of Regional Librarians Group to the Royal Commission on the NHS.) Nursing Mirror, 144, 5 May 1977, 37.

23 National Library of Medicine National Library of Medicine classification: a scheme for the shelf arrangement of books in the field of medicine and its related sciences. 4th ed. Bethesda, Md.: U.S. Dept. of Health, Education and Welfare, 1978.

24 Olaleye, C.A. The organisation and administration of libraries including library resources. Nigerian Nurse, 10 (2), Apr/Jun 1978, 32-36.

25 Pattinson, Michael Library and information services to the Cheshire Area Health Authority. Cheshire AHA, 1975.

26 Pentelow, G.M. A shush of librarians. (Work of medical librarians.) British Medical Journal, 1, 21 Apr 1979, 1055-1057.

27 Phinney, Eleanor, editor The librarian and the patient: an introduction to library services for patients in health care institutions. Chicago: American Library Association, 1977.

28 Picciano, J.L. Continuing information, continuing education. (Advice on using libraries and literature, with some reference to the American system of regional medical libraries.) American Journal of Maternal Child Nursing, 3 (5), Sep/Oct 1978, 269, 307-308.

29 Robinson, W. The new King's Fund Centre. (Building, functions and staff.) Nursing Mirror, 145, 17 Nov 1977, 7-9.

30 Roth, B.G. Health information for patients: the hospital library's role. Bulletin of the Medical Library Association, 66 (1), Jan 1978, 14-18.

31 Shanks, K. Warning: library usage may be habit forming. (With reference to its role in continuing education.) Journal of Continuing Education in Nursing, 10 (2), Mar/Apr 1979, 19-21.

32 Slater, A. Nursing librarians. (Letter from spokesman for North Western Librarians' Group.) Nursing Times, 74, 2 Nov 1978, 1810.

33 Smith, B. British Library. Lending Division and research abroad. Nursing Mirror, 142, 22 Jan 1976, 67-68.

34 Stewart, C.C. Your hospital library—an awakening giant. Hospital Topics, 53 (3), May/Jun 1975, 6, 46-47.

35 Tabor, R.B. Professional knowledge and the nurse. (Need for better library services for nurses.) Nursing Times, 75, 15 Nov 1979, 1983-1984.

36 Van Gieson, W.R. The hospital library in transition. (New roles for library serving staff of all disciplines.) Hospital Progress, 59 (6), Jun 1978, 66-69.

37 Wessex Regional Library and Information Service Libraries for health: the Wessex experience. Edited by R.B. Tabor. Southampton: WRLIS, 1978.

38 Yeoh, J.W. The planning stages of building a new or remodeled hospital library. Hospital Topics, 58 (2), Mar/Apr 1980, 53-54, 10.

2　BIOGRAPHY

1 Brian, V.A. The man behind the name. Nursing Times, 72.
Thomas Addison. 19 Aug 1976, 1281.
Richard Bright. 9 Dec 1976, 1937.
Abraham Colles. 14 Oct 1976, 1604.
Harvey Cushing. 10 Mar 1977, 356.
Robert Graves. 25 Nov 1976, 1855.
Thomas Hodgkin. 16 Sep 1976, 1451.
James Parkinson. 5 Aug 1976, 1201.

2 Dopson, L. Faces for the 80s. (Profiles of six nurses who may be leaders of their fields of nursing in the 1980s.) Nursing Times, 76, 3 Jan 1980, 19-21.

3 Abel-Smith, B. The Secretary of State's special adviser. (Professor Brian Abel-Smith.) Lancet, 1, 4 Feb 1978, 287-288.

4 Altschul, A.T. Interview. Annie T. Altschul. The recently appointed professor of nursing studies at the University of Edinburgh talks to Nursing Times, 73, 13 Jan 1977, 50-51.

5 ANDERSON, E.G. Evans, H. Elizabeth Garrett Anderson: a 'first' in medicine. (First woman to qualify as a doctor in Britain.) Nursing Mirror, 146, 22 Jun 1978, 7-8.

6 ANSTEY, O. Dunn, A. and Dopson, L. Olive Anstey—international nurse. (Interview with the president of the International Council of Nurses, Australia's Olive Anstey, MBE, during the Rcn congress last month in Guernsey.) Nursing Times, 75, 24 May 1979, 862-863.

7 ASHTON, R. Allen, M. Weathering the storm. (Profile of Ruth Ashton, new General Secretary of the RCM.) Nursing Mirror, 150, 20 Mar 1980, 24-25.

8 ASHTON, R. Fleischmann, C. Miss Ruth Ashton: a profile. (General Secretary of the RCM.) Midwife, Health Visitor and Community Nurse, 16 (5), May 1980, 209.

9 AULD, M. Cowper-Smith, F. Interview: Margaret Auld. Nursing Times, 73, 10 Mar 1977, 332-333.

10 BAILEY, H. Church, O.M. and Buckwalter, K.C. Harriet Bailey—a psychiatric nurse pioneer. Perspectives in Psychiatric Care, 18 (2), Mar/Apr 1980, 62-66.

11 BEDFORD FENWICK, E. Mrs. Bedford Fenwick SRN 1. (Article marking the occasion of the presentation of a silver badge to SRN 500,000, Carol Green.) Nursing Times, 72, 22 Jan 1976, 90.

12 BEDFORD FENWICK, E. Famous nurses: Mrs. Bedford Fenwick. Nursing Mirror, 148, 22 Mar 1979, 35.

13 Beaumont, Winifred A detail on the Burma front. British Broadcasting Corporation, 1977.

14 BENDALL, E. Robinson, W. Not disillusioned—deeply concerned. (Interview with Eve Bendall on nursing care today.) Nursing Mirror, 143, 14 Oct 1976, 36.

15 BICKERDYKE Litvin, Martin The young Mary 1817-1861: early years of Mother Bickerdyke, America's Florence Nightingale, and patron saint of Kansas. Galesburg, Illinois: Log City Books, 1977.

16 BLENKINSOP, D. Allen, M. Geordie girl on the go. (Profile of Dorothy Blenkinsop, Northern Region RNO.) Nursing Mirror, 149, 30 Aug 1979, Supplement ix-x, xii.

17 BRECKENRIDGE, M. Ernst, E.K.M. Tomorrow's child. (Life of Mary Breckenridge who founded the Frontier Nursing Service in USA in 1925 providing midwifery care.) Journal of Nurse-Midwifery, 24 (5), Sep/Oct 1979, 7-12.

18 Brook, F.F. Nursing in many fields. Johnson, 1977. (Personal memoirs of a nurse.)

19 CARTER, L. Shubin, S. A conversation with Lillian Carter, RN. Nursing, 8 (9), Sep 1978, 62-66.

20 CARTWRIGHT, A. Clode, D. The one woman diagnosis team. (The work of Ann Cartwright.) Health and Social Service Journal, 88, 6 Oct 1978, 1134-1135.

21 CAVELL, E. in Fraser, Antonia editor Heroes and heroines. Weidenfeld and Nicolson, 1980.

22 CAVELL, E. Gordon, J.E. Distinguished British nurses of the past. 8. Edith Cavell—pioneer nurse and wartime martyr. Midwife, Health Visitor and Community Nurse, 12 (11), Nov 1976, 361-366.

23 CLARK, J. Allen, M. Green is June's valley. (Profile of June Clark.) Nursing Mirror, 148, 19 Apr 1979, Supplement iv-vi, viii.

24 CLAY, T. Darby, C. A man in the middle. (A day with Trevor Clay, ANO Camden and Islington.) Nursing Mirror, 148, 3 May 1979, 21-23.

25 CRUICKSHANK, J. Famous nurses: Dame Joanna Cruickshank: founder of the RAF Nursing Service. Nursing Mirror, 148, 25 Jan 1979, 24.

26 DARLING, V. Alison Dunn talks to Vera Darling. (Interview with principal officer designate of JBCNS.) Nursing Times, 74, 26 Oct 1978, 1752-1753.

27 DIX, D. Famous nurses: Dorothea Dix. Nursing Mirror, 148, 1 Mar 1979, 25.

28 Dock, L.L. Lavinia L. Dock self portrait. (Autobiographical letter to Mrs. Stevens—a member of the American Journal of Nursing staff.) Nursing Outlook, 25 (1), Jan 1977, 22-26.

29 DOCK, L.L. Monteiro, L.A. Lavinia L. Dock (1947) on nurses and the cold war. (Lavinia Dock's protest against exclusion of Russian nurses from ICN meeting in New Jersey owing to

Truman doctrine of anti-communism.) Nursing Forum, 17 (1), 1978, 46-54.

30 GARDENER, M. Marjorie Gardener. (Interview with Alison Dunn and tributes from colleagues on her retirement from the Joint Board of Clinical Nursing Studies.) Nursing Times, 75, 1 Feb 1979, 182-184.

31 GARDENER, M. Thompson, S. Growing opportunities. (Interview with Marjorie Gardener to mark her retirement from the JBCNS.) Nursing Mirror, 148, 26 Apr 1979, 20-21.

32 GOODALL, F. Death of Frances Goodall. (Obituary.) Nursing Times, 72, 29 July 1976, 1142.

33 GORDON, E. In loving memory. (Appreciation of Elise Gordon with obituary and photograph on p.35.) Nursing Mirror, 144, 10 Feb 1977, 33, 35; Nursing's tribute to Elise Gordon, 14 Apr 1977, 38.

34 GREGORY, A. Famous nurses: Alice Gregory. (One of the founders of the British Hospital for Mothers and Babies in Woolwich.) Nursing Mirror, 148, 26 Apr 1979, 37.

35 HALL, C.M. Allen, M. Confessions of a workaholic. (Profile of Catherine Hall, Rcn General Secretary with brief review of the Rcn's recent history.) Nursing Mirror, 151, 11 Sep 1980, 20-23.

36 HALL, C.M. Dopson, L. Rcn Congress Preview. The Rcn's CMH. A private person in a public role. (Catherine Mary Hall, CBE.) Nursing Times, 76, 15 May 1980, 855-857.

37 HALL, C.M. Stevenson, J. Catherine Hall; the years of change. Nursing Mirror, 143, 16 Sep 1976, 37.

38 HARVEY, W. Solman, F. William Harvey. Nursing Mirror, 146, 6 Apr 1978, 7-8.

39 HENDERSON, V. Darby, C. Who's afraid of Virginia Henderson? (Interview during her visit to England to deliver Battersea Memorial Lecture.) Nursing Mirror, 145, 17 Nov 1977, 4.

40 HILL, J. McDougall, Jim Angel of the snow: the story of Judy Hill. (Nurse killed in air crash in Northern Canada.) Muller, 1977.

41 Holford, Ida M. But the nights are long. (A nurse's memoirs.) Hale, 1977.

42 HUNT, A. Famous nurses: Dame Agnes Hunt. Nursing Mirror, 148, 29 Mar 1979, 37.

43 JONES, A.E. Famous nurses: Agnes Elizabeth Jones. Workhouse infirmary reformer. Nursing Mirror, 148, 8 Feb 1979, 34.

44 JOSEPH Holland, M.M. and Dean, L. Mother Joseph: founder, architect, beggar. (Sister of Providence who founded hospitals and schools.) Hospital Progress, 61 (4), Apr 1980, 69-73.

45 LAMBIE, M. Campbell, Helen Mary Lambie: a biography. Wellington: New Zealand Nursing Education and Research Foundation, 1976.

46 LEES, F. Gordon, J.E. Distinguished British nurses of the past. 7. Florence Lees—Mrs. Dacre Craven—pioneer of district nursing, 1841-1922. Midwife, Health Visitor & Community Nurse, 12 (5), May 1976, 159-163.

47 LEES, F. Famous nurses: Florence Lees. Nursing Mirror, 148, 22 Feb 1979, 34.

48 Long, H. Change into uniform: an autobiography 1939-1946. Lavenham: Dalton, 1978. (Memoirs of a V.A.D.)

49 LUCKES, E. Famous nurses: Eva Luckes. Matron of the London Hospital and creator of the sister tutor. Nursing Mirror, 148, 15 Mar 1979, 33.

50 MAASS, C. Cunningham, John T. Clara Maass: a nurse, a hospital, a spirit. Rev.ed. Belleville, New Jersey: Rae Publishing Co., 1976.

51 MAASS, C. Clara Maass stamp is issued. RN Magazine, 38 (10), Oct 1976, 46-48.

52 McFARLANE OF LLANDAFF Jean McFarlane appointed to Royal Commission. Nursing Times, 72, 13 May 1979, 714.

53 McFARLANE OF LLANDAFF Allen, M. Enter the leading lady. (Interview with Jean McFarlane, first Professor of Nursing at an English university and first nurse to be made a peer.) Nursing Mirror, 149, 26 Jul 1979, 18-20.

54 MANNERHEIM, S. Famous nurses: Baroness Sophie Mannerheim. Nursing Mirror, 148, 8 Mar 1979, 32.

55 Markham, Joan The lamp was dimmed: the story of a nurse's training. Hale, 1975.

56 MEE, B. Andrews, A. A tribute to Brenda Mee. (Address at service of thanksgiving by Agnes Andrews, President of RCM and appreciation by Margaret Farrer, vice-president of RCM.) Nursing Times, 75, 4 Oct 1979, 1698-1699; See also Midwives Chronicle, 92, Oct 1979, 330-331, 346.

57 MEREDITH DAVIES, B. Smith, F. 'He has set up a unique link for two related hostile professions.' (The work of Dr. Brian Meredith Davies.) Health and Social Service Journal, 86, 26 Nov 1976, 2110-2111.

58 Moore, A. Silver Jubilee Year—a personal report. (A nurse's experiences over the last 25 years.) Nursing Mirror, 144, 2 Jun 1977, 19-21.

59 NIGHTINGALE, F. Two letters reproduced from originals given to the Archives at St. Bartholomew's Hospital. Nursing Mirror, 143, 1 Jul 1976, 68.

60 NIGHTINGALE, F. Florence Nightingale Commemoration Service. (Mainly illustrations.) Nursing Mirror, 140, 5 Jun 1975, 45-46; 142, 27 May 1976, 39-41; 144, 19 May 1977, 7-9.

61 NIGHTINGALE, Florence in Fraser, Antonia, editor Heroes and heroines. Weidenfeld and Nicolson, 1980.

62 NIGHTINGALE, F. Grier, B. and Grier, M. Contributions of the passionate statistician. Information available about the mathematical and statistical training of Florence Nightingale. Research in Nursing and Health, 1 (3), Oct 1978, 103-109.

63 NIGHTINGALE, F. Kopf, E.W. Florence Nightingale as statistician. (Reprinted from Journal of the American Statistical Association 1916.) Research in Nursing and Health, 1 (3), Oct 1978, 93-102.

64 NIGHTINGALE, F. May, T.R. and May, W.J. The light still shines in Elora. (Short

account of love affair between Florence Nightingale and her cousin John Smithurst.) Canadian Nurse, 76 (5), May 1980, 42.

65 NIGHTINGALE, F. **Nelson, J.** Florence, the legend. Nursing Mirror, 142, 13 May 1976, 40-41.

66 NIGHTINGALE, F. **Palmer, Irene Sabelberg** Florence Nightingale: founder of modern nursing. Boston, Massachusetts: Boston University Libraries Nursing Archive, 1976.

67 NIGHTINGALE, F. **Palmer, I.S.** Florence Nightingale: reformer, reactionary, researcher. Nursing Research, 26 (2), Mar-Apr 1977, 84-89.

68 NIGHTINGALE, F. **Palmer, I.S.** Florence Nightingale and the Salisbury incident. (Florence Nightingale: astute handling of theft from the Free Gifts Stores by Charlotte Salisbury in the Crimean War.) Nursing Research, 25 (5), Sep/Oct 1976, 370-377.

69 NIGHTINGALE, F. **Parker, P.** Florence Nightingale: first lady of administrative nursing. Supervisor Nurse, 8 (3), Mar 1977, 24-25.

70 NIGHTINGALE, F. **Seymer, L.** The writings of Florence Nightingale. (Oration delivered at ICN congress in 1947.) Nursing Journal of India, 70 (5), May 1979, 121-128.

71 NIGHTINGALE, F. **Thompson, J.** The passionate humanist: from Nightingale to the new nurse. (An examination of Miss Nightingale's beliefs and actions as they relate to the nurse's position within the present health care system.) Nursing Outlook, 28 (5), May 1980, 290-295.

72 NIGHTINGALE, F. **Verney, R.** Florence Nightingale by her god-daughter Ruth Verney. (Talk given in the Royal Commonwealth Society Library, October 4, 1960.) Nursing Times, 73, 3 Feb 1977, CNF Supplement 50-51.

73 NIGHTINGALE, F. **Verney, R.** Florence Nightingale. (By her god-daughter, with introduction by Donald Simpson.) Nursing Journal of India, 68 (5), May 1977, 123-125.

74 OXLADE, Z. **Dunn, A.** Zena Oxlade. (Report and interview with the new chairman of the GNC about her nursing career.) Nursing Times, 74, 9 Feb 1978, 218-219.

75 PAGET, R. **Gordon, E.** Distinguished British nurses of the past. 9. Dame Rosalind Paget, 1855-1948. Midwife, Health Visitor & Community Nurse, 13 (4), Apr 1977, 105-107, 110-111.

76 PAGET, R. Famous nurses: Dame Rosalind Paget: pioneer midwife. Nursing Mirror, 148, 1 Feb 1979, 29.

77 PALMER, S.F. **Christy, T.E.** Portrait of a leader: Sophia F. Palmer. Nursing Outlook, 23 (12), Dec 1975, 746-751.

78 PATTISON, D. **Ginger, D.** The saintly yet so-human Sister Dora. (Account of Sister Dora's work with photograph of statue in Walsall.) Nursing Mirror, 149, 20/27 Dec 1979, 36-37.

79 PATTISON, D. **Watkin, B.** Sister Dora of Walsall. (Dorothy Pattison, with two photographs from the T.V. drama series.) Nursing Mirror, 144, 23 Jun 1977, 7-9.

80 PEMBREY, S. **Thompson, S.** Artichokes

and the art of nursing. (Interview with Sue Pembrey.) Nursing Mirror, 148, 19 Apr 1979, Supplement xiv-xv.

81 PEPLAU, H.E. **Gregg, D.E.** Hildegard E. Peplau: her contributions. Perspectives in Psychiatric Care, 16 (3), May/Jun 1978, 118-121.

82 PEPLAU, H.E. **Sills, G.M.** Hildegard E. Peplau: leader, practitioner, academician, scholar, and theorist. Perspectives on Psychiatric Care, 16 (3), May/Jun 1978, 122-128.

83 POTTER, M. Famous nurses: Mary Potter. (Mother General of the Little Company of Mary, who influenced nurse training in Italy.) Nursing Mirror, 148, 5 Apr 1979, 40.

84 POWELL, M. Famous nurses: Dame Muriel Powell. Nursing Mirror, 148, 3 May 1979, 36.

85 POWELL, M. The nurse of our times. (Three tributes to Muriel Powell.) Nursing Times, 75, 11 Jan 1979, 52-53.

86 POWELL, M. **Young, P.** Dame Muriel Powell. (Interview.) Nursing Mirror, 143, 11 Nov 1976, 39.

87 PRENTICE, W. Winifred Prentice yearns for unity. (Interview.) Nursing Mirror, 143, 25 Nov 1976, 37.

88 PRIME, A. **Kingman, S.** Digging up the NHS seedling before the roots have grown. (Interview with Audrey Prime, former NALGO national officer for the health service.) Health and Social Service Journal, 90, 4 Jan 1980, 18-21.

89 SENIOR, E. **Darby, C.** A lonely life at the top. (A day in the life of Edith Senior, Regional Nursing Officer for Trent.) Nursing Mirror, 148, 26 Apr 1979, 22-24.

90 STILL, A.L. Famous nurses: Alicia Lloyd Still. (Matron of St. Thomas'.) Nursing Mirror, 148, 19 Apr 1979, 26.

91 STOREY, M. **Darby, C.** Maude Storey: the new face at the top. Nursing Mirror, 144, 24 Mar 1977, 35.

92 STOREY, M. **Dunn, A.** Maude Storey— Interview. (New registrar of the GNC.) Nursing Times, 73, 25 Aug 1977, 1306-1307.

93 STOREY, M. **Ellis, S.** Meet Miss Storey. (Interview with Maude Storey, registrar of the GNC.) Nursing Times, 75, 22 Mar 1979, 476-477.

94 STRONG, R. Famous nurses: Rebecca Strong. (A Scottish Nightingale trainee.) Nursing Mirror, 148, 12 Apr 1979, 33.

95 TERROT, S.A. **Richardson, Robert G.,** editor Nurse Sarah Anne: with Florence Nightingale at Scutari. Murray, 1977.

96 TORROP, H.M. Hilda M. Torrop 1892-1978. (Nurse involved in development of practical nursing as a profession.) Journal of Practical Nursing, 27 (7), Jul 1978, 14-17.

97 WARDROPER, S. Famous nurses: Sarah Wardroper. (Matron of St. Thomas' Hospital, London, she was the first superintendent of the training school there.) Nursing Mirror, 148, 15 Feb 1979, 30.

98 WHITAKER, M. **Morris, P.** Why Mollie likes to keep her gloves on. (Interview with new

chairman of NATN, Mollie Whitaker.) Nursing Mirror, 147, 2 Nov 1978, Supplement xxiii.

99 Wilkinson, M. Four score and ten. 3 parts. (Memoirs of Canadian nurse 1909-1959, including war service 1914-1918.) Canadian Nurse, 73 (10), Oct 1977, 25-28; (11), Nov 1977, 14-23; (12), Dec 1977, 16-23.

3 BRIGGS REPORT

a GENERAL

1 **Arnold, N.** Briggs: the lost horizon? (See also editorial on p.1815.) Nursing Times, 73, 24 Nov 1977, 1822-1823.

2 **Bendall, E.** The worst of both worlds. (A personal view of the proposals on the Briggs report in HC(76)22.) Nursing Times, 72, 3 Jun 1976, 838-839.

3 **British Medical Journal** Is Briggs alive? (Editorial comment on the proposals and the implementation of the report.) British Medical Journal, 1, 22 May 1976, 1237-1238.

4 **Chapman, C.** A philosophy of nursing practice and education. (In relation to the Briggs report.) Nursing Times, 74, 23 Feb 1978, 303-305.

5 **Collins, S.M.** The philosophy of 'Briggs'. Nursing Times, 73, 16 Jun 1977, Occ. papers, 85-87.

6 **Croft, J.C.** Briggs will not mean nurses will lose jobs. (Letter from Secretary to the Briggs Coordinating Committee.) Nursing Mirror, 147, 26 Oct 1978, 10.

7 **Croft, J.C.** Proposed statutory framework. (Letter commenting on Nursing Times article 8 Dec 1977, 1900-1901.) Nursing Times, 73, 22-29 Dec 1977, 2007.

8 **Department of Health and Social Security** Proposals on aspects of the Briggs report on nursing: a) Relationship between service and education. b) The statutory framework. The Department, 1976. (Health Circular (76) 22).

9 **Hunt, S.** No Briggs Bill this Parliamentary session. (News item.) Nursing Mirror, 146, 16 Mar 1978, 2.

10 **Kratz, C.** So I told the working party... (Personal evidence to Briggs Co-ordinating Committee Working Group Four.) Nursing Times, 74 (6), 9 Feb 1978, Community Outlook, 49, 51.

11 **Lancet** Commentary from Westminster. Briggs on the shelf. (Brief comment.) Lancet, 1, 25 Mar 1978, 674; More delay on Briggs, 9 Oct 1976, 812-813.

12 **Moyle, R.** Interview with Roland Moyle. (Minister of Health, chairman of a co-ordinating committee set up to prepare for the Briggs Bill.) Nursing Times, 73, 5 May 1977, 644-645.

13 **NATNews** Briggs Co-ordinating Committee—Working Group 4. (Evidence in support of a specialist committee for theatre nurses.) NATNews, 15 (3), Mar 1978, 8, 14.

14 **Nursing Mirror** AHAs and colleges to share student nurse training. (Comments on the

modified Government proposals for the implementation of Briggs in HC(76)22.) Nursing Mirror, 142, 27 May 1976, 35.

15 Nursing Mirror Parliamentary Correspondent New suggestion on Briggs Report proposals. Nursing Mirror, 143, 4 Nov 1976, 40; Hopes of early Briggs raised in Commons, 17 Nov 1977, 2.

16 Nursing Times Briggs proposals. (Comments on HC(76) 22.) Nursing Times, 72, 27 May 1976, 794; 3 Jun 1976, 831.

17 Nursing Times Briggs proposals. News items.
GNC poses Briggs dilemmas. 72, 23 Sep 1976, 1457.
DHSS sets high-speed schedule on Briggs steering committee. 73, 3 Feb 1977, 144.
Chairman resigns from key Briggs working group. (Maude Storey). 74, 16 Feb 1978, 256.
Compromise reached on Briggs. (Coordinating Committee). 74, 2 Mar 1978, 340-341.
Briggs Bill postponed—again. (With comments from organisations). 74, 16 Mar 1978, 428-429.

18 Nursing Times No Briggs until at least 1980. (Comments on 'Priorities for health and personal social services.') Nursing Times, 72, 1 Apr 1976, 474-475.

19 Nursing Times Nursing Times explains... (Statutory and standing committees and mandatory training in the context of the Briggs Bill.) Nursing Times, 73, 1 Dec 1977, 1856; 8 Dec 1977, 1900-1901.

20 Price, C. Briggs—what are the chances? Nursing Times, 73, 31 Mar 1977, 440-441.

21 Royal College of Nursing Rcn argues for mental, district and OH nurses. (Report on evidence to Briggs working group 4.) Nursing Times, 74, 19 Jan 1978, 84.

22 Royal College of Nursing Rcn comments on health circular HC(76)22 and attached papers (a) and (b): Proposals on aspects of the Briggs report on nursing. Rcn, 1976.

23 Royal College of Nursing Submission to Working Group 4, Briggs Co-ordinating Committee. Rcn, 1977.

24 Royal College of Nursing. Society of Occupational Health Nursing (Submission to Working Group 4, Briggs Co-ordinating Committee.) The need for statutory recognition of occupational health nursing. Rcn, 1977.

25 Royal College of Nursing Society of Primary Care Nursing (Submission to Working Group 4, Briggs Co-ordinating Committee.) Rcn, 1977.

26 Royal College of Nursing Society of Psychiatric Nursing (Submission to Working Group 4, Briggs Co-ordinating Committee.) The case for a statutory standing committee of the Central Council. Rcn, 1977.

27 Walker, K. Before Briggs and beyond. Nursing Mirror, 143, 11 Nov 1976, 71-72.

28 Watkin, B. Briggs one step nearer (after the publication of HC(76)22.) Nursing Mirror, 142, 3 Jun 1976, 42.

29 White, R. Questioning Briggs. Nursing Mirror, 143 (8), 19 Aug 1976, 62.

b LEGISLATION

1 Allen, M. Can nurses now show a more united front on the Briggs Bill? Nursing Mirror, 148, 18 Jan 1979, 7.

2 Batley, N. The Briggs legislation—is this what is wanted? (Personal view by Director of the CETHV). Nursing Times, 74, 12 Oct 1978, 1668-1671.

3 Briggs, A., Lord Maiden speech on the Briggs Bill. Nursing Times, 75, 22 Feb 1979, 304; 1 Mar 1979, 344-345.

4 Briggs, A., Lord Quick, quick, slow of the Bill a minister wanted immediately. (Comment on the Briggs report's recommendations.) Nursing Mirror, 147, 23 Nov 1978, 8-9.

5 British Medical Journal Nursing reform: shadow or substance? (The Briggs bill). British Medical Journal, 2, 2 Dec 1978, 1517.

6 Brown, A. From Briggs to eternity. (Implications of Nurses, Midwives, and Health Visitors Act regarding changes in nursing's governing bodies.) Nursing Mirror, 151, 11 Sep 1980, 26-27.

7 Darby, C. Long-awaited Briggs Bill offers new freedom to nurses. (The differences between original Briggs report and the bill, with summary of recent developments.) Nursing Mirror, 147, 16 Nov 1978, 9.

8 Dunn, A. Tales of mystery and suspence OR how the Briggs Bill reached the Statute Book. 1. Personalities. (Interviews with David Rye, Sheila Jack and Mary Jones.) Nursing Times, 75, 31 May 1979, 908-911.

9 Fenney, R. Tales of mystery and suspense OR how the Briggs Bill reached the Statute Book. 2. Organisations. (The Central Midwives Board, GNC for Scotland and the CETHV.) Nursing Times, 75, 7 Jun 1979, 952-955.

10 Moyle, R. Tales of mystery and suspense OR how the Briggs Bill reached the Statute Book. 3. The minister's tale. (How he helped steer bill through Parliament.) Nursing Times, 75, 14 Jun 1979, 991-992.

11 Nazer, G. The Briggs debate. Chasms open as the Briggs dust settles in Parliament. Nursing Mirror, 148, 26 Apr 1979, 6.

12 Nursing Mirror Progress of Briggs Bill. Nursing Mirror, 148, 25 Jan 1979, 4; 1 Feb 1979, 4; 15 Feb 1979, 2, 4; 22 Feb 1979, 2; 22 Mar 1979, 5.

13 Nursing Times Long wait for Briggs is over. (Report on its progress in Parliament. See also editorial on p.1821.) Nursing Times, 74, 9 Nov 1978, 1822. Second reading of Briggs Bill, 23 Nov 1978, 1921-1923.

14 Nursing Times Progress of Briggs Bill. Nursing Times, 75, 4 Jan 1979, 4; 25 Jan 1979, 137; 1 Feb 1979, 178; 15 Feb 1979, 265; 22 Mar 1979, 470.

15 Parliament Nurses, midwives and health visitors act 1979. HMSO, 1979 (Chapter 36).

16 Parliament Nurses, midwives and health visitors act 1979. Hansard.
Action on. 5 Nov 1979, WA 50-1.
Central Council set up. 6 Nov 1979, WA 166.
First chairman of Central Council. 14 Jul 1980, WA 430.

Composition of Central Council and national boards. 21 Jul 1980, WA 93-95.
Welsh Board. 7 Aug 1980, WA 246.

17 Parliament Nurses, midwives and health visitors bill. HMSO, 1978.

18 Parliament Nurses, midwives and health visitors bill. Hansard references.
Absence from Queen's speech.
Question from Mr. Jenkins. 4 Nov 1977, 252.
Question from Mr. Pavitt. 4 Nov 1977, 200.
Reply by Mr. Ennals. 4 Nov 1977, 268.
Planned for this session. 7 Feb 1978, WA 530.
Not possible this session. 15 Mar 1978, WA 232.
Introduction. Queen's speech. 1 Nov 1978, 8.
Queen's speech proposal. Lords, 7 Nov 1978, 273.

19 Parliament Nurses, midwives and health visitors bill. Hansard.
House of Commons.
1st reading. 2 Nov 1978, 198.
2nd reading. 13 Nov 1978, 35-126.
3rd reading. 7 Feb 1979, 413-509.
Report stage. 27 Mar 1979, 1473-1496.
Lords amendments considered. 4 Apr 1979, 1351-1357.
House of Lords.
1st reading. 13 Feb 1979, 1086.
2nd reading. 19 Feb 1979, 1643-1681.
Committee stage. 13 Mar 1979, 504-557.
3rd reading. 2 Apr 1979, 1729.
Royal assent. 4 Apr 1979, 1954.

20 Price, C. The politics of Briggs. (By a Labour MP.) Nursing Times, 75, 8 Feb 1979, 226.

21 Raybould, E. After the Act: an opportunity within our grasp. Nursing Times, 75, 16 Aug 1979, 1389-1390.

22 Raybould, E. Pushing the slow boat to progress. (Comment on the Briggs report and the Nurses, Midwives and Health Visitors Act.) Nursing Mirror, 149, 25 Oct 1979, 40-41.

23 Royal College of Midwives A letter on the Briggs legislation. Midwives Chronicle, 91, Apr 1978, 79-80.

24 Vaughan, G. Westminster. (Discussion of the Briggs Bill by Tory health spokesman.) Nursing Mirror, 147, 26 Oct 1978, 12.

25 Wells, R. The Salmon leaps to preserve Briggs. (Comment on developments in nursing during 1970s.) Nursing Mirror, 150, 3 Jan 1980, 16-17.

4 HISTORY

a GENERAL

1 Abu-Saad, H. Nursing: a world view. St. Louis: Mosby, 1979.

2 American Nursing Association ANA convention highlights the need for historical research. Nursing Research, 25 (5), Sep-Oct 1976, 323.

3 Ashley, J. Foundations for scholarship: historical research in nursing. Advances in Nursing Science, 1 (1), Oct 1978, 25-36.

4 Baly, M.E. A definitive nursing history textbook. (Letter suggesting methods of researching and teaching nursing history.) Nursing Times, 76, 3 Jan 1980, 32.

5 **Baly, M.** Nursing. Batsford, 1977. (Past into present series.)

6 **Baly, M.E.** Nursing and social change. 2nd ed. Heinemann Medical, 1980.

7 **Bingham, S.** Ministering angels. Osprey, 1979.

8 **Broadley, M.E.** It's different now. (London Hospital fifty years ago.) Nursing Times, 72, 11 Mar 1976, 365-366; 18 Mar 1976, 416-417; 25 Mar 1976, 465-467; 1 Apr 1976, 494-495; 8 Apr 1976, 540-541; 15 Apr 1976, 589-591; 22 Apr 1976, 629-631.

9 **Broadley, M.E.** Patients come first: nursing at 'the London' between the two World Wars. Tunbridge Wells: Pitman Medical for The London Hospital Special Trustees, 1980.

10 **Bullough, V. and Bullough, B.** The care of the sick: the emergence of modern nursing. Croom Helm, 1979.

11 **Davidson, E.** A career in nursing a century ago. (Author's grandmother's training in Bradford and work in Kendal.) Nursing Mirror, 146, 13 Apr 1978, 58.

12 **Davies, C.** Four events in nursing history: a new look. 1. (Sociological analysis of three events and their consequences: establishing a professional organisation 1915-1925, the Nurse Registration Act 1919 and the Rcn's (1944) document 'The place of nursing in the NHS'.) Nursing Times, 74, 22 Jun 1978, Occ. papers, 65-68.

13 **Davies, C.** Four events in nursing history: a new look. 2. Case 4. Education and management: options for change in the mid-1960s. Nursing Times, 74, 29 Jun 1978, Occ. papers, 69-71.

14 **Davies, C., editor** Rewriting nursing history. Croom Helm, 1980.

15 **Davies, C.** Where next for nursing history? Nursing Times, 76, 22 May 1980, 920-922.

16 **Deloughery, Grace L.** History and trends of professional nursing. 8th ed. St. Louis: Mosby, 1977.

17 **Dolan, J.A.** Nursing in society: a historical perspective. 14th ed. Philadelphia: Saunders, 1978.

18 **Ferguson, M.** Reflections on teaching a history of nursing. (Reason for, content of and associated problems with, and report of questionnaire survey of institutions with undergraduate courses.) Nursing Times, 75, 15 Nov 1979, Occ. papers, 117-120; 22 Nov 1979, Occ. papers, 121-122.

19 **Friend, P.** 30 years of the NHS. From where I sit: personal impression of the NHS. Nursing Mirror, 147, 6 Jul 1978, 12-14.

20 **Gordon, E.** Pioneers of British nursing. A clutch of queens. (Evidence of nursing by royalty.) Nursing Mirror, 143, 9 Dec 1976, 73.

21 **Gordon, E.** Pioneers of British nursing. Edeva of Barts. (Sisters at Barts from 1192 onwards.) Nursing Mirror, 144, 10 Feb 1977, 70.

22 **Gordon, E.** Pioneers of British nursing. The housewife nurse. (The nurse-role of the mother in the household from the Middle Ages.) Nursing Mirror, 144, 5 May 1977, 62.

23 **Harris, J.** Caring for the sick: a look back at the voluntary tradition. (History of nursing and the voluntary hospital in the nineteenth century.) New Society, 49, 9 Aug 1979, 287-290.

24 **Henderson, V.** Nursing—yesterday and tomorrow. Nursing Times, 76, 22 May 1980, 905-907.

25 **Hilton, A.** Fireside reflections. Memories of Ann Hilton who was trainee nurse during the blitz—with photograph.) Nursing Times, 74 (3), 19 Jan 1978, 122.

26 **Hollis, P., compiler** Women in public 1850-1900: documents of the Victorian women's movement. Allen & Unwin, 1979. Contains: Nursing, 95-99; Nursing of the poor, 249-251.

27 **Howie, W.B. and Black, S.A.B.** Hospital life a century ago. (Margaret Mathewson's record of her experiences as a patient in the Edinburgh Royal Infirmary in 1877.) British Medical Journal, 2, 28 Aug 1976, 515-517.

28 **Huveneers, A.** The Nurses' Memorial Chapel, Westminster Abbey. Nursing Times, 74, 21/28 Dec 1978, 2092-2093.

29 **Jarman, F.L.** The development of conception of nursing professionalism among general hospital nurses, 1860-1895. MA thesis, University of Warwick, 1980.

30 **Maggs, C.** Aspects of recruitment, training and post-certification experiences of general hospital nurses in England, 1881-1914. PhD thesis, University of Bath, 1980.

31 **Maggs, C.J.** Towards a social history of nursing. 2 parts. Nursing Times, 74, 18 May 1978, Occ. papers, 53-56; 25 May 1978, Occ. papers, 57-58.

32 **Nursing Times** Nursing histories. (Correspondence from J.M. Hunt, S. Davidson, D.M. Toyne.) Nursing Times, 73, 14 Jul 1977, 1080.

33 **Pickstone, J.** Yes, but what was it *really* like? (Importance of archives and records for historical research in nursing.) Journal of Community Nursing, 3 (9), Mar 1980, 20-22.

34 **Royal College of Nursing Library** A history workshop. (Comment on first meeting of historical group organised by Rcn library.) Nursing Times, 73, 8 Dec 1977, 1893. Also reported in Nursing Standard, 68, Jan 1978, 7.

35 **Safier, G.** What is oral history? What are the advantages and disadvantages of oral history? How can it be used in nursing history? Nursing Research, 25 (5), Sep/Oct 1976, 383-385.

36 **Terton, A.** Memories of the festive season in a cottage hospital of 1902. (From 'Lights and Shadows in a hospital' by a cottage hospital matron, published in 1902.) Health and Social Service Journal, 80, 19/26 Dec 1980, 1620-1622.

37 **Watkin, B.** Memories, memories... (Comment on listening to elderly people's (including nurses') experiences as historical method.) Nursing Mirror, 145, 22 Dec 1977, 9.

38 **White, R.** Approaches to history. (Letter commenting on Celia Davies' article in 22 May issue, with references.) Nursing Times, 76, 3 Jul 1980, 1177.

39 **White, R.** The development of the Poor Law Nursing Service 1848-1948: a discussion of the historical method and a summary of some of the findings. International Journal of Nursing Studies, 14 (1), 1977, 19-27.

40 **White, R.** Social change and the development of the nursing profession: a study of the poor law nursing service 1848-1948. Kimpton, 1978.

41 **White, R.** Some political influences surrounding the Nurses Registration Act 1919 in the United Kingdom. Journal of Advanced Nursing, 1 (3), May 1976, 209-217.

42 **Whyte, B.** Constant change is here to stay: important events and developments in the hospital nursing service over the past 25 years. Nursing Mirror, 144, 2 Jun 1977, 17-18.

43 **Winstead-Fry, W.** The need to differentiate a nursing self. (Challenging the myths and assumptions of nursing history.) American Journal of Nursing, 77 (9), Sep 1977, 1452-1454.

b OVERSEAS COUNTRIES

1 **Australian Nurses Journal** Royal Children's Hospital, Brisbane celebrates centenary. (Includes photograph of nurse in early 20th century uniform.) Australian Nurses Journal, 8 (4), Oct 1978, 12-13.

2 **Carew, H.M.** Approve ANA 85???—yes. (History of nursing in USA from 1904.) Occupational Health Nursing, 27 (10), Oct 1979, 22-23.

3 **Christy, T.E.** Entry into practice: a recurring issue in nursing history. American Journal of Nursing, 80 (3), Mar 1980, 485-488.

4 **Day, P.E.** Nursing history in the States. (Symposium of nursing in America.) Nursing Mirror, 143, 8 Jul 1976, 46-48.

5 **Elmore, J.A.** Nurses in American history. Black nurses: their service and their struggle. American Journal of Nursing, 76 (3), Mar 1976, 435-437.

6 **Erickson, E.H.** The nursing service director, 1880-1980. (Historical survey.) Journal of Nursing Administration, 10 (4), Apr 1980, 6-13.

7 **Fitzpatrick, L.M.** Nurses in American history. Nursing and the Great Depression. American Journal of Nursing, 75 (12), Dec 1975, 2188-2190.

8 **Fitzpatrick, M.L., editor** Historical studies in nursing: papers presented at the 15th annual Stewart Conference on Research in Nursing, March 1977, New York: Columbia University, Teachers College Press, 1978.

9 **Gabrielson, R.C.** Two centuries of advancement: from untrained servant to skilled practitioner. (History of nursing in America.) Journal of Advanced Nursing, 1 (4), Jul 1976, 265-272.

10 **Harrison, P.H.** Salute to some nursing pio-neers. (From 18th century.) Curationis, 2 (2), Sep 1979, 53-55.

11 **Ingles, T.** The physician's view of the evolving nursing profession 1873-1913. Nursing Forum, 15 (2), 1976, 123-164.

12 **Kalisch, B.J. and Kalisch, P.A.** Is history of nursing alive and well? (Nationwide survey on the status of the history of nursing content in

nursing education.) Nursing Outlook, 24 (6), Jun 1976, 362-366.

13 Martin, S. The after-nursing of abdominal sections, 1903. (Extracts from a lecture by Fourness Barrington, Honorary Surgeon to Lewisham Hospital for Women and Children to members of ATNA.) Lamp, 35 (11), Nov 1978, 19-24.

14 Martin, S. A day with the visiting nurse. May 16, 1910. (Extract from Canadian Nurse.) Lamp, 36 (2), Mar 1979, 10-12.

15 Martin, S. Nursing heart cases. (From an address given in 1905.) Lamp, 35 (12), Dec/Jan 1978/1979, 41-45.

16 Nursing Research Archives-historical researchers' treasures. (Editorial outlining nursing archive collections in USA.) Nursing Research, 27 (2), Mar/Apr 1978, 83.

17 O'Connor, R. American hospitals: the first 200 years. (With illustrations of nurses uniforms.) Hospitals, 50 (1), 1 Jan 1976, 62-72.

18 Safier, G. Contemporary American leaders in nursing: an oral history. New York: McGraw-Hill, 1977.

19 Shamansky, S.L. and Hamilton, W.M. Is the public health nurse's bag an anachronism? (With history of nurses based at Henry Street Settlement in New York and list of contents of their bags in circa 1906 and 1980.) Nursing Outlook, 28 (6), Jun 1980, 379-381.

20 Sticker, A. The beginnings of professional nursing organization in Germany. (The work of Agnes Karll.) International Nursing Review, 24 (1), Jan/Feb 1977, 15-17.

21 Watson, J. The evolution of nursing education in the United States; 100 years of a profession for women. Journal of Nursing Education, 16 (7), Sep 1977, 31-38.

22 Zimmerman, A. Nurses in American history. ANA: its record on social issues. American Journal of Nursing, 76 (4), Apr 1976, 588-590.

c SPECIAL AREAS

1 AORN Journal Issue devoted to the history of operating room nursing. AORN Journal, 24 (1), Jul 1976.

2 Besser, F.S. Great Ormond Street anniversary. (Developments over the last 125 years.) Nursing Mirror, 144, 10 Feb 1977, 60-63.

3 Bowman, M. Pointers to the need for change. (History of nurse education to the present.) Nursing Mirror, 150, 28 Feb 1980, 40-42.

4 Brian, V.A. Eighteenth century Dr. Spock. (Hugh Smith, doctor, who wrote 'Letters to Married Women' on baby care.) Nursing Mirror, 145, 10 Nov 1977, 28.

5 Brian, V. Scenes through the centuries. (History of the operating theatre.) Nursing Mirror, 148, 15 Mar 1979, Supplement i, iii-iv, vii, ix.

6 Charley, I.H. The birth of industrial nursing: its history and development in Great Britain. Baillière Tindall, 1978. 1954 edition reprinted and reissued.

7 Connolly, M.P. Health visiting: a review. 1. 1850-1900. 2. 1900-1910. Midwife, Health Visitor and Community Nurse, 16 (7), Jul 1980, 282, 284-285; (9), Sep 1980, 375-376, 378.

8 Davidson, J. Unfit to rule? (Medical history of monarchs and famous people.) Nursing Times, 72, 2 Jun 1977, 814-818.

9 Duncombe, J. 1927 and all that. (Account of political and social issues in year Journal first appeared.) Health Visitor, 50 (10), Oct 1977, 324-326.

10 Gill, Maud F. District nursing in Brighton 1877-1974. The author, 120 Ditchling Road, Brighton BN1 4SG, (1977).

11 Godfrey, H. One hundred years of industrial nursing. (Centenary of appointment of first industrial nurse by J. and J. Colman, with photographs.) Nursing Times, 74, 30 Nov 1978, 1966-1969.

12 Gordon, J.E. Pioneers of British nursing. The psychiatric nurse. (With particular reference to the work at the Bethlem Hospital, pioneered by Robert Baron and his wife Avice, in the fourteenth century.) Nursing Mirror, 144, 21 Apr 1977, 67-68.

13 Graham, Sarah Little urchins: sick children in the Victorian era. (Articles from Nursing Times.) Macmillan Journals, 1977.

14 Graham, S. Little victims. (Sick children of the Victorian age.) Nursing Times, 73.
1. Illness remembered. 4 Aug 1977, 1188-1192.
2 and 3. Children and hospitals. 11 Aug 1977, 1246-1248; 18 Aug 1977, 1289-1291.
4. The bighouse. (Victorian nannies.) 25 Aug 1977, 1329-1331.
5. Back streets and cottages. 1 Sep 1977, 1372-1373.
6. Illness at boarding school. 8 Sep 1977, 1409-1411.
7. Early gathered. (Children's deaths seen in Victorian literature.) 15 Sep 1977, 1450-1451.
8. The call to health. (Promotion of health in Victorian schools.) 22 Sep 1977, 1485-1488.

15 Greene, J. Steps along the way. (History of psychiatric nursing from the 1800s.) Nursing Mirror, 150, 26 Jun 1980, Supplement v-vii.

16 Health Visitor Twenty-five years of health visiting. (Editorial outlining developments.) Health Visitor, 50 (6), Jun 1977, 179; Golden anniversary issue, 50 (10), Oct 1977, 323-330.

17 Hill, P. Nurse in the 1920s: the life of a district nurse during the 1920s described by her daughter. Nursing Mirror, 142, 29 Apr 1976, 70-71.

18 Hospital Administration in Canada The evolution of O.R. (Photographs of past and present operating theatres, showing nurses' uniforms.) Hospital Administration in Canada, 20 (4), Apr 1978, 38-39.

19 Keywood, O. It used to be so different. (Reminiscences of district nursing in 1948.) Nursing Mirror, 146, 25 May 1978, 36-37.

20 Lindsay, G. The doctor and the district nurse. (History of village midwife and nurse in Somerset village in 19th century.) Nursing Times, 75, 9 Aug 1979, Community Outlook, 235-236.

21 Loudon, I.S.L. John Bunnell Davis and the Universal Dispensary for Children. (First major

institution devoted solely to the care of sick children.) British Medical Journal, 1, 5 May 1979, 1191-1194.

22 Martin, S. Some experiences of a private nurse on board a sailing ship, 1904. Lamp, 36 (4), May 1979, 17-18.

23 Mattingly, S.T. Looking back 50 years... The nurse in industry. (Paper presented in 1928 to nursing students describing nurses' work.) Occupational Health Nursing, 26 (1), Jan 1978, 17-18.

24 Morley, J.M. Training in the forties. (Author's memoirs.) Nursing Mirror, 146, 4 May 1978, 20-21.

25 Nursing Times Beer, beef bagatelle and bandages: an extract from the diary of a patient awaiting treatment for an eye condition in a London hospital in the summer of 1889. Nursing Times, 74, 16 Mar 1978, 456.

26 Occupational Health 100 years of occupational nursing. (Centenary of appointment of first industrial nurse with photographs.) Occupational Health, 30 (10), Oct 1978, 482-488.

27 Peterson, E. Forty years on. (Letter describing nurse training in 1937.) Nursing Mirror, 145, 14 Jul 1977, 11.

28 Queen's Nursing Journal Reading's mobile nurses. (Photographs of Queen's nurses at the beginning of the century and 1952 and district nurses in 1977, showing methods of transport.) Queen's Nursing Journal, 19 (15), Jun 1977, 431.

29 Roberts, A. A history of the plague in England—1. The coming of the plague—The Black Death. 2. Tudor epidemics and the Great Plague. 3. Coping with the plague. Nursing Times, 75, 10 May 1979, 777-779; 17 May 1979, 826-829; 24 May 1979, 869-871.

30 Schrader, E.S. From apron to gown: a history of OR attire (in the United States, including caps, gloves and masks.) AORN Journal, 24 (1), Jul 1976, 53-67.

31 Spray, W. Obituary at Nottingham. (Nurse's memories of nursing at Nottingham Children's Hospital with two photographs.) Nursing Mirror, 150, 27 Mar 1980, 27-28.

32 Stringer, M. Ninety years of district nursing. Nursing Mirror, 146, 13 Apr 1978, 63, 65-66.

33 THOUGHTS of 100 years of nurse training at the Hospital for Sick Children, Great Ormond Street, London: 1878-1978. The Hospital, 1978.

34 Underwood, E.A. The cliff top barrier. (History of health visiting and problems of professional identity.) Nursing Mirror, 148, 11 Jan 1979, 40-42.

35 West, C. How to nurse sick children. Hospital for Sick Children, Great Ormond Street, 1977. (Facsimile of 1854 edition.)

d WAR NURSING

1 Bullough, B. Nurses in American history. The lasting impact of World War 2 on nursing. American Journal of Nursing, 76 (1), Jan 1976, 118-120.

2 Canadian Nurse 1914-1976. (Unveiling in 1926 of monument honouring Canadian nurses who died in 1914-1918 war.) Canadian Nurse, 72 (11), Nov 1976, 48-49.

3 **Edwards, G.** New place of pride for the Army's angels. (QARANC museum at Aldershot with photograph of nurse in Boer War-style uniform.) Reprinted from the Hampshire Telegraph, Portsmouth, England. Australasian Nurses Journal, 3 (4), Oct 1977, 20-21.

4 **Farmborough, Florence** Russian album 1908-1918, edited by John Jolliffe. Salisbury: Michael Russell, 1979.

5 **Fisher, L.** A wartime memento. (Autograph book of Sister Smith, (now Mrs. Lilian Fisher) to which the soldiers whom she nursed in the First World War contributed drawings and poems.) Nursing Times, 75, 19 Apr 1979, 681.

6 **Haynes, E.** Down memory lane. Off to war. (Work in Brittany during World War Two.) Nursing Mirror, 149, 6 Sep 1979, 20-21.

7 **Hinton, J.** The VADs' service. (Letter outlining training of VADs after the war.) Nursing Times, 74, 30 Nov 1978, 1979-1980.

8 **Kalisch, B.J. and Kalisch, P.A.** Nurses in American history. The Cadet Nurse Corps—in World War II. American Journal of Nursing, 76 (2), Feb 1976, 240-244.

9 **Kalisch, P.A.** Heroines of '98. Female Army nurses in the Spanish-American War. Nursing Research, 24 (6), Nov-Dec 1975, 411-429.

10 **Kalisch, P.A.** How Army nurses became officers. A discussion of the World War I experiences of nurses in the U.S. Army, the nation's first large all graduate nursing service. (Includes illustrations of army uniforms.) Nursing Research, 25 (3), May/Jun 1976, 164-177.

11 **Kalisch, P.A. and Kalisch, B.J.** Nurses under fire. The World War II experiences of nurses on Bataan and Corregidor.(Philippines.) Nursing Research, 25 (6), Nov-Dec 1976, 409-442.

12 **Kalisch, P.A. and Kalisch, B.J.** Untrained but undaunted: the women nurses of the Blue and the Gray. (Role of nurses in the American Civil War.) Nursing Forum, 15 (1), 1976, 4-33.

13 **Keatinge, G.** A midwife at war. Midwife, motorist, volunteer nurse in the First World War. (Life and career of Baroness de T'Serclaes. (Mrs. Knocker).) Midwives Chronicle, 90, Oct 1977, 242-243.

14 **McBryde, B.** A nurse's war. (World War II.) Chatto and Windus, 1979. Extracts in Nursing Times, 75, 28 Jun 1979, 1084-1086; 5 Jul 1979, 1150-1152.

15 **McCausland, E. and Hancock, E.M.** A short history of the Princess Mary's Royal Air Force Nursing Service. (With 1927 and 1975 photographs.) PMRAFNS Magazine, 1 (1), Jun 1978, 5-8.

16 **McClelland, M.** Army nurse in Japan. (World War 2 experiences.) Nursing Times, 73, 26 May 1977, 771-773.

17 **McClelland, M.** Army nurse in the Raj. (Personal experiences of a member of the Queen Alexandra's Imperial Military Nursing Service.) Nursing Times, 72, 15 Jan 1976, 69-71.

18 **MacDonald, L.** The roses of no man's land. Joseph, 1980.

19 **Martin, S.** Nursing a typhoid epidemic at Coonamble in 1903. (In South Africa during the Boer War.) Lamp, 35 (10), Oct 1978, 17-18.

20 **Marwick, Arthur** Women at war 1914-1918. Croom Helm, 1977. Extract in Nursing Times, 73, 31 Mar 1977, 444-446.

21 **Nursing Mirror** The doctor poet and the poppies of Flanders. (John McCrae, doctor in World War I who inspired idea of poppy as symbol.) Nursing Mirror, 147, 9 Nov 1978, 16-17.

22 **Princess Mary's Royal Air Force Nursing Service** Diamond jubilee for RAF nurses. (History of PMRAFNS with photographs.) Nursing Mirror, 146, 1 Jun 1978, 7-9.

23 **Queen Alexandra's Royal Army Nursing Corps** War nurses relive history. (QARANC nurses celebration of 75 years of service.) Nursing Mirror, 145, 24 Nov 1977, 4; Nursing Times, 73, 24 Nov 1977, 1824.

24 **Rogers, B.** Nurses at war reflected in the pages of Nursing Mirror 1888-1978. Nursing Mirror, 146, 6 Apr 1978, 13-16.

25 **S.A. Nursing Journal** These women died in uniform. (South African Military Nursing Service.) S.A. Nursing Journal, 44 (8), Aug 1977, 19.

26 **Wilkinson, M.** Four score and ten. (Story of Canadian nurses involved in First World War. See also cover photo and caption p.1.) Canadian Nurse, 73 (11), Nov 1977, 14-23.

5 NURSING AS A PROFESSION

a GENERAL

1 **Advances in Nursing Science** Politics of care. Advances in Nursing Science, 2 (3), Apr 1980, 1-107.

2 **Altschul, A.T.** Commitment to nursing. (The Battersea Memorial Lecture 1978.) Journal of Advanced Nursing, 4 (2), Mar 1979, 123-135.

3 **Altschul, A.** Professing nursing. Lecture given by the new Professor of Nursing Studies, Edinburgh University. Nursing Mirror, 145, 8 Sep 1977, 7-9; 15 Sep 1977, 27-30.

4 **Anstey, O.E.** The watchword 'accountability': international and national implications for nursing. New South Wales College of Nursing, 1978 (26th annual oration, 20 Sep 1978). Reprinted in Australian Nurses Journal, 8 (8), Mar 1979, 28-31.

5 **Austin, R.** Professionalism and the nature of nursing reward. Journal of Advanced Nursing, 3 (1), Jan 1978, 9-23.

6 **Bandman, B. and Bandman, E.** Do nurses have rights? (The two authors give opposing views.) American Journal of Nursing, 78 (1), Jan 1978, 84-86.

7 **Bond, J. and Bond, S.** In touch with reality. (Sociology of occupations with reference to nursing as semi-profession.) Nursing Mirror, 150, 28 Feb 1980, 27-30.

8 **Brooker, R.** Professionalism/elitism and nursing education. Australian Nurses Journal, 7 (8), Mar 1978, 26-28, 49.

9 **Bullough, Bonnie and Bullough, Vern, editors** Expanding horizons for nurses. New York: Springer, 1977.

10 **Chapman, C.M.** Concepts of professionalism. Journal of Advanced Nursing, 2 (1), Jan 1977, 51-55.

11 **Chapman, C.M.** The rights and responsibilities of nurses and patients. Journal of Advanced Nursing, 5 (2), Mar 1980, 127-134.

12 **Chaska, N.L., editor** The nursing profession: views through the mist. New York: McGraw-Hill, 1978.

13 **Christman, L.** Nursing practice—whose responsibility? Australian Nurses Journal, 7 (11), Jun 1978, 38-40.

14 **Conservative Women's National Advisory Committee** The 'Cinderella' service? Report on the nursing profession presented by a working party. WNAC, 1977.

15 **Cowden, P.** Dissatisfaction and the changing meaning and purpose of the nurse's work. (With reference to professionalisation.) Nursing Forum, 17 (2), 1978, 202-209.

16 **Cowper-Smith, F.** Open forum. (Modern trends in nursing. Nursing Mirror Forum 1976.) Nursing Mirror, 142, 8 Apr 1976, 54-55.

17 **Cox, L.** To whom are we accountable? (Protection of patients both physically and emotionally.) Australian Nurses Journal, 8 (10), May 1979, 35-36, 44.

18 **Crompton, M.** Nursing in the 80s. (Prediction of trends and issues.) Nursing Times, 76, 3 Jan 1980, 23-25.

19 **Dachelet, C.Z.** Nursing's bid for increased status. Nursing Forum, 17 (1), 1978, 18-45.

20 **Davies, C.** Continuities in the development of hospital nursing in Britain. (Sociological analysis of developments in the nursing profession.) Journal of Advanced Nursing, 2 (5), Sep 1977, 479-493.

21 **Davies, C.** Experience of dependency and control in work: the case of nurses. (The development of nursing in Britain in the light of an assumption that professional groups will seek to gain autonomy and control over others.) Journal of Advanced Nursing, 1 (4), Jul 1976, 273-282.

22 **Davies, L.** What makes nursing so special? (Winner of Nursing Mirror essay competition.) Nursing Mirror, 149, 13 Dec 1979, 18-19.

23 **Earnshaw, B.** A profession must constantly strive to increase its knowledge and repute. (Essay by winner of 1977 Dettol Nursing Award.) Occupational Health, 29 (12), Dec 1977, 526-527.

24 **Ellis, B.** Nursing profession undergoes intensive scrutiny and adjustment. (Review of 1976 U.S. nursing literature.) Hospitals, 51 (7), 1 Apr 1977, 139-140, 142, 144.

25 **Ellis, J.R. and Hartley, C.L.** Nursing in today's world: challenges, issues and trends. Philadelphia: Lippincott, 1980.

26 **Ferguson, M.** The dilemma of professionalism and nursing organisation. Nursing Mirror, 143, 16 Dec 1976, 61-64.

27 **Gamer, M.** The ideology of profession-

alism. Nursing Outlook, 27 (2), Feb 1979, 108-111.

28 Germaine, A. A question of accountability. (Limits of nurses' responsibilities.) Hospital Administration in Canada, 19 (11), Nov 1977, 12-13.

29 Graham, J.A.G. On the state of the profession. (Criticism by a community physician of various aspects of nursing education, management and care with recommendations for improvement.) Nursing Times, 76, 31 Jan 1980, 186-187.

30 Gray, G. The tradition of nursing. (How handing down of opinions, beliefs and customs hinders application of problem-solving approach to nursing care.) Australian Nurses Journal, 8 (7), Feb 1979, 42-43.

31 Gunderson, K. and others How to control professional frustration. American Journal of Nursing, 77 (7), Jul 1977, 1180-1183.

32 Hancock, C. Focus on nursing. (Need for integration of clinical nurses, nurse managers and nurse teachers.) Nursing Focus, 1 (1), Sep 1979, 29, 32-33.

33 Hassenplug, L.W. Nursing can move from here to there. (A massive resocialization program is needed for the presentation of an effective, unified, professional front.) Nursing Outlook, 25 (7), Jul 1977, 432-438.

34 Hegyvary, S.T. Nursing in transition: issues and challenges. Sydney: New South Wales College of Nursing, 1979. (27th annual oration, 19 Sep 1979).

35 Hegyvary, S.T. and Haussman, R.K.D. Nursing professional review. (Proposal for developing a nursing professional review with the issues and problems related to this process.) Journal of Nursing Administration, 6 (9), Nov 1976, 12-16.

36 Hockey, L. Challenges for nursing. Nursing Times, 76, 22 May 1980, 908-911.

37 Hoy, R. and Robbins, J. The profession of nursing. New York: McGraw-Hill, 1979. (McGraw-Hill nursing studies series.)

38 Hungler, B. and others Professionalism in nursing master's graduates. (Research study using Flexner's criteria for professionalism.) Journal of Advanced Nursing, 4 (2), Mar 1979, 193-203.

39 Journal of Advanced Nursing Janforum. The nursing profession: ritualized, routinized or research-based? (With contributions from the Netherlands, Canada, U.K., Israel and India.) Journal of Advanced Nursing, 4 (1), Jan 1979, 87-98.

40 Journal of Advanced Nursing Janforum. Professionalism and nursing. (Opinions of seven top teachers, administrators and researchers from several countries.) Journal of Advanced Nursing, 5 (1), Jan 1980, 103-112.

41 Kelly, L.Y. The revolt of the nurses. (Independence and assertiveness as a professional group.) Nursing Outlook, 26 (10), Oct 1978, 661.

42 Labelle, H. Nursing authority. Four factors associated with authority, namely, (1) extensive knowledge of one's field, (2) accountability, (3) interpersonal relationships, and (4) power. (Based on ICN congress paper 1977.)

Journal of Advanced Nursing, 3 (2), Mar 1978, 145-154.

43 Leaf, A. and Roberts, K. The professional socialization of the nurse in contemporary society. Lamp, 34 (2), Feb 1977, 5, 7, 9, 11, 13.

44 Lewis, E.P. The right to inform. (Editorial on professional accountability of nurses. See also letter on p.546.) Nursing Outlook, 25 (9), Sep 1977, 561.

45 McClure, M.L. The long road to accountability. Nursing Outlook, 26 (1), Jan 1978, 47-50.

46 McFarlane, J.K., Baroness McFarlane of Llandaff A charter for caring. (Rcn Nursing Lecture 1975.) Journal of Advanced Nursing, 1 (3), May 1976, 187-196.

47 McFarlane, J.K., Baroness McFarlane of Llandaff Essays on nursing. King's Fund Centre, 1980. (KF project paper; RC2.)

48 McFarlane, J.K., Baroness McFarlane of Llandaff My eight aims for the 1980s. Nursing Mirror, 150, 10 Jan 1980, 14.

49 McFarlane, J.K. The science and art of nursing. (A paper given at the 23rd annual oration, New South Wales College of Nursing.) Australian Nurses Journal, 5 (6/7), Dec/Jan 1976, 28-30; Nursing Mirror, 142, 24 Jun 1976, 64-66.

50 MacQueen, J. A phenomenology of nursing. Nursing Papers, 6 (3), Fall 1974, 9.

51 Miller, M.H. and Flynn, B.C., editors Current perspectives in nursing: social issues and trends. Volume 1. St. Louis: Mosby, 1977. (Mosby's current practice and perspectives in nursing series.)

52 National League for Nursing Political, social and educational forces on nursing: impact of political forces. New York: NLN, 1978.

53 New Society Nurses. (Two letters on professional status of nurses.) New Society, 49, 27 Sep 1979, 696.

54 Notter, Lucille E. and Spalding, Eugenia Kennedy Professional nursing: foundations, perspectives and relationships. 9th ed. Philadelphia: Lippincott, 1976.

55 Nursing Mirror Into the 1980s. (Aspirations of nineteen leading figures in the field of nursing and the health service.) Nursing Mirror, 150, 3 Jan 1980, 18-28.

56 Nursing Mirror Modern trends in nursing. (Nursing Mirror Forum 1976. University of Edinburgh 26 Mar 1976.) Nursing Mirror, 142, 1 Apr 1976, 47-59; 8 Apr 1976, 49-55.

57 Nursing Mirror New year, new hopes— what will 1979 bring? (Views of 21 politicians, union leaders and influential nurses.) Nursing Mirror, 147, 28 Dec 1978, 16-23.

58 Nuttall, P. Nursing in the year AD 2000. (Address to the Association of Integrated and Degree Courses in Nursing.) Journal of Advanced Nursing, 1 (2), Mar 1976, 101-110.

59 O'Brien, D. Professionalism in perspective. (Occupational status of nursing.) Nursing Times, 74, 15 Jun 1978, 990.

60 O'Dwyer, E.M. Concept of professionalism. World of Irish Nursing, 4 (12), Dec 1975, 9.

61 Osborne, J. What makes nursing so special? (Runner-up in essay competition by SEN.) Nursing Mirror, 150, 10 Jan 1980, 22-23.

62 Patten, M.E. The rights of nurses: some of the fundamental issues underlying the 'rights of nurses' in the context of the declaration of a belief in the inalienable rights of all members of society. (Rights as a profession and as individuals.) Australian Nurses Journal, 6 (12), Jun 1977, 30-32, 37; Journal of Advanced Nursing, 3 (5), Sep 1978, 419-426.

63 Peplau, H.E. The changing view of nursing: (towards a higher professionalism and greater unity among all nurses.) International Nursing Review, 24 (2), Mar/Apr 1977, 43-45.

64 Pilkington, P. The illusion of final authority. (In relation to the nursing profession and accountability.) Australian Nurses Journal, 7 (11), Jun 1978, 51-53.

65 Poulin, M.A. Accountability: a professional imperative. Canadian Nurse, 73 (2), Feb 1977, 30-33.

66 Powell, Dame M. Address of welcome. (Nursing Mirror Forum 1976.) Nursing Mirror, 142 (14), 1 Apr 1976, 47-48.

67 Rhodes, B. Occupational orientations in nursing in Britain. (Identification of three orientations in nursing at Ward Sister level— professional, paramedical and bureaucratic— and the development of scale instruments to measure them.) International Journal of Nursing Studies, 17 (4), 1980, 235-245.

68 Roberts, K.L. Nursing: profession or pretender? (Suggests it is a semi-profession.) Australian Nurses Journal, 9 (10), May 1980, 33-35, 51.

69 Roberts, L. Job lot. (Challenge to the concept of professionalism in nursing.) Nursing Times, 73, 21 Jul 1977, 1105.

70 Robinson, D.E. Accountability—lip service or reality? Australian Nurses Journal, 9 (1), Jul 1979, 37-39, 55.

71 Robinson, W. The Queen and nursing: the role of the Royal Family in the nursing service of today. Nursing Mirror, 144, 2 Jun 1977, 7-9.

72 Royal College of Nursing Accountability in nursing: the report of a seminar for fellows of the Royal College of Nursing held at Leeds Castle, Kent, 15-18 April 1980. Rcn, 1980.

73 Royal College of Nursing Nursing—what price professionalism? (Rcn York and Northallerton Centre Conference.) Queen's Nursing Journal, 19 (6), Sep 1976, 181.

74 Ruch University Presbyterian-St.Luke's Medical Center Proceedings: the dedication of the John L. and Helen Kellogg National Center for Excellence in Nursing. Chicago: the Center, 1980.

75 Schrock, R.A. On political consciousness in nurses. (The welfare state, social thought and the politics of health care used as examples to demonstrate the kind of critical understanding nurses need to acquire.) Journal of Advanced Nursing, 2 (1), Jan 1977, 41-50.

76 Schrock, R.A. Politics and professionalism. Nursing Times, 73, 5 May 1977, 671-673.

77 Searle, C. The criteria for professionalism

in nursing in South Africa. Curationis, 1 (1), Jun 1978, 4-8.

78 Searle, C. The future of nursing. S.A. Nursing Journal, 43 (5), May 1976, 15-18.

79 Shryock, R.H. Nursing emerges as a profession: the American experience. *In* Leavitt, J.W. and Numbers, R.L., editors Sickness and health in America... Madison: University of Wisconsin Press, 1978. Ch.15, 203-215, bibliog.

80 Smith, J. Nursing needs rebirth in 1980. Nursing Mirror, 150, 10 Jan 1980, 24-27.

81 Smith, J. Rights, responsibilities and professionalization. (Editorial.) Journal of Advanced Nursing, 5 (2), Mar 1980, 123-126.

82 Solman, F. The next 90 years of nursing. (A personal forecast of the future.) Nursing Mirror, 146, 20 Apr 1978, 10-11.

83 Staunton, M. New dimensions of professional responsibility. International Nursing Review, 26 (3), May/Jun 1979, 84-85.

84 Storey, M. Setting the seal of courage. (Nursing as a profession.) Nursing Mirror, 148, 19 Apr 1979, Supplement xxix, xxxi-xxxii.

85 Taaffe, T.C. A concept of professionalism: accountability and responsibility. World of Irish Nursing, 4 (11), Nov 1975, 1-2.

86 Tucker, R.W. The value decisions we know as science. Advances in Nursing Science, 1 (2), Jan 1979, 1-12.

87 Wang, R.Y. and Watson, J. The professional nurse: roles, competencies and characteristics. (Review of literature.) Supervisor Nurse, 8 (6), Jun 1977, 69-71.

88 Wells, J.C.A. "Nursing: a profession that dislikes innovation"—an investigation of the reasons why. MA thesis, Brunel University, Department of Government, 1980.

89 White, R. Accountability—a necessity for survival? 2 parts. (Professional, managerial and intra-professional accountability.) Nursing Mirror, 145, 17 Nov 1977, 25-27; 24 Nov 1977, 30-31.

90 Williamson, S.B. Our professional heritage—philosophical perspectives. S.A. Nursing Journal, 43 (10), Oct 1976, 23, 26, 31.

91 Young, P. A new era in Scotland. (Interviews with Margaret Auld, CNO, Scottish Home and Health Department, and Annie Altschul, Professor of Nursing Studies, Edinburgh University.) Nursing Mirror, 145, 1 Sep 1977, 7-9.

92 Young, P. 1970...1980...1990. (Review of events in nursing in 1970 and suggestions for key posts in 1990.) Nursing Times, 76, 3 Jan 1980, 14-18.

93 Zimmerman, A. Toward a unified voice: individual and collective responsibility of nurses. (In relation to the development of appropriate health care systems to meet health needs of all individuals with special reference to primary health care.) Journal of Advanced Nursing, 3 (3), Sep 1978, 475-483.

b ATTITUDES

1 American Journal of Nursing Becoming an assertive nurse. (Two articles on assertiveness training and techniques.) American Journal of Nursing, 78 (10), Oct 1978, 1710-1713.

2 Briant, N.J. Prejudice in nursing. Canadian Nurse, 72 (6), Jun 1976, 26-30.

3 Bush, M.A. and Kjervik, D.K. The nurse's self-image. By being assertive, nurses will no longer grossly underrate their abilities. (Extract from Kjervik, D.K. and Martinson, I.M. eds. (1979) Women in stress—a nursing perspective. Appleton-Century-Crofts.) Nursing Times, 75, 26 Apr 1979, 697-701.

4 Chapman, R.W. Differences between nurses in two specialist clinical fields of general nursing. MSc (Occupational Behaviour) dissert., CNAA, North East London Polytechnic, 1980.

5 Clark, C.C. Assertiveness issues for nursing administrators and managers. Journal of Nursing Administration, 9 (7), Jul 1979, 20-24.

6 Donnelly, G.F. RN's assertiveness workbook. 'That role's not in my repertoire!' You can say 'no' to rigid sex-linked bit parts. RN, 42 (7), Jul 1979, 49-51.

7 Donnelly, G.F. RN's assertiveness workbook. When assertiveness exacts a price. RN, 42 (10), Oct 1979, 29-31.

8 Greenleaf, N.P., editor The politics of self-esteem. Wakefield, Massachusetts: Nursing Digest Inc., 1978.

9 Hauser, M.J. Assertiveness techniques: origins and uses. Journal of Psychiatric Nursing, 17 (12), Dec 1979, 15-17.

10 Herman, S.J. Becoming assertive: a guide for nurses. New York: Van Nostrand, 1978.

11 Hughes, E. Self-reliance. (Need for nurses to be assertive.) Nursing Leadership, 2 (1), Mar 1979, 14-20.

12 Hutchings, H. and Colburn, L. An assertiveness training program for nurses. Nursing Outlook, 27 (6), Jun 1979, 394-397.

13 Marriner, A. Assertive behaviour for nursing leaders. Nursing Leadership, 2 (4), Dec 1979, 14-20.

14 Pardue, S.F. Assertiveness for nursing. The myths and realities of assertive behavior in nursing. Supervisor Nurse, 11 (2), Feb 1980, 47-48, 50.

15 Partridge, K.B. Nursing values in a changing society. Nursing Outlook, 26 (6), Jun 1978, 356-360.

16 Rawnsley, M.M. The six "A's" of assertiveness. Journal of Continuing Education in Nursing, 11 (1), Jan/Feb 1980, 15-18.

17 Redfern, S.J. Hospital sisters: work, attitudes, perceptions and wastage. (Research study.) Journal of Advanced Nursing, 5 (5), Sep 1980, 451-466.

18 Rottkamp, B.C. Survey of nurse attitudes toward professional nursing practice. (New York State Nurses Association definition.) Journal of Nursing Education, 19 (5), May 1980, 32-38.

19 Schirger, M.J. Introspection: a prerequisite for emancipation. (Attitudes of nurses towards nursing and need for self-awareness in order to function independently as professionals.) Nursing Forum, 17 (3), 1978, 317-328.

20 Ugweugbu, D.C.E. and Ogundeyin, W.M. Self-image and job satisfaction of the Nigerian nurse: a comparative study. Journal of Advanced Nursing, 2 (1), Jan 1977, 29-39.

21 Vestal, K.W. Assertiveness: it's a two-way street. Journal of Practical Nursing, 30 (11), Nov/Dec 1980, 28-29, 56.

22 Walbek, B.H. and Gordon, V.C. Concurrent validity of three self-report measures of assertiveness. (Research study using 88 student nurses.) Research in Nursing and Health, 3 (4), Dec 1980, 159-162.

23 Wilson, M. Beliefs and values: some lessons to be learnt from the British National Health Service about the effects of beliefs and values on the practice of nursing. New Zealand Nursing Journal, 70 (7), Jul 1977, 21-22.

c ETHICS

1 Advances in Nursing Science Issue on ethics and values. Advances in Nursing Science, 1 (3), Apr 1979, 1-103.

2 American Association of Occupational Health Nurses Code of ethics. RN Magazine, 39 (8), Aug 1976, 20; Occupational Health Nursing, 25 (3), Mar 1977, 28.

3 American Journal of Nursing Symposium on ethics in nursing. American Journal of Nursing, 77 (5), May 1977, 845-876.

4 American Nurses' Association Code for nurses with interpretive statements. Kansas City: ANA, 1976.

5 American Nurses' Association Committee on Ethics. Ethics in nursing: references and resources. Kansas City: ANA, 1979.

6 American Nurses' Association Committee on Ethics. Ethics in nursing practice and education. Missouri: ANA, 1980.

7 Aroskar, M.A. Anatomy of an ethical dilemma. (Two articles on theory and practice.) American Journal of Nursing, 80 (4), Apr 1980, 658-663.

8 Aroskar, M.A. Ethics of nurse-patient relationships. (Four possible models of ethical nurse-patient relationships and how ethical issues can be taught.) Nurse Educator, 5 (2), Mar/Apr 1980, 18-20.

9 Barker, P. Bioethics and informed consent in American health care delivery. (With survey of ten nurses' perceptions of informed consent.) Journal of Advanced Nursing, 4 (1), Jan 1979, 23-28.

10 Barker, P. Ethics, nursing and behaviour modification. Nursing Times, 76, 29 May 1980, 976-978.

11 Bergman, R. Evolving ethical concepts for nursing. (Changes in the new Code of Ethics adopted by the ICN in 1973 compared with the Code approved in 1953.) International Nursing Review, 23 (4), Jul/Aug 1976, 116-117.

12 Berry, M. The Royal College of Nursing (Rcn) code of conduct. (Letter criticising some aspects.) Journal of Medical Ethics, 3 (4), Dec 1977, 194.

13 Boyd, K. The nature of ethics. (Symposium on moral dilemmas in nursing.) Nursing Mirror, 145, 21 Jul 1977, 14-16.

14 Boyd, K. and others Teaching medical ethics: University of Edinburgh. (Includes description of research study of how nursing students learn about medical ethics.) Journal of Medical Ethics, 4 (3), Sep 1978, 141-145.

15 Bliss, B.P. and Johnson, A.G. Communicating ethics during medical training. (Ethical discussions introduced in clinical reading programme.) Nursing Mirror, 136, 16 Feb 1973, 23-26.

16 Brearly, P. Confidentiality—the need for a code of practice. Nursing Times, 74, 23 Mar 1978, 505.

17 Canadian Nurses Association Code of ethics: an ethical basis for nursing in Canada. Canadian Nurse, 76 (5), May 1980, (7) between 36 and 37.

18 Canadian Nurses Association Convention '78. Ethical issues in nursing. Canadian Nurse, 74 (7), Jul/Aug 1978, 8-12.

19 Chalmers, H. Return to basics. 5. Ethics. Nursing Mirror, 145, 4 Aug 1977, Nursing care supplement series 5 i-iv.

20 Churchill, L. Ethical issues of a profession in transition. (Nursing.) American Journal of Nursing, 77 (5), May 1977, 873-875.

21 Clarke, D.D. and Clarke, D.M. Analysis: an introduction to ethical concepts. Definitions and ethical decisions. Journal of Medical Ethics, 3 (4), Dec 1977, 186-188.

22 Curtin, L. Nursing ethics: theories and pragmatics. Nursing Forum, 17 (1), 1978, 4-11.

23 Curtin, L. A proposed model for critical ethical analysis. Nursing Forum, 17 (1), 1978, 12-17.

24 Davis, A.J. and Aroskar, M.A. Ethical dilemmas and nursing practice. New York: Appleton-Century-Crofts, 1978.

25 Davis, A.J. and Krueger, J.C., editors Patients, nurses, ethics. New York: American Journal of Nursing, 1980.

26 Fenner, K.M. Ethics and law in nursing: professional perspectives. New York: Van Nostrand, 1980.

27 Finch, J. Law and the nurse: not so strictly confidential. (Legal and ethical codes governing disclosure of information.) Nursing Mirror, 151, 2 Oct 1980, 28-29.

28 Hays, P.I. Nurses and doctors. (Letter commenting on the Rcn 'Code of Professional Conduct for Nurses'.) British Medical Journal, 1, 12 Mar 1977, 714-715.

29 Health Visitors Association Guide for health visitors on confidentiality. Health Visitor, 53 (1), Jan 1980, 30.

30 Hide, S.E.I.M. Teaching ethics to student nurses. MA(Educ), University of London, Institute of Education, 1980.

31 Hostler, J. Analysis: an introduction to ethical concepts. The right to life. Journal of Medical Ethics, 3 (3), Sep 1977, 143-145.

32 Hughes-Ford, Nurse The importance of ethics and etiquette to the nursing profession. Lamp, 33 (1), Jan 1976, 17-18.

33 International Council of Nurses Bibliography on ethical concepts in nursing. Geneva: ICN, 1977.

34 International Council of Nurses Guidelines for member associations in regard to the ethical issues raised by the mechanical maintenance of life, interruption of life and genetic counselling and the moral dilemmas these pose for nurses. Geneva: ICN, 1980.

35 International Council of Nurses ICN guidelines to nurses as practitioners, educators, administrators and citizens concerning their action in safeguarding the human environment. International Nursing Review, 24 (5), Sep/Oct 1977, 158-159.

36 International Council of Nurses The nurse's dilemma: ethical considerations in nursing practice. Geneva: ICN, 1977.

37 Jarvis, P. Some comments on the Rcn code of professional conduct. Nursing Mirror, 145, 24 Nov 1977, 27-28.

38 Juliana, Sister Ethical and moral responsibilities of the operating room nurse. Australasian Nurses Journal, 6 (12), Jul 1977, 42, 44.

39 Kaserman, I. A nursing committee and the code for nurses. (Tennessee Nurses Association Ethics Committee and American Nurses' Association Code for Nurses.) American Journal of Nursing, 77 (5), May 1977, 875-876.

40 Ladd, John, editor Ethical issues relating to life and death. New York, Oxford: Oxford University Press, 1979.

41 Levine, M.E. Nursing ethics and the ethical nurse. American Journal of Nursing, 77 (5), May 1977, 845-849.

42 Mahon, K.A. and Everson, S.J. Moral outrage—nurses' right or responsibility: ethics rounds for nurses. (Discussion of cases causing ethical dilemmas.) Journal of Continuing Education in Nursing, 10 (3), May/Jun 1979, 4-7.

43 Mellor, P.D. The ethics of psychiatric nursing. Mind Out, 29, Jul/Aug 1978, 18-19.

44 Mellor, P.D. Moral dilemmas in psychiatric nursing. (Symposium on moral dilemmas in nursing.) Nursing Mirror, 145, 21 Jul 1977, 20-22.

45 National League for Nursing Ethical issues in nursing and nursing education. New York: NLN, 1980.

46 Nelson, L. Professionally speaking. Ethics and morals in nursing. American Journal of Maternal Child Nursing, 2 (6), Nov/Dec 1977, 343-347.

47 Nursing Clinics of North America Symposium on bioethical issues in nursing. Nursing Clinics of North America, 14 (1), Mar 1979, 1-91.

48 Nursing Mirror A symposium on moral dilemmas in nursing. Articles based on papers read at the Rcn Association of Nursing Students conference, March 1977. Nursing Mirror, 145, 21 Jul 1977, 13-16.

49 Nursing Times Professional code. (Comments on the Rcn code of professional conduct.) Nursing Times, 72, 30 Sep 1976, 1504-1505.

50 Rabb, J.D. Implications of moral and ethical issues for nurses. Nursing Forum, 15 (2), 1976, 168-179.

51 Rogan, J. Ethics and nurses. Nursing Mirror, 143, 21 Oct 1976, 75-76.

52 Romanell, P. Ethics, moral conflicts and choice. American Journal of Nursing, 77 (5), May 1977, 850-855.

53 Rousin, S. Commentary on professional ethics. Perspectives in Psychiatric Care, 14 (1), Jan-Mar 1976, 12-13.

54 Royal College of Nursing Rcn code of professional conduct: a discussion document. RCN, (1976).

55 Royal College of Nursing Royal College of Nursing (Rcn) code of professional conduct: a discussion document. (Full text with commentaries by the Assistant Secretary of the British Medical Association, a lawyer, A.T. Altschul, and student nurses.) Journal of Medical Ethics, 3 (3), Sep 1977, 115-123.

56 Rule, J.B. The professional ethic in nursing. Journal of Advanced Nursing, 3 (1), Jan 1978, 3-8. Reported in Nursing Mirror, 144, 12 May 1977, 34-35.

57 Sampson, C. The student's dilemma. (Symposium on moral dilemmas in nursing.) Nursing Mirror, 145, 21 Jul 1977, 16-17.

58 Schrock, R.A. A question of honesty in nursing practice. Journal of Advanced Nursing, 5 (2), Mar 1980, 135-148.

59 Sharples, J. At Halifax seminar: some ethical considerations for health care personnel. Hospital Administration in Canada, 17 (6), Jun 1975, 55-56

60 Shelly, J.A. Dilemma: a nurse's guide for making ethical decisions. Illinois: Intervarsity Press, 1980.

61 Shepherd, B.J. That's the ticket. (Professional ethics—supplement on safe practice in the operating theatre.) Nursing Times, 74, 2 Nov 1978, Theatre Nursing 11-12.

62 Smith, O. Dilemmas in hospital nursing practice. (Symposium on moral dilemmas in nursing.) Nursing Mirror, 145, 21 Jul 1977, 22-24.

63 Smith, S.J. and Davis, A.J. Ethical dilemmas: conflicts among rights, duties and obligations. American Journal of Nursing, 80 (8), Aug 1980, 1463-1466.

64 Steele, S.M. and Harmon, V.M. Values clarification in nursing. New York: Appleton-Century-Crofts, 1979.

65 Supervisor Nurse Ethics in a profession. 2. (Editorial quoting 1976 revision of the code for nurses.) Supervisor Nurse, 9 (6), Jun 1978, 7.

66 Swaffield, L. Seeking the meaning. European Congress of Catholic Nurses. Nursing Times, 72, 16 Sep 1976, 1422-1423.

67 Uustal, D.B. Exploring values in nursing. (Two articles.) AORN Journal, 31 (2), Feb 1980, 183-193.

68 Weber, L.J. Should physicians and nurses give moral advice? Hospital Progress, 57 (1), Jan 1976, 68-69, 80.

d IMAGE

1 Alexander, J.W. How the public perceives nurses and their education. (Survey in South Carolina.) Nursing Outlook, 27 (10), Oct 1979, 654-656.

2 AORN Journal Maybe nurses need to blow their own horns. (Calls for nurses to improve public's image of nurses by describing their work in professional journals.) AORN Journal, 26 (4), Oct 1977, 633-634.

3 AORN Journal What future for nursing? (Collection of views of nurses in the United States.) AORN Journal, 24 (2), Aug 1976, 217-235.

4 Benton, D.W. You want to be a what? (Image of nursing and vocational information gap.) Nursing Outlook, 27 (6), Jun 1979, 388-395.

5 Bergman, R. and others Opinion on nursing. Part 3: Social work students. (A study of how key members of the health team view nursing. For earlier parts, see International Nursing Review, 18 (3), 1971, and 19 (2), 1972.) International Nursing Review, 23 (1), Jan/Feb 1976, 15-24.

6 Brandner, P. Are nurses unique? Supervisor Nurse, 7 (11), Nov 1976, 34, 37-38.

7 Chapman, C.M. Image of the nurse. (ICN congress paper.) International Nursing Review, 24 (6), Nov/Dec 1977, 166-167, 170.

8 Clark, J. 'Speak up speak out'. (Advice on public speaking.) Nursing Times, 76, 15 May 1980, 858-859.

9 Elms, R.R. and Moorehead, J.M. Will the 'real' nurse please stand up. (With reference to nurses as shown in films and TV.) Nursing Forum, 16 (2), 1977, 112-127.

10 Fromm, L. The problem in nursing: nurses! (Attitudes of nurses hinder professional image of nursing.) Supervisor Nurse, 8 (10), Oct 1977, 15-16.

11 Hott, J.R. Updating Cherry Ames. (Changes in nursing's image since 1943.) American Journal of Nursing, 77 (10), Oct 1977, 1580-1583.

12 Hughes, L. The public image of the nurse. Advances in Nursing Science, 2 (3), Apr 1980, 55-72.

13 Kerrane, T. Why this annual circus is so demeaning. (Criticism of Nurse of the Year competition.) Health and Social Service Journal, 88, 16 Jun 1978, 701.

14 Lee, A.A. How nurses rate with the public. We want you, we need you... (Results of survey.) RN, 42 (6), Jun 1979, 25-39.

15 Lee, A.A. Nursing's shopworn image: how it hurts you...how it helps. (RN survey of doctors and the public.) RN, 42 (8), Aug 1979, 42-47.

16 Minnigerode, F.A. and others Masculinity and femininity in nursing. (Concept of the 'ideal nurse' was rated by male and female nursing students.) Nursing Research, 27 (5), Sep/Oct 1978, 299-302.

17 Nursing Mirror What you think of 'Angels'. (Prize-winning letters commenting on the BBC-TV series.) Nursing Mirror, 146, 11 May 1978, 12.

18 RN Magazine The public's love affair with nurses. (Brief account of survey in Maryland where nurses were rated highest among eight professionals.) RN, 42 (11), Nov 1979, 11, 13.

19 Robinson, B. A study of consumer perceptions to nursing. (Market research-type survey of 300 people's perception of ideal and actual nurse's function.) Nursing Leadership, 1 (1), Jun 1978, 14-18.

20 Roper, N. An image of nursing for the 1970s. Nursing Times, 72, 29 Apr 1976, Occ. papers, 61-64; 6 May 1976, Occ. papers, 65-66.

21 Sharma, R.L. Nurse and society: towards a better professional image. (With reference to India.) Nursing Journal of India, 68 (9), Sep 1977, 223-224.

22 Simmons, H. and Stinson, S.M. Nursing: image in conversation. (With a mental health consultant who has worked with public health nurses.) Nursing Papers, 12 (3), Aug 1980, 40-44.

23 Swaffield, L. The making of 'Angels'. (BBC-TV series based on nurses.) Nursing Times, 75, 6 Sep 1979, 1521-1527.

24 Watts, C.A.H. Making a speech. (Advice.) Nursing Mirror, 147, 3 Aug 1978, 34-35.

25 Weightman, G. When is a nurse not a nurse? (Image of the nurse and problems in recruitment.) New Society, 45, 20 Jul 1978, 130-132.

26 Williams, L.J. 'Ideal nurse' and 'real nurse'. (Pilot study to examine self-concepts and concepts of ideal nurse as perceived by trained nurses and students.) Australian Nurses Journal, 7 (9), Apr 1978, 44-46.

27 Winstead-Fry, W. The need to differentiate a nursing self. (Challenging the myths and assumptions of nursing history.) American Journal of Nursing, 77 (9), Sep 1977, 1452-1454.

e LAW: GENERAL

1 Cazalas, M.W. Nursing and the law. 3rd ed. Germantown, Md: Aspen Systems Corporation, 1978.

2 Finch, J. Law and the nurse. When are you liable for negligence? Nursing Mirror, 151, 4 Sep 1980, 22-24.

3 Hargreaves, M. Practical law for nurses. Tunbridge Wells: Pitman Medical, 1979.

4 Hemelt, M.D. and Mackert, M.E. Dynamics of law in nursing and health care. Reston: Reston Publishing Co., 1978.

5 Hospital and Health Services Review Notes for students. Privacy, professional confidence and the law. Hospital and Health Services Review, 74 (11), Nov 1978, 417-420; (12), Dec 1978, 457-460.

6 McCartney, M.L. In the witness box: how to give nursing testimony. Nursing, 77 (4), Apr 1977, 11-12.

7 Martin, A.J. The liability of nurses for professional negligence. Nursing Mirror, 142, 13 May 1976, 69-71.

8 Martin, A. The nurse and the law. The role of the coroner. Journal of Community Nursing, 3 (11), May 1980, 8, 10.

9 Mumme, J.L. Seven surefire ways to lose a malpractice case. RN Magazine, 40 (11), Nov 1977, 61-64.

10 Nursing (U.S.) Your legal guide to nursing practice. Nursing (U.S.), 9 (10), Oct 1979, 57-64; 9 (11), Nov 1979, 57-64; 9 (12), Dec 1979, 49-56.

11 Observer, pseud Knowledge of professional nursing legislation. Nursing Times, 73, 5 May 1977, 674-676.

12 Penberth, M. HELP with legal aspects of nursing practice: a management guide. Chapel Hill, NC: Ganong, Healthcare Management Consultants, 1979. (HELP management guide series; 18).

13 Perry, S.E. Managing to avoid malpractice. (Advice for nurse managers to help ensure delivery of safe patient care.) Journal of Nursing Administration, 8 (8), Aug 1978, 43-47; 8 (9), Sep 1978, 16-22.

14 Regan, W.A. Bicentennial forecast. Nursing and the law. RN Magazine, 39 (1), Jan 1976, 25-26, 30.

15 Royal College of Nursing Watchdog: for the record. Rcn, 1978.

16 Sheffield, R. Complex medicolegal issues surround modern nursing practice. (Conference findings and recommendations.) Hospitals, 52 (9), 1 May 1978, 105-106, 108-109.

17 Speller, S.R. Law notes for nurses; with supplement for Scotland by R.A. Bennett. 8th ed. Rcn, 1976.

18 Speller, S.R. Law relating to hospitals and kindred institutions; edited by J. Jacob. 6th ed. Lewis, 1978.

19 Thomas, B. Legal implications. (Symposium on moral dilemmas in nursing.) Nursing Mirror, 145, 21 Jul 1977, 24-26.

20 Warren, G. Quality assurance: insurance against malpractice. International Nursing Review, 26 (2), Mar/Apr 1979, 49-51.

21 Whincup, M. Doing one's best. (paper at an occupational health refresher course on legal responsibility in medicine and nursing.) Nursing Times, 72, 20 May 1976, 763.

22 Whincup, M.H. Legal aspects of medical and nursing service. 2nd ed. Beckenham: Ravenswood Publications, 1978. (Studies in law and practice for health service management Vol.5).

23 Whincup, M.H. Legal rights and duties in medical and nursing service. Beckenham: Ravenswood Publications, 1976. (Studies in health service management law and practice. Vol.5).

24 Whincup, M. The nurse and the law. Occupational Health, 28 (5), May 1976, 250-252.

f LAW: SPECIAL AREAS

1 Andrews, A.P. Disclosing what law

permits. (Legal principles of confidentiality of medical records.) Health and Social Service Journal, 90, 19 Sep 1980, 1230-1231.

2 Bailey, E. Legal notes. Vicarious liability. Nursing Focus, 2 (1), Sep 1980, 21-22.

3 Barkes, P. Bioethics and informed consent in American health care delivery. (With survey of ten nurses' perceptions of informed consent.) Journal of Advanced Nursing, 4 (1), Jan 1979, 23-38.

4 Besch, L.B. Informed consent: a patient's right. Nursing Outlook, 27 (1), Jan 1979, 32-35.

5 British Medical Journal Briefing. Confidentiality. British Medical Journal, 1, 10 Mar 1979, 698-699.

6 Clothier, C.M. Consent to medical experiment. Lancet, 1, 19 Mar 1977, 642-643.

7 Davis, R.W. and Hooker, J.E. If the patient is a suspected criminal. (Advice to accident and emergency nurses.) American Journal of Nursing, 79 (7), Jul 1979, 1250, 1252.

8 Dixon, E. The legal aspects of surgery. (Questionnaire and correct answers from research project.) NATNews, 17 (9), Sep 1980, 18-20, 22.

9 Farndale, W.A.J. Law on hospital consent forms. Beckenham: Ravenswood Publications, 1979. (Studies on health service management law and practice. Vol.8).

10 Farndale, W.A.J. The law relating to medical records. Nursing Times, 74, 13 Jul 1978, 1163-1164.

11 Finch, J. Law and the nurse. Why patients must consent to treatment. Nursing Mirror, 151, 11 Sep 1980, 24-25.

12 Gallop, M.R. Confidentiality of medical records. Occupational Health Nursing, 25 (11), Nov 1977, 13-15.

13 Godber, P. The health visitor in court. Health Visitor, 53 (3), Mar 1980, 83-84; (5), May 1980, 162, 164; (6), Jun 1980, 206, 209.

14 Holgate, P. Strictly between ourselves. (Confidentiality of medical records and information with reference to OH nurses.) Occupational Health, 30 (4), Apr 1978, 156-159.

15 Holgate, P. What can OH nurses prescribe? (Outline of laws and regulations.) Occupational Health, 31 (7), Jul 1979, 345-348.

16 Jones, R.V.H. and Richards, S.J. Confidentiality and medical records. (See also editorial on 131-132.) Journal of the Royal College of General Practitioners, 28, Mar 1978, 137-140.

17 Kelly, K. and McLelland, E. Signed consent: protection or constraint? Nursing Outlook, 27 (1), Jan 1979, 40-42.

18 Martin, A.J. Confidentiality — its nature in law. Nursing Times, 74, 23 Mar 1978, 503-504.

19 Martin, A.J. Consent to treatment. (A guide for nurses.) Nursing Times, 73, 2 Jun 1977, 810-811.

20 Martin, A. The nurse and the law. Confidentially speaking — don't! (With reference to

community nursing.) Journal of Community Nursing, 3 (2), Aug 1979, 15.

21 Martin, A. The nurse and the law. Donors and death. (Transplants.) Journal of Community Nursing, 3 (12), Jun 1980, 8.

22 Martin, A. The nurse and the law. In defence of oneself. (Assaults on nurses.) Journal of Community Nursing, 3 (5), Nov 1979, 32.

23 Martin, A. The nurse and the law. Professionals cannot slip up. (With reference to district nurses and accidents in patients' homes.) Journal of Community Nursing, 3 (7), Jan 1980, 26.

24 Martin, A. The nurse and the law. When help is not to hand. (When the patient's need for specialised services is diagnosed by the nurse but they are not available.) Journal of Community Nursing, 3 (10), Apr 1980, 8, 29.

25 Martin, A. Nurses and the law. Nursing Times 74.
1. Wills and gifts. 13 Apr 1978, 625.
2. Euthanasia. 11 May 1978, 800.
3. Negligence. 8 Jun 1978, 961-962.
4. Consent to treatment. (Patients with physical illness.) 13 Jul 1978, 1170.
10. Assault. (Right of self-defence.) 8 Feb 1979, 250-251.
12. Confidentiality. 12 Jul 1979, 1193.
13. Life and death. (Abortion, brain death, transplants and inquests.) 9 Aug 1979, 1372.

26 Martin, A. Nursing law. (Problems district nurses may face.) Community View, 5, May 1980, 11.

27 Peeke-Vout, L.K. The psychiatric nurse and the law. Canadian Journal of Psychiatric Nursing, 16 (6), Nov/Dec 1975, 11.

28 Rogers, C. Professional negligence in malpractice. (Vulnerability of the nurse — in particular the theatre nurse — to malpractice suits.) UNA Nursing Journal, 74 (4), Jul-Aug 1976, 24-28.

29 Royal College of Nursing. Working Party on Confidentiality in Nursing RCN
Statement on confidentiality. 1977.
Draft document. 1978.
Guidelines on confidentiality in nursing. 1980.

30 Simpson, R. Psychiatry under review. 9. Confidentiality in psychiatric nursing. Nursing Times, 76, 8 May 1980, 835-836.

31 Sklar, C.L. Legal consent and the nurse. Canadian Nurse, 74 (3), Mar 1978, 34-37.

32 Sklar, C.L. You and the law: unwarranted disclosure. (Confidentiality.) Canadian Nurse, 74 (5), May 1978, 6-8.

33 Walker, E. Nurses and the law of Scotland. Wills. Nursing Times, 74, 10 Aug 1978, 1344-1345.

34 Walshe-Brennan, K.S. The nurse and confidentiality. Nursing Mirror, 146, 20 Apr 1978, 32.

g ORGANISATIONS: GENERAL

1 Bolitho, B. and others The potential political power of nursing. Australian Nurses Journal, 9 (9), Apr 1980, 48-50.

2 Carey, S. The professional association — toward the 21st Century. (Its role and value.)

New Zealand Nursing Journal, 70 (8), Aug 1977, 12-13.

3 Cooper, S. Getting the most out of a conference. Journal of Continuing Education in Nursing, 7 (5), Sep/Oct 1976, 11-17.

4 Hott, J.R. Nursing and politics. The struggles inside nursing's body politic. Nursing Forum, 15 (4), 1976, 325-340.

5 Kalisch, B.J. and Kalisch, P.A. A discourse on the politics of nursing. Journal of Nursing Administration, 6 (3), Mar/Apr 1976, 29-34.

6 Nursing Administration Quarterly Issue on politics and power. (Eleven articles.) Nursing Administration Quarterly, 2 (3), Spring 1978, 1-99.

7 Powell, D.J. Nursing and politics. The struggles outside nursing body's politic. (To become an autonomous and self-regulating profession in the US.) Nursing Forum, 15 (4), 1976, 341-362.

8 University of Edinburgh. Nursing Studies Association Nurses in the political arena. (Annual conference, including contribution from Baroness McFarlane.) Nursing Times, 76, 29 May 1980, 946.

h ORGANISATIONS: INDIVIDUAL (alphabetically by title)

ASSOCIATION OF NURSE ADMINISTRATORS

1 Queen's Nursing Journal The Association of Nurse Administrators. (Annual general meeting report.) Queen's Nursing Journal, 18 (9), Dec 1975, 258.

2 Greene, J. Birth of an association. (Formation of the Association of Nurse Administrators in 1919.) Nursing Mirror, 149, 30 Aug 1979, Supplement xxi-xxii, xxiv-xxv.

COUNCIL FOR THE EDUCATION AND TRAINING OF HEALTH VISITORS

3 Wilkie, E. A history of the Council for the Education and Training of Health Visitors: an account of its establishment and field of activities 1962-1975. Allen and Unwin, 1979.

GENERAL NURSING COUNCIL FOR ENGLAND AND WALES

4 General Nursing Council for England and Wales Annual reports. GNC, 1975/76, 1976; 1976/77, 1977; 1977/78, 1979.

HEALTH VISITORS ASSOCIATION

5 Allen, M. After 21 years, still a healthy association. (Interview with Jane Wyndham-Kaye, General Secretary of the Health Visitors Association, with two photographs.) Nursing Mirror, 149, 25 Oct 1979, 28-30.

QUEEN'S NURSING INSTITUTE

6 Queen's Nursing Journal The Queen's Nursing Institute. (Survey of the year's work.) Queen's Nursing Journal, 18 (9), Dec 1975, 238, 240, 245.

7 Queen's Nursing Institute The beginnings. Queen's Nursing Journal, 19 (15), Jun 1977, 421.

8 Queen's Nursing Journal Queen's Nursing

Institute. (Functions of the Institute with illustrations and a history of the building.) Queen's Nursing Journal, 18 (10), Jan 1976, 275-278.

9 Stringer, M. Community nursing. Full circle. (History of Queen's Nursing Institute from 1887.) Nursing Mirror, 144, 30 Jun 1977, 43.

ROYAL COLLEGE OF NURSING
General (including Trade Union status)

10 British Medical Journal Nurses and trade unionism. (Report on a debate at the Royal College of Nursing Conference 1976.) British Medical Journal, 1, 17 Apr 1976, 973-974.

11 Chisholm, M. Why we should join. (Issues involved in union or Rcn membership for nurses.) Nursing Mirror, 143, 21 Oct 1976, 73-74.

12 Clark, J. Harrogate in retrospect. Appraisal of the Rcn Congress in Harrogate from April 6 to 9. Nursing Mirror, 142, 22 Apr 1976, 38-39.

13 Clark, J. Why I chose the Rcn. Nursing Mirror, 143, 16 Sep 1976, 39-40.

14 Grant, N. Inevitable decision: where the Rcn stands on trade union certification. Nursing Times, 72, 5 Aug 1976, 1186-1187.

15 Hall, C.M. Any questions? (Interview with Catherine Hall on the Rcn Council's decision to seek certification as a trade union.) Nursing Times, 72, 26 Aug 1976, 1301-1303.

16 Hall, C.M. Rcn: professional body and trade union? Comments on the leading article and news feature in Nursing Times, August 5. Nursing Times, 72, 26 Aug 1976, 1300.

17 Nursing Mirror Rcn Diamond Jubilee. (With congratulations from Founder Members.) Nursing Mirror, 142, 1 Apr 1976, 39-40. Editorial—Sixty glorious years, 33.

18 Nursing Mirror Whistle stop tour to convince members 'Rcn should become a union.' Nursing Mirror, 143 (12), 16 Sep 1976, 36.

19 Nursing Times Celebrating sixty years. (Rcn Diamond Jubilee.) Nursing Times, 72, 1 Apr 1976, 481-484.

20 Nursing Times Rcn and trade union certification. Nursing Times, 72, 29 Jul 1976, 1140, 1147; 5 Aug 1976, 1179; 2 Dec 1976, 1860.

21 Nursing Times Rcn to seek trade union certification? Members will decide at November annual general meeting. Nursing Times, 72, 29 Jul 1976, 1140.

22 Royal College of Nursing Charter and bye-laws 1978. Rcn, 1979.

23 Royal College of Nursing The implications of trade union status. Rcn, 1977.

24 Royal College of Nursing The Rcn tomorrow: professional organisation and trade union. Rcn, 1976.

25 Royal College of Nursing What the Rcn stands for. (A statement of policy issued in September by the Royal College of Nursing.) Rcn, (1976). Reprinted in Nursing Mirror, 143, 18 Nov 1976, 54-57.

26 Royal College of Nursing Congress 1976 Rcn Diamond Jubilee Congress 1976. Nursing Mirror, 142, 8 Apr 1976, 34-35; 15 Apr 1976, 35-36; Nursing Times, 72, 8 Apr 1976, 514-516; 15 Apr 1976, 559-562.

27 Royal College of Nursing Congress 1977 Professional Conference. Politics, prejudices and professionalism? (Report.) Nursing Times, 73, 12 May 1977, 678-679.

28 Royal College of Nursing Congress 1978 Harrogate, 5-9 June. Report. (Including paper by June Clark and interview with David Ennals.) Nursing Mirror, 146, 1 Jun 1978, Supplement 1, 3, 5-7, 9, 13, 15, 17, 19; 8 Jun 1978, 2-3; 15 Jun 1978, 4-7; Nursing Times, 1 Jun 1978, Rcn supplement 1, 3-4, 7, 11, 14, 17-19, 21; 8 Jun 1978, 938-939; 15 Jun 1978, 984-987.

29 Royal College of Nursing Congress 1978 The week: a personal view of medicopolitical events. (Rcn congress especially June Clark's contribution.) British Medical Journal, 1, 17 Jun 1978, 1632.

30 Simpson, H.M. The Rcn 1916-1976. Role and action in a changing health service. (Nursing lecture for Diamond Jubilee Year.) Royal College of Nursing, 1976. (Nursing Lecture 1976) Reprinted in Nursing Mirror, 143, 2 Dec 1976, 39-41.

31 Young, P. The Rcn today. (Rcn Diamond Jubilee Supplement.) Nursing Mirror, 143, 18 Nov 1976, i-viii. Highlights from the history of the Rcn (Photographs), 50-51.

ROYAL COLLEGE OF NURSING
Industrial Action

32 Bolger, T. and Fogg, D. Reasons for rocking the boat. (Views of Basildon and Thurrock Rcn Centre on pay problems and industrial action.) Nursing Times, 75, 5 Jul 1979, 1122-1123.

33 Carr, A. Professional industrial action? (With reference to possible decision by Rcn Council to authorise limited action.) Nursing Times, 75, 8 Feb 1979, 224-225.

34 Clark, J. and Hall, C.M. A critical professional issue. (Possible industrial action by Rcn.) Nursing Times, 75, 15 Feb 1979, 270-271.

35 Dunn, A. Excuse me, your pay slip is showing. (Editorial on lack of professionalism in possible proposed industrial action by Rcn.) Nursing Times, 75, 25 Jan 1979, 131.

36 Ellis, S. Where is the silent majority? (Low response to Rcn vote on limited industrial action.) Nursing Times, 75, 8 Mar 1979, 391.

37 McCarthy, M. My staff come first. (Why author would vote 'Yes' to limited industrial action.) Nursing Mirror, 148, 22 Feb 1979, 8-9.

38 McCarthy, M. The Rcn vote: a case of professional genocide? Nursing Mirror, 148, 8 Mar 1979, 6.

39 Nursing Times Industrial action—Rcn moves a step closer to the brink. (Report RRB.) Nursing Times, 76, 29 May 1980, 940.

40 Nursing Times Professional principles. (Correspondence on the Rcn's possible decision to approve limited industrial action.) Nursing Times, 75, 22 Feb 1979, 310.

41 Wells, R. and Plant, J. Views for and against a change in the Rcn's rules to allow limited industrial action. Nursing Mirror, 148, 22 Feb 1979, 4-5.

ROYAL COLLEGE OF NURSING
TUC Affiliation

42 Carr, A. Counting the cost of TUC affiliations. (Reasons against the Rcn affiliating to the TUC.) Nursing Mirror, 149, 11 Oct 1979, 10.

43 Clay, T. TUC debate. Why I will be voting in favour. Nursing Mirror, 148, 19 Apr 1979, Supplement x.

44 Darby, C. College membership to debate affiliation to TUC. (Report and editorial.) Nursing Mirror, 147, 21 Sep 1978, 1-2.

45 Darby, C. To affiliate to the TUC or not? —that is the question for the Rcn. (Summary of Rcn document with some comment.) Nursing Mirror, 147, 5 Oct 1978, 9.

46 Darby, C. New row as Rcn is barred from talks. (Camden and Islington AHA.) Nursing Mirror, 147, 20 Jul 1978, 1.

47 Dyson, R. Nursing and the TUC. (Boundary between professional and trade union activity and issues facing the Rcn regarding TUC affiliation.) Nursing Standard, 79, Dec 1978, 10.

48 Dyson, R. The Rcn and the TUC. (Comment on Rcn discussion document and examination of the implications of TUC affiliation for it and other health professions' organisations.) British Medical Journal, 2, 11 Nov 1978, 1380-1381.

49 Health and Social Service Journal Coming to the crunch. (Comment on Rcn's decision to discuss TUC affiliation.) Health and Social Service Journal, 88, 13 Oct 1978, 1156.

50 Health Services Manpower Review Viewpoint. (Editorial on Rcn debate on TUC affiliation.) Health Services Manpower Review, 4 (4), Nov 1978, 2.

51 Holder, S.J. TUC affiliation—a most important matter. (Letter on some of its implications for the Rcn.) Nursing Mirror, 147, 9 Nov 1978, 10.

52 Holder, S.J. TUC debate. A time to say 'no'. Nursing Mirror, 148, 19 Apr 1979 Supplement xi-xii.

53 Lightowlers, J. Organ music. (Comment on Rcn's discussion of TUC affiliation.) Journal of Community Nursing, 2 (5), Nov 1978, 20.

54 Morgan, K.E. Why I say 'yes' to joining the TUC. (Rcn affiliation.) Nursing Mirror, 149, 25 Oct 1979, 14.

55 Nursing Mirror Should the Rcn join the TUC? (Views of Rcn members in NM poll.) Nursing Mirror, 147, 26 Oct 1978, 16-17.

56 Nursing Times What is the TUC? (Advantages of TUC affiliation with particular reference to nursing organisations such as Rcn.) Nursing Times, 73, 12 May 1977, 684-685.

57 Philpot, T. When is a union not a union? (Dispute in Camden/Islington AHA over Rcn's non-affiliation to TUC.) Nursing Mirror, 146, 15 Jun 1978, 3.

58 Royal College of Nursing Debate on TUC affiliation. Nursing Times, 73, 19 May 1977, 718-722.

59 Royal College of Nursing The Rcn and affiliation to the TUC. (Discussion document.)

RCN, 1978. Also in Nursing Standard, 77, Oct 1978, 8-11.

60 Young, P. The great debate. (Over Rcn TUC affiliation.) Nursing Times, 75, 19 Apr 1979, 653.

i WOMEN AND NURSING

1 Austin, R. Sex and gender in the future of nursing. The feminine image of nursing and the possible effects of the increasing number of men in senior posts. Nursing Times, 73, 25 Aug 1977, Occ. papers, 113-116; 1 Sep 1977, Occ. papers, 117-119.

2 Bermosk, L.S. and Porter, S.E. Experiences of women as nurses in the health care system. In Bermosk, L.S. and Porter, S.E. Women's health and human wholeness. New York: Appleton-Century-Crofts, 1979.

3 Canadian Nurse Is there sex discrimination in health care? (Results of questionnaire among Canadian nurses.) Canadian Nurse, 71 (12), Dec 1975, 15-22.

4 Fasano, N.F. Credit for consciousness raising. (Course at University of Texas School of Nursing, to promote a career oriented attitude towards nursing, based on women's studies.) Journal of Nursing Education, 6 (8), Oct 1977, 3-6.

5 Greenleaf, N.P. Sex-segregated occupations: relevance for nursing. Advances in Nursing Science, 2 (3), Apr 1980, 23-27.

6 Hector, W. Women as nurses and nurses as women. (Review of 'Women in Nursing' by L. Hockey.) British Medical Journal, 1, 2 Apr 1977, 894-895.

7 Hockey, Lisbeth Women in nursing: a descriptive study. (In four areas of Scotland.) Hodder and Stoughton, 1976.

8 Kjervik, D.K. Influencing sex role opinions of undergraduate nursing students. (Description of course on women's studies and sex roles with evaluation of changes in students' opinions.) Journal of Nursing Education, 18 (8), Oct 1979, 43-49.

9 Keller, M.C. The effect of sexual stereotyping on the development of nursing theory. American Journal of Nursing, 79 (9), Sep 1979, 1584-1586

10 Kritek, P. and Glass, L. Nursing: a feminist perspective. (Course for student nurses.) Nursing Outlook, 26 (3), Mar 1978, 182-186.

11 Lytle, N.A., editor Nursing of women in the age of liberation. Dubuque: Brown, 1977.

12 Moore, D.S. and others Baccalaureate nursing students' identification with the women's movement. Nursing Research, 27 (5), Sep/Oct 1978, 291-295.

13 Schirm, V.M. Women in work: nontraditional occupations and the nursing profession. Occupational Health Nursing, 25 (12), Dec 1977, 13-21.

14 Shockley, J.S. Perspectives in femininity. Implications for nursing. (Reprinted from the Journal of Obstetric, Gynecologic and Neonatal Nursing, 3 (6), Nov/Dec 1974, 36-40.) Nursing Digest, 3 (6), Nov/Dec 1975, 49-52.

15 Yeaworth, R.C. Women and nurses: evolving roles. Occupational Health Nursing, 24 (8), Aug 1976, 7-9.

6 NURSE'S ROLE

a GENERAL

1 Akinsanya, J. The unique function of the nurse. (The caring role, providing continuous care 24 hours a day for the whole patient.) Nursing Times, 76, 28 Feb 1980, 360-361.

2 American Journal of Nursing Civil Service moves up 4,800 nurses to Grade 9 in major reclassification. (Standards revision that recognises nurses' expanded job functions.) American Journal of Nursing, 77 (5), May 1977, 757, 760, 764.

3 American Nurses' Foundation A cross-cultural study of the nursing role in ten countries. Nursing Research Report, 11 (3), 1976, 10-12.

4 Appelbaum, A.L. Commission leads way to joint practice for nurses and physicians. (Work of the National Joint Practice Commission in defining new roles and relationships for the two professions.) Hospitals, 52 (14), 16 Jul 1978, 78-81.

5 British Medical Journal Extending the role of the clinical nurse. (Comment on recent research and circular.) British Medical Journal, 2, 11 Nov 1978, 1320.

6 Bullough, B. Influences on role expansion (of registered nurses in the United States). American Journal of Nursing, 76 (9), Sep 1976, 1476-1481.

7 Bullough, B., editor The law and the expanding nursing role. New York: Appleton-Century-Crofts, 1975.

8 Canadian Nurses Association Development of a definition of nursing practice and standards for nursing practice. (Project report with draft standards.) Canadian Nurse, 76 (5), May 1980, 11-15.

9 Chaska, N.L. Status consistency and nurses' expectations and perceptions of role performance. (Analysis of effects of education, position and income.) Nursing Research, 27 (6), Nov/Dec 1978, 356-364.

10 Ciesla, J.H. Nursing practice acts. (Review of legislation in various states which defines role of professional nurses.) Occupational Health Nursing, 25 (10), Oct 1977, 13-17.

11 Clark, J. Diagnosis and prescribing by nurses. (Argues that competence should be the criterion for deciding who can diagnose and who can prescribe.) Occupational Health, 30 (1), Jan 1978, 12-15.

12 Clark, J. Janforum. Should nurses diagnose and prescribe? Journal of Advanced Nursing, 3 (5), Sep 1978, 485-488.

13 Clark, J. When should nurses prescribe? (Expansion and application of principles outlined in paper in previous issue.) Occupational Health, 30 (2), Feb 1978, 60-63.

14 Clark, N.M. and Lenburg, C.B. Knowledge-informed behavior and the nursing culture: a preliminary study. (Pilot study which

identified six intersecting roles and nine categories of behaviour.) Nursing Research, 29 (4), Jul/Aug 1980, 244-249.

15 Colliere, M.F. Nursing: thoughts on nursing service and identification of the service offered. International Nursing Review, 27 (2), Mar/Apr 1980, 49-52; (3), May/Jun 1980, 79-87; (4), Jul/Aug 1980, 114-118.

16 Congalton, A.A. The functions of a nurse. (Discussions and statement by Nurse Education Board of New South Wales.) Nursing Times, 73, 9 Jun 1977, Occ. papers, 81-83.

17 Coombes, P.T. and others Crumbs from the doctors. (Letter criticising aspects of the extended role of the nurse involving 'medical' tasks. For letter replying to this see Nursing Times, 6 April, 594.) Nursing Times, 74, 16 Mar 1978, 459.

18 Department of Health and Social Security The extending role of the clinical nurse: legal implications and training requirements. DHSS, 1977. (HC(77)22). (Summary in Nursing Times, 73, 14 Jul 1977, 1056.)

19 Ellis, B. Future evolution of nursing role contingent on legislation. (Nurse practice acts in the various states of the USA.) Hospitals, 52, 1 Feb 1978, 81-82.

20 Eriksson, K. Nursing—skilled work or a profession? (Study of the functions of the nurse carried out by a working group of the Northern Nurses Federation.) International Nursing Review, 23 (4), Jul/Aug 1976, 118-120.

21 Federation of Speciality Nursing Organisations and American Nurses' Association Nursing care statement issued by the Federation. (Statement on role and responsibilities of the professional nurse.) American Journal of Nursing, 77 (11), Nov 1977, 1754.

22 Friss, L. What do nurses do? (Role and four core functions of nursing; assisting, interviewing, informing and co-ordinating.) Journal of Nursing Administration, 7 (8), Oct 1977, 24-28.

23 Germaine, A. A question of accountability. (Limits of nurses' responsibilities.) Hospital Administration in Canada, 19 (11), Nov 1977, 12-13.

24 Greene, J. Extending the role of the nurse. Pushing forward the frontiers. (How Gloucestershire Area Health Authority approached the subject and made policy recommendations.) Nursing Mirror, 147, 26 Oct 1978, 34-36; Nursing Times, 73, 15 Sep 1977, 1424-1425.

25 Habeeb, M.C. and McLaughlin, F.E. Health care professionals' role expectations and patient needs. (Research study.) Nursing Research, 26 (4), Jul/Aug 1977, 288-298.

26 Health and Social Service Journal Britain's 'barefoot' doctors? (At BUPA medical centre nurses carry out screening procedures formerly done by doctors.) Health and Social Service Journal, 86, 28 Feb 1976, 400-401.

27 Hunt, G.J. Anatomy of a proposition. (Suggests that nurses should be allowed to prescribe certain appliances and substances.) Nursing Times, 76, 13 Mar 1980, 450-451.

28 Jayalakshmi, D. Nurses' role performance —a research study. Nursing Journal of India, 71 (3), Mar 1980, 63-68.

29 Koehne-Kaplan, N.S. and Tilden, V.P. The process of clinical judgment in nursing practice: the component of personality. (A study which shows the effects of the extended role of nurses and the increasing numbers of men and older women entering nursing on nurses' personality profile and the nursing process.) Nursing Research, 25 (4), Jul/Aug 1976, 268-272.

30 Kratz, C. Roles and realities. (Nurses' problems in defining their role.) Nursing Times, 72, 17 Jun 1976, 923.

31 Kraus, I. The role of the nurse in the hospital setting of the 1980s. (The author is a nurse and the first woman chairman of the American Hospital Association.) World Hospitals, 15 (2), May 1979, 132-135.

32 Lambertsen, E.C. The extended role of the nurse in providing health care. (Symposium paper.) SA Nursing Journal, 43 (9), Sep 1976, 11-16.

33 Lindars, M.E. Professional practice. The precise role of the nurse. Nursing Mirror, 146, 12 Jan 1978, 37.

34 Logan, J. The expanded role of the handmaiden. (The nursing profession in relation to other health professions.) Canadian Nurse, 76 (1), Jan 1980, 34-35.

35 MacGuire, J. The expanded role of the nurse. King's Fund Centre, 1980. (KF project paper, RC3).

36 Minehan, P.L. Nurse role conception. (Comparison of two scales measuring role conception showed differences between nurses in the 50s and the 70s.) Nursing Research, 26 (5), Sep/Oct 1977, 374-379.

37 New South Wales. Nurses Education Board The functions of a registered nurse. Lamp, 34 (1), Jan 1977, 20-21.

38 Nursing Journal of India Issue on the expanding role of the nurse. Nursing Journal of India, 68 (1), Jan 1977, 2-25.

39 Nursing Mirror What price progress? (Editorial on health circular on extending role of the clinical nurse.) Nursing Mirror, 145, 28 Jul 1977, 1.

40 Nursing Times Doctors back nurses' extended role. (Report of resolution at BMA junior medical staff's annual conference.) Nursing Times, 76, 17 Jul 1980, 1245.

41 Oda, D. Specialized role development: a three phase process. Nursing Outlook, 25 (6), Jun 1977, 374-377.

42 Oselladore, Y. The nurse within the bureaucracy. (The nurse's role in relation to the patient and other health professionals.) Australian Nurses Journal, 7 (10), May 1978, 46-48.

43 Registered Nurses' Association of British Columbia The nurse's role in health assessment and promotion. An official position paper. Canadian Nurse, 73 (3), Mar 1977, 40-41.

44 Reifsteck, S.W. Expanding R.N. roles. At the grass-roots level. RN Magazine, 38 (5), May 1975, 91-93, 97, 98.

45 Royal College of Nursing The duties and position of the nurse. Rev.ed. Rcn, 1978.

46 Royal College of Nursing The extended clinical role of the nurse. Rcn, 1979.

47 Royal College of Nursing The extending role of the nurse. (Report of Northallerton and York Rcn Centre's symposium.) Nursing Mirror, 145, 15 Sep 1977, 3.

48 Royal College of Nursing 'We are over-nursing and under-caring.' (Report of conference on the extended role of the nurse organised by the Rcn and Bristol Health District.) Nursing Times, 74, 13 Apr 1978, 610.

49 Rozovsky, L.E. Should the nurse's role be defined by law? Dimensions in Health Service, 53 (3), Mar 1976, 9-11.

50 Saint-Yves, I.F.M. Patient care in time and space. (Suggests extended use of paramedical personnel (HV and DN) as 'barefoot doctors' in the health service.) Royal Society of Health Journal, 98 (5), Oct 1978, 238-239.

51 Searle, C. Panel discussion. The extended role of the nurse in hospital. (Symposium report.) SA Nursing Journal, 43 (9), Sep 1976, 17-20.

52 Simms, S. Nursing's dilemma—the battle for role determination. (Role conflict of nurses.) Supervisor Nurse, 8 (9), Sep 1977, 29-31, 33.

53 Stoller, E.P. Preconceptions of the nursing role: a case study of an entering class. Journal of Nursing Education, 17 (6), Jun 1978, 2-14.

54 Trandel-Korenchuk, D.M. and Trandel-Korenchuk, K.M. How state laws recognise advanced nursing practice. Nursing Outlook, 26 (11), Nov 1978, 713-719.

55 Turner, M. Points for doctors. (Paper at Rcn meeting on the nurse's role in screening and prescribing including vaccination and immunisation.) Nursing Times, 73, 28 Jul 1977, 1144-1145.

56 Watson, J. Role conflict in nursing. (Review of literature.) Supervisor Nurse, 8 (7), Jul 1977, 40-41, 45-47, 50.

57 White, S. The expanded role for nurses. (Report (by journalist) of research study of nurses' and doctors' views on acceptable tasks for nurses.) Nursing, 7 (10), Oct 1977, 16-19.

58 Wilson-Barnett, J. Reflections on progress. (The need for identifying nursing tasks and skills to prevent erosion of the role of the nurse.) Nursing Times, 72, 24 Jun 1976, 962.

59 World of Irish Nursing Working Party on the Role of the Nurse. (Terms of reference and outline of work.) World of Irish Nursing, 9 (7/8), Jul/Aug 1980, 1.

b CHANGE

1 Aragon, L.M. The nurse as a health worker—new horizons. Philippine Journal of Nursing, 46 (3/4), Jul/Dec 1977, 152-161, 214.

2 Auld, M. Nursing in a changing society. (Technological, demographic, social and disease-pattern changes in British society. Rcn Nursing Lecture 1978.) Journal of Advanced Nursing, 4 (3), May 1979, 287-298.

3 Birckhead, L.M. Nursing and the technetronic age. (The effect of technology on nursing.) Journal of Nursing Administration, 8 (2), Feb 1978, 16-19.

4 Bolton, G. Preparing for the next decade. (Implications of increased use of technology on nursing and need for greater emphasis on education to prepare nurses more effectively.) Nursing Times, 73, 3 Jan 1980, 26-28.

5 Bronzino, J.D. Technology for patient care: applications for today, implications for tomorrow. St. Louis: Mosby, 1977.

6 Calton, S. Keeping pace with the times: the relationship between patterns of illness and the development of health care, in particular the role of the nurse. Nursing Mirror, 150, 31 Jan 1980, 36-37.

7 Corish, B. The future role of the nurse. World of Irish Nursing, 6 (1), Jan 1977, 1.

8 Dingwall, R. Are you ready for the microchip? What has the new technological revolution to do with nursing? Nursing Times, 75, 7 Jun 1979, 975-976.

9 Fagerhaugh, S. and others The impact of technology on patients, providers, and care patterns. Nursing Outlook, 28 (11), Nov 1980, 666-672.

10 Farmer, E. The impact of technology on nursing. (Report of study in a Scottish teaching hospital.) Nursing Mirror, 147, 28 Sep 1978, 17-20.

11 Fashina, E.M. The changing role of the nurse. Nigerian Nurse, 7 (4), Oct-Dec 1975, 16-17.

12 Henderson, V. Preserving the essence of nursing in a technological age. Nursing Times, 75, 22 Nov 1979, 2012-2013; 29 Nov 1979, 2056-2058; Journal of Advanced Nursing, 5 (3), May 1980, 245-260.

13 Hockey, L. The future nurse: selection and training: autonomy; should her health-care role be modified for future patient demands? Journal of Advanced Nursing, 3 (6), Nov 1978, 571-582.

14 Hockey, L. A nurse's contribution to care in a changing setting. (Based on a paper presented to the Ciba Foundation Symposium 'Health Care in a Changing Setting: the UK Experience' published 1976 by Elsevier/Excerpta Medica, 59-74.) Journal of Advanced Nursing, 2 (2), Mar 1977, 147-156.

15 International Council of Nurses ICN statement to UN conference on science and technology for development. International Nursing Review, 27 (3), May/Jun 1980, 96.

16 Kangori, S.W. Medicine for tomorrow and the role of the nurse. Kenya Nursing Journal, 7 (12), Dec 1978, 29-31.

17 Katz, F.M. and others Stepping out: nurses and their new roles. Kensington: New South Wales University Press, 1976.

18 Kerrane, T. Challenge of changing patterns in nursing. (A critical look at the changing role of the nurse.) Health and Social Service Journal, 87, 2 Sep 1977, 1244-1245.

19 Philip, M., Sister Health services and nursing: changing patterns. (Changing role of nurse.) Australian Nurses Journal, 2 (3), Sep 1972, 33-34.

20 Pinker, R. A nurse for all seasons? (An address on the future role of the nurse given at an

Rcn research conference.) Nursing Mirror, 146, 25 May 1978, 31-34.

21 Singh, R.N. Nurses as agents of change. (With reference to India.) Nursing Journal of India, 68 (7), Jul 1977, 183-184.

22 Smith, G. The changing role of the nurse. (Towards role of monitor and counsellor in health-oriented care rather than sickness-oriented care.) International Nursing Review, 25 (1), Jan/Feb 1978, 9, 13.

23 Steiner-Freud, J. and others Changing attitudes to health and illness: the effects on nursing practice. (With reference to Israel.) International Nursing Review, 25 (5), Sep/Oct 1978, 143-145.

24 Walker, B. Technological change: issues and impacts. Lamp, 37 (10), Oct 1980, 59-62.

c CONCEPTS AND PHILOSOPHY

1 Advances in Nursing Science ANS open forum. (Discussion by four nurses on actions needed to promote research and theory development in nursing.) Advances in Nursing Science, 1 (1), Oct 1978, 85-95.

2 Advances in Nursing Science Issue on holistic health. Advances in Nursing Science, 2 (4), Jul 1980, 1-92.

3 Anna, D.J. and others Implementing Orem's conceptual framework. (Based on assisting man with self-care practices, and its testing in a clinical setting.) Journal of Nursing Administration, 8 (11), Nov 1978, 8-11.

4 Arakelian, M. An assessment and nursing application of the concept of locus of control. Advances in Nursing Science, 3 (1), Oct 1980, 25-42.

5 Association of Integrated and Degree Courses in Nursing Developing a theory of nursing: report of the 4th open conference, University of Hull, 9-11 July, 1976. The Association, 1976.

6 Bartlett, A. Is nursing more of an art than a science? (Joint runner-up in competition.) Nursing Mirror, 151, 11 Dec 1980, 26-27.

7 Beckstrand, J. A critique of several conceptions of practice theory in nursing. Research in Nursing Health, 3 (2), Jun 1980, 69-79.

8 Bermosk, L.S. and Porter, S.E. Nursing and the search for human wholeness. In Bermosk, L.S. and Porter, S.E. Women's health and human wholeness. New York: Appleton-Century-Crofts, 1979.

9 Bohny, B.J. Theory development for a nursing science. Nursing Forum, 19 (1), 1980, 50-67.

10 Brodt, D.E. A re-examination of the synergistic theory of nursing. Nursing Forum, 19 (1), 1980, 85-93.

11 Broncatello, K.F. Auger in action: application of the model. (Auger's behavioural systems model.) Advances in Nursing Science, 2 (2), Jan 1980, 13-23.

12 Brower, H.F.T. and Baker, B.J. The Roy Adaptation Model: using the adaptation model in a practitioner curriculum. (To identify areas of nursing care in geriatric patients.) Nursing Outlook, 24 (11), Nov 1976, 686-689.

13 Bush, H.A. Models for nursing. (The concept of model, the relationship between models and theories and their use in nursing.) Advances in Nursing Science, 1(2), Jan 1979, 13-21.

14 Byrne, M.L. and Thompson, L.F. Key concepts for the study and practice of nursing. 2nd ed. St. Louis: Mosby, 1978.

15 Cantor, M.M. Philosophy, purpose and objectives: why do we have them? Wakefield, MA: Contemporary Publishing, 1977. (Contemporary nursing review, no.R1).

16 Carper, B.A. Fundamental patterns of knowing in nursing. Advances in Nursing Science, 1 (1), Oct 1978, 13-23.

17 Chapman, C.M. The use of sociological theories and models in nursing. Journal of Advances Nursing, 1 (2), Mar 1976, 111-127.

18 Chinn, P.L. and Jacobs, M.K. A model for theory development in nursing. Advances in Nursing Science, 1 (1), Oct 1978, 1-11.

19 Colliere, M.F. Nursing: thoughts on nursing service and identification of the service offered. Part 2. (Nursing theory.) International Nursing Review, 27 (3), May/Jun 1980, 79-87; (4), Jul/Aug 1980, 114-118.

20 Constantino, R.E.B. Conceptualizing general systems theory for nursing students and clinicians. Philippine Journal of Nursing, 49 (1), Jan/Mar 1979, 21-25.

21 Craig, S.L. Theory development and its relevance for nursing. Journal of Advanced Nursing, 5 (4), Jul 1980, 349-355.

22 Crawford, G. and others Evolving issues in theory development. Nursing Outlook, 27 (5), May 1979, 346-351.

23 Fawcett, J. A declaration of nursing independence: the relation of theory and research to nursing practice. Journal of Nursing Administration, 10 (6), Jun 1980, 36-39.

24 Fawcett, J. A framework for analysis and evaluation of conceptual models of nursing. Nursing Education, 5 (6), Nov/Dec 1980, 10-14.

25 Fenner, K. Developing a conceptual framework. (Use of Orem's self-care theory as a base for curriculum development.) Nursing Outlook, 27 (2), Feb 1979, 122-126.

26 Flaskerud, J.H. and Halloran, E.J. Areas of agreement in nursing theory development. Advances in Nursing Science, 3 (1), Oct 1980, 1-7.

27 Fuller, S.S. Holistic man and the science and practice of nursing. (Knowledge and concepts essential to nursing are defined by the nature of the human being.) Nursing Outlook, 26 (11), Nov 1978, 700-704.

28 Gortner, S.R. Nursing science in transition. Nursing Research, 29 (3), May/Jun 1980, 180-183.

29 Graham, D. A philosophy of nursing. Australian Nurses Journal, 6 (3), Sep 1976, 24.

30 Griffin, A.P. Philosophy and nursing. (The concept of caring, political consciousness in nurses, implications of a systems approach to the nursing process and an analysis of nursing theory

and research.) Journal of Advanced Nursing, 5 (3), May 1980, 261-272.

31 Grypdonck, M. and others Integrating nursing: a holistic approach to the delivery of nursing care. (Research study to develop model based on integration of physical and psycho-social components of nursing care.) International Journal of Nursing Studies, 16 (2), 1979, 215-230.

32 Gudmundsen, A.M. The conduct of inquiry into nursing. (Theoretical base of nursing.) Nursing Forum, 18 (1), 1979, 52-59.

33 Haase, P.T. and others A workbook on the environments of nursing: theoretical framework, Part I; by Patricia T. Haase, Mary Howard Smith and Barbara B. Reitt. Atlanta: Southern Regional Education Board, 1974. (Pathways to practice, vol.3.)

34 Hagemeier, D. and Hunt, C. Do new graduates use conceptual frameworks? (Research study to measure effectiveness of teaching the theory of nursing.) Nursing Outlook, 27 (8), Aug 1979, 545-548.

35 Hamilton, G.A. Miller's living systems: a theory critique. (Analysis of general systems theory and some discussion of its relevance to nursing practice.) Advances in Nursing Science, 1 (2), Jan 1979, 41-52.

36 Hardy, M.E. Perspectives on nursing theory. Advances in Nursing Science, 1 (1), Oct 1978, 37-48.

37 Hardy, M.E. and Conway, M.E. Role theory: perspectives for health professionals. New York: Appleton-Century-Crofts, 1978.

38 Harrison, O.A. and Hoffmeister, J.L. A statistical method for development of subconcepts in nursing. Nursing Research, 26 (6), Nov/Dec 1977, 448-451.

39 Henderson, V. The concept of nursing. (Paper read as the 3rd Battersea Memorial Lecture in November 1977.) Journal of Advanced Nursing, 3 (2), Mar 1978, 113-130. Reported in Nursing Mirror, 145, 10 Nov 1977, 2; Nursing Times, 73, 10 Nov 1977, 1731.

40 Hennessey, J. and Brown, A. Conceptual framework for nursing practice. Maternal-Child Nursing Journal, 9 (2), Summer 1980, 65-71.

41 Jacobs, M.K. and Huether, S.E. Nursing science: the theory-practice linkage. Advances in Nursing Science, 1 (1), Oct 1978, 63-73.

42 Jones, P.S. An adaptation model for nursing practice. (Based on Selye's theory of stress.) American Journal of Nursing, 78 (11), Nov 1978, 1900-1906.

43 Kearney, B.Y. and Fleischer, B.J. Development of an instrument to measure exercise of self-care agency. (Using Orem's concept.) Research in Nursing Health, 2 (1), Mar 1979, 25-34.

44 Ketefian, S. editor Translation of theory into nursing practice and education, with a bibliography on change: proceedings of the 7th annual clinical sessions. New York University, 1975.

45 Lanara, V.A. Philosophy of nursing and current nursing problems. International Nursing Review, 23 (2), Mar/Apr 1976, 48-54.

46 LaRocco, S.A. An introduction to role theory for nurses. Supervisor Nurse, 9 (12), Dec 1978, 41-45.

47 Leydon, I. Concepts basic to nursing. World of Irish Nursing, 5 (3), Mar 1976, 7.

48 Maas, M. and others Nurse autonomy: reality not rhetoric. (Development of a professional model of nursing practice including authority and accountability to enable nurses to control nursing care at Iowa Veterans Home.) American Journal of Nursing, 75 (12), Dec 1975, 2201-2208.

49 McFarlane, E.A. Nursing theory: the comparison of four theoretical proposals. (Those of Imogene King, Dorothea Orem, Martha Rogers and Sister Calista Roy.) Journal of Advanced Nursing, 5 (1), Jan 1980, 3-19.

50 Mastal, M.F. and Hammond, H. Analysis and expansion of the Roy adaptation model: a contribution to holistic nursing. Advances in Nursing Science, 2 (4), Jul 1980, 71-81.

51 Matejski, M.P. A framework for nursing: a concept for practice. (Based on the influence of stress on the rhythmic patterns of the individual as they affect his mobility.) Journal of Nursing Education, 18 (5), May 1979, 49-58.

52 Miller, J.F. The dynamic focus of nursing: a challenge to nursing administration. (Model of nursing practice based on patient's progression on illness-to-health continuum.) Journal of Nursing Administration, 10 (1), Jan 1980, 13-18.

53 Mitchell, P.M. Concepts basic to nursing. 2nd ed. New York: McGraw-Hill, 1977.

54 National League for Nursing Theory development: what, why, how? New York: NLN, 1978.

55 Newman, M.A. Theory development in nursing. Philadelphia: Davis, 1979.

56 Nursing Clinics of North America Symposium on the self-care concept of nursing. Nursing Clinics of North America, 15 (1), Mar 1980, 129-217.

57 Nursing Development Conference Group Concept formalization in nursing: process and product. 2nd ed. Boston: Little, Brown, 1979.

58 Orem, D.E. Nursing: concepts of practice. 2nd ed. New York: McGraw-Hill, 1980.

59 Paterson, J.G. and Zderad, L.T. Humanistic nursing. New York: Wiley, 1976.

60 Putt, A.M. General systems theory applied to nursing. Boston: Little, Brown and Co., 1978.

61 Ride, T. Developing a theory of nursing. (Association of Integrated and Degree Courses in Nursing Conference.) Nursing Mirror, 143 (4), 22 Jul 1976, 37.

62 Riehl, J.P. and Roy, C. Conceptual models for nursing practice. New York: Appleton-Century-Crofts, 2nd ed. 1980.

63 Rigley, A. 'Martha Rogers—challenging ideas for nursing'. (Her theory of nursing.) Lamp, 37 (2), Feb 1980, 20-22.

64 Roch, J. The uses and limitations of the concept of role for nurse education. Nursing Times, 76, 8 May 1980, 837-841.

65 Roper, N. A model for nursing and nursology. (A model for nursing care based on activities of daily living and its application for nurse training programmes.) Journal of Advanced Nursing, 1 (3), May 1976, 219-227.

66 Roy, C. Introduction to nursing: an adaptation method. Englewood Cliffs: Prentice-Hall, 1976.

67 Roy, C. The Roy Adaptation model. Comment. (The creator's reaction to practical experiments in the use of a theoretical model of nursing practice.) Nursing Outlook, 24 (11), Nov 1976, 690-691.

68 Schaefer, J. A forum for discussion: is nursing an adjective or a noun? Nursing Leadership, 3 (2), Jun 1980, 9-17.

69 Scottish National Nursing and Midwifery Consultative Committee. Working Group A new concept of nursing. Nursing Times, 72, 8 Apr 1976, Occ. papers, 49-52; 15 Apr 1976, Occ. papers, 53-56; 22 Apr 1976, Occ. papers, 57-60.

70 Smith, J.P. Towards a concept of care. (Need for nurses and nurse teachers to develop the role of care.) Journal of Community Nursing, 2 (9), Mar 1979, 11, 13, 15.

71 Spicker, S.F. and Gadow, S. editors Nursing: images and ideals: opening dialogue with the humanities. New York: Springer, 1980.

72 Stevens, B.J. Nursing theory: analysis, application, evaluation. Boston: Little, Brown and Co., 1979.

73 Towell, D. A 'social systems' approach to research and change in nursing care. (The development of a conceptual framework.) International Journal of Nursing Studies, 16 (1), 1979, 111-121.

74 Tumilty, E. Is nursing more of an art than a science? (Joint runner-up in competition.) Nursing Mirror, 151, 4 Dec 1980, 20-21.

75 Wagner, P. The Roy Adaptation Model: testing the adaptation model in practice. (Students at DePaul University). Nursing Outlook, 24 (11), Nov 1976, 682-685.

76 Watson, J. Nursing: the philosophy and science of caring. Boston: Little, Brown and Co., 1979.

77 Zbilut, J.P. Epistemologic constraints to the development of a theory of nursing. (Letter.) Nursing Research, 27 (2), Mar/Apr 1978, 128-129.

d PSYCHOSOCIAL ASPECTS

1 Bond, J. and Bond, S. Sociology. Nursing Mirror, 150.
1. From the public point of view. 14 Feb 1980, 26-29.
2. A concept for life. 21 Feb 1980, 28-31.
3. In touch with reality. 28 Feb 1980, 27-30.
4. Changing images. 6 Mar 1980, 28-31.
5. A taboo of our times. (Death and dying.) 13 Mar 1980, 23-26.

2 Chapman, C.M. Sociology for nurses. Baillière Tindall, 1977. (Nurses' aids series.)

3 Clarke, M. Psychology. Nursing Mirror 150.
1. Know your patient. 10 Apr 1980, 28-30.

2. Behave yourself. (Psychology of learning.) 17 Apr 1980, 20-21.
3. The whys and the wherefores. (Motivation, emotion and stress.) 24 Apr 1980, 28-30.
4. A sense of perception. 12 Jun 1980, 41-43.
5. Is anyone there? (Art of communication.) 19 Jun 1980, 29-31.
6. Acting on attitudes. (With reference to doctors and nurses.) 26 Jun 1980, 30-32.

4 Cohen, J. and Clark, J.H. Medicine, mind and man: an introduction to psychology for students of medicine and allied professions. Reading: W.H. Freeman, 1979.

5 Congalton, A.A. The individual in society: an introduction to sociology for nurses. New York: Wiley, 1976.

6 Cox, C.A. Who cares? Nursing and sociology: the development of a symbiotic relationship. Journal of Advanced Nursing, 4 (3), May 1979, 237-252.

7 Crow, R.A. A fresh look at psychology in nursing. (The contribution of psychology to the scientific basis of nursing care.) Journal of Advanced Nursing, 1 (1), Jan 1976, 51-62.

8 Dingwall, R. and McIntosh, J. editors Readings in the sociology of nursing. Churchill Livingstone, 1978.

9 Folta, J.R. and Deck, E.S. editors A sociological framework for patient care. 2nd ed. New York: Wiley Medical, 1979.

10 Hutchings, J. and Gathercole, C. Community nursing and psychology: 1. Where is the link? (What psychology can contribute to community nursing.) Journal of Community Nursing, 1 (9), Mar 1978, 4-5.

11 Preston, R.P. The dilemmas of care: social and nursing adaptation to the deformed, the disabled and the aged. New York: Elsevier, 1979.

12 Smith, J.P. Sociology and nursing. Churchill Livingstone, 1976. (Livingstone nursing texts.)

13 Thompson, L.F. and others Sociology: nurses and their patients in a modern society. 9th ed. St. Louis: Mosby, 1975.

7 HEALTH AND WELFARE

a SICKNESS AND ABSENCE

1 American Journal of Nursing Paraplegic nurse directs rehab services. (Nurse who was paraplegic on entering nurse training school.) American Journal of Nursing, 77 (10), Oct 1977, 1664, 1671.

2 Barr, E. Caring for the theatre team. (With reference to sickness absence.) NATNews, 16 (6), Jun 1979, 13-15, 18.

3 Barry-Zed, M. Why are your nurses absent today? (Survey of 450-bed hospital over three month period.) Health Care Can, 21 (7), Jul 1979, 15.

4 Belanger, C. and others The nurses' health study: current findings. (On relationship between hair dyes and cancer, oral contraceptives and myocardial infarction and positive family history and increased risk of breast cancer.) American Journal of Nursing, 80 (7), Jul 1980, 1333.

5 Brewer, C. Why nurses? (Study by the British Pregnancy Advisory Service which showed a high incidence of nurses having repeat abortions.) Nursing Times, 72 (49), 9 Dec 1976, 1909.

6 Butler, E.A. and Hay, H.J. The passionate statistician: a computerised record of nursing sickness and absence. 2 parts. (In St. Thomas's Health District.) Nursing Times, 73, 24 Nov 1977, Occ. papers, 149-152; 1 Dec 1977, Occ. papers, 153-156.

7 Clark, J.M. and Redfern, S.J. Absence and wastage in nursing. 1. (The relevance of absence and wastage to the organisation and association between the two); 2. Collecting and using information. Nursing Times, 74, 20 Apr 1978, Occ. papers, 41-44; 27 Apr 1978, Occ. papers, 45-48.

8 Clarke, S. and Hussey, D.G. Sickness absence amongst nursing staff at two hospitals. (Qualified staff including midwives in Leicester.) Journal of the Society of Occupational Medicine, 29 (4), Oct 1979, 126-130.

9 Davies, N. Both sides of the sheets. (How man with multiple sclerosis has become a nurse.) Nursing Mirror, 150, 12 Jun 1980, 50-52.

10 Diabetic nurses Correspondence in Nursing Times, 75, 24 May 1979, 875-876; 14 Jun 1979, 1009. Letter from E. Bagshaw describing survey of attitudes in schools of nursing, British Medical Journal, 280, 17 May 1980, 1227. Correspond-ence from the British Diabetic Association and a students' health service doctor, British Medical Journal, 280, 28 Jun 1980, 1616.

11 Elwood, J.M. and Hislop, T.G. Breast diseases in nurses, a 30-year study. (Study of nursing students at Vancouver General Hospital from 1945.) Canadian Nurse, 76 (11), Dec 1980, 38-39.

12 Farrant, E.M. Why do nurses go 'off sick'? Nursing Focus, 1 (1), Sep 1979, 20, 22, 24.

13 French, G.J. The problem of shoes. Nursing Mirror, 142, 29 Apr 1976, 50-54.

14 Gault, P.A. Mixed connective tissue disease. (Account of living with a chronic illness by a nurse who has this disease.) American Journal of Nursing, 77 (11), Nov 1977, 1818-1820.

15 Gibson, G. I was supposed to die two years ago. (Living with an incurable disease (aplastic anaemia) has given this young nurse an unenviable opportunity to improve the care she gives and evaluate the care she receives.) RN Journal, 40 (10), Oct 1977, 46-48.

16 Hefferin, E.A. and Hill, B.J. Analyzing nursing's work related injuries. (Study of a year's hospital records at the Veterans Administration Wadsworth Hospital showing back and leg injuries to be most serious.) American Journal of Nursing, 76 (6), Jun 1976, 924-927.

17 Hughes, F. Short term absence—another view. (With brief report of small study.) Nursing Focus, 1 (11), Jul 1980, 437-438.

18 Jamil, H.J. Sickness absence among employees of an area health authority. (Salford.) PhD thesis, Manchester University, Department of Occupational Health, 1978.

19 Leopoldt, H. and others Nursing staff accidents in a psychiatric hospital: a six-month survey of nursing staff accidents in a psychiatric hospital showing that most were caused by aggressive acts of patients. Nursing Times, 74, 26 Oct 1978, Occ. papers, 121-123.

20 Lysaght, E. A report on health problems of theatre nurses. (By chairman of a committee set up by Auckland Theatre Nurses Special Interest Section, based on questionnaire survey.) New Zealand Nursing Journal, 72 (1), Jan 1979, 24-26.

21 Pacey, N. Who cares for the caring profession? (Problems of the chronically sick or disabled nurse.) Nursing Times, 72, 7 Oct 1976, 1574-1575.

22 Panteleo, N. Nurse, do you take care of yourself? (Survey of attitudes to health care among nurses at the Illinois Masonic Medical Center, Chicago.) AORN Journal, 25 (1), Jan 1977, 54-59.

23 Perry, S.E. How to make a sick nurse a happy patient. RN Magazine, 40 (6), 15 Jun 1977, 42-44.

24 Peters, D. Job perils in the nursing service. (Report of questionnaire survey into hazards faced by hospital nurses and their attitudes to health and safety.) Occupational Safety and Health, 9 (2), Feb 1979, 23-24, 42.

25 Phillipson, P.A.J. and Geddes, N. The reasons learners go absent. (Survey of absenteeism rates among student and pupil nurses at South Tyneside School of Nursing.) Nursing Mirror, 146, 8 Jun 1978, 12-15.

26 Poole, F.T. Mobility of nurses—a factor in Court of Appeal decision. (The need for nurses who are injured in the course of their employment to bring claims as quickly as possible.) Nursing Mirror, 144 (77), 28 Apr 1977, 68.

27 Quattrucci, J. Beginning research. The hygiene of stethoscopes. (Study to test whether ear pieces contribute to ear complaints experienced by nurses.) Nursing Times, 73, 10 Feb 1977, 193-195.

28 Quinn, L.B. 'It's worth the effort—I know.' (Experiences of a nurse after leg amputation.) RN Magazine, 38 (10), Oct 1976, 57-63.

29 Redfern, S.J. Absence and wastage in trained nurses: a selective review of the literature. Journal of Advanced Nursing, 3 (3), May 1978, 231-249.

30 REHABILITATION nurse. (Nurse born with only one arm and leg.) Nursing, 7 (10), Oct 1977, 84, 85.

31 RN Magazine Happy nurses don't call in sick. RN Magazine, 41 (4), Apr 1978, 33-34.

32 Sadik, A.M. Absentees. (Letter describing author's research.) Nursing Times, 74, 1 Jun 1978, 926.

33 Simon, M.A.S. No one should face cancer alone—not even a nurse. (Nurse with cancer of the thyroid describes her experiences.) RN Magazine, 41 (3), Mar 1978, 79, 84, 86.

b ADDICTION

1 Bonney, J. How can nurses stop smoking? Nursing Mirror, 151, 21 Aug 1980, 18.

2 Canfield, T.M. Drug addiction of health professionals. AORN Journal, 24 (4), Oct 1976, 665-671.

3 Darity, M. Drugs: facing up to a problem on your staff. (Drug abuse by nurses.) RN Magazine, 42 (11), Nov 1979, 21-26.

4 Department of Health and Social Security Smoking and professional people. DHSS, 1977.

5 Elkind, A.K. Nurses' smoking behaviour: review and implications. (World-wide picture and implications for nurse's role in health education and nursing as a profession.) International Journal of Nursing Studies, 17 (4), 1980, 261-269.

6 Elkind, A.K. Nurses, smoking and cancer prevention. (Survey of nurses' smoking in a Northern hospital.) International Journal of Health Education, 12 (2), Apr/Jun 1979, 92-101.

7 General Nursing Council and others Smoking and nurses: the report of a symposium held in the Royal College of Physicians of Edinburgh, 26 Feb 1979. Edinburgh: Action on Smoking and Health, 1979.

8 Hawkins, L.H. and others Stress, smoking and nursing. (Aims of University of Surrey research study.) Nursing Times, 76, 4 Sep 1980, 1555.

9 Isler, C. The alcoholic nurse: what we try to deny. RN Magazine, 41 (7), Jul 1978, 48-55.

10 Kolesar, G. It could happen to you. (Problems of nurse abusers of drugs and alcohol.) Canadian Nurse, 76 (10), Nov 1980, 20-22.

11 Kushner, J.A. Why do so many nurses smoke so much? Journal of Community Nursing, 1 (7), Jan 1978, 24-25.

12 Leathar, D.S. Smoking among student nurses: an exploratory study into the reasons underlying nurses' smoking habits. (By Scottish Health Education Unit.) Nursing Times, 76, 3 Apr 1980, 589-590.

13 Neil, J.V. and others The smoking patterns and attitudes of student nurses and student teachers. (Research study.) Australian Nurses Journal, 9 (8), Mar 1980, 47-48.

14 Noll, C.E. Nurses' behavior, beliefs, and attitudes toward smoking and health. Chicago: University of Chicago, National Opinion Research Center, 1969. (Health professionals and the problems of smoking and health; 5).

15 Nursing Mirror Do you smoke? Why? (Ten nurses' views on their smoking habits.) Nursing Mirror, 150, 10 Apr 1980, 6-7.

16 Peirce, S.M. When the addict is a nurse. AORN Journal, 24 (4), Oct 1976, 655-664.

17 Ross, T. Why do you smoke, nurse? (Review of research with ten nurses' views, 6-7.) Nursing Mirror, 150, 10 Apr 1980, 18-19.

18 Small, W.P. and Tucker, L. The smoking habits of hospital nurses. (Survey of nurses in Edinburgh.) Nursing Times, 74, 16 Nov 1978, 1878-1879.

19 Stuart, A.M. The nurse who smokes. Nursing, 7, Nov 1979, 300.

c BACK PROBLEMS

1 Cust, G. Low back pain in nurses. Queen's Nursing Journal, 19 (1), Apr 1976, 6-8.

2 Harris, C.M.T. The mechanics of lifting. (Symposium paper.) Nursing Mirror, 144, 13 Jan 1977, 60-61.

3 Iveson-Iveson, J. Prevention: how to stay healthy. 8. Back strain. Nursing Mirror, 149, 1 Nov 1979, 22.

4 Muller, G.M. Disc problems and the district nurse. Queen's Nursing Journal, 19 (1), Apr 1976, 18-19, 23.

5 Northwick Park Hospital. Nursing Practice Research Unit and others Prevention of back pain in nursing: proceedings of the conference... held at Northwick Park Hospital, Harrow, Middlesex on Friday, 26th September, 1980. The Unit, 1980.

6 Poole, F.T. Industrial injuries. Account of an employee who received industrial benefit from an accident she had before going on duty. (Back injury.) Nursing Mirror, 142, 22 Apr 1976, 72.

7 Royal College of Nursing Avoiding low back injury among nurses: report of an Rcn working party. Rcn, 1979.

8 Troup, J.D.G. The causes, prevention and treatment of low back pain. (Symposium paper.) Nursing Mirror, 144, 13 Jan 1977, 46-49.

d COUNSELLING, WELFARE AND STRESS

1 Alhadeff, G. Anxiety in a new graduate. (Includes chart on treating reality shock.) American Journal of Nursing, 79 (4), Apr 1979, 687.

2 Annandale-Steiner, D. The nurse counsellor's role at Guy's. Nursing Times, 75, 9 Aug 1979, 1345.

3 Ashton, K. Counselling course breaks new ground. (Course for nurses at the North East London Polytechnic.) Nursing Times, 73, 31 Mar 1977, 437.

4 Ashton, K. Sharing the burden. (The need for counselling of nurses and patients.) Nursing Times, 75, 9 Aug 1979, 1340-1343.

5 Aston, G. When no home means no job. (Accommodation for hospital staff.) Health and Social Service Journal, 89, 12 Oct 1979, 1310-1311.

6 Beland, I.L. The burnout syndrome in nurses. In Werner-Beland, J.A. editor Grief responses to long-term illness and disability. Reston, 1980.

7 Bendall, E. Discipline—and welfare. (General Nursing Council Welfare Service.) Queen's Nursing Journal, 19 (6), Sep 1976, 163-164.

8 Birch, J.A. Anxiety in nurse education (with particular reference to the report of the Committee on Nursing.) PhD thesis, Newcastle-upon-Tyne University, 1978. Reported by C. Darby in Nursing Mirror, 147, 14 Dec 1978, 2.

9 Birch, J.A. The anxious learners. (Report of research study with first and second year learners.) Nursing Mirror, 148, 8 Feb 1979, 17-22.

10 Blainey, C.G. Anxiety in the undergraduate medical-surgical clinical student. Journal of Nursing Education, 19 (8), Oct 1980, 33-36.

11 Bloch, R.G. Two ways to retain staff. The nurses' ombudsman. American Journal of Nursing, 76 (10), Oct 1976, 1631-1633.

12 Bossenmaier, M. Students evaluate academic advising. (Research study of counselling on educational and vocational concerns.) Nursing Outlook, 27 (12), Dec 1979, 787-791.

13 Burke, S. Stress. (Among nurses.) Lamp, 37 (11), Nov 1980, 5-6.

14 Cardwell, C. Stresses and strains. (The need for a professional counselling service for students.) Nursing Times, 72, 19 Aug 1976, 265.

15 Clark, C.C. Burnout: assessment and intervention. (In nurse managers.) Journal of Nursing Administration, 10 (9), Sep 1980, 39-42.

16 Claus, K.E. and Bailey, J.T. editors Living with stress and promoting well-being: a handbook for nurses. St. Louis: Mosby, 1980.

17 Cohn, L. Coping with anxiety: a step-by-step guide. Nursing (US), 9 (12), Dec 1979, 34-37.

18 Conard, A.M. The nurse's spouse. A helper in patient care. (A husband of a nurse describes how he can provide emotional and practical support.) American Journal of Nursing, 77 (11), Nov 1977, 1821.

19 Coombe, E.I. Tuning in on stress signals (of student nurses.) Journal of Nursing Education, 15 (4), Jul 1976, 16-21.

20 Dartington, T. and Wilson, M. Preparing nurses for counselling. (Part-time counselling courses at the Rcn Institute of Advanced Nursing Education.) Nursing Mirror, 144, 27 Jan 1977, 54-56.

21 Davis, R.C. and Fricke, N. Crisis in nursing students. (Acute stress.) Nursing Forum, 16 (1), 1977, 56-70.

22 Dawar, A. Hygiene rules: OK? (Need for nurses to aim for positive health through leisure activities.) Nursing Mirror, 150, 19 Jun 1980, 26-27.

23 Donnelly, G.F. Why you 'just can't take it anymore!' . . . and some preliminary hints on what to do about it. (Advice to nurses on coping with stress.) RN Magazine, 43 (5), May 1980, 34, 36-37.

24 Dopson, L. Flats for nurses in an Aberdeen church. Nursing Times, 76, 1 May 1980, 793-794.

25 Edelwich, J. and Brodsky, A. Burnout: stages of disillusionment in the helping professions. New York: Human Sciences Press, 1980.

26 Faulker, I. and Martin, K. Counselling for ward managers. (Short course at Sheffield Polytechnic.) Health and Social Service Journal, 86, 4 Mar 1977, 386.

27 Fletcher, J. and others Food intake of hospital nurses under rationing and pay-as-you-eat. (Survey at the West Middlesex Hospital.) Nutrition, 29 (1), Jan/Feb 1975, 25-32.

28 Fordham, M. and others Physiological measurements of work stress in medical nursing. (Summary of paper read at research seminar in 1977.) Journal of Advanced Nursing, 3 (1), Jan 1978, 78-80.

29 Francis, B. A nursing network to battle burnout. (Support groups enabling nurses to share and express their feelings.) Journal of Practical Nursing, 30 (11), Nov/Dec 1980, 25-27.

30 Garrett, A. and others Stressful experiences identified by student nurses. (Research study.) Journal of Nursing Education, 15 (6), Nov 1976, 9-21.

31 Gilbert, G. A counselling service for nurses in training. (At Guy's Group Hospitals.) British Journal of Guidance and Counselling, 4 (2), Jul 1976, 224.

32 Gilbert, G. Nurse counselling service, Guy's Group of Hospitals, London contained in Watts, A.G. editor Counselling at work... Bedford Square Press, 1977, 39-44.

33 Grant, J.M. The nurse in crisis. (Stress in nurses.) New Zealand Nursing Journal, 71 (7), Jul 1978, 18-21.

34 Hartl, D.E. Stress management and the nurse: stress as a personal experience. (Advice for nurses on maintaining their own health.) Advances in Nursing Science, 1 (4), Jul 1979, 91-106.

35 Hathaway, D. When the honeymoon is over: dealing with the real world of nursing. (Advice on coping with 'reality shock' and 'burnout'.) Journal of Practical Nursing, 30 (7), Jul 1980, 32-33, 41-42.

36 Hawkins, K. We need looking after, too! (Problems of new learners.) Nursing Mirror, 148, 17 May 1979, 10.

37 Humphrey, J. Counselling. (Description of Rcn part-time counselling course.) Nursing Times, 75, 29 Nov 1979, 2086-2087.

38 Ivancevich, J.M. and Matteson, M.T. Nurses and stress: time to examine the potential problem. (Research study into job factors creating stress in trained nurses.) Supervisor Nurse, 11 (6), Jun 1980, 17-20, 22.

39 Johnson, J. Jean Johnson researches stress reduction. (Report on her various research projects and the implementation of their findings in nursing.) American Journal of Nursing, 78 (1), Jan 1978, 128-129.

40 Jones, D. The need for a comprehensive counselling service for nursing students. (Research study with fifty nursing students.) Journal of Advanced Nursing, 3 (4), Jul 1978, 359-368.

41 Journal of Nursing Education Stress and stress management: an overview. (Eleven articles with five on intensive care and bibliography, 58-63.) Journal of Nursing Education, 19 (6), Jun 1980, 5-63.

42 Latimer, J. Stress and the student nurse. Nursing, 10, Feb 1980, 449-450.

43 Layden, M. Responsibility to self: first step to leadership. (How nurses can develop self-awareness with Nurse Personal Inventory.) Nursing Leadership, 2 (3), Sep 1979, 26-29.

44 Leatt, P. and Schneck, R. Differences in stress perceived by headnurses across nursing specialties in hospitals. (Survey of headnurses from nine specialties.) Journal of Advanced Nursing, 5 (1), Jan 1980, 31-46.

45 Lewis, J. Stresses in paediatric nursing. Australasian Nurses Journal, 4 (10), Apr 1976, 51-53.

46 McKay, S.R. A review of student stress in nursing education programs. Nursing Forum, 17 (4), 1978, 376-393.

47 MacMaster, E. Sources of stress in university nursing students. (Research study.) Nursing Papers, 11 (4), Winter 1979, 87-96.

48 Maher, J. Struck off! It could never happen to me—or could it? (The role of the GNC Nurses' Welfare Service in giving support to those struck off the Register or Roll.) Nursing Mirror, 148, 26 Apr 1979, 30-31.

49 Manning, M. Nursing under stress. (With reference to district nurses.) Community View, 7, Sep 1980, 8-9.

50 Meredith, L. and Weatherhead, R. Psychiatric consultation liaison nursing: 18 months later. (Scheme to help reduce anxiety of nurses through discussion of problems related to care of particular patients.) Lamp, 37 (6), Jun 1980, 19-20.

51 Mohl, P.C. and Booth, K. Psychiatric liaison groups with neurosurgery nurses. (Group psychotherapy led by psychiatrists to reduce stress and frustration in nurses.) Journal of Neurosurgical Nursing, 11 (2), Jun 1979, 114-117.

52 National League for Nursing Stress: making it work for you. New York: NLN, 1977.

53 Nurse, G. Counselling and the nurse: an introduction. 2nd ed. Aylesbury: HM and M, 1980. (Topics in community health series.)

54 Olsen, M. OR nurses' perception of stress. (Study of 104 nurses in Seattle hospitals.) AORN Journal, 25 (1), Jan 1977, 43-48.

55 Parkes, K.R. Occupational stress among student nurses. 1. A comparison of medical and surgical wards. 2. A comparison of male and female wards. Nursing Times, 76, 30 Oct 1980, Occ. papers, 113-116; 6 Nov 1980, Occ. papers, 117-119.

56 Patrick, P.K.S. Burnout: job hazard for health workers. Hospitals, 53 (22), 16 Nov 1979, 87-88, 90.

57 Queen's Nursing Institute New look announced for QNI. Institute will offer welfare services for all nurses. Nursing Times, 72 (38), 23 Sep 1976, 1456.

58 Royal College of Nursing Rcn orders high suicide rate probe. (Investigation of high suicide rate among nurses by Rcn Society of Psychiatric Nursing.) Nursing Mirror, 146, 23 Feb 1978, 2.

59 Royal College of Nursing. Association of Nursing Students Focus on nurses' residences. Rcn, 1978. Comment on survey in Nursing Times, 9 Nov 1978, 1824-1825.

60 Royal College of Nursing. Institute of

Advanced Nursing Education Counselling in nursing: report of a working party. Rcn, 1978. (Chairman: E.L. Perry).

61 Royal College of Nursing. Welfare Advisory Service A helping hand. An appraisal of the work of the Rcn's Welfare Advisory Service. Nursing Mirror, 142, 25 Mar 1976, 40-41.

62 Salvage, J. Home squalid home. (Conditions in nurses homes.) Nursing Mirror, 150, 10 Apr 1980, 8-10.

63 Sanders, M.M. Stressed? Or burnt out? (Review of literature.) Canadian Nurse, 76 (9), Oct 1980, 30-33.

64 Sandroff, R. Nurse/mother: how to cope with a double career. (RN survey.) RN Magazine, 43 (7), Jul 1980, 53-57.

65 Scully, R. Stress in the nurse. American Journal of Nursing, 80 (5), May 1980, 912-915.

66 Sellek, T. Satisfying and anxiety creating incidents as identified by student nurses during the process of becoming a state registered nurse. MSc thesis, University of Manchester, 1977.

67 Selye, H. A code for coping with stress (for operating room nurses.) AORN Journal, 25 (1), Jan 1977, 35-42.

68 Sherwood Jones, D. Counselling facilities. (Letter describing what is being done in Liverpool and elsewhere.) Nursing Times, 72, 25 Nov 1976, 1857.

69 Shubin, S. Burnout: the professional hazard you face in nursing. (Advice on dealing with stress.) Nursing (US), 8 (7), Jul 1978, 22, 24-25, 27.

70 Skinner, K. Burn-out: is nursing dangerous to your health? (Advice on coping with emotional exhaustion.) Journal of Nursing Care, 12 (12), Dec 1979, 8-9, 30.

71 Smith, J. How nurses can help themselves. (Lack of counselling services for nurses in spite of official approval, with some reference to schemes at Guy's and St. Thomas' Hospitals.) Nursing Mirror, 147, 9 Nov 1978, 18-20.

72 Smith, R.L. 'Those people aren't people anymore...they are mere bodies moving by me.' (Professional burn-out.) Hospital Topics, 57 (6), Nov/Dec 1979, 14-15.

73 Sobol, E.G. Self-actualization and the baccalaureate nursing student's response to stress. Nursing Research, 27 (4), Jul/Aug 1978, 238-244.

74 Spicer, J.G. Help for the staff nurse in crisis. (Stress and role of nurse managers.) Supervisor Nurse, 9 (9), Sep 1978, 82-83.

75 Storlie, F.J. Burnout: the elaboration of a concept. (With special reference to intensive care nurses.) American Journal of Nursing, 79 (12), Dec 1979, 2108-2111.

76 Tierney, M.J.G. and Strom, L.M. Stress: Type A behaviour. American Journal of Nursing, 80 (5), May 1980, 915-918.

77 Townsend, I. and Linsley, W. Creating a climate for careers. (Co-counselling, with some reference to its usefulness for nurses.) Nursing Times, 76, 3 Jul 1980, 1188-1190.

78 Turner, J. Sunny stories. (New accommo-

dation for nurses at the Evelyn Nursing Home, Cambridge.) Nursing Times, 72, 14 Oct 1976, 1588-1589.

79 Vachon, M.L.S. Care for the caregiver. (Advice to nurses on dealing with stress.) Canadian Nurse, 76 (9), Oct 1980, 28-33.

80 Vachon, M.L.S. Enforced proximity to stress in the client environment. (Advice to nurses on coping.) Canadian Nurse, 72 (9), Sep 1976, 40-43.

81 Van-Altaan, M. A counselling course. (Report by HV.) Health Visitor, 53 (3), Mar 1980, 93, 96.

82 Van Emden, J. Driving under stress. (With reference to community nurses.) Journal of Community Nursing, 1 (8), Feb 1978, 28.

83 Walsh, M. Within these walls. (Suggestions for the improvement of nurses' homes.) Nursing Mirror, 142, 10 Jun 1976, 68-69.

84 Watkin, B. Out of their minds. (Comment on recent case of nurses' dismissal owing to history of psychiatric illness.) Nursing Mirror, 146, 6 Apr 1978, 10. See also 146, 23 Feb 1978, 5.

85 Wilkins, M. A suicidal R.N.'s crisis. (Nurse's experiences in a psychiatric unit and comment by psychiatric nurses.) RN Magazine, 40 (9), Sep 1977, 55-58.

86 Willis, R.W. Options in managing stress. (In nursing.) Pediatric Nursing, 5 (1), Jan/Feb 1979, 24-27.

e RETIRED NURSES

1 Nursing Times Another Jubilee. (Golden Jubilee of National Gardens Scheme, which raises funds for retired district nurses. History of district nursing outlined, with photographs.) Nursing Times, 73, 8 Sep 1977, 1384-1387.

2 Robinson, W. Nurses in retirement. (At Howard House, Gerrards Cross, in Bucks, home for retired nurses.) Nursing Mirror, 146, 13 Apr 1978, 43, 44, 46, 48.

8 SALARIES AND CONDITIONS

a GENERAL

1 Adie, D. Maternity rights and employment in the National Health Service. Nursing Focus, 1 (12), Aug 1980, 474-475.

2 Bateman, J.M. Nursing staff, annual leave and public holidays. (A method of calculating holiday entitlement for use by health administrators.) Health and Social Service Journal, 86, 3 Jul 1976, 1208-1209.

3 Beletz, E.E. and Meng, M.T. The grievance process. American Journal of Nursing, 77 (2), Feb 1977, 256-260.

4 Beletz, E.E. Some pointers for grievance handlers. Whatever a nurse's position in the hierarchy, she should learn how to handle grievances. Supervisor Nurse, 8 (8), Aug 1977, 12-14.

5 **Brown, A.** Ten years on—still low pay and long hours. (Review of events affecting nurses during 1970s.) Nursing Mirror, 150, 3 Jan 1980, 13-15.

6 **Dimond, B.** The rights way to motherhood. (Maternity rights for nurses under the Employment Protection Act and Whitley Council provisions.) Nursing Mirror, 149, 6 Dec 1979, 28-30.

7 **Dixon, M.** Is there a case for compensating nurses? (for injuries.) Nursing Mirror, 144, 6 Jan 1977, 55-56.

8 THE EMPLOYMENT Protection Act 1975. (Outline of main provisions.) Midwives Chronicle, 91, Dec 1978, 360-362.

9 **General Nursing Council** Basic explanation of GNC's disciplinary responsibilities. (Circular 77/13.) Nursing Times, 73, 1 Sep 1977, Occ. papers, 120. See also Professional discipline. Nursing Times, 73, 4 Aug 1977, 1184.

10 **Hospital and Health Services Review** Rising expectations. (Grievances of nurses concerning salaries and conditions.) Hospital and Health Service Review, 70 (6), 1974, 185-187.

11 **International Labour Organisation** ILO adopts convention and recommendation for nursing personnel. International Nursing Review, 24 (5), Sep/Oct 1977, 156-157.

12 **International Labour Organisation** Convention concerning employment and conditions of work and life of nursing personnel. Geneva: ILO, 1977.

13 **International Labour Organisation** Recommendation concerning employment and conditions of work and life of nursing personnel. Geneva: ILO, 1977. (Recommendation 157. Summary in WHO Chronicle, 31 (6), Jun 1977, 252.

14 **International Labour Organisation** International Labour Conference, 63rd, 1977. Employment and conditions of work and life of nursing personnel. Geneva: ILO, 1976.

15 **Jacox, I.** An underestimated problem in nursing: the effect of the economic and social welfare of nurses on patient care. Geneva: ICN, 1977.

16 **Lloyd, P.** ILO charter of justice for nurses. (New standards to improve working conditions and pay.) Occupational Health, 29 (10), Oct 1977, 440.

17 **McMullan, D.** The role of the nurse as employee: a case of mutual responsibilities. New York: NLN, 1976.

18 **Martin, A.** Nurses and the law. 11. Accidents at work. Nursing Times, 75, 14 Jun 1979, 1008.

19 **Morris, P.** The balance of injustice. (Position of nurse complaining about treatment of patients and danger of reprisals.) Nursing Mirror, 148, 5 Apr 1979, 24-26.

20 **Nazer, G.** What happens to lost sheep who go astray. (GNC disciplinary committee.) Nursing Mirror, 148, 5 Apr 1979, 6.

21 **Occupational Health** Industrial relations 'machinery'. (Employment Protection Act.) Occupational Health, 28, Jan 1976, 21-23.

22 **Parliament** Employment Act, 1980. HMSO, 1980.

23 **Poole, F.T.** Ill health and unfair dismissal. Occupational Health, 29 (1), Jan 1977, 32-33.

24 **Pyne, R.H.** The professional disciplinary function of the statutory body and the role of the nurses' welfare service. Royal Society of Health Journal, 99 (1), Feb 1979, 12-16, 22.

25 **Pyne, R.H. and Darby, C.** The price of sin goes up for bogus nurses. (Interview with Reginald Pyne, Deputy Registrar of the GNC on forthcoming legislation.) Nursing Mirror, 145, 25 Aug 1977, 4-5.

26 **University of Aston in Birmingham. Department of Safety and Hygiene** Employment protection. Occupational Health, 28 (6), Jun 1976, 310-313.

27 **Walsh, M.** Victimisation. Nursing Mirror, 143, 26 Aug 1976, 39-40.

28 **Whincup, M.** Dismissing for dishonesty. (With case reports.) Health Services Manpower Review, 3 (4), Nov 1977, 3-5.

29 **Whincup, M.** Workers—new laws for old. (Summary and implications of Employment Act.) Health and Social Service Journal, 90, 5 Sep 1980, 1166-1168.

30 **Wiley, L.** Good patient care. Can you give it in the real world? (Problems over conditions of work.) Nursing, 7 (9), Sep 1977, 5-6.

b LABOUR RELATIONS: UK

1 **Allen, M.** David Williams is no Jay-bird. (Interview with COHSE Assistant General Secretary.) Nursing Mirror, 148, 7 Jun 1979, 19-20.

2 **Ashton, K.** Interview. Take two young men. (Ray Rowden and Steve Grant, regional officers of Rcn and COHSE respectively.) Nursing Times, 74, 31 Aug 1978, 1436-1437.

3 **Carr, A.** Let strikers suffer the consequences. (Comment on GNC statement on nurses and industrial action.) Nursing Mirror, 149, 13 Sep 1979, 12.

4 **Carr, A.** Professional industrial action? (With reference to possible decision by Rcn council to authorise limited action.) Nursing Times, 75, 8 Feb 1979, 224-225.

5 **Carpenter, M.** Unity in action. (History of COHSE.) Nursing Times, 76, 10 Jul 1980, 1204-1205. See also Nursing Mirror, 151, 10 Jul 1980, 8.

6 **Clark, J.** The right to strike. (Comment on GNC's statement on nurses and industrial action.) Nursing Mirror, 149, 23 Aug 1979, 20-21.

7 **Clode, D.** Contradictions which hit Nalgo's solidarity. (The evolution of the Association of National and Local Government Officers to its present status.) Health and Social Service Journal, 87, 22 Jul 1977, 1078-1080.

8 **Confederation of Health Service Employees** COHSE Annual Conference in Scarborough. Nursing Mirror, 146, 22 Jun 1978, 2; 29 Jun 1978, 4-7; Nursing Times, 74, 22 Jun 1978, 1028; 29 Jun 1978, 1064-1071.

9 **Confederation of Health Service Employees** Annual conference 1977. Nursing Mirror, 144, 23 Jun 1977, 3-4; Nursing Times, 73, 23 Jun 1977, 924-928.

10 CURRENT trends in industrial relations—areas of concern. Midwives Chronicle, 91, Jul 1978, 170.

11 **Department of Employment** Certification office—the first year. (Interview with Mr. John Edwards, who is responsible for determining the independence of trade unions.) Department of Employment Gazette, 85 (5), May 1977, 439-442.

12 **Dimmock, S. and Mercer, G.** The membership of trade unions and professional associations in general nursing. Health and Social Service Journal, 28 Apr 1978, Centre eight papers F25-F28.

13 **Dolton, W.D.** Managing the industrial action with particular reference to admissions policies and the use of volunteers. (With reference to agreement reached in Liverpool in January 1979.) Health Services Manpower Review, 5 (3), Aug 1979, 25-26.

14 **Dworkin, G.** Strikes and the National Health Service: some legal and ethical issues. Journal of Medical Ethics, 3 (2), Jun 1977, 76-84.

15 **Dyer, B.** Industrial relations—what now? (Effect of recent legislation on the nursing profession.) Nursing Times, 72, 8 Jul 1976, 1038-1039.

16 **Dyson, R.** Industrial relations and nursing organisations. Nursing Focus, 1 (5), Jan 1980, 186-188.

17 **Dyson, R.** Industrial relations in the NHS. (Review of recent developments including question of Rcn affiliation to TUC.) Midwife, Health Visitor and Community Nurse, 15 (1), Jan 1979, 7-8.

18 **Felgate, R.V.R.** The emergence of militancy in the nursing profession 1960-1972. PhD thesis, Surrey University, 1977.

19 **Fusco, L.** One union, one front for all battles. (Plea for one union for all health service workers.) Health and Social Service Journal, 89, 15 Jun 1979, 735-736.

20 **General Nursing Council** Alleged professional misconduct and industrial action. (Statement and related comment.) GNC circular 79/21 + enclosure 79/21/A, Jul 1979.

21 **Gostin, L.** Industrial action: is the target management or patients? The right of the nursing profession to take industrial action when confronted with violent patients. Nursing Mirror, 147, 12 Oct 1978, 15-17.

22 **Gourlay, J.R. and Johnson, P.M.** Union membership agreements (UMAs). (For Whitley Council staff.) Health Services Manpower Review, 3 (3), Aug 1977, 14-18.

23 **Gray, M.** Angels with no muscle. (The need for nurses to unite in one exclusive union to fight NHS cuts.) Health and Social Service Journal, 86, 29 Oct 1976, 1934.

24 **Greene, J.** The right to strike. (Comment on GNC statement.) Nursing Mirror, 149, 13 Sep 1979, 20.

25 **Hardie, M.** The right to strike. (By Director of Labour Relations of the RCM.) Nursing Mirror, 149, 27 Sep 1979, 18.

26 Health Visitors' Association The General Nursing Council: alleged professional misconduct and industrial action. (Comments on GNC circular.) Health Visitor, 52 (10), Oct 1979, 442.

27 Heller, T. Nurses unite. (The role of the trade union movement in the NHS.) Nursing Times, 73, 5 May 1977, 640-641.

28 Hennel, J. To strike or not to strike? (The case for.) Nursing Mirror, 148, 31 May 1979, 10.

29 Jarvis, P. Nursing and the ethics of withdrawing professional services. Nursing Mirror, 146, 16 Feb 1978, 30-31.

30 Jones, B. The right to strike. (Comment on GNC's statement on nurses and industrial action by national officer of NUPE.) Nursing Mirror, 149, 30 Aug 1979, 12.

31 Kaye, V. Giving their skeleton some healthy muscle. (Confederation of Health Service Employees.) Health and Social Service Journal, 87, 29 Jul 1977, 1104-1107.

32 Kaye, V. Inside engine room of NUPE powerhouse... (Past and present.) Health and Social Service Journal, 87, 15 Jul 1977, 1042-1045.

33 Lancet Nurses and industrial action. (Comment on GNC circular and response to it.) Lancet, 2, 18 Aug 1979, 375.

34 Lawrence, V. Taking action. (Account of nurses' strike in Ireland.) Nursing Times, 76, 19 Jun 1980, 1078.

35 McConnell, T.C. The incentive argument for the unionisation of medical workers. Journal of Medical Ethics, 5 (4), Dec 1979, 182-184.

36 McKay, H. New industrial relations training. (For shop stewards and staff representatives.) Nursing Times, 74, 2 Nov 1978, 1813-1814.

37 Martin, A. The nurse and the law. The legal risk of striking. Journal of Community Nursing, 3 (9), Mar 1980, 4, 38.

38 Morgan, M. The right to strike. (Comment on GNC statement.) Nursing Mirror, 149, 6 Sep 1979, 16-17.

39 Morris, P. GNC: a reminder that the patient must come first. (Comment on GNC statement on nurses and industrial action.) Nursing Mirror, 149, 9 Aug 1979, 6.

40 Northamptonshire Area Health Authority Union membership agreements. (The document outlines the policy and principles to be followed when concluding union membership agreements between the Northamptonshire Area Health Authority and appropriate independent recognised staff organisations.) Health Services Manpower Review, 3 (4), Nov 1977, 11-14.

41 Nursing Mirror Peaceful co-existence. (Editorial on trades union and professional organisations.) Nursing Mirror, 142, Feb 1976, 33.

42 Nursing Mirror Would you take industrial action? (Views of fourteen nurses.) Nursing Mirror, 148, 22 Feb 1979, 6-7.

43 Prentice, G. What is an independent trade union? Personnel Management, 9 (1), Jan 1977, 27-30.

44 Ride, T. Legal right or moral conflict? (In relation to nurses and strike action.) Nursing Times, 75, 10 May 1979, 774.

45 Rye, D. The right to strike. (Comment on GNC statement.) Nursing Mirror, 149, 20 Sep 1979, 18.

46 Sabel, C. How to break the strife. (Inadequacies of dispute procedures.) Health and Social Service Journal, 89, 13 Apr 1979, 419-420.

47 Spanswick, A. Why nurses should join a trade union. Nursing Mirror, 143, 9 Sep 1976, 39-40.

48 Stevenson, O. Unintended consequences. (Effects of social workers' strike on their public image and comparison with image of nurses.) Health and Social Service Journal, 90, 7 Mar 1980, 326-327.

49 Storey, M. The right to strike. (Comment on GNC circular by GNC Registrar.) Nursing Mirror, 149, 4 Oct 1979, 16.

50 Swaffield, L. Marking time. (COHSE annual conference.) Nursing Times, 72 (27), 8 Jul 1976, 1036-1037.

51 THEATRE of the absurd. (Comment on the Dulwich dispute.) Hospital and Health Services Review, 74 (5), May 1978, 148-149.

52 THE TRADE Union and Labour Relations Acts (1974 and 1976). Midwives Chronicle, 91, Sep 1978, 244-245.

53 UNION membership agreements. (In general and in the NHS.) Midwives Chronicle, 91, Mar 1978, 56.

54 Watkin, B. The nursing officer's guide to management. 6. Industrial relations. Nursing Mirror, 146, 29 Jun 1978, Supplement iii-iv.

55 Webb, N. Why the closed shop oils the wheel of freedom... (Union view of blueprint pioneered in Northamptonshire AHA to facilitate union management agreements.) Health and Social Service Journal, 88, 24 Mar 1978, 342-345.

56 Wells, R. Nurses in unions spells CONFLICT. Nursing Mirror, 148, 29 Mar 1979, 11.

57 Whitehead, T. United unions for a healthier service. (Role of trade unions in the mental health service.) Mind Out, 25, Nov/Dec 1977, 12-15.

58 Williams, D. The right to strike. (Comment on GNC statement by Assistant General Secretary COHSE.) Nursing Mirror, 149, 16 Aug 1979, 16.

59 Williams, D. Interview with David Williams, assistant general secretary of COHSE. Nursing Times, 73, 27 Oct 1977, 1661.

c LABOUR RELATIONS: OVERSEAS

1 Adler, J. and others When a nursing staff organizes: management rights and collective bargaining. (Programmed instruction.) American Journal of Nursing, 78 (4), Apr 1978, P.I. 1-12.

2 American Association of Occupational Health Nurses Occupational health nurses and collective bargaining. Occupational Health Nursing, 25 (1), Jan 1977, 15-16.

3 Atkinson, P.J. and Goodwin, L. The role of the nurse administrator in collective bargaining. Nursing Clinics of North America, 13 (1), Mar 1978, 111-118.

4 Beason, C. Nursing's labor relations crisis. Will nurses wait for their traditional associations to get serious about collective bargaining? Or will they take action on their own? RN Magazine, 42 (2), Feb 1979, 21-22, 24, 26, 28, 32-33.

5 Bentivegna, G. Labour relations: union activity increases among professionals. (Review of 1978 literature.) Hospitals, 53 (7), 1 Apr 1979, 131-132, 134, 136, 138-139.

6 Bloom, B.I. Collective action by professionals poses problems for administrators. (Collective bargaining among physicians, nurses and pharmacists.) Hospitals, 51 (6), 16 Mar 1977, 167-168, 170, 174.

7 Brown, J.A. Core issues of unionization: your ten most frequently asked questions answered. AANA J, 48 (1), Feb 1980, 26-30.

8 Crooks, E. Nurses' associations and collective bargaining: wave of the past? (U.S. situation.) RN Magazine, 42 (4), Apr 1979, 83-84, 88.

9 Curtin, L.L. Quoth the raven, 'Nevermore'. (Editorial on trends towards unionisation of nurses in the USA.) Supervisor Nurse, 10 (1), Jan 1979, 6.

10 Denton, J.A. Attitudes toward alternative models of unions and professional associations. (A study of 75 nurses to investigate the relationship between motivation for entering nursing and attitudes towards unions.) Nursing Research, 25 (3), May/Jun 1976, 178-180.

11 Donovan, L. Is nursing ripe for a union explosion? (Results of a survey.) RN Magazine, 41 (5), May 1978, 63-65.

12 Fralic, M.F. The nursing director prepares for labor negotiations: practical information and perspective. Journal of Nursing Administration, 7 (6), Jul/Aug 1977, 4-8.

13 Gideon, J. Unions: choice and mandate. AORN Journal, 31 (7), Jun 1980, 1201-1207.

14 Hanson, D.J. Why are we on strike? (Article by nurse in form of a letter to a fellow-striker.) American Journal of Nursing, 80 (5), May 1980, 954-955.

15 Herzog, T.P. The National Labor Relations Act and the ANA: a dilemma of professionalism. Journal of Nursing Administration, 6 (8), Oct 1976, 34-36.

16 Hopping, B. Professionalism and unionism: conflicting ideologies. Nursing Forum, 15 (4), 1976, 372-383.

17 Jacox, I. Welfare of nurses and patient care. (Role of collective action in the nursing profession.) Nursing Journal of India, 49 (5), May 1978, 105-111.

18 Korn, R. Nurses united! One staff's decision to strike. (New York City, February 1980.) American Journal of Nursing, 80 (12), Dec 1980, 2218-2221.

19 Kruger, D.H. Labor-management issues for the future. New York: National League for Nursing, 1979.

20 Lawrence, V. Taking action. (Account of nurses' strike in Ireland.) Nursing Times, 76, 19 Jun 1980, 1078.

21 Lockhart, C.A. and Werther, W.B., editors Labor relations in nursing. Wakefield, Mass.: Nursing Resources, 1980. (Management anthology series 5).

22 McClure, K. I lost my job by defending nurses' rights. (Owing to union activities.) RN Magazine, 40 (12), Dec 1977, 35-37.

23 Makotoko, J. On strike. (Nurse describes her experiences during strike in Ontario in December 1977.) Canadian Nurse, 74 (4), Apr 1978, 30-32.

24 METHODIST nurses ratify contract after five days on picket lines. (Report of fourth nurses' strike against New York voluntary hospitals.) American Journal of Nursing, 80 (5), May 1980, 841.

25 Metzger, N. Hospital labor scene marked by union issues. (Nurses and the National Labor Relations Board (NLRB).) Hospitals, 54 (7), 1 Apr 1980, 105-106, 108, 111-112.

26 Miller, M.H. and Dodson, L. Work stoppage among nurses. (Study of incidents of nurse work stoppage in the U.S.A. from 1960-1974.) Journal of Nursing Administration, 6 (10), Dec 1976, 41-45.

27 Miller, R.U. Collective bargaining: a nursing dilemma. AORN Journal, 31 (7), Jun 1980, 1195-1200.

28 Natonski, J. Why a union contract didn't work at our hospital. RN Magazine, 41 (5), May 1978, 69-71.

29 O'Connor, M. How the Irish strike affected patients. (Letter.) Nursing Times, 76, 17 Jul 1980, 1263.

30 Patten, M.E. The nurse and corporate action. (With reference to the activities of RANF.) Australian Nurses Journal, 8 (8), Mar 1979, 43-45.

31 RN Magazine Public nurses take on New York's tough antistrike law — and win. RN Magazine, 41 (3), Mar 1978, 22, 24.

32 Reece, D.A. Union decertification and the salaried approach: a workable alternative. Journal of Nursing Administration, 7 (6), Jul/Aug 1977, 20-24.

33 Roach, D.L. and others Hospitals stand firm, ensure care in lengthy areawide nurses' strike. (10 week strike in Seattle in 1976.) Hospitals, 51 (15), 1 Aug 1977, 49-51.

34 Rowsell, G. Nurses unions, professional associations and YOU. 1. Nurses take the union route. 2. The role of the nurse manager in labor relations. Canadian Nurse, 76 (7), Jul/Aug 1980, 44-45; (8), Sep 1980, 30-32.

35 Samaras, J.T. Administrative attitudes on collective bargaining in hospitals. (Report of a small research study among hospital administrators.) Supervisor Nurse, 9 (1), Jan 1978, 56, 59.

36 Sargis, N.M. Will nursing director's attitudes affect future collective bargaining? (Survey of attitudes of top nursing managers in 216 US hospitals.) Journal of Nursing Administration, 8 (12), Dec 1978, 21-26.

37 Supervisor Nurse To strike or not to strike: a debate on the ethics of strikes by nurses. Supervisor Nurse, 10 (1), Jan 1979, 52, 55-59.

38 Trained Nurses' Association of India TNAI policy with regard to strikes by nurses. (Policy statement.) Nursing Journal of India, 69 (1), Jan 1978, 5-6.

39 Wenham, D. To strike or not to strike? — The R.P.N. and collective bargaining. Canadian Journal of Psychiatric Nursing, 15 (2), Mar/Apr 1974, 8-9.

40 Werther, W.B. Unions do not happen, they are caused. New York: National League for Nursing, 1978.

41 Wynne, D. A union contract was the only language our hospital would understand. RN Magazine, 41 (5), May 1978, 66-68.

d HOURS OF WORK

1 Bajnok, I. The 12 hour shift: it's good for nurses, but is it good for the patients? (Experiment at University Hospital, London, Ontario.) Hospital Administration in Canada, 17 (10), Oct 1975, 25-26.

2 Bissett, E.M. and Graham, J. Flextime in nursing. 1. Preparing a questionnaire. 2. Views of nurses. (Feasibility study at Leith Hospital, Edinburgh, to solve staff shortage problem.) Nursing Times, 73, 13 Jan 1977, 68-71; 20 Jan 1977, 100-102.

3 Boyarski, R.P. Nursing workweek equalizes shifts, time off: analysis of two years experience at Mercy Medical Center, Dubuque, Ia. Hospital Progress, 57 (7), Jul 1976, 36-37, 40, 45.

4 Cales, A.D. A twelve hour schedule experiment. Supervisor Nurse, 7 (6), Jun 1976, 71-72, 74, 76.

5 Carr, A. Reduction in the working hours of nurses. Nursing Focus, 1 (9), May 1980, 345.

6 Crump, C.K. and Newson, E.F.P. Implementing the 12 hour shift: a case history. (Results of a study conducted at the University Hospital in London, Ontario.) Hospital Administration in Canada, 17 (10), Oct 1975, 20-24.

7 Donovan, L. Is there a 7-day work week in your future? (Progress report on schedules in various USA hospitals.) RN Magazine, 41 (3), Mar 1978, 62-67.

8 Ganong, W.L. and others The 12 hour shift: better quality, lower cost. (Study of staffing, seven days on, seven days off at Medical Park Hospital, North Carolina, since 1971.) Journal of Nursing Administration, 6 (2), Feb 1976, 17-29.

9 General Nursing Council 37½ hour week. (Guidance.) GNC Circular no.80/10 + enclosure 80/10/1, Mar 1980.

10 Godfrey, M.A. The part-time question and the hospital's answer. Part 2. (Results of questionnaire.) Nursing (US), 10 (11), Nov 1980, 65-72.

11 Katz, E. Flexible scheduling using part-time nurses. Dimensions in Health Service, 55 (3), Mar 1978, 18-19.

12 Nursing Times Reduced working week. Ennals supports reduced working week. (Letter urging RHAs to increase intake of learner nurses to reduce nurses' working week by 1981.) Nursing Times, 74, 1 Jun 1978, 900. Cost of reducing nurses' working week as estimated by Anthony Carr. 4 May 1978, 732.

13 Shaw, P. The 10-hour day in the 4-day week. (Implementation of alternative to 8-hour shift.) Supervisor Nurse, 9 (9), Oct 1978, 47-53, 56.

14 Shevas, A. Unions win 37½-hour week. (Agreement allowing AHAs to introduce shorter week from April 1980.) Nursing Mirror, 150, 20 Mar 1980, 4.

15 Stuart, A.J. An experiment in innovative staffing. (Using twelve hour shift, with discussion of why it was not a success.) Canadian Nurse, 75 (8), Sep 1979, 45-46.

16 Tyler, G. Flexible hours for regional staff. (Plantime monitoring equipment used at Trent RHA.) Health and Social Service Journal, 86, 28 Aug 1976, 1559.

e NIGHT DUTY AND SHIFT-WORKING

1 Altnagelvin Hospital, Northern Ireland Survey of night nursing services. Reported in Nursing Times, 75, 15 Nov 1979, 1960; Health and Social Service Journal, 90, 4 Jan 1980, 25.

2 Barnes, H. Night work for nurses 'living upside down'. (Survey of nurses by Department of Labour based on questionnaire.) New Zealand Nursing Journal, 73 (5), May 1980, 22-23, 27-29, 43.

3 Carr, A.J. Hospital night staffing. (Letter describing situation at the Royal Victoria Infirmary, Newcastle.) British Medical Journal, 1, 14 Feb 1976, 400.

4 Carr, A.J. Work load and staffing on night duty. (Visits to Newcastle General Infirmary and the Royal Victoria Infirmary to assess the staffing situation.) Nursing Times, 72 (30), 29 Jul 1976, Occ. papers, 105-108.

5 Eaves, D. Time for a change. (Circadian rhythm disturbances experienced by nurses on night duty.) Nursing Mirror, 150, 7 Feb 1980, 22-24.

6 Felton, G. and Ward, J.H. Regression models in the study of circadian rhythms in nursing research. (Effect on nurses' sleep patterns.) International Journal of Nursing Studies, 14 (3), 1977, 151-161.

7 Fitzpatrick, L. How do you feel about.... working nights? (Survey by CN. See also editorial on page 3.) Canadian Nurse, 93 (9), Sep 1977, 34-39. Questionnaire used in Canadian Nurse, 72 (10), Oct 1976, 15-17.

8 Hamilton, M. Eskimo's had no circadian rhythms. (Summary of a research project at Northwick Park Hospital to investigate physiological adaptation of nurses to night duty.) Occupational Health, 29 (3), Mar 1977, 109.

9 Hawkins, L.H. and Armstrong-Esther, C.A.

Circadian rhythms and night shift working in nurses. (Pilot study measuring short-term memory and body temperature.) Nursing Times, 74, 4 May 1978, Occ. papers, 49-52.

10 **Lyons, B.** Keep in step with your circadian rhythms. (With a brief reference to the effect of night duty on nurses in New South Wales.) Australian Nurses' Journal, 5 (5), Nov 1975, 22-23.

11 **Salvage, J.** A necessary evil. (Night duty and ways in which it could be improved.) Nursing Mirror, 150, 7 Feb 1980, 24.

12 **Vousden, M.** Sleep well, night nurse! (Aspects of the work and status of night nurses.) Nursing Mirror, 149, 6 Sep 1979, 12.

f SALARIES AND SUPERANNUATION

1 **Ashton, K.** Why we have waited. (Speakman review of top nurses' salaries.) Nursing Times, 74, 2 Nov 1978, 1790.

2 **Ball, D.** Defusing that minefield at the top. (Progress of Whitley Council review of top posts.) Health and Social Service Journal, 88, 31 Mar 1978, 364-366.

3 **Bosanquet, N.** Third time lucky? (Comment on methods and findings of Clegg Commission.) Nursing Times, 76, 17 Jan 1980, 98-99.

4 **Bullough, B.** The struggle for women's rights in Denver: a personal account. (Account of legal hearing of case brought by ten nurses against the City and County of Denver over low pay.) Nursing Outlook, 26 (9), Sep 1978, 566-567.

5 **Carr, A.** After Clegg—what next for nurses. (Evaluation of the position of senior nurses.) Nursing Focus, 1 (7), Mar 1980, 271-272.

6 **Cole, A.** Not-so-goodbye? (Comment on value of Prof Clegg's work with nurses' pay.) Nursing Times, 76, 14 Aug 1980, 1424.

7 **Cole, A.** The shape of things to come? (Evidence to Clegg commission by the government and Staff Side.) Nursing Times, 75, 22 Nov 1979, 2011.

8 **Cole, A.** When it comes to the crunch... will Clegg bring nurse conflicts to a head? (Report of Roger Dyson's speech on industrial relations in nursing at a King's Fund Centre conference of nurse managers.) Nursing Times, 75, 27 Sep 1979, 1653.

9 **Dopson, L.** Clegg's conundrum. (How the comparability commission is doing its work and some of the issues raised.) Nursing Times, 75, 8 Nov 1979, 1917-1918.

10 **Dunn, A.** The curate's Clegg. (Editorial on findings of the Clegg report.) Nursing Times, 76, 10 Jan 1980, 47.

11 **Dyson, R. and Long, A.** Health service pay. (Includes nurses.) Health Services Manpower Review, 5 (2), May 1979, 3-6.

12 **Field, F.** Nurses' pay: together we stand. (Three-point plan of action to raise pay and develop a fairer spread of differentials, by director of the Low Pay Unit.) Nursing Mirror, 147, 23 Nov 1978, 20-22.

13 **George, J.S.** Comparability—some of the issues. Hospital and Health Service Review, 75 (6), Jun 1979, 201-203.

14 **Halpern, S.** Report from the conference of the Association of Nurse Administrators. (With details of speeches of Gerard Vaughan and Barry Curnow of HAY management consultants on Clegg report.) Health and Social Service Journal, 90, 4 Apr 1980, 438-439.

15 **Hansard** Nurses' pay. Pay Comparability Report. Parliamentary references in Hansard. Statement on report. 15 Jan 1980, WA 713. PM's satisfaction with findings. 29 Jan 1980, WA 558-0.

16 **Health Services** Clegg Commission on nurses' pay. (COHSE's oral evidence and problems of nurses' pay generally.) Health Services, Nov 1979, 6-7.

17 **Heywood Jones, I.** Wages through the ages. Nursing Times, 76, 17 Jul 1980, 1279-1280.

18 **Hospital and Health Services Review** Speakman at last. (Comment on top posts review with special reference to nurses' salaries.) Hospital and Health Service Review, 75 (8), Aug 1979, 261-263.

19 **Howell, L.C.** Nursing salaries. Fairer system for nurses' pay. (Based on professional development.) Health and Social Service Journal, 90, 5 Sep 1980, 1171-1173.

20 **Hyde, A.** Bottom line on the top people—by Speakman. (Comment on review of top posts.) Health and Social Service Journal, 89, 13 Jul 1979, 858-859.

21 **Klein, R.** Incomes: vive la difference. (Comparison of the salaries of different professions including doctors and nurses.) British Medical Journal, 2, 10 Jul 1976, 126-127.

22 **Knight, L.** It's a struggle to cope. (Financial problems of two nurses with dependent relatives.) Nursing Mirror, 148, 1 Mar 1979, 18-19.

23 **Knight, L.** A singular problem over pay. (Problems faced by three single nurses with children.) Nursing Mirror, 148, 15 Feb 1979, 16-18.

24 **Knight, L.** A treat is a bag of chips for two. (Problem of nurses' low pay illustrated by three male nurses with families.) Nursing Mirror, 148, 22 Feb 1979, 20-22.

25 **Link, C.R. and Settle, R.F.** Labor market competition and nurses' earnings: an economic analysis. Research in Nursing and Health, 2 (4), Dec 1979, 141-149.

26 **Midwives Chronicle** Superannuation—the new regulations. (Explanation of 'contracting out'.) Midwives Chronicle, 91, Jan 1978, 6.

27 **Morris, P.** Clegg finds his job rather tougher than he expected. (Comparability study and nurses' pay.) Nursing Mirror, 149, 2 Aug 1979, 5.

28 **Nursing Mirror** What do you think about the Clegg Report. (Views of June Clark, Anthony Carr, Paul Sykes, Shirley Goodwin, Harry Packham and Sylvia Winterbottom and others.) Nursing Mirror, 150, 17 Jan 1980, 6-7, 8-12; 24 Jan 1980, 8-9; 31 Jan 1980, 8-9.

29 **Nursing Times** Clegg Report. 19.6%. But it's still not nearly enough. (Background, summary and reactions.) Nursing Times, 76, 10 Jan 1980, 48-49.

Thumbs down all round! (Views of nurses at Queen Elizabeth Hospital, Birmingham.) 17 Jan 1980, 96-97.
Clegg: the aftermath. (Readers' letters and Professor Clegg's replies to some criticisms.) 24 Jan 1980, 140-143.

30 **Nursing Times** A suitable case for special treatment... (Background to current pay claim with comparative salary scales for other occupations.) Nursing Times, 75, 18 Jan 1979, 94-95.

31 **Philpot, T.** Nursing Mirror campaign: nurses are worth more. (Nurses' views, p.14-16.) Nursing Mirror, 147, 5 Oct 1978, 17-20.

32 **Royal College of Nursing** Submission to the Standing Commission on Pay Comparability. Sep 1979. Rcn, 1979.

33 **Sabel, C.** Does the answer lie in the merit money minefield? (Suggestions for a comprehensive new pay policy for the health service.) Health and Social Service Journal, 87, 29 Jul 1977, 1102-1103.

34 **Smith, J.** Nurses' 100-year battle against low pay. (Historical background.) Nursing Mirror, 148, 22 Mar 1979, 16-17.

35 **Spanswick, A.** Protecting the low paid. (Nurses' salaries, by General Secretary of COHSE.) Nursing Mirror, 147, 16 Nov 1978, 24-25.

36 **Speakman, A.J.** Top posts in the National Health Service: report to the Nurses and Midwives, the Administrative and Clerical and the Professional and Technical (B) Whitley Councils. DHSS, 1979.

37 **Standing Commission on Pay Comparability** Report no.3: nurses and midwives. HMSO, 1980. (Chairman: Professor H.A. Clegg. Cmnd.7795).

38 **Wilson, D.** Clegg-opportunity or catastrophe? (Comment.) Journal of Community Nursing, 3 (8), Feb 1980, 20.

39 **Wyndham-Kaye, J.** A pay research unit for NHS nurses and midwives? Nursing Mirror, 142, 6 May 1976, 40-41.

g WHITLEY COUNCIL

1 **Brown, A.** Which way for Whitley? (Possible alternatives for negotiating nurses' pay.) Nursing Mirror, 151, 3 Jul 1980, 9.

2 **Cowie, V.** Making Whitley work. Health Services Manpower Review Special Series (1), 1977, 11-12.

3 **Dyson, R.** Can Whitley be made to work? Health Services Manpower Review Special Series (1), 1977, 2-5.

4 **Dyson, R.** Implications of the McCarthy report. With particular reference to the future of the NHS professional associations. British Journal of Occupational Therapy, 40 (2), Feb 1977, 31-32.

5 **Dyson, R.** Making Whitley work: a progress report. British Medical Journal, 1, 10 Jun 1978, 1567-1568.

6 **Farnham, D.** Sixty years of Whitleyism. Personnel Management, 10 (7), Jul 1978, 29-32.

7 Fisher, A. A trade union view of the McCarthy report. Health Services Manpower Review Special Series (1), 1977, 8-10.

8 Health Services Manpower Review The McCarthy report. Health Services Manpower Review Special Series (1), Feb 1977, 2-14.

9 Health Visitors Association Association News. The McCarthy Report. (HVA comments on the proposals.) Health Visitor, 50 (12), Dec 1977, 405-407.

10 Hospital and Health Service Review The McCarthy report: a progress report on developments. Hospital and Health Service Review, 74 (4), Apr 1978, 133-134.

11 Hospital and Health Service Review The McCarthy report recommendations. Hospital and Health Service Review, 73 (1), Jan 1977, 25-27. A better Whitley? (Comments on the Report.) 1-3.

12 Howell, L.C. Retaining the Whitley system. Nursing Times, 72, 19 Aug 1976, 1288-1289.

13 Klein, R. The National Health Industry: costs of complexity. (Comments on McCarthy Report.) British Medical Journal, 2, 11 Dec 1976, 1461, 1464.

14 McCarthy, W.E.J. Making Whitley work: a review of the operation of the National Health Service Whitley Council System. DHSS, 1976.

15 McCarthy Report 'Making Whitley Work'. A review of the operation of the NHS Whitley Council system by Lord McCarthy. Nursing Mirror, 143, 9 Dec 1976, 39-41; Midwives Chronicle, 90, Jan 1977, 6.

16 Nixon, C. Lord McCarthy recommends major overhaul of Whitley Council system. British Journal of Occupational Therapy, 40 (1), 1977, 3-6.

17 Pethyridge, F. The McCarthy report. Health Services Manpower Review Special Series (1), 1977, 6-7.

18 Royal College of Midwives Comments on the McCarthy report 'Making Whitley Work.' Midwives Chronicle, 90, Aug 1977, 189-190.

19 Royal College of Midwives Review of the NHS Whitley machinery. (Comments sent to DHSS.) Midwives Chronicle, 88, Nov 1975, 379.

20 Royal College of Nursing (Summary of) 'Making Whitley work': the McCarthy Report. Rcn, 1976.

21 'STAFF side is too big.' Comments invited on McCarthy proposals for Whitley. Nursing Times, 72 (49), 9 Dec 1976, 1903.

22 Vulliamy, C. Major problems in loosening the Treasury's grip on wages. (A review of the McCarthy Report on Whitley.) Health and Social Service Journal, 89, 10 Dec 1976, 2188-2189.

23 Watkin, B. Whitleyism. Nursing Mirror, 142, 10 Jun 1976, 42.

24 Wells, R. The way out of the stop-go cycle. (Call for different negotiating machinery for nurses' salaries.) Nursing Mirror, 147, 19 Oct 1978, 16-17.

25 Williams, D. Making Whitley work. Health Services Manpower Review Special Series (1), 1977, 13-14.

h UNIFORMS

1 Baker, J. Uniforms: keeping up the quality. (Visit to Boyd-Cooper, uniform specialists.) Nursing Times, 76, 17 Jan 1980, 109-110.

2 Bell, R. What do nurses think of the national uniform? (Views of nurses.) Nursing Times, 76, 17 Jan 1980, 118.

3 Below the belt? (News items on nurses at the Royal East Sussex Hospital who want to keep their belts and buckles instead of new uniform.) Health and Social Service Journal, 88, 24 Mar 1978, 338.

4 Berglas, C. Farewell to caps: an account of how nurses caps have survived laments, controversy and resistance. Nursing Mirror, 142, 20 May 1976, 66.

5 Bevan-Pritchard, J. Caps on duty? (Letter objecting to discarding of caps in Bucks.) Nursing Times, 74 (1), 5 Jan 1978, 29.

6 Brennan, M. It's not all uniform! (Eight photographs of various aspects of nurses' uniforms.) Nursing Times, 76, 17 Jan 1980, 114-115.

7 Ellis, S. Where did you get that hat? (Social status of nurses' caps.) Nursing Times, 74, 21/28 Dec 1978, 2094.

8 Fifty years ago. (Letter on uniforms in 1927.) Nursing Times, 73, 25 Aug 1977, 1301.

9 Hawkins, K. Uniform or mufti? (Discussion of value and drawbacks of nurses' uniforms.) Nursing Mirror, 148, 29 Mar 1979, 12.

10 Heywood Jones, I. Uniforms: a history. Nursing Times, 76, 17 Jan 1980, 105-108.

11 Heywood Jones, I. Uniforms: serving the profession for over a century. (History of Garroulds, formerly a department store, now supplier of many types of uniforms.) Nursing Times, 76, 17 Jan 1980, 111-113.

12 Hughes, E. and Proulx, J. You are what you wear. Uniforms and professional roles are frequently tied in the minds of both staff and patient, so it may be advisable to return to greater use of uniforms by hospital professional staffs. Hospitals, 55 (16), Aug 1979, 113-114, 116-118.

13 Meglaughlin, J. Hospital badges. (Seven badges with descriptions.) Nursing Times, 76, 17 Jan 1980, 116-117.

14 Nursing Mirror Changing uniforms over 90 years. (Photographs and drawings.) Nursing Mirror, 146, 13 Apr 1978, 60-61.

15 RN Magazine Key to nursing pins on RN's cover. (Photographs of 80 nursing badges dating from 1924.) RN Magazine, 40 (12), Dec 1977, 20-21.

16 Tootal Workwear 'Design a nurse's dress competition' A uniform fit for the 80s. (Nine designs chosen as finalists in competition.) Nursing Times, 76, 27 Mar 1980, 540-545. Prizewinners and comments. Nursing Times, 76, 22 May 1980, 896-897; Nursing Mirror, 142, 24 Jun 1976, 37.

17 Watson, G. The uniform that brings confidence. (The case for and against nurses' uniforms.) Nursing Mirror, 147, 20 Jul 1978, 34.

i UNIFORMS: PSYCHIATRIC

1 Llewelyn, S.P. A change for the better? (Research study by psychologist into attitudes of patients, visitors and nurses towards uniform for psychiatric nurses.) Nursing Mirror, 149, 16 Aug 1979, 27-29.

2 Malcomson, K. and others An evaluation of the effect of nurses wearing street clothes on socialization patterns. (Of psychiatric patients.) Journal of Psychiatric Nursing and Mental Health Services, 15 (1), 18-21.

3 Meade, H.A.C. Or no uniform at all? (Advantages and disadvantages of psychiatric nurses' wearing uniforms.) Nursing Times, 76, 24 Jan 1980, 147-148.

MANPOWER AND MANAGEMENT

9 MANPOWER

a GENERAL

1 Abel, P.M. and others Nursing manpower. A sound statistical base for policy making. (An outline of Scottish Home and Health Department studies.) Nursing Times, 72, 1/8 Jan 1976, Occ. papers, 1-4; 15 Jan 1976, Occ. papers, 5-7.

2 Allen, A.S., editor Introduction to health professions. 2nd ed. St. Louis: Mosby, 1976.

3 Arnold, N. A nursing view. Where have all the nurses gone? (Factors involved and recommendations for improving staff situation.) British Medical Journal, 280, 19 Jan 1980, 199-201; Correspondence, 9 Feb, 406; 16 Feb, 486; 1 Mar, 480.

4 Beard, T.C. Observations on the shortage of trained nurses. Medical Journal of Australia, 1975, 2, 26 Jul 1975, 137-140. (Reprint file.)

5 Boam, T.V. A question of balance: tactics and strategy of nurse manpower planning. Nursing Times, 73, 6 Jan 1977, Occ. papers, 5-8; 20 Jan 1977, Occ. papers, 9-12.

6 Borgmeyer, W.A.E. Charting manpower. (Techniques of manpower planning for nursing administrators.) Health and Social Service Journal, 85, 20/27 Dec 1975, 2788.

7 Butler, A.M. Manpower planning for quality nursing care. (Research studies by the Auckland Hospital Board.) New Zealand Nursing Journal, 69 (3), Mar 1976, 26-30.

8 Canadian Nurses Association CNA research study reveals few key changes in nursing employment, education patterns since 1966. Canadian Nurse, 73 (3), Mar 1977, 12-13.

9 Clode, D. Circling the pyramid by camel— via the needle's eye. (Manpower problems in the nursing and medical professions.) Health and Social Service Journal, 89, 3 Aug 1979, 972-975.

10 Donovan, L. The shortage: good jobs are going begging these days, so why not be choosy? (RN nationwide survey of staffing shortage.) RN Magazine, 43 (6), Jun 1980, 21-27.

11 Emerton, A. Nurse staffing problems unlikely to change by 1978. (Royal Society of Health conference paper.) Nursing Mirror, 142, 22 Jan 1976, 36.

12 Gray, J.A.M. More nurses. (Letter stressing shortage of nurses as the most serious threat to the health service.) Lancet, 2, 9 Oct 1976, 796-797.

13 Hakim, C. Sexual divisions within the labour force: occupational segregation. (With table showing percentage of women in the nursing profession.) Department of Employment Gazette, 86 (11), Nov 1978, 1264-1268, 1278-1279.

14 Hayar, B.L. and Supta, S.S. Education and administration: need for research (for planning nursing manpower in India). Nursing Journal of India, 68 (1), Jan 1977, 14-16.

15 Howell, L.C. An experiment in the use of a model for a nurse manpower planning in the commissioning of a new district general hospital. MSc thesis in Public Sector Management, University of Aston in Birmingham, 1977.

16 Hunt, S. The facts and myths about nurse unemployment. (NM special report on current situation.) Nursing Mirror, 146, 9 Mar 1978, 3.

17 Johnson, W. Trends in nursing education and projections of the supply of nurses. Contained in: Hiestand, D.L. and Ostow, M. Health manpower information for policy guidance. Cambridge, Mass.: Ballinger, 1976. Chapter 5, 47-59.

18 Kalisch, B. and Kalisch, P. Nursing shortage? Yes. (Throughout the US.) American Journal of Nursing, 79 (3), Mar 1979, 469-480.

19 Keane, M.C. Manpower planning. World of Irish Nursing, 6 (1), 1977, 4-5.

20 LeBourdois, E. RNAO urges nursing alternatives. (Registered Nurses' Association of Toronto conference on the problems of nurse unemployment.) Dimensions in Health Service, 53 (7), Jul 1976, 18.

21 Lee, J.M. Nurse bank scheme. (In hospitals and the community in Romford, Essex.) Nursing Times, 73, 8 Dec 1977, 1926-1927.

22 Lewis, B.R. Personality profiles for qualified nurses: possible implications for recruitment and selection of trainee nurses. (Research at UMIST.) International Journal of Nursing Studies, 17 (4), 221-234.

23 Long, A. and Mercer, G. Nurses down the drain? How bad planning wastes resources. (The effect of demographic factors on manpower planning in nursing.) Nursing Mirror, 147, 23 Nov 1978, 16-19.

24 McCullough, D.M. Nursing manpower planning. World of Irish Nursing, 6 (1), Jan 1977, 7-8.

25 Monaghan, G. The market for nurses— we've come a long way. (Shortage of and now unemployment among Canadian nurses.) Canadian Nurse, 72 (12), Dec 1976, 38-41.

26 Moses, E. and Roth, A. Nursepower: what do statistics reveal about the nation's nurses? (Results of 1977 National Sample Survey of Registered Nurses.) American Journal of Nursing, 79 (10), Oct 1979, 1745-1756.

27 NURSING shortages in NHS hospitals. British Medical Journal, 2, 15 Jul 1978, 222-223.

28 Nursing Times Rcn survey highlights desperate shortage of specialist nurses. (Geriatric and mental handicap nurses, and those working in theatres, intensive care and coronary care.) Nursing Times, 76, 4 Dec 1980, 2128.

29 Philippines. Overseas Employment Development Board Employment opportunities and the nursing profession. (Problems of Filipino nurses working in other countries and suggested remedies.) Philippine Journal of Nursing, 49 (1), Jan/Mar 1979, 26-28.

30 Roth, A.V. Trends in the distribution of nursing manpower. Contained in: Hiestand, D.L. and Ostow, M. editors. Health manpower information for policy guidance. Cambridge, Mass.: Ballinger, 1976. Chapter 6, 61-73.

31 Sandroff, R. The shortage: how it's changing nursing what you can expect. (Results of survey.) RN Magazine, 43 (11), Nov 1980, 55-59, 86, 88, 90.

32 Scott, J.M. and Levine, E. Nursing manpower analysis: its past, present and future. Contained in: Hiestand, D.L. and Ostow, M. editors. Health manpower information for policy guidance. Cambridge, Mass.: Ballinger, 1976. Chapter 4, 25-46.

33 Scottish Home and Health Department The movements of hospital nursing staff in Scotland. Edinburgh: The Department, 1975. (Nursing manpower planning report no.5.)

34 Scottish Home and Health Department Nurse staffing (hospital) survey: book of tables. Edinburgh: The Department, 1975. (Nursing manpower planning report no.3.)

35 Scottish Home and Health Department A profile of qualified nurses working in the Scottish hospital service in 1972. The Department, 1976. (Nursing manpower planning report no.6.)

36 Slack, P. Staff shortages in London. (Accommodation and transport problems.) Nursing Times, 76, 1 May 1980, 791-792.

37 Taaffe, T.C. Manpower planning. World of Irish Nursing, 5 (11) & (12), Nov/Dec 1976, 1-2.

38 Tun, A. Aspects of nurse manpower planning with particular reference to the non-participation of married nurses in the labour force. PhD thesis, UMIST, Department of Management Sciences, 1977.

39 United States Department of Health, Education and Welfare. Bureau of Health Resources Development Division of Medicine International migration of physicians and nurses: an annotated bibliography. USDHEW, 1975.

40 World Health Organization Multinational study of the international migration of physicians and nurses: country specific migration statistics. Geneva: WHO, 1976.

41 Yett, Donald E. An economic analysis of the nurse shortage. Lexington, Mass.: Lexington Books, 1975.

b NURSING AS A CAREER

1 Adam, E. To be a nurse. Toronto: Saunders, 1980.

2 Ainslie, D.S. Vocational development of health professionals. (Survey of university students entering nursing, medicine, social work and health administration to investigate what led to their career choice.) Hospital Administration in Canada, 17 (11) & (12), Nov/Dec 1975, 51-53.

3 American Hospital Association Career goals of hospital school of nursing seniors: report of a survey. Chicago: The Association, 1975.

4 Bristow, S. Career opportunities. Choosing a course. Nursing Times, 72, 10 Jun 1976, 884-887.

5 CAREERS in nursing and other health service professions. New Opportunity Press, 1979.

6 Dowdall, P. Fears of the hospital trained nurse, her future mobility and international recognition. (As opposed to the nurse with degree or diploma.) Australian Nurses Journal, 8 (7), Feb 1979, 39-41, 48-49.

7 Everest, R. and others What happens to Maudsley nurses? A follow-up study. (Investigation of work history of nurses who trained at the Maudsley School of Nursing between 1959 and 1970.) International Journal of Nursing Studies, 16 (3), Aug 1979, 253-266.

8 International Council of Nurses ICN statement on career mobility in nursing. International Nursing Review, 24 (5), Sep/Oct 1977, 155.

9 Krzyzak, K., editor Careers in nursing and other health service professions 1975. Classic Publications, 1975.

10 Lenburg, C., editor Open learning and career mobility in nursing. St. Louis: Mosby, 1975.

11 Logan, W. The migration of nursing personnel. International Nursing Review, 27 (4), Jul/Aug 1980, 119-122.

12 Loree, D.J. and Leckie, I. Why nursing? Occupation and career perceptions of nursing students in New Brunswick. (Research study.) Canadian Nurse, 73 (12), Dec 1977, 30-33.

13 Moss, S. Careers in nursing and allied professions. Kogan Page, 1979.

14 Nash, P.M. Evaluation of employment opportunities for newly licensed nurses: health

manpower references. U.S. Department of Health, Education and Welfare, 1975.

15 National League for Nursing Your career in nursing. New York: The League, 1976.

16 Nuttall, P.D. Working as a nurse. Batsford, 1978. (Careers series).

17 Story, D.K. Career mobility: implementing the ladder concept in associate degree and practical nursing curricula. St. Louis: Mosby, 1974.

18 White, R. Career cycle. (Relationship of a nurse's career cycle to the family life cycle.) Nursing Mirror, 143, 16 Sep 1976, 67.

19 Young, D. More emphasis on attitude. (Need for flexibility in developing a nursing career structure including progression in the clinical field.) Nursing Focus, 2 (4), Dec 1980, 124-125.

c RECRUITMENT

1 Australian Nurses Journal Catch 22. Editorial. (Unemployment among nurses in Australia.) Australian Nurses Journal, 8 (3), Sep 1978, 5.

2 Brown, B.J. How to succeed in recruiting. (Campaign at the Family Hospital, Milwaukee using posters, advertisements, community seminars and nurse to nurse communication.) American Journal of Nursing, 76 (4), Apr 1976, 604-605.

3 Buckley, J. Faculty commitment to retention and recruitment of black students. Nursing Outlook, 28 (1), Jan 1980, 46-50.

4 Byatt, J. The greatest happiness. (Findings of survey in Hillingdon AHA to study factors affecting recruitment and retention of nursing staff.) Health and Social Service Journal, 86, 25 Feb 1977, 343.

5 Cooper, C.L. and others Personality profiles for long serving senior nurses: implications for recruitment and selection. (Study at the University of Manchester Institute of Science and Technology.) International Journal of Nursing Studies, 13 (4), 1976, 251-257.

6 Feldman, D.C. Organizational socialization of hospital employees. A comparative view of occupational groups. (Ways in which employees, including nurses, are attracted to, recruited by, and developed and trained within hospitals.) Medical Care, 15 (10), Oct 1977, 799-813.

7 Fisher, R.F. Recruitment. 14. Initiatives in nursing recruitment. (Report of South East Thames RHA's working conference to consider the best methods of recruiting psychiatric nurse.) Nursing Times, 76, 18/25 Dec 1980, 2252-2254.

8 Harrison, F. Where are the nurses coming from? (Suggests that learner recruitment and education should be redirected at mature women.) Nursing Times, 76, 18 Sep 1980, 1648-1650.

9 Hughes, J. Recruitment. 13. Women, work and the part-time community nurse in London. (Ways in which trained nurses could be attracted to community nursing in London.) Nursing Times, 76, 11 Dec 1980, 2202-2205.

10 Lewis, B.R. The marketing of nursing. PhD thesis, Manchester University, 1979.

11 Lewis, B. Recruitment of trainee nurses—the role of schools of nursing. (Survey of 125 schools of nursing.) Nursing Times, 76, 25 Sep 1980, 1694-1696.

12 Lewis, B.R. Personality profiles for qualified nurses: possible implications for recruitment and selection of trainee nurses. (Research at the University of Manchester Institute of Science and Technology.) International Journal of Nursing Studies, 17 (4), 1980, 221-234.

13 Pearson, R. Assessing the labour market for nurses. (Issues to consider in recruitment campaigns with sources of information.) Nursing Times, 76, 18 Sep 1980, 1650-1652.

14 Public Service Public Service looks at nurse recruitment. (Two articles.) Public Service, 52 (7), May 1978, 8-9.

15 Shevas, A. Everything you wanted to know about nursing... ('Please nurse?' recruitment campaign in Northern RHA.) Nursing Mirror, 150, 7 Feb 1980, 9.

16 Wishart, C. and Hall, J.N. Obtaining student nurses. 2. Conclusions. Nursing Times, 76, 4 Dec 1980, Occ. papers, 125-126.

17 Wong, S. and Wong, J. Representation of racial minority students in selected Canadian university schools of nursing. Journal of Advanced Nursing, 5 (1), Jan 1980, 83-90.

d RETURN TO NURSING

1 BRIDGING the back-to-work gap in Newcastle-upon-Tyne. (Nurse bank scheme operating from Job Centre.) Nursing Times, 74, 17 Aug 1978, 1358-1360.

2 Cleland, V. and others Social and psychologic influences on employment of married nurses. Nursing Research, 25 (2), Mar-Apr 1976, 90-97.

3 Feldman, R. Working mothers: employed nurses and their children's anxiety levels. (Pilot study.) Occupational Health Nursing, 26 (7), Jul 1978, 16-19.

4 Field, P.M. The setting up of a nurse bank. (In Doncaster AHA.) Nursing Times, 76, 28 Feb 1980, 388-389.

5 Hospital and Health Services Review As it seems. (Comments on 'Reality Shock: why nurses leave nursing', by M. Kramer.) Hospital and Health Services Review, 72 (3), Mar 1976, 80-81.

6 Hume, B. American nurses. (Employment of married nurses.) Nursing Times, 72, 15 Jul 1976, 1100-1101.

7 Karseras, P. Bank statement. (Experiences of a bank nurse—member of a nurse bank.) Nursing Mirror, 144, 3 Feb 1977, 59.

8 Karseras, P. A fresh perspective on nursing. (Personal experiences of a return to nursing after 11 years.) Nursing Mirror, 143, 22 Jul 1976, 50.

9 Link, C.R. and Settle, R.F. Financial incentive and labor supply of married professional nurses: an economic analysis. Nursing Research, 29 (4), Jul/Aug 1980, 238-243.

10 May, J. Polishing my lamp. (Experiences

of a return to nursing.) Nursing Mirror, 143, 19 Aug 1976, 63.

11 **Michel, R.P.** Returning to nursing. (An experience in theatre nursing after ten years absence.) Nursing Mirror, 142, 20 May 1976, 65.

12 **Murray, S.** (1978) Back to nursing. (Nurse describes her experiences and need for courses.) Nursing Times, 74, 1 Jun 1978, 904-905.

13 **Nelson, J.** No interest from this bank. (Critical comments on the system of nurse banks compared with agencies.) Nursing Mirror, 146, 30 Mar 1978, 34.

14 **Scheffer, B.** Refresher perspectives. (Issues in training nurses returning to the profession.) Canadian Nurse, 72 (8), Aug 1976, 43-46.

15 **Taylor, V. and Cruden, G.** Bringing people back to nursing: the hospitals of today need the nurses of yesterday. (Course in Grampian Health Board (South District).) Nursing Times, 75, 19 Jul 1979, 1237-1238.

e WASTAGE AND TURNOVER

1 **Annandale-Steiner, D.** Unhappiness is the nurse who expected more. (Survey by nurse counsellor of reasons why nurses leave nursing.) Nursing Mirror, 149, 29 Nov 1979, 34-36.

2 **Aydelotte, M.K.** The determinates of nursing turnover. (Summary of ongoing study.) Nursing Research Report, 12 (2), May 1977, 5-6.

3 **Campbell, W.** Looking at the when and why of staff turnover. A four year study of staff turnover in a psychiatric unit. (At John Conolly Hospital, Birmingham.) Health and Social Service Journal, 87, 9 Sep 1977, 1272-1273.

4 **Clark, J.M. and Redfern, S.J.** Absence and wastage in nursing. 1. The relevance of absence and wastage to the organisation and association between the two. 2. Collecting and using information. Nursing Times, 74, 20 Apr 1978, Occ. papers, 41-44; 27 Apr 1978, Occ. papers, 45-48.

5 **Cunningham, C.V.** Staff nurses and their reasons for leaving. MPhil thesis, Edinburgh University, Department of Nursing Studies, 1979.

6 **Donehue, A.** Wastage in nursing training. (With reference to Australia.) Australian Nurses Journal, 7 (10), May 1978, 42-45.

7 **Gartside, G.** Save it. (Need to investigate and prevent wastage among nurses.) Nursing Times, 76, 14 Feb 1980, 274.

8 **Hallas, G.G.** Why nurses are giving it up. (Survey in Florida of reasons for wastage.) RN Magazine, 43 (7), Jul 1980, 17-21.

9 **Hawkins, K.** Why I'm giving up nursing. (By a third year student.) Nursing Mirror, 149, 22 Nov 1979, 10.

10 **Hutcheson, J.D. and others** Antecedents of nursing school attrition: attitudinal dimensions. Nursing Research, 28 (1), Jan/Feb 1979, 57-62.

11 **Knopke, H.J.** Predicting student attrition in a baccalaureate curriculum. (Longitudinal study of enrolment data at University of Wisconsin Madison School of Nursing.) Nursing Research, 28 (4), Jul/Aug 1979, 224-227.

12 **Mercer, G.** The employment of nurses: nursing labour turnover in the NHS. Croom Helm, 1979.

13 **Mercer, G. and others** Nurses on the move. (Survey of turnover in West Yorkshire hospitals carried out by the Department of Sociology, Leeds University.) Nursing Times, 72, 25 Mar 1976, 441-443; Health and Social Service Journal, 86, 7 Aug 1976, 1432-1433.

14 **Mercer, G. and Long, A.** The turnover of labour in nursing. Health Services Manpower Review, 3 (3), Aug 1977, 8-13; (4), Nov 1977, 6-10.

15 **Mercer, G. and Mould, C.** An investigation into the level and character of labour turnover amongst trained nurses. Leeds University Department of Sociology, 1977. (Summary of a report for the DHSS.)

16 **Montgomery, J.S. and Palmer, P.E.** Reducing attrition in an ad program. (Associate degree program.) Nursing Outlook, 24 (1), Jan 1976, 49-51.

17 **National League for Nursing** Promoting student retention in a nursing program. New York: NLN, 1978.

18 **Reres, M.E.** Turnover among hospital nurses: a suggested model. (As a basis for the collection of data on reasons for leaving.) Journal of Nursing Administration, 6 (8), Oct 1976, 55-58.

19 **Rotenberg, A.** Attitudes and beliefs versus study results: exemplified by attrition in a school of nursing in Israel during 1968-1974. Journal of Advanced Nursing, 3 (5), Sep 1978, 427-432.

20 **Rotenberg, A.** Local studies — the way to solve local problems. (Research study of attrition in a school of nursing in Israel.) International Nursing Review, 25 (2), Mar/Apr 1978, 53-54.

21 **Salvage, J.** A crisis of morale? Causes which lead to a nurse's decision to quit nursing. Nursing Mirror, 149, 13 Dec 1979, 14.

22 **Seybolt, J.W. and others** Turnover among nurses: it can be managed. (Predictive model based on data from an attitude survey.) Journal of Nursing Administration, 8 (9), Sep 1978, 4-9.

23 **Strilaeff, F.** How work organisation affects nursing turnover. (Research study of organisation of work in hospital wards including team nursing and task allocation.) Dimensions in Health Service, 55 (5), May 1978, 28, 30-31.

24 **Strilaeff, F.** Shift work and turnover of general duty nurses. (Study of the reasons for the turnover of nurses employed in four hospitals in Western Canada.) Dimensions in Health Service, 53 (8), Aug 1976, 36-38.

25 **Strilaeff, F.** Supervision and turnover of general staff nurses. (Study of three hospital wards with high, medium and low turnover rates.) Dimensions in Health Service, 53 (11), Nov 1976, 36-39.

26 **Twyman, S.** The junior nurse's dilemma. (Need for student nurse to conform and possible reason for leaving training.) Nursing Mirror, 149, 11 Oct 1979, 21-22.

27 **Watson, L.A.** Keeping qualified nurses. (Research study of nurses' reasons for leaving positions and which factors would encourage them to stay.) Supervisor Nurse, 10 (10), Oct 1979, 29, 32-34.

28 **Wilkinson, R.** How do you stop them leaving? (Turnover of nurses and other employees.) Nursing Mirror, 150, 19 Jun 1980, 43.

29 **Wilson, H.S. and Levy, J.** Why RN students drop out. Nursing Outlook, 26 (7), Jul 1978, 437-441.

f AGENCY NURSES

1 **Amenta, M.M.** Staffing through temporary help agencies. (Use and abuse of agency nurses.) Supervisor Nurse, 8 (12), Dec 1977, 19-20, 23, 25-26.

2 **Esson, E.** What makes a good nursing agency? (Prize-winning essay.) Nursing Mirror, 147, 23 Nov 1978, 22-23.

3 **Federation of Personnel Services of Great Britain** Agency nurses: a national survey of attitudes, comments and statistics. The Federation, 1975.

4 **MacLeod, A.** Agency experience is good experience. (Based on a prize essay.) Nursing Mirror, 147, 13 Jul 1978, 24.

5 **Prescott, P.A. and Langford, T.L.** Supplemental nursing service: boon or bane? (Pilot study of use of agency nurses.) American Journal of Nursing, 79 (12), Dec 1979, 2140-2144.

6 **Statutory Instruments 1978** 1443. The nurses agencies amendment regulations 1978.

g AUXILIARIES

1 **Bacon, F.** First impressions. (Of a part-time nursing auxiliary at Pembury Hospital, Kent.) Nursing Times, 74, 23 Feb 1978, 312.

2 **Bergman, R.** Health auxiliaries and the health team. Nursing education and the evolving role of the nurse. World Hospitals, Feb 1978, 30-31.

3 **Brief, A.P. and others** A study: the impact of task characteristics on employee response in hospital nursing. (Survey with nursing aides and assistants.) Nursing Administration Quarterly, 2 (4), Summer 1978, 107-114.

4 **Courtney, Z.P.** Training for the job. (In-service training scheme at Southmead Hospital, Bristol, for nursing auxiliaries.) Nursing Times, 74, 26 Jan 1978, 164-165.

5 **Cowper-Smith, F.** Untrained nurse, unsolved problem. (Current usage, aims and objectives of Nursing Auxiliaries Association and SHHD's suggested training and duties.) Nursing Times, 74, 23 Feb 1978, 306-309.

6 **Department of Health** Health circular HC 78. Instruction of nursing auxiliaries and nursing assistants. The Department, 1978.

7 **Donovan, J.E. and others** The nurse assistant. 2nd ed. New York: McGraw-Hill, 1978.

8 **Hameister, D.R.** A design of inservice education for nurses aides in a nursing home setting. Journal of Continuing Education in Nursing, 8 (2), Mar/Apr 1977, 6-12.

9 **Hardie, M.** Auxiliaries in nursing: implications for the division of nurses' labour. PhD thesis, University of Edinburgh, 1980.

10 **Hardie, M.** Assisting the nurse in Denmark. (Work of nursing auxiliaries examined by a Winston Churchill Travelling Fellow.) Nursing Mirror, 142, 29 Jan 1976, 63-64.

11 **Hardie, M.** The nurses' aide in Sweden. (Winston Churchill Travelling Fellowship 1975.) Nursing Mirror, 142 (5), 5 Feb 1976, 67-69.

12 **Hardie, M.** The nurses' helper in Holland. (Work of the nursing auxiliary described by a Winston Churchill Travelling Fellow 1975.) Nursing Mirror, 142 (4), 22 Jan 1976, 63-64.

13 **Hardie, M.** You and research. Multidisciplinary aides in the community. (Application of an American home help scheme — the Kaiser Permanente Medical Care System Portland.) Social Work Today, 7 (8), 8 Jul 1976, 241.

14 **Hardie, M. and Hockey, L., editors** Nursing auxiliaries in health care. Croom Helm, 1978.

15 **Hennel, J.** Don't call them 'nurses'. (Argues against formalisation of training for auxiliaries.) Nursing Mirror, 149, 20 Sep 1979, 14. For comment see 4 Oct 1979, 10; 11 Oct 1979, 9; 25 Oct 1979, 12. Expanded version of article appears in Nursing Mirror, 150, 3 Jan 1980, 10-11.

16 **Hospital Research and Education Trust** Being a nursing aide. 2nd ed. Chicago: the Trust, 1978.

17 **International Workshop on Nursing Auxiliaries** Are auxiliaries getting a rough deal? (Report of workshop.) Nursing Mirror, 145, 17 Nov 1977, 3.

18 **Johnson, M.L.** Nursing auxiliaries and nurse professionalisation. Nursing Times, 74, 23 Feb 1978, 313.

19 **Kaskubar, J.P.** Levels of nursing assistants. (Continuing education to advance position.) Supervisor Nurse, 9 (5), May 1978, 26, 28, 30, 32-34.

20 **Keywood, O.** Will our auxiliaries become assistant nurses? (History of recognition of SENs and possible repetition of demand for recognition by auxiliaries.) Nursing Mirror, 146, 16 Mar 1978, 39.

21 **Marshall, J.R. and Schau, E.** An evaluation process for nursing assistants. (Seattle Veterans Administration Hospital.) Journal of Nursing Administration, 6 (8), Oct 1976, 37-40.

22 **Martin, N.** When auxiliaries became official. (Letter on history and training of auxiliaries by general secretary of their organisation.) Nursing Mirror, 149, 11 Oct 1979, 9.

23 **National Association of Auxiliaries** Auxiliaries. The Southmead scheme. (Policy statement and schedule of training prepared by Education Committee of NAA which formed basis for Southmead scheme.) Nursing Times, 74, 23 Feb 1978, 310-311.

24 **Scottish Home and Health Department** Training and duties of nursing auxiliaries and nursing assistants. (NHS circular no.1977 (Gen)35.) Edinburgh: The Department, 1977.

25 **Skeet, M. and Elliott, K.** Health auxiliaries and the health team. Croom Helm, 1978.

26 **Skeet, M.** Nursing aides, auxiliaries and assistance. (Paper delivered at the International Hospital Federation in Tokyo.) Nursing Times, 73, 17 Nov 1977, Occ. papers, 145-148.

27 **Smith, J.P.** Training of nursing auxiliaries: the British Red Cross Society can help. Queen's Nursing Journal, 19 (2), May 1976, 46.

28 **Sparrow, H.E.** Nursing auxiliaries. (Duties and training in the Southampton district nursing service.) Queen's Nursing Journal, 19 (4), Jul 1976, 99.

29 **Walsh, M.** Do we still need auxiliaries? Nursing Mirror, 144, 31 Mar 1977, 41.

30 **Watkin, B.** Independent Trade Union no.51 OT. (Nursing Auxiliaries Association.) Nursing Mirror, 144, 30 Jun 1977, 10.

h GRADUATES

1 **Adebo, E.O. and Chokrieh, A.C.** As we see ourselves: a study in the self-image of the nurse. (Survey of career patterns of graduates of nursing degree course in Ibadan, Nigeria and their attitudes towards their training and performance.) International Nursing Review, 27 (2), Mar/Apr 1980, 41-48.

2 **Bergman, R. and others** Worklife of the graduates of schools for practical nurses in Israel. (Personal and professional characteristics and reasons for leaving nursing.) International Journal of Nursing Studies, 14 (4), 1977, 167-198.

3 **Darby, C.** Is the Open University a career ladder? (Career prospects for nurses with OU degrees.) Nursing Focus, 1 (4), Dec 1979, 156-157.

4 **Davenport, N.J.** The nurse scientist — between two worlds. (Value of nurses with higher degrees in the biological sciences to do research.) Nursing Outlook, 28 (1), Jan 1980, 28-31.

5 **Grey, J.E. and others** Do graduates of technical and professional nursing programs differ in practice? (Survey at University of Vermont School of Nursing.) Nursing Research, 26 (5), Sep/Oct 1977, 368-373.

6 **Kirby, P.** Problems of graduate nurses. Nursing Mirror, 143, 15 Jul 1976, 57.

7 **Marsh, N.** Summary report of a study on the career patterns of diplomates/graduates of the undergraduate nursing course in the University of Manchester, England. Journal of Advanced Nursing, 1 (6), Nov 1976, 539-542.

8 **Meleis, A.I.** The graduate dilemma: the Kuwaiti experience. (Graduates of a newly established junior college programme, including 'reality shock' and employers' refusal to employ them.) International Journal of Nursing Studies, 16 (4), 1979, 337-343.

9 **Nursing Outlook** Nursing: a career for college graduates. (Series of three articles.) Nursing Outlook, 24 (2), Feb 1976, 88-103.

10 **POLYTECHNIC's** first nursing graduates prepare for their careers. (Wellington Polytechnic.) New Zealand Nursing Journal, 69 (2), Feb 1976, 15-16.

11 **Ratcliffe, J.** Past developments. (Symposium on the graduate nurse.) Nursing Mirror, 144, 10 Feb 1977, 47-48.

12 **Reichow, R.W. and Scott, R.E.** Study compares graduates of two, three and four year programs. (A study in Kansas to compare employers' attitudes to nurses with different systems of educational preparation.) Hospitals, 50 (14), 16 Jul 1976, 95-97, 100.

13 **Scott Wright, M. and others** The nurse/graduate in nursing; preliminary findings of a follow-up study of former students of the University of Edinburgh Degree/nursing programme. Health Bulletin, 35 (6), Nov 1977, 317-323. See also 34 (4), Jul 1976, 188-189.

14 **Searle, C.** The academic in the nursing profession. S.A. Nursing Journal, 43 (1), Jan 1976, 15-17.

15 **Smith, R.A.** Nursing: a career for college graduates. Why college graduates choose nursing. (Survey at the University of Massachusetts.) Nursing Outlook, 24 (2), Feb 1976, 88-91.

16 **Tierney, A.J.** Present trends. (Symposium on the graduate nurse.) Nursing Mirror, 144, 10 Feb 1977, 49-50.

17 **Toman, J.** A course to pursue. (Report of the annual conference of the Association of Health Careers Advisers with discussion and summary of C. Armstrong-Esther's paper on degrees for nurses.) Nursing Times, 75, 26 Apr 1979, 694-695.

18 **University of Edinburgh** A symposium on the graduate nurse from the University of Edinburgh. Nursing Mirror, 144, 10 Feb 1977, 45-58.

19 **Williamson, L.** Future prospects. (Symposium on the graduate nurse.) Nursing Mirror, 144, 10 Feb 1977, 50-51.

i LICENSED PRACTICAL NURSES (US)

1 **Becker, B.G. and Fendler, D.T.** Vocational and personal adjustments in practical nursing. 3rd ed. St. Louis: Mosby, 1978.

2 **Journal of Practical Nursing** A page for your thoughts. (Questionnaire survey by journal of the work of licensed practical nurses.) Journal of Practical Nursing, 29 (12), Dec 1979, 13-17, 32-33.

3 **National Federation of Licensed Practical Nurses** Nursing practice standards for the licensed practical vocational nurse. Journal of Nursing Care, 12 (12), Dec 1979, 21-22.

4 **Sandiford, J.** Practical nursing: the future is in your hands. (Current situation of this section of the profession.) Journal of Practical Nursing, 29 (1), Jan 1979, 14-17.

5 **Sandiford, J.** Practical nursing: where are we headed? (Its future in the light of attempts in Ohio and New York to phase out practical nurse programmes.) Journal of Practical Nursing, 28 (2), Feb 1978, 36-39.

j MALE NURSES

1 **Bergman, R.** Sex discrimination in nursing in Israel; male or female lib? (Effect of male

nurses on the profession.) Journal of Advanced Nursing, 2 (5), Sep 1977, 533-541.

2 Bush, P.J. The male nurse: a challenge to traditional role identities. Nursing Forum, 15 (4), 1976, 390-405.

3 Butler, J. Mr Nightingale? (Differences in proportion of male nurses in hospital and district nursing who are charge nurse II grade, with request for information on male district nurse's work.) Nursing Times, 76, 10 Jan 1980, Community outlook, 9.

4 Carlini, A. Men in nursing are struggling with a particular set of problems. (By a male nurse.) Australasian Nurses Journal, 6 (10), May 1977, 6-7, 9.

5 Ellis, S. Nursing—a question of sex. (Report of author's survey into attitudes to male nurses.) Nursing Times, 74, 9 Nov 1978, 1830-1831.

6 Greene, J. Fighting for men's lib. (History of Chief Male Nurses' Association.) Nursing Mirror, 151, 13 Nov 1980, 18.

7 Gumley, C.J.G. and others Personality correlates in a sample of male nurses in the British Royal Air Force. Journal of Advanced Nursing, 4 (4), Jul 1979, 355-364.

8 Hass, S. The role of the man in nursing. Australian Nurses Journal, 7 (1), Jul 1977, 52-53, 80.

9 JANFORUM. The male/female dichotomy in the nursing profession in a time of social change: more male nurses, but increasing numbers of female patients—an international perspective. (Comments by nurses from seven countries.) Journal of Advanced Nursing, 3 (1), Jan 1978, 65-72.

10 Jones, E.M. The vanishing male nurse. (Study of key personnel in nurse education, general education and the careers advisory service to discover their attitudes towards men in nursing and the kind of careers advice available to boys.) Nursing Mirror, 149, 23 Aug 1979, 28-29.

11 Joyson, Graham Royal Melbourne Hospital. First male director of nursing. Australasian Nursing Journal, 5 (1), Jul 1976, 25.

12 Lyons, H.A. Sex discrimination in health authorities—does it exist? (Based on a research study.) Health and Social Service Journal, 86, 7 Feb 1976, 250-251.

13 Nelson, J. Men only. (Influence and effect of male nurse managers.) Nursing Mirror, 145, 28 Jul 1977, 27.

14 Nelson, J. Personal viewpoint. Male domination ahead? Nursing Mirror, 142 (16), 15 Apr 1976, 69.

15 NURSE Fred. (Research in New York into female nurses' reactions to male colleagues. Reported in the Journal of Health and Social Behaviour, 17 (2), 98.) New Society, 38, 11 Nov 1976, 312.

16 Nursing Mirror Does nursing need more men? (Views of fourteen nurses.) Nursing Mirror, 147, 14 Dec 1978, 16-17.

17 Nursing Times The best person for the job. (Relative position of male nurses since reorganisation.) Nursing Times, 72, 15 Jan 1976, 39.

18 Nursing Times Embarrassment of male nurses. (Problems in female psychogeriatric wards at Warlingham Park Hospital.) Nursing Times, 76, 27 Mar 1980, 533. Males nursing females. (Two letters on lack of problems.) 24 Jul 1980, 1304.

19 Pomfret, I. Men under the microscope—a worm's eye view. (Value of male nurses, by a male district nurse.) Journal of Community Nursing, 2 (3), Sep 1978, 18.

20 Schoemaker, A. and others Men nursing students: how they perceive their situation... Conflict between expectations and reality. Reports of two independent university studies. Nursing Outlook, 24 (5), May 1976, 298-305.

21 Sharpe, D. Male nurses on female psychiatric wards. (Problems experienced.) Nursing Times, 75, 11 Oct 1979, 1773-1774.

22 Vousden, M. An age of intimate concern. (Potential problems in elderly ladies' attitudes to male nurses.) Nursing Mirror, 151, 17 Jul 1980, 12.

k OVERSEAS NURSES IN BRITAIN

1 Akinsanya, J.A. Qualified Nigerian nurses in Britain. Nigerian Nurse, 7 (3), Jul-Sep 1975, 40-42.

2 Bristow, S. UKCOSA's annual meeting and conference. The new schemes to improve our treatment of overseas students. Nursing Mirror, 143, 12 Aug 1976, 39-40.

3 Bristow, S. The work of UKCOSA. Nursing Times, 72, 26 Aug 1976, 1314-1315.

4 CHANNEL-ling help to foreign students. Nursing Times, 72, 19 Feb 1976, 243.

5 Clarke, M. and Lee, T.R. The impressions of a sample of British and overseas student nurses of some social aspects of their training. (A study to investigate the extent of friendship between British and overseas nurses.) Journal of Advanced Nursing, 1 (1), Jan 1976, 37-49.

6 Department of Health and Social Security. Statistics and Research Division Overseas born student and pupil nurses and pupil midwives in training in National Health Service hospitals in England and Wales, 31 Dec 1976. DHSS, 1978.

7 Edwards, P.J. Listening comprehension test for nurses. (Language test designed to predict what an overseas student's performance will be in the hospital situation and to indicate the need for further help.) International Nursing Review, 23 (3), May/Jun 1976, 88-91.

8 Edwards, P. Problems of communication facing overseas nurses. (In training in England and Wales. Research study involving interviews, questionnaire survey and participant observation.) Nursing Times, 74, 30 Nov 1978, Occ. papers, 133-136.

9 Journal of Nursing Education Four articles on problems foreign nurses face on going to USA and taking courses there. Journal of Nursing Education, 19 (1), Jan 1980, 4-32.

10 Lee, H. Overseas nursing trainees. Research study into the problems of pre-registration overseas student and pupil nurses in the UK. 5 parts. Nursing Mirror, 143, 21 Oct 1976, 71-72; 28 Oct 1976, 69-70; 4 Nov 1976, 68-70; 11 Nov 1976, 67-68; 18 Nov 1976, 69-70.

11 Mair, J. Finding a friendly face. (Work of CHANNEL, Centre of Help and Advice for Newcomers to Nursing Education and Life in the U.K.) Nursing Standards No.85, 22 Mar 1979, 6.

12 Morris, P. When getting the best means having to move into Europe... (Recent recruitment of five German student nurses by Brent and Harrow School of Nursing.) Nursing Mirror, 149, 23 Aug 1979, 7.

13 Parkinson, J. English for doctors and nurses. Evans, 1978.

14 PLIGHT of immigrant nurses. (Effects of NHS cuts.) Nursing Mirror, 143, 12 Aug 1976, 33.

15 Raven, K. 'Trust the Allied Medical Group.' (Views of the Allied Medical Group on the controversial plan to train Iranian nurses in Britain.) Nursing Times, 72 (50), 16 Dec 1976, 1946.

16 Thompson, S. Overseas nurses deserve better protection. (Problems faced by overseas nurses working in Britain and the steps being taken to help them.) New Psychiatry, 1 (1), 19 Sep 1974, 22-23.

17 Royal College of Nursing Passport and employment guidelines when assisting overseas nurse learners (basic and post-basic) and nurses trained overseas. Rcn, 1977.

18 Schenk, K. Nursing abroad in an undergraduate programme. (One-term course for American nursing students at Harlaxton Manor in Lincolnshire.) International Nursing Review, 27 (4), Jul/Aug 1980, 108-111.

19 Shanley, E. Overseas nurses—effective therapeutic agents? (Problems faced by immigrant nurses which inhibit their effectiveness as psychiatric nurses.) Journal of Advanced Nursing, 5 (5), Sep 1980, 539-543.

20 STRANGERS in no-man's land. (CHANNEL, a counselling and problem-solving service for overseas nurses.) Nursing Times, 74, 27 Jul 1978, 1234-1237.

21 Sulco, C.D. An American nurse at The London Hospital. Nursing Outlook, 24 (8), Aug 1976, 504-508.

22 United Kingdom Council for Overseas Student Affairs UKCOSA Weekend Workshop for Nursing Personnel. Call to quantify problems of immigration and employment. Nursing Mirror, 143, 11 Nov 1976, 36.

23 United Kingdom Council for Overseas Student Affairs and Royal College of Nursing of the United Kingdom Nurses in training from overseas guidance leaflets. DHSS, 1976.

24 Walsh, S. Meet the British. (Work of CHANNEL—an organisation for overseas nurses.) Nursing Times, 72, 15 Jan 1976, 46-47.

25 Walsh, S. Overseas nurses: training for a caring profession. A study identifying the needs of, resources available to, and the employment expectations of overseas nurses whilst training in the N.H.S. CHANNEL, 1979.

l STATE ENROLLED NURSES

1 Bodington, M. Why the SEN must be the patient's friend. (The role of the SEN in the

residential care of the physically handicapped.) Nursing Mirror, 147, 23 Nov 1978, 40-42.

2 **Bristow, S.** Career opportunities. Enrolled nurses. Nursing Times, 72, 10 Jun 1976, 896-897.

3 **Carr, A.J.** The state enrolled nurse in the community. (Summary of recent report of the Working Party on the Education and Training in District Nursing for the State Enrolled Nurse.) Journal of Community Nursing, 3 (12), Jun 1980, 14-15.

4 **Ellerton, E.** Her future's assured! (SEN describes her observations of different districts' use of SENs in the community based on visits done through scholarship award.) Journal of Community Nursing, 3 (12), Jun 1980, 26, 28.

5 **Hardie, M. and Macmillan, M.** The nurse-in-the-middle. (The position of the SEN with reference to authors' research on nursing auxiliaries.) Nursing Times, 76, 17 Apr 1980, 678-680.

6 **Isaacs, B.** Rubbish! SENs are not second class. Nursing Mirror, 149, 18 Oct 1979, 14.

7 **Jefferies, P.M.** The role of the state enrolled nurse. (Summary of research study by working group in the King's Health District.) Nursing Times, 76, 17 Apr 1980, 681-683.

8 **Lightowlers, J.** Will SEN training be on the right tack? (Working party investigating SEN training for work in the community.) Journal of Community Nursing, 1 (9), Mar 1978, 16.

9 **Lloyd, P.V.** SENs future in industry assured. (Letter from Rcn's nurse advisor.) Occupational Health, 32 (7), Jul 1980, 375.

10 **Nursing Times** The search for racial equality. (Suggests that overseas SENs' feeling that they are treated unfairly may have some foundation.) Nursing Mirror, 151, 28 Aug 1980, 12.

11 **Royal College of Nursing. Professional Nursing Department** Post-basic training opportunities for state enrolled nurses. Rcn, 1976.

12 **Royal College of Nursing Working Party**...on the Senior State Enrolled Nurse in the Community. Report. Rcn, 1978.

13 **Wyley, B.** The Ad Hoc report...and after. (Committee to examine the role, preparation and career structure of the enrolled nurse in the New Zealand health service.) New Zealand Nursing Journal, 71 (9), Sep 1978, 15-16.

10 MANAGEMENT

a GENERAL

1 **Adebo, E.O.** The administrative functions of professional nurses in nursing services. Nigerian Nurse, 9 (3), Jul/Sep 1977, 21-28.

2 **Akiwumi, A.** Administrative controls in hospital nursing service. (The systems approach.) International Nursing Review, 24 (6), Nov/Dec 1977, 176-181.

3 **Alexander, E.L.** Nursing administration in the hospital health care system. 2nd ed. St. Louis: Mosby, 1978.

4 **Andrews, M. and others** A nursing management model. (Dual posts of patient care specialist and nurse manager at head nurse level.) Supervisor Nurse, 10 (12), Dec 1979, 28-30.

5 **Association of Nurse Administrators** 'All pull together' Dyson advises professional nursing organisations. (Report of Autumn conference.) Nursing Mirror, 143 (17), 21 Oct 1976, 35.

6 **Association of Nurse Administrators** Annual conference report. Put nursing back into administration. Nursing Mirror, 142, 8 Apr 1976, 36.

7 **Auld, M.** Effective management through partnership. Objective thinking at the top. (Nursing Mirror Forum 1976.) Nursing Mirror, 142 (15), 8 Apr 1976, 49-51.

8 **Brown, B.** Clinical nursing: a basis for administrative excellence. (Clinical components of nurse manager's role with report of group discussion on p.26-28). Nursing Administration Quarterly, 3 (4), Summer 1979, 19-28.

9 **Carpenter, Michael** The new managerialism and professionalism in nursing. Contained in Stacey, Margaret, editor Health and the division of labour. Croom Helm, 1977, 165-193.

10 **Carr, A.** Management: a word of many meanings... (Need to revalue nursing management.) Nursing Mirror, 149, 6 Sep 1979, 30-31.

11 **Carr, A.J.** Nursing administration—looking to the future. Nursing Focus, 1 (1), Sep 1979, 9-11.

12 **Carr, A.** Nursing is a two-sided coin. (Suggested new management structure with separation of clinical and management sides.) Nursing Mirror, 151, 21 Aug 1980, 12.

13 **Chaska, N.L.** Nursing: many issues raised, many unresolved, many neglected. (Review of 1978 literature, with special reference to nursing management.) Hospitals, 53 (7), 1 Apr 1979, 158-162.

14 **Clark, C.C. and Shea, C.A.** Management in nursing: a vital link in the health care system. New York: McGraw-Hill, 1979.

15 **Clark, J.** Authority patterns in nursing management structures. Nursing Times, 73, 12 May 1977, Occ. papers, 65-68.

16 **Cristman, L.** Nursing care administration. Nurses seek to influence care. (1975 literature review.) Hospitals, 50 (7), 1 Apr 1976, 97-98, 100.

17 **Department of Health and Social Security** Management services and the nurse: papers given at or prepared after a seminar held at the NHS Training and Studies Centre, Harrogate, 27-28 Sept 1979. Hebburn: DHSS Central Management Services, 1980.

18 **Field, E.R.** Authority: a select power. Advances in Nursing Science, 3 (1), Oct 1980, 69-83.

19 **Flint, J.W.** The nursing systems analyst: are you ready for her? (To analyse, design and improve nursing work systems and methods.) Supervisor Nurse, 11 (1), Jan 1980, 55-56.

20 **Frey, M.** Planning for nursing service. Hospital Progress, 57 (10), Oct 1976, 78, 80-81.

21 **Gagneaux, V. and Shaver, D.V.** Distrac-

tions at nurses' stations during intershift report. Nursing Research, 26 (1), Jan-Feb 1977, 42-46.

22 **Ganong, W. and Ganong, J.** Strengthening the nursing service organization. (Situational analysis, including objective and subjective feedback from personnel performance indicators and unit profiles.) Journal of Nursing Administration, 7 (7), Sep 1977, 14-15, 52.

23 **Germaine, A.** Developing a nursing service department. Hospital Administration in Canada, 17 (11) & (12), Nov/Dec 1975, 46, 48.

24 **Gugenheim, A.M.** Health care leaders examine role of nursing service administrator. (American Hospital Association conference.) Hospitals, 53 (2), 16 Jan 1979, 109-111.

25 **Harris, C. and Morgan, M.** Unit management: preparing to share new common ground. (Within the restructured NHS. Two articles.) Health and Social Service Journal, 90, 14 Nov 1980, 1474-1476.

26 **Kerrane, T.A.** The nurse philosophers. (A comparison of organisation, the motivation attitudes of American and British nurse administrators.) Nursing Mirror, 143, 8 Jul 1976, 51-53.

27 **Kimbro, C.D. and Gifford, A.J.** The nursing staff organization: a needed development. Nursing Outlook, 28 (10), Oct 1980, 610-616.

28 **LaViolette, S.** Hospital pressures trigger increased democracy in nursing departments. (Decentralisation of authority.) Modern Healthcare, 9 (5), May 1979, 62-63.

29 **Lloyd, T.** Now let's use Speakman! (Comment on top posts review.) Nursing Mirror, 149, 16 Aug 1979, 10.

30 **McClure, M.L.** The administrative component of the nurse administrator's role. (Conference paper with report of group discussion on p.13-17.) Nursing Administration Quarterly, 3 (4), Summer 1979, 1-17.

31 **Marriner, A.** Development of management thought. (History of management theories with some discussion of their implications for nurse managers.) Journal of Nursing Administration, 9 (9), Sep 1979, 21-31.

32 **Moffett, M.** Structures can strangle. (Conference paper on the organizational structure of nursing departments.) Australian Nurses' Journal, 5 (6) & (7), Dec/Jan 1976, 25-27.

33 **Nelson, E.G. and Blenkinsop, D.** Managing the system: a theoretical and practical review of a case of managerial development in a hospital nursing service. Northern Regional Health Authority, 1976.

34 **Nursing Clinics of North America** Symposium on nursing administration and supervision. Nursing Clinics of North America, 13 (1), Mar 1978, 85-153.

35 **O'Donovan, T.R.** The department head and health care delivery. (The unique role of the middle manager.) Journal of Nursing Administration, 6 (1), Jan 1976, 32-36.

36 **Oribabor, P.E.** The organisation of work and occupational strategies of hospital nurses. PhD thesis, Keele University, 1979.

37 **Pati, B.** Nursing consultation: a collabor-

ative process. Journal of Nursing Administration, 10 (11), Nov 1980, 33-37.

38 Phillips, M.S. A nursing practice committee. Can enhance the management efficiency of a nursing department. (Clarke Institute of Psychiatry, Toronto.) Hospital Administration in Canada, 18 (6), Jun 1976, 76-78.

39 Porter-O'Grady, T. The organization of nursing services: a model for the future. (The matrix model.) Supervisor Nurse, 9 (7), Jul 1978, 30, 32-38.

40 Pyves, M.G. A study on the nurse staff officer's role. (Personal assistant to a district nursing officer.) Nursing Times, 74, 23 Nov 1978, Occ. papers, 129-132.

41 Raybould, E., editor A guide for nurse managers. Blackwell, 1977.

42 Ross, M. Accountability for nursing care —towards a new structure. (With unit sister responsible for clinical leadership, teaching and management within unit.) Nursing Times, 75, 30 Aug 1979, 1478-1480.

43 Rotkovitch, R. The heartbeat of nursing services: Standard 4. (Comments on American Nurses Association Standard 4. 'The nursing care program is integrated into the total program of the health care organization.) Journal of Nursing Administration, 6 (4), May 1976, 32-35.

44 Shaw, M. and Heyman, B. Constructs of relationships and issues of authority in nursing. Journal of Advanced Nursing, 5 (2), Mar 1980, 187-198.

45 Shiflett, N. and McFarland, D.E. Power and the nursing administrator. (Personality aspects, organizational context and professional values.) Journal of Nursing Administration, 8 (3), Mar 1978, 19-23.

46 Slack, P. Portrait of a team. (Visit to Birmingham South's DNO and nursing management team.) Nursing Times, 76, 13 Mar 1980, 473-477.

47 Smith, J. Rumbling it—then tumbling it. (Suggests change of structure for the organisation of nursing care and nursing administration.) Nursing Times, 74, 9 Mar 1978, 390.

48 Stevens, B.J. The nurse as executive. 2nd ed. Wakefield, Mass: Nursing Resources, 1980.

49 Watkin, A. The nurse manager in 1979. (Role in providing high standards and caring environment.) Nursing Mirror, 148, 17 May 1979, 19-22.

50 Watkin, B. The job of the nurse manager. (Comments on Rosemary White's article 'Management of the Nursing Service' in Nursing Mirror, October 28.) Nursing Mirror, 143, 16 Dec 1976, 42.

51 Watt, E. Lengthy look at way forward for nursing. (Review of findings of Wessex RHA's study of the management of nursing units.) Health and Social Service Journal, 88, 10 Feb 1978, 160-162.

52 Wessex Regional Health Authority The management of 120-bed clinical nursing units: an account of research carried out in the five years 1970-1974. Parts 1 and 2. Winchester: Wessex RHA, 1977.

53 White, R. Management of the nursing

service. (A personal comment.) Nursing Mirror, 143, 28 Oct 1976, 67-68.

54 Wilkinson, J. The nurse administrator's role in the 1980s. (With some reference to Australia.) Australian Nurses Journal, 9 (9), Apr 1980, 32-36.

b TECHNIQUES AND TEXTBOOKS

1 Alexander, E.L. Nursing administration in the hospital health care system. 2nd ed. St. Louis: Mosby, 1978.

2 Arndt, C. and Huckabay, L.M.D. Nursing administration: theory for practice with a systems approach. St. Louis: Mosby, 1975. 2nd ed. 1980.

3 Bailey, J.T. and Claus, K.E. Decision making in nursing: tools for change. St. Louis: Mosby, 1975.

4 Beardon, A. Who wants to be a manager? (With description of how a good manager works.) Nursing Times, 76, 3 Jul 1980, 1161-1162.

5 Bell, M.L. Management by objectives. (With examples of its use in staff evaluation and patient care planning.) Journal of Nursing Administration, 10 (5), May 1980, 19-26.

6 Berger, M.S. and others, editors Management for nurses: a multidisciplinary approach. 2nd ed. St. Louis: Mosby, 1980.

7 Beyers, M. and Phillips, C. Nursing management for patient care. 2nd ed. Boston: Little, Brown, 1979.

8 Bollock, M.J. Nursing management. Strategies. Hospital Topics, 57 (5), Sep/Oct 1979, 21-23.

9 Bopp, W.J. and Rosenthal, W.P. Participatory management. (In nursing at University of Miami/Jackson Memorial Medical Center.) American Journal of Nursing, 79 (4), Apr 1979, 671-672.

10 Brunner, N.A. Communications in nursing service administration. Journal of Nursing Administration, 7 (8), Oct 1977, 29-32.

11 Calboun, G. and Perrin, M. Management, motivation and conflict. Topics in Clinical Nursing, 1 (3), Oct 1979, 71-80.

12 Carr, A. Cost-effective nursing. (Ways of keeping costs of nursing care down.) Nursing Times, 74, 1 Jun 1978, 906-907.

13 Cassell, R. and Shilling, M. Study projects nursing staff needs, budget. Hospitals, 53 (14), 16 Jul 1979, 108, 114, 118, 122.

14 Clark, C.C. and Shea, C.A. Management in nursing: a vital link in the health care system. New York: McGraw-Hill, 1979.

15 Clode, D. Of fleas and smaller fleas... (Schemes that make monitoring as management tool a constructive exercise.) Health and Social Service Journal, 89, 25 May 1979, 628-631.'

16 Conway, R. Points system helps financial control plus job satisfaction. An efficient and rewarding system of staff budgeting for nurse managers. Health and Social Service Journal, 87, 8 Jul 1977, 1014-1015.

17 Davies, T. Beating out pathways towards better nurse management. (System of participative management in Nottingham health district.) Health and Social Service Journal, 88, 18 Aug 1978, 933-934.

18 Diekelmann, N.L. and Broadwell, M.M. How to get the job done by someone else. (Management skills.) Nursing, 7 (9), Sep 1977, 13-16.

19 Divincenti, M. Administering nursing service. 2nd ed. Boston: Little, Brown and Co., 1977.

20 Dixon, N. Choice errors—some hazards of decision-making. Nursing Mirror, 144, 17 Feb 1977, 59-61.

21 Donovan, H.M. Nursing service administration: managing the enterprise. St. Louis: Mosby, 1975.

22 Douglass, L.M. The effective nurse: leader and manager. St. Louis: Mosby, 1980.

23 Douglass, L.M. and Bevis, E.O. Nursing management and leadership in action. 3rd ed. St. Louis: Mosby, 1979.

24 Edelstein, R.R.G. Self-management in American nursing. (Employee participation in decision-making.) International Nursing Review, 26 (3), May/Jun 1979, 78-83.

25 Elliott, M.K. and Fisher, R.H. Management audit—the Exeter method. (Separation from staff appraisal system and use as educational aid for nurses.) Nursing Times, 75, 16 Aug 1979, Occ. papers, 89-92.

26 Flook, J. Creating a system with high degree of sensitivity. (Standard costing system for the nursing service to produce more efficient use of nursing manpower resources.) Health and Social Service Journal, 87, 9 Dec 1977, 1678.

27 Flook, J. A standard costing system for nursing services. Nursing Times, 74, 30 Mar 1978, 547-548.

28 Ford, J.A.G. and others Applied decision making for nurses. St. Louis: Mosby, 1979.

29 Franck, P. and Price, M. Nursing management: a programmed text. 2nd ed. New York: Springer, 1980. (Programmed text)

30 Fritz, R. How do you rate as a nursing manager? (Nursing management skills profile.) Nursing (U.S.), 10 (12), Dec 1980, 17-21.

31 Fuller, M.E. The budget. (Comments on American Nurses Association Standard 5. 'Nursing administration determines the budget necessary to carry out the nursing care program and administers the approved budget.) Journal of Nursing Administration, 6 (4), May 1976, 36-38.

32 Ganong, J.M. and Ganong, W.L. Nursing management. 2nd ed. Rockville, Md.: Aspec, 1980.

33 Greiner, D. and Mason, J.T. Secrets in administrative systems. (Communication between nurse managers and staff nurses.) Topics in Clinical Nursing, 1 (3), Oct 1979, 81-88.

34 Harper, R.W. and Rhodes, M.A. Development and application of flow-charting techniques in nursing practice. Journal of Nursing Administration, 7 (5), May/Jun 1977, 11-19.

35 **Hela, N.** Management audit. S.A. Nursing Journal, 43 (3), Mar 1976, 14-15, 13.

36 **Herrod, C.D.** Participation—a style of management. (Project sponsored by DHSS at St. Mary's Hospital, Burghill, Herefordshire.) Nursing Times, 74, 16 Mar 1978, 466-468.

37 **Hill, B.S.** Participative management: a valid alternative to traditional organizational behavior. Supervisor Nurse, 7 (3), Mar 1976, 19-21.

38 **Huczynski, A.** Nursing management audit: the reaction of users. (Evaluation research project into Doncaster scheme.) Journal of Advanced Nursing, 2 (5), Sep 1977, 521-531.

39 **Huczynski, A.A.** Practical issues in the implementation of nursing management audit. (Doncaster Nursing Management Audit.) Nursing Times, 76, 7 Feb 1980, Occ. papers, 13-16.

40 **Hunt, J.M.** A comparative study to determine the most effective method of communicating nursing instructions: final report. The author, 1979.

41 **Journal of Nursing Administration** The techniques of nursing management: a reader. Wakefield, Mass.: Contemporary Publishing, 1975.

42 **Karch, A.M.** Concurrent nursing audit. Thorofare, N.J.: Charles B. Slack, 1980.

43 **Kepler, T.L.** Mastering the people skills. (In nursing management.) Journal of Nursing Administration, 10 (11), Nov 1980, 15-20.

44 **King's Fund Centre** The Doncaster system of audits for the nursing service. The Centre, 1977. (King's Fund project paper.)

45 **La Monica, E. and Finch, F.E.** Managerial decision making. (The Vroom and Yetton managerial decision-making model.) Journal of Nursing Administration, 7 (5), May/Jun 1977, 20-28.

46 **Lemin, B.** First line nursing management. Pitman, 1977.

47 **Lewis, J.H.** Conflict management. (Procedures for stimulating constructive conflict.) Journal of Nursing Administration, 6 (10), Dec 1976, 18-22.

48 **McWilliams, C.A.** Systems analysis can solve nursing management problems. Supervisor Nurse, 11 (5), May 1980, 17-20, 22-26.

49 **Marcus, J. and Marcus, R.** 'Nursing' the organization. (Use of nurse consultant to aid problem-solving in nursing administration.) Supervisor Nurse, 8 (10), Oct 1977, 8, 10, 12.

50 **Marriner, A.** Budgets. An introductory overview of budgeting and the types of budgets. Supervisor Nurse, 8 (4), Apr 1977, 53-56.

51 **Marriner, A.** Conflict resolution. Supervisor Nurse, 10 (5), May 1979, 46, 49, 52-54.

52 **Marriner, A. editor** Current perspectives in nursing management. St. Louis: Mosby, 1979. (Mosby's current practice and perspectives in nursing series; 1).

53 **Marriner, A.** Guide to nursing management. St. Louis: Mosby, 1980.

54 **Marriner, A.** Organizational concepts— Part 1. Charts, span of control and flat vs tall structures. Supervisor Nurse, 8 (9), Sep 1977, 40-44.

55 **Marriner, A.** Time management. (Ways in which the nurse manager can maximise her time.) Journal of Nursing Administration, 9 (10), Oct 1979, 16-18.

56 **Miller, P.W.** Open minds to new ideas: an injunction for nursing leaders. (Participative management.) Supervisor Nurse, 7 (4), Apr 1976, 18-22.

57 **Moores, B.** Making use of the tools which are available. (Use of statistics in nursing and health service management.) Health and Social Service Journal, 90, 2 May 1980, 578-582.

58 **Moores, Y.** When it comes to the crunch. (Decision-making by management teams with reference to ANO's role.) Nursing Mirror, 149, 20 Sep 1979, 35-36.

59 **Mrazek, M.** Nursing information system. (Used at Misericordia Hospital, Edmonton to monitor the nursing management model.) Dimensions in Health Service, 56 (11), Nov 1979, 12-14.

60 **Myrtle, R.C. and Glogow, E.** How nursing administrators view conflict. Nursing Research, 27 (2), Mar/Apr 1978, 103-106.

61 **National League for Nursing** Conflict management: flight, fight, negotiate? New York: NLN, 1977.

62 **National League for Nursing** Management perspectives. New York: NLN, 1979.

63 **Nicholls, B.** Dealing with conflict. Journal of Continuing Education in Nursing, 10 (6), Nov/Dec 1979, 24-27.

64 **Nursing Administration Quarterly** Issue on cost effectiveness for nursing. (Eight articles.) Nursing Administration Quarterly, 3 (1), Fall 1978, 1-87.

65 **Nursing Unit Administration (Canada)** (Nursing unit administration program textbook.) Ottawa: the Author, 1980.

66 **Pellet, J.** Are you making delegation work for you? (A discussion of delegation as a management tool.) AORN Journal, 25 (5), Apr 1977, 865-868.

67 **Porter-O'Grady, T.** Financial planning: budgeting for nursing. Supervisor Nurse, 10 (8), Aug 1979, 35-38; (9), Sep 1979, 25-30.

68 **Quinn, S.** What is a co-ordinator? (Discussion of concept in relation to teams and consensus management.) Nursing Times, 76, 19 Jun 1980, 1079.

69 **Rowland, H.S. and Rowland B.** Nursing administration handbook. Germantown, Md.: Aspen, 1980.

70 **Schmied, E.** Allocation of resources: preparation of the nursing department budget. Journal of Nursing Administration, 7 (7), Sep 1977, 31-36.

71 **Schmied, E. editor** Maintaining cost effectiveness. Wakefield, Mass.: Nursing Resources, 1979. (Management anthology series, 3.)

72 **Schweiger, J.L.** The nurse as manager. New York: Wiley, 1980.

73 **Sheehy, E.** Functional budgeting: and the nurse manager. (Description of system in Enfield district.) Nursing Times, 74, 20 Apr 1978, 683.

74 **Smith, J.P.** Nursing management audit. (Report of a King's Fund Centre conference.) Nursing Mirror, 146, 26 Jan 1978, 9.

75 **South Glamorgan Area Health Authority (Teaching)** Nursing audit. Cardiff: the AHA, 1976.

76 **Stevens, B.J.** The nurse as executive. Wakefield, Mass.: Contemporary Publishing, 1975. 2nd Ed. 1980.

77 **Stevens, W.F.** Management and leadership in nursing. New York: McGraw-Hill, 1978.

78 **Stone, S. and others, editors** Management for nurses: a multidisciplinary approach. St. Louis: Mosby, 1976.

79 **Swansburg, Russell C.** Management of patient care services. St. Louis: Mosby, 1976.

80 **Swansburg, R.C.** The nursing budget. Supervisor Nurse, 9 (6), Jun 1978, 40-42, 44-47.

81 **Taylor, A.G.** Decision making in nursing: an analytical approach. Journal of Nursing Administration, 8 (11), Nov 1978, 22-30; (12), Dec 1978, 39-42.

82 **Volk-Tebbitt, B.** Time: who controls yours? (Advice for nurse managers on efficient use of time.) Supervisor Nurse, 9 (4), Apr 1978, 17-19, 21-22.

83 **Wiley, L.** The ABCs of time management. (Planning work on basis of allotting time to priority tasks first, with reference to a nurse's afternoon.) Nursing, 8 (9), Sep 1978, 6-8.

84 **Wilkinson, R.** Effective meetings: get ready for a get together. Nursing Mirror, 150, 14 Feb 1980, 40.

85 **Wilkinson, R.** How to win a paper war. (Advice to managers on delegating and improving efficiency.) Nursing Mirror, 150, 7 Feb 1980, 32.

86 **Zegeer, L.J.** Calculating a nurse staffing budget for a 20 bed unit at 100% occupancy. Journal of Nursing Administration, 7 (2), Feb 1977, 11-14.

c COMPUTERS AND AUTOMATION

1 **Barber, B. and Scholes, M.** Learning to live with computers. (In nursing and other parts of the health service.) Nursing Mirror, 149, 5 Jul 1979, 22-24.

2 **Birckhead, L.M.** The need for nurses support systems in affecting computer systems. Journal of Nursing Administration, Mar 1978, 51-53.

3 **Brown, R.L.** Computerised nursing. Nursing Mirror, 142, 12 Feb 1976, 56.

4 **Farlee, C.** The computer as a focus of organisational change in the hospital. (The potential impact of automated systems on nursing and hospital administration.) Journal of Nursing Administration, 8 (2), Feb 1978, 20-26.

5 **Hannah, K.J.** The computer and nursing practice. Nursing Outlook, 24 (9), Sep 1976, 555-558.

6 **Hannah, K.J.** Computers and nursing. Hospital Administration in Canada, 20 (5), May 1978, 20-23.

7 **Henney, C.R.** The nurse and the computer. (Ward computer project at Ninewells Hospital, Dundee, involving computer-generated nursing care plans based on ward patient file.) Nursing Mirror, 145, 17 Nov 1977, 13-14.

8 **Hughes, S.J.** Installing a computer-based patient information system. Journal of Nursing Administration, 10 (5), May 1980, 7-10.

9 **Journal of Nursing Administration** Two articles on how computers work. Journal of Nursing Administration, 8 (2), Feb 1978, 4-15.

10 **McNeill, D.G.** Developing the complete computer-based information system. (Problem-oriented medical information system for planning and reviewing patient care.) Journal of Nursing Administration, 9 (11), Nov 1979, 34-46.

11 **Monaco, R.J. and Smith, T.T.** How supervisors can put systems to work in day to day management. (Use of computer in nursing and hospital administration.) Hospital Topics, 55 (5), Sep/Oct 1977, 34, 36-41.

12 **Parsons, R.** The future of the nursing profession: computer technology and clinical nursing practice. Lamp, 33 (6), Jun 1976, 24, 34; S.A. Nursing Journal, 43 (10), Oct 1976, 9-11; (11), Nov 1976, 17-19, 21, 12.

13 **Pocklington, D.B. and Guttman, L.** Computer technology in nursing: a comprehensive bibliography. Hyattsville, Md.: United States Department of Health and Human Services, 1980. (Nurse planning information series; 16.)

14 **Scholes, M.** An overview of the use of computers in nursing. Royal Society of Health Journal, 99 (1), Feb 1979, 8-9.

15 **Scholes, M. and Barber, B.** The role of computers in nursing. Nursing Mirror, 143, 23 Sep 1976, 46-48.

16 **Zielstorff, R.D.** Automation in nursing: designing automated information systems. (Systems approach to problem-solving and decision making.) Journal of Nursing Administration, 7 (4), Apr 1977, 14-18.

17 **Zielstorff, R.D. editor** Computers in nursing. Wakefield, Mass.: Nursing Resources, 1980.

18 **Zielstorff, R.D.** Nurses can affect computer systems. (Through active participation in planning and developing.) Journal of Nursing Administration, 8 (3), Mar 1978, 49-51.

19 **Zielstorff, R.D.** Orienting personnel to automated systems. Journal of Nursing Administration, 6 (3), Mar/Apr 1976, 14-16.

d LEADERSHIP AND SUPERVISION

1 **Bailey, J.T. and Claus, K.E.** Preparing nurse leaders for the world of tomorrow. (Development of post-basic programme in leadership.) Nursing Leadership, 1 (1), Jun 1978, 19-28.

2 **Baker, W.G.** Changes in life goals as related to success in a nursing leadership role. (Study revealed major differences in life goals of successful nurses.) Nursing Research, 28 (4), Jul/Aug 1979, 234-236.

3 **Blenkinsop, D.** Challenge for the 21st century. (Leadership in nursing management.) Nursing Mirror, 149, 11 Oct 1979, 26-27.

4 **Bottitta Stagnitto, M.R.E.** Nursing supervision: leadership or police work? Supervisor Nurse, 10 (1), Jan 1979, 17-19.

5 **Bowman, M.** Leading qualities. (Leadership in nursing management and education.) Nursing Mirror, 150, 17 Apr 1980, 37-39.

6 **Brooten, D.A. and others** Leadership for change: a guide for the frustrated nurse. Philadelphia: Lippincott, 1978.

7 **Buzzell, M.** Nurse supervision: patient care or paper pushing? (Roles of nurse managers including the ward sister and the clinical nurse specialist.) Australian Nurses Journal, 7 (2), Aug 1977, 32-34.

8 **Calkin, J.D.** Using management literature to enhance new leadership roles. (How knowledge of leadership characteristics and other management concepts can help in selection of nurse managers.) Journal of Nursing Administration, 10 (4), Apr 1980, 24-30.

9 **Carr, A.J.** Nurse managers look for leaders. (Abridged version of paper given at Rcn Association of Nursing Management conference.) Nursing Standard, 93, 17 May 1979, 7.

10 **Claus, K.E. and Bailey, J.T.** Power and influence in health care: a new approach to leadership. St. Louis: Mosby, 1977.

11 **Colton, M.R.** Nursing's leadership vacuum. The anatomy of a changing profession as seen through examples of the defects of 'leaders' and suggestions for what qualifications nursing leaders must have in the future. Supervisor Nurse, 7 (10), Oct 1976, 29-30, 33, 37.

12 **Davis, L.A.** How do you follow up? (To ensure subordinates' effective work performance.) Journal of Nursing Administration, 10 (2), Feb 1980, 25-30.

13 **Douglass, L.M.** Review of leadership in nursing. 2nd ed. St. Louis: Mosby, 1977.

14 **Ellis, B.** Nurses told of need for more influence. American Society of Nursing Service Administrators seeks to develop leadership role in resolving current nursing and health care issues. Hospitals, 54 (3), 1 Feb 1980, 57-58.

15 **Feeley, E. and Tarr, J.** Alternative leadership experiences for senior students in an acute care setting. (Scheme to prepare students for team leading, with peers and with junior level students.) Journal of Nursing Education, 18 (2), Feb 1979, 25-28.

16 **Fine, R.B.** Application of leadership theory: integrating thought and action. Nursing Clinics of North America, 13 (1), Mar 1978, 139-153.

17 **Garnett, J.** What is leadership? Nursing Mirror, 143, 30 Sep 1976, 40-41.

18 **Heimann, C.G.** Four theories of leadership. (Style, trait, situation, now superseded by interaction theory which combines all three.) Journal of Nursing Administration, 6 (5), Jun 1976, 18-24.

19 **Hersey, P. and others** A look at your supervisory style. (Tools to measure leadership behavior.) Supervisor Nurse, 7 (6), Jun 1976, 27-31, 35-36, 38-40.

20 **Hersey, P. and others** A situational approach to supervision: leadership theory and the supervising nurse. Supervisor Nurse, 7 (5), May 1976, 17-20.

21 **Lambertsen, E.C.** Nursing team leadership. (Symposium paper.) S.A. Nursing Journal, 43 (9), Sep 1976, 33-38.

22 **McNally, J.M.** Leadership—the needed component. Nursing Leadership, 2 (3), Sep 1979, 6-12.

23 **McNally, J.M.** Loneliness and alone-ness in the administrator: an essay on distinctions. Supervisor Nurse, 9 (1), Jan 1978, 28-29.

24 **Marriner, A.** Theories of leadership. Nursing Leadership, 1 (3), Dec 1978, 13-17.

25 **Oermann, M.** Diagnostic supervision. (Staff development as part of ward sister's role.) Supervisor Nurse, 8 (11), Nov 1977, 9-11, 14.

26 **Ogundeyin, W.M.** The nature of nursing supervision. Nigerian Nurse, 10 (2), Apr/Jun 1978, 17-20.

27 **Placey, R.J.** The nursing supervisor—barrier or help? (Between the nursing administrator and the head nurse.) Supervisor Nurse, 7 (6), Jun 1976, 21-22, 25-26.

28 **Plaszczynski, L.** A systematic approach to leadership selection. Journal of Nursing Administration, 9 (3), Mar 1979, 6-15.

29 **Schuldt, S.** Supervision and the informal organization. (Network of personal and social relations within nursing department.) Journal of Nursing Administration, 8 (7), Jul 1978, 21-25.

30 **Shores, L.** Staff development for leadership. Nursing Clinics of North America, 13 (1), Mar 1978, 103-109.

31 **Spennrath, S.** Nurses need leadership skills. (Leadership development workshops for staff nurses.) Canadian Nurse, 75 (6), Jun 1979, 33-38.

32 **Stevens, B.J. editor** The delicate art of nursing supervision and leadership. Wakefield, Mass.: Contemporary Publishing, 1977. (Nursing Digest, vol.5, no.3.)

33 **Trainor, M.A.** A helping model for clinical supervision. The supervisor's relationship with the staff nurse parallels that of the nurse with the patient. Supervisor Nurse, 9 (1), Jan 1978, 30, 32-36.

34 **Wilson, J.S.** Leadership: a review of the literature and theoretical framework for nursing courses. Nursing Leadership, 3 (2), Jun 1980, 32-38.

35 **Yura, H. and others** Nursing leadership: theory and process. New York: Appleton-Century-Crofts, 1976.

36 **Zorn, J.M.** Nursing leadership for the 70s and 80s. (Ten leadership strategies for the nurse manager.) Journal of Nursing Administration, 7 (8), Oct 1977, 33-35.

e MANAGEMENT TRAINING

1 Bacon, L.F. Backing into a shake-up. (Development of middle management workshops for head nurses.) Supervisor Nurse, 8 (10), Oct 1977, 24-25.

2 Baldwin, B.A. and others Out of the desk and onto the stage: an experiment in assertive role playing. (For senior students on management courses.) Journal of Nursing Education, 18 (7), Sep 1979, 38-42.

3 Beardon, A. Whose job is staff care? (First line management courses in the NHS by a tutor, with an appreciation by some of his students.) Nursing Times, 74, 9 Feb 1978, 234-236.

4 Blair, E.M. Needed: nursing administration leaders. (Master's programme in nursing administration at the University of Colorado School of Nursing.) Nursing Outlook, 24 (9), Sep 1976, 550-554.

5 Blenkinsop, D. A study of the training and criteria of effectiveness of two grades of nurse managers. (Sister and nursing officer.) MPhil thesis, Durham University, 1978.

6 Blenkinsop, D. We must train nurses to manage. (Reasons for resistance to management training and ways of meeting management training needs for nurses, with reference to National Staff Committee for Nurses and Midwives scheme.) Nursing Mirror, 149, 23 Aug 1979, 30-32.

7 Brock, A.M. Impact of a management-oriented course on knowledge and leadership skills exhibited by baccalaureate nursing students. Nursing Research, 27 (4), Jul/Aug 1978, 217-221.

8 Browne, S.E. Group leadership experiences for students. Three models of exposure to group process were tried—co-leader, observer, and initiator—with subsequent evaluation by both instructor and students. Nursing Outlook, 28 (3), Mar 1980, 166-169.

9 Carruthers, L.J. and others The management training needs of senior nursing officers. (Survey in an Area Health Authority.) Nursing Times, 73, 17 Mar 1977, Occ. papers, 37-38.

10 Carter, K.A. Managerial role development in the nursing supervisor. Supervisor Nurse, 11 (7), Jul 1980, 26-28.

11 Chenevert, M. Special techniques in assertiveness training for women in the health professions. St. Louis: Mosby, 1978.

12 Cox, A. and others Time to look again at role-based training for nurse managers. (Investigation into needs of senior nursing officers and senior tutors in line management posts by group of senior nurse managers at South West Thames Regional Health Authority.) Nursing Times, 75, 13 Sep 1979, 1580-1585.

13 Dimarco, N. and Kuehl, C. Predictors of management. Training effectiveness for nursing supervisors. Journal of Continuing Education in Nursing, 7 (4), Jul/Aug 1976, 39-46.

14 Eckvahl, V.R. On the job management training. Journal of Nursing Administration, 6 (3), Mar/Apr 1976, 38-40.

15 Elliott, T.G. and others Communication: a program design. (Course to improve communication skills for all nurses including nurse managers.) Supervisor Nurse, 10 (2), Feb 1979, 12, 14-18.

16 Fagan, A. From Arica to Inuvik. (Nursing administration courses established in developing countries by grants from the Canadian International Development Agency.) Dimensions in Health Service, 54 (1), 1977, 8-10.

17 Frawley, A.M. Change for the better. (Changes in nurses' attitudes after first line management course.) Health and Social Service Journal, 86, 15 Oct 1976, 1858.

18 Frawley, A. Curing nurses' prejudice. (Attitudes of nurses and tutors to first line management training.) Health and Social Service Journal, 86, 1 Oct 1976, 1759.

19 Frawley, A.M. Management de-mystified. (Identification of training needs for management courses.) Health and Social Service Journal, 86, 8 Oct 1976, 1810.

20 Frawley, A.M. On the spot training. (Multidisciplinary first line management training in the Wessex Region.) Health and Social Service Journal, 86, 24 Sep 1976, 1710.

21 Gerschefske, L. Assessment and development for head nurse positions. Measuring managerial potential among head nurse candidates. (Through assessment exercises.) Supervisor Nurse, 11 (2), Feb 1980, 21-22, 24-25.

22 Gilliss, C.L. Teaching group skills to nurse managers. Journal of Continuing Education in Nursing, 10 (3), May/Jun 1979, 19-30.

23 Hardy, A.M. No one told me... (Need for better management courses for nurses with reference to author's attendance at a business course.) Nursing Times, 76, 4 Dec 1980, 2136-2137.

24 Hunt, C.D. A course for sisters and charge nurses. (In St. Thomas' Health District.) Nursing Times, 76, 4 Dec 1980, 2145-2146.

25 Hyde, P. First-line management training: the setting up of a programme within Warwickshire AHA. Nursing Times, 75, 12 Jul 1979, 1194-1195.

26 Kennedy, R. and Vose, A.B. Preparing the nurse manager to assume new accountabilities. (Programme of staff development for nurse managers.) Hospitals, 52, 1 Jan 1978, 66-69.

27 Lees, S. Developing effective institutional managers in the 1980s. 1. A current analysis. 2. Some new directions. Journal of Advanced Nursing, 5 (2), Mar 1980, 209-220; (3), May 1980, 329-339.

28 Lindeman, B.Z. and Bone, L.I. Getting a degree. A degree in management for the working nurse. Supervisor Nurse, 7 (9), Sep 1976, 49-51.

29 Macmillan, P. Case studies for nursing management courses. Pitman, 1975.

30 Maisey, P. Beyond the sausage machine. (Training and selection of top nursing managers.) Health and Social Service Journal, 87, 22 Jul 1977, 1082.

31 Neuman, M.M. Developing a nurses' ability to manage: a program design. Journal of

Continuing Education in Nursing, 4 (6), Nov-Dec 1973, 28-33.

32 Nursing Administration Quarterly Nursing education. Part 2. Preparation of nurse administrators. (Proceedings of conference at Boston University School of Nursing.) Nursing Administration Quarterly, 3 (4), Summer 1979, 45-112.

33 Pain, D. Role-based training: an evaluation. (Of experimental workshop for senior nursing officers and senior tutors in SW Thames RHA.) Nursing Times, 75, 8 Nov 1979, 1947-1948.

34 Pethybridge, F. Training for management. The need for a change of direction. (Includes nurses.) Hospital and Health Services Review, 74 (2), Feb 1978, 41-43.

35 Rotkovitch, R. A clinical component in education for nursing administration? (Argues against it.) Nursing Outlook, 27 (10), Oct 1979, 668-671.

36 Smyth, M. Site-based first-line management training. (In North Camden Health District.) Nursing Times, 76, 4 Dec 1980, 2143-2144.

37 Stevens, B. Education in nursing administration. Nursing Research Report, 11 (3), 1976, 14-17.

38 Strong, P.G. A locally-based first-line management course. (Experimental non-residential six-month modular course in Salop AHA.) Nursing Times, 74, 23 Nov 1978, 1931-1933.

39 Tomlinson, F. Who wants management courses? (For NHS staff, including nurses.) Health Services Manpower Review, 4 (1), Feb 1978, 16-20; (2), May 1978, 14-19.

40 Walton, M.J. The basic management workshop. (Experimental series of multidisciplinary first-line management workshops in Swindon Health District.) Nursing Times, 76, 4 Dec 1980, 2140-2142.

41 Watkin, B. One option: some thoughts on management eeducation for the NHS. Hospital and Health Services Review, 74 (9), Sep 1978, 300-303.

42 Wheeler, A. Participative management. (Trial exercise following DHSS training course in Ipswich Health District.) Nursing Times, 74, 16 Mar 1978, 469-470.

43 White, D. Management development: problems and progress. Nursing Focus, 1 (9), May 1980, 354, 356.

44 White, D. Some thoughts on the development of 'upper middle' managers in the NHS. Health Services Manpower Review, 4 (2), May 1978, 19-23.

f NON-NURSING DUTIES

1 Harris, G.A. Non-nursing duties. Nursing Mirror, 144, 17 Feb 1977, 66.

2 Lamp Non-nursing duties schedule 5 hospitals. (Guidelines drawn up by a committee.) Lamp, 33 (1), Jan 1976, 7, 9.

3 Rambo, B.J. Ward clerk skills. New York: McGraw-Hill, 1978. (Nursing and allied health series).

g NURSING OFFICER

1 Carr, A.J. The work of the nursing officer. (Survey of work over eight days and nights.) Nursing Times, 74, 24 Aug 1978, Occ. papers, 89-92; 31 Aug 1978, Occ. papers, 93-98.

2 Darcy, P.T. Exclusion from the care-giving process. (Lack of clinical involvement by nurse managers and suggestion that nursing officers should be given patient caseloads.) Nursing Times, 76, 10 Jan 1980, 54.

3 Heyman, B. and Shaw, M. Nurses' perceptions of the British hospital nursing officer. (Views of 170 nurses of various grades in two general, one psychiatric and one mental subnormality hospital.) Journal of Advanced Nursing, 5 (6), Nov 1980, 613-623.

4 Howell, L.C. Organisation of nursing services. 2. Strength in integration. (Development of the role of the nursing officer.) Health and Social Service Journal, 90, 22 Aug 1980, 1104-1106.

5 Ongley, V.M. Nursing officer: clinical specialist or administrator? (An activity analysis of a nursing officer's work during a four-week period to define the time spent in the clinical situation.) Nursing Mirror, 142 (6), 12 Feb 1976, 57-61.

6 Pyves, M.G. A study of staff officers (nursing) at district level. MSc thesis, University of Aston in Birmingham, Management Centre, 1977.

7 Ramadas, P. Leadership role of the nursing officer. Nursing Journal of Singapore, 15 (2), Nov 1975, 100-101.

8 Schurr, M.C. The role of the nursing officer—what is it? Nursing Mirror, 143 (9), 26 Aug 1976, 59-60.

9 Smith, J.P. The unit nursing officer: manager of nursing care. Journal of Advanced Nursing, 2 (6), Nov 1977, 571-588.

10 Towler, B. Nursing officers and supplies. Nursing Focus, 2 (4), Dec 1980, 127-128.

11 Watkin, B. Number seven. (Comments on 'Nursing officer—clinical specialist or administrator', by V. Ongley, Nursing Mirror, 12 Feb 1976.) Nursing Mirror, 142, 25 Mar 1976, 42.

12 Watkin, B. The nursing officer's guide to management. 1. What the job entails. 2. Work planning and staff deployment. Nursing Mirror, 146, 15 Jun 1978, Supplement i-iv.

13 Watkin, B. The nursing officer's guide to management. 3. Leadership and making decisions. Nursing Mirror, 146, 22 Jun 1978, Supplement i-ii.

14 Watkin, B. The nursing officers' guide to management. 7. Communication skills... 8. Numbers and management. Nursing Mirror, 147, 13 Jul 1978, Supplement i-iv.

15 Watkin, B. The nursing officers' guide to management. 9. The wider setting. 10. Money matters. Nursing Mirror, 147 20 Jul 1978, Supplement i-iv.

16 Watkinson, H. The nursing officer. 2. A review of the literature. 3. A questionnaire for learners. Nursing Times, 75, 21 Jun 1979, 1043-1046; 28 Jun 1979, 1101-1105.

17 Wilson-Barnett, J. and Hancock, C. A future for ward-based nursing officers? (Research study to evaluate experimental post of nursing officer based on one ward with managerial responsibility for the other wards of a unit.) Nursing Mirror, 147, 30 Nov 1978, 27-29.

h POLICY AND PLANNING

1 Bryant, Y. The role of the nurse in systems design. Royal Society of Health Journal, 99 (1), Feb 1979, 9-11, 27.

2 Clarke, H.F. Challenging the status quo: the nurse's role in health care delivery planning. (Registered Nurses Association of British Columbia promotes nurses' participation in planning.) Canadian Nurse, 73 (1), Jan 1977, 40-42.

3 Flint, J.W. The nursing systems analyst: are you ready for her? (To analyse, design and improve nursing work systems and methods.) Supervisor Nurse, 11 (1), Jan 1980, 55-56.

4 Garant, C.A. The process of effecting change in nursing. Nursing Forum, 17 (2), 1978, 152-167.

5 Manez, J. The untraditional nurse manager; agent of change and changing agent. Hospitals, 52, 1 Jan 1978, 62-65.

6 Nelson, E.G. Management implications of organisational change: an investigation of the management requirements of hospital nursing. MSc thesis, Business School, Durham University, 1969.

7 Stevens, B.J. Management of continuity and change in nursing. Journal of Nursing Administration, 7 (4), Apr 1977, 26-31.

8 Swansburg, R.C. Planning—a function of nursing administration. Supervisor Nurse, 9 (4), Apr 1978, 25-28; (5), May 1978, 77-80.

i SALMON REPORT

1 Auld, M. The reality of Salmon. Nursing Mirror, 142, 27 May 1976, 57-58.

2 Dunn, A. Madness of back-seat driving. (Interview with Brian Salmon about his work on nursing management structure and supplies.) Health and Social Service Journal, 90, 4 Jan 1980, 17-19.

3 Gordon, D. Salmon: will it sink or swim? (Report on NHS supplies.) Health and Social Service Journal, 88, 7 Jul 1978, 754-755.

4 Greene, J. An episode of nursing history. (Salmon report and its achievements.) Nursing Mirror, 142 (25), 17 Jun 1976, 60-62.

5 Hulme, M. Well, should matron come back? (Review of advantages and disadvantages of the Salmon structure.) Nursing Mirror, 150, 7 Feb 1980, 28-29.

6 Illsley, R. Why are we the harlot in reverse. (Progress in nurse management in the light of the Salmon report and suggestion for future developments.) Health and Social Service Journal, 89, 4 May 1979, 520-521.

7 Plant, J. Making Salmon work. (The author, a DNO describes implementation of the Salmon structure in North Tees district and the importance of cooperation between nurses and doctors.) British Medical Journal, 1, 25 Mar 1978, 800-802.

8 Salmon, B. Salmon after ten years. (Interview with Brian Salmon who gives his thoughts on the effectiveness of the management structure.) Nursing Mirror, 142 (21), 20 May 1976, 39-41.

j WARD MANAGEMENT

1 Castledine, G. Adding the icing to the cake. (The role of the ward sister and need for a clinical career structure.) Nursing Mirror, 149, 30 Aug 1979, 8.

2 Curationis Special issue on the ward sister. Curationis, 3 (1), Jun 1980, 3-43. Includes Cremer, L.M. Dealing with conflict, 22-25.

3 Gilbertson, D.W. The ward sister—a vital role in the health care team. New Zealand Nursing Journal, 69 (7), Jul 1976, 5-10.

4 Gilbertson, D.W. and others The ward sister: a suitable case for treatment. (Review of her role in the New Zealand Health Service.) International Nursing Review, 24 (4), Jul/Aug 1977, 108-113.

5 Hinkle, M.T. and Hinkle, B.J. Priorities of the charge nurse. (Aspects of the ward sister's role.) Supervisor Nurse, 8 (11), Nov 1977, 47-49, 53-54; 8 (12), Dec 1977, 41-45.

6 Hockey, L. and others Patterns of ward organisation. (Research supported by the Leverhulme Trust Fund.) The Author, 1978.

7 King's Fund Centre Current thinking on written ward policies: report of a conference held at the King's Fund Centre on 12th June 1979. Reported by Bernadette Fallon. The Centre, 1979. (KFC 79/171)

8 Markham, G. 'You're always so busy, sister'. (Range of work of ward sisters.) Nursing Mirror, 151, 4 Sep 1980, 38-40.

9 Nursing Times Quandary—1. Problems of conscience. (Case of a ward sister in conflict with nursing management.) Nursing Times, 72 (43), 28 Oct 1976, 1675.

10 Ogier, M.E. A study of the leadership style and verbal interactions of ward sisters with nurse learners. PhD thesis, Department of Occupational Psychology, Birkbeck College, London University, 1980. (Published as 'An ideal sister', RCN, 1982.)

11 Pembrey, S. A nursing view. Deference, authority, flirtation and stealth. (Need to bring back status of ward sister through structural change and career development.) British Medical Journal, 279, 1 Dec 1979, 1450-1451; Correspondence, 280, 12 Jan 1980, 117.

12 Pembrey, S. Teamwork in the ward. (Nursing Mirror Forum 1976.) Nursing Mirror, 142, 8 Apr 1976, 52-53.

13 Pembrey, S.E.M. The ward sister—key to nursing: a study of the organisation of individualised nursing. Rcn, 1980. (Based on 'The role of the ward sister in the management of nursing'. PhD thesis, Edinburgh University, 1978.)

14 Perry, E.L. Ward management and teaching. 2nd ed. Baillière Tindall, 1978.

15 Redfern, S.J. The charge nurse: job attitudes and occupational stability. PhD thesis, University of Aston, 1979.

16 Redfern, S.J. Hospital sisters: work attitudes, perceptions and wastage. (Research study.) Journal of Advanced Nursing, 5 (5), Sep 1980, 451-466.

17 Runciman, P.J. Ward sisters' perceptions of problems in their work role. MPhil thesis, University of Edinburgh, 1980.

18 Searle, C. The ward sister—some aspects of her role and function. Curationis, 3 (1), Jun 1980, 4-9.

19 Sheahan, J. Ward sister—manager, nurse, or teacher? (Based on prize-winning essay in Baillière Prize for Nursing Studies 1977 competition.) Nursing Mirror, 146, 18 May 1978, 18-21.

20 Ward, A. The ward sister—nurse, manager or teacher? Nursing Times, 74, 9 Feb 1978, 220-221.

k UNIT MANAGEMENT AND HEAD NURSE (US)

1 Boissoneau, R. and others The supervisory relationship between unit managers and ward clerks in a nursing department. Hospital Topics, 55 (4), Aug 1977, 30-34.

2 Byers, H.J. and Klink, J.A. The role of clinical supervisors and head nurses in management. Nursing Clinics of North America, 13 (1), Mar 1978, 119-129.

3 Courtade, S. The role of the head nurse: power and practice. Supervisor Nurse, 9 (12), Dec 1978, 16-17, 20-23.

4 Doona, M.E. A nursing unit as a political system. (Analysis of staff dissatisfaction in a medical geriatric unit resulting in the development of committees hearing staff demands.) Journal of Nursing Administration, 7 (1), Jan 1977, 28-32.

5 Farrell, N.L. and LaCosta, C. Unit administration updated. Hospitals, 51 (4), 16 Feb 1977, 75-76, 78.

6 Ganong, J.W. and Ganong, W.L. Help for the head nurse: a management guide. 2nd ed. Chapel Hill: W.L. Ganong Co., 1974.

7 Germaine, A. Old habits are hard to break. Operation of an efficient health unit is hindered by antiquated, illogical and traditional reasons for promotion. Hospital Administration in Canada, 19 (4), Apr 1977, 43-44.

8 Heiman-Elkind, H. Nursing administration in an Israeli hospital. (Reorganisation involving making supervisors in charge of one aspect of administration instead of specific units.) Nursing Times, 76, 20 Mar 1980, Occ. papers, 36.

9 Jones, N.K. and Jones, J.W. The head nurse: a managerial definition of the activity role set. Nursing Administration Quarterly, 3 (2), Winter 1979, 45-47.

10 McPhail, A. From head nurse to nurse manager. (Combination of the roles of head nurse and supervisor to create new role of middle manager/patient care coordinator in charge of a unit.) Canadian Nurse, 74 (1), Jan 1978, 32-39.

11 Pinkerton, S.E. A model for head nurse development. (Orientation of new staff through analysis of functions and use of model to solve problems.) Supervisor Nurse, 8 (4), Apr 1977, 83, 86-88.

12 SURVEY of perceived relationships between chief operating officers and directors of nurses. (A survey of the role of the director of nursing carried out in Pennsylvania hospitals.) Hospital Topics, 55 (2), Mar/Apr 1977, 38-40.

11 STAFFING

a GENERAL

1 Bahr, J. and others Innovative methodology enhances nurse deployment, cuts costs. Computerized self-updating system evaluates staffing requirements in a dynamic environment. Hospitals, 51 (8), 16 Apr 1977, 104, 105, 109.

2 Ballantyne, D.J. A computerized scheduling system with centralized staffing. Journal of Nursing Administration, 9 (3), Mar 1979, 38-45.

3 Clark, E.L. A model of nurse staffing for effective patient care. Journal of Nursing Administration, 7 (2), Feb 1977, 22-27.

4 Germaine, A. Staffing patterns and mobility of nursing personnel. Hospital Administration in Canada, 17 (5), May 1975, 46, 48, 50.

5 Hope, M. Nurse utilisation study. (Use of the American Resource Monitoring System for assessing staffing requirements in three Sydney hospitals, April to September 1973.) Lamp, Dec 1975, 14-17, 28.

6 Horoshak, I. This team of floaters flies high. (System at University Hospital, Los Angeles—nurses who may be assigned to any department depending on needs.) RN Magazine, 39 (11), Nov 1976, 85-86, 91-92.

7 Journal of Nursing Administration Staffing: a reader. Wakefield: Mass.: Contemporary Publishing. 2. 1975; 3. 1976.

8 Lancashire Area Health Authority Report of independent review team on the needs of nurse staffing at Calderstones Hospital. Preston: Lancashire AHA, 1977.

9 McConnell, E. Staffing should be spelled $taffing or how many staff nurses are enough? (Assessing staff needs and costs.) Nursing, 7 (11), Nov 1977, 17-19.

10 Moriuchi, J. and others Juggling staff to reduce costs. (Computerised system of allocation of staff.) Dimensions in Health Service, 55 (4), Apr 1978, 13-14.

11 National League for Nursing Concerns in the acquisition and allocation of nursing personnel. New York: NLN, 1978.

12 Nursing Administration Quarterly Issue on staffing: (Part 2). Nursing Administration Quarterly, 2 (1), Fall 1977, 1-96.

13 Nyberg, J. and Simler, M. Developing a framework for an integrated nursing department. (Including job description for and performance appraisal of staff nurse and patient classification system.) Journal of Nursing Administration, 9 (11), Nov 1979, 9-15.

14 Parkes, M. Nurse staffing patterns in Australian hospitals. (Research study to test hypothesis that when hospital nursing staff are organised as a stable work team the quality and quantity of nursing care provided would increase.) Australian Nurses Journal, 8 (7), Feb 1979, 29-33.

15 Scottish Association of Nurse Administrators Getting the manpower question right. (Conference report including contribution from M. Auld.) Nursing Times, 72, 25 Aug 1977, 1279.

16 Somers, J.B. Purpose and performance: a system analysis of nurse staffing. Journal of Nursing Administration, 7 (2), Feb 1977, 4-9.

17 Thomas, A. and Kataria, M. Manpower planning in inpatient units. Nursing Journal of India, 68 (2), Feb 1977, 54-56.

b INTER-PROFESSIONAL RELATIONSHIPS

1 Banks, S. Integrated ward discussions. Nursing Times, 72, 19 Feb 1976, 272.

2 Bergman, R. Interpersonal relations in health care delivery. International Nursing Review, 24 (4), Jul/Aug 1977, 104-107.

3 Bickford, J. The crisis. (Use of crisis-meeting to attempt to resolve conflicts among staff.) Supervisor Nurse, 10 (1), Jan 1979, 28-29.

4 Brunner, N.A. and Singer, L.E. A joint practice council in action. (Developed at a community hospital to provide forum for nurse/doctor discussion of roles and practice.) Journal of Nursing Administration, 9 (2), Feb 1979, 16-20.

5 Devine, B.A. Nurse-physician interaction: status and social structure within two hospital wards. (In USA.) Journal of Advanced Nursing, 3 (3), May 1978, 287-295.

6 Dudley, H.A.F. Professional relationships. (A doctor discusses relationships with nursing staff.) Nursing Mirror, 142, 6 May 1976, 65-66.

7 Frost, W. Doctor and nurse—the changing relationship. (Changes in the role of the nurse and attitudes to nursing by doctors.) Midwife, Health Visitor and Community Nurse, 14 (12), Dec 1978, 433, 436-437.

8 Glaser, I. and Horvath, K. A tool for dealing with nursing problems: the nursing group seminar proved therapeutic for both patients and staff. Supervisor Nurse, 10 (4), Apr 1979, 46-47, 51-52.

9 Gliddon, T. Interprofessional communication. (Between health professionals.) Australian Nurses Journal, 9 (3), Sep 1979, 50-53.

10 Goodwin, L. and Taylor, N. Doing away with the 'Doctor-nurse game'. (Overcoming problems in doctor/nurse communication via discussion on case management.) Supervisor Nurse, 8 (6), Jun 1977, 25-26.

11 Heineken, J. The team scapegoat. (Channelling of tension and anxiety on to vulnerable members of the group.) Supervisor Nurse, 11 (2), Feb 1980, 36-37.

12 Jacobs, M.K. Equilibrium theory applied to small nurse groups. (Research study to test certain propositions of an equilibrium theory of interpersonal relationships in a natural work setting.) Advances in Nursing Science, 1 (2), Jan 1979, 23-29.

13 Johnson, M.N. Interpersonal relationships in nursing. Nigerian Nurse, 7 (4), Oct-Dec 1975, 22-26, 31.

14 Kalisch, B.J. and Kalisch, P.A. An analysis of the sources of physician-nurse conflict. Journal of Nursing Administration, 7 (1), Jan 1977, 51-57.

15 Kramer, M. and Schmalenberg, C.R. Conflict: the cutting edge of growth. (A survey among 200 new hospital staff nurses of job conflict—defined as the tension generated by disagreements among individuals related to incompatible activities and interests.) Journal of Nursing Administration, 6 (8), Oct 1976, 19-25.

16 Lancet Round the world. North America. (Relationship between physician and nurse in North America.) Lancet, 2, 2 Aug 1980, 251.

17 Lee, A.A. How nurses rate with MDs: still the handmaiden. (RN survey of 536 American doctors' attitudes to nursing.) RN Magazine, 42 (7), Jul 1979, 21-30.

18 Leopoldt, H. Responsibility and the doctor/nurse relationship. Nursing Mirror, 144, 3 Feb 1977, 60-61.

19 McGee, A.D. and Martin, W.B.W. The games nurses play. (In doctor-nurse and nurse-nurse interactions.) Canadian Nurse, 74 (7), Jul/Aug 1978, 49-52.

20 Marco, N.D. Measures of transactional analysis ego states for nurses. (Used in studying communication among nurses.) Nursing Research, 28 (5), Sep/Oct 1979, 295-298.

21 Mullins, A.C. and Barstow, R.E. Care for the caretakers. (Nurses' need for support from their peers.) American Journal of Nursing, 79 (8), Aug 1979, 1425-1427.

22 Munn, H.E. Communications between patients, nurses, physicians and surgeons. Hospital Topics, 55 (2), Mar/Apr 1977, 6-7.

23 Northouse, P.G. Interpersonal trust and empathy in nurse-nurse relationships. Nursing Research, 28 (6), Nov/Dec 1979, 365-368.

24 Park, J. Negotiating ambiguity: an aspect of the nurse-doctor relationship. New Zealand Nursing Journal, 72 (11), Nov 1979, 14-16, 36.

25 Phillips, J.R. Health care provider relationships: a matter of reciprocity. (Task, authority deference and affect dimensions in the nurse-doctor relationship.) Nursing Outlook, 27 (11), Nov 1979, 738-741.

26 Portnoy, F.L. Observations on conflict: a nurse sociologist analyses a hospital conflict. (Group of nursing supervisors confront the hospital management.) Supervisor Nurse, 7 (3), Mar 1976, 32-33.

27 Rogers, A. Nursing care of the young doctor. (The new houseman's point of view.) Nursing Mirror, 143, 30 Dec 1976, 51-52.

28 Royal College of Physicians of Edinburgh Co-operation between medical and other health professions: a series of six report. The College, 1977.

29 Shubin, S. Communicating (or make that noncommunicating) with doctors. (Discussions with six nurses.) Nursing (U.S.), 9 (2), Feb 1979, 12-16.

30 Sills, G.M. Nursing, medicine and hospital administration. (Relationship between organizational triad of administrator, doctor and nurse.) American Journal of Nursing, 76 (9), Sep 1976, 1432-1434.

31 Smith, C.M. Identifying blocks to communication in health care settings and a workshop plan. Journal of Continuing Education in Nursing, 8 (2), Mar-Apr 1977, 26-32.

32 Trop, J.L. Consultation to groups in conflict: some aspects of group design. (Solving the problem of conflict between a ward sister and her staff nurses.) Journal of Psychiatric Nursing and Mental Health Services, 13 (6), Nov/Dec 1975, 11-15.

33 Vine, M. The 'Doctor Fell' syndrome. (Maladjustment of working relationships by illogical compulsive dislike.) Nursing Mirror, 143, 9 Dec 1976, 53.

34 Wilson-Barnett, J. Why do nurses hate doctors? (Exploitation of nurses by the medical profession and need for nurses to concentrate on nursing priorities not medical ones.) Midwife, Health Visitor and Community Nurse, 14 (6), Jun 1978, 172-175.

c JOB DESCRIPTIONS AND JOB EVALUATION

1 Brockenshire, A. and Hattstaedt, M.J.O. Revising job descriptions: a consensus approach. Supervisor Nurse, 11 (3), Mar 1980, 16, 18-20.

2 Carpenter, M. A worthwhile job? (Aims and methods of job evaluation with reference to recent DHSS report.) Nursing Times, 73, 6 Oct 1977, 1542-1543.

3 Cowie, V. and Gains, R.C. Job evaluation for nurses and midwives. Nursing Mirror, 142, 25 Mar 1976, 39-40.

4 Department of Health and Social Security Job Evaluation Unit Report…into the grading structure for nurses and midwives. DHSS, 1977.

5 Grimshaw, H. Closed minds? (Letter on job evaluation report from secretary of North Western Group of Area Nurses.) Nursing Times, 74 (2), 12 Jan 1978, 71-72.

6 Health Visitor Association Job evaluation. (Comments on the DHSS report.) Health Visitor, 51 (2), Feb 1978, 48.

7 Jacob, D. Failed criteria: a verdict on the job evaluation document. (Views of a management consultant on the DHSS report.) Nursing Times, 73, 13 Oct 1977, 1579.

8 Kratz, C. Forgive us for asking. (Comment on DHSS Job Evaluation report.) Nursing Times, 73, 13 Oct 1977, Community Outlook 83.

9 Kratz, C. What's the moral? (Comment on findings and criticisms of the DHSS Job Evaluation report. Letter.) Nursing Times, 73, 8 Dec 1977, 1913.

10 Newey, M.A. Job evaluation: some of the questions answered. (By member of the DHSS Job Evaluation Unit. See also editorial on p.1.) Nursing Mirror, 146, 19 Jan 1978, 6-8.

11 Newey, M.A. Understanding job evaluation. (Answers to most commonly asked questions about the DHSS report.) Nursing Times, 74, 26 Jan 1978, 133-134.

12 Norton, D. and others Job evaluation. (Letter criticising methodology of DHSS report.) Nursing Times, 73, 24 Nov 1977, 1845-1846.

13 Nursing Times Background to evaluation. (Progress of the Nurses' and Midwives' Whitley Council job evaluation.) Nursing Times, 72, 25 Mar 1976, 438-439.

14 Nursing Times Job evaluation. (Three letters (one from Rcn Research Society) criticising methodology of DHSS report.) Nursing Times, 73, 4 Nov 1977, 1711-1712.

15 Pantall, John Job descriptions for nurse managers. Cheadle: the Author. (7 Balmoral Ave, Cheadle Hulme, Cheshire SK8 5EQ), 1980.

16 Samaras, J.T. and others Wage evaluation methods: a model for nurse administrators. (Involving sixteen weighted job factors which can be used to determine wages according to the demands of any nursing post.) Journal of Nursing Administration, 8 (6), Jun 1978, 13-21.

17 Wallace, R. and Williams, D. Understanding job evaluation. (Letter from the chairmen of the Management and Staff Sides of the Nurses and Midwives Whitley Council, followed by answers by Maurice Newey to the questions commonly asked about the DHSS job evaluation report.) Nursing Times, 74, 26 Jan 1978, 132-134.

18 Watkin, B. Easier said than done. (Comment on recent report by DHSS Job Evaluation Unit.) Nursing Mirror, 140, 20 Oct 1977, 10.

19 White, R. Job evaluation: report. (Comment on recent DHSS report.) Nursing Mirror, 145, 29 Sep 1977, 31. Further comment under title 'Complaisant, compliant or conned?', 10 Nov 1977, 7; 'Where do we go from here?', 146, 9 Feb 1978, 9.

d JOB SATISFACTION

1 Arne, S. and others Staff motivation through a self help design: a practical application of motivational theory. Supervisor Nurse, 7 (10), Oct 1976, 65-66, 68.

2 Blalack, R.A. and Davis, H.J. Job strain and satisfaction among unit managers. Hospital Topics, 55 (1), Jan/Feb 1977, 30-35.

3 Brosan, J. and Johnston, M. Stressed but satisfied: organizational change in ambulatory care. (Effect of change measured through job satisfaction and role tension questionnaires.) Journal of Nursing Administration, 10 (11), Nov 1980, 43-46.

4 Cronin-Stubbs, D. Job satisfaction and dissatisfaction. Among new graduate staff nurses. (Research study.) Journal of Nursing Administration, 7 (10), Dec 1977, 44-49.

5 Donovan, L. What nurses want (and what they're getting). (Survey of 1051 nurses' job satisfaction.) RN Magazine, 43 (4), Apr 1980, 22, 24-30.

6 Everly, G.S. and Falcone, R.L. Perceived dimensions of job satisfaction for staff registered nurses. Nursing Research, 25 (5), Sep/Oct 1976, 346-348.

7 Gerberich, S.G. and others Motivation via an evaluation tool. (Pilot study using evaluation tool to measure staff motivation.) International Nursing Review, 25 (3), May/Jun 1978, 72-77.

8 Heinen, B. Job satisfaction for the float staff. (Research study.) Supervisor Nurse, 10 (1), Jan 1979, 48-51.

9 Johnston, R. Nurses and job satisfaction: a review of some research findings. Australian Nurses' Journal, 5 (11), May 1976, 23-27.

10 Joshi, H.B. and Dubey, B.L. Personality dimensions and job satisfaction of nurses. (Study at Nehru Hospital, Chandigarh.) Nursing Journal of India, 48 (9), Aug 1976, 191-192.

11 Kistler, J.F. and Kistler, R.C. Motivation and morale in the hospital. Generating loyalty and commitment is the test of the successful manager. Supervisor Nurse, 11 (2), Feb 1980, 26, 28-29.

12 Marriner, A. Motivation of personnel: a review of motivational theory. Supervisor Nurse, 7 (10), Oct 1976, 60, 62-63.

13 Marriner, A. and Craigie, D. Job satisfaction and mobility of nursing educators in baccalaureate and higher degree programs in the West. Nursing Research, 26 (5), Sep/Oct 1977, 349-360.

14 Nursing Job satisfaction or should that be dissatisfaction: how nurses feel about nursing. (Responses to survey by journal by M.A. Godfrey.) Nursing, 8 (4), Apr 1978, 13-25; (5), May 1978, 17-27; (6), Jun 1978, 65-73.

15 Pablo, R.Y. Job satisfaction in a chronic care facility. (Survey of 86 nursing and non-nursing staff at Parkwood Hospital, London, Ontario.) Dimensions in Health Service, 53 (1), Jan 1976, 36-39.

16 Slavitt, D.B. and others Nurses' satisfaction with their work situation. (Development of Index of Work Satisfaction and its use with hospital nurses and nurses in a private group practice setting.) Nursing Research, 27 (2), Mar/Apr 1978, 114-120.

17 Stamps, P.L. and others Measurement of work satisfaction among health professionals. (Research study of doctors, nurses and support staff in both institutional and ambulatory care settings.) Medical Care, 16 (4), Apr 1978, 337-352.

18 Stember, M.L. and others Job satisfaction research—an aid in decision making. Nursing Administration Quarterly, 2 (4), Summer 1978, 95-105.

19 Ullrich, R.A. Herzberg revisited: factors in job dissatisfaction. (Research study of trained nurses showing dissatisfaction with intrinsic as well as extrinsic factors.) Journal of Nursing Administration, 8 (10), Oct 1978, 19-24.

20 Wallis, D. and Cope, D. Job satisfaction and organisational change in hospitals: final report on the nursing staff project in Wales. Cardiff: UWIST, Department of Applied Psychology, 1980.

e STAFF APPRAISAL

1 Aime, D.B. Employee evaluations: what's the difference. (Study of discrepancy between employee self-evaluation scores and scores given

them by their supervisors.) Supervisor Nurse, 10 (6), Jun 1979, 52, 54-57, 59-60.

2 Benglas, C. Evaluation. Nursing Mirror, 142, 25 Mar 1976, 64.

3 Beveridge, W.E. Can appraisal systems work? (General discussion.) Nursing Focus, 1 (1), Sep 1979, 17-18.

4 Breeden, S.A. Participative employee evaluation. Journal of Nursing Administration, 8 (5), May 1978, 13-19.

5 Brief, A.P. Developing a usable performance appraisal system. Journal of Nursing Administration, 9 (10), Oct 1979, 7-10.

6 Broderick, M.E. and Ammentorp, W. Information structures: an analysis of nursing performance. (Investigation of decision-making behaviour of expert nurses.) Nursing Research, 28 (2), Mar/Apr 1979, 106-110.

7 Carr, A. How to turn a rebel into a friend. (How managers can discipline employees effectively.) Nursing Mirror, 149, 15 Nov 1979, 10.

8 Cook, P.A. Painless performance evaluations—that work. RN Magazine, 42 (10), Oct 1979, 75-76, 80, 82, 84-85.

9 Council, J.D. and Plachy, R.J. Performance appraisal is not enough. Journal of Nursing Administration, 10 (10), Oct 1980, 20-26.

10 Craig, J. Anecdotal records. (To serve as basis for assessment of performance or learning.) Canadian Nurse, 74 (5), May 1978, 25-27.

11 Crooks, E. Supervisor, nurse jointly appraise performance. (With performance appraisal form.) AORN Journal, 28 (1), Jul 1978, 128, 130, 132, 136, 138, 140, 144, 146.

12 Dau, C.J. The appraisal process. Supervisor Nurse, 7 (8), Aug 1976, 39-42.

13 Del Bueno, D.J. Implementing a performance evaluation system. Supervisor Nurse, 10 (2), Feb 1979, 48, 51-52.

14 Del Bueno, D.J. Performance evaluation, when all is said and done, more is said than done. Journal of Nursing Administration, 7 (10), Dec 1977, 21-23.

15 Dickson, B. Maintaining anonymity in peer evaluation. Supervisor Nurse, 10 (5), May 1979, 21-23, 26-29.

16 Dracup, K. Improving clinical evaluation. (Staff appraisal.) Supervisor Nurse, 10 (6), Jun 1979, 24-27.

17 Gauerke, R.D. Appraisal as a retention tool. Properly conceived and executed, staff evaluation should cut turnover rates. Supervisor Nurse, 8 (6), Jun 1977, 34, 36-37.

18 Gerberich, S.G. and others (1978) Motivation via an evaluation tool. (Pilot study using evaluation tool to measure staff motivation.) International Nursing Review, 25 (3), May/Jun 1978, 72-77.

19 Germaine, A. Problem solving and 'others.' Some thoughts and views on discipline and reprimand—and how they relate to effectiveness, productivity, job satisfaction and staff development. Hospital Administration in Canada, 19 (1), 1977, 38, 41.

20 Golightly, C. MBO and performance appraisal. (How nursing staff were involved in analysing problems with performance appraisal using management by objectives.) Journal of Nursing Administration, 9 (9), Sep 1979, 11-20.

21 Haar, L.F. and Hicks, J.H. Performance appraisal: derivation of effective assessment tools. Journal of Nursing Administration, 6 (7), Sep 1976, 20-29.

22 Hagen, B.L.W. How to get rid of a bad apple. (Problems in dealing with unprofessional behavior in nursing staff.) RN Magazine, 40 (5), May 1977, 52, 54-57.

23 Hatton, J. Performance evaluation in relation to psychosocial needs. (Analysis of nurse-patient interaction.) Supervisor Nurse, 8 (7), Jul 1977, 30, 32, 35.

24 Jarvis, J. Staff appraisal. (Scheme for community nurses introduced in Roehampton Health District.) Nursing Mirror, 145, 3 Nov 1977, 47-48.

25 Jones, D. Training—the key to effective appraisal. (Illustrated by a report of the Polytechnic of Central London's study of the National Nursing Staff Committee appraisal scheme.) Health Services Manpower Review, 3 (1), 15-20.

26 Jones, D. and Rogers, A. Nursing staff appraisal: a study of the system. (Summary of report to the National Staff Committee for Nurses and Midwives.) Polytechnic of Central London, 1976.

27 Jones, D. and Rogers, A. Nursing staff appraisal in the health service: a study of the system. Final report to the National Staff Committee for Nurses and Midwives. Polytechnic of Central London, 1976. Summary in Nursing Mirror, 144, 3 Feb 1977, 57-58.

28 Katz, F.M. and Snow, R. Assessing health workers' performance: a manual for training and supervision. Geneva: WHO, 1980. (Public health papers, 72.)

29 Kehoe, D.M. and Harker, T. Principles of assessing nursing skills. Tunbridge Wells: Pitman Medical, 1979.

30 Kramer, M. and Schulenberg, G. The first job...a proving ground. Basis for empathy development. (Appraisal methods for the new graduate nurse.) Journal of Nursing Administration, 7 (1), Jan 1977, 12-20.

31 Lawson, B.N. Evaluation—a sorry procedure. (Staff appraisal including chart of highly acceptable, acceptable and non-acceptable behaviour.) Supervisor Nurse, 9 (9), Oct 1978, 32-34.

32 Leopoldt, H. Controversy corner. Cost effectiveness and staff appraisal. Nursing Mirror, 142, 1 Apr 1976, 41.

33 MacKinnon, H.A. and Eriksen, L. C.A.R.E. A four track professional nurse classification and performance evaluation system. Journal of Nursing Administration, 7 (4), Apr 1977, 42-44.

34 Marriner, A. Evaluation of personnel: a discussion of the tools available for performance appraisal. Supervisor Nurse, 7 (5), May 1976, 36-39.

35 Marshall, J.R. and Schau, E. An evaluation process for nursing assistants. (Seattle

Veterans Administration Hospital.) Journal of Nursing Administration, 6 (8), Oct 1976, 37-40.

36 Mulholland, R.C. A performance appraisal scheme for health visitors. Nursing Times, 72, 22 Jul 1976, Occ. papers, 101-104.

37 National Staff Committee for Nurses and Midwives A report on NHS staff development and performance review: nurses, midwives, health visitors and tutorial staff. HMSO, 1977.

38 Nursing Times Staff development and performance review. Nursing Times, 74, 20 Apr 1978.
Introduction. 654-
The appraisal interview. 657-658.
The problems of measuring performance, by A.M. Stewart, 659-661.
Preparation for success by J.C. Gardner. 661-662.
Implementing the scheme. (At the Royal Marsden) by L. Burdge and K. Kay. 663-664.

39 Parkinson, R. Recipe for a realistic appraisal system. Personnel Management, 9 (11), Nov 1977, 37-40.

40 Partridge, R. Evaluating performance of nursing personnel. Nursing Leadership, 2 (3), Sep 1979, 18-22.

41 Phillips, M. Performance appraisal—a participative approach. (Experimental procedures with administrative nursing staff at the Clarke Institute of Psychiatry, Toronto.) Hospital Administration in Canada, 19 (6), Jun 1977, 68, 70.

42 Rosen, H. and Marella, M. Basic quantitative thinking for nurse managers. (Use of numerical ratings to evaluate nurses' performance quantitatively.) Journal of Nursing Administration, 7 (5), May/Jun 1977, 6-10.

43 Saarmann, S.M.V.L. Peer review in quality assurance. (The examination and evaluation of an individual's clinical nursing practice by colleagues.) American Journal of Nursing, 78 (12), Dec 1978, 2094-2096.

44 Schneider, H.L. Evaluation of nursing competence. Boston, Mass.: Little, Brown, 1979.

45 Schwirian, P.M. Evaluating the performance of nurses: a multidimensional approach. (Development of the Six-Dimension Scale of Nursing Performance for use in staff appraisal or research.) Nursing Research, 27 (6), Nov/Dec 1978, 347-351.

46 South, J.C. The performance profile: a technique for using appraisals effectively. Journal of Nursing Administration, 8 (1), Jan 1978, 27-31.

47 Stevens, B.J. Employee performance appraisal. Wakefield, Mass.: Contemporary Publishing, 1977. (Contemporary nursing review, no.R.4.)

48 Stevens, B.J. Performance appraisal: what the nurse executive expects from it. Journal of Nursing Administration, 6 (8), Oct 1976, 26-31.

49 Taylor, J.W. Outcome criteria as a measurement of nurse performance. (Reprinted from the Journal of the New York State Nurses' Association.) Nursing Digest, 3 (5), Sep/Oct 1975, 41-45.

50 Thompson, D.J.C. Staff development and performance review. A case of cart before the horse? (New appraisal schemes approved by the National Staff Committees for nurses and administrative and clerical staff.) Hospital and Health Services Review, 74 (1), Jan 1978, 16-20.

51 Thompson, D.J.C. Staff development and performance review. (Strengths of new National Staff Committee for Nurses and Midwives scheme, with outline of problems and some solutions.) Nursing Times, 75, 1 Mar 1979, 25-28.

52 West, N. and others An objective appraisal instrument for minimizing subjectivity in performance evaluation. Supervisor Nurse, 10 (3), Mar 1979, 32, 34-38.

f STAFF SELECTION AND DEVELOPMENT

1 Belanger, C. Staff development—a living growing organism. A design for staff development progressing from orientation to safe practice to skilled practice. Supervisor Nurse, 9 (6), Jun 1978, 16, 18-19, 21-22, 23-25.

2 Carr, A. How it may be just the job! (Advice on being interviewed for nursing management posts.) Nursing Mirror, 150, 26 Jun 1980, 12.

3 Everly, G.S. and Schabdach, G.M. A 'professional development' approach to the supervision of staff nurses. Supervisor Nurse, 7 (12), Dec 1976, 31-32, 34-35.

4 Francis, G. Nursing personnel functions study: who is doing what in hospital? (Survey. See also p.18-20 for article on implementing policy changes.) Supervisor Nurse, 8 (4), Apr 1977, 66, 68-69.

5 Francis, J. The function of the personnel nurse. (In an integrated personnel department serving staff of all disciplines.) Nursing Times, 75, 20 Sep 1979, 1614-1616.

6 Germaine, A. Nursing administration. Effective staff hiring calls for special skills. Hospital Administration in Canada, 19 (3), Mar 1977, 20-21, 23, 25.

7 Gourlay, J.R. The personnel nurse. Quo vadis? Nursing Times, 75, 20 Sep 1979, 1613-1614.

8 Hall, D.C. Nursing personnel systems. Journal of Advanced Nursing, 1 (1), Jan 1976, 79-87.

9 Iveson-Iveson, J. Staff development for better care. Report on a recent regional conference run by the Brent and Harrow AHA on the revised staff development and performance review. (By the National Staff Committee for Nurses and Midwives.) Nursing Mirror, 146, 5 Jan 1978, 6-7.

10 Kaiser, P. Ten steps to interviewing job applicants. (With tips for applicants as well.) American Journal of Nursing, 78 (4), Apr 1978, 627-630.

11 Kowalski, K.E. Job interviewing: an effective tool for hiring staff nurses. Journal of Nursing Administration, 5 (1), Jan 1975, 28-32.

12 Marriner, A. The selection of personnel. Supervisor Nurse, 7 (1), Jan 1976, 18-22.

13 Mondy, R.W. and Mills, H.N. Interviewing and selecting staff: choice not chance in nurse selection. (Includes Job Descriptive Index of job satisfaction.) Supervisor Nurse, 9 (11), Nov 1978, 35-38.

14 Speakman, J. Area nurse (personnel) officer: to be or not to be? Nursing Times, 75, 20 Sep 1979, 1611-1612.

15 Tebbitt, B.V. Preparing the interviewer: a program for preparing supervisors and head nurses to participate in hiring their own staff members. Supervisor Nurse, 8 (4), Apr 1977, 44, 46-48.

16 Tobin, H.M. and others The process of staff development: components for change. 2nd ed. St. Louis: Mosby, 1979.

17 Watkin, B. The nursing officer's guide to management. 4. Recruitment and selection of staff. Nursing Mirror, 146, 22 Jun 1978, Supplement iii-iv.

18 Watkin, B. The nursing officer's guide to management. 5. Training and development of staff. Nursing Mirror, 146, 29 Jun 1978, Supplement i-ii.

19 Wherry, C. The nurse personnel officer: the lost voice of the staffing specialist. (At district and area level.) Nursing Mirror, 147, 9 Nov 1978, 36-37.

g WORKLOAD, ESTABLISHMENT AND PATIENT DEPENDENCY

1 Addenbrooke's Hospital Patient nurse dependency analysis moved into the computer world. (Three year experiment at Addenbrooke's Hospital, Cambridge, to evaluate the use of computers in analysing dependency information.) Nursing Mirror, 142, 26 Feb 1976, 37.

2 Audette, M.C.L. and Tilquin, C. Patient classification by care required. (Analysis of existing systems and a proposed classification.) Dimensions in Health Service, 54 (9), Sep 1977, 32-34, 36.

3 Auld, M.G. How many nurses? A method of estimating the requisite nursing establishment for a hospital. Rcn, 1976 (Research Series). Summaries in Nursing Times, 73, 4 Aug 1977, Occ. papers, 108.

4 Berry, V.I. and Reichelt, P.A. Using routinely collected data for staffing decisions. Hospitals, 51, 16 Nov 1977, 89-90, 91.

5 Bethell, P. Counting the cost of care. (Report of conference on dependency and establishments organised by Rcn and North Western RHA.) Health and Social Service Journal, 90, 16 May 1980, 628.

6 Bihldorff, J.P. and others An approach to patient classification...and some results. (McMaster University Medical Centre.) Hospital Administration in Canada, 18 (2), Feb 1976, 22-25.

7 Butler, A.M. Towards a staffing formula: a staffing system for general and obstetric wards. 2 parts. New Zealand Nursing Journal, 73 (2), Feb 1980, 33-37; (3), Mar 1980, 8-10.

8 Cabban, P.T. Patient dependency classification. (Introduction of system developed by Trevedi and published by Griffith and others in 1976.) Lamp, 37 (7), Jul 1980, 12-18.

9 Cameron, J. The Aberdeen Formula: revision of nursing workload per patient as a basis for staffing. Nursing Times, 75, 6 Dec 1979, Occ. papers, 131-132.

10 Chagnon, M. and others A patient classification system by level of nursing care requirements. (Description of classification scheme and instrument to measure workload.) Nursing Research, 27 (2), Mar/Apr 1978, 107-112.

11 Chagnon, M. and others Validation of a patient classification through evaluation of the nursing staff degree of occupation. (Index indicates how busy the staff is during a given shift on a particular unit.) Medical Care, 16 (6), Jun 1978, 465-475.

12 Charles, S.T. and Gillott, M. Equating ward staff with work loads. (Development of a method of determining nursing establishment.) Nursing Times, 73, 24 Feb 1977, Occ. papers, 29-32.

13 Chia, M. and others A nursing management project at Toa Payoh Hospital, Singapore. Phase 11B—categorisation of patients and the evaluation of workload. (Patient dependency project.) Nursing Journal of Singapore, 17 (1), May 1977, 25-27, 28-32.

14 Crompton, M. and others The Aberdeen formula (for determining nursing establishment.) Nursing Times, 72, 26 Aug 1976, Occ. papers, 121-124; 2 Sep 1976, Occ. papers, 125-128.

15 Curtis, C. A system of measurement of patient dependency and nurse utilization. Australian Nurses Journal, 6 (10), Apr 1977, 36-38, 42.

16 Curtis, C. What is the use of patient dependency studies? (With dependency rating sheet used at the Royal North Shore Hospital.) Lamp, 37 (7), Jul 1980, 6-11.

17 Des Ormeaux, S.P. Implementation of the C.A.S.H. patient classification system for staffing determination. Supervisor Nurse, 8 (4), Apr 1977, 29-30, 33-35.

18 Friend, J.H. A reorganised medical division. (Reorganisation of medical wards to provide three areas offering different levels of care: a high dependency unit, an intermediate area and a planned investigation unit.) British Medical Journal, 1, 24 Jun 1978, 1676-1678.

19 Garrod, N. The development of mathematical programming based algorithms to assist in the more effective deployment of various grades of nursing personnel. PhD thesis, Manchester University, Department of Management Sciences, 1980.

20 Giovannetti, P. Understanding patient classification systems. Journal of Nursing Administration, 9 (2), Feb 1979, 4-9.

21 Gloucester Health District The Gloucester project: a total care nursing dependency study of the tower block of the Gloucestershire Royal Hospital. The Health District, 1978.

22 Goldstone, L. Choosing the right use for the formula. (Comment on uses of the Aberdeen formula and suggestion that it is more useful for region-wide planning than day-to-day management.) Health and Social Service Journal, 90, 20 Jun 1980, 808-811.

23 Grant, N.K. Time to care: a method of calculating nursing workload based on individualised patient care. Rcn, 1979.

24 Halevi, H.S. and Ron, R. Medical patient/ nurse dependency in Israel. (An analysis of the staffing needs of procedures such as bathing and feeding and a comparison with similar studies in New Zealand and Switzerland.) Journal of Advanced Nursing, 1 (1), Jan 1976, 63-78.

25 Hancock, C. Finding the right level. (Comment on recent research on patient dependency and use of workload indices with implications for nurse managers.) Nursing Mirror, 150, 10 Jan 1980, 37-38.

26 Hancock, C. Finding the right level. (Comment on Senior's research on dependency and establishments.) Nursing Mirror, 150, 24 Apr 1980, 42.

27 Harman, R.J. Nursing services information system. (A method of gathering and reporting patient census, workload indices, staffing figures to improve quality of patient care in nursing units.) Journal of Nursing Administration, 7 (3), Mar 1977, 14-20.

28 Harrison, S. and Rathwell, T. The use of staffing norms—a cautionary view. (With some reference to the Aberdeen formula and the Auld method.) Health Services Manpower Review, 6 (4), Nov 1980, 9-10.

29 Henney, C.R. and Bosworth, R.N. A computer-based system for the automatic production of nursing workload data. (Based on Aberdeen formula.) Nursing Times, 76, 10 Jul 1980, 1212-1217.

30 Howarth, M.H. Activity sampling in nursing. (Use in a work study of ward and departmental staff 1969-1970.) International Journal of Nursing Studies, 13 (1), 1976, 47-53.

31 Iuliano, A.B. Developing a medical intermediate care area. (For patients who needed more than average nursing care but not intensive care.) Supervisor Nurse, 11 (4), Apr 1980, 61-63.

32 Kuhn, B.G. Prediction of nursing requirements from patient characteristics. 2 parts. (Research study into dependency of neurological patients.) International Journal of Nursing Studies, 17 (1), 1980, 5-15; (2), 1980, 69-78.

33 Levine, H.D. and Phillip, P.J. Factors affecting staffing levels and patterns of nursing personnel. U.S. Department of Health Education and Welfare, 1975.

34 Macrae, R. Changing patterns of management. (Need for good planning and reassessment of type of care needed by different types of patients.) Nursing Times, 76, 3 Jan 1980, 22-23.

35 MacGuire, J. Nurse/patient dependency measures: a management tool. King's Fund Centre, 1973. (KFC reprint; 776).

36 Mackley, B. and others The Aberdeen formula: evaluation on the larger scale. (Pilot scheme in South Tyneside Area Health Authority to evaluate nurse staffing establishments based on the formula.) Nursing Times, 75, 15 Mar 1979, Occ. papers, 29-32; 22 Mar 1979, Occ. papers, 33-36; 29 Mar 1979, Occ. papers, 37-39.

37 Marcus, R.T. Nursing shortages in NHS hospitals. (Letter from surgeon suggesting points system for staffing based on criteria of skill and experience.) British Medical Journal, 2, 12 Aug 1978, 497-498.

38 Marriner, A. Variables affecting staffing. (Review of factors including patient classification systems, staffing formulas and ways of meeting fluctuating needs.) Supervisor Nurse, 10 (9), Sep 1979, 62-65.

39 Melia, K.M. A sociological approach to the analysis of nursing work. (Analysis based on research of the work of hospital ward nurses with description of multi-skilled and single skilled work roles.) Journal of Advanced Nursing, 4 (1), Jan 1979, 57-67.

40 Meyer, D. Work load management system ensures stable nurse-patient ratio. (Research study of GRASP System of adjusting work load to staffing in which patient care units (PCUs) are estimated for all incoming admissions, the goal being an even distribution of work load among nursing units.) Hospitals, 52 (5), Mar 1978, 81-82, 84-85.

41 Miller, E.A. Staffing with the aid of dependency indices. A logical method for the utilisation of patient dependency indices in the distribution and rostering of available staff, and as an aid to the estimation of required staff. Nursing Times, 72, 12 Aug 1976, Occ. papers, 113-115.

42 Miller, J.F. The dynamic focus of nursing: a challenge to nursing administration. (Model of nursing practice based on patient's progression on illness-to-health continuum.) Journal of Nursing Administration, 10 (1), Jan 1980, 13-18.

43 Mitchell, M. and Smith, J. The Aberdeen Formula: a trial in SE Thames. Nursing Times, 73, 2 Jun 1977, 839-840.

44 Moores, B. and Moult, A. Patterns of nurse activity. (Research study of nurses' activity and interactions with patients in medical, surgical and orthopaedic wards of three hospitals.) Journal of Advanced Nursing, 4 (2), Mar 1979, 137-149.

45 Moores, B. and Moult, A. The relationship between the level of nurse staffing and the patterns of patient care and staff activity. Journal of Advanced Nursing, 4 (3), May 1979, 299-306.

46 Moult, A.P. A study of different nurse staffing levels and their relationship with nurse activity and patterns of patient care. MSc thesis, UMIST, Department of Management Sciences, May 1977.

47 Nimmo, A.W. Nursing workload: results and analysis of a short survey in the Peterhead area. Aberdeen: Grampian Health Services Information Unit, 1975. (Report no.26)

48 Norby, R.B. and others A nurse staffing system based upon assignment difficulty. (Including an instrument that measures quality of care and unit to unit monthly management reports based upon information gathered in daily monitoring of staffing needs.) Journal of Nursing Administration, 7 (9), Nov 1977, 2-24.

49 Overton, P. and others Patient classification by types of care. (For patients in the community as well as hospital.) Dimensions in Health Service, 54 (8), Aug 1977, 27-30.

50 Pable, R.Y. Patient care classification in a long term care and rehabilitation hospital. (At the University of Saskatchewan for assessing nursing needs and developing a work load index.) Hospital Administration in Canada, 19 (2), Feb 1977, 38-42.

51 Pace, A.J. and Grimshaw, E. Regional

nurse staffing: a system for recording the utilisation of nursing staff. (And measuring nursing work load. See also letter on p.1567 of 21 Sep issue from Dorset AHA ANO on progress of the scheme.) Nursing Times, 74, 7 Sep 1978, Occ. papers, 101-104; 21 Sep 1978, Occ. papers, 105-108.

52 Plummer, J. Patient classification proves staffing needs. (Kingston General Hospital, Ontario.) Dimensions in Health Service, 53 (5), May 1976, 36-38.

53 Rhys Hearn, C. Comparison of Rhys Hearn method of determining nursing staff requirements with the Aberdeen formula. International Journal of Nursing Studies, 16 (1), 1979, 95-103.

54 Rhys Hearn, C. and Potts, D. The effect of patients' individual characteristics upon activity times for items of nursing care. (Patient dependency study for calculating workload.) International Journal of Nursing Studies, 15 (1), 1978, 23-30.

55 Roehrl, P.K. Patient classification: a pilot test. (System at Medical Center Hospital of Vermont utilising a modification of the Veterans Administration classification system.) Supervisor Nurse, 10 (2), Feb 1979, 21-22, 25-27.

56 Senior, O.E. Dependency and establishments: nursing establishments in general hospital wards — the changeover from a non-teaching to a teaching hospital. Rcn, 1979. (Royal College of Nursing Research Series.)

57 Senior, O.E. Nursing establishments in general hospital wards. MPhil thesis, University of Nottingham, Dec. 1977.

58 Senior, O.E. RNO tackles staffing problems. (Report of address at meeting of Institute of Practitioners in Work Study, Organisation and Methods on methods of calculating nursing establishments in general wards.) Nursing Mirror, 145, 24 Nov 1977, 5.

59 Slack, P. How many nurses? Rcn Association of Nurse Management and the North Western RHA conference on 'Assessment of nursing establishments'. Nursing Times, 76, 15 May 1980, 853. (See also Health and Social Service Journal, 90, 16 May 1980, 628.)

60 Stewart, W. A systems approach to nurse allocation. (In Southampton.) Nursing Mirror, 148, 10 May 1979, Supplement i-xii.

61 Telford, W.A. Determining nursing establishments. (Description of system developed by author.) Health Service Manpower Review, 5 (4), Nov 1979, 11-17.

62 Tilquin, C. and others Determining nursing team size and composition. (PRN system used in Montreal based on each patient's level of need.) Dimensions in Health Service, 55 (12), Dec 1978, 12, 14-16.

63 Tilquin, C. Patient classification does work. (Classification according to patient care demand with an example used in a Montreal hospital.) Dimensions in Health Service, 53 (1), Jan 1976, 12-13, 16.

64 United States. Department of Health, Education and Welfare. Health Resources Administration Methods for studying nurse staffing in a patient unit: a manual to aid hospitals in making use of personnel. Hyattsville, Md.: USDHEW, 1978.

65 Vaughan, R.G. and MacLeod, V. Nurse staffing studies: no need to reinvent the wheel. (Need to standardise principles and terminology of patient classification and nursing workload systems.) Journal of Nursing Administration, 10 (3), Mar 1980, 9-15.

66 Williams, M.A. Quantification of direct nursing care activities. (Measurement of observable nursing activities as basis for staffing.) Journal of Nursing Administration, 7 (8), Oct 1977, 15-18.

67 Williams, M.A. and Murphy, L.N. Subjective and objective measures of staffing adequacy. (Comparison of charge nurses' views with assessment based on patient classification.) Journal of Nursing Administration, 9 (11), Nov 1979, 21-29.

68 Wilson-Barnett, J. A review of patient-nurse dependency studies. DHSS, 1978.

69 Youell, L. Patient classification program. (Used at Misericordia Hospital, Edmonton.) Dimensions in Health Service, 56 (11), Nov 1979, 17-18.

NURSE AND PATIENT

12 PATIENT CARE

a GENERAL

1 American Nurses' Association ANA clinical sessions, 1974. New York: Appleton-Century-Crofts, 1975.

2 American Nurses' Association Clinical conference papers, 1973. Kansas City: The Association, 1975.

3 Aspy, V.H. 'We've always done it that way.' (Ways to change traditional practices in nursing.) Supervisor Nurse, 8 (5), May 1977, 27-29.

4 Auger, Jeanine Roose Behavioural systems and nursing. Englewood Cliffs: Prentice-Hall, 1976.

5 Beswetherick, M. Staffing assignment: a review of past and current systems of nursing care delivery. (From 1900, of methods including team nursing and primary nursing.) Canadian Nurse, 75 (5), May 1979, 18-22.

6 Beyers, M. and Phillips, C. Nursing management for patient care. 2nd ed. Boston: Little, Brown and Co., 1979.

7 Bickerton, J. and others Nursing: theory and practice. New York: McGraw-Hill, 1979.

8 Burgess, A.W. Nursing: levels of health intervention. Englewood Cliffs: Prentice Hall, 1978.

9 Castledine, G. Helping ourselves to care. (Concept of selfcare in nursing.) Nursing Mirror, 148, 8 Mar 1979, 12.

10 Champion, M.R. The contribution of the trained nurse to patient care. MSc thesis, University of Wales, Welsh National School of Medicine, Department of Advanced Nursing Studies, 1979.

11 Chapman, C.M. Nursing—rhyme or reason? (An examination of the assumptions that nursing is patient centred, training is learner centred.) Nursing Times, 72, 5 Aug 1976, Occ. papers, 109-112.

12 Colledge, M.M. and Jones, D., editors Readings in nursing. Edinburgh: Churchill Livingstone, 1979.

13 De Young, L. The foundations of nursing as conceived, learned, and practiced in professional nursing. 3rd ed. St. Louis: Mosby, 1976.

14 Dicken, A. Why patients should plan their own recovery. (Goal-setting for patients with physical and psychiatric disorders.) RN Magazine, 41 (3), Mar 1978, 52-55.

15 Du Gas, B.W. Introduction to patient care: a comprehensive approach to nursing. 3rd ed. Philadelphia: Saunders, 1977.

16 Efionayi, K.M. Worklist: a useful directive for nursing care. (Used in Ibadan University College Hospital as an attainable job directive.) Journal of Advanced Nursing, 2 (4), Jul 1977, 373-382.

17 Ellis, J.R. and Nowlis, E.A. Nursing: a human needs approach. 2nd ed. Boston: Houghton Mifflin, 1977.

18 Ford, L.C. Unification of nursing practice, education and research. International Nursing Review, 27 (6), Nov/Dec 1980, 178-183, 192.

19 Given, B. and others Relationships of processes of care to patient outcomes. (Effect of diagnosis and therapy by nurse and patient's compliance behaviour on patient's functional status, clinical health status and perception of health and care.) Nursing Research, 28 (2), Mar/Apr 1979, 85-93.

20 Grier, M.R. and Schnitzler, C.P. Nurses' propensity to risk. (Descriptive study to assess nurses' willingness to take risks and gain information about how nurses make decisions about health care.) Nursing Research, 28 (3), May/Jun 1979, 186-191.

21 Hamilton, J. Changes in clinical nursing. International Nursing Review, 26 (3), May/Jun 1979, 75-77.

22 THE HEALTH profile. A new approach to patient care based on health rather than illness. (Model for identifying nursing care needs.) Nursing Times, 75, 18 Jan 1979, Health Profile 1-12.

23 Johnson, M.M. and Davis, M.L.C. Problem solving in nursing practice. 2nd ed. Dubuque: Brown, 1975.

24 Kinlein, L.M. A self-care concept. (A nursing approach.) American Journal of Nursing, 77 (4), Apr 1977, 598-601.

25 Lelean, S.R. The communication of instructions for nursing care in medical wards. PhD thesis, Surrey University, Department of Human Biology and Health, 1977.

26 Longo, D.C. and Williams, R.A., editors Clinical practice in psychosocial nursing: assessment and intervention. New York: Appleton-Century-Crofts, 1978.

27 McEvoy, M.D. and Egan, E.C. The process of developing a nursing intervention model.

(To provide framework for nursing practice, illustrated by model for patients dying of cancer.) Journal of Nursing Education, 18 (4), Apr 1979, 19-25.

28 Myer, E.M. How far should patients decide on their own treatment? Nursing Times, 72, 18 Nov 1976, 1818-1819.

29 New Zealand Nurses Association Resolutions for action by the professional services committee. (Brief guidelines and selected bibliography on patient assignment and the nursing process.) New Zealand Nursing Journal, 70 (6), Jun 1977, 23.

30 Norris, C.M. Self-care. American Journal of Nursing, 79 (3), Mar 1979, 486-489.

31 O'Connor, M.P. Implementing change in the organisation of nursing care. New Zealand Nursing Journal, 69 (4), Apr 1976, 8-11.

32 Pepper, R.J. Professionalism, training and work: a study of nursing in a general hospital. PhD thesis, Kent University, 1977.

33 Roper, N. An image of nursing for the 1970s. (Survey to show how nursing activities relate to clinical areas, diagnostic labels and secondary symptoms in individual patients.) Nursing Times, 72, 29 Apr 1976, Occ. papers, 61-64; 6 May 1976, Occ. papers, 65-66.

34 Rouhani, G.C. Holistic health: the challenge to nursing. (Whole health of body, mind and spirit with reference to self-care.) Australian Nurses Journal, 9 (5), Nov 1979, 42-45.

35 Skeet, M. Notes on nursing: the science and the art. Edinburgh: Churchill Livingstone, 1980. Issued as a two volume set with 'Notes on nursing' by Florence Nightingale.

36 Smith, J.P. Towards a concept of care. (Need for nurses and nurse teachers to develop the role of career.) Journal of Community Nursing, 2 (9), Mar 1979, 11, 13, 15.

37 Tiffany, R. Mobilizing nursing skills. (Basing nursing care on the 'nursing model' with reference to personalised patient care at the Royal Marsden Hospital.) Journal of Advanced Nursing, 4 (1), Jan 1979, 3-8.

38 Webber, D.L. and Malley, P. Behavioural programmes and patient management for first year nursing students. (Application of behavioural science to planning of patient care.) International Journal of Nursing Studies, 15 (1), 1978, 31-36.

39 Whitson, B.J. and others Complemental nursing. A form of independent practice tailor-made for the patient, as conceived by its originator, experienced by a patient, and practiced by a complemental nurse. (Viewpoints of originator, patient and nurse.) American Journal of Nursing, 77 (6), Jun 1977, 984-988.

b NURSING PROCESS

1 Ashworth, P. Problems and solutions. (Advantages of nursing process and reasons given by nurses reluctant to implement it.) Nursing Mirror, 151, 4 Sep 1980, 34-36.

2 Ashworth, P. A way to better care. (The nursing process.) Nursing Mirror, 151, 28 Aug 1980, 26-27.

3 Bartos, L.T. and Knight, M.R. Documentation of nursing process. (With discussion on nursing records generally.) Supervisor Nurse, 9 (7), Jul 1978, 41-43, 46-48.

4 Bradshaw, P.L. Patient care: the nursing process in operation. (Nursing care plan for patient with Hodgkin's disease at home.) Journal of Community Nursing, 1 (3), Sep 1977, 21, 23-25.

5 Browning, M.H. compiler The nursing process in practice. New York: American Journal of Nursing Co., 1974.

6 Butherus, G.C. The nursing process. 1. Assessment and planning. 2. Implementation and evaluation. Journal of Practical Nursing, 28 (10), Oct 1978, 15-18, 40; (11), Nov 1978, 31-32, 39.

7 Buxton, S. The nursing process: an approach to patient centered care. (Describes its implementation.) Australasian Nurses Journal, 8 (9), Jul 1979, 34-38.

8 Chavasse, J. The nursing process. (General description.) World of Irish Nursing, 7 (1), Jan 1978, 1-2.

9 Clark, M.O. Why do we need the nursing process? 2. For professional reasons. Nursing Times, 74, 30 Nov 1978, 1986-1987.

10 Cormack, D.F.S. The nursing process: an application of the SOAPE model. (Extension of SOAPE model involving problem oriented medical records to include evaluation of care, with reference to non-physical aspects of care illustrated by plan for psychogeriatric patient.) Nursing Times, 76, 3 Apr 1980, Occ. papers, 37-40.

11 Cowper-Smith, F. What is the point of the nursing process? (Report of conference on the nursing process organised by nursing degree students.) Nursing Times, 74, 4 May 1978, 738-739.

12 Crow, J. The nursing process: articles from the 'Nursing Times'. Macmillan Journals, 1977.

13 Crow, J. The nursing process—1. Theoretical background. 2. How and why to take a nursing history. 3. A nursing history questionnaire for two patients. (Care studies p.983-984 and care plans on centre pages.) Nursing Times, 73, 16 Jun 1977, 892-896; 23 Jun 1977, 950-957; 30 Jun 1977, 978-982.

14 Darcy, P.T. The nursing process—a base for all nursing developments. (Abridged version of prize-winning essay.) Nursing Times, 76, 20 Mar 1980, 497-501.

15 Davis, B.D. Why do we need the nursing process? 3. For professional reasons. Nursing Times, 74, 30 Nov 1978, 1987-1988.

16 Deininger, J.M. The nursing process implementation and evaluation. Journal of Practical Nursing, 25 (12), Dec 1975, 18, 32.

17 Duberley, J. How will the change strike me and you...? (Problems in implementing the nursing process in nursing care.) Nursing Times, 73, 10 Nov 1977, 1736-1738.

18 French, P. A myth, a model, a necessity. (The nursing process.) Nursing Times, 76, 21 Aug 1980, 1468.

19 Goodwin, J.O. A cross-cultural approach to integrating nursing theory and practice. (Application of nursing process to existing nursing theories and to French culture and nursing practice.) Nursing Education, 5 (6), Nov/Dec 1980, 15-20.

20 Hammond, M. The nursing process. (Outline of its five phases.) Curationis, 1 (3), Dec 1978, 19-23.

21 Hegyvary, S.T. Nursing process: the basis for evaluating the quality of nursing care. International Nursing Review, 26 (4), Jul/Aug 1979, 113-116.

22 Hegyvary, S.T. and Haussman, R.K.D. The relationship of nursing process and patient outcomes. (Results of survey.) Journal of Nursing Administration, 6 (9), Nov 1976, 18-21.

23 Holt, D. and others Making a new record. (Implementation of nursing process at the Royal Alexandra Hospital in Rhyl.) Nursing Mirror, 151, 21 Aug 1980, 32-33.

24 Humphris, M.R. The nursing process: an application of scientific method. Australian Nurses Journal, 9 (4), Oct 1979, 30-31.

25 Hunt, J.M. Prescription for nursing care. (Research project at the London Hospital to implement the nursing process and introduce written care plans.) Nursing Times, 74, 30 Nov 1978, Supplement 14-18.

26 Jones, C. The nursing process—individualised care. (Brief outline of the four phases.) Nursing Mirror, 145, 13 Oct 1977, 13-14.

27 Jasmin, S. and Trygstad, L.N. Behavioral concepts and the nursing process. St. Louis: Mosby, 1979.

28 Joseph, L.S. Self-care and the nursing process. (With reference to patient teaching.) Nursing Clinics in North America, 15 (1), Mar 1980, 131-143.

29 Kirwin, B. From the ivory tower to the ward floor. (Assessment of the fate of the nursing process in the U.S.A. and England based on visits.) Nursing Mirror, 150, 28 Feb 1980, 36-38.

30 Kratz, C.R. The nursing process. (Introduction to series of articles by J. Crow.) Nursing Times, 73, 9 Jun 1977, 854-855.

31 Kratz, C.R. editor The nursing process. Baillière Tindall, 1979.

32 La Monica, E.L. The nursing process: a humanistic approach. Menlo Park, Cal.: Addison-Wesley, 1979.

33 Lancet The nursing process. (Editorial comment.) Lancet, 2, 29 Jul 1978, 248.

34 McClure, E. and Warwick, J. The nursing process studied in Toronto. (Eight week study tour of students from the University of Edinburgh.) Nursing Mirror, 144, 10 Feb 1977, 55-57.

35 McGilloway, F.A. The nursing process: a problem-solving approach to patient care. (Discussion and literature review.) International Journal of Nursing Studies, 17 (2), 1980, 79-90.

36 MacMillan, P. Please don't throw out the baby with the bathwater. (Criticism of nursing process.) Nursing Times, 75, 8 Nov 1979, 1923-1924.

37 Marks-Maran, D. In the process of better care. (Discusses reasons why nursing process is not being implemented.) Nursing Mirror, 149, 12 Jul 1979, 12.

38 Marks-Maran, D. Patient allocation v task allocation in relation to the nursing process. Nursing Times, 74, 9 Mar 1978, 413-416.

39 Marriner, A. The nursing process: a scientific approach to nursing care. 2nd ed. St. Louis: Mosby, 1979.

40 Measures, A. The nursing process—a useful step? (How it can provide better patient care and greater job satisfaction.) Nursing Mirror, 148, 14 Jun 1979, 20-21.

41 Murchison, I. and others Legal accountability in the nursing process. St. Louis: Mosby, 1978.

42 Neilson, A.F. Why do we need the nursing process? 1. For legal reasons. Nursing Times, 74, 30 Nov 1978, 1984-1985.

43 Nursing Times Rediscovering the patient. (Supplement on how the nursing process has been introduced at Manchester Royal Infirmary and the London Hospital.) Nursing Times, 74, 30 Nov 1978, Supplement 2-24.

44 Nursing Times Why do we need the nursing process? (Three articles on the legal, practical and professional reasons.) Nursing Times, 74, 30 Nov 1978, 1984-1988.

45 Royal College of Nursing Implementing the nursing process. Rcn, 1979.

46 Royal College of Nursing. Association of Nursing Education Introducing the nursing process. (Report of first conference.) Nursing Times, 73, 26 May 1977, 763.

47 Rubel, M. Coming to grips with the nursing process. Supervisor Nurse, 7 (2), Feb 1976, 30-32, 34, 36, 38-39.

48 Scottish National Nursing and Midwifery Consultative Committee The process of nursing. (A concept and model of nursing which embodies the principles of progression developed by the Briggs Committee.) Nursing Mirror, 143, 1 Jul 1976, 55-57.

49 Sofaer, B. Spreading the word. Seminar approach to disseminating information on the nursing process at Bangour General Hospital, Broxburn, West Lothian, Scotland. Nursing Times, 76, 27 Mar 1980, 567-568.

50 Sundeen, S.J. and others Nurse-client interaction: implementing the nursing process. St. Louis: Mosby, 1976.

51 Tucker, E.R. The nursing process. (Its

value and applications.) Nursing Mirror, 146, 9 Mar 1978, 22-23.

52 **West, A.** Patient into person. (Implementation of the nursing process in an acute neurosurgical ward at Atkinson Morley Hospital.) Nursing Mirror, 150, 21 Feb 1980, 32-34.

53 **Whelton, B.J.** An operationalization of Martha Rogers' theory throughout the nursing process. (Rogers' theory of the individual is put forward in 'An introduction to the theoretical basis of nursing,' 1970.) International Journal of Nursing Studies, 16 (1), 1979, 7-20.

54 **World Health Organisation. Regional Office for Europe** The nursing process. (Meeting at Nottingham University to examine aspects of the nursing process.) Nursing Times, 73, 6 Jan 1977, 11.

55 **World Health Organisation. Regional Office for Europe** Nursing process workbook. Copenhagen: WHO, 1976.

56 **Yura, H. and Walsh, M.B. editors** Human needs and the nursing process. New York: Appleton-Century-Crofts, 1978.

57 **Yura, H. and Walsh, M.B.** The nursing process: assessing, planning, implementing, evaluating. 2nd ed. New York: Appleton-Century-Crofts, 1973.

NURSING PROCESS — TEACHING

58 **Alexander, M.** Teaching the nursing process: adapting the nursing process for use in a surgical unit. Nursing Times, 75, 23 Aug 1979, 1443-1447.

59 **Carter, S.L.** Teaching the nursing process: the nurse educator. (With reference to two philosophical schools of thought, humanism and behaviourism. Reprinted from Nursing Outlook, Sep 1978.) Nursing Times, 75, 2 Aug 1979, 1315-1317.

60 **Clarke, M.** Who's afraid of the nursing process? (Teaching of concept through handouts, flip chart and cartoons.) Nursing Times, 76, 12 Jun 1980, Community Outlook, 175-176, 178, 180.

61 **Crow, J.** Teaching the nursing process. The nursing process — a framework for care studies. (Guidelines used by author in helping students prepare care studies.) Nursing Times, 75, 9 Aug 1979, 1362-1365.

62 **Grubb, M.** Teaching the nursing process: a clinical teacher's view. Nursing Times, 75, 23 Aug 1979, 1448-1449.

63 **Heath, J.** A new kind of nurse — 3. It's a taxing process. (Taxonomy of objectives devised around the nursing process as framework for curriculum planning.) Nursing Mirror, 149, 23 Aug 1979, 24-27.

64 **Hollingworth, S.** Teaching the nursing process: a challenge for nurse teachers. Nursing Times, 75, 26 Jul 1979, 1263.

65 **Jeroes, M.C.** Nursing process: a tool to quality nursing. (With reference to the care of a dying patient who subsequently recovered.) Philippines Journal of Nursing, 49 (1), Jan/Mar 1979, 12-15.

66 **Kershaw, J.E.M.** Teaching the nursing process. Standard care plans. (For giving the

necessary basic care common to all patients with the same condition.) Nursing Times, 75, 16 Aug 1979, 1413-1416.

67 **Luker, K.A.** Teaching the nursing process. A framework for the nursing process: problem-oriented recordings. Nursing Times, 75, 30 Aug 1979, 1488-1490.

68 **Mallick, M.J.** Do nursing educators preach what they want practiced? (Recommends that the nursing process should form the framework of all nursing education.) Nursing Outlook, 25 (4), Apr 1977, 244-247.

69 **Newall, E.** The nursing process and nursing care studies. (How learners at Canterbury and Thanet Hospital are given project of care study based on nursing process.) Nursing Times, 76, 10 Jul 1980, 1235-1236.

70 **Reed, J.C. and Haynes, V.** (1978) Management: an experimental approach. (Experimental teaching procedure to integrate the nursing process, nursing care plans, the research process and management principles.) Journal of Nursing Education, 17 (6), Jun 1978, 20-25.

71 **Sculco, C.D.** Development of a taxonomy for the nursing process. (To differentiate the various levels of teacher expectations and students' ability in applying process.) Journal of Nursing Education, 17 (6), Jun 1978, 40-48.

72 **Spicer, J.** Bringing the system home. (How the nursing process is taught to district nursing students.) Nursing Mirror, 151, 11 Sep 1980, Supplement iv, vi, vii-ix.

c EVALUATION AND STANDARDS

1 **American Nurses Association** Evaluation research: assessment of nursing care. (16 papers given at the June 1979 conference.) Nursing Research, 29 (2), Mar/Apr 1980, 69-133.

2 **American Nurses Association** Guidelines for review of nursing care at the local level. Kansas City: The Association, 1977.

3 **American Nurses Association** Quality assurance workbook. Kansas City: The Association, 1976.

4 **Ashton, K.** Falling over falling standards. (Interview with Eileen Oxley, nursing auxiliary who is secretary of local COHSE branch.) Nursing Times, 74, 20 Jul 1978, 1190.

5 **Barba, M. and others** The evaluation of patient care through use of ANA's standards of nursing practice. Supervisor Nurse, 9 (1), Jan 1978, 42, 45-46, 49-50, 53-54.

6 **Blank, D.** Standards: are they really necessary? Canadian Nurse, 74 (8), Sep 1978, 24-27.

7 **Bloch, D.** Criteria, standards, norms — crucial terms in quality assurance. Journal of Nursing Administration, 7 (7), Sep 1977, 20-30.

8 **Byrd, J.M.** Peer review for quality charting. (Committee of registered nurses to improve record keeping through teaching and audit to establish and implement standards of patient care.) Supervisor Nurse, 8 (7), Jul 1977, 25-27.

9 **Canadian Nurses Association** A definition of nursing practice/standards for nursing practice. Ottawa: the Association, 1980.

10 **Canadian Nurses Association** Develop-

ment of a definition of nursing practice and standards for nursing practice. (Project report with draft standards.) Canadian Nurse, 76 (5), May 1980, 11-15.

11 **Canto, M.M.** Achieving nursing care standards: internal and external. Wakefield, Mass.: Nursing Resources Inc., 1978.

12 **Carr, A.** Well, are standards of care falling? (Need for more realistic assessment of individual care needed.) Nursing Mirror, 149, 13 Dec 1979, 12.

13 **Carter, J.H. and others** Standards of nursing care: a guide for evaluation. 2nd ed. New York: Springer, 1976.

14 **Chapman, C.** Rising standards of care. Nursing — a cost benefit analysis. (Importance of research to improve the quality of care.) Royal Society of Health Journal, 96 (5), Oct 1976, 208-211.

15 **Chow, R.K.** Assuring the quality of care: a personal perspective from tailoring to outcome measurement. (Use of PACE measuring instrument-Patient Appraisal and Care Evaluation.) Nursing Leadership, 1 (2), Sep 1978, 11-22.

16 **Christman, L.** Nursing practice — whose reponsibility? Australian Nurses Journal, 7 (11), Jun 1978, 38-40.

17 **Clinton, J. and others** Developing criterion measures of nursing care: case study of a process. (Description of patient outcome criteria to measure effectiveness of nursing care.) Journal of Nursing Administration, 7 (7), Sep 1977, 41-45.

18 **Cohen, A.G.** An on-going internal audit of nursing care. (Nursing care evaluation tool.) Hospital Topics, 58 (4), Jul/Aug 1980, 24-31.

19 **Cortazzi, D.** Crisis cartoons. (Multidisciplinary groups explore what goes wrong with patient care by drawing incidents.) Nursing Mirror, 143 (3), 15 Jul 1976, 46-48.

20 **Curtis, C.** Determining the quality of nursing care. (General review with definitions.) Lamp, 37 (8), Aug 1980, 9-13.

21 **Davidson, S. and others** Nursing care evaluation: concurrent and retrospective review criteria. St. Louis: Mosby, 1977.

22 **Davis, A.I.** Development of a blueprint for a quality assurance program. Supervisor Nurse, 8 (2), Feb 1977, 17-22, 25-26.

23 **Devaneson, B.A. and Bhanimathi, P.P.** The challenge of innovations. (Evaluation of a system of patient care in one hospital with solutions to particular problems.) Nursing Journal of India, 57 (10), Oct 1976, 243-244, 247.

24 **Diddie, P.J.** Quality assurance — a general hospital meets the challenge. Journal of Nursing Administration, 6 (6), Aug 1976, 6-8, 12-16.

25 **Dimarco, N. and others** Nursing resources on the nursing unit and quality of patient care. (A study of the relationship between grades of staff available and quality of care.) International Journal of Nursing Studies, 13 (3), 1976, 139-152.

26 **Donald, R.L. and Southern, R.M.** Quality care — commonplace or chimera. (With some

reference to nursing.) Journal of Medical Ethics, 4 (4), Dec 1978, 186-194.

27 Duke University Hospital Nursing Services Quality assurance: guidelines for nursing care. Philadelphia: Lippincott, 1980.

28 Eichhorn, M.L. and Fervert, E.I. Evaluation of a primary nursing system using the quality patient care scale. (QualPaCS). Journal of Nursing Administration, 9 (10), Oct 1979, 11-15.

29 Ethridge, P.E. and Packard, R.W. An innovative approach to measurement of quality through utilization of nursing care plans. Journal of Nursing Administration, 6 (1), Jan 1976, 25-31.

30 Evenson, B.O. Teaching quality assurance. Nurse Educator, 5 (2), Mar/Apr 1980, 8-12.

31 Felton, G. and others Pathway to accountability: implementation of a quality assurance program. Journal of Nursing Administration, 6 (1), Jan 1976, 20-24.

32 Fifer, W.R. Quality assurance: debate persists on goals, impact, and methods of evaluating care. (Review of 1978 literature.) Hospitals, 53 (7), 1 Apr 1979, 163-167.

33 Finkelman, A.W. The standards of nursing practice and the supervisor. (Using the American Nurses Association Standard.) Supervisor Nurse, 7 (5), May 1976, 31-34.

34 Froebe, D.J. and Bain, R.J. Quality assurance programs and controls in nursing. St. Louis: Mosby, 1976.

35 Gallant, B.W. and McLane, A.M. Outcome criteria: a process for validation at the unit level. (Research study to devise method for evaluating nursing care.) Journal of Nursing Administration, 9 (1), Jan 1979, 14-21.

36 Gassett, H. 'Q' for 'Q' — Quest for quality assurance. (Evaluation of nursing care at Presbyterian Hospital, Albuquerque.) Supervisor Nurse, 8 (2), Feb 1977, 29-31, 35.

37 Gray, G. Measurement of care — it's a long path. (Review of methods of measuring quality of nursing care.) Australian Nurses Journal, 8 (4), Oct 1978, 34-37, 43.

38 Grayshon, J. Nurse could you care more? (Observations by a nurse who is ex-patient.) Nursing Times, 75, 8 Nov 1979, 1919.

39 Haussmann, R.K.D. and others Monitoring quality of nursing care. 2. Assessment and study of correlates. 3. Professional review for nursing: an empirical investigation. Bethesda, Md.: US Department of Health, Education and Welfare, 1976-1977.

40 Haussmann, R.K. and Hegyvary, S.T. Monitoring the quality of nursing care (by continuous assessment of the nursing process). Australian Nurses Journal, 5 (8), Feb 1976, 29-32, 36.

41 Hegedus, K.S. A patient outcome criterion measure. (Research study to evaluate the Volicer Hospital Stress Rating Scale as measure of effectiveness of nursing care.) Supervisor Nurse, 10 (1), Jan 1979, 40-45.

42 Hegyvary, S.T. and Haussmann, R.K.D. Correlates of the quality of nursing care. (Study

of 102 patient care units in 19 hospitals in the U.S.A.) Journal of Nursing Administration, 6 (9), Nov 1976, 22-27.

43 Hegyvary, S.T. and Haussmann, R.K.D. Monitoring nursing care quality. (Method focusing on the nursing process and delivery of nursing care pilot tested in two hospitals.) Journal of Nursing Administration, 6 (9), Nov 1976, 3-9.

44 Hegyvary, S.T. and Haussmann, R.K.D. Nursing professional review. (Proposal for development and issues and problems involved.) Journal of Nursing Administration, 6 (9), Nov 1976, 12-16.

45 Hill, B.S. The missing ingredient in quality assurance programs. (Satisfying factors — responsibility, creativity, achievement/recognition and growth). Supervisor Nurse, 10 (11), Nov 1979, 19, 22.

46 Hofford, E.C. Standards of nursing care. (Changes during the last 10 years and the resulting quality of care.) Nursing Times, 72, 16 Sep 1976, 1439-1442.

47 Horswill, K. A study of nursing quality assurance programs in Wisconsin. Wisconsin Regional Medical Program, 1975.

48 Hover, J. and Zimmer, M.J. Nursing quality assurance: the Wisconsin system. (Defines its population groups broadly, thus reducing the number of criteria sets needed.) Nursing Outlook, 26 (4), Apr 1978, 242-248.

49 Jacobs, C.M. and others Measuring the quality of patient care: the rationale for outcome audit. Cambridge, Mass.: Ballinger, 1976.

50 Journal of Nursing Administration Quality control and performance appraisal: a reader. Wakefield, Mass.: Contemporary Publishing, 1976.

51 Joyce, A. Systematic review: you can afford it. (Review of nursing care conducted by senior staff, based on individual care plans and interviews with patients and staff.) Supervisor Nurse, 8 (9), Sep 1977, 13-18.

52 Kinross, N.J. Evaluating the quality of nursing care. New Zealand Nursing Journal, 70 (3), Mar 1977, 3-5.

53 Kneedler, J.A. and others From standards into practice. (Seven articles on the standards relating to each step in the planning and evaluation of care.) AORN Journal, 28 (4), Oct 1978, 603-637, 640, 642.

54 Laros, J. Deriving outcome criteria from a conceptual model. (A nursing model as a means of evaluating the quality of care.) Nursing Outlook, 25 (5), May 1977, 333-336.

55 Lenburg, C.B. Criteria for developing clinical performance evaluation. New York: NLN, 1976.

56 Lindeman, C.A. Measuring quality of nursing care. 2 parts. (Research procedures and current projects.) Journal of Nursing Administration, 6 (5), Jun 1976, 7-9; (7), Sep 1976, 16-19.

57 McClure, M.L. ANA standards for nursing services: considerations in evaluation. Supervisor Nurse, 7 (8), Aug 1976, 27, 30-31.

58 McClure, M.L. Quality assurance and

nursing education: a nursing service director's view. Nursing Outlook, 24 (6), Jun 1976, 367-369.

59 McFarlane, J.K. Take aim and shoot for goal. (Standards of nursing care, evaluation and the nursing process.) Nursing Mirror, 148, 19 Apr 1979 Supplement xx, xxiii-xxiv, xxvi, xxviii-xxix.

60 Majesky, S.J. and others Development of a research tool: Patient Indicators of Nursing Care. (List of physiological indicators showing complications accountable to nurses, eg skin ulceration.) Nursing Research, 27 (6), Nov/Dec 1978, 365-371.

61 Marriner, A. The research process in quality assurance. (Methods of evaluating quality of nursing care with ANA's Standards of Nursing Practice.) American Journal of Nursing, 79 (12), Dec 1979, 2158-2161.

62 Martin, N.S. Clinical management models: staff education curriculum for quality assurance. Supervisor Nurse, 10 (11), Nov 1979, 24, 26, 28.

63 Martin, P.J. Quality assurance in Australia. Australian Nurses Journal, 9 (7), Feb 1980, 45-49.

64 Mason, E.J. How to write meaningful nursing standards. New York: Wiley, 1978.

65 Mayers, M.G. and others Quality assurance for patient care: nursing perspectives. New York: Appleton-Century-Crofts, 1977.

66 National League for Nursing Pathways to quality care. New York: NLN, 1976.

67 National League for Nursing. Department of Baccalaureate and Higher Degree Programs. Quality assurance: models for nursing education. New York: NLN, 1976.

68 New Zealand Nurses' Association Standards for nursing services. New Zealand Nursing Journal, 71 (8), Aug 1978, 7-9.

69 Nicholls, M.E. and Wessells, V.G. editors Nursing standards and nursing process. Wakefield, Mass.: Contemporary Publishing Co., 1977.

70 Nursing Times Nurse could you care more? (Account by a nurse of poor standard of care given to her husband while hospitalised.) Nursing Times, 74, 7 Dec 1978, 2009.

71 Nursing Times Nurse could you care more? (Instances of nurses' thoughtless actions described by two clinical teachers.) Nursing Times, 75, 10 May 1979, 776.

72 Nursing Times Nurse could you care more? (Comment by nurse on ways in which nursing care is lacking, with checklist of points to improve care.) Nursing Times, 74, 16 Nov 1978, 1882-1883.

73 Pembrey, S. Standards in nursing. Address to the Rcn professional conference in Guernsey. Nursing Times, 75, 17 May 1979, 814-815.

74 Phaneuf, M.C. Model for quality: a matrix. AORN Journal, 23 (5), Apr 1976, 759-765.

75 Phaneuf, M.C. Quality assurance: a nursing view. (Reprinted from Hospitals, 47, 16

Oct 1973, 62-68.) New Zealand Nursing Journal, 69 (2), Feb 1976, 9-11.

76 Pitts, A. Standards for nursing—their impact on quality care. (New Zealand Nursing Association standards.) New Zealand Nursing Journal, 73 (3), Mar 1980, 3-7.

77 Plant, J. Various approaches proposed to assess quality in long-term care. Appraisal methods range from patient questionnaire to survey of setting, patients, staff and records. Hospitals, 51, 1 Sep 1977, 93-94, 96-98.

78 Potter, A. Standards of nursing care. (Role of nurse manager.) Nursing Focus, 1 (2), Oct 1979, 85, 87, 89.

79 Prescott, P.A. Cost-effectiveness: tool or trap? (One aspect of measurement of quality of care.) Nursing Outlook, 27 (11), Nov 1979, 722-728.

80 Prescott, P.A. Evaluation research: issues in evaluation of nursing programs. Nursing Administration Quarterly, 2 (4), Summer 1978, 63-80.

81 Ring, D.S. What can we do better? Our professional performance committee is finding plenty of answers. (On ways to improve patient care and nursing standards.) RN Magazine, 40 (10), Oct 1977, 60-61.

82 Rinneard, B. Nurses need written standards. Hospital Administration in Canada, 19 (11), Nov 1977, 35.

83 Royal College of Nursing. Working Committee on Standards of Nursing Care
Standards of nursing care. Rcn, 1980. Chairman: S.M. Quinn. Towards standards: a discussion document. Second report of the Working Committee. 1981.

84 Rule, J.B. Raising standards of care—what can we afford? What needs? Who cares? Royal Society of Health Journal, 96 (5), Oct 1976, 204-208.

85 Schmadl, J.C. Quality assurance: examination of the concept. Nursing Outlook, 27 (7), Jul 1979, 462-465.

86 Selvaggi, L.M. and others Implementing a quality assurance program in nursing. (Jackson Memorial Hospital, Florida.) Journal of Nursing Administration, 6 (7), Sep 1976, 37-43.

87 Shetland, M.L. Nursing standards: who, why, what and how? Wellington: New Zealand Nursing Education and Research Foundation, 1976.

88 Shetland, M.L. On nursing standards (in the context of social change.) New Zealand Nursing Journal, 68 (12), Dec 1975, 11-14.

89 Shetland, M.L. On nursing standards. (Seminar paper.) New Zealand Nursing Journal, 69 (2), Feb 1976, 4-8.

90 Smith, B.J. Standards of nursing. (Correspondence.) Hospital and Health Services Review, 72 (9), Sep 1976, 317-318.

91 Smith, J.P. Editorial. Evaluation in nursing. (Review of recent studies in practice and education, with short bibliography.) Journal of Advanced Nursing, 3 (2), Mar 1978, 111-112.

92 Stevens, B.J. ANA's standards for nursing services: how do they measure up? Journal of Nursing Administration, 6 (4), May 1976, 29-31.

93 Sweatingen, D. and others Improving patient care through measurement; goal importance and achievement scaling. (Goal-oriented record keeping and procedure for quantifying judgments of goal importance and achievement.) Journal of Psychiatric Nursing and Mental Health Services, 15 (9), Sep 1977, 30-36.

94 Taylor, G. Quality assurance programs in nursing: an overview. Lamp, 35 (2), Feb 1978, 4-7.

95 Tescher, B.E. and Colavecchio, R. Definition of a standard for clinical nursing practice. (Developed at the University of California, San Francisco. Includes job descriptions of clinical nurses.) Journal of Nursing Administration, 7 (3), Mar 1977, 32-34.

96 Tucker, S.M. and others Patient care standards. St. Louis: Mosby, 1975. 2nd ed. 1980.

97 University of Wisconsin-Extension Department of Nursing. Health Services Unit
Quality assurance: scripts from a series of tapes developed for nursing dial access. The University, 1975.

98 Ventura, M.R. and Crosby, F. Preparing the nurse observer to use the quality patient care scale: a modular approach. Journal of Continuing Education in Nursing, 9 (6), Nov/Dec 1978, 37-40.

99 Ventura, M.R. and others Interrater reliabilities for two measures of nursing care quality. (QualPacs and Rush-Medicus instrument.) Research in Nursing and Health, 3 (1), Mar 1980, 25-32.

100 Wandelt, M.A. and Ager, J.W. Quality patient care scale. New York: Appleton-Century-Crofts, 1974.

101 Watson, A. and Mayers, M. Evaluating the quality of patient care through retrospective chart review. Journal of Nursing Administration, 6 (3), Mar/Apr 1976, 17-21.

102 Weinstein, E.L. Developing a measure of the quality of nursing care (at the Hospital for Sick Children in Toronto.) Journal of Nursing Administration, 6 (6), Aug 1976, 1-3.

103 Williams, L.J. Observations on the use of a quality monitoring instrument. (Rush-Medicus quality monitoring tool.) Australian Nurses Journal, 9 (9), Apr 1980, 25-27.

104 Williams, L.J. Which tool for measuring quality of care? (Review of methods.) Australian Nurses Journal, 9 (11), Jun 1980, 47-49.

105 World Health Organization. Working Group on the Evaluation of Inpatient Nursing Practice Summary report, Regensburg 18-21 Oct 1977. Geneva: WHO, 1977.

106 World Health Organization. Regional Office for Europe Evaluation of inpatient nursing practice: report on a Working Group. Geneva: WHO, 1979. (EURO reports and studies, 4.)

d NURSING AUDIT

1 Benedikter, H. From nursing audit to multi-disciplinary audit. New York: NLN, 1977.

2 Davidson, S.V.S. editor PSRO: utilization and audit in patient care. St. Louis: Mosby, 1976.

3 Deets, C. and Schmidt, A. Process criteria based on standards. (Conceptual framework for developing criteria to evaluate nursing care by audit.) AORN Journal, 26 (4), Oct 1977, 685-686, 688, 691.

4 Doughty, D.B. and Mash, N.J. Nursing audit. Philadelphia: Davis, 1977.

5 Dunham, C.W. A quality of patient care project. (An audit model developed by the California Nurses, Medical and Hospital Associations.) Supervisor Nurse, 7 (4), Apr 1976, 34-36, 38.

6 Foster, W. and others Hospital/community/education nursing audit—a research enterprise. (In South Glamorgan, of all grades of nursing staff with paramedical and medical staff involved.) Nursing Mirror, 145, 8 Dec 1977, 26-28.

7 Galton, M. and Reilly, M. Evaluation of nursing care through a nursing audit: a research project. Australian Nurses Journal, 6 (11), May 1977, 34-37.

8 Hanna, K.K. Nursing audit at a community hospital. (A model for evaluating nursing care used in a California hospital.) Nursing Outlook, 24 (1), Jan 1976, 33-37.

9 Holmes, A. McD. Problem-oriented medical records, nursing audit and accountability. Supervisor Nurse, 11 (4), Apr 1980, 40, 42-43.

10 Hurwitz, L.S. and Tasch, V. Developing a quality assurance program in nursing. (Description of program which progressed from nursing audit to interdisciplinary audit.) Supervisor Nurse, 8 (6), Jun 1977, 50-51, 54-55, 58-59.

11 Joyce, A. Systematic review: you can afford it. (Review of nursing care conducted by senior staff, based on individual care plans and interviews with patients and staff.) Supervisor Nurse, 8 (9), Sep 1977, 13-18.

12 Karch, A.M. Concurrent nursing audit. Thorofare, N.J.: Charles B. Slack, 1980.

13 King, B. Continuing nursing audit. (To measure quality of nursing care.) Australian Nurses Journal, 8 (7), Feb 1979, 36-38.

14 Kneedler, J.A. Corrective action completes audit cycle. (Implementation of audit information.) AORN Journal, 26 (3), Sep 1977, 485-494.

15 Langill, G. and Finch, E. A computer assisted nursing audit program. Dimensions in Health Service, 55 (3), Mar 1978, 36-37.

16 McNally, F. Nursing audit: evolution without pain. (Objectives outlined and explanation of terminology in nursing language.) Supervisor Nurse, 8 (6), Jun 1977, 40, 45, 46.

17 Martin, P.J. Haste, resistance and the nursing audit. (Conference paper.) Australian Nurses Journal, 9 (2), Aug 1979, 39-42.

18 Martin, P.J. One meter stick—the nursing audit. (Critical evaluation of its value with reference to nursing in Australia.) Journal of Advanced Nursing, 5 (2), Mar 1980, 199-208.

19 Middleton, G. Special audit of critical

incidents. (And the nursing action taken.) Dimensions in Health Service, 56 (8), Aug 1979, 22.

20 Moore, K.R. What nurses learn from nursing audit. (Evaluating quality of care with individual patients.) Nursing Outlook, 27 (4), Apr 1979, 254-258.

21 Nadolny, M.D. The patient care audit. What is it? When did it start? Why? Where is it going? Hospital Topics, 57 (6), Nov/Dec 1979, 30-33.

22 Padilla, G.V. Incorporating research in a service setting. (Recommends nursing audit as institutional mechanism for implementing and sustaining research activities.) Journal of Nursing Administration, 9 (1), Jan 1979, 44-49.

23 Phaneuf, M.C. The nursing audit: self-regulation in nursing practice. 2nd ed. New York: Appleton-Century-Crofts, 1976.

24 Schmidt, A. and Deets, C. Responsibility for audit criteria. (Which professional group is responsible for achievement of each criterion.) AORN Journal, 27 (4), Mar 1978, 657-662.

25 Schmidt, A. and Deets, C. Writing measurable nursing audit criteria. AORN Journal, 26 (3), Sep 1977, 495-499.

26 Trussell, P.M. and Strand, N. A comparison of concurrent and retrospective audits on the same patients. Journal of Nursing Administration, 8 (5), May 1978, 33-38.

27 Ventura, M.R. Correlation between the quality patient care scale and the Phaneuf Audit. (Research study.) International Journal of Nursing Studies, 17 (3), 1980, 155-162.

28 Wiseman, J. A nursing audit of basic care, or Nursing A.B.C. (Blackpool Nursing Service Audit.) Nursing Times, 42, 2 Dec 1976, Occ. papers, 169-172; 9 Dec 1976, Occ. papers, 173-176.

29 Wiseman, J. A nursing audit of basic care. Further developments and a critical evaluation. (Of the Blackpool system.) Nursing Times, 73, 27 Oct 1977, Occ. papers, 137-140; 3 Nov 1977, Occ. papers, 141-143.

e NURSING CARE PLAN

1 Baldwin, S.M. Made to measure care. (Planning nursing care based on scientific principles and the setting of objectives.) Nursing Times, 72 (12), 25 Mar 1976, 468-469.

2 Bowens, B. and Rodgers, T. Patient care planning through the phases of hospitalization. (Four phases—admission, diagnostic, therapeutic and convalescent/discharge.) Journal of Neurosurgical Nursing, 11 (1), Mar 1979, 48-52.

3 Bower, F.L. The process of planning nursing care: a model for practice. 2nd ed. St. Louis: Mosby, 1977.

4 Bryant, R.B. Problem-oriented nursing care plans. (In use at Royal Adelaide Hospital.) Australian Nurses Journal, 10 (1), Jul 1980, 35-36.

5 Caruso, M.M. and Thompson, M. POR and nursing care plan: an integrated system. (With example of standard care plan used in rehabilitation institute.) AORN Journal, 4 (4), Jul/Aug 1979, 8-9.

6 Christensen, J.C. Planning nursing care. New Zealand Nursing Journal, 69 (4), Apr 1976, 3-7.

7 Clarke, M. Planning nursing care: recent past, present and future. (Review focusing on the planning of nursing care as part of the role of the nurse.) Nursing Times, 74, 16 Feb 1978, Occ. papers, 17-20.

8 Dincher, J.R. and Stidger, S.L. Evaluation of a written simulation format for clinical nursing judgment: a pilot study. Nursing Research, 25 (4), Jul/Aug 1976, 280-285.

9 Eaton, C. Nursing care plans and the private duty home care patient. (Care study of private patient nursed at home, with care plan.) Canadian Nurse, 76 (1), Jan 1980, 25-27.

10 Forman, M. Building a better nursing care plan. American Journal of Nursing, 79 (6), Jun 1979, 1086-1087.

11 Grier, M.R. Decision making about patient care. (Study to establish nurses' ability to quantify decisions about patient care in four situations.) Nursing Research, 25 (2), Mar-Apr 1976, 105-110.

12 Hunt, J. and Marks-Maran, D. Nursing care plans: the nursing process at work, Aylesbury, HM&M, 1980. Recipe for change. (Interview with Alison Dunn.) Nursing Times, 76, 18 Sep 1980, 1646-1647.

13 Jackson, C. and others Promoting written care plans: a small study of the use of 'verbal and nonverbal feedback'. Supervisor Nurse, 9 (8), Aug 1978, 43-47.

14 Janz, N. and others How shared nursing rounds pay off. (Nurses in different units meet to discuss nursing care problems.) RN Magazine, 40 (3), Mar 1977, 45-48.

15 Jones, E.S. A patient allocation trial. (Based on the nursing care plan Kardex used by the North Lothian Group of Hospitals.) Nursing Times, 73, 17 Mar 1977, 390-392.

16 Little, D.E. and Carnevali, D.L. Nursing care planning. 2nd ed. Philadelphia: Lippincott, 1976.

17 McCloskey, J.C. The nursing care plan, past, present and the uncertain future—a review of the literature. Nursing Forum, 14 (4), 1975, 364-382.

18 Mackie, L. Teaching the nursing process: revitalising the nursing care plan. (Reintroduction of nursing care plans on trial ward and later whole surgical unit.) Nursing Times, 75, 23 Aug 1979, 1440-1442.

19 Malloy, J.L. Taking exception to problem oriented nursing care. (Planning nursing care by defining behavioural objectives compared with the problem approach.) American Journal of Nursing, 76 (4), Apr 1976, 582-583.

20 Marks-Maran, D. Introducing individual care plans. (As part of a research project on the implementation of the nursing process at the London Hospital.) Nursing Times, 74, 30 Nov 1978 Supplement 18-19.

21 Marks-Maran, D. Problem oriented nursing care plans. Medical Record, 20 (2), May 1979, 501-509.

22 Mayers, M.G. A systematic approach to

the nursing care plan. 2nd ed. New York: Appleton-Century-Crofts, 1978.

23 Nichols, E.G. and Barstow, R.E. Do nurses really use standard care plans? (Research study.) Journal of Nursing Administration, 10 (5), May 1980, 27-31.

24 Palmer, M.E. The nursing care plan: a tool for staff development. Wakefield, Mass.: Contemporary Publishing, 1977. (Contemporary nursing review, no.R.2.)

25 Porter, S.F. JCAH Nursing Standard IV. (Joint Commission on Accreditation of Hospitals standard on nursing care plans and documentation of nursing care.) Supervisor Nurse, 10 (11), Nov 1979, 32-33, 35.

26 Rehman, J.E. Writing patient care plans: a reference guide for nurses. San Diego: Professional Lecture Series Inc., 1976.

27 Schurr, M.C. Planning patient care. (Team nursing and patient allocation.) World of Irish Nursing, 7, (2/3), Feb/Mar 1978, 1-2, 5-6.

28 Silverthorn, A. Nursing care plans: a vital tool. (With example.) Canadian Nurse, 75 (3), Mar 1979, 36-41.

29 Sklar, C.L. The legal significance of charting. Canadian Nurse, 74 (3), Mar 1978, 10-11.

30 Snyder, P.J. Goal setting. (Nursing care plans including discharge planning.) Supervisor Nurse, 9 (9), Sep 1978, 61-62, 64.

31 Vitale, B.A. and others A problem solving approach to nursing care plans: a program. St. Louis: Mosby, 1974. 2nd ed. 1978.

f NURSING RECORDS

1 Baggaley, S. Deficiencies in traditional reporting and recording techniques. (Research study.) Australian Nurses Journal, 8 (9), Apr 1979, 30-31.

2 Baumann, B.A. The integrated progress record. (Record of patient's progress from admission to discharge with doctors' and nurses' notes on same record.) Supervisor Nurse, 8 (8), Aug 1977, 29-35.

3 Bernhardt, J.H. Record keeping—key to professional accountability. (In OH nursing.) Occupational Health Nursing, 26 (8), Aug 1978, 22-28.

4 Billings, C.V. Documentation—the supervisor's dream. (Auditing of charts to establish standards for nursing records.) Supervisor Nurse, 9 (9), Oct 1978, 16-17, 20.

5 Blount, M. and others Documenting with the problem-oriented record system. (Description of forms developed to implement system.) American Journal of Nursing, 78 (9), Sep 1978, 1539-1542.

6 Castledine, G. Keeping our records straight. (Reasons for improving nursing records.) Nursing Mirror, 148, 3 May 1979, 12.

7 DOCUMENTING patient care responsibly. Horsham: International Communications, 1978.

8 Gassett, H. Participative planned charge. (Project introducing the keeping of nursing records by the patients' bedside proposed and implemented by an all-professional nursing group.) Supervisor Nurse, 7 (3), Mar 1976, 34-35, 39-40.

9 Germaine, A. and Rinneard, B. How effectively do you use your incident/accident report? (The importance to nursing departments.) Hospital Administration in Canada, 18 (8), Aug 1976, 24-26.

10 Gwynne, A.L. The legal importance of nursing notes. Nursing Times, 74, 13 Jul 1978, 1161-1162.

11 Hanchett, E.S. The problem oriented system: a literature review. United States Department of Health, Education and Welfare, 1978. (Nurse planning information series, no.3.)

12 Harris, R.J. Facilitating change to the problem-oriented medical record system. (Report of interdisciplinary project and obstacles encountered.) Journal of Nursing Administration, 8 (8), Aug 1978, 35-38.

13 Hill, P. Resurrecting untapped wealth. (Medical and nursing records.) Health and Social Service Journal, 89, 8 Jun 1979, 694-697.

14 Holdich, R.J. The importance of patient care records. (Medical records, including automation and problems of confidentiality.) Nursing Times, 74, 13 Jul 1978, 1159-1161.

15 Lee, P. No half measures. (Problems in using standardised nursing history sheet.) Nursing Times, 76, 26 Jun 1980, 1121.

16 McGugin, M.B. and others An andragogical approach to teaching the problem-oriented method of recording (POR). (Andragogy—the art and science of helping adults learn.) Journal of Continuing Education in Nursing, 10 (1), Jan/Feb 1979, 7-11.

17 Mancini, M. Documenting clinical records. (Legal aspects of record-keeping.) American Journal of Nursing, 78 (9), Sep 1978, 1556, 1561.

18 Pepper, G.A. Bedside report: would it work for you? (Change-of-shift report at bedside and involving patient.) Nursing, 8 (6), Jun 1978, 74-75.

19 Peterson, G. The SOAP revolution. 2 parts. (Problem oriented nursing and medical records.) Journal of Practical Nursing, 27 (8), Aug 1977, 36-38; (9), Sep 1977, 32-35.

20 Prendergast, J.A. Implementing problem-oriented records in a primary nursing system. Nursing Clinics of North America, 12 (2), Jun 1977, 235-246.

21 Schreiber, L.A. and Van Den Heever, K.D. Have you tried the 'Problem oriented nursing record?' (Objectives and value, with example.) S.A. Nursing Journal, 44 (8), Aug 1977, 9-11.

22 Steckel, S.B. Utilization of reinforced contracts to increase written evidence of the nursing assessment. (Setting goals to encourage nurses to write more detailed nursing records.) Nursing Research, 25 (1), Jan-Feb 1976, 58-61.

23 Supervisor Nurse Issue on problem oriented record and nursing care plans. Supervisor Nurse, 8 (1), Jan 1977, 12-32.

24 Ulisse, G.C. POMR: application to nursing records. Menlo Park: Addison-Wesley, 1978.

25 Vaughan-Wrobel, B.C. and Henderson, B. The problem-oriented system: a workbook. St. Louis: Mosby, 1976.

26 Walter, J.B. and others, editors Dynamics of problem-oriented approaches: patient care and documentation. Philadelphia: Lippincott, 1976.

27 Woolley, F.R. and Kane, R.L. Telling it like it is through problem orientation. (Problem oriented records and nursing audit.) Nursing Care, 9 (6), Jun 1976, 25-27.

g NURSING DIAGNOSIS

1 Advances in Nursing Science Issue on nursing diagnosis. Advances in Nursing Science, 2 (1), Oct 1979, 1-100.

2 Aspinall, M.J. Nursing diagnosis—the weak link. (Learning the skill of nursing diagnosis to effect adequate nursing care.) Nursing Outlook, 24 (7), Jul 1976, 433-437.

3 Aspinall, M.J. Use of a decision tree to improve accuracy of diagnosis. Nursing Research, 28 (3), May/Jun 1979, 182-185.

4 Aspinall, M.J. and others The why and how of nursing diagnosis. MCN, 2 (6), Nov/Dec 1977, 355-358.

5 Baer, E.D. and others How to take a health history. American Journal of Nursing, 77 (7), Jul 1977, 1190-1193.

6 Bircher, A.U. On the development and classification of diagnoses. Nursing Forum, 14 (1), 1975, 10-29.

7 Byers, V.B. Nursing observation. 3rd ed. Dubuque: Brown, 1977. (Foundations of nursing series).

8 Campbell, C. Nursing diagnosis and intervention in nursing practice. New York: Wiley, 1978.

9 Chalmers, H. Return to basics. 3. Look and see. (Observation of patients.) Nursing Mirror, 145, 21 Jul 1977 Nursing care supplement series 5, i-iv.

10 Dossey, B. Perfecting your skills for systematic patient assessments. Nursing (U.S.), 9 (2), Feb 1979, 42-45.

11 Eggland, E.T. How to take a meaningful nursing history. Nursing, 77 (7), Jul 1977, 22-30.

12 Fitzsimons, V.M. and Gallagher, L.P. Physical assessment skills: a historical perspective. Nursing Forum, 17 (4), 1978, 344-355.

13 Fuhs, M.F. How nursing diagnosis helps focus your care: 'it seems like acute respiratory dysfunction'.... RN Magazine, 42 (10), Oct 1979, 51-54.

14 Gordon, M. Nursing diagnosis: looking at its use in the clinical area. (Evaluation from discharge records of use of nursing diagnosis.) American Journal of Nursing, 80 (4), Apr 1980, 672-674.

15 Gordon, M. Nursing diagnoses and the diagnostic process. American Journal of Nursing, 76 (8), Aug 1976, 1298-1300.

16 Gordon, M. Predictive strategies in diagnostic tasks. (Factors affecting nurses' ability to take nursing histories and make nursing diagnoses.) Nursing Research, 29 (1), Jan/Feb 1980, 39-45.

17 Henderson, B. Nursing diagnosis: theory and practice. Advances in Nursing Science, 1 (1), Oct 1978, 75-83.

18 Jackson, B.S. and Mantle, D.D. Teaching patient assessment: the pros and cons of clinical rounds. Journal of Nursing Education, 16 (2), Feb 1977, 24-29.

19 Jarvis, C.M. Perfecting physical assessment. Nursing, 77 (5), May 1977, 28-37; (6), Jun 1977, 38-45.

20 Kesler, A.R. Pitfalls to avoid in interviewing outpatients. (Advice on taking a health history.) Nursing, 7 (9), Sep 1977, 70-73.

21 Larkin, P.D. and Backer, B.A. Problem-oriented nursing assessment. New York: McGraw-Hill, 1977.

22 Lash, A.A. A re-examination of nursing diagnosis. Nursing Forum, 17 (4), 1978, 332-343.

23 McVan, B. Odors. What the nose knows. (Use of olfactory sense in identifying diseases.) Nursing, 77 (4), Apr 1977, 46-49.

24 Mahoney, E.A. and others How to collect and record a health history. Philadelphia: Lippincott, 1976.

25 Malasanos, L. and others Health assessment. St. Louis: Mosby, 1977.

26 Oermann, M. Diagnostic supervision. (Staff development as part of charge nurse's role.) Supervisor Nurse, 8 (11), Nov 1977, 9-11, 14.

27 Price, M.R. How nursing diagnosis helps focus your care: the patient is starving but why? RN Magazine, 42 (11), Nov 1979, 45-48.

28 Price, M.R. Nursing diagnosis: making a concept come alive. American Journal of Nursing, 80 (4), Apr 1980, 668-671.

29 Roberts, A. Systems of life. No.63. Systems and signs: introduction. (Ways of assessing patient's condition by looking, feeling etc.) Nursing Times, 76, 6 Mar 1980 (4).

30 Ross, M. Learning to observe. (Evaluation of course on learning observational skills.) Nursing Papers, 11 (1/2), 1979, 46-54.

31 Wheeler, R. and others Nursing assessment. New York: Wiley, 1977. (Wiley nursing concept modules).

32 Wilson, G. Nursing diagnosis (assessment) and changing accountability. Australian Nurses Journal, 9 (10), May 1980, 36-38.

h PATIENT ASSIGNMENT

1 Corry, M.F. Will patient assignment improve nursing care? New Zealand Nursing Journal, 69 (2), Feb 1976, 24-26.

2 Jones, W.J. Management by crisis or by objectives? 2 parts. (Experiences of patient allocation in a 24 bed female medical ward.) Nursing Times, 73, 10 Mar 1977, 342-343; 73, 17 Mar 1977, 388-390.

3 Plumpton, M. Experiments in nurse-patient

allocation. (Subjective assessment of success of various methods at the London Hospital.) Nursing Times, 74, 9 Mar 1978, 417-419.

i PATIENT CENTRED CARE

1 Barham, V. A patient oriented nursing system starting as an interdisciplinary project on the postsurgical service. Journal of Nursing Administration, 6 (2), Feb 1976, 40-42.

2 Collett, P. Why patient-centred care? (Team nursing and patient assignment.) New Zealand Nursing Journal, 70 (6), Jun 1977, 25-27.

3 Ellis, B. The all-RN staff: why not? (Evidence shows that patient-centred care produces higher standard of care than team nursing and is now an increased trend.) Hospitals, 52 (20), 16 Oct 1978, 107-108, 110, 112.

4 Isler, C. Rx for a sick hospital: primary nursing care. (With comments from other nurses, p.67.) RN Magazine, 39 (2), Feb 1976, 60-65.

5 Journal of Nursing Administration Primary nursing. Wakefield, Mass.: Contemporary Publishing, 1977.

6 Mackay, C. and Ault, L.D. A systematic approach to individualizing nursing care. (Transition from a task oriented approach to care at the Veterans Administration Hospital, Palo Alto.) Journal of Nursing Administration, 7 (1), Jan 1977, 39-48.

7 Parkin, M.M.W. Primary nursing — an American experience. (Description of implementation on author's ward.) Australian Nurses Journal, 9 (1), Jul 1979, 35-36.

8 Riutta, S. Patient centered procedures. (Drawing up a procedure manual on the basis of patient centred, as opposed to task oriented delivery of care.) Supervisor Nurse, 7 (4), Apr 1976, 30-31.

j TEAM NURSING

1 Daulby, C.N. A study in staffing. (Pilot staffing scheme in a 32 bed surgical ward to introduce team nursing.) Australian Nurses Journal, 7 (5), Dec 1977, 2-6.

2 Graham, J.C. and others Involvement attitudes in medical service organizations. (Survey to measure the team approach to patient care.) Supervisor Nurse, 7 (8), Aug 1976, 9-11, 14-16.

3 Kelly, P.A. and Lambert, K.L. The effect of a modified team approach: on nurse-patient interaction and job satisfaction. (Report and evaluation of year-long experiment with permanent teams.) Journal of Nursing Administration, 7 (4), Apr 1978, 3-9.

4 Lewis, M. Teamwork and morale. Nursing Mirror, 148, 24 May 1979, 32.

5 Pearson, S. Team spirit. (Introduction of team nursing on a surgical ward at Brompton Hospital.) Nursing Mirror, 142 (16), 15 Apr 1976, 62-64.

k TOTAL PATIENT CARE
(Primary Nursing Care)

1 Allen, P. Joint practice in a large, urban

hospital. (Sharing of responsibility between doctors and nurses in a scheme which involves primary nursing.) AORN Journal, 29 (7), Jun 1979, 1257-1262.

2 Anderson, M. Primary nursing in day by day practice. American Journal of Nursing, 76 (5), May 1976, 802-805.

3 Anderson, M. and Choi, T. Primary nursing in an organizational context. (One-to-one nurse/patient relationship analysed from administrative point of view.) Journal of Nursing Administration, 10 (3), Mar 1980, 26-31.

4 Andrews, G.A. and others Complete nursing care. 2. (Views of ward sister, student nurses, NO and SNO on implementation of total patient care. For Part 1 see Morland.) Nursing Times, 76, 21 Aug 1980, 1484-1487.

5 Bartels, D. and others The role of the head nurse in primary nursing. Canadian Nurse, 73 (3), Mar 1977, 26-30.

6 Baskin, P. Primary nursing: Australia's emerging patterns. Australian Nurses Journal, 9 (9), Apr 1980, 28-31.

7 Beltran, H. and others An adaptation of primary nursing. (Including non-professional personnel.) Supervisor Nurse, 10 (7), Jul 1979, 16-19.

8 Brooker, R. There is a better way. (Evaluation of staff's and patients' attitudes to and costs of implementation of primary nursing in Concord, New South Wales.) Australian Nurses Journal, 9 (3), Sep 1979, 54-57.

9 Carey, R.G. Evaluation of a primary nursing unit. (Personalised patient care including primary nursing, decentralisation of services and unit management.) American Journal of Nursing, 79 (7), Jul 1979, 1253-1255.

10 Castledine, G. 'My nurse' — and 'my patient'. (Author describes his experience of implementing primary nursing.) Nursing Mirror, 151, 7 Aug 1980, 14.

11 Ciske, K.L. Accountability: the essence of primary nursing. American Journal of Nursing, 79 (5), May 1979, 890-894.

12 Ciske, K.L. editor Primary nursing: advanced seminar. Nursing Dimensions, 7 (4), Winter 1980, 1-69.

13 Corn, F. and others Salvaging primary nursing. (Research study to determine if patient assignment improves health care and satisfaction of patients and job satisfaction of nurses.) Supervisor Nurse, 8 (5), May 1977, 19-21, 24-25.

14 Corpuz, T. Primary nursing meets needs, expectations of patients and staff. (Modular nursing, where an RN and a nursing assistant work as a collaborative unit to provide care for 8-10 patients.) Hospitals, 51 (11), 1 Jun 1977, 95-96, 98, 100.

15 Dahlen, A.L. 'With primary nursing we have it all together'. (Description of system at Meridian Park Hospital, Oregon.) American Journal of Nursing, 78 (3), Mar 1978, 426-429.

16 Dean, L.P. The change from functional to primary nursing. Nursing Clinics of North America, 14 (2), Jun 1979, 357-364.

17 Eichhorn, M.L. and Frevert, E.I. Evaluation of a primary nursing system using the

quality patient care scale. (QualPaCS). Journal of Nursing Administration, 9 (10), Oct 1979, 11-15.

18 Fairbanks, J. Primary nursing: what's so exciting about it? 2 parts. Nursing (U.S.), 10 (11), Nov 1980, 55-57; (12), Dec 1980, 58-61.

19 Flynn, K.T. Modes of delivery of patient care: primary or team nursing. Hospital Topics, 57 (6), Nov/Dec 1979, 34-40.

20 Frank-Stromborg, M. and Stromborg, P. Primary care assessment and management skills for nurses: a self-assessment manual. Philadelphia: Lippincott, 1979.

21 Giovannetti, P. A comparison of team and primary nursing care systems. Nursing Dimensions, 7 (4), Winter 1980, 96-100.

22 Hood, G.H. and Dincher, J.R. Total patient care: foundations and practice. St. Louis: Mosby. 5th ed. 1980.

23 Isler, C. Rx for a sick hospital: primary nursing care. (With comments from other nurses, p.67.) RN Magazine, 39 (2), Feb 1976, 60-65.

24 Journal of Nursing Administration Primary nursing: a selection of articles. Wakefield, Mass.: Contemporary Publishing, 1977.

25 Kachel, P. Primary nursing at Concord (R.G.H.) — it really does work. (Author describes implementation of scheme.) Australian Nurses Journal, 9 (10), May 1980, 48-50.

26 Keiser, G.J. and Bickle, I.M. Attitude change as a motivational factor in producing behavior change related to implementing primary nursing. Nursing Research, 29 (5), Sep/Oct 1980, 290-294.

27 Kocher, P. Should primary nursing replace team nursing? (Primary nursing defined as caring for patients on a one to one basis.) Nursing Care, 9 (2), Feb 1976, 32-33.

28 Kratz, C. Letter from Australia 2. Primary nursing. (Project at the Sir Charles Gairdner Hospital in Perth.) Nursing Times, 75, 18 Oct 1979, 1790-1791.

29 LaViolette, S. Does primary nursing offer solutions or cause problems? Modern Health Care, 9 (8), Aug 1979, 50-51.

30 Lee, M.E. Towards better care: 'primary nursing'. Nursing Times, 75, 20/27 Dec 1979, Occ. papers, 133-135.

31 McCarthy, D. and Schifalacqua, M.M. Primary nursing: its implementation and six month outcome. Journal of Nursing Administration, 8 (5), May 1978, 29-32.

32 McGreevy, M.E. and Coates, M.R. Primary nursing implementation using the project nurse and the nursing process framework. (Change from team nursing.) Journal of Nursing Administration, 10 (2), Feb 1980, 9-15.

33 Machiavelli, N. An assessment of primary nursing. (Study of effectiveness of total patient care according to six objectives.) Dimensions in Health Service, 55 (11), Nov 1978, 18, 20-22.

34 Manfredi, C. Primary nursing and change: a case study. Nursing Leadership, 3 (3), Sep 1980, 8-15.

35 Manthey, M. The practice of primary

nursing. Boston, Oxford: Blackwell Scientific, 1980.

36 Manthey, M. A theoretical framework for primary nursing. Journal of Nursing Administration, 10 (6), Jun 1980, 11-15.

37 Marram, G. The comparative costs of operating a team and primary nursing unit. (Study in a Boston hospital.) Journal of Nursing Administration, 6 (4), May 1976, 21-24.

38 Marram, G. and others Cost-effectiveness of primary and team nursing. Wakefield, Mass.: Contemporary Publishing, 1976.

39 Marram, G. and others Primary nursing: a model for individualized care. 2nd ed. St. Louis: Mosby, 1979.

40 Mathews, K. Deployment of registered nurses for primary nursing in the hospital setting. (Patient allocation to one nurse throughout patient's stay.) Australian Nurses Journal, 8 (1), Jul 1978, 34-35, 38.

41 Mayer, G.G. Adapting the patient care conference to primary nursing. Journal of Nursing Administration, 9 (6), Jun 1979, 7-10.

42 Moritz, D.A. Primary nursing: implications for curriculum development. Journal of Nursing Education, 18 (3), Mar 1979, 33-37.

43 Morland, R. Complete nursing care. 1. (Implementation of total patient care based on teams of nurses caring for 12 patients.) Nursing Times, 76, 14 Aug 1980, 1426-1429.

44 Munson, F. and Clinton, J. Defining nursing assigment patterns. (Method of measuring the assignment pattern in a unit, eg functional, team or primary nursing.) Nursing Research, 28 (4), Jul/Aug 1979, 243-249.

45 Munzig, N.C. Primary nursing—futurist nursing here today. (Research study of patients', nurses' and doctors' perceptions of primary nursing in a haemodialysis unit.) Journal of the American Association of Nephrology Nurses and Technicians, 6 (4), 1979, 200-207.

46 National League for Nursing Primary nursing: one nurse-one client planning care together. New York: NLN, 1977.

47 National League for Nursing The realities of primary nursing care: risk, roles, research. New York: NLN, 1978.

48 Nenner, V.C. and others Primary nursing. (Patient allocation from admission to discharge.) Supervisor Nurse, 8 (5), May 1977, 14-16.

49 Nursing Clinics of North America Symposium on primary nursing. (Nursing care of specific patient under the continuous guidance of one nurse from admission to discharge.) Nursing Clinics of North America, 12 (2), Jun 1977, 185-255.

50 Nursing Dimensions Primary nursing: advanced seminar. (19 articles.) Nursing Dimensions, 7 (4), Winter 1980, 1-69.

51 Nursing Dimensions Primary nursing: descriptive, analytical, and experimental research studies. (Seven articles edited by G.C. Mayer.) Nursing Dimensions, 7 (4), Winter 1980, 73-103.

52 Nursing Times Rediscovering the patient.

Macmillan Journals, 1978. (Supplement to Nursing Times, 30 Nov 1978).

53 Ojeda, M. Primary nursing for shortened stay surgical patients. Supervisor Nurse, 7 (9), Sep 1976, 42, 45, 48.

54 Osinski, E. and Gerhardt Powals, J. The all-RN staff three years later. (Measurement of patient, nurse and doctor satisfaction with primary nursing.) Supervisor Nurse, 9 (9), Oct 1978, 25-27.

55 Osinski, E.G. and Morrison, W.H. The all-RN staff. Primary nursing is logically complete when only professional nurses do the nursing. Supervisor Nurse, 9 (9), Sep 1978, 66, 69-70, 73-74.

56 Parkin, M.M.W. Primary nursing: an American experience. (Description of implementation on author's ward.) Australian Nurses Journal, 9 (1), Jul 1979, 35-36.

57 Raskin, P. Primary nursing: Australia's emerging patterns. Australian Nurses Journal, 9 (9), Apr 1980, 28-31.

58 Roberts, L.E. Primary nursing. (Pilot project at Victoria General Hospital Winnipeg to compare effectiveness with team nursing.) Canadian Nurse, 76 (11), Dec 1980, 20-23.

59 Spitzer, R. Making primary nursing work. Supervisor Nurse, 10 (1), Jan 1979, 12-14.

60 Tiffany, R. Mobilizing nursing skills. (Basing nursing care on the 'nursing model' with reference to personalised patient care at the Royal Marsden Hospital.) Journal of Advanced Nursing, 4 (1), Jan 1979, 3-8.

61 Urquhart, J.M. Primary nursing. A return to 'old fashioned nursing' with many new twists. How does it compare to team nursing? Journal of Practical Nursing, 28 (16), Oct 1978, 12-14.

62 Van Servellen, G.M. Primary nursing—the adoption of a nursing care modality. (Study to establish extent to which it is implemented in U.S.) Nursing and Health Care, 1 (3), Oct 1980, 144-149, 157.

63 Watson, J. Patient evaluation of a primary nursing project. (Survey of patients in wards using traditional nurse-patient assignment and primary nursing units.) Australian Nurses Journal, 8 (5), Jan 1979, 30-33, 49.

64 Watson, J. Primary nursing—nursing care can be patient centred. (Review of research studies and discussion of its implications.) Australian Nurses Journal, 7 (2), Aug 1977, 35-39, 54.

65 Williams, F.G. and Stewart, M.T. Pilot unit shifts to primary nursing. (From team nursing.) Hospitals, 54 (2), 16 Jan 1980, 112-115.

66 Zander, K.S. Primary nursing won't work ...unless the head nurse lets it. Journal of Nursing Administration, 7 (8), Oct 1977, 19-23.

67 Zander, K.S. Primary nursing: development and management. Germantown: Aspen Systems, 1980.

1 LONG TERM CARE

1 American Academy of Nursing Long-term care: some issues for nursing. Papers presented at

the annual meeting Sep 22-23, 1975. Kansas City: the Academy, 1976.

2 Benoliel, J.Q. and others Development of a social dependency scale. (In chronically ill patients.) Research in Nursing and Health, 3 (1), Mar 1980, 3-10.

3 Cang, S. and Clarke, F. Home care of the sick—an emerging general analysis based on schemes in France. Community Health, 9 (3), Feb 1978, 167-172.

4 Dodick, M. Individualised patient care. (At a hospital for chronic care and rehabilitation.) Health Care in Canada, 21 (4), Apr 1979, 48-49.

5 Kratz, C. Planning nursing care for the chronic sick. (Review of some of the variables underlying the care of the chronic sick.) Nursing Times, 74, 26 Jan 1978, Occ. papers, 9-12.

6 Lafek, E.V. and others Sample standard nursing care plans for residents in extended care units: a working document. Vancouver: Registered Nurses' Association of British Columbia, 1977.

7 McBrien, M. Long-term health care. (In Scotland.) Nursing Mirror, 146, 4 May 1978 Supplement ix-xi.

8 McCarthy, M. and Millard, P.H., editors Management of chronic illness: papers from a seminar. King Edward's Hospital Fund for London, 1979.

9 Patterson, K. Nursing care study. Care in chronic illness using a health profile. 2 parts. (Care by student nurse during period of district nursing experience.) Nursing Times, 76, 7 Aug 1980, 1387-1390; 14 Aug 1980, 1430-1435.

13 NURSING PRACTICE

a TEXTBOOKS

1 Arkhangelsky, G.V. editor Manual for nurses: nervous and psychic diseases, skin and venereal diseases, diseases of the nose, throat and ear, eye diseases, translated from the Russian by Ludmila Aksenova. Moscow: MIR Publishers, 1978.

2 Bell, B.M. Integrated basic theory and practice of nursing. Melbourne: Pitman Medical, 1979.

3 Bendall, E.R.D. and Raybould, E. Basic nursing. 4th ed. Lewis, 1977.

4 Beyers, M. and Dudas, S. The clinical practice of medical-surgical nursing. Boston: Little, Brown and Co., 1977.

5 Britten, J.D. Practical notes on nursing procedures; revised by M.A. Priest. 7th ed. Churchill Livingstone, 1979.

6 Broadwell, L. and Milutinovic, B. Medical-surgical nursing procedures. New York: Van Nostrand Reinhold, 1977.

7 Brunner, L.S. and others Textbook of medical-surgical nursing. Philadelphia: Lippincott. 3rd ed. by L.S. Brunner and D.S. Suddarth, 1975. 4th ed. 1980.

8 Burrowes, P.M. and Reakes, M.E. First level general nursing. New York: McGraw-Hill, 1979. (McGraw-Hill nursing studies series.)

9 **Chapman, C.M.** Medical nursing. 9th ed. Baillière Tindall, 1977. (Nurses' aids series.)

10 **Chilman, A.M. and Thomas, M.** Understanding nursing care. Churchill-Livingstone, 1978.

11 **Clarke, M.** Practical nursing. 12th ed. Baillière Tindall, 1977. (Nurses' aids series.)

12 **Corbett, N.A. and Beveridge, P.** Clinical simulations in nursing practice. Philadelphia: Saunders, 1980.

13 **Crispin, M.E.** Handbook of practical nursing. Baillière Tindall, 1976.

14 **Dison, N.** Clinical nursing techniques. 4th ed. St. Louis: Mosby, 1979.

15 **Du Gas, B.W.** Introduction to patient care: a comprehensive approach to nursing. 3rd ed. Philadelphia: Saunders, 1977.

16 **Elhart, D. and others** Scientific principles in nursing. 8th ed. St. Louis: Mosby, 1978.

17 **Ellis, J.R. and Nowlis, E.A.** Nursing: a human needs approach. Boston: Houghton Mifflin, 1977.

18 **Emerton, M.D.** Principles and practice of nursing. St. Lucia, Qld.: University of Queensland Press, 1976.

19 **Fream, W.C.** Notes on medical nursing. 2nd ed. Churchill Livingstone, 1977.

20 **Glass, M. and Atchison, E.** Integrated studies in patient care. New York: Van Nostrand Reinhold, 1978.

21 **Gration, H.M. and Holland, D.L.** A ward pocket-book for the nurse; revised by Joan Brotton. Faber, 1978.

22 **Hazzard, M.E.** Medical-surgical nursing review. New York: Arco, 1980. (Arco nursing review series.) 2nd ed. 1980.

23 **Hector, W.** Modern nursing: theory and practice. 6th ed. Heinemann, 1976.

24 **Henderson, V. and Nite, G.** Principles and practice of nursing. 6th ed. Macmillan, 1978.

25 **Johnson, R.W.H. and Johnson, D.W.** Introduction to nursing care. New York: McGraw-Hill, 1976. (Nursing and allied health series.)

26 **Johnston, D.F. and Hood, G.H.** Medical-surgical nursing workbook for practical nurses. 4th ed. St. Louis: Mosby, 1976.

27 **Jones, D.A. and others** Medical-surgical nursing: a conceptual approach. New York: McGraw-Hill, 1978.

28 **Kennedy, M.S. and Pfeifer, G.M.** Current practice in nursing care of the adult: issues and concepts. St. Louis: Mosby, 1979. (Mosby's current practice and perspectives in nursing series; 1.)

29 **Kintzel, K.C. editor** Advanced concepts in clinical nursing. 2nd ed. Philadelphia: Lippincott, 1977.

30 **Kozier, B. and Erb, G.** Fundamentals of nursing: concepts and procedures. Menlo Park: Addison-Wesley, 1979.

31 **Kurtz, R.B. and Miller, N.F.** Clinical workbook in medical-surgical nursing. Philadelphia: Saunders, 1978.

32 **Lee, E.R.** Concepts in basic nursing: a modular approach. Philadelphia: Saunders, 1980.

33 **Lewis, L.W.** Fundamental skills in patient care. Philadelphia: Lippincott, 1976.

34 **Lippincott** manual of nursing practice. 2nd ed. Philadelphia: Lippincott, 1978.

35 **Luckmann, J. and Sorensen, K.C.** Medical-surgical nursing: a psychophysiologic approach. 2nd ed. Philadelphia: Saunders, 1980.

36 **McGraw-Hill** handbook of clinical nursing; edited by Margaret E. Armstrong and others. New York: McGraw-Hill, 1979.

37 **Morgan, W. and Whyte, B.** Pupil nurse's workbook. New York: McGraw-Hill, 1975.

38 **Mosby's** comprehensive review of nursing. 7th ed. St. Louis: Mosby, 1978.

39 **Mosby's** review of practical nursing. 7th ed. St. Louis: Mosby, 1978.

40 **Murray, M.** Fundamentals of nursing. Englewood-Cliffs, N.J.: Prentice-Hall, 1976.

41 **Murray, R.B. and Zentner, J.P.** Nursing assessment and health promotion through the life span. 2nd ed. Englewood Cliffs, N.J.: Prentice-Hall, 1979.

42 **Murray, R.B. and Zentner, J.P.** Nursing concepts for health and promotion. 2nd ed. Englewood Cliffs, N.J.: Prentice-Hall, 1979.

43 **Nichols, A.O. and Day, J.** Pearls for nursing practice: a choice collection of tips, hints, timesavers... Philadelphia: Lippincott, 1979.

44 **Pearce, E.** A general textbook of nursing. 20th ed. Faber, 1980.

45 **Phipps, W.J. and others, editors** Medical-surgical nursing: concepts and clinical practice. St. Louis: Mosby, 1979.

46 **Readey, H.** Introduction to nursing essentials: a handbook. St. Louis: Mosby, 1977.

47 **Rines, A.R. and Montag, M.L.** Handbook of fundamental nursing techniques. New York: Wiley, 1976.

48 **Rines, A.R. and Montag, M.L.** Nursing concepts and nursing care. New York: Wiley, 1976.

49 **Shafer, K.N. and others** Medical-surgical nursing. 6th ed. St. Louis: Mosby, 1979. 7th ed. 1980.

50 **Sorensen, K.C. and Luckmann, J.** Basic nursing: a psychophysiologic approach. Philadelphia: Saunders, 1979.

51 **Spencer, M. and Tait, K.M.** Introduction to nursing. 4th ed. Blackwell, 1976.

52 **Story, D.K.** Principles and practice of nursing care. New York: McGraw-Hill, 1976.

53 **Vander Salm, T.J. editor** Atlas of bedside procedures. Boston: Little, Brown, 1979.

54 **Watson, J.E.** Medical-surgical nursing and related physiology. 2nd ed. Philadelphia: Saunders, 1979.

55 **Welsh, E.M. and others** An outline of basic nursing care. 2nd ed. Heinemann, 1978. (Modern practical nursing series parent volume)

56 **Wolff, L. and others** Fundamentals of nursing: the humanities and the sciences in nursing. 6th ed. Philadelphia: Lippincott, 1979.

57 **Wood, L.A. and Rambo, B.J. editors** Nursing skills for allied health services. Revised ed. 2 vols. Philadelphia: Saunders, 1977.

b PROCEDURES

1 **Bateman, J.M.** Rudiments of care. 1. Helping the patient with eating and drinking. Nursing Times, 75, 7 Jun 1979, 957-959.

2 **Billing, D.H.M.** Practical procedures for nurses. 2nd ed. Baillière Tindall, 1976. (Nurses' aids series.)

3 **Chalmers, H.** Return to basics. 2. The care of the patient in bed. Nursing Mirror, 145, 14 Jul 1977, Nursing care supplement series 5, i-iv.

4 **Dann, T.C.** Preinjection skin swabbing. (Letter with references stating lack of need for this procedure.) British Medical Journal, 2, 16 Sep 1978, 834.

5 **Dickie, H.M.** Trays, trolleys and treatments: a nurse's guide. 6th ed. Churchill Livingstone, 1977. (Previous edition entitled Tray and trolley setting.)

6 **Gasennelwe, K.** A study of relationship of theory to practice in some basic nursing skills. MSc thesis, University of Manchester, Department of Nursing, Oct 1979.

7 **Gormlie, H.E.C.** Improved kaolin poultice. (Designed by a nurse at Gartnavel General Hospital, Glasgow.) Nursing Times, 72, 28 Oct 1976, 1679.

8 **Hogstel, M.** How to give a safe and successful cleansing enema. American Journal of Nursing, 77 (5), May 1977, 816-817.

9 **Itty, A. and others** Intramuscular injections: an investigation into possibilities of reducing pain. Nursing Journal of India, 68 (10), Oct 1977, 251-252.

10 **Jungreis, S.W.** Exercises for expediting mobility (and decreasing disability) in bedridden patients. Nursing, 7 (8), Aug 1977, 47-51.

11 **King, E.M. and others** Illustrated manual of nursing techniques. Philadelphia: Lippincott, 1977.

12 **Kinnes, C.F.** Injecting an iron idea. (Describes how intramuscular injections of flupenthixol (Depixol) can leak and therefore advises technique of pulling the skin to one side.) Nursing Mirror, 151, 4 Dec 1980, 11.

13 **Kruszewski, A.Z. and others** Effect of positioning on discomfort from intramuscular injections in the dorsogluteal site. (Patients in prone position with hips internally rotated to relax gluteus.) Nursing Research, 28 (2), Mar/Apr 1979, 103-105.

14 **Lang, S.H. and others** Reducing dis-

comfort from IM injections. American Journal of Nursing, 76 (5), May 1976, 800-801.

15 McConnell, E.A. 10 problems with naso-gastric tubes. . .and how to solve them. Nursing (U.S.), 9 (4), Apr 1979, 78-81.

16 Niederbaumer, L. Rethinking the pro-cedure manual. (An evaluation of its useful-ness.) Supervisor Nurse, 8 (4), Apr 1977, 59-60, 63.

17 Nursing Clinics of North America Sym-posium on bio-instrumentation for nurses. Nursing Clinics of North America, 13 (4), Dec 1978, 559-640.

18 Osler, E.J. Venepuncture. (Illustrations of 34 steps in procedure.) Nursing Times, 76, 8 May 1980, Community Outlook 135-137.

19 Pepler, C.J. Your fingers on the pulse: evaluating what you feel. Nursing (U.S.), 10 (11), Nov 1980, 33-39.

20 Registered Nurses' Association of British Columbia. Steering Committee to Identify Essential Manual Skills Essential manual skills for a new graduate. Ottawa: the Association, 1978.

21 Sandham, G. and Reid, B. Some Q's and A's about suctioning, with an illustrated guide to better techniques. Nursing, 7 (10), Oct 1977, 60-65.

22 Savage, J.H. Removing hypodermic needles. (Safe disposal of thermoplastic syringes.) Nursing Mirror, 144, 19 May 1977, 34-36.

23 Schwertner, T. and Scibek, T.S.S. Nurs-ing care guidelines. (Work of a Nursing Practice Committee in planning and implementing nursing procedures.) Supervisor Nurse, 7 (3), Mar 1976, 23-26.

24 Thomas, S. Passing tubes and catheters. (Ryle's tube, stomach washout, urinary catheter, colonic washout and enema.) Nursing Mirror, 148, 29 Mar 1979, 32-34.

25 Thomas, S. Pulse, respiration and blood pressure. (Significance and how to measure and record.) Nursing Mirror, 148, 10 May 1979, 24-27.

26 Wells, T.J. Clinical nursing: 'curiouser and curiouser'. (How nursing practice is based on trial and error, custom and commonsense rather than research.) American Journal of Nursing, 79 (10), Oct 1979, 1757-1760.

27 Wright, M.L. A lesson in procedure writing. (Producing a procedure manual.) Supervisor Nurse, 8 (4), Apr 1977, 26-27.

c LIFTING PATIENTS

1 Back Pain Association Lifting: instructors manual. Teddington: the Association, 1978.

2 Chartered Society of Physiotherapy Lifting. (Supplement designed as pull-out booklet.) Physiotherapy, 65 (9), Sep 1979, 281-292.

3 Lawson, S. Bathing without back injury. (Survey of bathing routine and use of hoists at Etwall Hospital, Derbyshire.) Nursing Mirror, 148, 14 Jun 1979, 22-24.

4 Leinweber, E. Belts to make moves smoother. (Method of helping patients walk and transferring patients to and from beds and chairs.) American Journal of Nursing, 78 (12), Dec 1978, 2080-2081.

5 Long, B.C. and Buergin, P.S. The pivot transfer. How patients who can bear weight on only one leg can be helped in and out of bed. American Journal of Nursing, 77 (6), Jun 1977, 980-982.

6 Rantz, M.J. and Courtial, D. Lifting, moving and transferring patients: a manual. St. Louis: Mosby, 1977.

d TEMPERATURES

1 Abbey, J. and others How long is that thermometer accurate? (Research study to discover if thermometers become inaccurate over a period of time, in use or in storage.) American Journal of Nursing, 78 (8), Aug 1978, 1375-1376.

2 Aird, E. Thermography. (Diagnostic use of measuring temperature distribution.) Nursing Mirror, 144, 3 Feb 1977, 66-67.

3 Angerami, E.L.S. Epidemiological study of body temperature in patients in a teaching hospital. International Journal of Nursing Studies, 17 (2), 1980, 91-99.

4 Brislen, W. and others Assessment of a single use clinical thermometer. (A study at Ham Green Hospital, Bristol, to compare the use of a glass/mercury thermometer with a disposable chemical dot thermometer 'Temtake'.) Nursing Times, 72 (6), 12 Feb 1976, 235-237.

5 British Medical Journal Errors in using clinical thermometers. British Medical Journal, 1, 20 Mar 1976, 692.

6 Efionayi, K.M. and others A new use for the temperature chart. (Experiment at University College Hospital, Ibadan, scoring drug dosages on temperature charts.) Nursing Times, 72 (35), 2 Sep 1976, 1364-1368.

7 Erickson, R. Oral temperature differences in relation to thermometer and technique. Nursing Research, 29 (3), May/Jun 1980, 157-164.

8 Erickson, R. Thermometer placement for oral temperature measurement in febrile adults. (Study carried out on 50 patients.) International Journal of Nursing Studies, 13 (4), 1976, 199-208.

9 Felton, C.L. Hypoxemia and oral temper-atures. (Report of survey on ICU patients receiv-ing oxygen therapy to investigate best method of temperature measurement.) American Journal of Nursing, 78 (1), Jan 1978, 56-57.

10 Fitzpatrick, J.J. and Donovan, M.J. A follow up study of the reliability and validity of the motor activity rating scale. (For observing and recording body positions and body move-ments.) Nursing Research, 28, May/Jun 1979, 179-181.

11 Hoskins, C. Level of activation, body temperature, and interpersonal conflict in family relationships. Nursing Research, 28 (3), May/Jun 1979, 154-160.

12 Jackson, B.S. and others Energy expend-iture, heart rate, rhythm and blood pressure in normal female subjects engaged in common

hospitalized patient positions and modes of patient transfer. International Journal of Nursing Studies, 15 (3), 1978, 115-128.

13 Kirkpatrick, M. and Stanley, S.M. Evaluation of a new single use thermometer. (Study to ascertain the accuracy and depend-ability of a single use thermometer and to evaluate its use in industrial practice.) Occupational Health Nursing, 24 (12), Dec 1976, 9-18.

14 Litsky, B.Y. A study of temperature taking systems. (A microbiological comparison of three commonly used thermometer systems and a recent thermometer sheath system.) Supervisor Nurse, 7 (5), May 1976, 48-49, 51-53.

15 Moorat, D.S. The cost of taking temper-atures. (Study of three methods carried out at Cumberland Infirmary, Carlisle.) Nursing Times, 72 (20), 20 May 1976, 767-770.

16 Purves, R. Digital thermometers. (Letter reporting evaluation project on use of electronic thermometer.) Nursing Times, 74, 12 Oct 1978, 1688.

17 Sims-Williams, A.J. Temperature taking with glass thermometers: a review (of the literature.) Journal of Advanced Nursing, 1 (6), Nov 1976, 481-493.

18 Stronge, J.L. and Newton, G. A costly rise in efficiency? (Clinical trial of glass and electronic thermometers.) Nursing Mirror, 151, 21 Aug 1980, 29.

19 Thomas, S. Temperatures. (Ranges and methods of taking temperatures.) Nursing Mirror, 148, 3 May 1979, 32-33.

14 CLINICAL NURSE SPECIALIST

a GENERAL

1 Adderley, B.V. and Hill, M.H. Janforum: the contribution of clinical nurse specialists to the education of student nurses. Journal of Advanced Nursing, 4 (3), May 1979, 327-329.

2 Alterman, S.K. Clinical nurse specialist bibliography. AORN Journal, 23 (4), Mar 1976, 600-602.

3 Ashton, K. Clinical nurse specialists? (Rcn seminar at Leeds Castle.) Nursing Times, 72 (28), 15 Jul 1976, 1072.

4 Ashworth, P. The role of the clinical nurse consultant. (Symposium paper.) Nursing Mirror, 142 (20), 13 May 1976, 46-48.

5 Blake, P. The clinical specialist as nurse consultant. (One of range of roles for clinical specialist.) Journal of Nursing Administration, 7 (10), Dec 1977, 33-36.

6 British Medical Journal Nurse consultants. (Letter from D. Eyre-Walker expressing surprise that a nurse should be called a 'consultant'.) British Medical Journal, 2, 4 Dec 1976, 1386. Letter in reply from Jean Kelly, 1, 1 Jan 1977, 49 and subsequent correspondence from D. Eyre Walker and Robert Tiffany, 1, 22 Jan 1977, 232.

7 Burdge, L. The clinical nurse specialist-5. The role of the clinical nursing officer. (With

reference to the Royal Marsden Hospital.) Nursing Times, 74, 3 Aug 1978, 1299-1300.

8 Buzzell, M. Perspectives in clinical specialties. (Role of the clinical nurse specialist.) Australian Nurses Journal, 6 (9), Mar 1977, 43-46, 49.

9 Cahoon, M.C. Developing clinical specialist roles. Nursing Mirror, 144, 24 Mar 1977, 66-68.

10 Colerick, E.J. and others Evaluation of the clinical nurse specialist role: development and implementation of a dual purpose framework. Nursing Leadership, 3 (3), Sep 1980, 26-34.

11 Cowper-Smith, F. Why does the nurse specialist threaten sister? Report on a study day at the Royal Marsden Hospital which highlighted some of the working problems between the nurse specialist and the generalist. Nursing Times, 73, 15 Dec 1977, 1942-1943.

12 Cox, S. The clinical nurse specialist-1. The introduction of nurse specialists. (With reference to their work at the Royal Marsden Hospital.) Nursing Times, 74, 6 Jul 1978, 1125.

13 Disch, J.M. The clinical nurse specialists in a large peer group. (Where hospitals employ a large number of CNS.) Journal of Nursing Administration, 8 (12), Dec 1978, 17-20.

14 Duberley, J. The clinical nurse specialist. (The role needs to grow out of that of ward sister to improve patient care.) Nursing Times, 72 (46), 18 Nov 1976, 1794-1795.

15 Grabow, R. The clinical nurse specialist-2. The staging unit. (Her work in this unit at the Royal Marsden Hospital where progress of the disease is monitored.) Nursing Times, 74, 13 Jul 1978, 1168-1169.

16 Gregory, C.L. and Lang, S.H. Role modelling: the nurse clinician's challenge. (Formation and sharing of effective approaches to patient care.) Supervisor Nurse, 8 (8), Aug 1977, 51-54.

17 Hamric, A.B. and others Staff evaluation of clinical leaders. (Clinical nurse specialist and head nurse.) Journal of Nursing Administration, 8 (1), Jan 1978, 18-26.

18 Haynor, P. Career ladder: back to the bedside. (New post of advanced staff nurse at Thomas Jefferson University Hospital, Philadelphia.) Supervisor Nurse, 9 (2), Feb 1978, 33-36.

19 Hooker, E.Z. and O'Rourke, T.W. Extending roles in nursing. (Nurse midwife, physician's assistant, nurse practitioner and clinical nurse specialist.) Public Health Reviews, 3 (2), Apr/Jun 1974. (Reprint file.)

20 Keithley, J.K. and others Help at hand: using the nurse consultant. Nursing (U.S.), 9 (11), Nov 1979, 9-12.

21 Kinross, N. and others The nurse specialist. From the Massey University Nursing Studies Unit. New Zealand Nursing Journal, 69 (1), Jan 1976, 9-11.

22 Knable, J. and Petre, G. Resistance to role implementation. (Problem facing clinical nurse specialist.) Supervisor Nurse, 10 (2), Feb 1979, 31-34.

23 Kohnke, M.F. The case for consultation in

nursing: designs for professional practice. New York: Wiley, 1978.

24 Kratz, C.R. The clinical nurse consultant. Queen's Nursing Journal, 19 (7), Oct 1976, 190-191. Nursing Times, 72, 18 Nov 1976, 1792-1793.

25 Lange, F.M. The multifaceted role of the nurse consultant. Journal of Nursing Education, 18 (9), Nov 1979, 30-34.

26 Larkin, M. and Crowder, N.E. Nurse consultation: the instilling of hope. Nurse consultants can provide the specialized expertise needed by generalists. Supervisor Nurse, 7 (11), Nov 1976, 54, 57-58.

27 McMullan, D. Preparation of the nurse specialist. New York: National League for Nursing, 1977.

28 Meintel, P. and Rhodes, D. Clinical career ladder rewards RNs. (Guidelines devised by Mercy Hospital, Des Moines after a year's project to define levels of expertise and to provide incentives.) Hospital Progress, 58 (8), Aug 1977, 36, 38, 40-41, 44, 46, 48.

29 Murphy, J.F. and Schmitz, M. The clinical nurse specialist: implementing the role in a hospital setting. Journal of Nursing Administration, 9 (1), Jan 1979, 29-31.

30 Nelson, C.A. and Arford, P.H. Strategy for clinical advancement. (Organisational structure for clinical nursing to complement administrative one.) Journal of Nursing Administration, 7 (4), Apr 1977, 46-51.

31 Niessner, P. The clinical specialist's contribution to quality nursing care. Nursing Leadership, 2 (1), Nov 1979, 21-30.

32 Norman, J. The clinical specialist as performance appraiser. (Suggests that enhanced quality of care is dependent on performance appraisal by clinicians.) Supervisor Nurse, 9 (7), Jul 1978, 61-64.

33 Nursing Administration Quarterly Issue on maximizing nursing practice. (Eight articles with three on the clinical nurse specialist and two on the nurse practitioner.) Nursing Administration Quarterly, 4 (1), Fall 1979, 1-95.

34 Nursing Mirror A symposium on the clinical nurse consultant. Nursing Mirror, 142 (20), 13 May 1976, 45-58.

35 Padilla, G.V. editor The clinical nurse specialist and improvement of nursing practice. Wakefield, Mass.: Nursing Resources, 1979. (Nursing Digest; 6 (4), 1979.)

36 Passeri, A.J. and Patten, C.S. Delineating privileges for clinical nurses. (Nurse's special skills established by qualification and competence and approved by committee.) Hospital Topics, 58 (2), Mar/Apr 1980, 4-7.

37 Pembrey, S. Vision of the future. (Analysis of recent developments in nursing and roles of clinical nurse specialist and ward sister.) Nursing Mirror, 149, 30 Aug 1979, Supplement xxxi-xxxii.

38 Piazza, D. and Jackson, B.S. Clinical nurse specialists: issues, power and freedom. (Their role in the U.S. health service and modern society.) Supervisor Nurse, 9 (12), Dec 1978, 47-51.

39 Robinson, C.R. Rediscovering clinical nursing. (Experiences on returning to nursing as clinical nurse specialist.) American Journal of Nursing, 77 (5), May 1977, 839.

40 Rotkovitch, R. editor Quality patient care and the role of the clinical nursing specialist. New York: Wiley, 1976.

41 Royal College of Nursing New horizons in clinical nursing: report of a seminar held at Leeds Castle, Kent, 14-17 October 1975. Rcn, 1976

42 Smoyak, S.A. Specialization in nursing from then to now: clinical specialists need to assess their role against the perspective of its historical development and the obstacles to its implementation. Nursing Outlook, 24 (11), Nov 1976, 676-681.

43 Stevens, B.J. Accountability of the clinical specialist: the administrator's viewpoint. Journal of Nursing Administration, 6 (2), Feb 1976, 30-32.

44 Stevens, B.J. The use of consultants in nursing service. (To solve management problems or help implement new schemes.) Journal of Nursing Administration, 8 (8), Aug 1978, 7-15.

45 Wiles, V.A. The practice of nursing. Clinical specialisation. (Implications of the Australian 'Goals in nursing education' report for clinical practitioner.) Australian Nurses Journal, 5 (3), Sep 1975, 6-9.

b NURSE PRACTITIONER

1 Austin, R. The nurse practitioner in health care. (With discussion of role of nurse generally.) International Nursing Review, 25 (3), May/Jun 1978, 82-88.

2 Bliss, A.A. and Cohen, E.D. editors The new health professionals: nurse practitioners and physician's assistants. Germantown: Aspen Systems Corporation, 1977.

3 Bracken, R.L. and Christman, L. An incentive program designed to develop and reward clinical competence. (Separate career pathway for staff nurses to become nurse practitioners.) Journal of Nursing Administration, 8 (10), Oct 1978, 8-18.

4 British Medical Journal Making better use of our nurses. (Nurse practitioner course at McMaster University, Canada and their role here.) British Medical Journal, 1977, 1, 21 May 1977, 1306.

5 British Medical Journal Using auxiliaries. (Use of physician's assistants and nurse practitioners in the U.S.A., with discussion of nurse's role here.) British Medical Journal, 2, 12 Aug 1978, 454.

6 Canadian Nurse Nurse practitioners—the national picture. (Four articles on their development, education and work in various parts of Canada.) Canadian Nurse, 74 (4), Apr 1978, 13-27.

7 Celentano, D.D. New health professional practice patterns. (Comparison of health associates and nurse practitioners.) Medical Care, 16 (10), Oct 1978, 831-849.

8 Christensen, M.G. and others Professional development of nurse practitioners as a function of need motivation, learning style, and focus of control. Nursing Research, 28 (1), Jan/Feb 1979, 51-56.

9 Diers, D. and Molde, S. Some conceptual and methodological issues in nurse practitioner research. Research in Nursing and Health, 2 (2), Jun 1979, 73-84.

10 Edgecombe-Green, B. Extending the role of the clinical nurse. (Letter describing work of nurse practitioners in Northern Canada.) British Medical Journal, 1, 10 Mar 1979, 688.

11 Edmunds, M.W. Gender and the nurse practitioner role. Nurse Practitioner, 5 (6), Nov/Dec 1980, 42, 44.

12 Edmunds, M.W. 'Junior doctoring'. The tendency for a nurse practitioner to identify with the physician as a role model may cause the nurse to develop a role much like a physician assistant. Nurse Practitioner, 4 (5), Sep/Oct 1979, 38, 40-41, 46.

13 Ferguson, M.C. Nursing at the crossroads: which way to turn? (A look at the model of a nurse practitioner.) Journal of Advanced Nursing, 1 (3), May 1976, 237-242.

14 Ford, L.C. A nurse for all settings: the nurse practitioner. (Review of functions and need for assessment of their long-term impact.) Nursing Outlook, 27 (8), Aug 1979, 516-521.

15 Gibbs, J. The education role of the nurse practitioner. (Nurse practitioners are defined here as qualified nurses in direct care situations and the community.) Australian Nurses Journal, 10 (1), Jul 1980, 37-39.

16 Jelinek, D. The longitudinal study of nurse practitioners: report of phase 2. (Results of questionnaire survey about their work.) Nurse Practitioner, 3 (1), Jan-Feb 1978, 17-19.

17 Kapadia, K.B. and Julius, R.K. Nurse practitioner programme. (Educational preparation in India.) Nursing Journal of India, 47 (7), Jul 1976, 173-174.

18 Kettel, L. and others Admissions nurse practitioners make a difference. (Scheme at Tucson Veterans Administration Hospital using nurse practitioners to take health history and order diagnostic tests.) American Journal of Nursing, 78 (4), Apr 1978, 648-649.

19 Kilmon, C. and others Clinical objectives for nurse practitioner students. Journal of Nursing Education, 19 (8), Oct 1980, 37-41.

20 King, C. The PNP movement enters graduate school. (Present role and progress of the nurse practitioner movement.) Journal of Nursing Education, 15 (4), Jul 1976, 27-32.

21 Klaus, B.J. Protocols handbook for nurse practitioners. New York: Wiley, 1979.

22 Knafl, K.A. How nurse practitioner students construct their role. (Refers to what the nurse's role is as opposed to the doctor's.) Nursing Outlook, 26 (10), Oct 1978, 650-653.

23 Komaroff, A.L. and others Nurse practitioner management of common respiratory and genitourinary infections, using protocols. (Comparison of treatment by a nurse guided by protocols with traditional physician examination.) Nursing Research, 25 (2), Mar-Apr 1976, 84-89.

24 Lawrence, R.S. and others Physician

receptivity to nurse practitioners: a study of the correlates of the delegation of clinical responsibility. (Survey in North Carolina in 1973.) Medical Care, 15 (4), Apr 1977, 298-310.

25 Levine, E. What do we know about nurse practitioners? (Forces affecting present numbers and future requirements.) American Journal of Nursing, 77 (11), Nov 1977, 1799-1803.

26 Levine, J.I. and others The nurse practitioner: role, physician utilization, patient acceptance. Nursing Research, 27 (4), Jul/Aug 1978, 245-254.

27 Lewis, M.A. Managing nurse practitioners in ambulatory care: what are the issues? Journal of Nursing Administration, 10 (6), Jul 1980, 11-17.

28 Linn, L.S. and Lewis, M.A. RAP Sessions: for nurse practitioner students. (Staff student consultation to overcome personal, learning and role related problems.) American Journal of Nursing, 76 (5), May 1976, 782-784.

29 Little, M. Physicians' attitudes toward employment of nurse practitioners. 2 parts. Nurse Practitioner, 3 (4), Jul/Aug 1978, 27-30; (6), Nov/Dec 1978, 15, 35-36.

30 McAtee, P.R. and Silver, H.K. What about a national nurse-practitioner program? (Proposals for training nurse practitioners.) RN Magazine, 38 (12), Dec 1975, 22-26.

31 McTavish, M. The nurse practitioner: an idea whose time has come. (Need to revive interest in this concept.) Canadian Nurse, 75 (8), Sep 1979, 41-44.

32 Mauksch, I.G. Critical issues of the nurse practitioner movement. (History and current role.) Nurse Practitioner, 31 (6), Nov/Dec 1978, 15, 35-36.

33 Miller, M.H. Self perception of nurse practitioners: changes in stress, assertiveness, and sex role. (Research study.) Nurse Practitioner, 2 (5), May/Jun 1977, 26-29.

34 O'Connell, A.L. and Bates, B. The case method in nurse practitioner education. Nursing Outlook, 24 (4), Apr 1976, 243-246.

35 Paxton, C.S. and Scoblic, M.A. Defining and developing protocols for the nurse practitioner. Nursing Forum, 17 (3), 1978, 268-283.

36 Reedy, B.L. The new health practitioners in America: a comparative study. King Edward's Hospital Fund for London, 1978.

37 Roos, P.D. Nurse practitioner employment, unemployment, re-employment. (Survey of graduates of one course and comment on their employment status, reasons for unemployment and changes in employment.) Nursing Research, 28 (6), Nov/Dec 1979, 348-353.

38 Roy, C. and Obloy, M. The practitioner movement—toward a science of nursing. American Journal of Nursing, 78 (10), Oct 1978, 1698-1702.

39 Shimo, M. Occupational consciousness in the nurse practitioner. (Discussion of her role.) Supervisor Nurse, 8 (9), Sep 1977, 54-55, 57-59.

40 Siegel, M.A. and Bullough, B. Constructing and adapting protocols. (Outlined steps for nurse practitioners to diagnose and treat given

conditions.) American Journal of Nursing, 77 (10), Oct 1977, 1616-1618.

41 Sparks, S.M. and others Teaching of interpersonal skills to nurse practitioner students. Journal of Continuing Education in Nursing, 11 (3), May/Jun 1980, 5-16.

42 Stoner, M.H. and others The real S.O.A.P. on a core curriculum. (Development of curriculum for nurse practitioners based on the problem-oriented recording system.) Journal of Nursing Education, 18 (8), Oct 1979, 50-55.

43 Sultz, H.A. Nurse practitioners: USA. Lexington, Mass.: Lexington Books, 1979.

44 United States. Department of Health, Education and Welfare. Division of Nursing The nurse practitioner in an adult outpatient clinic. Washington: USDHEW, 1976.

45 University of North Carolina. Department of Epidemiology Assessing the clinical skills of nurse practitioners. Hyattsville, Md.: US Department of Health, Education and Welfare, 1978.

46 Webster-Stratton, C. The nurse practitioner in private practice. (In Alaska.) Pediatric Nursing, 4 (1), Jan/Feb 1978, 24-30.

c PHYSICIAN'S ASSISTANT

1 Baudry, J. The nurse and the medical assistant—functions and status. (Research study in the six WHO administrative regions of their educational background and preparation and functions.) International Nursing Review, 25 (4), Jul/Aug 1978, 108-112.

2 Christman, L. Janforum: the relationship of the physician's assistant to nursing. (With some reference to the expanding role of the nurse.) Journal of Advanced Nursing, 4 (2), Mar 1979, 215-218.

15 NURSE AND PATIENT

a NURSE/PATIENT RELATIONSHIP

1 Almore, M.G. Dyadic communication. (Interpersonal perception between two people.) American Journal of Nursing, 79 (6), Jun 1979, 1076-1078.

2 American Journal of Nursing Working with the confused or delirious patient. (Four articles.) American Journal of Nursing, 78 (9), Sep 1978, 1491-1512.

3 Anderson, N.D. Human interaction for nurses. (With importance of non-verbal communication between nurse and patient.) Supervisor Nurse, 10 (10), Oct 1979, 44, 48-50.

4 Armitage, S. Non-compliant recipients of health care. (Concepts of patient role and 'good' or 'bad' patients and the effect of these definitions on nursing care and patient outcome.) Nursing Times, 76, 3 Jan 1980, Occ. papers, 1-3.

5 Barcock, D.E. Transactional analysis. (Use of a social psychological technique in nursing.) American Journal of Nursing, 76 (7), Jul 1976, 1152-1155.

6 **Bayer, M. and Brandner, P.** Nurse/patient peer practice. (Recognition of patients' intelligence in an equal partner relationship.) American Journal of Nursing, 77 (1), Jan 1977, 86-90.

7 **Beard, J.M.** What is your attitude saying? (Nurses' attitudes towards patients.) AORN Journal, 24 (4), Oct 1976, 782, 784, 786, 788.

8 **Bergman, R.** Interpersonal relations in health care delivery. International Nursing Review, 24 (4), Jul/Aug 1977, 104-107.

9 **Bhanumathi, P.P.** Nurses' conception of 'sick role' and 'good patient' behaviour: a cross-cultural comparison. International Nursing Review, 24 (1), Jan/Feb 1977, 20-24.

10 **Browne, G.** Patient/professional interaction and its relationship to patients' psychological distress and frequent use of health services. (Research study of interactions between patients and either family doctors or nurse practitioners.) Nursing Papers, 11 (1/2), 1979, 28-45.

11 **Burton, G.** Interpersonal relations: a guide for nurses. 4th ed. New York: Springer, 1977.

12 **Carlson, C.E. and Blackwell, B. editors** Behavioral concepts and nursing intervention. 2nd ed. Philadelphia: Lippincott, 1978.

13 **Chalmers, H.** Return to basics. 7. First impressions stick. (Helping patients to settle into ward on admission.) Nursing Mirror, 145, 7 Jul 1977, Nursing care supplement series 5, i-iv.

14 **Chapman, C.M.** Social exchange Part 2. The meeting of needs. (Nurse/patient interaction.) World of Irish Nursing, 6 (7/8), Jul/Aug 1977, 1-2.

15 **Cox, L.** To whom are we accountable? (Protection of patients both physically and emotionally.) Australian Nurses Journal, 8 (10), May 1979, 35-36, 44.

16 **Efthymiou, G.** Management of attention seeking patients. Nursing Times, 72, 16 Sep 1976, 1452-1453; 23 Sep 1976, 1490-1491.

17 **Flaskerud, J.H. and others** Avoidance and distancing: a descriptive view of nursing. (Five nursing theorists examine the role of the nurse and the nurse/patient relationship.) Nursing Forum, 18 (2), 1979, 158-174.

18 **Forsyth, G.L.** Analysis of the concept of empathy: illustration of one approach. Advances in Nursing Science, 2 (2), Jan 1980, 33-42.

19 **Forsyth, G.L.** Exploration of empathy in nurse-client interaction. (Research study with appendix describing the Hogan Empathy Scale and the Barrett-Lennard Relationship Inventory.) Advances in Nursing Science, 1 (2), Jan 1979, 53-61.

20 **Germaine, A.** On behalf of some of our patients. (Nurses attitudes towards patients should show sensitivity and courtesy.) Hospital Administration in Canada, 18 (4), Apr 1976, 34, 36.

21 **Gerrard, B.A. and others** Interpersonal skills for health professionals. Reston, Va: Reston, 1980.

22 **Gladstone, T.U. and McKegney, F.P.** Relationship between patient behaviors and nursing staff attitudes. (Research study using various scales, with some reference to unpopular

patients.) Supervisor Nurse, 11 (6), Jun 1980, 32-35.

23 **Gordy, H.E.** Gift giving in the nurse-patient relationship. American Journal of Nursing, 78 (6), Jun 1978, 1026-1028.

24 **Hall, B.A. and Mitsunaga, B.K.** Education of the nurse to promote interpersonal attraction. (Promoting good nurse/patient relationships even with 'unpopular' patients.) Journal of Nursing Education, 18 (5), May 1979, 16-21.

25 **Harris, J.** Advantages of the nurse-patient contract. (With four types of contracts outlined.) Nursing Papers, 10 (3), Fall 1978, 56-59.

26 **Hart, C.** All in a day's work. (Aspects of nurse/patient and staff/staff relationships which adversely affect patient care.) Nursing Times, 74, 19 Oct 1978, 1704-1705.

27 **Hein, E. and Leavitt, M.** Providing emotional support to patients. Nursing, 77 7 (5), May 1977, 39-41.

28 **Hughes, J.** Manipulation: a negative element in care. (Characteristics of 'the helping personality' and how both career and patient can manipulate and be manipulated.) Journal of Advanced Nursing, 5 (1), Jan 1980, 21-29.

29 **James, B.** Trends in medical care and the nurse/patient relationship. New Zealand Nursing Journal, 70 (5), May 1977, 11-12.

30 **Jungman, L.B.** When your feelings get in the way. (Nurses' emotional responses to patients.) American Journal of Nursing, 79 (6), Jun 1979, 1074-1075.

31 **Keane, B.** The management of the anxious patient in the general hospital ward. Australian Nurses Journal, 7 (9), Apr 1978, 47-49.

32 **King, E.S.** Should we get emotionally involved? Hell yes! (Nurse-patient relationships.) RN Magazine, 40 (6), 15 Jun 1977, 49-54.

33 **Kraus, V.L.** Preinformation—its effect on nurses' descriptions of a patient. Journal of Nursing Education, 15 (5), Sep 1976, 18-26.

34 **Langford, T.** Establishing a nursing contract. If patients are to understand and cooperate with nurses, they may need to discuss and agree about their own and the nurses' expectations. Nursing Outlook, 26 (6), Jun 1978, 386-388.

35 **Larson, P.A.** Influence of patient status and health condition on nurse perceptions of patient characteristics. (Research with nurses using slides and notes about patients.) Nursing Research, 26 (6), Nov/Dec 1977, 416-421.

36 **McGilloway, F.A.** Dependency and vulnerability in the nurse/patient situation. (A theoretical study.) Journal of Advanced Nursing, 1 (3), May 1976, 229-236.

37 **McGreevy, A.D. and Heukelem, J.** Crying: the neglected dimension. (Nursing care of the crying patient.) Canadian Nurse, 72 (1), Jan 1976, 19-21.

38 **McIntosh, J.B.** The nurse-patient relationship. (Topics and tactics of communication and interaction with patients.) Nursing Mirror, 148, 25 Jan 1979 Supplement i-ii, iv-v, viii, x-xi.

39 **McWilliams, R.M.** The balance of caring.

(Sensitivity and response to human needs as vital components of caring.) AORN Journal, 24 (2), Aug 1976, 314-317, 320.

40 **Malden, H.** Caring in crisis. (The importance of emotional and spiritual development of nurses for solving problems in the patient/client situation.) Australian Nurses Journal, 6 (5), Nov 1976, 24-26.

41 **Marshall, J.** Reassurance. (Value of human approach by nurses to patients.) Nursing Times, 75, 4 Oct 1979, 1723-1724.

42 **Miller, A.E.** Nurses' attitudes towards their patients. (Includes review of research.) Nursing Times, 75, 8 Nov 1979, 1929-1933.

43 **Miller, G.A.** Patient knowledge and nurse role strain in three hospital settings. Medical Care, 14 (8), Aug 1976, 662-673.

44 **Mooney, J.** Attachment/separation in the nurse-patient relationship. Nursing Forum, 15 (3), 1976, 259-264.

45 **Purtilo, R.** Health professional/patient interaction. 2nd ed. Philadelphia: Saunders, 1978.

46 **Rawnsley, M.M.** Toward a conceptual base for effective nursing. (Need for investigation of responsiveness to distress and empathy.) Nursing Outlook, 28 (4), Apr 1980, 244-247.

47 **Rieder, K.A. and Wood, M.J.** Problem-orientation: an experimental study to test its heuristic value. (Research study to explore the effect of problem-orientation on a nursing staff's ability to identify underlying patient problems.) Nursing Research, 27 (1), Jan/Feb 1978, 25-29.

48 **RN Magazine** Handling the difficult patient. (Three case histories.) RN Magazine, 38 (5), May 1975, 41-47.

49 **Robinson, L.** A therapeutic paradox—to support intimacy and regression or privacy and autonomy. (Nurses' responses to patients who need privacy or intimacy.) Journal of Psychiatric Nursing, 17 (10), Oct 1979, 19-23.

50 **Rosenbaum, M.S.** Mrs. Reynolds still needs a nurse. (Advice on dealing with the demanding patient.) Nursing, 7 (12), Dec 1977, 32, 34-35.

51 **Rosenthal, C.J. and others** Nurses, patients and families. Croom Helm, 1980.

52 **Sainsbury, M.J.C.** The bedside manner. (Importance of psychological care of patients and relatives.) Nursing Mirror, 146, 4 May 1978, 40-41.

53 **Sanders, S.H. and others** Analysis of nurses' knowledge of behavioral methods applied to chronic and acute pain patients. (Ways of decreasing negative and increasing positive behaviour.) Journal of Nursing Education, 19 (4), Apr 1980, 46-50.

54 **Scheideman, J.M.** Problem patients do not exist. American Journal of Nursing, 79 (6), Jun 1979, 1082-1084.

55 **Seeger, P.A.** Self-awareness and nursing. (Nurse-patient relationship.) Journal of Psychiatric Nursing and Mental Health Services, 15 (8), Aug 1977, 24-26.

56 **Smith, L.** Limit-setting. (Placing by nurses

of boundaries to mark acceptable or tolerable behaviour from patients in general and psychiatric hospitals.) Nursing Times, 74, 29 Jun 1978, 1074-1075.

57 **Sparling, S.L. and Jones, S.L.** Setting: a contextual variable associated with empathy. (Research study to compare nurses in psychiatric and non-psychiatric settings to see if they differed in empathic skills.) Journal of Psychiatric Nursing and Mental Health Services, 15 (4), Apr 1977, 9-12.

58 **Turner, V.** How the nurse can help preserve a patient's individuality. (Second prizewinner of Baillière's prize for nursing students.) Nursing Mirror, 144, 20 Jan 1977, 60-64; 27 Jan 1977, 59-62.

59 **Uys, L.R.** Towards the development of an operational definition of the concept 'therapeutic use of self'. (Ability of the nurse to employ herself as a tool for promoting health.) International Journal of Nursing Studies, 17 (3), 1980, 175-180.

60 **Wallston, K.A. and others** Increasing nurses' person-centerdness. (Research study measuring nurses' responses to audiotaped statements from simulated patients.) Nursing Research, 27 (3), May/Jun 1978, 156-159.

61 **Williamson, Y.M.** Methodologic dilemmas in tapping the concept of patient needs. (Problems in constructing questionnaires to measure patients' needs and nurses' perceptions of them.) Nursing Research, 27 (3), May/Jun 1978, 172-177.

62 **Wilting, J.** People, patients and nurses: a guide for nurses toward improved interpersonal relationships. Edmonton: University of Alberta Press, 1980.

63 **Woolf, J.** Nurse could you care more? (How a dehumanising process can take place in the nurse/patient relationship as the sick person becomes a 'patient'.) Nursing Times, 75, 7 Jun 1979, 946-947.

64 **Wylie, N.** Nurse-patient relationships in chronic illness. Nursing Journal of Singapore, 15 (2), Nov 1975, 93-95.

b COMMUNICATION AND COUNSELLING

1 **Abrams, N.** A contrary view of the nurse as patient advocate. Nursing Forum, 17 (3), 1978, 258-267.

2 **Archer, R.** Breaking the sound barrier. (Ways of listening more carefully to patients.) Community View, 5, May 1980, 6-7.

3 **Ashton, K.** Patient counselling and education. (Report on papers read at international conference on patient counselling.) Nursing Times, 75, 9 Aug 1979, 1347-1349.

4 **Billings, C.** Can you hear between the lines? (Active listening skills to improve nurse-patient communication.) RN Magazine, 41 (9), Sep 1978, 117-118, 120, 122.

5 **Bechervaise, M.D.** Nursing care study. The riddle of communication—1. (Patient with carcinoma of the bronchus and hypertrophic pulmonary osteoarthropathy who eventually died, with reference to 'conspiracy of silence' over prognosis.) Nursing Times, 75, 23 Aug 1979, 1434-1436.

6 **Breckman, B.** A personal view of counselling. Journal of Community Nursing, 2 (4), Oct 1978, 8-9.

7 **Brockway, B.F. and others** Effect of nursing reassurance on patient vocal stress levels. Nursing Research, 25 (6), Nov-Dec 1976, 440-446.

8 **Carpenter, K.F. and Kroth, J.A.** Effects of videotaped role playing on nurses' therapeutic communication skills. Journal of Continuing Education in Nursing, 7 (2), Mar/Apr 1976, 47-53.

9 **Chisholm, M.** Communications—choke or channel? (The part the nurse can play in relation to the patient.) Nursing Mirror, 142, 18 Mar 1976, 70-71.

10 **Clarke, M.** Psychology. 5. Is anyone there? (Communication with reference to nurses and patients.) Nursing Mirror, 150, 19 Jun 1980, 29-31.

11 **Collins, M.** Communication in health care: understanding and implementing effective human relationships. St. Louis: Mosby, 1977.

12 **Crews, N.E.** Developing empathy for effective communication. AORN Journal, 30 (3), Sep 1979, 536, 540, 542-545, 548.

13 **Curtin, L.L.** The nurse as advocate: a philosophical foundation for nursing. Advances in Nursing Science, 1 (3), Apr 1979, 1-10.

14 **Daubenmire, M.J. and others** A methodologic framework to study nurse-patient communication. (Study of communicative interaction patterns using synchronology.) Nursing Research, 27 (5), Sep/Oct 1978, 303-310.

15 **Donahue, M.P.** The nurse: a patient advocate? Nursing Forum, 17 (2), 1978, 143-151.

16 **Enelow, A.J. and Swisher, S.N.** Interviewing and patient care. 2nd ed. New York: Oxford University Press, 1979.

17 **Faulkner, A.** Communication and the nurse. (Research study with second-year student nurses to find out if nurses perceived themselves as having a role in giving information to patients.) Nursing Times, 76, 4 Sep 1980, Occ. papers, 93-95.

18 **Faulkner, A.** Monitoring nurse-patient conversation in a ward. (Tape recording with discussion of method and some of research study's findings.) Nursing Times, 75, 30 Aug 1979, Occ. papers, 95-96.

19 **Fay, P.** Sounding board: in support of patient advocacy as a nursing role. (Assisting patients in learning about, protecting and asserting their rights within the health care context.) Nursing Outlook, 26 (4), Apr 1978, 252-253.

20 **French, H-P.** Reassurance: a nursing skill? (Discussion of definition of reassurance and outline of behaviours which may be employed to achieve it.) Journal of Advanced Nursing, 4 (6), Nov 1979, 627-634.

21 **Givan, P.** Healing and creative skills in counselling. (With special reference to the role of the nurse.) Nursing Times, 73, 18 Aug 1977, 1279-1283.

22 **Hein, E.C.** Communication in nursing practice. 2nd ed. Boston: Little, Brown, 1980.

23 **Hennessy, D.** Nurse counselling as a career. S.A. Nursing Journal, 43 (2), Feb 1976, 6-7.

24 **Hodgkinson, P.** Counselling and the nurse. (Problems of acceptance as basic nursing skill and place in training.) Journal of Community Nursing, 4 (6), Dec 1980, 14-15, 17.

25 **Hopson, B. and Scally, M.** Counselling— a case for demystifying and deprofessionalising. Nursing Times, 74, 12 Jan 1978, 50-51.

26 **Jenny, J.** Patient advocacy—another role for nursing. (With American Hospital Association's 'A patient's bill of rights'.) International Nursing Review, 26 (6), Nov/Dec 1979, 176-181.

27 **Johnson, M.N.** Anxiety/stress and the effects on disclosure between nurses and patients. Advanced in Nursing Science, 1 (4), Jul 1979, 1-20.

28 **Journal of Practical Nursing** Five articles on nurse-patient communication, including the non-English speaking patient and the aphasic patient. Journal of Practical Nursing, 28 (4), Apr 1978, 16-26.

29 **Kopacz, M.S. and O'Connor, C.M.** Through a glass darkly. (Techniques for nurses counselling patients.) American Journal of Nursing, 75 (12), Dec 1975, 2159-2160.

30 **Kottler, J.A.** Promoting self-understanding in counselling: a compromise between the insight and action-oriented approaches. Journal of Psychiatric Nursing, 17 (12), Dec 1979, 18-23.

31 **Lawson, K.** Listening to patients. (Techniques of listening and asking questions.) Nursing Times, 76, 9 Oct 1980, 1784-1788.

32 **Lay, T.N.** Personal awareness: therapeutic communication. (Ten skills and qualities required in helping relationships.) Journal of Nursing Care, 12 (9), Sep 1979, 16-18.

33 **Macilwaine, H.** Breaking through the communication barrier. (Need for improved nurse/patient communication with reference to nursing theorists and American system of liaison nurse as consultant for patients with problems.) Nursing Mirror, 147, 7 Dec 1978, 19-21.

34 **Macilwaine, H.** Communication in the nurse/patient relationship. (Method of teaching skills by process recording used at Manchester University.) Nursing Mirror, 146, 16 Feb 1978, 32-34.

35 **Marsh, N.** The patient needs to talk. Nursing Mirror, 148, 28 Jun 1979, 16-18.

36 **Marson, S.N.** Nursing, a helping relationship? How to choose the appropriate training technique for developing communication skills. Nursing Times, 75, 29 Mar 1979, 541-544.

37 **Martin, I.C.A.** Clinical parable. A strident silence. (Advocates judicious use of silence in nurse/patient communication.) Nursing Times, 73, 19 May 1977, 754-755.

38 **Nichols, K.A.** A reason to worry. (A case for more detailed information for patients rather than general assurance from medical and nursing staff.) Nursing Times, 72 (51), 23/30 Dec 1976, 1990-1991.

39 **Nurse, G.** Counselling and helping skills: how can they be learned? 2 parts. (Part-time counselling course at Rcn's Institute of Advanced

Nursing Education; Courses and their evaluation.) Nursing Times, 76, 24 Apr 1980, 737-738; 1 May 1980, 789-790.

40 Nurse, G. There's no easy answer to clients' problems, warns Nurse. (Account of talk on counselling by nurses.) Nursing Mirror, 145, 15 Dec 1977, 3.

41 Nurse, G. What is counselling? Midwife, Health Visitor and Community Nurse, 14 (10), Oct 1978, 352, 354-355.

42 O'Brien, M.J. Communications and relationships in nursing. 2nd ed. St. Louis: Mosby, 1978.

43 Parsons, V. and Sanford, N. Inter-personal interaction in nursing: basic concepts in nurse-patient communication. Menlo Park, Ca.: Addison-Wesley, 1979.

44 Pluckhan, M.L. Human communication: the matrix of nursing. New York: McGraw-Hill, 1978.

45 Ramaekers, M.J. Communication blocks revisited. American Journal of Nursing, 1979, 79 (6), Jun 1979, 1079-1081.

46 Scott, M. and Cooper, G. Two views on the delivery of true counselling principles. Health and Social Service Journal, 88, 7 Jul 1978, 766-767.

47 Segall, J.J. Patient counselling. Com-munity Health, 9 (3), Feb 1978, 173-177.

48 Sierra-Franco, M.H. Therapeutic com-munication in nursing. New York: McGraw-Hill, 1978.

49 Smith, C.E. A decade of patient advocacy. Heart Lung, 8 (5), Sep/Oct 1979, 926-928.

50 Smith, L. Communication skills. Process recordings can be used to teach psychiatry students how to communicate. Nursing Times, 75, 31 May 1979, 926-929.

51 Smith, V. and Bass, T.A. Communication for health professionals. Philadelphia: Lippin-cott, 1979.

52 Stetler, C.B. Relationship of perceived empathy to nurses' communication. (Explor-atory analysis of verbal and vocal commun-icative behaviours of nurses using simulated nurse/patient interviews.) Nursing Research, 26 (6), Nov/Dec 1977, 432-438.

53 Stewart, B. Nursing and counselling—a conflict of roles? (Reprinted from Nursing Mirror, 140, 6 Feb 1975, 71-73.) Occupational Health, 30 (10), Oct 1978, 489-493.

54 Stewart, W. Health service counselling. Pitman Medical, 1979.

55 Swann, F. Rudiments of care. 5. Helping the patient communicate with others. Nursing Times, 75, 5 Jul 1979, 1148-1149.

56 Tetrault, A.I. Evaluation of develop-mental health counselling: healthfulness of self-support behavior. (Survey of patients attending long-term illness clinic.) Nursing Research, 26 (5), Sep/Oct 1977, 386-390.

57 Topics in Clinical Nursing Issue on com-munication. Topics in Clinical Nursing, 1 (3), Oct 1979, 1-100.

58 Turner, B. Fostering personal growth through small group interaction in a diploma school of nursing. (Counselling staff help students to develop communication skills.) Journal of Nursing Education, 15 (6), Nov 1976, 37-39.

59 Walke, M.A.K. When a patient needs to unburden his feelings. (Role of nurse.) American Journal of Nursing, 77 (7), Jul 1977, 1164-1166.

60 Wallston, K.A. and others Increasing nurses' person-centeredness. (Research study measuring nurses' responses to audiotaped statements from simulated patients.) Nursing Research, 27 (3), May/Jun 1978, 156-159.

61 Wells, R. A basic guide to nursing care. Who, what and when to tell? (Role of the nurse in ethical decisions about how much to tell the patient.) Nursing Mirror, 148, 19 Apr 1979, 22-23.

62 Wiedenbach, E. and Falls, C.E. Com-munication: key to effective nursing. New York: Tiresias Press, 1978.

63 Wilson, M. Should the patient be told the truth? (With some reference to nursing.) Patient Counseling and Health Education, 1 (2), Fall 1978, 70-74.

64 Yearwood-Grazette, H.S. An anatomy of communication. (Interpersonal communication with some reference to nurse-patient and nursing staff relationships.) Nursing Times, 74, 12 Oct 1978, 1672-1679.

c PATIENT TEACHING

1 Adair, L.P. Patient education. Nursing Care, 9 (4), Apr 1976, 29-31.

2 Alvey, G. How to begin a new job as patient education coordinator or tools for the beginning patient education coordinator. Hospital Topics, 56 (3), May/Jun 1978, 12-16.

3 Appelbaum, A.L. Patient education seen as integral part of patient care. Hospitals, 51, 16 Nov 1977, 113, 116, 118.

4 Bartlett, M.H. and Meyer, T.C. Patients receive current, concise health information by telephone. (Health-Line patient information service developed at the University of Wisconsin's Center for Health Sciences, Madison.) Hospitals, 50 (4), 16 Feb 1976, 79-80, 82.

5 Bille, D.A. A study of patients' knowledge in relation to teaching format and compliance. In-hospital teaching of patients must be individ-ualized to be effective. Supervisor Nurse, 8 (3), Mar 1977, 55-57, 60-62.

6 Brieger, W.R. A behavioural guide for eval-uating patient educators. International Journal of Health Education, 23 (1), 1980, 55-61.

7 Del Bueno, D.J. Patient education: planning for success. A comparison is made of the advantages and disadvantages of using a centralized or integrated organizational structure for patient education. Journal of Nursing Administration, 8 (6), Jun 1978, 3-7.

8 Fralic, M.A. Developing a viable inpatient education program—a nursing director's per-spective. (Braddock General Hospital, Pennsyl-vania.) Journal of Nursing Administration, 6 (7), Sep 1976, 30-36.

9 Frantz, R.A. Selecting media for patient education. Topics in Clinical Nursing, 2 (2), Jul 1980, 77-85.

10 Fuhrer, L.M. and Bernstein, R. Making patient education a part of patient care. (Illinois Masonic Medical Center.) American Journal of Nursing, 76 (11), Nov 1976, 1798-1799.

11 German, P.S. and Shwalow, A.J. Con-flicts in ethical problems of patient education: strategies for hypertension control explore contractual approach. (Study at Johns Hopkins Medical Institution Center of the use of health education of patients.) International Journal of Health Education, 14 (3), 1976, 195-201.

12 Gulko, C.S. and Butherus, C. Toward better patient teaching. Part 2. Journal of Practical Nursing, 28 (6), Jun 1978, 36-38.

13 Gusfa, A. and others Patient teaching: one approach. (Account of a 'Patient teaching programs manual', with instruction on indwell-ing urinary catheter, given as an example.) Supervisor Nurse, 6 (12), Dec 1975, 17, 19, 22.

14 Hautman, M.A. Assessment: one factor in effective client teaching. Nursing Forum, 18 (4), 1979, 405-414.

15 Hays, B.J. and Mockelstrom, N.R. Con-sumer survey: an approach to teaching consumer participation in community health. Journal of Nursing Education, 6 (8), Oct 1977, 30-34.

16 Herje, P.A. Hows and whys of patient contracting. (Method of patient teaching between nurse and patient about goals of behaviour for patient to achieve.) Nurse Educator, 5 (1), Jan/Feb 1980, 30-34.

17 Hinthorne, R.A. and Jones, R. Co-ordinating patient education in the hospital. (Through patient education committee to evaluate and co-ordinate work of different departments including library.) Hospitals, 52 (11), Jun 1978, 85-86, 88.

18 Iveson-Iveson, J. Prevention: how to stay healthy. 12. Everybody's business—but espec-ially the nurse's. (Nurse's teaching role.) Nursing Mirror, 149, 29 Nov 1979, 26.

19 Jenny, J. Patient teaching as a curriculum thread. Canadian Nurse, 74 (2), Feb 1978, 28-29.

20 Jenny, J. A strategy for patient teaching. Journal of Advanced Nursing, 3 (4), Jul 1978, 341-348.

21 Jones, P. 'Patient education—yes—no—'. A patient education form facilitates the docu-mentation of teaching. Supervisor Nurse, 8 (5), May 1977, 35, 38, 43.

22 Jones, P. and Oertel, W. Developing patient teaching objectives and techniques: a self-instructional program. Wakefield, Ma.: Nursing Digest Inc., 1977. Reprinted from Nurse Educ-ator, 2 (5), Sep/Oct 1977.

23 Kibbee, P. Puzzles for patients: a 'fun' approach to patient teaching. (Crossword puzzle and multiple-choice questions.) Journal of Practical Nursing, 30 (9), Sep 1980, 27-28, 37.

24 Kratzer, J.B. What does your patient need to know? (Use of Patient Education Assessment and Teaching Plan to provide outline for patient teaching.) Nursing, 7 (12), Dec 1977, 70-71.

25 Kuehnel, C. and Rowe, B. Patient educ-

ation and the audit: a new format developed for a teaching Kardex has been very successful as a means of documenting patient education. Supervisor Nurse, 11 (12), Dec 1980, 15-19.

26 Lee, E.A. and Garvey, J.L. How is inpatient education being managed? Survey assesses how hospitals plan, coordinate, finance, document and evaluate inpatient education. Hospitals, 51 (11), 1 Jun 1977, 75-76, 78, 80, 82.

27 Leighton, A.O. Ten steps to better patient teaching. RN Magazine, 38 (10), Oct 1976, 76-78.

28 Levin, L.S. Patient education and self-care: how do they differ? Nursing Outlook, 26 (3), Mar 1978, 170-175.

29 McCormick, R-M.D. and Gilson-Parkevich, T. editors Patient and family education: tools, techniques, and theory. New York: Wiley Medical, 1979.

30 McGowan, H.M. Partners in care. (Patient teaching as an integral part of the nursing process.) Supervisor Nurse, 10 (12), Dec 1979, 36, 38.

31 Miller, V. Rudiments of care 2. Helping the patient learn. Nursing Times, 75, 14 Jun 1979, 1016-1017.

32 Narrow, B.W. Patient teaching in nursing practice: a patient and family-centered approach. New York: Wiley Medical, 1979.

33 National League for Nursing Patient education. New York: NLN, 1976.

34 Nursing Administration Quarterly Patient teaching/patient rights. Nursing Administration Quarterly, 4 (2), Winter 1980, 1-115.

35 Nursing Digest Issue on patient teaching. Nursing Digest, 6 (1), Spring 1978, iv-viii, 1-87.

36 Redman, B.K. Curriculum in patient education. (Includes 'A patient's bill of rights' produced by the American Hospital Association.) American Journal of Nursing, 78 (8), Aug 1978, 1363-1366.

37 Redman, B.K. The process of patient teaching in nursing. 4th ed. St. Louis: Mosby, 1980.

38 RN Magazine A better way to calm the patient who fears the worst. (Patient teaching which includes information on sensory experiences the patient might have.) RN Magazine, 40 (4), Apr 1977, 47-54.

39 Ross Laboratories Patient education: the hospital's role. Journal of Nursing Care, 12 (10), Oct 1979, 15-20.

40 Salmond, S.W. Inservice and patient education. (Ten-step process to develop patient teaching programme and to train staff to teach patients.) Supervisor Nurse, 9 (5), May 1978, 95-97, 101.

41 Samborsky, V. Patient education with audio-tape self-confrontation. (Replay of taped interview which helps patients to come to terms with their health problems and reinforce their efforts to change health-related behaviour.) Journal of Gerontological Nursing, 5 (4), Jul/Aug 1979, 40-42.

42 Schenk, K. Teaching distributive nursing. (Teaching preventive medicine in an ambulatory care setting.) Nursing Outlook, 24 (9), Sep 1976, 574-577.

43 Shuler, C. Documenting patient teaching. Supervisor Nurse, 10 (6), Jun 1979, 43, 47-49.

44 Smith, C.E. Learning from sensations. (Teaching approaches illustrating the need to attend to patients' sensory experiences.) Journal of Nursing Education, 19 (2), Feb 1980, 31-33.

45 Steckel, S.B. Contracting with patient-selected reinforcers. (To achieve a specific health-related behaviour with the nurse's help.) American Journal of Nursing, 80 (9), Sep 1980, 1596-1599.

46 Sturdevant, B. Why don't adult patients learn? (Problems nurses face in teaching patients and how these may be overcome.) Supervisor Nurse, 8 (5), May 1977, 44, 46.

47 Sturdevant, B. and Patterson, R. Helping patients do their 'homework'. The nursing process provides the base for teaching patients and their families. Supervisor Nurse, 8 (4), Apr 1977, 72-73.

48 Swezey, A.M. and Kaufman, A.M. Library cart service provides information for clinic patients. (About arthritis.) Hospitals, 51, 1 Sep 1977, 65-67.

49 Taffa, P. The nursing role: an innovative approach. (Patient teaching.) Lamp, 35 (12), Dec/Jan 1978/1979, 30-33.

50 Veninga, R. Are you a successful communicator? (How effective patient education depends on good interpersonal communication.) Canadian Nurse, 74 (10), Nov 1978, 34-37.

51 Visintainer, M. and Wolfer, J. How rehearsing your patients can help them cope. (Going over patients' concerns about their illness using role-play, with reference to sex after a colostomy.) RN Magazine, 42 (1), Jan 1979, 57-62.

52 Whitehouse, R. Forms that facilitate patient teaching. (Record card including patient's acknowledgement of receipt of information.) American Journal of Nursing, 79 (7), Jul 1979, 1227-1229.

53 Williamson, K.C. and McCray, N. Putting together a patient education program that works. ('Teaching basket' of guidelines for nurses and booklets for patients.) RN Magazine, 40 (11), Nov 1977, 53-55.

54 Wise, P.S.Y. Barriers (or enhancers) to adult patient education. Journal of Continuing Education in Nursing, 10 (6), Nov/Dec 1979, 11-16.

55 Zander, K.S. and others, editors Practical manual for patient-teaching. St. Louis: Mosby, 1978.

56 Zonca, B.M. The role of the patient education coordinator. Supervisor Nurse, 11 (12), December 1980, 21-24, 26-27.

d THERAPEUTIC TOUCH

1 American Journal of Nursing Therapeutic touch. (Three articles on act of healing or helping akin to laying-on of hands.) American Journal of Nursing, 79 (4), Apr 1979, 660-665.

2 Blondis, M.N. and Jackson, B.E. Non-verbal communication with patients: back to the human touch. New York: Wiley, 1977.

3 Boguslawski, M. Therapeutic touch: a facilitator of pain relief. Topics in Clinical Nursing, 2 (1), Apr 1980, 27-37.

4 Boguslawski, M. The use of therapeutic touch in nursing. Journal of Continuing Education in Nursing, 10 (4), Jul/Aug 1979, 9-15.

5 Cooper, J. Actions really *do* speak louder than words. (Importance of non-verbal cues in nurse-patient interaction.) Nursing (U.S.), 9 (4), Apr 1979, 29-31.

6 Davis, A.J. Body talk. (Importance of non-verbal communication.) Supervisor Nurse, 9 (6), Jun 1978, 36-37.

7 Dunea, G. Healing by touching. (Chiropractors in the USA.) British Medical Journal, 1, 24 Mar 1979, 795-796.

8 Goodykoontz, L. Touch: attitudes and practice. (Review of research.) Nursing Forum, 18 (1), 1979, 4-17.

9 Goodykoontz, L. Touch: dynamic aspect of nursing care. Journal of Nursing Care, 13 (6), Jun 1980, 16-18.

10 Kittelson, Sister R. How to acquire the healing touch. (Religious healing.) Australian Nurses Journal, 7 (10), May 1978, 41.

11 Krieger, D. Alternative medicine. Therapeutic touch. Nursing Times, 72 (15), 15 Apr 1976, 572-574.

12 Krieger, D. The therapeutic touch: how to use your hands to help or to heal. Englewood Cliffs, N.J.: Prentice-Hall, 1979.

13 Lynch, J.L. The simple act of touching. (Research study in CCU and shock trauma unit to determine how human contact affects heart rhythm.) Nursing, 8 (6), Jun 1978, 32-36.

14 McCoy, P. Further proof that touch speaks louder than words. (Author's survey of the effects of touch on casualty patients.) RN Magazine, 40 (11), Nov 1977, 43-46.

15 Mason, A. Touch. (With reference to the nurse-patient relationship.) Nursing Times, 76, 5 Jun 1980, 999-1001.

16 Miller, L.A. An explanation of therapeutic touch: using the science of unitary man. Nursing Forum, 18 (3), 1979, 278-284, 286-287.

17 Montagu, A. Touching: the human significance of the skin. 2nd ed. New York: Harper and Row, 1978.

18 Sandroff, R. A sceptic's guide to therapeutic touch. (Method of paranormal healing.) RN Magazine, 43 (1), Jan 1980, 25-30, 82-83.

19 Ujhely, G.B. Touch: reflections and perceptions. Nursing Forum, 18 (1), 1979, 18-32.

20 Weiss, S.J. The language of touch. (Review of literature and discussion of conceptual framework.) Nursing Research, 28 (2), Mar/Apr 1979, 76-80.

21 Zefron, L.J. The history of the laying on of hands in nursing. Nursing Forum, 14 (4), 1975, 350-363.

e SEXUALITY

1 Anderson, M.L. Talking about sex—with less anxiety. Journal of Psychiatric Nursing, 18 (6), Jun 1980, 10-15.

2 Barnard, M.U. and others Human sexuality for health professionals. Philadelphia: Saunders, 1978.

3 Couldon, L. and Tayler, J. Sexual bias in nursing practice. (Study to test hypothesis that nurses prefer to nurse male patients.) Lamp, 34 (9), Sep 1977, 13-15.

4 Deer, B. Rights for gays in the face of NHS 'homophobia'. (Includes reference to course for health workers to dispel myths.) Health and Social Service Journal, 89, 25 May 1979, 618-619.

5 Gillan, P. Sex therapy. Midwife, Health Visitor and Community Nurse, 15 (5), May 1979, 182, 184, 186.

6 Gross, M.J.G. Two articles on homosexuality. (Attitudes towards it and a psychoanalytic view.) Perspectives in Psychiatric Care, 16 (2), Mar/Apr 1978, 70-79.

7 Hampton, P.J. Coping with the male patient's sexuality. Nursing Forum, 18 (3), 1979, 304-310.

8 Harland, P. Sexual deviation. Nursing Mirror, 142, 19 Feb 1976, 57-60.

9 Harris, J.K. Human sexuality: implications for occupational health nursing. Occupational Health Nursing, 25 (9), Sep 1977, 7-10.

10 Hicks, C. Taking the lid off . . . (Report of conference of Rcn's Association of Nursing Students on sexuality and the nurse.) Nursing Times, 76, 25 Sep 1980, 1681-1682.

11 Hogan, R.M. Nursing and human sexuality. Appleton-Century-Croft, 1980. Extract in Nursing Times, 76, 24 Jul 1980, 1296-1300.

12 Horowitz, J.A. Sexual difficulties as indicators of broader personal and inter-personal problems. Perspectives in Psychiatric Care, 16 (2), Mar/Apr 1978, 66-69.

13 Kjervik, D.K. and Palta, M. Sex-role stereotyping in assessments of mental health made by psychiatric-mental health nurses. Nursing Research, 27 (3), May/Jun 1978, 166-171.

14 Kolodny, R.C. and others Textbook of human sexuality for nurses. Boston: Little, Brown, 1979.

15 Kraemer, W.P. Homosexuality—is it an illness? Midwife, Health Visitor and Community Nurse, 12 (5), May 1976, 147, 149, 151, 153.

16 Kroll, U. Sexual counselling. SPCK, 1980. (Care and counselling.)

17 Krozy, R. Becoming comfortable with sexual assessment. (As part of health history-taking.) American Journal of Nursing, 78 (6), Jun 1978, 1036-1038.

18 Lanehan, C.C. Homosexuality: a different sexual orientation. Nursing Forum, 15 (3), 1976, 314-319.

19 Lawrence, J.C. Gay peer counselling. (Mental Health Clinic in Boston serving homosexual persons and their families.) Journal of Psychiatric Nursing and Mental Health Services, 15 (6), Jun 1977, 33-37.

20 Lawrence, J.C. Homosexuals, hospitalization and the nurse. Nursing Forum, 14 (3), 1975, 305-317.

21 Linken, A. and others Sexual attitudes factor: restructuring of sexual attitudes to help those who counsel others on sexual problems. Nursing Focus, 1 (9), May 1980, 358, 360.

22 Mindek, L. Inpatient psychiatric women's groups: the concept of sexuality. Journal of Psychiatric Nursing, 17 (4), Apr 1979, 36-39.

23 Mitchell, J.R. Male adolescents' concern about a physical examination conducted by a female. Nursing Research, 29 (3), May/Jun 1980, 165-169.

24 Payne, T. Sexuality of nurses: correlations of knowledge, attitudes and behavior. Nursing Research, 25 (4), Jul/Aug 1976, 287-292.

25 Pettyjohn, R.D. Health care of the gay individual. Nursing Forum, 18 (4), 1979, 367-393.

26 Roberts, L.A.M. Female homosexuality. (Theories of causation and implications for nursing.) Nursing Times, 73, 15 Sep 1977, 1426-1429.

27 Roznoy, M.S. The young adult. Taking a sexual history. American Journal of Nursing, 76 (8), Aug 1976, 1279-1282.

28 Schlesinger, B. From A to Z with adolescent sexuality. (Issues for nurses to consider.) Canadian Nurse, 73 (10), Oct 1977, 34-37.

29 Schofield, M. Why is homosexuality still something to hide? New Society, 47, 15 Feb 1979, 348-350.

30 Schrock, R.A. and Dunn, I. 'Homosexuality and the medical profession: a behaviourist's view' by John Bancroft. (Commentary on a paper which appeared in the Journal of Medical Ethics, vol.1, p.176.) Journal of Medical Ethics, 2 (1), Mar 1976, 24-27.

31 Topics in Clinical Nursing Issue on human sexuality. Topics in Clinical Nursing, 1 (4), Jan 1980, 1-106.

32 Whitley, M.P. Seduction and the hospitalized person. (The effect of illness on sexuality and how to cope with seductive behaviour from patients.) Journal of Nursing Education, 17 (6), Jun 1978, 34-39.

33 Whitley, M.P. and Willingham, D. Adding a sexual assessment to the health interview. Journal of Psychiatric Nursing and Mental Health Services, 16 (4), Apr 1978, 17-22, 27.

f SLEEP AND CIRCADIAN RHYTHMS

1 Adam, K. A time for rest and a time for play. (Value of sleep and factors affecting it.) Nursing Mirror, 150, 6 Mar 1980, 17-18.

2 Beardslee, C. The sleep of infants and young children: a review of the literature. Maternal-Child Nursing Journal, 5 (1), Spring 1976, 5-14.

3 Burrows, P.J. Biorhythms. (Internal cycles of physical, emotional and intellectual change.) Nursing Mirror, 144, 16 Jun 1977, 30-31.

4 Dodds, E.J. Slept well? A study of ward activity and nurse-patient interaction at night. MSc thesis, Surrey University, 1980.

5 Esson, E. Nurse could you care more? (How nurses on night duty can help patients sleep well.) Nursing Times, 75, 16 Aug 1979, 1387-1388.

6 Garner, H.G. You may have to leave the hospital to get well. The therapeutic value of sleep is unnecessarily denied the hospitalized patient. Supervisor Nurse, 9 (9), Sep 1978, 76-79.

7 Gillis, L. Sleeplessness can you help? (Research study of nurse-patient interaction regarding sleeplessness.) Canadian Nurse, 72 (7), Jul 1976, 32-34.

8 Hayter, J. The rhythm of sleep. American Journal of Nursing, 80 (3), Mar 1980, 457-461.

9 Hilton, A. Quantity and quality of patients' sleep and sleep disturbed factors in a respiratory intensive care unit. (Descriptive study.) Journal of Advanced Nursing, 1 (6), Nov 1976, 453-468.

10 Leddy, S. Sleep and phase shifting of biological rhythms. (Research study to determine the relationship between an abrupt 1 hr shift in the sleep portion of the sleep-wakefulness cycle and changes of phase in blood pressure and temperature in young women.) International Journal of Nursing Studies, 14 (3), 1977, 137-150.

11 Rader, J. and White, J. Circadian rhythms: how the patient's biological timetable affects your care. RN Magazine, 41 (9), Sep 1978, 100-102, 104, 106, 109-110.

12 Watts, C.A.H. Sleep and sleeplessness. Nursing Mirror, 145, 22 Sep 1977, 16-17.

13 Zelechowski, G.P. Helping your patient sleep: planning instead of pills. Nursing, 77 7 (5), May 1977, 63-65.

16 PATIENT

a PATIENT PSYCHOLOGY

1 Addison, C. Social implications of sudden facial disfigurement. (Following surgery for cancer.) Social Work Today, 9, 27 Jun 1978, 18-20.

2 Advances in Nursing Science Issue on stress and adaptation. Advances in Nursing Science, 1 (4), Jul 1979, 1-108.

3 Armitage, S. Non-compliant recipients of health care. (Concepts of patient role and 'good' or 'bad' patients and the effect these definitions may have on nursing care and patient outcome.) Nursing Times, 76, 3 Jan 1980, Occ. papers, 1-3.

4 Bond, J. and Bond, S. Changing images. (The concepts of the patient career, illness behaviour and the sick role.) Nursing Mirror, 150, 6 Mar 1980, 28-31.

5 Brink, P.J. Patientology: just another ology? (All aspects of the study of people as patients.) Nursing Outlook, 26 (9), Sep 1978, 574-575.

6 Brockway, B.F. Situational stress and

temporal changes in self-report and vocal measurements. (Using audio-recordings of speech.) Nursing Research, 28 (1), Jan/Feb 1979, 20-24.

7 Brown, M.S. Normal development of body image. New York: Wiley, 1977. (Wiley nursing concept module series.)

8 Bunch, B. and others Psychological care aided by RN counsellors. Three RNs working on master's degrees in counselling helped hospitalized patients and their families, nurses, and physicians deal with psychological aspects of illness. Hospitals, 53 (12), 16 Jun 1979, 125-126.

9 Clarke, M. Psychology. 1. Know your patient. Nursing Mirror, 150, 10 Apr 1980, 28-30.

10 Clough, D.H. and Derdiarian, A. A behavioral checklist to measure dependence and independence. (In patients.) Nursing Research, 29 (1), Jan/Feb 1980, 55-58.

11 Creighton, H. A curriculum investigation of patient anxieties. (New South Wales Nurses Education Board study.) Australian Nurses Journal, 6 (6 & 7), Dec 1976-Jan 1977, 12-13.

12 Dagsland, H. To be ill. (Need for the nursing profession to emphasise in education and practice the psychological needs of patients.) International Nursing Review, 25 (4), Jul/Aug 1978, 116-118.

13 Derdiarian, A. and Clough, D. Patients' dependence and independence levels on the pre-hospitalization-postdischarge continuum. (Effects of the stress of hospitalization and surgery.) Nursing Research, 25 (1), Jan-Feb 1976, 27-34.

14 Dingwall, R. Aspects of illness. Robertson, 1976. (Medicine in society series.)

15 Eggland, E.T. The anxious patient. Nursing Care, 9 (7), Jul 1976, 13-14.

16 Fisher, E.E. Psychology for nurses and the hospital team. 2nd ed. Cape Town: Juta, 1977. 3rd ed. 1979.

17 Gillis, L. Human behaviour in illness: psychology and interpersonal relationships. 3rd ed. Faber, 1980.

18 Guzzetta, C.E. and Forsyth, G.L. Nursing diagnostic pilot study: psychophysiologic stress. (Study to develop a typology of stress in patients with acute illness and assessment tool for nurses.) Advances in Nursing Science, 2 (1), Oct 1979, 27-44.

19 Hazzard, M.E. and Thorndal, M.L. Patient anxiety: teaching students to intervene effectively. Nursing Education, 4 (1), Jan/Feb 1979, 19-21.

20 Holderby, R.A. and McNulty, E.G. Feelings, feelings: how to make a rational response to emotional behavior. Nursing (U.S.), 9 (10), Oct 1979, 39-43.

21 Hover, J. and Juelsgaard, N. The sick role reconceptualized. Nursing Forum, 17 (4), 1978, 406-416.

22 Jarvis, J.M. and Gibson, J. Psychology for nurses. 4th ed. Blackwell, 1977.

23 Lake, G.M. Hospitalization and person-ality change: recognition vital to nursing care. Canadian Nurse, 73 (1), Jan 1977, 44-45.

24 Lawrence, S.A. and Lawrence, R.M. A model of adaptation to the stress of chronic illness. Nursing Forum, 18 (1), 1979, 33-42.

25 Lipe, H.P. The function of weeping in the adult. (Including nursing implications.) Nursing Forum, 19 (1), 1980, 26-44.

26 McGhie, A. Psychology as applied to nursing. 7th ed. Churchill Livingstone, 1979. (Churchill Livingstone nursing text series.)

27 McGilloway, F.A. One aspect of the social/psychological element of the illness state. (Exploration of situation of new patient in a general hospital ward.) International Journal of Nursing Studies, 16 (3), Aug 1979, 267-273.

28 MacLeod, A. Illness as a deviant role. A clue to the rejection of symptoms. (Research study of forty patients' attitudes before and after carotid artery reconstruction.) Nursing Times, 74, 24 Aug 1978, 1400-1401.

29 Marten, L. Self-care nursing model for patients experiencing radical change in body image. (With reference to care of patient after radical vulvectomy.) Journal of Obstetric, Gynecologic and Neonatal Nursing, 7 (6), Nov/Dec 1978, 9-13.

30 Matejski, M.P. A framework for nursing: a concept for practice. (Based on the influence of stress on the rhythmic patterns of the individual as they affect his mobility.) Journal of Nursing Education, 18 (5), May 1979, 49-58.

31 Newman, M.A. Movement tempo and the experience of time. (A survey to test the relationship between preferred rate of walking and the individual's estimate of time.) Nursing Research, 25 (4), Jul/Aug 1976, 273-279.

32 Nurses Education Board of New South Wales A curriculum investigation of patient anxieties. Sydney: the Board, 1976.

33 O'Brien, J. Mirror, mirror, why me? (The development of the body image and how nurses can help patients cope with traumatic changes such as stomas or mastectomy.) Nursing Mirror, 150, 24 Apr 1980, 36-37.

34 Pettit, E. Body image. Nursing, 16, Aug 1980, 690-692.

35 Rawnsley, M.M. The concept of privacy. Advances in Nursing Science, 2 (2), Jan 1980, 25-31.

36 Roberts, S.L. Behavioral concepts and nursing throughout the life span. Englewood Cliffs, N.J.: Prentice-Hall, 1978.

37 Roberts, S.L. Piaget's theory reapplied to the critically ill. (Alteration in patients' cognitive abilities with implications for nursing.) Advances in Nursing Science, 2 (2), Jan 1980, 61-78.

38 Rutter, D.M. Measurement of psychological factors in chronic illness. Rheumatology and Rehabilitation, 15 (3), Aug 1976, 174-178.

39 Saunders, S.J. The effects of ward rounds on patients. (Psychological effects.) S.A. Nursing Journal, 44 (10), Oct 1977, 24.

40 Saylor, D.E. Understanding patients' feelings of loss. (Due to the process of hospitalisation.) Hospital Progress, 58 (5), May 1977, 88-90, 92, 94.

41 Schneider, J.S. Hopelessness and helplessness. (Relevance to nursing care.) Journal of Psychiatric Nursing, 18 (3), Mar 1980, 12-21.

42 Schultz, E.D. Privacy: the forgotten need. Canadian Nurse, 73 (7), Jul 1977, 33-34.

43 Shontz, F.C. The psychological aspects of physical illness and disability. Collier Macmillan, 1975.

44 Sloboda, S. Understanding patient behavior. (Psychological assessment of patients.) Nursing, 7 (9), Sep 1977, 74-77.

45 Smith, D.W. Survivors of serious illness. (Study of patients in order to understand the survival experience and its effect on personal development so that nurses may help patients to cope.) American Journal of Nursing, 79 (3), Mar 1979, 441-446.

46 Snyder, C.C. and Wilson, M.F. Elements of a psychological assessment. (An assessment tool developed by psychiatric nurses which can be used for general patient assessment.) American Journal of Nursing, 77 (2), Feb 1977, 235-239.

47 Stanley, L. Does your own body image hurt patient care? (Nurses' reactions to nursing patients who are disfigured.) RN Magazine, 40 (12), Dec 1977, 52-53.

48 Starr, B.D. and Goldstein, H.S. Human development and behavior: psychology in nursing. New York: Springer, 1975.

49 Stephenson, C.A. Stress in critically ill patients. (Physiological effects.) American Journal of Nursing, 77 (11), Nov 1977, 1806-1809.

50 Stillman, M.J. Territoriality and personal space. (With reference to hospital patients and nursing care.) American Journal of Nursing, 78 (10), Oct 1978, 1670-1672.

51 Strongman, K.T. Psychology for the paramedical professions. Croom Helm, 1979.

52 Taggart, M. Body image: looking beyond the mirror. Part 1. Normal development. Part 2. Adjusting to alterations. (Patients' coping mechanisms and nursing care.) Journal of Practical Nursing, 27 (7), Jul 1977, 32-33; (8), Aug 1977, 25-28, 35.

53 Trust, D. Disfigurement therapy. Nursing Mirror, 143 (4), 22 Jul 1976, 62-66.

54 Volicer, B.J. and Burns, M.E. Pre-existing correlates of hospital stress. (Survey of medical and surgical patients.) Nursing Research, 26 (6), Nov/Dec 1977, 408-415.

55 Walker, F.A. Psychological stress associated with coming into hospital. New Zealand Nursing Journal, 70 (3), Mar 1977, 9-12.

56 Wilson-Barnett, J. and Carrigy, A. Factors influencing patients' emotional reactions to hospitalization. (Research study with medical ward patients.) Journal of Advanced Nursing, 3 (3), May 1978, 221-229.

57 Wilson-Barnett, J. In hospital: patients' feelings and opinions. (Research study to explore what factors are most likely to be associated with strong affective experiences of patients in hospital.) Nursing Times, 74, 16 Mar 1978, Occ. papers, 29-32; 23 Mar 1978, Occ. papers, 33-34.

58 Wilson-Barnett, J. Patients' emotional reactions to hospitalization: an exploratory study. (Interview with 200 medical patients.) Journal of Advanced Nursing, 1 (5), Sep 1976, 351-358.

59 Wilson-Barnett, J. Prevention and alleviation of stress in patients. Nursing, 10, Feb 1980, 432-436.

60 Wilson-Barnett, J. Stress in hospital: patients' psychological reactions to illness and health care. Edinburgh: Churchill Livingstone, 1979.

61 Zerubavel, E. Patterns of time in hospital life: a sociological perspective. Chicago: University of Chicago Press, 1979.

b SENSORY DEPRIVATION

1 Aiello, J. The concept of sensory deprivation. (With reference to intensive care.) Australian Nurses Journal, 7 (10), May 1978, 38-40.

2 Ashworth, P. Sensory deprivation. 2. The acutely ill. Nursing Times, 75, 15 Feb 1979, 290-294.

3 Association of Integrated and Degree Courses in Nursing Fundamental concepts in nursing: sensory deprivation. Report of 6th open conference, Nottingham University, 7-9 Jul 1978. The Association, 1978.

4 Smith, J. Sensory deprivation—a primary concept of nursing. (With reference to various types of patients including the elderly and acutely ill.) Nursing Mirror, 147, 3 Aug 1978, 7.

5 Wood, M. Clinical sensory deprivation: a comparative study of patients in single care and two-bed rooms. Journal of Nursing Administration, 7 (10), Dec 1977, 28-32.

c PATIENTS' VIEWS

1 Ashton, K. Home truths for hospital nurses. (Ex-patients describe the special needs of the long term sick and disabled in hospital and offer advice to nurses.) Nursing Times, 73, 5 May 1977, 642-643.

2 Breitung, J. What patients remember about their nurses. (Results of study by student nurses.) Journal of Practical Nursing, 30 (2), Feb 1980, 19-20.

3 Cosper, B. How well do patients understand hospital jargon? (Survey of patients.) American Journal of Nursing, 77 (12), Dec 1977, 1932-1934.

4 Croydon Community Health Council What the consumer really thinks. (Croydon CHC's questionnaire survey of patients at Mayday Hospital, Croydon including satisfaction with nursing care.) Health and Social Service Journal, 90, 28 Mar 1980, 411.

5 Doll, A. The things patients say about their nurses. (Comments on interpersonal skills but not skill or expertise.) Nursing (U.S.), 9 (5), May 1979, 18-23.

6 Fleming, G.V. Using consumer evaluations

of health care. (In hospitals.) Hospital Progress, 60 (8), Aug 1979, 54-60, 68.

7 Genvert, G. and others Isolation information booklet stimulates dialog, allays fears. (Patients' manual to supplement verbal explanations based on patients' questionnaire.) Hospitals, 53 (3), 1 Feb 1979, 72, 74-75.

8 Hawkins, C. Patients' reactions to their investigations: a study of 504 patients. (Study of what patients knew and anxiety and discomfort experienced.) British Medical Journal, 2, 15 Sep 1979, 638-640.

9 Kirchhoff, K.T. Let's ask the patient: consumer input can improve patient care. (Interviews with patients on transfer from intensive care to the medical unit to improve ICU care.) Journal of Nursing Administration, 6 (10), Dec 1976, 36-40.

10 Laing, G.P. Hospitalization: is it always a negative experience? (Survey of patients' reactions.) Canadian Nurse, 73 (11), Nov 1977, 35-37.

11 Machray, I.D. Do-it-yourself evaluation. (Report of working party at Sunnyside Royal Hospital in Scotland to obtain views of patients, staff and others on aspects of care.) Hospital and Health Service Review, 76 (9), Sep 1980, 300-301.

12 Pascoe, D.W. and others Patients' attitudes to health care: a literature review. World Hospitals, 14 (3), Aug 1978, 165-170.

13 Peach, H. and Pathy, M.S. Evaluation of patients' assessment of day hospital care. (Geriatric patients.) British Journal of Preventive and Social Medicine, 31 (3), Sep 1977, 209-210.

14 Price, J.L.W. The patient's morale. (Letter based on hospital experience.) Lancet, 1977, 1, 5 Mar 1977, 533.

15 Raphael, Winifred Patients and their hospitals: a survey of patients' views of life in general hospitals. 3rd ed. King Edward's Hospital Fund for London, 1977.

16 Reynolds, M. No news is bad news: patients' views about communication in hospital. (Survey of 133 patients by medical student.) British Medical Journal, 1, 24 Jun 1978, 1673-1676.

17 Royal Commission on the National Health Service Patients' attitudes to the hospital service. HMSO, 1978. (Research paper no.5)

18 Schwarz, K. The need and demand for medical care. (Definition of need and demand with reference to New Zealand and patient opinion survey of hospital stay.) Public Health, 93 (2), Mar 1979, 105-110.

19 Smith, R.B. Patient opinions help place hospital services in perspective. (Use of questionnaires, telephone surveys, inpatient 'hotline' and advisory board at Sacramento Medical Center, California.) Hospitals, 51 (16), 16 Aug 1977, 65-66, 68.

20 Steele, S.J. and Morton, D.J.R. The ward round. (Survey of patients' criticisms and authors' suggestions for improvement.) Lancet, 1, 14 Jan 1978, 85-86.

21 Stevenson, M.J. A CHC patient attitude survey. (Conducted by Stockport CHC in a long-

stay hospital.) Hospital and Health Services Review, 74 (7), Jul 1978, 224-225.

22 Tomson, P.R.V. Some books for the general practitioner. (Books illuminating patients' experiences.) Journal of the Royal College of General Practitioners, 26, Aug 1976, 588-590.

23 Williamson, Y.M. Methodologic dilemmas in tapping the concept of patient needs. (Problems in constructing questionnaires to measure patients' needs and nurses' perceptions of those needs.) Nursing Research, 27 (3), May/Jun 1978, 172-177.

d PATIENT WELFARE

1 Ball, D. Bridging the gap. (Two articles on the present state of medical social work.) Health and Social Service Journal, 88, 14 Apr 1978, 418-420.

2 Beckingham, C.R. What about the relatives? (Experience of caring for relatives, gained while studying in Oxford.) New Zealand Nursing Journal, 69 (11), Nov 1976, 14-15.

3 Berkeley, J.S. Patients' families and friends at home and in hospital. (Comparison of accessibility of cottage hospitals and general hospitals.) Practitioner, 222, May 1979, 593-596.

4 Branton, P. The big unisex wards controversy. Nursing Mirror, 147, 20 Jul 1978, 10-11.

5 Breu, C. and Dracup, K. Helping the spouses of critically ill patients. (Nursing care plan for spouse to relieve anxiety and provide support.) American Journal of Nursing, 78 (1), Jan 1978, 51-53.

6 Brown, A. Vital links. From one problem to another. (Work of medical social worker.) Nursing Mirror, 148, 3 May 1979, 26-27.

7 Calnan, J. Sex mix. (Advocates more mixed-sex wards.) World Medicine, 13, 8 Feb 1978, 45-46.

8 Castledine, G. Involving the family in patient care. (Aspects of basic care such as tube-feeding, administering eye-drops.) Nursing Mirror, 147, 14 Dec 1978, 14.

9 Central Health Services Council The organisation of the in-patient's day: report of a Committee. HMSO, 1976. (Chairman: Sir John Hanbury.)

10 Condon, T.B. and Korn, J.T. Patient support line provides instant response or aid. (Telephone link at Yale New Haven Hospital dealing with patients' problems.) Hospitals, 51 (6), 16 Mar 1977, 93-94, 98, 100.

11 Cooper, H. Is the patient a guinea-pig and secondary to all technology to which he is subjected? S.A. Nursing Journal, 44 (2), Feb 1977, 23-24.

12 Cooper, J.E. Pets in hospitals. British Medical Journal, 1976, 1, 20 Mar 1976, 698-700.

13 Cuming, M.W. The day in hospital. (Letter describing a King's Fund College visit to hospital wards to see if 'The pattern of the in-patient's day' had been implemented.) Nursing Times, 72 (6), 12 Feb 1976, 228-229.

14 Farrow, G. and MacMillan, P. Major implications. (Two comments on TV play 'Minor complications' in which a patient complaining of pain is treated as a difficult patient.) Nursing Times, 76, 4 Dec 1980, 2138-2139.

15 Garton, E.J. In praise of open visiting. Nursing Times, 75, 11 Oct 1979, 1747.

16 Gordon, P. CHC visiting: a guide to visiting long-stay hospitals and units. King's Fund Centre, 1979. (KF project paper; 23.)

17 Hamilton, Lady Dressed for a normal life. (Problems in the provision of personal clothing for long-stay patients.) Health and Social Service Journal, 87, 21 Oct 1977, 1476-1477.

18 Health and Social Service Journal Buttons and bows and a boutique for long stay patients. (Recent seminar on personalised clothing for long-stay patients.) Health and Social Service Journal, 89, 9 Nov 1979, 1444-1445.

19 Hospitals The human ingredient. (Three articles on humanistic care which enhances the dignity of patients and staff alike.) Hospitals, 53 (22), 16 Nov 1979, 75-82, 84.

20 Johnson, B.D.L. Mixing could be distressing. (Letter in criticism of mixed-sex wards by an anaesthetist.) Nursing Mirror, 147, 21 Dec 1978, 8.

21 Kingman, S. Where people are too ill to care whose company they keep: the mixed-sex wards controversy. Health and Social Service Journal, 89, 25 May 1979, 622-623.

22 Kinsella, P. The relative: forgotten member of the health care team. Hospital Administration in Canada, 18 (1), Jan 1976, 29.

23 Leonard, A.W. How the visitor is treated affects the patient. (Preparation of student nurses in helping visitors.) Journal of Psychiatric Nursing and Mental Health Services, 14 (4), Apr 1976, 20-23.

24 MacArthur, C. and Wakefield, J. Patients' acceptance of mixed-sex wards. (Survey in Manchester.) Health and Social Service Journal, 88, 26 May 1978, Centre eight papers, A21-A24.

25 MacMillan, P. Women of the world, unite. (Criticism of mixed sex wards.) Nursing Times, 75, 16 Aug 1979, 1391-1392.

26 Mann, J.K. and others The social worker on the critical care team. (Medical social worker as counsellor to patients' relatives.) Supervisor Nurse, 8 (9), Sep 1977, 62-64, 67-68.

27 Miller, S. Pets, people and health. 1 and 2. Health Visitor, 53 (3), Mar 1980, 89-90, 92; (4), Apr 1980, 127-128, 130.

28 Nazer, G. Time for stricter controls over the growth of mixed wards? Nursing Mirror, 148, 25 Jan 1979, 6.

29 Nursing Times Mixed accommodation. (In wards—letters.) Nursing Times, 73, 25 Aug 1977, 1320.

30 Nursing Times A tale of four teeth. (Experience of Alison Dunn, Nursing Times editor, in hospital for the removal of wisdom teeth, told by colleagues.) Nursing Times, 74, 7 Sep 1978, 1473.

31 Moran, M.E. and Sutter, J. Comfort, care for families who must wait. (Volunteers staff a special waiting room that extends humanistic care to meet the needs of families as they wait to learn the outcome of their relatives' surgery or tests.) Hospitals, 53 (22), 16 Nov 1979, 112.

32 Perrin, J. Guide to preparing a patient information booklet. Dimensions in Health Service, 53 (8), Aug 1976, 22, 25.

33 Roberts, A.C.M. A survey of patients' attitudes to mixed wards in Brook General Hospital, Greenwich Health District. SE Thames Regional Health Authority, 1979.

34 Royal College of Nursing. Association of Nursing Practice Mixed sex wards. (Policy document.) Rcn, 1978.

35 Rozovsky, L.E. Responsibility for patient's property. Dimensions in Health Service, 53 (6), Jun 1976, 8-9.

36 Sainsbury, M.J.C. The bedside manner. (Importance of physiological care of patients and relatives.) Nursing Mirror, 146, 4 May 1978, 40-41.

37 Smith, M.C. Patient responses to being transferred during hospitalization. (A study by 8 clinical nurse specialists and a nurse research consultant.) Nursing Research, 25 (3), May/Jun 1976, 192-196.

38 Sturdevant, B. The extra dimension in nursing care. (Patient activity hour in an adult ward to encourage social interaction among patients.) RN Magazine, 39 (1), Jan 1976, 44-45.

39 Toban, P.L. and Moore, R. Program ensures better treatment for patients. Training program for all employees with patient contact. Hospitals, 54 (11), 1 Jun 1980, 76-78.

40 Toynbee, P. Hospital. Hutchinson, 1977.

41 Verzillo, J.K. A program for caring. (Programme to make the hospital a kinder, more empathetic place.) Supervisor Nurse, 11 (7), Jul 1980, 10-12, 15-16.

42 Watkin, B. One for the road. (Discusses recent complaints about mixed-sex wards.) Nursing Mirror, 145, 7 Jul 1977, 6.

43 West Midlands Regional Health Authority Mixed sex wards. Birmingham: the Health Authority, 1978. Summary in Hospital and Health Services Review, 74 (3), Mar 1978, 98.

44 Whitaker, M. Identification of patients. (To prevent errors and to treat patients as individuals.) Nursing Times, 74, 2 Nov 1978, Theatre Nursing, 17-18.

45 Wilson, S.S. Mixed wards. (Letter from campaigner against them.) World Medicine, 13 (15), 3 May 1978, 69, 71.

46 Wright, N. and Jones, D. Patient referrals in the NHS. (A model showing the flow of patients between health care facilities.) Health and Social Service Journal, 86, 6 Mar 1976, 440-441.

e CULTURAL DIFFERENCES

1 Bonaparte, B.H. Ego defensiveness, open-closed mindedness, and nurses' attitude toward culturally different patients. (Survey of nurses representing four ethnic groups.) Nursing Research, 28 (3), May/Jun 1979, 161-165.

2 Branch, M.F. and Paxton, P.P. joint editors Providing safe nursing care for ethnic people of color. New York: Appleton-Century-Crofts, 1976.

3 Brink, P.J. editor Transcultural nursing: a book of readings. Englewood Cliffs, N.J.: Prentice-Hall, 1976.

4 Capotorti, F. Study on the rights of persons belonging to ethnic, religious and linguistic minorities. New York: United Nations, 1979.

5 Chappell Mitchell, A. Black skin: an historical, psychological and health care perspective. Journal of Continuing Education in Nursing, 10 (6), Nov/Dec 1979, 28-33.

6 Cottle, T. A wasted death? (Case study of West Indian woman with cancer who claims doctors and nurses gave her inadequate care because of her colour.) New Society, 41, 29 Sep 1977, 656-657.

7 Davis, M. Getting to the root of the problem: hair grooming techniques for black patients. Nursing, 77 7 (4), Apr 1977, 60-65.

8 Frenkel, S.I. and others Does patient contact change racial perceptions? (Research study of racial perceptions of student nurses.) American Journal of Nursing, 80 (7), Jul 1980, 1340-1342.

9 Henley, A. Asian patients in hospital and at home. King Edward's Hospital Fund for London, 1979.

10 Henley, A. Practical care of Asian patients. Nursing, 16, Aug 1980, 683-686.

11 Leininger, M. Transcultural nursing: concepts, theories and practices. New York: Wiley, 1978.

12 Long, R. A tale of two cultures. (Communication with Asian and Arab patients.) Nursing Times, 73, 4 Aug 1977, 1215-1216.

13 Lothian Community Relations Council Religions and cultures: a guide to patients' beliefs and customs for health service staff. Edinburgh: Lothian Community Relations Council, 1978.

14 Luckraft, D. editor Black awareness: implications for patient care. New York: American Journal of Nursing Company, 1976.

15 McDonald, C.J. and Kelly, A.P. Black skin problems. American Journal of Nursing, 79 (6), Jun 1979, 1092-1094.

16 Nursing Clinics of North America Symposium on cultural and biological diversity and health care. Nursing Clinics of North America, 12 (1), Mar 1977, 1-86.

17 Solman, F. Through the language barrier: the Language Card Service offered by the British Red Cross Society. Nursing Mirror, 146, 23 Feb 1978, 9.

18 Speck, P. East comes West. (Practical guide to the religious beliefs, dietary habits and social customs of Asian patients.) Nursing Times, 72, 29 Apr 1976, 662-664.

19 Spector, R.E. Cultural diversity in health and illness. New York: Appleton-Century-Crofts, 1979.

20 Spratlen, L.P. Introducing ethnic cultural factors in models of nursing: some mental health care applications. (Introduction of cultural

factors into the mental health curriculum.) Journal of Nursing Education, 15 (2), Mar 1976, 23-29.

21 Standeven, M.V. Social sensitivity in health care. (Multidisciplinary course to increase understanding of other health professions and patients from other cultural and social groups.) Nursing Outlook, 25 (10), Oct 1977, 640-643.

17 INTENSIVE CARE

a GENERAL

1 Apps, M.C.P. Intensive care—8. Metabolic problems. Nursing Times, 74, 6 Apr 1978, 591-593.

2 Ashworth, P. Ethics in the ITU. Nursing Times, 72 (44), 4 Nov 1976, Occ. papers, 153-156.

3 Cadmus, R.R. Intensive care reaches silver anniversary. (Development since 1954.) Hospitals, 54 (2), 16 Jan 1980, 98-99, 101-102.

4 CURRENT Practice in Critical Care. Volume 1. St. Louis: Mosby, 1979. (Mosby's current practice and perspectives in nursing series.)

5 Davis, A.J. Ethics rounds with intensive care nurses. Nursing Clinics in North America, 14 (1), Mar 1979, 45-55.

6 Ledingham, I. McA. editor Recent advances in intensive therapy. 1. Churchill Livingstone, 1977.

7 Lenihan, J. The history of intensive care. Nursing Focus, 1 (2), Oct 1979, 75-76.

8 Lewis, S. Intensive care—7. Physiotherapy in the intensive therapy unit. Nursing Times, 74, 30 Mar 1978, 534-537.

9 Payne, J.P. and Hill, D.W. editors The management of the acutely ill: a symposium held in July 1976 (at Chartridge, Bucks.) Stevenage: Peregrinus, 1977.

10 Sherwood Jones, E. Essential intensive care. Lancaster: MTP, 1978.

11 Skillman, J.J. Intensive care. Boston: Little, Brown and Co., 1975.

12 Stoddart, J.C. Intensive therapy. Blackwell, 1975.

13 Tinker, J. Intensive care—1. General intensive therapy. Nursing Times, 74, 16 Feb 1978, 266-268.

14 Tinker, J. Intensive care—2. Two methods of assessing the critically ill patient. (Central venous pressure (CVP) and pulmonary wedge pressure (PWP).) Nursing Times, 74, 23 Feb 1978, 318-320.

15 Tinker, J. Intensive care—4. Shock. Nursing Times, 74, 9 Mar 1978, 406-408.

b EQUIPMENT AND MONITORING

1 Christopherson, K.I. Microprocessor technology adds new dimension to patient monitoring systems. (Use for the intensive care unit, Henderson Hospital, Hamilton, Ontario.) Hospital Administration in Canada, 18 (5), May 1976, 50-51.

2 Johnson, D.S. and others A computerized alert program for acutely ill patients. (Computer-assisted medical decision-making with some application to primary nursing.) Journal of Nursing Administration, 10 (6), Jun 1980, 26-35.

3 Rithalia, S. Intensive care—11. Equipment in the ICU. Nursing Times, 74, 27 Apr 1978, 713-716.

4 Tolbert, S.H. and Pertuz, A.E. Study shows how computerization affects nursing activities in ICU. (Computer-based monitoring system.) Hospitals, 51, 1 Sep 1977, 79-82, 84.

5 Walleck, C. The neurosurgical nurse and computer work together. (Use of computers in intensive care.) Journal of Neurosurgical Nursing, 7 (2), Dec 1975, 102-106.

c MANAGEMENT, PLANNING AND STAFFING

1 Aitkenhead, A.R. and others An economical mobile intensive care unit. British Medical Journal, 17 May 1980, 1219-1221.

2 Baldwin, L. and Pierce, R. Mobile intensive care: a problem-oriented approach. St. Louis: Mosby, 1978.

3 Brown, A.J. Change in charting on critical-care units. (Towards problem-oriented records.) Nursing Clinics of North America, 14 (2), Jun 1979, 365-372.

4 Evans, S.K. and others Projecting staffing requirements for intensive care units. Journal of Nursing Administration, 10 (6), Jul 1980, 34-42.

5 Gibson, V.J. Rotation of critical care nursing personnel. Supervisor Nurse, 9 (5), May 1978, 15-17.

6 Goodwin, I.H. A guide to planning critical care units. Journal of Nursing Administration, 9 (6), Jun 1979, 20-25.

7 Ledingham, I. McA. and Banks, J.G. Movement of the critically ill patient. (Mobile intensive care unit developed at Western Infirmary Glasgow.) Hospital Update, 6 (1), Jan 1980, 43-45, 48-49.

8 Long, A. and others Staffing intensive therapy units. (Research study to discover problems in staffing.) Nursing Times, 73, 24 Nov 1977, 1836-1838.

9 McAlister, E. Managing an intensive care unit. Nursing Focus, 1 (2), Oct 1979, 67-69.

10 Mann, J.K. Nursing leadership in the critical care setting. Nursing Clinics of North America, 13 (1), Mar 1978, 131-138.

11 Savoy, J. Simplify your critical-care records. (Improved chart for intensive care patients' records.) Nursing, 7 (8), Aug 1977, 16-18.

12 Schmied, E. Intensive care. The planning process: a nurse's view. Hospital Topics, 54 (3), May/Jun 1976, 14-16, 18.

13 Silverston, P.P. A decade on the road. (Role of Mobile Intensive Care Nurse in USA.) Nursing Mirror, 150, 20 Mar 1980, 16-18.

d NURSING

1 Adler, D. Critical care nursing. (Symposium on nursing in America.) Nursing Mirror, 143 (2), 8 Jul 1976, 54-55.

2 American Association of Critical-Care Nurses Methods in critical care: the AACN manual. Philadelphia: Saunders, 1980.

3 Burrell, Z.L. and Burrell, L.O. Critical care. 3rd ed. St. Louis: Mosby, 1977.

4 Daly, B.J. Intensive care nursing. New York: Medical Examination Pub.Co.; Henry Kimpton, 1980. (Current clinical nursing series.)

5 Goodland, N.L. General intensive care. Bristol: Wright, 1978.

6 Hazzard, M.E. Critical care nursing. Kimpton, 1978. (Nursing outline series.)

7 Holloway, N.M. Nursing the critically ill adult. Menlo Park, Calif.: Addison-Wesley, 1979.

8 Houser, D.M. A study of nurses new to special care units: an evaluation of the factors which influence job performance. Supervisor Nurse, 8 (7), Jul 1977, 15-17, 20-22.

9 Hudak, C.M. and others Critical care nursing. 2nd ed. Philadelphia: Lippincott, 1977.

10 Jackson, T. and others Sample standard nursing care plans for patients in intensive and coronary care units: a working document. Vancouver: Registered Nurses' Association of British Columbia, 1977.

11 Meltzer, L.E. and others, editors Concepts and practices of intensive care for nurse specialists. 2nd ed. Bowie, Maryland: Charles Press, 1976.

12 MOSBY's manual of critical care, by L.F. Abels. St. Louis: Mosby, 1979.

13 Petersen, J. and others Nursing students' experience in critical care. (Study of 100 newly trained nurses.) Journal of Nursing Education, 16 (7), Sep 1977, 3-9.

14 Pierce, S.F. Clinical experience in the intensive care unit. (For student nurses.) Nursing Outlook, 25 (10), Oct 1977, 650-652.

15 Retsas, A. Socialization and the intensive care unit. (Sociological analysis of nurse's position within team.) Australian Nurses Journal, 9 (5), Nov 1979, 33-34.

16 Tinker, J. and Porter, S.W. A course in intensive therapy nursing. Arnold, 1980.

17 Williamson, J.A. and others Intensive care nursing continuing education review: 403 essay questions and referenced answers. Flushing: Medical Examination Publishing Co., 1977.

e NURSING EDUCATION AND TRAINING

1 Blowers, S. Total care teaching. (JBCNs course on intensive care nursing.) Nursing Focus, 1 (2), Oct 1979, 71-72.

2 Collins, B.E. Methods of clinical teaching in intensive care units. New Zealand Nursing Journal, 70 (6), Jun 1977, 17-18.

3 **Harrell, J.R.S.** Orienting the experienced critical care nurse. (Three week programme.) Supervisor Nurse, 11 (1), Jan 1980, 32-33.

4 **Joint Board of Clinical Nursing Studies** 6. General intensive care. Nursing Mirror, 143 (10), 2 Sep 1976, Nursing care supplement, series 2, i-iv.

5 **Lindstrom, S.R. and Archibald, E.J.** A critical care teaching method. (Self-paced modules in in-service education.) Supervisor Nurse, 11 (1), Jan 1980, 49.

6 **Purushotham, D.** The dilemma facing critical care nursing. (Should training for intensive care be in basic or post-basic programs?) Hospital Administration in Canada, 18 (2), Feb 1976, 32, 34.

7 **Sherer, B.K. and Thompson, M.A.** The process of developing a learning center in an acute care setting. (At El Camino Hospital in California.) Journal of Continuing Education in Nursing, 9 (1), Jan-Feb 1978, 36-44.

8 **Worthington, L.** On-going education in critical care. (Description of eight-day course organised by author.) Canadian Nurse, 74 (3), Mar 1978, 41-43.

f PSYCHOLOGICAL ASPECTS
(Staff, patients and family)

1 **Adams, M. and others** The confused patient: psychological responses in critical care units. American Journal of Nursing, 78 (9), Sep 1978, 1504-1512.

2 **Ashworth, P.** Care to communicate: an investigation into problems of communication between patients and nurses in intensive therapy units. Royal College of Nursing, 1980.

3 **Ashworth, P.** Communication in the intensive care unit. (Between nurse and patient.) Nursing Mirror, 146, 16 Feb 1978, 34-36.

4 **Cassem, N.H. and Hackett, T.P.** Stress on the nurse and therapist in the intensive and coronary-care units. Nursing Digest, 4 (4), Fall 1976, 76-79.

5 **Chilver, W.L.C.** On being a patient in an intensive therapy unit. (Author's experience of being attached to ventilator.) Nursing Mirror, 146, 6 Apr 1978, 33-35.

6 **Cowper-Smith, F.** Intensive care needed for all in ITUs. (Sources of stress in patients and staff.) Nursing Times, 74, 13 Jul 1978, 1158.

7 **Cowper-Smith, F.** Watch the patient—not his blood gases. (Report of conference of Nursing Intensive Care Group.) Nursing Times, 75, 9 Aug 1979, 1339.

8 **Dossett, S.M.** Stress—1. Nursing staff in high dependency areas. Nursing Times, 74, 25 May 1978, 888-889.

9 **Dossett, S.M.** Stress—2. The patient in the intensive therapy unit. Nursing Times, 74, 25 May 1978, 890-891.

10 **Eisendrath, S.J. and Dunkel, J.** Psychological issues in intensive care unit staff. (Study of psychological environment of ICU and staff/patient interaction.) Heart Lung, 8 (4), Jul/Aug 1979, 751-758.

11 **Haynes, G.** Intensive care—12. The problem of stress. (In patients and nurses.) Nursing Times, 74, 4 May 1978, 753-754.

12 **Hoover, M.J.** Intensive care for relatives. (Support provided by social workers and chaplains to assist nurses.) Hospitals, 53 (14), 16 Jul 1979, 219-220, 222.

13 **Huckaby, L.M.D. and Jagla, B.** Nurses' stress factors in the intensive care unit. (Research study.) Journal of Nursing Administration, 9 (2), Feb 1979, 21-26.

14 **Journal of Nursing Education** Stress and stress management: an overview. (Eleven articles with five on intensive care nurses and bibliography on p.58-63.) Journal of Nursing Education, 19 (6), Jun 1980, 5-63.

15 **Lai, S.K.** Psychological problems of intensive care. Nursing Journal of Singapore, 16 (2), Nov 1976, 86-87.

16 **Lochoff, R.V. and others** Is intensive care a stressful occupation? (Research study in two South African hospitals.) S.A. Nursing Journal, 44 (8), Aug 1977, 15-16.

17 **Melia, K.M.** The intensive care unit—a stress situation? (An examination of the concept of stress for nurses, patients, and relatives based on a small literature review and personal experience.) Nursing Times, 73, 3 Feb 1977, Occ. papers, 17-20.

18 **Nelson, J.** Intensive care. (Ways of reducing pressure on intensive care unit staff.) Nursing Mirror, 146, 19 Jan 1978, 20.

19 **Noble, M.A.** Communication in the ICU: therapeutic or disturbing? (Research study of nurse-patient and staff-staff communication.) Nursing Outlook, 27 (3), Mar 1979, 195-198.

20 **Oskins, S.L.** Identification of situational stressors and coping methods by intensive care nurses. (Research study.) Heart Lung, 8 (5), Sep/Oct 1979, 953-960.

21 **Roberts, S.L.** Behavioral concepts and the critically ill patient. Englewood-Cliffs, N.J.: Prentice-Hall, 1976.

22 **Rumpler, C.H. and Seigerman, C.** A behaviour modification approach to dealing with violent behaviour in an intensive care unit. Perspectives in Psychiatric Care, 16 (5/6), Sep/Dec 1978, 206-211, 245.

23 **Shircore, R.** Stress and intensive care staff. Health and Social Service Journal, 86, 14 Aug 1976, 1476-1477.

24 **Shubin, S.** Rx for stress—your stress. (Programme at a New York hospital to help ICU nurses deal with their stresses.) Nursing (U.S.), 9 (1), Jan 1979, 53-55.

25 **Skinner, K.** Support group for ICU nurses. (To help them cope with stress.) Nursing Outlook, 28 (5), May 1980, 296-299.

26 **Stillman, S.M. and Strasser, B.L.** Helping critical care nurses with work-related stress. (Weekly inservice small group programme.) Journal of Nursing Administration, 10 (1), Jan 1980, 28-31.

27 **Storlie, F.** The family: thirteen years of observation. (Family attitudes towards intensive care staff.) Supervisor Nurse, 7 (2), Feb 1976, 10-14.

28 **Sullon, G.** What happened to Mrs. Brown?: a study of acute psychotic reactions in patients nursed in Intensive Care Units. Lamp, Dec 1975, 26-27.

29 **Tomlin, P.J.** Psychological problems in intensive care. (Of patients and staff.) British Medical Journal, 2, 13 Aug 1977, 441-443.

30 **Tomlin, P.** Rescue the ITU nurses top consultant pleads. (A call for nurses working in intensive care to undergo psychological screening for their own safety. Nursing Mirror, 145, 18 Aug 1977, 3.

31 **West, N.D.** Stresses associated with ICUs affect patients, families, staff. Hospitals, 49 (24), 16 Dec 1975, 62-63.

32 **Woods, N.F. and Falk, S.A.** Noise stimuli in the acute care area. (Intensive care unit and recovery room.) Nursing Research, 23 (2), Mar/Apr 1974, 144-150.

18 SPIRITUAL CARE

a NURSING

1 **Association of Religious Nursing Sisters** Annual report 1975-1976. The Association, 1975-76.

2 **Baqui, M.A.** Muslim teaching concerning death. (A St. Joseph's Hospice occasional paper.) Nursing Times, 75, 5 Apr 1979, 43-44.

3 **Carson, V.** Meeting the spiritual needs of hospitalized psychiatric patients. Perspectives in Psychiatric Care, 18 (1), Jan/Feb 1980, 17-20.

4 **Carson, V. and Huss, K.** Prayer—an effective therapeutic and teaching tool. (Pilot project to teach student nurses how to meet spiritual needs of clients and evaluate methods including prayer.) Journal of Psychiatric Nursing, 17 (3), Mar 1979, 34-36.

5 **Darocy, C.** Religious considerations in patient care. (With outline of practices of various religions.) Journal of Practical Nursing, 29 (12), Dec 1979, 18-21, 31.

6 **Fichter, J.H.** Do suffering patients turn to God? (Data from Catholic hospitals.) Hospital Progress, 61 (3), Mar 1980, 52-55.

7 **Fish, S. and Shelly, J.A.** Spiritual care: the nurse's role. Downers Grove, Ill.: Intervarsity Press, 1978.

8 **Joyce, C.** The religious as group therapists. Attitudes and conflicts. (A nun describes her experiences.) Perspectives in Psychiatric Care, 15 (3), 1977, 112-117.

9 **Lally, M.M.** Last rites and funeral customs of minority groups. Midwife, Health Visitor and Community Nurse, 14 (7), Jul 1978, 224-225.

10 **Levenstein, M.** Jewish teaching concerning death. A St. Joseph's Hospice Occasional Paper. Nursing Times, 74, 23 Mar 1978, Occ. papers, 35-36.

11 **McGilloway, F.A. and Donnelly, L.** Religion and patient care: the functionalist approach. Journal of Advanced Nursing, 2 (1), Jan 1977, 3-13.

12 Nursing Issue on beliefs and behaviour. Nursing, 16, Aug 1980, 675-716.

13 Nursing Religion as a way of life. (Judaism, Jehovah's Witnesses and Christian Scientists.) Nursing, 16, Aug 1980, 687-688.

14 Nursing (U.S.) Recognizing your patients' spiritual needs. (With summaries of the beliefs of various religions regarding diet, birth and death, etc.) Nursing, 7 (12), Dec 1977, 64, 66-69.

15 Ormerod, Father B. Religious order that helps fill the gaps in the NHS. (Hospital Order of St. John of God, at Richmond, Yorkshire.) Nursing Mirror, 142 (26), 24 Jun 1976, 70-72.

16 Patey, E.H. The sacred and the secular. (Spiritual needs of patients.) Nursing Mirror, 145, 10 Nov 1977, 25-26.

17 Richards, F. What they believe and why. 1. Roman Catholics, Jehovah's Witnesses and Christian Scientists. 2. The Jewish faith. 3. Muslims, Hindus and Buddhists. Nursing Mirror, 144, 14 Apr 1977, 65-66; 21 Apr 1977, 64; 28 Apr 1977, 67.

18 St. Joseph's Hospice Christian teaching concerning death. (A St. Joseph's Hospice Occasional Paper on the Roman Catholic, Anglican and Non-conformist approaches.) Nursing Times, 74, 25 May 1978, Occ. papers, 58-60.

19 Saylor, D. The spiritual shelf. (Beliefs of various religions.) Journal of Practical Nursing, 27 (8), Aug 1977, 16-17, 30.

20 Simsen, B. Spiritual dimension (of nursing practice). New Zealand Nursing Journal, 69 (1), Jan 1976, 12-14.

21 Zumbro Valley Medical Society Medicine and religion committee Religious aspects of medical care: a handbook of religious practices of all faiths. 2nd ed. St. Louis: Catholic Hospital Association, 1978.

b HOSPITAL CHAPLAINS

1 ALL God's children. (Position of hospital chaplains in the recognised NHS.) Health and Social Service Journal, 88, 17 Mar 1978, 298.

2 Autton, N. The hospital chaplain. Nursing, 16, Aug 1980, 697-699.

3 Bowlby, R. Chaplains are different. British Medical Journal, 2 (20/27), Dec 1980, 1689.

4 Church Information Office A handbook on hospital chaplaincy. CIO Publishing, 1978.

5 Corrigan, A. Three-year growth of a pastoral care department. Hospital Progress, 60 (2), Feb 1979, 27-28.

6 Fives, B. Support your patient's family - with a chaplain. (Their role in an ED.) RN Magazine, 40 (3), Mar 1977, 58-59.

7 Grubb, G. The pastor's role in visiting the sick. Nursing Mirror, 144, 23 Jun 1977, 33.

8 Hospital Chaplaincies Council Directory of whole-time hospital chaplains, hospital church sisters and chaplain assistants in Great Britain. Hospital Chaplaincies Council, 1975. Revised ed. 1980.

9 Law, M. and others Exploring the work of a hospital chaplain in a psychiatric hospital. (Research study by chaplain and colleagues.) Nursing Times, 74, 7 Sep 1978, 1478-1482.

10 LeBourdais, E. Pastoral services rated important. (Survey of patients' attitudes to pastoral services by the Association of Hospitals of the Province of Quebec.) Dimensions in Health Service, 53 (5), May 1976, 18-19.

11 Lyall, D. Chaplaincy involvement in nurse education. (Scheme at North Lothian College of Nursing and Midwifery.) Nursing Times, 74, 15 Jun 1978, 1022-1023.

12 Murr, J.M. Patients and staff favor night ministry program. Hospitals, 52 (18), 16 Sep 1978, 72-74.

13 Potter, C. Bringing heaven right down to earth. (The success of a pilot course in Cardiff for training hospital chaplains.) Health and Social Service Journal, 89, 22 Feb 1979, 184-185.

14 Thompson, S. A ministry of calm. (A day spent with John Barton, chaplain of the Radcliffe group of hospitals, Oxford.) Nursing Mirror, 148, 31 May 1979, 22-23.

15 Woodyatt, G.W. Hospital chaplains. Hospital and Health Services Review, 74 (10), Oct 1978, 348-350.

16 Wright, P. Nurse and chaplain. (By nurse who is also chaplain at The London Hospital.) Nursing Times, 76, 24 Jul 1980, 1314-1316.

19 TERMINAL CARE AND DEATH

a GENERAL

1 Armstrong, M.E. Dying and death—and life experiences of loss and gain: a proposed theory. Nursing Forum, 14 (1), 1975, 95-104.

2 Barton, D. editor Dying and death: a clinical guide for caregivers. Baltimore: Williams and Wilkins, 1977.

3 Beauchamp, T.L. and Perlin, S. editors Ethical issues in death and dying. Englewood Cliffs, N.J.: Prentice-Hall, 1978.

4 Bond, J. and Bond, S. A taboo of our times. (The sociology of death and dying.) Nursing Mirror, 150, 13 Mar 1980, 23-26.

5 Bunch, B. and Zahra, D. Dealing with death: the unlearned role. American Journal of Nursing, 76 (9), Sep 1976, 1486-1488.

6 Christian, M.S. and others Confirmation of death. (Results of questionnaire and recommendations of working party concerning patients believed to be dead on arrival.) British Medical Journal, 281, 13 Sep 1980, 717-719.

7 Cliff, K.S. Recording death in the NHS. Health and Social Service Journal, 86, May 1976, 794.

8 Coggan, D. On dying and dying well: extracts from the Edwin Stevens lecture. Journal of Medical Ethics, 3 (2), Jun 1977, 57-60.

9 Hall, G. Death and dying—specifically related to intensive care areas. New Zealand Nursing Journal, 69 (12), Dec 1976, 20-23.

10 Hornby, A. Death, dying and bereavement. Nursing Mirror, 146, 16 Feb 1978, 18.

11 Kramer, J. Learning about care of the dying. (Doctor's experience based on four weeks' interviews with dying patients.) Australian Nurses Journal, 9 (4), Oct 1979, 34-36, 50.

12 Lynch, L. The experience of death: care of the dying and the bereaved. Liverpool Institute of Socio-Religious Studies, 1977. (Pastoral investigation of social trends working paper no.6.)

13 Pennington, E.A. Postmortem care: more than ritual. (Nursing care after death.) American Journal of Nursing, 78 (5), May 1978, 846-847.

14 Sell, I.L. Dying and death: an annotated bibliography. New York: Tiresias Press, 1977.

15 Siegler, M. The doctor and the dying role. Practitioner, 216, Jun 1976, 690-694.

16 Thompson, I. editor Dilemmas of dying: a study in the ethics of terminal care. Edinburgh: Edinburgh University Press, 1979. (Edinburgh Medical Group, moral issues on health care; 1.)

17 Tombleson, P.M.J. and Carsed, M.P. How do we cope with death? Journal of the Royal College of General Practitioners, 27, Jan 1977, 33-36.

18 THE undiscovered country. (Near-death experiences.) British Medical Journal, 2, 15 Dec 1979, 1530.

19 Weightman, G. Death and the doctors. (Doctors' reaction to the dying and the lack of medical education on the care of the dying.) New Society, 41, 4 Aug 1977, 222-224.

b BEREAVEMENT

1 Baker, B.S. and Lynn, M.R. Psychiatric nursing consultation: the use of an inservice model to assist nurses in the grief process. Journal of Psychiatric Nursing, 17 (5), May 1979, 15-19.

2 Bellis, G.H. Death is not the end of caring. (Care of bereaved relatives.) Midwife, Health Visitor and Community Nurse, 13 (4), Apr 1977, 101-102, 104.

3 Bowlby, J. 'How will mummy breathe and who will feed her?' (Children who mourn dead parents.) New Society, 51, 6 Mar 1980, 492-494.

4 Branson, H.K. Grieving...and growing. (Explaining death to children.) Journal of Practical Nursing, 26 (12), Dec 1976, 34.

5 Bruce, M. The family and the bereaved. (Counselling of relatives before and after a death. A St. Joseph's Hospice Occasional Paper.) Nursing Times, 74, 29 Jun 1978, Occ. papers, 71-72.

6 Castle, B. Coming to terms with the agony being alone. (Widowhood.) Times, 29 May 1980, 16.

7 Coles, P. Nursing care study. Distress therapy: breaking the grief barrier. A successful behavioural treatment of a patient with an unresolved grief reaction two years after the death of his mother. (By a nurse therapist.) Nursing Mirror, 148, 31 May 1979, 34-35.

8 Courtemanche, J. Death in emergency.

(Stages of grief of bereaved person.) Canadian Nurse, 74 (10), Nov 1978, 24-26.

9 **Craig, V.** Support for bereaved parents. (1976 Symposium on parental bereavement.) Health and Social Service Journal, 86, 19 Jun 1976, 1126-1127.

10 CRUSE The work of Cruse. (Charity aiming to provide support for all members of widowed family and those who work with dying and bereaved.) Health Visitor, 53 (3), Mar 1980, 92-93.

11 **DeCosta, L.** Brief intervention with bereaved adolescents. (Newham Child Guidance Clinic, Young People's Counselling Service.) Social Work Today, 8 (6), 9 Nov 1976, 13-14.

12 **Dracup, K.A. and Breu, C.S.** Using nursing research findings to meet the needs of grieving spouses. (Nursing care plan based on research findings for relatives of CCU patients.) Nursing Research, 27 (4), Jul/Aug 1978, 212-216.

13 **Family Welfare Association** Bereavement papers. The Association, 1978.

14 **Fell, J.** Grief reactions in the elderly following death of a spouse: the role of crisis intervention and nursing. Journal of Gerontological Nursing, 3 (6), Nov/Dec 1977, 17-20.

15 **Freihofer, P. and Felton, G.** Nursing behaviors in bereavement: an exploratory study. Nursing Research, 25 (5), Sep/Oct 1976, 332-337.

16 **Furman, E.** A child's parent dies: studies in childhood bereavement. New Haven: Yale University Press, 1974.

17 **Glauert, D.** Compassion—that's what friends are for. (Role of Compassionate Friends, a charity for bereaved parents.) Journal of Community Nursing, 3 (2), Aug 1979, 18-19.

18 **Hauser, M.J. and Feinberg, D.R.** An operational approach to the delayed grief and mourning process. Journal of Psychiatric Nursing and Mental Health Services, 14 (7), Jul 1976, 29-35.

19 **Hodgkinson, P.E.** Treating abnormal grief in the bereaved. (Using behaviour therapy.) Nursing Times, 76, 17 Jan 1980, 126-128.

20 **Leared, J.** The need for counselling. (After bereavement.) Social Service Quarterly, 52 (3), Spring 1979, 85-87.

21 **Levy, B.** A study of bereavement in general practice. (Study of forty-six bereaved relatives.) Journal of the Royal College of General Practitioners, 26, May 1976, 329-336.

22 **Lewis, E.** Inhibition of mourning by pregnancy: psychopathology and management. British Medical Journal, 2, 7 Jul 1979, 27-28.

23 **Marks, M.J.B.** Dealing with death: the grieving patient and family. American Journal of Nursing, 76 (9), Sep 1976, 1488-1491.

24 **Martin, I.C.A.** Many unhappy returns. (Stages of mourning in bereavement.) Nursing Times, 76, 24 Jul 1980, 1319-1321.

25 **Norman, M.** Grief and mourning. Health Visitor, 49 (11), Nov 1976, 357-358.

26 **Nuttall, D.** Attitudes to dying and the bereaved. (Work of Cruse, organisation to help the widowed.) Nursing Times, 73, 13 Oct 1977, 1605-1607.

27 **Nuttall, D.** Bereavement. Health Visitor, 53 (3), Mar 1980, 84-86.

28 **Parkes, C.M.** Bereavement counselling: does it work? British Medical Journal, 281, 5 Jul 1980, 3-6.

29 **Penson, J.M.** Care of the terminal patient —3. Helping the bereaved. Nursing Times, 75, 5 Apr 1979, 593-595.

30 **Pincus, L.** Death and the family: the importance of mourning. Faber, 1976.

31 **Riley, L. and Sheard, R.** A widows' befriending scheme. Social Work Today, 9, 13 Jun 1978, 17-19.

32 **Rinear, E.E.** The nurse's challenge when death is unexpected. (A patient care co-ordinator in an emergency department gives advice on how to help next of kin after a sudden death.) RN Magazine, 38 (12), Dec 1975, 50-55.

33 **Schiff, H.S.** The bereaved parent. Souvenir Press (E&A), 1979.

34 **Smith, K.** Help for the bereaved. Duckworth, 1978.

35 **Solomon, H.McF.** Grief and bereavement. International Journal of Social Psychiatry, 23 (3), Autumn 1977, 211-222.

36 **Speck, P.W.** Loss and grief in medicine. Baillière Tindall, 1978.

37 **Thompson, D.M.** Thoughts on bereavement. Nursing Times, 73, 25 Aug 1977, 1334-1335.

38 **Torrie, A.** When children grieve. Richmond: Cruse, 1978.

39 **Ward, A.W.M.** Mortality of bereavement. (Survey of the death rate of 87 widowers and 279 widows in Sheffield.) British Medical Journal, 1976, 1, 20 Mar 1976, 700-702.

40 **Willis, R.W.** Bereavement management in the emergency department. Journal of Emergency Nursing, 3 (2), Mar/Apr 1977, 35-39.

c EUTHANASIA

1 **Bandman, E.L.** The dilemma of life and death: should we let them die? (Euthanasia and role of nurse.) Nursing Forum, 17 (2), 1978, 118-132.

2 **Beauchamp, J.M.** Euthanasia and the nurse practitioner. Nursing Forum, 14 (1), 1975, 56-73.

3 **Berg, D.L. and Isler, C.** The right to die dilemma. How do you fit in? RN Magazine, 40 (8), Aug 1977, 48-55.

4 **Cawley, M.A.** Euthanasia: should it be a choice? American Journal of Nursing, 77 (5), May 1977, 859-861.

5 **Epstein, C.** Nursing implications (of euthanasia.) Nursing Digest, 4 (4), Fall 1976, 54-55.

6 **Forsyth, D.M.** The will to live and the right to die. (Research study with elderly patients to discover their attitudes.) Practitioner, 220, Mar 1978, 363-366.

7 **Husak, D.N.** Killing, letting die and euthanasia. Journal of Medical Ethics, 5 (4), Dec 1979, 200-202.

8 **Lancet** Choosing when to die and how. (EXIT's suicide booklet.) Lancet, 2, 13 Sep 1980, 571.

9 **Lappe, M.** Dying while living: a critique of allowing-to-die legislation. Journal of Medical Ethics, 4 (4), Dec 1978, 195-199.

10 **Lejeune, P.** When it's a voluntary decision. (Voluntary euthanasia, by spokesman for EXIT, The Society for the Right to Die with Dignity.) Nursing Mirror, 151, 11 Sep 1980, 12.

11 **Martin, A.** The nurse and the law. A right worth dying for? (EXIT's guide to suicide methods.) Journal of Community Nursing, 4 (6), Dec 1980, 25-26.

12 **Martin, A.** Nurses and the law—2. Euthanasia. Nursing Times, 74, 11 May 1978, 800.

13 **Parramore, J.** Suicide and assisted suicide —some aspects of personal involvement. (By secretary of Australian Voluntary Euthanasia Society.) Australian Nurses Journal, 8 (1), Sep 1978, 29-30.

14 **Rachels, J.** Active and passive euthanasia. Nursing Digest, 4 (4), Fall 1976, 52-54.

15 **RN Magazine** Are you *too* sure of your stand on the right to die? (Two case histories.) RN Magazine, 41 (12), Dec 1978, 74-76, 78, 82.

16 **Saunders, C.** Care of the dying. 1 and 2. The problem of euthanasia. Nursing Times, 72, 1 Jul 1976, 1003-1005; 8 Jul 1976, 1049-1051.

17 **Saunders, C.** Caring to the end. (Why author is opposed to euthanasia.) Nursing Mirror, 151, 4 Sep 1980, 52-53.

18 **Towers, B.** Report from America. The impact of the California Natural Death Act. (To enable competent adults to instruct their doctors to withdraw life-sustaining procedures.) Journal of Medical Ethics, 4 (2), Jun 1978, 96-98.

19 **Winget, C. and others** Attitudes towards euthanasia. (Survey of medical, nursing and college students and practising nurses and doctors at the University of Cincinnati Medical Center.) Journal of Medical Ethics, 3 (1), Mar 1977, 18-25.

20 **Wootton, B.** Death—whose right to choose? (Euthanasia.) Midwife, Health Visitor and Community Nurse, 16 (5), May 1980, 205-206.

21 **Wootton, B.** The right to die. (Voluntary euthanasia.) New Society, 46, 26 Oct 1978, 202-203.

d HOSPICE CARE

1 **Ames, R.P.** Starting a hospice requires tenacity, high standards. Hospital Progress, 61 (2), Feb 1980, 56-60.

2 **Cohen, K.P.** Hospice: prescription for terminal care. Germantown, Md.: Aspen Systems, 1979.

3 **Crail, R.B.** A pilot scheme in continuing care. (Ward in general practitioner-run cottage hospital at Weybridge offering hospice-type care.) Practitioner, 224, Feb 1980, 126-127.

4 Cunningham, R.M. When enough is enough. The goals of hospitals and hospices are not necessarily incompatible, and hospice care may be an opportunity for hospitals to further humanize their services. Hospitals, 53 (13), 1 Jul 1979, 63-65.

5 Helena Marie, Sr. Domiciliary night nursing for terminal patients. (St. Joseph's Hospice's home care service.) Midwife, Health Visitor and Community Nurse, 15 (4), Apr 1979, 152.

6 Hospital Progress The hospice alternative. (Special issue.) Hospital Progress, 60 (3), Mar 1979, 38-76.

7 INTERNATIONAL Hospice Conference Changing the face of death. (Conference to mark St. Christopher's Hospice's thirteenth year.) Lancet, 1, 21 Jun 1980, 1340-1341.

8 Isler, C. Approaching the final days. (Hospice unit at Bellin Memorial Hospital in Wisconsin for terminal care of cancer patients.) RN Magazine, 41 (4), Apr 1978, 63-65.

9 Kohn, J. Hospice building speaks on many emotional levels to patient, family. (New Haven Hospice, Connecticut.) Modern Healthcare, 6 (4), Oct 1976, 56-57.

10 Kohn, J. Hospice movement provides humane alternative for terminally ill patients. Modern Healthcare, 6 (3), Sep 1976, 26-28.

11 Kolbe, R. Inside the English Hospice. (Tarner Home, Brighton and St. Joseph's Hospice, London.) Hospitals, 51 (13), 1 Jul 1977, 65-67.

12 Lamerton, R. Nurse could you care more? (The emphasis on caring in hospices and the need for more nurses to staff them, especially the hospice domiciliary services.) Nursing Times, 75, 31 May 1979, 905-906.

13 Luxton, R.W. The modern hospice and its challenge to medicine. British Medical Journal, 2, 8 Sep 1979, 583-584.

14 Markel, W.M. and Sinon, V.B. The hospice concept. Journal of Practical Nursing, 29 (3), Mar 1979, 24-26, 28-29, 39.

15 Matthews, B. Setting up terminal care units. (Hospice-type care with home care service.) Journal of the Royal College of General Practitioners, 30, Aug 1980, 472-476.

16 Paige, R.L. and Looney, J.F. When the patient is dying. Hospice care for the adult. Integration of a hospice team within a hospital medical center. (St. Luke's Hospital Center, New York City.) American Journal of Nursing, 77 (11), Nov 1977, 1812-1815.

17 Paula, Sr. Care of the terminal patient—5. The work of the hospice. Nursing Times, 75, 19 Apr 1979, 667.

18 Philpot, T. Death—a part of life. (Care at St. Joseph's Hospice in East London.) Nursing Mirror, 151, 21 Aug 1980, 20-23.

19 Portington, J.M. Seven days at St. Luke's. (St. Luke's Nursing Home, Sheffield, hospice for the terminally ill.) Nursing Mirror, 143 (8), 19 Aug 1976, 64-65.

20 Robinson, W. Royal Hospital and Home for Incurables (Putney). Nursing Mirror, 145, 15 Sep 1977, 16-19.

21 Slack, P. The hospice comes of age. (Conference on hospice care at St. Christopher's Hospice.) Nursing Times, 76, 12 Jun 1980, 1034.

22 Stoddard, S. The hospice movement: a better way of caring for the dying. Cape, 1979.

23 Tanner, E.R. A time to die. (A St. Joseph's Hospice Occasional Paper.) Nursing Times, 74, 2 Feb 1978, Occ. papers, 16.

24 Walborn, K.A. A nursing model for the hospice: primary and self-care nursing. Nursing Clinics of North America, 15 (1), Mar 1980, 205-217.

25 Wald, F.S. and others The hospice movement as a health care reform. (Need to integrate with the US health care system.) Nursing Outlook, 28 (3), Mar 1980, 173-178.

26 Ward, B.J. Hospice home care program. (By multidisciplinary team at Overlook Hospital, Summit, New Jersey.) Nursing Outlook, 26 (10), Oct 1; 89, 646-649.

27 Watkin, B. Care of the dying. (Comment on the hospice approach.) Nursing Mirror, 147, 21 Sep 1978, 10.

28 Wentzel, K.B. The dying are the living. (Case study from St. Christopher's Hospice.) American Journal of Nursing, 76 (6), Jun 1976, 956-957.

29 West, T.S. Hospice care for a dying person and his family. (By Deputy Medical Director of St. Christopher's Hospice.) Patient Counseling and Health Education, 1 (2), Fall 1978, 65-69.

30 Worby, C.M. and others Hospice care: current status and future prospects. (In U.S.A.) Patient Counseling and Health Education, 1 (2), Fall 1978, 61-64.

e NURSING

1 Ainsworth-Smith, I. At the front line of dying. (Nursing care.) Journal of Community Nursing, 1 (4), Oct 1977, 11-12.

2 Anderson, J.L. Communicating with terminal cancer patients. (Method of teaching medical students.) Patient Counseling and Health Education, 2 (1), First Quarter 1980, 28-31.

3 Barnish, J. and Walsh, A. Parallels in care. (A district nurse and HV describe their roles in care of the terminally ill at home.) Journal of Community Nursing, 2 (12), Jun 1979, 25-26, 28.

4 Boccuzzi, N.K. Humanistic supervision for terminal care. (Support of staff by supervisor.) Supervisor Nurse, 8 (8), Aug 1977, 26-27.

5 Bodington, M. Concepts of nursing care at the RHHI. (Royal Hospital and Home for Incurables, Putney.) Nursing Mirror, 145, 8 Dec 1977, 17-19.

6 Boland, M. Care of the dying patient in intensive care areas. (Research study to find out what students are taught about the care of the dying.) Nursing Mirror, 145, 25 Aug 1977, 20-21.

7 Brimigion, J. Living with dying. (By director of a nursing home who has developed techniques including inservice training for staff and group therapy sessions for patients.) Nursing, 8 (9), Sep 1978, 76, 78-79.

8 Brown, E.A. Care of the terminal patient—2. Personal experience in the professional care of the dying. (How nurses could be trained to cope with emotional needs of the dying patient.) Nursing Times, 75, 29 Mar 1979, 545-546.

9 Chapman, C. Care of the terminal patient—1. What can I say? A Christian nurse's view of dying. Nursing Times, 75, 22 Mar 1979, 487-488.

10 Cohen, R.M. The bedside nurse in terminal care. (Seven articles.) Journal of Practical Nursing, 30 (6), Jun 1980, 17-25, 40.

11 Donner, G. Death and dying: a personal perspective. (With reference to crisis intervention.) Canadian Nurse, 74 (10), Nov 1978, 20-21.

12 Donovan, H. Mind-heart work: caring for the dying. (With reference to the nurse/patient relationship.) Supervisor Nurse, 10 (9), Sep 1979, 20-23.

13 Doyle, D. Why being prepared counts in home care of the dying. (Equipment needed in home and symptoms to be relieved.) Geriatric Medicine, 9 (10), Oct 1979, 77-78.

14 Earle, A.M. and others, editors The nurse as caregiver for the terminal patient and his family. New York: Columbia University Press, 1976.

15 Epstein, C. Nursing the dying patient: learning processes for interaction. Reston, Virginia: Reston Publishing Co., 1975.

16 Goffnett, C. Your patient's dying: now what? (Advice on terminal care nursing.) Nursing (U.S.), 9 (11), Nov 1979, 27-33.

17 Gray, G.I. Assessment of the nursing needs of the dying patient. MSc thesis, Faculty of Medicine, Victoria University of Manchester, Oct 1977.

18 JOINT Board of Clinical Nursing Studies. 4. Care of the dying. Nursing Mirror, 143 (8), 19 Aug 1976; Nursing care supplement series 2, i-iv.

19 Keck, V.E. and Walther, L.S. Nurse encounters with dying and nondying patients. (Measurement of duration of encounters during two-hour period showing more time was spent with the dying.) Nursing Research, 26 (6), Nov/Dec 1977, 465-469.

20 Keith, P.M. and Castles, M.R. Expected and observed behavior of nurses and terminal patients. (Study conducted in hospitals in three small midwestern communities.) International Journal of Nursing Studies, 16 (1), 1979, 21-28.

21 Khoo, O.T. The management of terminal illness. Nursing Journal of Singapore, 17 (1), May 1977, 12-17.

22 Lamerton, R. Care of the dying. Harmondsworth: Penguin. 2nd ed. 1980.

23 Lamerton, R. The care of the dying: a speciality. (Criticism of present standards of nursing care for the dying.) Nursing Times, 74, 16 Mar 1978, 436.

24 Lamerton, R. Going deeper into care of the dying. Nursing Mirror, 144, 3 Mar 1977, 64-65.

25 **Lamerton, B.** Resurrected by an enema. (Care of the dying patient.) Nursing Times, 72 (42), 21 Oct 1976, 1653.

26 **Lannie, V.J.** The joy of caring for the dying. Supervisor Nurse, 9 (5), May 1978, 66, 69, 72.

27 **Le Roux, R.S.** Communicating with the dying person. Nursing Forum, 16 (2), 1977, 145-155.

28 **McEver, D.H.** Death education: an inservice program. Nurse Educator, 2 (6), Nov/Dec 1977, 7-8.

29 **McGrory, A.** A well model approach to care of the dying client. New York: McGraw-Hill, 1978.

30 **McMahon, M. and Miller, P.** Behavioral cues in the dying process and nursing implications. Journal of Gerontological Nursing, 6 (1), Jan 1980, 16-20.

31 **Miller, P.** Doing away with 'inspired neglect'. (Role of the nurse in counselling dying patients.) Supervisor Nurse, 8 (9), Sep 1977, 21-23.

32 **Murphy, J.C.** Communicating with the dying patient. (Nurse describes her own experience.) American Journal of Nursing, 79 (6), Jun 1979, 1084.

33 **Nelson, J.** Live thoughts on dying patients. Nursing Times, 72 (15), 15 Apr 1976, 592-593.

34 **Nursing Mirror** The dark side of nursing. What happened to the man in bed 14? (Five articles about different aspects of nursing dying patients.) Nursing Mirror, 148, 5 Apr 1979, 14-20.

35 **Prichard, E.R. and others, editors** Home care: living with dying. New York: Columbia University Press, 1979.

36 **RN Magazine** The Lazarus syndrome. (Three articles on the nursing care of patients who've 'returned from the dead' after resuscitation.) RN Magazine, 41 (6), Jun 1978, 54-64.

37 **Ross, C.W.** Nurses' personal death concerns and responses to dying-patient statements. Nursing Research, 27 (1), Jan/Feb 1978, 64-68.

38 **Saunders, C.** Care of the dying—6. The nursing of patients dying of cancer. Nursing Times, 72 (31), 5 Aug 1976, 1203-1205.

39 **Saunders, C.** Care of the dying—7. The last achievement. Nursing Times, 72 (32), 12 Aug 1976, 1247-1249.

40 **Saunders, C.M. editor** The management of terminal disease. Arnold, 1978. (Management of malignant disease series no.1.)

41 **Schultz, C.** The dying person. (Nursing care with patient experiencing a slow death.) Journal of Nursing Education, 5 (3), May/Jun 1979, 12-16.

42 **Stott, M.** Nursing care study. Care of a dying patient. (With cancer.) Nursing Times, 76, 3 Jul 1980, 1178-1183.

43 **Ufema, J.K.** Dare to care for the dying. (Personal experiences of a nurse caring for dying patients.) American Journal of Nursing, 76 (1), Jan 1976, 88-90.

44 **Ufema, J.** Do you have what it takes to be a nurse-thanatologist? (Specialist in needs and care of dying patients.) Nursing, 77 7 (5), May 1977, 3, 5.

45 **Wald, F.S.** Terminal care and nursing education. (Hospice care.) American Journal of Nursing, 79 (10), Oct 1979, 1762-1764.

46 **West, T.S. and Holmes, P.M.** Specialised care. 9. Care of the dying. Introduction and Two Patients. (Case studies.) Nursing Mirror, 145, 17 Nov 1977, Nursing care supplement series 6, i-iv.

47 **Wilson, D.** Nurse typical, job unique. (District nurse who liaises between community and St. Luke's Sheffield, a nursing home specialising in terminal care.) Journal of Community Nursing, 1 (4), Oct 1977, 18-19.

f NURSING ATTITUDES

1 **Boyd, K.** Attitudes to death: some historical notes. Journal of Medical Ethics, 3 (3), Sep 1977, 124-128.

2 **Davidson, G.P.** Coming to terms with cancer. (Attitudes to dying.) New Zealand Nursing Journal, 71 (6), Jun 1978, 4-6.

3 **Denton, J.A. and Wisenbaker, V.S.** Death experience and death anxiety among nurses and nursing students. (Survey at Eastern Kentucky University, Richmond.) Nursing Research, 26 (1), Jan-Feb 1977, 61-64.

4 **Hopping, B.L.** Nursing students' attitudes towards death. (Survey using questionnaire.) Nursing Research, 26 (6), Nov/Dec 1977, 443-447.

5 **Kerr, J.C.** Dying in hospital. (General discussion on ethical issues and staff attitudes to death.) Canadian Nurse, 74 (10), Nov 1978, 17-19.

6 **Laube, J.** Death and dying workshop for nurses: its effect on their death anxiety level. (Research study.) International Journal of Nursing Studies, 14 (3), 1977, 111-120.

7 **Lewis, F.M.** A time to live and a time to die: an instructional drama. (Dramatic presentation about death and dying to educate hospital staff.) Nursing Outlook, 25 (12), Dec 1977, 762-765.

8 **Lewis, J.** How the nurses cope with grief. (Care of dying patients.) Australian Nurses Journal, 8 (4), Jan/Feb 1979, 16-17.

9 **Marie, H.** Reorienting staff attitudes toward the dying. (Courses for staff developed by the thanatology cooordinator.) Hospital Progress, 59 (8), Aug 1978, 74-76, 92.

10 **Millerd, E.J.** Health professionals as survivors. (Reactions to death and dying.) Journal of Psychiatric Nursing and Mental Health Services, 15 (4), Apr 1977, 33-37.

11 **Mood, D.W. and others** Attitudes of nursing personnel toward death and dying: 1. Linguistic indicators of avoidance. 2. Linguistic indicators of denial. Research in Nursing and Health, 2 (2), Jun 1979, 53-60; (3), Sep 1979, 95-99.

12 **Perks, G.S.** Some thoughts on death. 1. (General discussion followed by personal experiences of three nurses.) Nursing Times, 73, 28 Jul 1977, Occ. papers, 101-104.

13 **Perks, G.S.** Some thoughts on death. 2. (Views of a clinical teacher, charge nurse, tutor and housewife.) Nursing Times, 73, 4 Aug 1977, Occ. papers, 105-107.

14 **Pett, D.** Care of the terminal patient—6. Grief in hospital. Grief comes in various phases and the dying, their relatives and their nurses may not all be at the same stage. Nursing Times, 75, 26 Apr 1979, 709-712.

15 **Sonstegard, L. and others** Dealing with death: the grieving nurse. American Journal of Nursing, 76 (9), Sep 1976, 1490-1492.

16 **Stoller, E.P.** Effect of experience on nurses' responses to dying and death in the hospital setting. Nursing Research, 29 (1), Jan/Feb 1980, 35-38.

17 **Whitfield, S.A.** A descriptive study of student nurses' ward experiences with dying patients and their attitudes towards them. MSc thesis, University of Manchester, Department of Nursing, Oct 1979.

g PATIENT AND FAMILY

1 **Adams, R. and others** Informing the individual of impending death—yes or no? (Research study with forty-nine non-hospitalised patients.) New Zealand Nursing Journal, 71 (10), Oct 1978, 12-14.

2 **Autton, N.** Peace at the last: talks with the dying. SPCK, 1978. (Care and counselling series.)

3 **Burgess, K.E.** The influence of will on life and death. Nursing Forum, 15 (3), 1976, 239-258.

4 **Caughill, R.E. editor** The dying patient: a supportive approach. Boston: Little, Brown and Co., 1976.

5 **Clark, I.** Nursing care study. Terminal illness: time to be home with the family. Nursing Mirror, 148, 1 Mar 1979, 36-37.

6 **COMMUNITY Outlook** She died at home. (Two case studies showing different types of support by relatives and health professionals.) Nursing Times, 75, 14 Jun 1979, Community outlook, 169-170.

7 **Duncan, S. and Rodney, P.** Hope—a negative force. (Problem of 'institutional dissonance': dying patients in an environment oriented to treating and making well.) Canadian Nurse, 74 (10), Nov 1978, 22-23.

8 **Esberger, K.K.** Dying and the aged. Journal of Gerontological Nursing, 6 (1), Jan 1980, 11-15.

9 **Fradd, E.** When the patient is your parent. (Nurse describes care of dying father at home.) Nursing Mirror, 149, 13 Sep 1979, 38-39.

10 **Gray, A.** Dying at home. (Support needed by author when nursing her dying mother.) Nursing Times, 73, 11 Aug 1977, Community Outlook, 9-10.

11 **Griffiths, J.** When a patient talks about death. (By hospital chaplain.) Nursing Mirror, 149, 13 Sep 1979, 35-37.

12 **Hancock, S.** How do your patients want to die? The lessons she learned from the deaths of her mother and her husband. World Medicine, 11 (17), 2 Jun 1976, 17-20, 23-24.

13 **Hencher, J.H.**   Community care study. A health visitor's role in family care. (During terminal illness of father.) Nursing Times, 76, 10 Apr 1980, 647-649.

14 **Hockey, L.**   Dying at home. (Conference paper giving the viewpoint of the district nurse.) Nursing Times, 72 (9), 4 Mar 1976, 324-325.

15 **Jozefowski, J.**   Paula's legacy. (Video-taped interview made on the author's suggestion to describe young dying patient's feelings and improve communication with family.) RN Magazine, 40 (11), Nov 1977, 81-83.

16 **Lucas, M.A.**   Praying with the terminally ill. (And their bereaved relatives.) Hospital Progress, 59 (3), Mar 1978, 66-70.

17 **MacLean, U.**   Learning about death. (Review of research on patients' and doctors' attitudes to terminal illness.) Journal of Medical Ethics, 5 (2), Jun 1979, 68-70.

18 **Nursing Times**   Nurse could you care more? (A personal experience of the exclusion of relatives at the moment of death.) Nursing Times, 75, 26 Apr 1979, 696.

19 **Radford, C.**   Nursing care to the end. (Care of the terminally ill patient at home.) Nursing Mirror, 150, 24 Jan 1980, 30-31.

20 **Raven, R.W. editor**   The dying patient. Pitman, 1975.

21 **Reed, F.**   Meaning of care. (Experiences of a terminally ill nurse in hospital.) Nursing Times, 72 (42), 21 Oct 1976, 1624.

22 **Rogers, B.J. and Mengel, A.**   Communicating with families of terminal cancer patients. Topics in Clinical Nursing, 1 (3), Oct 1979, 55-61.

23 **Saunders, C.**   Care of the dying—3. Should a patient know...? Nursing Times, 72 (28), 15 Jul 1976, 1089-1091.

24 **Saunders, C.**   Care of the dying—5. Mental distress in the dying. Nursing Times, 72 (30), 20 Jul 1976, 1172-1174.

25 **Scott, M.**   There are more answers than a deadly silence. (Taboos affecting communication between the medical profession and terminally ill patients.) Health and Social Service Journal, 88, 27 Oct 1978, 1218-1219.

26 **Sheer, B.L.**   Help for parents in a difficult job—broaching the subject of death. (With bibliography of books for children about the concept of death.) American Journal of Maternal-Child Nursing, 2 (5), Sep/Oct 1977, 320-324.

27 **Shubin, S.**   Cancer widows: a special challenge. (Care of relatives of cancer patients during terminal illness.) Nursing, 8 (4), Apr 1978, 56, 59-60.

28 **Turner, J.**   Old people who die alone. New Society, 48, 12 Apr 1979, 82, 84.

29 **Wilkes, E.**   Quality of life. Effects of the knowledge of diagnosis in terminal illness. (Review of 500 patients.) Nursing Times, 73, 29 Sep 1977, 1504-1507.

30 **Yarling, R.R.**   Ethical analysis of a nursing problem: the scope of nursing practice in disclosing the truth to terminal patients. An Inquiry directed to the National Joint Practice

Commission of the AMA and the ANA. Part II. Supervisor Nurse, 9 (5), May 1978, 45-50; (6) Jun 1978, 28-34.

h PROLONGATION OF LIFE AND RESUSCITATION

1 **Alexander, M.**   A matter of life and death. (Nurse's viewpoint on resuscitation of the terminally ill.) Nursing Mirror, 149, 6 Dec 1979, 26-27.

2 **Dunea, G.**   Death with dignity. (The 'obscenity of modern death' due to sophisticated technology illustrated by the case of Karen Quinlan.) British Medical Journal, 1976, 1, 3 Apr 1976, 824-825.

3 **Gaskell, M.**   An investigation into the problem of deciding which hospital patients are/are not to be resuscitated. MSc thesis, Manchester University, Department of Nursing, 1977.

4 **Kennedy, I.M.**   Focus: current issues in medical ethics. The Karen Quinlan case: problems and proposals. Journal of Medical Ethics, 2 (1), Mar 1976, 3-7.

5 **Kucera, W.R.**   The right to privacy and the right to die. (The Karen Quinlan case.) AANA Journal, 44 (3), Jun 1976, 303-305.

6 **Lawler, J.**   The ethical dilemma of resuscitation. Lamp, 33 (12), Dec 1976, 27-30.

7 **Lestz, P.**   A committee to decide the quality of life. (Policy alternatives on who decides to withdraw medical care.) American Journal of Nursing, 77 (5), May 1977, 862-864.

8 **McCormick, R.A.**   Commentary on the Quinlan decision. The moral right to privacy. Hospital Progress, 57 (8), Aug 1976, 38-42.

9 **Melia, K.**   Saving life—a difficult decision. (Discussion on the quality of life.) Nursing, 15, Jul 1980, 631-632.

10 **O'Rourke, K.D.**   Some new perspectives on prolonging life. Active and passive euthanasia: the ethical distinction. Hospital Progress, 53 (11), Nov 1976, 68-73, 100.

i TERMINAL CARE

1 **Castledine, G.**   Hospitals make war, not love. (Inability of many hospitals to provide psychological and spiritual support for dying patients.) Nursing Mirror, 149, 1 Nov 1979, 12.

2 **COMFORT and counselling** for the dying and bereaved. (Terminal care health visitor in Brent Health District.) Geriatric Medicine, 9 (5), May 1979, 5-6.

3 **Doyle, D.**   Domiciliary terminal care. (Work of home care team in Edinburgh based on St. Columba's Hospice.) Practitioner, 224, Jun 1980, 575, 577, 579, 581-582.

4 **Doyle, D. editor**   Terminal care. Edinburgh: Churchill Livingstone, 1979.

5 **Ford, G.R. and Pincherle, G.**   Arrangements for terminal care in the NHS (especially those for cancer patients.) (Need for services, present provision and future developments.) Health Trends, 4 (10), Nov 1978, 73-76.

6 **Hinton, J.**   Comparison of places and policies for terminal care. (Acute hospital setting and hospices.) Lancet, 1, 6 Jan 1979, 29-32.

7 **INTERNATIONAL Work Group** on Death, Dying and Bereavement Assumptions and principles underlying standards for terminal care. American Journal of Nursing, 79 (2), Feb 1979, 296-297; Nursing Times, 75, 28 Jun 1979, Occ. papers, 69-70.

8 **Kassakian, M.G. and others**   The cost and quality of dying: a comparison of home and hospital. (Cancer patients.) Nurse Practitioner, 4 (1), Jan/Feb 1979, 18, 22-23.

9 **Kensington, Chelsea and Westminster Area Health Authority (Teaching)**   Report of the planning group: care of the dying. The AHA, 1977.

10 **Lewis, S.**   Chasing the shadow from our most sun-filled days. (First district general hospital-based support team for the dying at St. Thomas' Hospital, consisting of two doctors, two nurses, social worker, chaplain and secretary.) Health and Social Service Journal, 89, 6 Jul 1979, 838-839.

11 **Matthews, B.**   Setting up terminal care units. (With history and description of some of the 40-plus units in the British Isles. Reprinted from Journal of the Royal College of General Practitioners.) Nursing Times, 76, 18 Sep 1980, Occ. papers, 97-100.

12 **Parkes, C.M.**   Home or hospital? Terminal care as seen by surviving spouses. (Survey in South London.) Journal of the Royal College of General Practitioners, 28, Jan 1978, 19-22, 25-28, 30.

13 **Russo, P.M.**   Evolution of a terminal cancer scare facility. (At Calvary Hospital, New York City.) Hospital Progress, 58 (12), Dec 1977, 42, 44-45.

14 **Saunders, B.M.**   Care of the dying. (Letter describing project at St. Thomas' Hospital using a terminal care support team.) Nursing Times, 74, 13 Apr 1978, 637.

15 **Saunders, B.**   The terminal care support team. Nursing, 15, Jul 1980, 657-659.

16 **Simpson, M.A.**   Planning for terminal care. Lancet, 1976, 2, 24 Jul 1976, 192-193.

17 **STANDING Sub-committee** on Cancer. Working Group on Terminal Care National terminal care policy. (Shortened version of approved report.) Journal of Royal College of General Practitioners, 30, Aug 1980, 466-471.

j BRAIN DEATH

1 **Aplin, S.**   Brain death. (Tests used at the Royal Devon and Exeter Hospital to diagnose brain death.) Nursing Times, 76, 11 Dec 1980, 2186-2188.

2 **Black, P. McL.**   Criteria of brain death. Review and comparison. Nursing Digest, 4 (4), Summer 1976, 71-73.

3 **CONFERENCE of Medical Royal Colleges** and their Faculties in the United Kingdom Diagnosis of brain death. (Statement issued on 11 Oct 1976 including code of practice and diagnostic criteria.) British Medical Journal, 2, 13 Nov 1976, 1187-1188; Lancet, 2, 13 Nov 1976, 1069-1070 (Comments 1064-1066.)

4 CONFERENCE of Medical Royal Colleges and their Faculties in the United Kingdom Diagnosis of death. Memorandum issued by the honorary secretary of the Conference of Medical Royal Colleges and their Faculties in the United Kingdom on 15 January 1979. British Medical Journal, 1, 3 Feb 1979, 332.

5 DeMere, M. Developing a definition of death. (American Bar Association definition for legal purposes.) AORN Journal, 31 (5), Apr 1980, 930-932, 934.

6 Forrester, A.C. Brain death and the donation of cadaver kidneys. (Includes the recommendations in the 'Code of Practice for Brain Death' used in the Institute of Neurological Sciences, Glasgow, and Department of Surgical Neurology, University of Edinburgh.) Health Bulletin, 34 (4), Jul 1976, 199-204.

7 Jennet, B. Diagnosis of brain death. Journal of Medical Ethics, 3 (1), Mar 1977, 4-6.

8 Kaste, M. and others Diagnosis and management of brain death. (Criteria developed in Finland.) British Medical Journal, 1, 24 Feb 1979, 525-527.

9 Kennedy, I. The definition of brain death. Journal of Medical Ethics, 3 (1), Mar 1977, 5-6.

10 Searle, J. and Collins, C. A brain-death protocol. (Operation of Royal Colleges' protocol, including removal of organs for transplantation and dealing with relatives.) Lancet, 1, 22 Mar 1980, 641-643.

11 Skegg, P.D.G. The case for a statutory 'definition of death.' Journal of Medical Ethics, 2 (4), Dec 1976, 190-191.

20 NURSING EDUCATION

a GENERAL

1 Allen, H.O. Caring—the contribution of education. Nursing Focus, 1 (4), Dec 1979, 150-151.

2 Allen, M. Evaluation of educational programmes in nursing. Geneva: World Health Organization, 1977.

3 Altschul, A. Education and the role of nurses. In Black, Sir D. and Thomas, G.P., editors. Providing for the health services. Proceedings of Section X (General) of the British Association for the Advancement of Science... 1977. Croom Helm, 1978, 39-46. Nursing Times, 74, 25 May 1978, 885-887.

4 Altschul, A. A measure of education. (Paper delivered at conference of Rcn Association of Nursing Education.) Nursing Standard, 73, Jun 1978, 12.

5 Association of Integrated and Degree Courses in Nursing Nursing: an education or training? Report of the 3rd open conference, University of Surrey, 11-13 July 1975. The Association, 1975.

6 Bakutis, A. Writing a school philosophy. (Summary of five major philosophic schools of thought to aid nurse anaesthesia educators in developing their own educational philosophies.) American Association of Nurse Anesthetists Journal, 48 (3), Jun 1980, 248-256.

7 Bell, E.A. Nursing Mirror Forum 76. Clinical teamwork—the aim of education. Nursing Mirror, 143 (22), 25 Nov 1976, 45-58.

8 Bendall, E. The future of British nurse education. (Second Battersea Memorial Lecture.) Journal of Advanced Nursing, 2 (2), Mar 1977, 171-181.

9 Bowman, M. Pointers to the need for change. (History of nurse education to the present.) Nursing Mirror, 150, 28 Feb 1980, 40-42.

10 Boylan, A. Education—where are we going? Nursing Focus, 1 (9), Jun 1980, 393-394.

11 Brooker, R. Professionalism/elitism and nursing education. Australian Nurses Journal, 7 (8), Mar 1978, 26-28, 49.

12 Chapman, C. Present systems and future options. (Nursing Mirror Forum 76 paper discussing developments in nurse education.) Nursing Mirror, 143 (23), 2 Dec 1976, 49-51.

13 Combes, R.B. Educating the learner... (A defence of the present system of nurse education.) Nursing Times, 73, 13 Jan 1977, 46.

14 Congalton, A.A. Nurse education in the United Kingdom. Observations during a recent visit. Lamp, 34 (7), Jul 1977, 42-43.

15 Davies, C. Past and present in nursing education. Nursing Times, 76, 25 Sep 1980, 1703-1707.

16 Derdiarian, A.K. Education: a way to theory construction in nursing. (Issues facing nursing profession and relationship of education to them.) Journal of Nursing Education, 18 (2), Feb 1979, 36-47.

17 Fitzpatrick, M.L. editor Present realities/ future imperatives in nursing education. New York: Teachers College Press, 1977.

18 Gaevert, H.S. Striking a balance between content and method in nursing education: an idea from Alfred North Whitehead's Philosophy. Nursing Forum, 17 (3), 1978, 245-257.

19 General Nursing Council for England and Wales Educational policy 1977. GNC, 1977. (GNC circular 77/19 + enclosures A-D.)

20 Graham, J.E. The adaptation of principles to a variety of nursing care activities. (As a basis for teaching.) Lamp, 37 (11), Nov 1980, 7-9.

21 Green, D. A rethink on nurse education. (Current problems facing the nursing profession.) Nursing Times, 76, 25 Sep 1980, 1675.

22 Hall, D.C. The nature of nursing and the education of the nurse. Journal of Advanced Nursing, 5 (2), Mar 1980, 149-159.

23 Heath, J. A new kind of nurse—1. Tomorrow's approach to learning. (Factors affecting curriculum design and value of self-instructional methods of learning.) Nursing Mirror, 149, 9 Aug 1979, 22-23.

24 Journal of Nursing Education Issue on conflict. Journal of Nursing Education, 17 (5), May 1978, 7-52.

25 Lightowlers, J. New thinking on nurse education. (New Nursing Education Research Unit at Chelsea College.) Journal of Community Nursing, 1 (4), Oct 1977, 32.

26 Logan, W. Recent developments in nursing education. (In Scotland.) Nursing Mirror, 146, 4 May 1978, Supplement xiii-xv.

27 Marsh, N. Developing professionalism: teaching care to the careers. (Ensuring quality of caring as well as skills.) Nursing Mirror, 147, 2 Nov 1978, 20-22.

28 Mirin, S.K. editor Teaching tomorrow's nurse: a Nurse Education reader. Wakefield, Mass.: Nursing Resources, 1980.

29 National League for Nursing A judgment of merit: evaluation of programs in nursing. Applications. New York: NLN, 1979.

30 National League for Nursing A judgment of merit: evaluation of programs in nursing: methodology. New York: NLN, 1979.

31 National League for Nursing Program evaluation. New York: NLN, 1978.

32 Nursing Times Quest 1 (1). Education supplement. Nursing Times, 76, 25 Sep 1980, 1713-1720.

33 O'Donoghue, A. The need for a theory of nursing with particular reference to nurse education. 2 parts. World of Irish Nursing, 7 (8), Sep 1978, 7, 9; (9), Oct 1978, 2.

34 Rajabally, M.H. Nursing education: another tower of Babel? (Criticism of new conceptual frameworks in nursing.) Canadian Nurse, 93 (9), Sep 1977, 30-31.

35 Rassool, G.H. Social relationships in a classroom. (Use of sociometry.) Nursing Mirror, 145, 1 Sep 1977, 26-27.

36 Reilly, D.E. editor Teaching and evaluating the affective domain in nursing programs. Thorofare: Slack, 1978.

37 Roch, J. The uses and limitations of the concept of role for nurse education. Nursing Times, 76, 8 May 1980, 837-841.

38 Roy, C. Relating nursing theory to education: a new era. Nurse Educator, 4 (2), Mar/Apr 1979, 16-21.

39 Rule, J. A life of service in nurse education. (Interview with Miss J. Rule discussing the present state of nurse education, by W. Robinson.) Nursing Mirror, 143, 12 Aug 1976, 36.

40 Schaefer, M.J. Forecasting and resource allocation in educational administration. Nursing Outlook, 25 (4), Apr 1977, 265-270.

41 Sheahan, J. Education. 1. What is education? 2. Teaching concepts and values and learning to nurse. Nursing Times, 72, 26 Aug 1976, 1328-1329; 2 Sep 1976, 1366-1368.

42 Sheahan, J. The relevance of a philosophical perspective on education. (With brief reference to nursing education.) Journal of Advanced Nursing, 4 (4), Jul 1979, 429-438.

43 Williamson, J.A. editor Current perspectives in nursing education: the changing scene. 2 vols. St. Louis: Mosby, 1976. (Mosby's current practice and perspectives in nursing series.)

44 Wyatt, J. A look at nurse education— from the outside. (Changes affecting teacher and nurse education over the past few years.) Nursing Times, 74, 5 Jan 1978, 10-11.

b CURRICULUM: GENERAL

1 Allen, H.O. Curriculum planning. Nursing Times, 72, 20 May 1976, 790-791.

2 Allen, H.O. and Murrell, J. Nurse training: an enterprise in curriculum development at St. Thomas' Hospital, London. Macdonald and Evans, 1978.

3 Bevis, E.O. Curriculum building in nursing: a process. 2nd ed. St. Louis: Mosby, 1978.

4 Birchenall, P.D. Innovation in nurse education. (Obstacles in the way of implementing curriculum changes in schools of nursing.) Nursing Times, 76, 29 May 1980, 951-953; Correspondence from M. Gott, 19 Jun 1980, 1095; A. Townsend, 24 Jul 1980, 1306.

5 Bowman, M. The curriculum and the staff. Changing standards of nurse training. Nursing Mirror, 143 (11), 9 Sep 1976, 66-68.

6 Creighton, H. The present preparation of the student: is it meeting present needs? Findings of a curriculum workshop. Lamp, 33 (4), Apr 1976, 32-35.

7 Eisenhauer, L.A. and others Building a faculty team: (to design an integrated curriculum.) Nursing Outlook, 24 (7), Jul 1976, 437-440.

8 Farley, V.M. An evaluative study of an open curriculum/career ladder nursing program. New York: National League for Nursing, 1978.

9 Graham, L.E. The development of a useful conceptual framework in curriculum design. Nursing Papers, 9 (3), Fall 1977, 84-92.

10 Green, J.L. and Stone, J.C. Curriculum evaluation theory and practice, with a case study from nursing education. New York: Springer, 1977. (Springer series on the teaching of nursing vol.1.)

11 Haase, P.T. Pathways to practice. (The Southern Regional Education Board's curriculum study.) American Journal of Nursing, 76 (5), May 1976, 806-809; 76 (6), Jun 1976, 950-954.

12 Higgs, Z.R. Expectations and perceptions of the curricular leadership role of administrators of nursing education units. (Baccalaureate level education.) Nursing Research, 27 (1), Jan/Feb 1978, 57-62.

13 Hutchings, J. and Farrell, P. Community nursing and psychology, 10: it's often taught too soon…and badly. Journal of Community Nursing, 2 (11), May 1979, 15, 26.

14 Ketefian, S. Curriculum change in nursing education: sources of knowledge utilized. (A study of five current curricular innovations in the United States with a classification of the range of resources used to produce the change.) International Nursing Review, 23 (4), Jul/Aug 1976, 107-115.

15 Ketefian, S. Strategies of curriculum change. (With reference to baccalaureate nursing education in USA.) International Nursing Review, 25 (1), Jan/Feb 1978, 14-21, 24.

16 Kurian, A.P. An experiment in curriculum change. (Study of the implementation of the new curriculum proposed by the Indian Board of Nursing Education.) Nursing Journal of India, 68 (1), Jan 1977, 16-18.

17 Levine, L.B. Through the looking glass at the integrated curriculum. (History and development of the concept from 1923.) Journal of Nursing Education, 18 (7), Sep 1979, 43-46.

18 Llewelyn, S.P. The unexplored alliance. (How clinical psychologists could help nurses understand psychology through in-service training.) Nursing Mirror, 150, 26 Jun 1980, 34-36.

19 Marriner, A. and others Curriculum evaluation: wordfact, ritual, or reality. Nursing Outlook, 28 (4), Apr 1980, 228-232.

20 Meleis, A.I. The development of a conceptually based nursing curriculum: an international experiment. (Process used in developing a conceptual framework for a new college in Kuwait.) Journal of Advanced Nursing, 4 (6), Nov 1979, 659-671.

21 National League for Nursing Curriculum development and its implementation through a conceptual framework. New York: NLN, 1978.

22 National League for Nursing Selected readings from open curriculum literature: an annotated bibliography. 2nd ed. New York: NLN, 1977.

23 National League for Nursing. Division of Research Proceedings of the open curriculum conference IV, September 22-23, 1975, New York: a project of the NLN study of the open curriculum in nursing education. New York: NLN, 1976.

24 Nichols, R.S. and Bates, M.C. Non-traditional curriculum. (Designed to organise related subject matter into meaningful units at the Shepard Gill School of Practical Nursing.) Journal of Practical Nursing, 26 (4), Apr 1976, 27-29, 35.

25 Notter, L.E. and Robey, M. The open curriculum in nursing education: final report of the NLN open curriculum study. New York: NLN, 1979.

26 Ogundeyin, W.M. Principles of curriculum development. International Nursing Review, 23 (6), Nov/Dec 1976, 183-189.

27 Olade, R.A. Integration of mental health concepts into general nursing education in Nigeria: a survey of nurses' opinions. International Journal of Nursing Studies, 14 (2), 1977, 63-68.

28 Ozimek, D. Relating the open curriculum to accountability in baccalaureate nursing education. New York: National League for Nursing, 1976.

29 Parsons, M.A. and Collison, C.R. The process of change in curriculum evaluation. (A faculty's plan for systematic review.) Journal of Nursing Education, 19 (7), Sep 1980, 36-38.

30 Pepler, C. The practical aspects of using a conceptual framework. (Curriculum develop-

ment at the Faculty of Nursing, University of New Brunswick.) Nursing Papers, 9 (3), Fall 1977, 93-101.

31 Peterson, C.J. and others Competency-based curriculum and instruction. New York: National League for Nursing, 1979.

32 Peterson, C.J. Questions frequently asked about the development of a conceptual framework. (As basis for curriculum development.) Journal of Nursing Education, 16 (4), Apr 1977, 22-32.

33 Redman, B.K. On 'problems' with integrated curricula in nursing. Journal of Nursing Education, 17 (6), Jun 1978, 26-29.

34 Richards, M.A. One integrated curriculum. An empirical evaluation. (Students of a new course at Harris College of Nursing, Fort Worth, Texas, had more leadership ability but less critical thinking ability than students on a 'block' program.) Nursing Research, 26 (2), Mar-Apr 1977, 90-95.

35 Roberts, K.L. Curriculum planning and the sequence of learning. How much effect does the order in which learning experiences take place have upon the efficiency of the learning process? Australian Nurses Journal, 7 (8), Mar 1978, 40-42.

36 Ruffing, M.A. Literature by consumers for nursing. (Incorporation of non standard material into the curriculum to accentuate the humanistic foundations of nursing practice.) Nursing Forum, 14 (1), 1975, 87-94.

37 Sheahan, J. Curriculum development in nursing education. Nursing Mirror 144:
1. 20 Jan 1977, 53-55.
2. Objectives, 17 Feb 1977, 56-58.
3. Knowledge, 17 Mar 1977, 59-61.
4. Learning experiences, 14 Apr 1977, 58-60.
5. Evaluation, 19 May 1977, 29-31.

38 Sheahan, J. Some aspects of the teaching and learning of nursing. (Including curriculum theory and development. Has extensive bibliography.) Journal of Advanced Nursing, 5 (5), Sep 1980, 491-511.

39 Skeath, A. Nurse education and the curriculum. A good curriculum design should encompass both traditional and new approaches. Nursing Times, 76, 29 May 1980, 954-956.

40 Smith, J.P. Professing nursing through the curriculum. Journal of Advanced Nursing, 3 (4), Jul 1978, 331-332.

41 Styles, M.M. In the name of integration. (An examination of the process of taking 'the integrated approach' to curriculum development.) Nursing Outlook, 24 (12), Dec 1976, 738-744.

42 Sullivan, T.J. An experience with a systems approach to curriculum design. Journal of Nursing Education, 16 (3), Mar 1977, 25-34.

43 Thomas, B. Promoting creativity in nursing education. (Study of graduates of old and new curriculum designed to foster creativity.) Nursing Research, 28 (2), Mar/Apr 1979, 115-119.

44 Tubi, A.M. Now is the time: need for a review of the syllabus of the basic nursing education. Nigerian Nurse, 8 (1), Jan-Mar 1976, 22-24, 28.

45 Walker, D.J. An approach to curriculum evaluation at the master's level. Nursing Forum, 15 (1), 1976, 86-94.

46 Watson, M. Curriculum change: the process in a school of nursing. (Account of change at Newcastle Regional School of Nursing, N.S.W.) Lamp, 37 (7), Jul 1980, 29-32.

47 Weitzel, M.H. Philosophical base for the integrated nursing curriculum. Nursing Leadership, 3 (1), Mar 1980, 17-37.

48 White, M.B. and Coburn, D. The trials, tribulations, and triumphs of curriculum change. The faculty's experiences as they worked their way through to a totally revised curriculum. Nursing Outlook, 25 (10), Oct 1977 , 644-649.

49 Will, E.A. Curriculum evaluation in nursing. New Zealand Nursing Journal, 69, 9 Sep 1976, 3-5.

50 Wu, R.R. Designing a curriculum model. Journal of Nursing Education, 18 (3), Mar 1979, 13-21.

51 Zornow, R.A. A curriculum model for the expanded role. (Arizona State University College of Nursing.) Nursing Outlook, 25 (1), Jan 1977, 43-46.

c CURRICULUM: SPECIAL SUBJECTS

1 Akinsanya, J.A. and Hayward, J.C. The biological sciences in nursing education: the contribution of bionursing. (Exploration of concept of bionursing and results of a preliminary study on the definition of a biological basis for nursing practice.) Nursing Times, 76, 6 Mar 1980, 427-432.

2 Aroskar, M.A. Ethics in the nursing curriculum. Nursing Outlook, 25 (4), Apr 1977, 260-264.

3 Branch, M. Models for introducing cultural diversity in nursing curricula. Journal of Nursing Education, 15 (2), Mar 1976, 7-13.

4 Conners, V.L. Teaching affective behaviors. (To promote good nurse/patient communication.) Journal of Nursing Education, 18 (6), Jun 1979, 33-39.

5 Dexter, P. and Applegate, M. How to solve a math problem. (Need for and method of improving maths content in the curriculum.) Journal of Nursing Education, 19 (2), Feb 1980, 49-53.

6 Farrell, M. and others Teaching interpersonal skills: a systematic approach to developing and evaluating a course of basic communication skills for beginning nursing students. Nursing Outlook, 25 (5), May 1977, 322-325.

7 Fredette, S. and O'Connor, K. Nursing diagnosis in teaching and curriculum planning. Nursing Clinics in North America, 14 (3), Sep 1979, 541-552.

8 Fromer, M.J. Teaching ethics by case analysis. Nursing Outlook, 28 (10), Oct 1980, 604-609.

9 Grigsby, K. and Smith, R.N. Teaching basic nursing skills in a new curriculum. Journal of Nursing Education, 16 (3), Mar 1977, 17-21.

10 Hall, J.N. and Brooks, K.M. Teaching psychologists to teach psychology: the improvement of teaching skills in health service professions. (Using a short course in methods of teaching psychology to nurses as an example.) Medical Education, 10 (3), May 1976, 183-188.

11 Jaffee, M. and Flanagan, M.J. Specialist in an integrated curriculum: an odyssey. (Holistic approach to man and the environment.) Journal of Nursing Education, 18 (6), Jun 1979, 46-49.

12 Journal of Nursing Education Issue on the introduction of cultural content to the nursing curriculum. Journal of Nursing Education, 15 (2), Mar 1976, 3-34.

13 King, E.C. and Long, T.E. Competency based math curricula. Journal of Practical Nursing, 26 (6), Jun 1976, 28-30.

14 Koshi, P.T. Cultural diversity in the nursing curricula. Journal of Nursing Education, 15 (2), Mar 1976, 14-21.

15 Krawczyk, R. and Kudzma, E. Ethics: a matter of moral development. (Seminars in which students discuss specific ethical dilemmas rather than a formal course dealing with theoretical ethics.) Nursing Outlook, 26 (4), Apr 1978, 254-257.

16 Langham, P. Open forum: on teaching ethics to nurses. Nursing Forum, 16 (3, 4), 1977, 220-227.

17 McGivern, D.O. and others Teaching primary care in a baccalaureate program. Nursing Outlook, 24 (7), Jul 1976, 441-445.

18 Miller, P. Patient outcomes—the basis for nursing curriculum. (Preparing nurses to plan patient care.) Journal of Nursing Education, 16 (5), May 1977, 3-8.

19 Miller, S.R. Have we dichotomized theory and practice in nursing? (With reference to teaching students about family theories and practice.) Nursing Leadership, 1 (1), Jun 1978, 34-36.

20 Mitchell, C.A. and Avello, E.A. Hygiene made interesting: the case method. Journal of Nursing Education, 15 (5), Sep 1976, 11-13.

21 Murphy, J. Research Q. and A. Q: How can statistics be introduced effectively into the undergraduate nursing curriculum? Nursing Research, 26 (5), Sep/Oct 1977, 391-392.

22 O'Sullivan, S. and others A new way of teaching general nurses about human behaviour. (With details of curriculum.) Lamp, 36 (8), Sep 1979, 19-23.

23 Siegel, M. and Siegel, C. The use of literature in professional nursing education. (The arts and humanities as a means of communicating experience to students.) Nursing Forum, 16 (2), 1977, 157-164.

24 Ryden, M.B. An approach to ethical decision-making. (Students learn to explore with clients the probable outcomes of health-related actions and their value and risk to the client's well-being.) Nursing Outlook, 26 (11), Nov 1978, 705-706.

25 Valadez, A.M. and Heusinkveld, K.B. Teaching nursing students to teach patients. Journal of Nursing Education, 16 (4), Apr 1977, 10-14.

26 Voight, J.W. Physical assessment skills in the curriculum: a pilot project and follow-up. Journal of Nursing Education, 19 (2), Feb 1980, 26-30.

27 Zerr, S. The development of a teaching module for nursing students on drug use information. Nursing Papers, 12 (3), Aug 1980, 30-37.

d CURRICULUM: SEX EDUCATION

1 Boyd, J. Sex and psychiatric nursing—a view from the North. (Recent report on education and training of nurses.) Australian Nurses Journal, 9 (6), Dec/Jan 1980, 28-30.

2 deLemos, H. Changes in helping professionals' knowledge and attitudes following a human sexuality workshop led by a nurse. Journal of Psychiatric Nursing and Mental Health Services, 15 (7), Jul 1977, 11-21.

3 Fontaine, K.L. Human sexuality: faculty knowledge and attitudes. (Survey in Chicago schools of nursing to investigate the teaching of sexuality.) Nursing Outlook, 24 (3), Mar 1976, 174-176.

4 Kjervik, D.K. Influencing sex role opinions of undergraduate nursing students. (Description of course on women's studies and sex roles with evaluation of changes in students' opinions.) Journal of Nursing Education, 18 (8), Oct 1979, 43-49.

5 Mims, F.H. Human sexuality workshop: a continuing education program. (Evaluation of programme.) Journal of Continuing Education in Nursing, 9 (6), Nov/Dec 1978, 29-36.

6 Mims, F.H. and others Human sexuality course evaluation. (A three day program for medical, nursing and graduate psychology students at the University of Cincinnati.) Nursing Research, 25 (3), May/Jun 1976, 187-191.

7 Nelson, S.E. All about sex education for students. (To clarify their attitudes and respond to patients' problems.) American Journal of Nursing, 77 (4), Apr 1977, 611-612.

8 Pinch, W.J. Values exploration: a teaching model. (Using attitudes towards human sexuality as an example.) Journal of Nursing Education, 18 (8), Oct 1979, 56-59.

9 Santopietro, M.C.S. Effectiveness of a self-instructional module in human sexuality counselling. Nursing Research, 29 (1), Jan/Feb 1980, 14-19.

10 Woods, N.F. and Mandetta, A.F. Sexuality in the baccalaureate nursing curriculum. (Survey of curriculum content in 220 programs.) Nursing Forum, 15 (3), 1976, 294-313.

e EDUCATION: PRACTICE AND SERVICE NEEDS

1 Bendall, E. Learning for reality. (Research project to test the assumption that a student's written description of patient care is reflected in the actual care given.) Journal of Advanced Nursing, 1 (1), Jan 1976, 3-9.

2 Darwin, J. Obedience is not enough. (Methods of linking theory with practice in nurse education.) Nursing Mirror, 141, 2 Oct 1980, 32-34.

3 Dexter, P.A. and Laidig, J. Breaking the education/service barrier. After interviewing nursing service administrators, a faculty team recommended curricular changes regarding nursing care plans, discharge planning, and patient teaching. Nursing Outlook, 28 (3), Mar 1980, 179-182.

4 Esther, C.A.A. and Bryant, R.J. Educating the learner...to work on the ward. (Two research nurses advocate that the current system of nurse education be developed to unite theory and practice.) Nursing Times, 73, 13 Jan 1977, 47.

5 Gallagher, J. Educational planning and health. (Co-ordinating educational programmes for the health professions and health service needs.) WHO Chronicle, 30 (2), Feb 1976, 70-71.

6 GENERAL Nursing Council Education and service. (Three courses of action suggested by the GNC in evidence to the DHSS on 'The relationship between education and service.') Nursing Times, 72, 7 Oct 1976, 1546-1547.

7 Gugenheim, A.M. Nursing focus on education. (Review of 1979 nursing administration literature which gave extensive coverage to 'entry into practice' and service/education issues.) Hospitals, 54 (7), 1 Apr 1980, 151-155.

8 House, K.K. The new graduate looks at service and education. Supervisor Nurse, 7 (3), Mar 1976, 14-16.

9 Howarth, B. How can the vision of Janus help professional nursing? The problem of anxiety in relation to the clinical education of student nurses in Australian hospitals while cognizant of the hospital's primary task of providing quality care. Australian Nurses' Journal, 4 (11), Jun 1975, 31-33, 36.

10 Kergin, D.J. Issues in nurse education. The problems of separating education from practice. (With reference to Canada and methods of bridging the gap at McMaster University.) Medical Teacher, 2 (3), May/Jun 1980, 123-126.

11 Lynaugh, J. The 'entry into practice' conflict: how we got where we are and what will happen next. American Journal of Nursing, 80 (2), Feb 1980, 266-270.

12 Moores, B. The cost and effectiveness of nurse education. (Estimate of real cost to health service of employing a trainee nurse and nurses' attitudes to allocation programmes.) Nursing Times, 75, 21 Jun 1979, Occ. papers, 65-68; 28 Jun 1979, Occ. papers, 71-72.

13 Nayer, D.D. Unification: bringing nursing service and nursing education together. (Schemes at various hospitals.) American Journal of Nursing, 80 (6), Jun 1980, 1110-1114.

14 Nursing Papers Deviance and education for leadership. (Three articles on problems in educating nurses for differences between ideal nursing as taught and nursing as practised.) Nursing Papers, 10 (2), Summer 1978, 64-70.

15 Powers, M.J. The unification model in nursing. (Integration of service and education in the United States.) Nursing Outlook, 24 (8), Aug 1976, 482-487.

16 REALISM versus idealism — the tutor's dilemma. (Comment on gap between teaching and ward practice in nursing care.) Nursing Mirror, 145, 1 Dec 1977, 28.

17 Rodgers, J.A. Today's preparation for tomorrow's practice: the Lehman College nursing programme. (City University of New York.) Journal of Advanced Nursing, 1 (4), Jul 1976, 311-322.

18 ROYAL Society of Health Cost benefit research needed on nurse training. (Conference report.) Nursing Times, 72, 6 May 1976, 678.

19 Slater, P.V. Multi-level preparation for nursing impact on nursing practice. (Technical skill approach and professional approach.) Australian Nurses Journal, 7 (11), Jun 1978, 40-43.

20 Smith, D. Training in the NHS — doctors and nurses. Health and Social Service Journal, 87, 7 Oct 1977, F9-F12.

21 Weyman, A. The nurse and the system. (Problems arising from inadequate nurse training.) Health and Social Service Journal, 85, 20/27 Dec 1975, 2789.

f MODULAR SYSTEM

1 Copeland, W.L. and Miller, B.E. Development of a modular curriculum for nursing service orientation. Journal of Continuing Education in Nursing, 7 (4), Jul/Aug 1976, 10-15.

2 Cyrs, T.E. How to design learning modules. Journal of Practical Nursing, 26 (9), Sep 1976, 30-33.

3 Cyrs, T.E. Managing students through the use of learning modules. (Includes a detailed bibliography.) Journal of Practical Nursing, 26 (8), Aug 1976, 20-21, 32, 35.

4 Harrison, J. and others Integrating theory and practice in modular schemes for basic nurse education. Journal of Advanced Nursing, 2 (5), Sep 1977, 503-519.

5 Harrison, J. and others Some structural considerations in modular education for basic nursing students. Journal of Advanced Nursing, 2 (4), Jul 1977, 383-391.

6 Hackaby, L.M.S. Conditions of learning and instruction in nursing, modularized. St. Louis: Mosby, 1980.

7 Kochman, A.F. Are letter grades and modularized nursing programs compatible? The Nursing Department of California State University, Long Beach, is in the process of transitioning from conventional teaching to a modularized program. Journal of Nursing Education, 15 (3), May 1976, 25-27.

8 Mitchell, W. Psychiatric module in general training. Nursing Mirror, 142, 29 Jan 1976, 55-56.

9 Thompson, M.A. A systematic approach to module development. Journal of Nursing Education, 17 (8), Oct 1978, 20-26.

10 Wakeling, C.M. Fact or fantasy: a modular comprehensive educational programme for all nurse students and pupils. (Operated by the Highland Health Board.) Nursing Mirror, 146, 4 May 1978, Supplement xv-xvi.

11 Warcaba, B. An experimental scheme in nurse education. (Pilot modular system at St. Crispin's Hospital, Northampton, based on the recommendations of the Nurse Tutor Working

Party.) Journal of Advanced Nursing, 1 (3), May 1976, 243-252.

g OBJECTIVES

1 Bloom, R.S. Stating educational objectives in behavioral terms. Nursing Forum, 14 (1), 1975, 30-42.

2 Bowman, M. Specifically objective. (Need for aims and objectives in nursing education.) Nursing Mirror, 149, 6 Sep 1979, 28-29.

3 Curran, C.L. Behavioral objectives: a necessity for nurse educators. Journal of Continuing Education in Nursing, 8 (6), Nov/Dec 1977, 3-6.

4 Ellis, L. and others Implementing a conceptual framework. (Developing learning objectives with reference to Bloom's taxonomy.) Nursing Outlook, 27 (2), Feb 1979, 127-130.

5 Griffin, J.K. Writing and using behavioral objectives in nursing education. New York: National League for Nursing, 1977.

6 Kennedy, L. Educating nurses — for today and tomorrow. (Objectives and teaching methods.) Nursing Times, 74, 2 Feb 1978, 205-206.

7 Marson, S. A new kind of nurse — 2. Objectives: markers along the way. Nursing Mirror, 149, 16 Aug 1979, 17-19.

8 Nuttelman, D. Instructional objectives: how to write behavioral objectives, why and when. Supervisor Nurse, 8 (11), Nov 1977, 35, 38-40, 43-44.

9 Okunade, A. Formulating educational objectives. Nigerian Nurse, 8 (4), Oct-Dec 1976, 20-27.

10 Reilly, D.E. Behavioral objectives in nursing: evaluation of learner attainment. New York: Appleton-Century-Crofts, 1975.

11 Roberts, K.L. Behavioral objectives: panacea or pain? (In nursing education.) Australian Nurses Journal, 6 (12), Jun 1977, 35-37.

12 World Health Organization. Study Group Criteria for the evaluation of learning objectives in the education of health personnel. Geneva: WHO, 1977.

h PRENURSING COURSES

1 Greenwood, N.D. Pre-nursing education in a changing situation: the report of an investigation into pre-nursing education in England 1974-1977. Summary of main findings. The author, 1977.

2 Morton, J.M. Pre-nursing courses. (Course at West Kent College of Further Education, Tonbridge, for all entrants to the 'caring' professions.) Nursing Times, 72, 28 Oct 1976, 1692-1693.

3 Newell, J. and Thomas, P.A. Preparing to nurse. (Two articles on the pre-nursing course based at South Fields College, Leicester, describing the course's philosophy and hospital placement.) Nursing Times, 74, 13 Apr 1978, 639-641.

i SCHOOLS OF NURSING

1 Brueckner, S.J. and Blair, E. Cost of education in a department of nursing service at a University Medical Center. (Study at the University of Colorado to identify educational costs in order to allocate resources more effectively. Journal of Nursing Administration, 7 (3), Mar 1977, 21-27.

2 CHARLES Frears School of Nursing. Nursing Mirror, 142 (12), 18 Mar 1976, 56.

3 Corns, R.H. Development of an International Nursing Centre. (New Hodgson Woodruff School of Nursing, Emory University, Atlanta, Georgia.) International Nursing Review, 23 (3), May/Jun 1976, 84-87.

4 DEPARTMENT of Health and Social Security Directory of schools of nursing. HMSO. 3rd ed. 1977, 4th ed. 1980.

5 Dyck, M.H. The effect of organizational and group characteristics of faculty's perception of climate in schools of nursing. (Research study.) Nursing Papers, 11 (3), Fall 1979, 63-85.

6 Everest, P. Clerical support services in schools of nursing. 1. (Job evaluation survey of the South East Thames Region to investigate the adequacy of clerical services.) Nursing Times, 72, 10 Jun 1976, Occ. papers, 81-84.

7 Everest, P. Clerical support services in schools of nursing. 2. (Factors affecting the increased complexity of clerical tasks, the deployment of clerical staff, and job grading.) Nursing Times, 72, 17 Jun 1976, Occ. papers, 85-87.

8 Everest, P. Clerical support services in schools of nursing. 3. (Role specifications for 8 clerical functions identified by a job analysis including the library.) Nursing Times, 72, 24 Jun 1976, Occ. papers, 89-92.

9 Everest, P. Clerical support services in schools of nursing. 4. (Organisation and planning in suggestions for the calculation of staff numbers.) Nursing Times, 72, 1 Jul 1976, Occ. papers, 93-96.

10 Everest, P. Clerical support services in schools of nursing. 5. (The availability of resources, a six step plan as a guideline to the implementation of change, and a summary of the main findings.) Nursing Times, 72, 8 Jul 1976, Occ. papers, 97-99.

11 Ferguson, A.C. De-schooling nurses. Do we really need schools of nursing? Nursing Times, 42, 2 Dec 1976, 1864.

12 GENERAL Nursing Council Advice on contracts for student and pupil nurses. (Part of GNC series of advice notes on management in schools of nursing 76/5 and 77/1.) Nursing Times, 73, 19 May 1977, Occ. papers, 69-72; 73, 26 May 1977, Occ. papers, 73-76.

13 GENERAL Nursing Council Series of management advice notes: nurse training schools advised on admissions and dismissals. (Comment on the Trades Union and Labour Relations Act and the Employment Protection Act.) Nursing Mirror, 142, 26 Feb 1976, 36.

14 Morris, P. It's all a question of training. (North versus South for quality of nurse training.) Nursing Mirror, 148, 12 Apr 1979, 5-6.

15 Schaefer, M.J. Educational admin-istration: how should we organize? Journal of Nursing Administration, 6 (2), Feb 1976, 12-14.

16 Smith, M. Elizabeth Garrett Anderson. Beloved training school. Nursing Times, 72, 23 Sep 1976, 1479-1481.

17 Whyte, B.B. The Thomas Guy School of Nursing. Nursing Mirror, 142, 6 May 1976, 51-52.

18 Whyte, B.B. The Thomas Guy School of Nursing *contained in* Handler, Clive E. editor Guy's Hospital: 250 years. Guy's Hospital Gazette, 1976, 86-88.

19 Wilkinson, J.A. Hospital schools of nursing: profits counterpoise costs. (Advantages of clinical experience obtained in the hospital school compared with other nurse training establishments.) Hospitals, 50 (8), 16 Apr 1976, 95-98.

j NURSE TEACHERS

1 Andreoli, K.G. Faculty productivity. (Analysis of workload of teaching staff, with bibliography.) Journal of Nursing Administration, 9 (11), Nov 1979, 47-53.

2 Akinsanya, J.A. Preaching what you practise. (The problems of a two year training for nurse tutors with comments on an article by W.M. Watson, Nursing Times, 16 Sep 1976.) Nursing Times, 73, 3 Mar 1977, 314-315.

3 Armiger, B. The educational crisis in the preparation of Deans. Nursing Outlook, 24 (3), Mar 1976, 164-168.

4 Bower, D. and others Part-time faculty: responsibilities, opportunities, employment terms. (Survey of nursing schools with part time lecturers.) Nursing Outlook, 28 (1), Jan 1980, 43-45.

5 Bowman, M. The great charade. (The role of professionals in institutes of higher education.) Nursing Mirror, 150, 27 Mar 1980, 14.

6 Bowman, M. The teacher—manager and leader. (Important considerations in the preparation of nurse teachers.) Nursing Mirror, 149, 30 Aug 1979, Supplement xviii, xx-xxi.

7 Buzzell, M. Accent on learning. Nurse educators, whose needs are you meeting? Australian Nurses Journal, 6 (11), May 1977, 39-40.

8 Carter, S.L. The nurse educator: humanist or behaviorist? (Two types of learning theory.) Nursing Outlook, 26 (9), Sep 1978, 554-557.

9 Coetsee, M. Teacher effectiveness: an issue in educational administration. (Review of literature.) Curationis, 2 (3), Dec 1979, 4-7.

10 Conway, M.E. and Glass, L.K. Socialization for survival in the academic world. (Nurse teachers in university schools of nursing.) Nursing Outlook, 26 (7), Jul 1978, 424-429.

11 Crawshaw, C.A. Selected nurse tutors' perceptions of their actual and potential clinical involvement with their learners. MSc thesis, University of Manchester, 1977.

12 Dunlop, M.J. and Smith, K.R. Expect-ations of the ideal lecturer. (Research study of nurses on post-basic courses.) Australian Nurses Journal, 9 (4), Oct 1979, 49-50.

13 Everest, P. Role development workshop for administrators in schools of nursing. (In the South-East Thames Region.) Nursing Times, 74, 16 Nov 1978, Occ. Papers, 125-128.

14 Fitzpatrick, M.L. and Heller, B.R. Teach-ing the teachers to teach. (Issues facing American nurse education including lack of nurse teachers.) Nursing Outlook, 28 (6), Jun 1980, 372-373.

15 Forrest, I. and Dodds, M. A new venture in preparing nurse tutors. (A one year continuous assessment course at Huddersfield Polytechnic.) Nursing Times, 72, 19 Feb 1976, 276-277.

16 Gallego, A.P. and others The working life of the nurse teacher. (One-week study done by students of MA Curriculum Studies in Nursing Education course.) Nursing Times, 76, 7 Aug 1980, 1409-1411.

17 Gorecki, Y. Faculty peer review. (Evaluation of tutors' teaching performance by their colleagues.) Nursing Outlook, 25 (7), Jul 1977, 439-442.

18 Grandjean, B.D. and others Professional autonomy and the work satisfaction of nursing educators. (Study of satisfaction in four state university schools of nursing.) Nursing Research, 25 (3), May/Jun 1976, 216-221.

19 Green, M. Preparing the nurse teacher. (New Rcn diploma of nursing education.) Nursing Times, 74, 13 Apr 1978, 613.

20 Hawken, P.L. Growing our own: a way to prepare deans. (Training in nursing education administration through a year's experience as an administrative associate to the dean of school of nursing.) Nursing Outlook, 28 (3), Mar 1980, 170-172.

21 Holliman, J.M. Analyzing faculty workload. Nursing Outlook, 25 (11), Nov 1977, 721-723.

22 House, V. and Sims, A. Teachers of nursing in the United Kingdom: a description of their attitudes. (GNC survey of 2923 registered teachers.) Journal of Advanced Nursing, 1 (6), Nov 1976, 495-505.

23 Ketefian, S. A Paradigm for faculty eval-uation. (To delineate tutors' functions and evaluate their performance.) Nursing Outlook, 25 (11), Nov 1977, 718-720.

24 Malhotra, A.K. The role of nurse educator in the health team. Nursing Journal of India, 47 (6), Jun 1976, 129-130.

25 Marsh, N. Student teacher: a small experi-ment within the Manchester course. (On the organisation of practical work.) Nursing Times, 66, 10 Sep 1977, Occ. papers, 135.

26 Mercer, J. Teaching nurses to teach. (Teaching on a Practical Work Teachers course, Polytechnic of North London.) Queen's Nursing Journal, 19 (2), May 1976, 45-46.

27 Mitsunaga, B.K. and Hall, B.A. The deanship: manifest and latent identity. (Questionnaire survey to investigate their role perception, expectations and dissatisfaction.) Nursing Outlook, 24 (11), Nov 1976, 692-696.

28 Mooneyhan, E.L. Evaluating a potential employer in academia. (Criteria for prospective teachers to assess job in a school of nursing.) Nursing Outlook, 26 (11), Nov 1978, 697-699.

29 Morris, P. Wanted: 800 more teachers. (Shortage of nurse tutors and problems of unattractive salary.) Nursing Mirror, 150, 24 Jan 1980, 6.

30 Mutzebraugh, C.E. The teacher as a 'reinforcement machine' in the teaching-learning process. Journal of Nursing Education, 15 (5), Sep 1976, 27-33.

31 National League for Nursing Instructor accountability: issues, facts, impact. New York: NLN, 1976.

32 National League for Nursing Roles, rights and responsibilities: the educational administrator's 3 R's. New York: NLN, 1978.

33 Page, S. and Loeper, J. Peer review of the nurse educator: the process and development of a format. Journal of Nursing Education, 17 (9), Nov 1978, 21-29.

34 Perry, E. Educating the educators: the new Diploma in Nursing of the University of London. Nursing Times, 76, 25 Sep 1980, 1715-1717.

35 Plawecki, J.A. and Plawecki, H.M. Factors that influence attraction and retention of qualified nurse educators. (Survey of 92 faculty members in Iowa institutions.) Nursing Research, 25 (2), Mar-Apr 1976, 133-135.

36 Raybould, E. editor A guide for teachers of nurses. Blackwell, 1975.

37 Rimmer, T. Education evaluated. (Nurse teachers' case for pay parity with nurse managers.) Nursing Times, 75, 15 Nov 1979, 1962-1963.

38 Roberts, E. Becoming a nurse tutor. (Letter outlining various methods of preparation for tutor courses.) Nursing Times, 73, 17 Nov 1977, 1799-1780.

39 Royal College of Nursing Guidelines for the professional practical experience of student teachers: report of a Working Party. Rcn, 1976.

40 Schlotfeldt, R.M. Recruiting, appointing and renewing faculty: a shared responsibility. (Selection of nursing school personnel.) Nursing Outlook, 24 (3), Mar 1976, 148-154.

41 Sheahan, J. Continuous assessment in the preparation of teachers of nursing. (Course at Huddersfield Polytechnic.) Nursing Times, 72, 12 Feb 1976, Occ. papers, 21-23.

42 Sheahan, J. Educating teachers of nursing: the contribution of educational studies. (Account of the elements which may be studied in a certificate of education course.) Journal of Advanced Nursing, 3 (5), Sep 1978, 447-455.

43 Sheahan, J. Educating teachers of nursing: the contribution of pedagogical studies. (Pedagogy can be defined as the art and science of teaching or the way a curriculum is transmitted.) Journal of Advanced Nursing, 3 (6), Nov 1978, 515-524.

44 Sheahan, J. Educating teachers of nursing: a survey of the opinions of students. (Survey of how 1978-1979 tutor students at Huddersfield Polytechnic rated various aspects of their course.) Journal of Advanced Nursing, 5 (1), Jan 1980, 71-81.

45 Sims, A. Teachers of nursing in the United Kingdom: some characteristics of teachers and their jobs. (Report of a GNC study carried out in 1974-1975.) Journal of Advanced Nursing, 1 (5), Sep 1976, 377-389.

46 Smith, J.P. Role strain of US nurse tutors. (Report of King's Fund seminar.) Nursing Times, 75, 29 Mar 1979, 521.

47 Solomons, H.C. and others How faculty members spend their time. (Analysis of workload showed little time given to research.) Nursing Outlook, 28 (3), Mar 1980, 160-165.

48 Watson, M.W. New perspectives for nurse teachers. (Changes in nurse teacher preparation in the University of London and a suggested pattern of preparation for senior nurse educators.) Nursing Times, 72 (37), 16 Sep 1976, Occ. papers, 133-135.

49 Stafford, L. and Graves, C.C. Some problems in evaluating teaching effectiveness. (Evaluation of tutors' abilities and clinical competence with regard to promotion within educational institution.) Nursing Outlook, 24 (8), Aug 1978, 494-497.

50 Wigmore, H. A new approach to qualification as a teacher of nursing. (The new Diploma in Nursing Education at the Rcn's Institute of Advanced Nursing Education.) Nursing Times, 76, 25 Sep 1980, 1717-1719.

21 TEACHING AND LEARNING

a GENERAL

1 Arnold, J. Let's discuss teaching strategies. (Research study to discover the most effective teaching strategy in a first year degree course.) Journal of Nursing Education, 17 (1), Jan 1978, 15-20.

2 Baldonado, A. Creative teaching-learning strategies. Journal of Continuing Education in Nursing, 10 (3), May/Jun 1979, 11-16.

3 Bridgewater, S. Criteria for selection of nursing textbooks. Journal of Nursing Education, 15 (1), Jan 1976, 3-5.

4 Calnan, J. A lecture on lecturing. Medical Education, 10 (6), Nov 1976, 445-447.

5 Cason, C. and others Peer instruction in professional nurse education: a qualitative case study. Journal of Nursing Education, 16 (7), Sep 1977, 10-22.

6 Clark, C.C. Classroom skills for nurse educators. New York: Springer, 1978. (Springer series on the teaching of nursing, vol.4.)

7 CONFERENCE '79. (Report of conference on learning and teaching.) Nursing Times, 75, 8 Nov 1979, Community outlook 341-342, 345, 347-348, 350.

8 Connolly, A.C. and Hoozer, H.V. The systems approach: a basis for course redesign. When a lecture course seems to be unsatisfactory, a systematic analysis of its content, objectives, and learner characteristics is made. Nursing Outlook, 28 (11), Nov 1980, 695-698.

9 Crosby, M.H. Interest in teaching skills development: a survey of Virginia nurses. (To discover if nurses had received teaching skills instruction during basic or post basic nursing education.) Journal of Continuing Education in Nursing, 8 (4), Jul/Aug 1977, 35-36.

10 Crosby, M.H. Teaching strategies: a microteaching project for success in Virginia. (University of Virginia School of Nursing.) Nursing Research, 26 (2), Mar-Apr 1977, 144-147.

11 Dixon, J.K. and Koerner, B. Faculty and student perceptions of effective classroom teaching in nursing. Nursing Research, 25 (4), Jul/Aug 1976, 300-305.

12 Hansell, H.N. and Foster, S.B. Critical care nursing orientation: a comparison of teaching methods. (Comparative study of classroom teaching and programmed instruction showing advantages of the latter method.) Heart Lung, 9 (6), Nov/Dec 1980, 1066-1072.

13 Hardy, L.K. Keeping up with 'Mrs Chase': an analysis of nursing skill-learning. Journal of Advanced Nursing, 5 (3), May 1980, 321-327.

14 Huckaby, L.M. and others Effect of specific teaching techniques on cognitive learning, transfer of learning, and affective behavior of nurses in an in-service education setting. Nursing Research, 26 (5), Sep/Oct 1977, 380-385.

15 Iversen, S.M. Microcounseling: a model for teaching the skills of interviewing. (Using videotaped or live role play.) Journal of Nursing Education, 17 (7), Sep 1978, 12-16.

16 Iveson-Iveson, J. Students' forum: how to get the most out of studying. (With multiple choice and long answer questions on cardiology.) Nursing Mirror, 150, 14 Feb 1980, 20-25.

17 Koshy, K.R. How to study effectively. Nursing Mirror, 145, 27 Dec 1977, 19.

18 Krawczyk, R.M. Peer participatory conference: a dynamic method of nursing instruction. (Involving each member's presentation of case study of patient currently nursed.) Journal of Nursing Education, 17 (8), Oct 1978, 5-8.

19 Lenburg, C.B. Non-traditional approaches to learning. (In continuing education.) AORN Journal, 26 (1), Jul 1977, 48-53.

20 Maury-Hess, S. and others Textbook selection for associate degree nursing programs (an evaluative study). (Includes assessing readability of textbooks.) Journal of Nursing Education, 18 (1), Jan 1979, 11-16.

21 Miltz, R.J. Nurses improve their personal communication. (Training seminar using microteaching.) Supervisor Nurse, 8 (12), Dec 1977, 13-15.

22 Moser, D.H. and Kondracki, M.R. Comparison of attitudes and cognitive achievement of nursing students in three instructional strategies. (Lecture methods, black and white television, and colour televised instruction via a Dial Access Information and Retrieval System.) Journal of Nursing Education, 16 (1), Jan 1977, 14-28.

23 National League for Nursing Concepts and components of effective teaching. New York: NLN, 1978.

24 National League for Nursing Evaluation of teaching effectiveness. New York: NLN, 1977.

25 National League for Nursing Generating effective teaching. New York: NLN, 1978.

26 National League for Nursing Teaching-learning strategies in baccalaureate nursing education. New York: NLN, 1976.

27 Norman, E.M. and Haumann, L. A model for judging teaching effectiveness. (With annotated bibliography.) Nursing Education, 3 (2), Mar/Apr 1978, 29-35.

28 Perry, S.E. Teaching strategy and learner performance. (With reference to modules and programmed instruction units where students know how well they perform.) Journal of Nursing Education, 18 (1), Jan 1979, 25-27.

29 Pugh, E.J. Dynamics of teaching learning interaction. Nursing Forum, 15 (1), 1976, 47-58.

30 Samuel, S.A. Teaching learning process in nursing. Nursing Journal of India, 48 (8), Aug 1976, 183-184.

31 Sheahan, J. Education. Nursing Times 72.
1. What is education. 26 Aug 1976, 1328-1329.
2. Teaching concepts and values and learning to nurse. 2 Sep 1976, 1366-1368.
3. Method learning: planning for teaching. 9 Sep 1976, 1405-1407.
4. Lectures and forum teaching methods. 16 Sep 1976. 1448-1450.
5. Discovery methods of teaching and team teaching. 23 Sep 1976, 1487-1489.
6. Teaching skills and teaching aids. 30 Sep 1976, 1526-1528.
7. Communication skills and assessment learning. 7 Oct 1976, 1570-1572.

32 Shipley, R.H. Applying learning theory to nursing practice. Nursing Forum, 16 (1), 1977, 83-94.

33 Spencer, M. Did the student learn? A comparison of different study methods. (Pilot study of 18 student nurses using formal lecture, tape/slide package and guided study sheets with text books.) Nursing Times, 75, 4 Jan 1979, 35-37.

34 Stevens, B.J. The teaching-learning process. (Review of types of learning and methods of teaching.) Nursing Education, 1 (1), May/Jun 1976, 9, 12-15, 18-20.

35 Sullivan, P.A. and Beeler, J.L. Methods of teaching—revisited: a format for discussion. Journal of Continuing Education in Nursing, 10 (5), Sep/Oct 1979, 15-17.

36 Tibbitts, G.E. and others Nurse training: how much of it is education? (A comparison of five teaching methods: reading, lectures, audio-lecture, programmed instruction and multi-media.) International Journal of Nursing Studies, 13 (3), 1976, 187-193.

37 World Health Organization Annotated bibliography of teaching-learning materials for schools of nursing and midwifery. Geneva: WHO, 1975. (WHO offset publication no.19.)

b AUDIOVISUAL AND LEARNING RESOURCE CENTRES

1 Bauman, K. and Kunka, A.K. Overhead transparencies: the overlooked medium. Nurse Educator, 4 (4), Jul/Aug 1979, 21-25.

2 Beaton-Mamak, M. Education that 'turns on' staff. (Use of an audio-visual department in a large hospital.) Dimensions in Health Service, 53 (7), Jul 1976, 40-41.

3 Blatchley, M.E. and others The media center. It's great, but... (Suggestions for effective use.) Journal of Nursing Education, 17 (1), Jan 1978, 24-28.

4 Brain, E.A. and Bidwell, C.M. How to do it: construct an audiovisual programme. British Medical Journal, 1, 10 Feb 1979, 394-396.

5 Burns, E. and Brooker, R. The use and further application of film triggers in nursing education and research. (Filmed nursing situations.) Australian Nurses Journal, 8 (3), Sep 1978, 40-41, 51.

6 Cooper, S.S. Methods of teaching—revisited. The overhead projector. Journal of Continuing Education in Nursing, 11 (3), May/Jun 1980, 56, 71-72.

7 Cooper, S.S. Methods of teaching—revisited. Slides and slide-sound presentations. Journal of Continuing Education in Nursing, 11 (5), Sep/Oct 1980, 52-55.

8 Crabb, R. The learning resources centre. The law of copyright. Nursing Times, 73, 21 Apr 1977, 585-587.

9 Dahmer, J. and others Evaluation of an integrated multi media learning system. Medical Education, 10 (6), Nov 1976, 491-496.

10 Dalgarno, J. A guide to the overhead projector. 1 and 2. Nursing Times, 76, 21 Aug 1980, 1482-1483; 18 Sep 1980, 1669-1670.

11 Dalgarno, J. The learning resources centre. The audio-visual aids technician. Nursing Times, 73, 21 Apr 1977, 581-583.

12 Davies, V.J. Complementary communications: making a tape-slide sequence. (Detailed advice.) Journal of Human Nutrition, 31 (5), 348-351.

13 Donaldson, M.L. Instructional media as a teaching strategy. Nurse Educator, 4 (4), Jul/Aug 1979, 18-20.

14 Dubin, G. and others Story boarding—a teaching tool. (Sequence of cards with pictures and text, to organise ideas and as preparation for illustrated lecture.) Canadian Nurse, 72 (6), Jun 1976, 42-44.

15 Evans, A.D. and others Speech compression: options for speeding nursing education. (Research study of use of compressed speech audiotapes.) Journal of Nursing Education, 19 (5), May 1980, 20-26.

16 Forsyth, D.McN. Assisting in the development of a slide tape: a learning experience. Journal of Nursing Education, 19 (4), Apr 1980, 42-45.

17 Graves, J. and Graves, V. Designing a tape-slide programme. (ASME Medical education booklet no.9.) Medical Education, 13 (2), Mar 1979, 135-143.

18 Graves, J. and Graves, V. 20 years later. (Development of Medical Recording Service Foundation.) Nursing Mirror, 145, 27 Oct 1977, 27-28.

19 Gustafson, M.B. The blackboard/chalkboard revisited. (Suggestions for maximising and varying use.) Supervisor Nurse, 8 (5), May 1977, 57, 59, 61.

20 Gustafson, M.B. Methods of teaching—revisited. Be your own tour guide? Journal of Continuing Education in Nursing, 11 (2), Mar/Apr 1980, 51-53.

21 Heath, J. The learning resources centre. A practical approach to curriculum development. Nursing Times, 73, 21 Apr 1977, 576-578.

22 Hoose, D.C. A model for a nursing media center. (University of Wisconsin-Milwaukee School of Nursing.) Nursing Outlook, 24 (2), Feb 1976, 104-106.

23 Iveson-Iveson, J. Looking at educational technology today. Nursing Mirror, 142, 11 Mar 1976, 41.

24 Lange, C.M. The media center. Adapting media for independent study. Nursing Outlook, 24 (9), Sep 1976, 546.

25 Lange, C.M. The media center. Future directions. (In the use of audio-visual media.) Nursing Outlook, 25 (12), Dec 1977, 753.

26 Lange, C.M. The media center. Modifying media for individual instruction. Nursing Outlook, 24 (8), Aug 1976, 477.

27 Lange, C.M. The media center. Using the overhead projector. Nursing Outlook, 24 (3), Mar 1976, 145.

28 Lange, C.M. Using media in evaluation. (Of students.) Nursing Outlook, 25 (4), Apr 1977, 241.

29 Lewis, J. Making tape-slide programmes. (In nurse education.) Nursing Times, 74, 20 Apr 1978, 673-675.

30 McGinn, H.P. Constructing a media center. Journal of Practical Nursing, 26 (10), Oct 1976, 28-30.

31 Marson, S.N. and Townsend, I. Educational technology...a movement for change: the future of educational technology in British nurse education. Journal of Advanced Nursing, 1 (2), Mar 1976, 155-162.

32 Marson, S.N. The learning resources centre. Nursing education and educational technology. Nursing Times, 73, 21 Apr 1977, 574-576.

33 Marson, S.N. NHS Learning Resources Unit. Nursing Times, 73, 24 Feb 1977, 276-277.

34 Miles, I.M. Educational technology and resource-based learning as applied to nursing education. (With reference to use of modules for ward-based self-instruction for study between blocks of classroom study.) Curationis, 1 (2), Sep 1978, 36-41.

35 Miles, I.M. A medical and nursing tape recording service. (Medical Tape Recording Unit, College of General Practitioners of South Africa following the example of the Medical Recording Service Foundation, England.) S.A. Nursing Journal, 43 (5), May 1976, 10-11.

36 Milio, N. A broad perspective on health: a teaching learning tool. (A chart illustrating the effects of the environment and personal health services on health.) Nursing Outlook, 24 (3), Mar 1976, 160-163.

37 **Monks, J.** Economical slide-making. (With reference to use in developing countries.) Nursing Times, 74, 17 Aug 1978, 1381.

38 **Murray, T.S.** How to do it: use an overhead projector. British Medical Journal, 1, 3 Mar 1979, 602-603.

39 **NATIONAL** Health Service Learning Resources Unit. National Centre for Developments in Nurse Education Education and training technology: a bibliography. Sheffield: the Unit, (1979).

40 **Olson, G.R.** The instructional media service framework: a user-oriented organizational structure for instructional media operations. (Audio-visual aids.) Journal of Nursing Education, 16 (6), Jun 1977, 36-41.

41 **Pearson, B.D.** Evaluation of the nursing process through visual motion media. (Problems in evaluation by audio-visual aids of clinical competence and the application of abstract thinking processes such as the nursing process.) International Nursing Review, 25 (4), Jul/Aug 1978, 119-120.

42 **Podratz, R.O.** Audio visual project: an alternative learning experience in pediatrics. Journal of Nursing Education, 15 (6), Nov 1976, 33-36.

43 **Rollo, J.** A new approach to learning: the mobile teaching unit. (A mobile cabinet incorporating audio-visual aids designed at Westminster Hospital.) Nursing Times, 72 (36), 9 Sep 1976, Occ. papers, 129-132.

44 **Schmalenberg, C.** Making and using slides. Nurse Educator, 4 (4), Jul/Aug 1979, 12-15.

45 **Shepherd, B.J.** Learning by looking. (Audio-visual aids for teaching student nurses in theatre.) Nursing Times, 73, 6 Oct 1977, Theatre Nursing, 9-10, 12.

46 **Simonds, A.** Preparing students in an OR skills lab. (Use of learning laboratory and audiovisual programmes.) AORN Journal, 32 (5), Nov 1980, 830-831, 834.

47 **Skarratt, R.** The learning resources centre. Building a centre on a shoestring. Nursing Times, 73, 21 Apr 1977, 583-584.

48 **Slack, P.** Taking the slog out of searching! (A.V. MINE, information service on audiovisual aids for nurse education at NHS Learning Resources Unit in Sheffield.) Nursing Times, 76, 17 Apr 1980, 698.

49 **Sparks, S.M.** Pooling audiovisual instructional resources. (Among several nursing schools.) Nursing Outlook, 25 (10), Oct 1977, 625.

50 **Stephen, S.** The learning resources centre. Audio-visual aids and the librarian's role. Nursing Times, 73, 21 Apr 1977, 579-580.

51 **Stroud, J.** Making the most of audio-visual aids. (Work of the National Committee for Audio-Visual Aids in Education and the Educational Foundation for Visual Aids.) Health and Social Service Journal, 86, 29 May 1976, 987.

52 **Stroud, J.** Medical Recording Service Foundation. Health and Social Service Journal, 86, 28 Feb 1976, 398.

53 **Stroud, J.** Training with films. (Work of Camera Talks Ltd.) Health and Social Service Journal, 86, 19 Jun 1976, 1133.

54 **Townsend, I.** Are we using our educational resources efficiently? (Audio-visual media.) Nursing Times, 74, 30 Mar 1978, 549-550.

55 **Townsend, I.** The audio-visual revolution: do we really need it? (In nurse education.) Journal of Advanced Nursing, 4 (2), Mar 1979, 181-192.

56 **Townsend, I.** Caring to learn: the evolution and practice of resource-based learning in nurse education. MA thesis, University of York, Department of Education, 1978.

57 **Townsend, I.** Choosing and using tape-slide packages. Nursing Times, 74, 20 Apr 1978, 675-676.

58 **Townsend, I.** Educational media information services. Information resources in the general teaching aids field which can be used by nurse educators. Nursing Mirror, 144, 3 Feb 1977, 64-65.

59 **Townsend, I.** The learning resources movement: its relationship to nurse education. (Based on experience and a research project and outlining how learning resources have not been used to their full potential.) Journal of Advanced Nursing, 5 (5), Sep 1980, 513-529.

60 **Townsend, I.** Machine made transparencies. Nursing Mirror, 143 (9), 26 Aug 1976, 64-65.

61 **Townsend, I.** The resource centre revisited. (Review of literature and findings of research project into attitudes of staff and progress made towards setting up centres.) Nursing Mirror, 151, 25 Sep 1980, 29-32.

62 **Townsend, I.** Talking about innovation—1. Setting up a learning resources centre. Nursing Times, 73, 31 Mar 1977, 460-461.

63 **Townsend, I.** Talking about innovation—2. A selection of books available (for organising a learning resources centre.) Nursing Times, 73, 7 Apr 1977, 495.

64 **Townsend, I.** Talking about innovation—3. A utopian view of the centre and its role in the nurse training school. Nursing Times, 73, 14 Apr 1977, 533-534.

65 **Townsend, I.** Talking about innovation—4. Space and equipment requirements (in a learning resources centre.) Nursing Times, 73, 28 Apr 1977, 617-618.

66 **Townsend, I.** Talking about innovation—5. Who does what? (in the resource centre.) Nursing Times, 73, 5 May 1977, 657-658.

67 **Townsend, I.** Talking about innovation—6. A selected bibliography (of the general literature on resource centres.) Nursing Times, 73, 12 May 1977, 713-715.

68 **Townsend, I.** Talking about innovation—7. Results of surveys by the NHS Learning Resources Unit. (Into tutors' interest in and demand for resource-based learning courses.) Nursing Times, 73, 19 May 1977, 751-753.

69 **Townsend, I.** Talking about innovation—8. A blueprint for the future. (Of resource centres.) Nursing Times, 73, 26 May 1977, 793-794.

70 **Townsend, I.** Tips for teaching transparencies. Nursing Mirror, 143 (8), 19 Aug 1976, 56.

71 **Townsend, I.** Using audio-visual equipment. (How to handle and use equipment properly.) Nursing Times, 72 (23), 10 Jun 1976, 904-905.

72 **Townsend, I.** What's new in overhead projectors. Nursing Mirror, 143 (7), 12 Aug 1976, 59.

73 **U.S.** school develops simulaids for nursing practice. (Manikins for use in teaching nursing skills.) International Nursing Review, 27 (4), Jul/Aug 1980, 123-124.

74 **Vogt, R.B.** Enhancing students' experience through the use of tape recordings. (Tape recording by students of care plans of various patients.) Journal of Nursing Education, 19 (4), Apr 1980, 42-45.

75 **Waddington, L.R.** The use and transmission of audio-visual material in overseas schools of nursing and medicine. Lamp, 37 (3), Mar 1980, 24-35.

76 **Williams, A.R.** Visual aids for nurses. (Visual media and visual presentation of information.) Nursing Mirror, 145, 28 Jul 1977, 13-16.

77 **Wolfe, H. and Erickson, R.** The assessment man. (A schematic drawing of the human body outlining major areas of assessment to help students in observing patients.) Nursing Outlook, 25 (2), Feb 1977, 103-107.

c AUDIOVISUAL: TELEVISION

1 **Connolly, J. and Bird, J.** Video tape in teaching and examining clinical skills: a short case format. Medical Education, 11 (4), Jul 1977, 271-275.

2 **Dalgarno, J.** Producing a programme on videotape and taking care of the equipment. Nursing Times, 76, 18/25 Dec 1980, 2250-2251.

3 **Finley, B. and others** Maximizing video-taped learning of interpersonal skills. Journal of Nursing Education, 18 (1), Jan 1979, 33-41.

4 **Holland, J.A.S.** Videotaping clinical experience. (Learning tool for nursing students.) Nursing Outlook, 25 (5), May 1977, 337-338.

5 **Memmer, M.K.** Television replay: a tool for students to learn to evaluate their own proficiency in using sterile technique. Journal of Nursing Education, 18 (8), Oct 1979, 35-42.

6 **Miles, I.M.** A multimedia approach to education. (An analysis of investigations into the use of television outside South Africa.) S.A. Nursing Journal, 42 (7), Jul 1975, 13-15.

7 **Paduano, M.A.** Bringing about learning in the college laboratory. (Videotaping of children's behaviour to teach child development.) Journal of Nursing Education, 17 (6), Jun 1978, 30-33.

8 **Pfeiffer, I.L. and Dunlap, J.** Microteaching to micropreaching. (Videotaping of teacher students to analyse and improve performance, with reference to theological students.) Visual Education, Jan 1979, 29-31.

9 Shaffer, M.K. and Pfeiffer, I. Television can improve instruction. Journal of Nursing Education, 15 (6), Nov 1976, 3-8.

10 Shaffer, M.K. and Pfeiffer, I.L. Videotape as a method for staff development of nurses. Journal of Continuing Education in Nursing, 9 (6), Nov/Dec 1978, 19-24.

11 Townsend, I. Educational television: legal aspects, choice and versatility of audio-visual equipment for education. Nursing Mirror, 143 (1), 1 Jul 1976, 67-68.

d CLINICAL TEACHING AND WARD LEARNING

1 Anderson, M.H. Clinical instructor training program: trainers manual. Revised ed. University Extension, University of California, Los Angeles: Allied Health Professions Publications, 1978.

2 Buchanan, D. Doing is best. A course on teaching in the wards. (In service training for ward sisters and charge nurses.) Nursing Times, 73, 13 Oct 1977, 1608-1609.

3 Carr, A.J. Clinical nurse teaching: programme for the practising nurse. (Day release at Newcastle AHA for City and Guilds Further Education Teachers Course.) Nursing Times, 73, 27 Jan 1977, Occ. papers, 13-14.

4 Clarke, M. Psychology. 2. Behave yourself! (Psychology of learning with some reference to clinical teaching, patient teaching and operant learning.) Nursing Mirror, 150, 17 Apr 1980, 30-32.

5 Crowther, E. A clinical teacher looks at nurse education. Nursing Mirror, 146, 6 Apr 1978, 29-30.

6 Duff, P. Teaching in the practical situation. 4. The role of the nursing officer. Queen's Nursing Journal, 19 (14), May 1977, 393-394.

7 Fletcher, S.W. and Oseasohn, C.S. Picking up the cues. (Project at McGill University to teach baccalaureate students to perform physical assessments of patients.) Canadian Nurse, 74 (1), Jan 1978, 40-43.

8 Ford, J. and others A pilot course on ward teaching methods. (Planning and evaluation of course for ward managers in Bromley AHA.) Nursing Times, 75, 1 Feb 1979, Occ. papers, 13-16.

9 Fretwell, J.E. An inquiry into the ward learning environment. (With objective of identifying and describing wards with good learning environments and observation of teaching and learning in different wards.) Nursing Times, 76, 26 Jun 1980, Occ. papers, 69-75.

10 Fretwell, J.E. Socialisation of nurses: teaching and learning in hospital wards. PhD thesis, University of Warwick, Department of Sociology, 1978.

11 Greaves, F. Teaching nurses in clinical settings. (Detailed guidance for teachers including example of teaching notes.) Nursing Mirror, 148, 22 Feb 1979, Supplement i, iii-iv, vii, x-xii, xiv-xv; 1 Mar 1979, Supplement i-ii, iv, vi-viii, x-xii.

12 Hinchliff, S.M. editor Teaching clinical nursing. Churchill Livingstone, 1979.

13 Kilpack, V. The head nurse creates a new order for clinical learning. (Structuring a climate for care.) Journal of Nursing Administration, 6 (8), Oct 1976, 41-46.

14 Kirkwood, L. The clinical teacher. (Study of role based on results of questionnaire sent to clinical teachers, ward sisters and tutors.) Nursing Times, 75, 3 May 1979, Occ. papers, 49-51.

15 Malasanos, L. and Tichy, A.M. The bedside clinic—nursing rounds as a teaching strategy. Journal of Nursing Education, 16 (6), Jun 1977, 10-15.

16 Martin, J.L. Learning through experience. (Controlling the clinical environment by developing models to implement the curriculum.) Nursing Times, 72 (14), 8 Apr 1976, 546-548.

17 Orton, H.D. Ward learning climate and student nurse response. MPhil thesis, Sheffield City Polytechnic, Department of Health Studies, 1979.

18 Perry, E. and Nurse, G. Clinical teaching survey (of students who have completed the Rcn Clinical Teachers Course.) The authors, (1976.)

19 Schweer, J.E. and Gebbie, K.M. Creative teaching in clinical nursing. 3rd ed. St. Louis: Mosby, 1976.

20 Smith, D.W. Perspectives on clinical teaching. 2nd ed. New York: Springer, 1977. (Springer series on the teaching of nursing, vol.2.)

21 Unsworth, G. Whither education, or whithered education? (Participation of ward staff in nursing education.) Nursing Mirror, 142, 6 May 1976, 56.

22 Wong, S. and Wong, J. The effectiveness of clinical teaching: a model for self-evaluation. (Three-step model including preparation of objectives and evaluating students' performance.) Journal of Advanced Nursing, 5 (5), Sep 1980, 531-537.

e COMPUTER LEARNING

1 Bitzer, M.D. and Bitzer, D.L. Teaching nursing by computer: an evaluative study. Computers in Biology and Medicine, 3 (3), Oct 1973, 187-204. (Reprint file.)

2 Buchholz, L.M. Computer-assisted instruction for the self-directed professional learner? Journal of Continuing Education in Nursing, 10 (1), Jan/Feb 1979, 12-14.

3 Corcoran, S. Should a service setting be used as a learning laboratory? An ethical question. Nursing Outlook, 25 (12), Dec 1977, 771-776.

4 Huckaby, L.M.D. and others Cognitive, affective, and transfer of learning consequences of computer-assisted instruction. (Comparison of effect of computer-assisted with lecture-discussion method of teaching.) Nursing Research, 28 (4), Jul/Aug 1979, 228-233.

5 Kirchhoff, K.T. and Holzemer, W.L. Student learning and a computer-assisted instructional program. (Research study.) Journal of Nursing Education, 18 (3), Mar 1979, 22-30.

6 Kuramoto, A.M. Computer-assisted instruction: will it be used? (Its uses and limitations.) Nursing Leadership, 1 (1), Jun 1978, 10-13.

7 Marsh, P. Rise of the teaching machine. (Computer-assisted learning.) New Scientist, 82, 3 May 1979, 354-356.

8 Meadows, L.S. Nursing education in crisis: a computer alternative. (Uses of computers in nursing education.) Journal of Nursing Education, 16 (5), May 1977, 13-21.

9 Porter, S.F. Application of computer-assisted instruction to continuing education in nursing: review of the literature. Journal of Continuing Education in Nursing, 9 (6), Nov/Dec 1978, 5-9.

10 Ronald, J.S. Computers and undergraduate nursing education: a report on an experimental introductory course. (Teaching students about the use of computers and technology.) Journal of Nursing Education, 18 (9), Nov 1979, 4-9.

f GROUP METHODS

1 Browne, S.E. Group leadership experiences for students. (Three models—co-leader, observer and initiator—with evaluation by instructor and students.) Nursing Outlook, 28 (3), Mar 1980, 166-169.

2 Choi-Lao, A.T.H. The sleep assignment: a way to learn problem solving. (Group experiment with student nurses.) Canadian Nurse, 72 (8), Aug 1976, 34-35.

3 Clark, C.C. The nurse as group leader. New York: Springer, 1977. (Springer series on the teaching of nursing, vol.3.)

4 Hannon, J. Group process-success in one graduate nursing program. (Method of introducing students to understanding of self and interpersonal skills.) Journal of Nursing Education, 19 (1), Jan 1980, 46-52.

5 Jensen, J.L. The use of group techniques to increase learning of psychiatric concepts. (By nursing students.) Journal of Nursing Education, 16 (4), Apr 1977, 33-37.

6 Little, R.L. (1977) Group methods for learning in nursing education. S.A. Nursing Journal, 44 (12), Dec 1977, 29-30.

7 Ruddock, R. Working with groups. The effect group relationships and expectations have on the learning process. Nursing Mirror, 146, 2 Mar 1978, 38-40.

g SELF-DIRECTED LEARNING

1 Birmingham, J.J. The problem-oriented record: a self-learning module. New York: McGraw-Hill, 1978.

2 Blatchley, M.E. and others Effects of self-study on achievement in a medical-surgical nursing course. Nursing Outlook, 26 (7), Jul 1978, 444-447.

3 Bouchard, J. and Steels, M. Contract learning: the experience of two nursing schools. (Self-directed learning with more responsibility placed on student.) Canadian Nurse, 76 (1), Jan 1980, 44-48.

4 Cowart, M.E. and Burge, J.M. Evaluation

by jury. Students completing this self-paced learning nursing curriculum must meet terminal objectives evaluated by a panel of nurses at the end of the program. (Florida State University.) Nursing Outlook, 27 (5), May 1979, 329-333.

5 **Cudney, S.A.** Mediated self-instruction of basic nursing skills. Nurse Education, 1 (2), Jul/Aug 1976, 14-15.

6 **Donohue, J.D. and others** PSI: an innovative approach to teaching nursing technologies. (Personalised system of instruction — an individualized learning technique used at Georgetown University School of Nursing.) Journal of Nursing Education, 15 (4), Jul 1976, 7-12.

7 **Gentine, M.** Methods of teaching — revisited. Self-learning packages. Journal of Continuing Education in Nursing, 11 (3), May/Jun 1980, 57-59.

8 **Gregg, D.E. and others** Individual supervision: a method of teaching psychiatric concepts in nursing education. Perspectives in Psychiatric Care, 14 (3), Jul-Sep 1976, 115-119.

9 **Hogstel, M.O.** A system for personalized instruction. (Self-paced learning with help from student proctors.) Nursing Outlook, 24 (2), Feb 1976, 110-114.

10 **Huckabay, L.C. and Arndt, G.** Effect of acquisition of knowledge on self evaluation and the relationship of self evaluation to perception of real and ideal self concept. (A study of 69 graduate nursing students to compare the effect of mastering learning — a student centred learning concept — with traditional lectures and discussion groups.) Nursing Research, 25 (4), Jul/Aug 1976, 244-251.

11 **Lewis, L.C.** Independent/individualized learning: the process and the processors. Nursing Forum, 17 (1), 1978, 84-95.

12 **Luther, D.C. and Wolfe, M.J.** Toward a partnership in learning: the heart of this teaching/learning tool is a personal interview in which teacher and learner share information and plan ways to meet mutual goals. Nursing Outlook, 28 (12), Dec 1980, 745-750.

13 **Paduano, M.A.** Introducing independent study into the nursing curriculum. Journal of Nursing Education, 18 (4), Apr 1979, 34-37.

14 **Pensivy, B.A.** Traditional versus individualized nursing instruction: comparison of state board examination scores as a result of these two methods of nursing instruction. Journal of Nursing Education, 16 (2), Feb 1977, 14-18.

15 **Scott, L.P.** Self-instruction and review in nursing. Vol.1. Body structure and function, nutrition and food management, basic pharmacology and drug therapy. 2nd ed. New York: Macmillan, 1979.

16 **Sheahan, J.** An evaluation of a workshop for teachers of nursing on an individualized teaching and learning strategy. (Keller Plan.) Journal of Advanced Nursing, 4 (6), Nov 1979, 647-658.

17 **Skarratt, R.** Student-centred learning in nurse education. A preliminary report on an innovation of an educational method in one school of nursing. Nursing Times, 76, 29 May 1980, 953.

18 **Sommerfield, D.P. and Hughes, J.R.** How independent should independent learning be? (Clinical placements in final year of study backed up by group seminars, videotapes and log keeping.) Nursing Outlook, 28 (7), Jul 1980, 416-420.

19 **Swanson, E.A. and Dalsing, C.W.** Independent study: a curriculum expander. Journal of Nursing Education, 19 (9), Nov 1980, 11-15.

20 **Yunek, M.** Self-assessment of learning needs: a tool to assist nurses in self-directed learning. Journal of Continuing Education in Nursing, 11 (5), Sep/Oct 1980, 30-33.

h OTHER METHODS

1 **Anderson, N.E.** The use of the seminar as a teaching technique with senior undergraduate nursing students. Journal of Nursing Education, 19 (2), Feb 1980, 20-25.

2 **Baker, J. and others** An alternative to process recording. (Observation of student-client interviews for teaching psychosocial nursing skills.) Nursing Outlook, 24 (2), Feb 1976, 115-118.

3 **Barrett, J.E.** Values clarification as a teaching strategy in nursing. Journal of Nursing Education, 17 (2), Feb 1978, 12-18.

4 **Becker, C.** An overview of simulation games and comments on their use in baccalaureate nursing education. Nursing Papers, 12 (2), Summer 1980, 32-44.

5 **Bradshaw, C.E.** Concentrated experimental learning laboratories. (Method of exploring students' feelings about topics such as sexuality.) Journal of Nursing Education, 17 (2), Feb 1978, 32-35.

6 **Clark, C.C.** Simulation gaming: a new teaching strategy in nursing education. Nurse Educator, 1 (4), Nov/Dec 1976, 4-9.

7 **Cooper, S.S.** Methods of teaching — revisited. Journal of Continuing Education in Nursing. Part 1, 9 (4), Jul/Aug 1978, 24-26.
Brainstorming. 9 (6), Nov/Dec 1978, 16-18.
Dramatic representation: skits. 10 (6), Nov/Dec 1979; 34-35.
Field trips and study tours. 11 (2), Mar/Apr 1980, 50, 60-61.
Formal discussion: the debate. 10 (4), Jul/Aug 1979, 58, 71.
Formal discussion: the seminar. 10 (3), May/Jun 1979, 39-40.
Games and simulation. 10 (5), Sep/Oct 1979, 14, 47-48.
Informal discussion. 9 (5), Sep/Oct 1978, 14-16.
Nursing care conference. 10 (1), Jan/Feb 1979, 28-30.
Panel discussion; symposium; colloquy. 10 (2), Mar/Apr 1979, 36-38.
Role playing. 11 (1), Jan/Feb 1980, 36, 57-58.

8 **Crancer, J. and Maury-Hess, S.** Games: an alternative to pedagogical instruction. Journal of Nursing Education, 19 (3), Mar 1980, 45-52.

9 **Davidson, M.E. and McArdle, P.E.** PAIR: peer analysis of interpersonal responsiveness and plan for encouraging effective reshaping. Journal of Nursing Education, 19 (2), Feb 1980, 8-12.

10 **Eaton, S. and others** Discussion stoppers in teaching. If the student participation needed to make a class come alive isn't forthcoming, could one of the teacher behaviors in this list be responsible? Nursing Outlook, 25 (9), Sep 1977, 578-583.

11 **French, P.** A place for simulation in nurse education. (Includes role-play and academic gaming.) Nursing Focus, 1 (11), Jul 1980, 445-446.

12 **Garner, A.E. and Thillen, C.** Is your school of nursing ready to implement interdisciplinary team teaching? Journal of Nursing Education, 16 (7), Sep 1977, 27-30.

13 **Gendron, D.** An experience developing and using written simulations as a method of teaching. (Clinical nursing situations.) Nursing Papers, 9 (1), Spring 1977, 20-26.

14 **Gendron, D.** Show me. (Use of role play with learners to show effective patient teaching.) Canadian Nurse, 74 (11), Dec 1978, 10-13.

15 **Grexton, E.M.** Telephone communication network seminars in nursing education. (State University of New York at Buffalo.) Journal of Nursing Education, 15 (3), May 1976, 28-32.

16 **Gustafson, M.B.** Methods of teaching — revisited: try Haiku. (Japanese poetry-form to provide creative form of verbal expression and to increase sensitivity to topics.) Journal of Continuing Education in Nursing, 10 (4), Jul/Aug 1979, 59-60.

17 **Hayter, J.** How good is the lecture as a teaching method? Nursing Outlook, 27 (4), Apr 1979, 274-277.

18 **Hogstel, M.O. and Ackley, N.L.** Making team teaching work. Nursing Outlook, 27 (1), Jan 1979, 48-51.

19 **Jeffers, J.M. and Christensen, M.G.** Using simulation to facilitate the acquisition of clinical observational skills. (Research study on the effect of simulated nursing rounds.) Journal of Nursing Education, 18 (6), Jun 1979, 29-32.

20 **Lincoln, R. and others** Using simulated patients to teach assessment. Nursing Outlook, 26 (5), May 1978, 316-320.

21 **Martin, P. and Tremlett, R.** Physiology at play: the nephron. (Board game for learners.) Nursing Mirror, 147, 21 Dec 1978, 26-29.

22 **Page, G.G. and Saunders, P.** The role of simulation in the health professions. (Method of teaching and evaluating clinical problem-solving skills.) Journal of Nursing Education, 17 (4), Apr 1978, 29-32.

23 **Pullen, B. and Plant, S.M.** Spot on! — that's the name of the game. (Board game on nursing problems for use with learners.) Nursing Mirror, 147, 7 Dec 1978, 26-29.

24 **Reakes, J.C.** Behavior rehearsal revisited: a multi-faceted tool for the instructor. (Use of role play in group learning experiences for nursing students.) Journal of Nursing Education, 18 (2), Feb 1979, 48-51.

25 **Schroy, I.J.** TA: a useful tool in the teaching-learning process. (Transactional analysis.) Journal of Nursing Education, 18 (1), Jan 1979, 28-32.

26 **Spruck, M.** An approach to analysis of a symptom: an educational experience. (Training students in interviewing through role play and problem identification.) Journal of Nursing Education, 19 (7), Sep 1980, 45-48.

27 Stevens, B.J. The successful workshop: how to bring it off! (Educational experience of one to five days length.) Nurse Educator, 11 (1), Jan/Feb 1977, 16-20.

28 Sullivan, K. and others From learning modules to clinical practice. (Role-playing exercise involving students as patients in simulated hospital day.) Nursing Outlook, 25 (5), May 1977, 319-321.

29 Tarpey, K.S. and Chen, Shu-Pi Team teaching: is it for you? Journal of Nursing Education, 17 (2), Feb 1978, 36-39.

30 Taylor, A.P. Clinical simulations in nursing. (Project to develop units for use by nurse learners to improve efficiency and accuracy of decision-making skills.) Nursing Times, 76, 10 Jul 1980, 1217-1218.

31 Welch, L.B. Team teaching: is it effective? Nursing Forum, 18 (4), 1979, 394-404.

32 Williams, L.V. Patient role-playing by learners. (Exercise at Bury St. Edmunds District School of Nursing to help learners understand what it is like to be blind, wheelchair-bound or partially paralysed.) Nursing Times, 74, 24 Aug 1978, 1402-1406.

33 Wise, P.S.Y. Methods of teaching—revisited. Character play and role play. Journal of Continuing Education in Nursing, 11 (1), Jan/Feb 1980, 37-38.

34 Wolf, M.S. and Duffy, M.E. Simulation/ games: a teaching strategy for nursing education. New York: National League for Nursing, 1979.

35 Yeaw, E.M.J. Problem solving as a method of teaching strategies in classroom and clinical teaching. Journal of Nursing Education, 18 (7), Sep 1979, 16-22.

22 SELECTION AND ASSESSMENT

a SELECTION AND PSYCHO-LOGICAL TESTS

1 Ainslie, B.S. and others Predictive value of selected admission criteria for graduate nursing education. (Survey of 193 graduates of a masters degree program.) Nursing Research, 25 (4), Jul/Aug 1976, 296-299.

2 Beale, A.V. and McCutcheon, A.F. On becoming a nurse. (Research study in Virginia of factors considered important in selecting nursing students.) Journal of Nursing Education, 19 (4), Apr 1980, 28-32.

3 Belbin, R.M. and Toye, J. Trainability tests and the recruitment of student nurses. (Description and evaluation of test with student nurses at five London hospitals.) Journal of Advanced Nursing, 3 (3), May 1978, 277-285.

4 Bersch, M.C. Group discussion: a tool for student selection. (Used by the Bon Secours School of Nursing, Geneva.) International Nursing Review, 26 (2), Mar/Apr 1979, 52.

5 Chang, A.M. An investigative look at the entrance standard for the basic nursing course. (Research study to discover if educational qualifications achieved at school are associated with success with the theoretical aspects of the nursing

course.) Australian Nurses Journal, 8 (1), Jul 1978, 36-38.

6 Clemence, B.A. and Brink, P.J. How predictive are admissions criteria? (Research study in bachelors course in UCLA School of Nursing, Los Angeles.) Journal of Nursing Education, 17 (4), Apr 1978, 5-10.

7 Fong, M.L. and Leton, J.B. The group interview: a tool for nursing student selection. Journal of Nursing Education, 17 (7), Sep 1978, 35-40.

8 Lewis, B.R. and Cooper, C.L. Personality measurement among nurses: a review. (Use as predictors of success and wastage in training.) International Journal of Nursing Studies, 13 (4), 1976, 209-229.

9 Marsh, M. Summary report of the school educational attainment, General Nursing Council test scores and performance in university examinations of Manchester University's undergraduate nursing students. Journal of Advanced Nursing, 2 (2), Mar 1977, 209-212.

10 National League for Nursing Trends, issues and implications in student selection. New York: NLN, 1978.

11 Quine, S. A preliminary study to investigate the relationship between educational entry level and later nursing ability. (In New South Wales.) Australian Nurses Journal, 6 (10), Apr 1977, 47-50.

12 Reeve, P.E. The selection interview in the assessment of suitability for nurse training. (An outline of work done on identifying a 'personality mix or constellation' and ways of exploring and assessing it.) Journal of Advanced Nursing, 3 (2), Mar 1978, 167-179.

13 Rotenberg, A. Psychological tests in selection of students to schools of nursing in Israel. (Report of three research studies.) Curationis, 1 (2), Sep 1978, 47-49.

14 SCOTTISH National Nursing and Midwifery Consultative Committee. Working Group A new concept of nursing. 3. (Importance of selection with regard to Briggs recommendations.) Nursing Times, 72 (16), 22 Apr 1976, Occ. papers, 57-60.

15 Thomas, B. Differential utility of predictors in graduate nursing education. (Problems of predicting success of students at the University of Iowa.) Nursing Research, 26 (2), Mar-Apr 1977, 100-102.

16 Ventura, M.R. Use of Torrance Test of Creative Thinking to measure differences between student nurses. (In different nursing education programmes in USA.) Australasian Nurses Journal, 9 (2), Dec 1979, 26-28.

b ASSESSMENT

1 Adderley, B.V. and Brock, A.M. Evaluating clinical performance in nursing. (Of nursing students.) Journal of Advanced Nursing, 2 (4), Jul 1977, 355-363.

2 Angus, M.D. Analysis of student performance ratings. (Five scales of knowledge and judgment, conscientiousness, skill in human relations, organisational ability and observational ability.) Nursing Papers, 12 (1), Spring 1980, 5-16.

3 Argue, Z. and Fencott, L. Development of a learning tool at WASON. (Method of evaluation of students in the clinical area at the Western Australian School of Nursing.) Australian Nurses Journal, 9 (7), Feb 1980, 35-37.

4 Castledine, G. Assessing ward assessments. Nursing Mirror, 148, 5 Apr 1979, 10.

5 Exton-Smith, J. Management of ward based assessments. (Method developed at Bedford General Hospital for student assessment.) Nursing Times, 72 (9), 4 Mar 1976, 349-350.

6 Frederickson, K. and Mayer, G.G. Problem solving skills: what effect does education have. (Research study with nursing students.) American Journal of Nursing, 77 (7), Jul 1977, 1167-1169.

7 Frisbie, D.A. Evaluating student achievement: principles, trends and problems. New York: National League for Nursing, 1979.

8 Gillies, D.A. and Alyn, I.B. Saunders tests for self-evaluation of nursing competence. Philadelphia: Saunders. 3rd ed. 1980.

9 Gould, E. O'G. Satisfactory/unsatisfactory grading in the evaluation of clinical performance in nursing: its effect on student motivation as perceived by nursing students. Journal of Nursing Education, 17 (8), Oct 1978, 36-47.

10 Grant, J.M. Evaluation of student nurses —is it worth the effort? (Research to investigate the relationship between academic achievement and clinical competence.) New Zealand Nursing Journal, 69 (8), Aug 1976, 8-11.

11 Gustafson, D.D. Student peer evaluation: a successful adaptation for observed home visits. Journal of Nursing Education, 19 (2), Feb 1980, 4-7.

12 Harrington, D.C. Continual assessment of student nurses. (Methods.) Curationis, 2 (4), Mar 1980, 27-32.

13 Huckabay, L.M. Cognitive and affective consequences of formative evaluation in graduate nursing students. (Formative evaluation refers to the assessment of the learner's continuous progress in learning and the effectiveness of instruction.) Nursing Research, 27 (3), May/Jun 1978, 190-194.

14 Huckabay, L.M.D. Cognitive-affective consequences of grading versus nongrading of formative evaluations. Nursing Research, 28 (3), May/Jun 1979, 173-178.

15 Jefferies, P.M. and Tibbles, H.J. Continuous assessment within the King's Health District. (Of practical skills in general and specialised areas of care.) Nursing Times, 76, 21 Aug 1980, Occ. papers, 89-92.

16 Kehoe, D.M. and Hartker, T. Principles of assessing nursing skills. Tunbridge Wells: Pitman Medical, 1979.

17 King, E.C. Classroom evaluation strategies. St. Louis: Mosby, 1979.

18 Kirby, S. Assessing general nursing students at the bedside. (Project to investigate feasibility of implementing the clinical skills assessment tests.) Lamp, 35 (6), Jun 1978, 42-45.

19 Krumme, U.S. The case for criterion referenced measurement. (To evaluate clinical nursing performance with particular reference to students.) Nursing Outlook, 23 (12), Dec 1975, 764-770.

20 **Layton, J.M.** The use of modelling to teach empathy to nursing students. (Evaluation of learning using Empathy Test, Barrett-Leonard Relationship Inventory and Carkhuff Empathy Scale.) Research in Nursing and Health, 2 (4), Dec 1979, 163-176.

21 **Lenburg, C.B.** The clinical performance examination: development and implementation. New York: Appleton-Century-Crofts, 1979.

22 **Litwack, L.** A system for evaluation. Nursing Outlook, 24 (1), Jan 1976, 45-48.

23 **Long, P.** Judging and reporting on student nurse clinical performance: some problems for the ward sister. (A GNC survey of practical assessment forms with specific reference to a form produced by the United Liverpool Hospitals.) International Journal of Nursing Studies, 13 (2), 1976, 115-121.

24 **Long, P.** Student nurse assessment. (General Nursing Council research projects evaluating the ward progress report and 'critical incident technique.') Nursing Times, 72 (14), 8 Apr 1976, 552-555.

25 **Loustau, A. and others** Evaluating students' clinical performance: using videotape to establish rater reliability. Journal of Nursing Education, 19 (7), Sep 1980, 10-17.

26 **Lynch, E.A.** Evaluation: principles and processes. New York: National League for Nursing, 1978.

27 **McCaffrey, C.** Performance check lists: an effective method of teaching, learning and evaluating. Nurse Educator, 3 (1), Jan/Feb 1978, 11-13.

28 **McLane, A.M.** Core competencies of masters-prepared nurses. (Survey using a Process Competency Scale.) Nursing Research, 27 (1), Jan/Feb 1978, 48-53.

29 **Miller, C.L.** Factors in graduate nursing student performance. (Development of method based on criterion rating scale and using critical incidents to assess students for admission to post-baccalaureate doctoral programmes.) International Journal of Nursing Studies, 17 (1), 1980, 39-45.

30 **Miller, C.L. and Applegate, M.** Guided study student achievement. (Study to measure change in student achievement by comparing students in an Associate Degree 'Guided Study' program with other Associate Degree students in the same group.) International Journal of Nursing Studies, 13 (4), 1976, 231-241.

31 **Miller, G.E.** Continuous assessment. Medical Education, 10 (2), Mar 1976, 81-86.

32 **Morgan, B. and others** Evaluating clinical proficiency. (Design and administration of three assessments in a baccalaureate programme.) Nursing Outlook, 27 (8), Aug 1979, 540-544.

33 **Morle, K.M.F.** Examination of the evaluation procedures used in student nurse training with particular regard to prediction of success. MSc thesis, University of Manchester, Department of Nursing, 1978.

34 **Morton, J. and others** A clinical evaluation tool for student nurses. (Description of its development.) Canadian Nurse, 72 (6), Jun 1976, 37-41.

35 **National League for Nursing** Evaluation of students in baccalaureate nursing programmes. New York: NLN, 1977.

36 **National League for Nursing** Measurement and evaluation in nursing education: papers presented at a conference at the St. Luke's College of Nursing, Tokyo, 12-14 Jan 1979. New York: NLN, 1980.

37 **Nelson, L.F.** Competence of nursing graduates in technical, communicative and administrative skills. (Baccalaureate, diploma and associate degree nursing program graduates.) Nursing Research, 27 (2), Mar/Apr 1978, 121-125.

38 **Nichols, E.G. and Heyman, A.H.** Staff participation in student evaluation. Supervisor Nurse, 7 (10), Oct 1976, 74, 76, 78-79.

39 NURSING: pretest self-assessment and review. New York: McGraw-Hill, 1980. (Multiple choice questions.)

40 **Reese, J.L. and others** Evaluating physical assessment skills. Nursing Outlook, 27 (10), Oct 1979, 662-665.

41 **Rezler, A.G. and Stevens, B.J. editors** The nurse evaluator in education and service. New York: McGraw-Hill, 1978.

42 **Roberts, K.L.** Formal evaluation and the student nurse. (General discussion of the value of assessment.) Australian Nurses Journal, 8 (1), Jul 1978, 45-47.

43 **Rogers, S.** Testing the RN student's skills. (Evaluation techniques developed at Salem State College, Massachusetts.) Nursing Outlook, 24 (7), Jul 1976, 446-449.

44 **Sampson, C.** Ward based practical assessments — the student's view. Nursing Mirror, 143, 25 Nov 1976, 40.

45 **Schneider, H.L.** Evaluation of nursing competence. Boston: Little, Brown, 1979.

46 **Scott, B.M.** Clinical assessment and identifying learning difficulties. (Development of competency-based checklist. Has bibliography of 33 items.) Australian Nurses Journal, 9 (4), Oct 1979, 32-33.

47 **Sheahan, J.** Assessing project work. Nursing Mirror, 145, 1 Dec 1977, 24-27.

48 **Sheahan, J.** Education — 8. Assessment by supply tests and by recognition tests. Nursing Times, 72 (41), 14 Oct 1976, 1612-1614.

49 **Sheahan, J.** Education — 9. Continuous assessment, guiding and supporting. Nursing Times, 72 (42), 21 Oct 1976, 1650-1652.

50 **Sheahan, J.** Measurement in nursing education. (Outline of evaluation programmes.) Journal of Advanced Nursing, 4 (1), Jan 1979, 47-56.

51 **Sims, A.** The critical incident technique in evaluating student nurse performance. (A GNC pilot study examining the use of the technique in eight general hospitals.) International Journal of Nursing Studies, 13 (2), 1976, 123-130.

52 **Steele, S.** Educational evaluation in nursing. Thorofare: Slack, 1978.

53 **Sweeney, M.A.** Evaluating the nonverbal communication skills of nursing students.

Journal of Nursing Education, 16 (3), Mar 1977, 5-11.

54 **Turner, L.** Discussion of a project on peer evaluation in the faculty of nursing, University of Toronto, Canada. Journal of Advanced Nursing, 3 (5), Sep 1978, 457-473.

55 **Ventura, M.R.** Use of Torrance Test of Creative Thinking to measure differences between student nurses. (In different nursing education programmes in USA.) Australasian Nurses Journal, 9 (2), Dec 1979, 26-28.

56 **Wolff, L.V. and others** Student self-evaluation manual in fundamentals of nursing. Philadelphia: Lippincott, 1979.

57 **Woolley, A.S.** The long and tortured history of clinical evaluation. (Of nursing students. Review.) Nursing Outlook, 25 (5), May 1977, 308-315.

58 **Wyman, J. and Fernau, K.** Developing a criterion-referenced tool. (To assess self-paced learning.) Nursing Outlook, 25 (9), Sep 1977, 584-586.

59 **Young, A.P.** Progress and problems of continuous assessment. (Evaluation of scheme at the Thomas Guy School of Nursing.) Nursing Times, 76, 20 Mar 1980, Occ. papers, 33-35.

60 **Young, A.P. and Morgan, W.** Continuous assessment for nurses in the Thomas Guy School of Nursing. 2 parts. Nursing Times, 74, 21/28 Dec 1978, Occ. papers, 141-144; 75, 4 Jan 1979, Occ. papers, 1-3.

c EXAMINATIONS

1 **American Journal of Nursing** A new licensing exam for nurses. (Questions and answers on new examination to be introduced in July 1982.) American Journal of Nursing, 80 (4), Apr 1980, 723-725.

2 **Babajide, O.** The need to overhaul the current system of the final practical examination of the Nursing Council of Nigeria. Nigerian Nurse, 8 (2), Apr/Jun 1976, 40-43.

3 **Barr, D.W.** A realistic assessment of examination scores. (Ways of obtaining standardised scores to reflect student's performance more sensitively than raw scores do.) Australian Nurses Journal, 8 (7), Feb 1979, 34-35.

4 **Behm, R.J. and Warnock, F.N.** State board examinations and degree program effectiveness. Nursing Research, 27 (1), Jan/Feb 1978, 54-56.

5 **Bell, J.A. and Martindill, C.F.** A cross validation study for predictors of scores on State Board Examinations. Nursing Research, 25 (1), Jan-Feb 1976, 54-57.

6 **Bendall, E.** Assessing nursing knowledge. (Evaluation of objective tests in the new GNC examination.) Nursing Mirror, 143 (21), 18 Nov 1976, 40-41.

7 **Bevan, J.** State final questions and answers for nurses. 6th ed. Faber, 1976.

8 **Boreham, N.C.** The use of case histories to assess nurses' ability to solve clinical problems. (A method of making written examinations more relevant to the clinical situation.) Journal of Advanced Nursing, 2 (1), Jan 1977, 57-66.

9 Castle, W.M. Multiple choice examinations: lessons learnt. Medical Education, 10 (2), Mar 1976, 97-104.

10 Chandler, J.M. and Hunter, M.L. Teaching by testing. (Experiment allowing students to see test questions before the examination at Evanston Hospital School of Nursing.) Nursing Outlook, 24 (6), Jun 1976, 386-388.

11 Cheung, P. Put test questions on a computer! (Computerised objective test bank set up at Southampton School of Nursing.) Nursing Mirror, 149, 1 Nov 1979, 26-28.

12 Cobb, B.A. and Williams, D.D. Medical-surgical nursing: 1,503 multiple choice questions with referenced explanatory answers. Garden City: Medical Examination Publishing Co., 1978. (Nursing study and series.)

13 Copcutt, L. Multiple choice: our system from (A) to (Z). (Queen Elizabeth School of Nursing in Birmingham.) Nursing Focus, 1 (9), Jun 1980, 396-398.

14 Cundey, B.E. Effective preparation for examinations. Nursing Mirror, 142 (20), 13 May 1976, 66-68.

15 Dalgarno, J. Question and answer board. (Method of testing knowledge with light showing when correct button is pressed.) Nursing Times, 75, 27 Sep 1979, 1684-1686.

16 Dean, N.R. Effect of free time the day prior to mastery testing on nursing students' scores. (Comparison of scores of students who spent a day before test in clinical laboratory with those who had free time for study.) Nursing Research, 28 (1), Jan/Feb 1979, 40-42.

17 Deardorff, M. and others Selected National League for Nursing achievement test scores as predictors of State Board examination scores. Nursing Research, 25 (1), Jan-Feb 1976, 35-38.

18 Dennison, E.M. Examination techniques: how to answer multiple choice questions. Nursing Times, 75, 5 Apr 1979, 596-597.

19 Dietrich, G. The Diploma approach to psychology. (Advice on answering examination questions in the psychology paper in Part A of the Diploma of Nursing.) Nursing Mirror, 146, 18 May 1978, 32-35.

20 Di Marco, N. and others Predictors of practical nursing state board examination scores. (Research study.) International Journal of Nursing Studies, 16 (1), 1979, 59-63.

21 Ercolano, N.H. Review of medical nursing. New York: McGraw-Hill, 1979.

22 Forrest, I.S. A guide to examination techniques. (Advice on answering examination questions.) Nursing Times, 74, 5 Oct 1978, 1654-1655.

23 GENERAL Nursing Council GNC changes state finals. (Introduction of objective tests and multiple choice.) Nursing Mirror, 142 (17), 22 Apr 1976, 34; Nursing Times, 72, 22 Apr 1976, 600; 26 Aug 1976, 1295.

24 GENERAL Nursing Council GNC answers complaints on multiple-choice tests. (Objections from Patients Association and others.) Nursing Times, 72 (36), 9 Sep 1976, 1374.

25 GENERAL Nursing Council for England and Wales Progress towards changes in the written examination for the general part of the register. GNC, 1979. (Circular 79/34.)

26 Hadler, C.A.S. and Hewett, J.P. The renal, genito-urinary, reproductive and alimentary systems. Heinemann Medical, 1980. (MCQ tutor for nurses; 2.)

27 Hull, E.J. and Isaacs, B.J. Quizzes and questions for nurses. Baillière Tindall, 1976: Book A: medical nursing and paediatric nursing. Book B: surgical nursing and geriatric nursing.

28 Hume, N. Objective testing for S.R.N.: a textbook study guide. Rickmansworth: Penn Central Books, 1977.

29 Isaacs, B. It's not the examiners' fault if you fail.... (Reasons for failure in state registration examinations.) Nursing Mirror, 149, 15 Nov 1979, 12.

30 Jefferson, E. and Birchenall, P. A course for potential examiners. (Course organised by Durham AHA to encourage training of practical examiners and assessors in both general and psychiatric nursing.) Nursing Times, 75, 1 Nov 1979, 1904-1905.

31 Jeyam, W. and Gengasamy, K. Prescription for success. (Advice on answering examination questions.) Nursing Mirror, 146, 2 Mar 1978, 21-24.

32 Kapoor, S.D. Focusing the spotlight on nursing. (Review of the organisation of practical examinations at Hawkes Bay School of Nursing.) New Zealand Nursing Journal, 69 (12), Dec 1976, 16-17.

33 Kirby, S. On your mark... A guide to the interpretation to test statistics. (Objective tests with multiple choice questions.) Lamp, 34 (4), Apr 1977, 5, 7, 9.

34 Knox, J.D.E. How to use modified essay questions. (Series of events in the evolution of a case study.) Medical Teacher, 2 (1), Jan/Feb 1980, 20.

35 McCloskey, D.I. and Holland, R.A.B. A comparison of student performances in answering essay-type and multiple-choice questions. Medical Education, 10 (5), Sep 1976, 382-385.

36 MULTIPLE choice questions, book 3: psychology for nurses by A. Altschul, pharmacology for nurses, by R.E. Bailey. Baillière Tindall, 1980. (Nurses' aids series.)

37 Murphy, S.A. Improving teacher-made tests in an integrated curriculum. Journal of Nursing Education, 18 (9), Nov 1979, 41-45.

38 Pearce, C. The art of passing the state final examination: some points to remember when sitting the written examination. Nursing Times, 76, 24 Jan 1980, 167-168.

39 Ross, G.R. and Ross, M.C. Using the computer to prepare multiple choice examinations: a simplified system. Journal of Nursing Education, 16 (5), May 1977, 32-39.

40 Rowe, W. and others A fresh slant on the dropout. (A study to identify the relationship between reading skills and successful examination performance of 99 students in Sydney hospitals.) Australian Nurses Journal, 5 (3), Sep 1975, 31-32.

41 Ryden, M.B. The predictive value of a clinical examination of interpersonal relationship skills. (Research study.) Journal of Nursing Education, 16 (5), May 1977, 27-31.

42 Walshe-Brennan, K.S. Examination psychology. Nursing Mirror, 142 (3), 15 Jan 1976, 53-54.

43 Ward, J.A. and Griffin, J.M. Improving instructions through computer-graded examinations. Nursing Outlook, 25 (8), Aug 1977, 524-529.

44 Westwick, C.R. Item analysis (of achievement tests to determine the success of a particular item.) Journal of Nursing Education, 15 (1), Jan 1976, 27-32.

45 Wolfle, L.M. and Bryant, L.W. A casual model of nursing education and state board examination scores. Nursing Research, 27 (5), Sep/Oct 1978, 311-315.

46 Wood, V. and Wladyka, J. Grading student nurses. (Review of research.) Canadian Nurse, 76 (6), Jun 1980, 30-32.

23 PRACTICAL EXPERIENCE

a GENERAL AND ALLOCATION

1 Alexander, M.F. Nurse education: an experiment in integration of theory and practice in nursing. PhD thesis, University of Edinburgh, 1980.

2 Brennan, A. Theory and practice correlation. (Planning of a student centred programme of clinical experience.) New Zealand Nursing Journal, 69 (1), Jan 1976, 15-18.

3 Butler, E. and Howarth, M. A computer system for student nurse allocation during training. (At St. Thomas' Hospital, London.) Nursing Times, 76, 10 Jul 1980, 1208-1212.

4 Castledine, G. Bridging the classroom gap. (Description of scheme at Manchester Royal Infirmary involving author and colleague as 'clinical lecturers' combining teaching and ward sister/charge nurse role.) Nursing Mirror, 147, 19 Oct 1978, 12.

5 Chen, S-P.C. and others Documented clinical experiences of primary care RN students: a preliminary report. (Analysis of records of nurse-patient encounters suggested need for classification scheme for health problems.) Nursing Research, 26 (5), Sep/Oct 1977, 342-348.

6 Cosper, B. Coping with an increased student faculty ratio. A teacher shares four techniques she has found helpful in guiding a large group of students through their clinical experience. American Journal of Nursing, 76 (10), Oct 1976, 1642-1644.

7 Duff, P. Teaching in the practical situation — 4. The role of the nursing officer. Queen's Nursing Journal, 19 (14), May 1977, 393-394.

8 Duncan, M.J. Report on study tour of the U.S.A., Canada, the U.K. and South Africa. Part 1. (Planning, implementation, supervision and evaluation of clinical practice components of basic nursing courses.) Lamp, 36 (1), Feb 1979, 10-18.

9 Dunlop, D. and others Crisis intervention in basic nursing education. (Course for student nurses while obtaining experience in accident and emergency department.) Journal of Nursing Education, 17 (4), Apr 1978, 37-41.

10 Fuhr, M.T. Clinical experience record and nursing care planning: a guide for student nurses. 2nd ed. St. Louis: Mosby, 1978.

11 Gott, M. Student nurses: introductory course preparation and work world expectations. Report of a pilot study. (Research study to investigate relationship between practical instruction in school and practical activity on the wards and adequacy for ward work.) International Journal of Nursing Studies, 16 (4), 1979, 307-317.

12 Hall, M.B. How do students learn on a primary nursing care unit? (Patient assignment.) Nursing Outlook, 25 (6), Jun 1977, 370-373.

13 Hogan, R. Making clinical assignments. Nursing Outlook, 24 (8), Aug 1976, 496-498.

14 Holm, K. and others A teaching-learning experience: nursing rounds. Journal of Nursing Education, 17 (4), Apr 1978, 33-36.

15 Kelly, E.M. Bolton's introductory course. (Scheme where learners spend most of eight-week course on the wards.) Nursing Times, 76, 31 Jan 1980, 213-214.

16 Kreagel, J.M. A model for areawide co-ordination of pediatric clinical experiences. (A centralized system in Milwaukee which matches patients' care needs with students' learning needs.) Nursing Outlook, 24 (11), Nov 1976, 697-703.

17 Lee, L.A. An investigation of the effects of clinical experience on cognitive gains. Journal of Nursing Education, 18 (7), Sep 1979, 27-37.

18 Mackay, E. A student nurse in out-patients. (Author's experience of student placement and assessment of its value.) Nursing Times, 74, 10 Aug 1978, 1346-1347.

19 Moores, B. and Wood, I. Nursing allocation using a time-shared computer. Nursing Times, 73, 18 Aug 1977, Occ. papers, 109-112.

20 Porter, K.K. and Feller, C.M. The relationship between patterns of massed and distributive clinical practicum and student achievement. (Concentration of clinical hospital experience followed by community health experience or fewer hours per week of both types of experience over longer period.) Journal of Nursing Education, 18 (8), Oct 1979, 27-34.

21 Roe, A.K. and Sherwood, M.C. Learning experience guide for nursing students. Vol.1. 3rd ed. New York: Wiley, 1978.

22 Roper, N. Clinical experience in nurse education: a survey of the available nursing experience for general student nurses in a school of nursing in Scotland. Edinburgh: Churchill Livingstone, 1976. (University of Edinburgh Department of Nursing Studies monograph no.5.)

23 Saxon, J. Multiple assignments—try them! (Assigning 3 students to each patient with practitioner, researcher and observer roles.) American Journal of Nursing, 75 (12), Dec 1975, 2183-2184.

24 Skeath, B. Back to the grass roots. (Nurse tutor who worked on a ward for a week to rediscover problems of learning.) Nursing Mirror, 151, 14 Aug 1980, 36-37.

25 Skeath, W.A. and others Criteria to be used in the selection of clinical areas for basic nurse training. Journal of Advanced Nursing, 4 (2), Mar 1979, 169-180.

26 Stewart, W. compiler Nurse allocation handbook. King's Fund Centre, 1979.

27 Stewart, W. A systems approach to nurse allocation. (In Southampton.) Nursing Mirror, 148, 10 May 1979, Supplement i-xii.

28 Stewart, W. The way forward in nurse allocation: a reappraisal of the role of the allocation officer. Nursing Times, 75, 27 Sep 1979, 1676-1678.

29 Strohmann, R. Improving student clinical experiences. Nursing Outlook, 25 (7), Jul 1977, 460-462.

30 Van Den Berg, E.L. The multiple assignment: an effective alternative for laboratory experiences. (Study to test the efficacy of assigning a group of students to one patient.) Journal of Nursing Education, 15 (3), May 1976, 3-12.

31 Waltz, C.F. Faculty influence on nursing students' preferences for practice. (Indirect/direct involvement in patient care.) Nursing Research, 27 (2), Mar/Apr 1978, 89-97.

b COMMUNITY

1 Beer, D. and others A caring approach. (The approach to the community care option in Calderdale AHA.) Nursing Times, 75, 9 Aug 1979, Community Outlook 232.

2 Cousins, M. Chasing rainbows. Experiences when on community care secondment in second year of nurse training: searching for the ideal and finding the facts of human predicament. Nursing Mirror, 142 (14), 1 Apr 1976, 77.

3 Frapwell, C. EEC directives relative to community experience for student nurses. Health Visitor, 52 (1), Jan 1979, 7, 9.

4 Gustafson, M.R. Let's broaden our horizons about the use of contracts. (Proposals for extending the use of contracts developed in American schools of nursing as a method of linking students with families and patients.) International Nursing Review, 24 (1), Jan/Feb 1977, 18-19, 24.

5 Harrison, J. Community nursing services. (Observations while undertaking a GNC research project to evaluate community care experience.) Nursing Times, 73, 24 Mar 1977, 415-417.

6 Harrison, J. and Murray, L. Community care courses for student nurses: some differences between 'modular' and polytechnic based courses. General Nursing Council Research Unit, 1977.

7 Jemmott, A. What's happening in Kent? (Organisation of community care programmes for student nurses.) Queen's Nursing Journal, 18 (12), Mar 1976, 329-330.

8 Kratz, C. Worthwhile experience. Report on survey of community care options for general nursing students. (By Rcn Community Health Tutors' Forum.) Nursing Times, 73, 10 Nov 1977, Community Outlook, 111-112.

9 Pridham, K.F. and Hurie, H.R. A day care health program: linking health services and primary care nursing education. (Providing learning experiences for nursing students in day-nursery-type facilities for children.) International Journal of Nursing Studies, 17 (1), 1980, 55-62.

10 Royal College of Nursing Community care experience in basic nurse education, and the community tutor. Rcn, 1979.

11 Royal College of Nursing Community Health Tutors' Forum Community experience for student nurses. Results of a questionnaire sent to DNEs by the Rcn Association of Nursing Education. Nursing Mirror, 145, 10 Nov 1977, 8-9.

12 Zaweckis, C. and Westfall, U.E. A reason to integrate. Description of two elements within a nursing course. (Integration of teaching-learning and community assessment and diagnosis.) Journal of Nursing Education, 15 (3), May 1976, 13-19.

c THEATRE

1 AORN Journal Special issue on student experience in the operating theatre. AORN Journal, 32 (5), Nov 1980, 755.

2 Armitage, P.A. Nursing students return to the operating room. AORN Journal, 31 (4), Mar 1980, 710, 712, 714-716.

3 Burridge, C.M. The implementation of teaching programmes for learners in operating departments. (Research study.) NATNews, 17 (6), Jun 1980, 17-18, 20-22.

4 Dixon, E. The student nurse in the operating department. (Objectives and teaching programme for three-week placement.) NATNews, 15 (7), Jul 1978, 16-17, 20-21.

5 Dodge, G.H. OR staff nurses serve as models for nursing students. AORN Journal, 26 (1), Jul 1977, 27-28, 30.

6 Farley, M. Continuing study on the training of students in the operating theatres in Australia. (Report of study tour and survey.) NATNews, 16 (2), Feb 1979, 14-15, 17-18.

7 Farley, M. The objectives of student nurse training in the operating theatres. NATNews, 15 (10), Oct 1978, 8-12, 15.

8 Greaves, J. and others Education in the operating department for the student and pupil nurse. (Report of session at 1977 NATN Congress, including research project by Margaret Farley.) NATNews, 15 (1), Jan 1978, 17, 19-20, 22-23.

9 Hazzard, M.E. Linking the OR to curriculum goals. AORN Journal, 32 (5), Nov 1980, 807-814.

10 Hodgkin, F.C. Plan for teaching students in OR. (New curriculum at DeKalb Community College, Clarkson, Georgia.) AORN Journal, 24 (3), Sep 1976, 437-441.

11 Ilch, E.V. Workshops introduce students to OR. (To attract new theatre staff.) AORN Journal, 26 (1), Jul 1977, 69-70.

12 Marcus, C. Will OR experience be part of nurses' undergraduate program? Hospital Administration in Canada, 18 (6), Jun 1976, 42-43, 46.

13 National Association of Theatre Nurses Recommended syllabus for student and pupil nurse training in the operating theatre. Harrogate: NATN, 1977.

14 Nolan, M.G. O.R. clinical experience: catalyst for student learning. Enthusiastic response to a 12 hour operating room experience that involved active participation on a scrub team. Nursing Outlook, 24 (6), Jun 1976, 378-383.

15 Pank, P.A. Student nurses in the operating theatre. (Structuring and evaluation of two-week experience including writing of care study.) NATNews, 17 (7), Jul 1980, 15-16, 18.

16 Richardson, A.M. The two week student nurse in the operating theatre—and the clinical teacher. (Modular training at University College Hospital.) NATNews, 11 (5), Jul 1974, 17-18, 20.

17 Rumsey, J.M. A learner in theatre. A study of theatre experience for student nurses. (Synopsis of award-winning project based on research.) NATNews, 14 (6), Aug 1977, 8, 10-11.

18 Sanders, S. An experiment in 'live' theatre. (Use of the pre-operative interview as a learning tool for students.) Australian Nurses Journal, 5 (6 & 7), Dec/Jan 1976, 31-32.

19 Shankland, M.T. Teaching OR nursing as part of total care. (Programme for students in each year of educational course.) AORN Journal, 28 (5), Nov 1978, 978-980, 982, 984, 986.

20 Shaw, H. ...And then there were none. (Education of theatre training for student and pupil nurses.) NATNews, 13 (7), Sep 1976, 21.

21 Shepherd, B.J. Training of learners in the theatre unit. Nursing Times, 72 (42), 21 Oct 1976, Theatre nursing supplement, 7-10.

22 Stentiford, C. Practical assessment for learners. (Programme of learning and assessment in operating theatre.) Nursing Times, 73, 10 Nov 1977, 1762-1763.

23 Sykes, P. The end of the week. (Address at 1978 annual congress of NATN on the student's view of theatre nursing and nursing generally.) NATNews, 16 (1), Jan 1979, 16-19.

24 Sykes, P. Nurse could you care more? (Learners' fear in operating department.) Nursing Times, 75, 12 Apr 1979, 614.

25 Tenzer, I.E. Nursing students learn OR skills. (Programme at San Jose State University, California.) AORN Journal, 26 (1), Jul 1977, 62-68.

24 DEGREE AND EXPERI-MENTAL COURSES

a DEGREE COURSES

1 Altschul, A. Bachelors and masters of nursing. (The history, work and future prospects of Edinburgh University Dept. of Nursing Studies.) Nursing Mirror, 146, 11 May 1978, 7-8.

2 Association of Integrated and Degree Courses in Nursing Care: the purpose of it all: report of the 5th open conference, Brighton Polytechnic, 8-10 July 1977. The Association, 1977.

3 Bashford, A.J. Nursing and the Universities: a student's view (University of Edinburgh Dept. of Nursing Studies.) Nursing Times, 66 (42), 15 Oct 1970, 1340-41.

4 Battersby, J.L. and Read, M.C. No preferential treatment. (Outline of Liverpool University's BSc/SRN course in response to criticisms.) Nursing Mirror, 147, 17 Aug 1978, 12.

5 Clarke, M. A degree of nursing. (Opportunities for qualified SRN's to take degrees in allied subjects.) Nursing Mirror, 142, 20 May 1976, 60-61.

6 Darby, C. Is the Open University a career ladder? (Career prospects for nurses with OU degrees.) Nursing Focus, 1 (4), Dec 1979, 156-157.

7 Dopson, L. What went wrong? (Closure of Newcastle Polytechnic's degree course in nursing.) Nursing Times, 76, 28 Feb 1980, 358. Correspondence, 76, 10 Apr 1980, 643; 1 May 1980, 783.

8 Dunn, A. Professor Jack Hayward. (Biography and report of interview, with details of Chelsea College nursing degree and research unit.) Nursing Times, 74, 30 Nov 1978, 1961-1963.

9 Eaves, D. A better deal for graduates, please. (Criticism of content of two-year course for graduates.) Nursing Mirror, 147, 7 Dec 1978, 13.

10 Edwards, J. The plight of the undergraduate nurse. (Personal experience after one year of a combined nursing degree course.) Nursing Mirror, 142, 15 Jan 1976, 42.

11 Emblin, R. and Hill, M.J. Degree courses in nursing. (Research into degree courses opportunities and a guide for young people contemplating nursing as a career.) Nursing Times, 72 (40), 7 Oct 1976, Occ. papers, 141-144; 14 Oct 1976, Occ. papers, 145-148; 72, 28 Oct 1976, Occ. papers, 149-152.

12 Hayward, J. A growing partnership. (Inaugural lecture of Chelsea College's professor of nursing studies on undergraduate education in nursing.) Nursing Times, 74, 7 Dec 1978, 2028-2033. Short report in Nursing Mirror, 147, 2 Nov 1978, 2.

13 House, V.G. Attitudes to degree courses and shortened courses for graduates: interviews with ward sisters/charge nurses. Nursing Times, 73, 31 Mar 1977, Occ. papers, 41-44.

14 House, V. A degree of care: a study of differential perceptions and expectations of methods of preparation of the degree nurse for the profession. Summary. GNC Research Unit, 1977.

15 House, V.G. Problems facing the undergraduate nurse. (The move from a relatively informal organisation to a hierarchical formal institution.) Nursing Times, 72, 9 Dec 1976, 1935-1936.

16 Jarvis, A.H.B. Degree programme in Scotland. (Scotland's first bachelor of science degree in nursing at Dundee College of Technology.) Nursing Times, 72, 1 Jul 1976, 1021.

17 Jones, D.C. and Keighley, A.C. Applications to undergraduate nursing courses. (Survey to ascertain demand for courses showed downward trend in suitable applications in 1975 and 1976.) Journal of Advanced Nursing, 4 (1), Jan 1979, 79-85.

18 Journal of Advanced Nursing Janforum. The interface between an academic department of nursing, the nursing profession, and society: international viewpoints from nursing academics. (Including Margaret Scott-Wright, Jack Hayward and Annie Altschul and contributions from Nigeria, Jamaica, Ireland and USA.) Journal of Advanced Nursing, 3 (4), Jul 1978, 383-390.

19 Journal of Advanced Nursing Objectives of undergraduate/baccalaureate nursing education: an international review. Journal of Advanced Nursing, 2 (4), Jul 1977, 405-413.

20 Kratz, C. Progress at the poly. (Nursing education at the South Bank Polytechnic.) Nursing Times, 76, 17 Jul 1980, 1277-1278.

21 Lee, P. Why nursing needs graduates. (Shortened courses for graduates in other disciplines.) Nursing Mirror, 148, 25 Jan 1979, 10.

22 Marsh, N. Development of the undergraduate nursing course in the University of Manchester. Journal of Advanced Nursing, 3 (3), May 1978, 297-313.

23 Myer, E.M. The Open University: a student's point of view. Nursing Times, 72, 9 Sep 1976, 1384-1386.

24 Nursing Times Open University degrees for nurses? Working party will sound out course possibilities. (Organised by Open Medicine Trust.) Nursing Times, 71, 25 Sep 1975, 1521.

25 Rhodes, B. Attitudes to higher education. (Problems registered nurses face in trying to study for BSc in nursing studies at Leeds Polytechnic.) Nursing Times, 76, 10 Jul 1980, 1224.

26 Rhodes, B. Nursing degree course for registered nurses. (CNAA day-release course over four academic years, at Leeds Polytechnic.) Nursing Times, 74, 3 Aug 1978, 1303.

27 Ross, T. The best of both worlds. (Report of visit to Edinburgh to meet students and graduates of the degree course in nursing.) Nursing Mirror, 148, 22 Mar 1979, 18-21.

28 Shore, H. A new look at degree nurses. (A look at available courses and experiences of participants.) Nursing Week, 3/10 Jan 1976, 8-9.

29 Smith, G. and Todd, F. Inter-relating nursing care and the social sciences: specialist disciplines in an applied course. (Description of CNAA degree in nursing course at Leeds Polytechnic.) International Journal of Nursing Studies, 15 (3), 1978, 143-151.

30 Smith, J.P. The realities of care. (Report on fifth annual conference of the Association of Integrated and Degree Courses in Nursing.) Nursing Mirror, 145, 14 Jul 1977, 3.

31 Strehlow, M.S. The Open University: opportunities for nurses. (Introduction—what is the OU? 1382). Nursing Times, 72, 9 Sep 1976, 1383-1384.

32 Thomas, M.C. Achievement and conflict in undergraduate nurses. (Review of research into academic and vocational under-achievement in women with reference to the differing educational philosophies of university and hospital-based learning.) Nursing Times, 75, 30 Aug 1979, Occ. papers, 93-95.

33 Thomas, M.C. Study difficulties in undergraduate nursing students—a British perspective. International Journal of Nursing Studies, 16 (4), 1979, 200-305.

34 Young, P. History of the Department of Nursing Studies at the University of Edinburgh, scene of the second Nursing Mirror forum. Nursing Mirror, 142, 11 Mar 1976, 40.

b DEGREE COURSES: OVERSEAS COUNTRIES

1 Adebo, E.O. and Schokrieh, A.C. The measurement and comparison of the democratic versus autocratic attitudinal change of the BSc (Nursing) students of the University of Ibadan during the 1972/3 academic session. International Journal of Nursing Studies, 13 (2), 1976, 103-113.

2 Australian Nurses Journal Major confrontation over bans on degree in nursing course. (At Western Australian Institute of Technology.) Australian Nurses Journal, 7 (6), Dec/Jan 1978, 11-12.

3 Banks, M.E. and others Nursing electives—a survey of available options. (Optional courses in baccalaureate degree programme.) International Nursing Review, 25 (5), Sep/Oct 1978, 138-142, 153.

4 Bauer, F.W. Failure of nurse graduate programmes. (Letter describing low standard of nursing skills in graduate nurses compared with RNs trained under previous system.) Lancet, 1, 2 Feb 1980, 262.

5 Christensen, J.C. After three years. (Degree course at Wellington Polytechnic.) New Zealand Nursing Journal, 69 (3), Mar 1976, 23-24.

6 Cleland, V. Developing a doctoral program. Nursing Outlook, 24 (10), Oct 1976, 631-635.

7 Cleveland, T.L. The intercollegiate center for nursing education. (Involving four higher education institutions, in Spokane, Washington.) Nursing Outlook, 25 (10), Oct 1977, 653-657.

8 Diers, D. Nursing: a career for college graduates. A combined basic graduate program for college graduates. (Yale University.) Nursing Outlook, 24 (2), Feb 1976, 92-98.

9 Downs, F.S. Doctoral education in nursing: future directions. Nursing Outlook, 26 (1), Jan 1978, 56-61.

10 Downs, F.S. Doctoral preparation in nursing: is it worth it? (Follow up study of graduates from the New York University doctoral program 1964-1974.) Nursing Outlook, 24 (6), Jun 1976, 375-377.

11 Fields, S.K. Nurses earn their B.S. Degrees—on the job. (Pilot project at the State University of New York, Stony Brook.) Nursing Outlook, 24 (3), Mar 1976, 169-173.

12 Grace, H.K. The development of doctoral education in nursing: in historical perspective.

Journal of Nursing Education, 17 (4), Apr 1978, 17-27.

13 Harte, C.C. Tertiary undergraduate nursing in N.S.W. Cumberland sets out. (Cumberland College of Health Sciences.) Australian Nurses Journal, 5 (9), Mar 1976, 20-22.

14 Hayter, J. A follow-up study of a master's program. (Survey as means of curriculum evaluation.) Nursing Outlook, 26 (6), Jun 1978, 380-385.

15 Hendry, M.N. Change of scene. (Nursing degree student's experience on a one year exchange in Philadelphia.) Nursing Times, 74, 23 Feb 1978, 336-337.

16 Hillsmith, K.E. From RN to BSN: student perceptions. (Research study of RNs who returned to college to take baccalaureate degree nursing course.) Nursing Outlook, 26 (2), Feb 1978, 98-102.

17 Hipps, O.S. Nursing electives: how many and of what nature? (Appropriateness of optional courses in baccalaureate nursing program including special projects and topics and independent study.) Nursing Outlook, 25 (9), Sep 1977, 570-574.

18 Hughes, B. University education for nurses: the first phase. (Collapse of diploma of nursing course at University of Otago in 1926 and subsequent developments.) New Zealand Nursing Journal, 71 (12), Dec 1978, 8-12.

19 Hurd, J.M.L. Nursing and the degree mystique. 1. (With reference to split between professional and technical nurses.) 2. Nursing now has a place on the university campus but has it freed itself from the shackles of its hospital past? Canadian Nurse, 75 (4), Apr 1979, 36-39; (5), May 1979, 36-38.

20 Jones, J.W. United States undergraduate nursing education: a system pathology. (Study of the development of the present system, analysing the reasons for the difficulty of the transition from student to professional nurse and the need for new policies.) International Journal of Nursing Studies, 16 (1), 1979, 123-133.

21 Kelley, L.K. Women in nursing and academic tenure. (Nurses' position in the U.S. academic system.) Journal of Nursing Education, 19 (2), Feb 1980, 41-48.

22 Kinross, N.J. Nursing studies at university level. (Courses at Massey and Victoria Universities.) New Zealand Nursing Journal, 71 (10), Oct 1978, 4-10.

23 Kirwin, B. Nurse education in the USA: training an army of generals. (Critical assessment of degree programme for nurses.) Nursing Mirror, 150, 21 Feb 1980, 38-39.

24 Leininger, M. Doctoral programs for nurses: trends, questions and projected plans. (Includes a list of all existing and proposed programs in the United States.) Nursing Research, 25 (3), May/Jun 1976, 201-210.

25 Lenburg, C.B. The external degree in nursing: the promise fulfilled. (State University of New York.) Nursing Outlook, 24 (7), Jul 1976, 422-429.

26 McClure, M.L. Entry into professional practice: the New York proposal. (The proposal that the baccalaureate degree becomes the

minimal educational requirement for nursing by 1985.) Journal of Nursing Administration, 6 (5), Jun 1976, 12-17.

27 McGriff, E. and Simms, L. Two New York nurses debate the NYSNA 1985 proposal. (The New York State Nurses Association proposal that a baccalaureate degree will be required for licensure.) American Journal of Nursing, 76 (6), Jun 1976, 930-935.

28 National League for Nursing The community college and associate degree nursing, 1952-1980. New York: NLN, 1980.

29 National League for Nursing Developing a master's program in nursing. New York: NLN, 1978.

30 National League for Nursing Strategies in administration and teaching in associate degree nursing education. New York: NLN, 1976.

31 National League for Nursing. Council of Baccalaureate and Higher Degree Programs Current issues affecting nursing as a part of higher education: papers presented at the 15th conference of the Council, March 1976. New York: NLN, 1976.

32 National League for Nursing. Division of Associate Degree Programs Competencies of the associate degree nurse on entry into practice. New York: NLN, 1978.

33 New Zealand Nursing Journal Nature and purpose of nursing courses. (University of Wellington BA Degree.) New Zealand Nursing Journal, 69 (12), Dec 1976, 18-19.

34 Nursing Outlook Focus on associate degree nursing. (In U.S.A. Five articles.) Nursing Outlook, 25 (8), Aug 1977, 496-518.

35 Ohlson, V.M. Baccalaureate nursing education in the United States. International Nursing Review, 24 (6), Nov/Dec 1977, 168-170.

36 Peterson, C.J. Development of competencies in associate degree nursing: a new perspective. New York: National League for Nursing, 1978.

37 Quiring, J.D. and Gray, G.T. Is baccalaureate education based on a patchwork curriculum? (Research study.) Nursing Outlook, 27 (11), Nov 1979, 708-713.

38 Rotkovitch, R. The AD nurse: a nursing service perspective. (The objectives of the associate degree program.) Nursing Outlook, 24 (4), Apr 1976, 234-236.

39 Searle, C. Doctoral programmes in nursing in South Africa. S.A. Nursing Journal, 44 (3), Mar 1977, 42-43.

40 Searle, C. Extra mural and external nursing degree courses. A query and an answer. (University of South Africa.) Rhodesian Nurse, 8 (4), Dec 1975, 15-23.

41 Seivwright, M.J. Up to date information about advanced nursing education at the University of the West Indies. Jamaican Nurse, 15 (2), Aug 1975, 12-14, 24.

42 Trussell, P.M. Establishing a graduate nursing program: the Arkansas experience. Hospitals, 49 (23), 1 Dec 1975, 43-44.

43 Westbrook, M.T. and others Nurses graduating with Diplomas of Applied Science:

their attitudes toward their training and careers. (Study of twelve graduates of Cumberland College of Health Sciences, N.S.W.) Lamp, 37 (3), Mar 1980, 5-11.

44 Williams, M.A. and others Values and value changes of graduate nursing students: their relationship to faculty values and to selected educational factors. Nursing Research, 27 (3), May/Jun 1978, 181-189.

45 Wilson, H.S. and others The second step model of baccalaureate education for registered nurses. The students' perspective. (Degree course for registered nurses.) Journal of Nursing Education, 16 (6), Jun 1977, 27-35.

46 Woodward, E.S. Reflections of an external degree graduate. Nursing Outlook, 24 (7), Jul 1976, 429-432.

c EXPERIMENTAL AND INTER-DISCIPLINARY COURSES

1 Attwood, M. An interdisciplinary teacher education experience. A group of health instructors who attended a summer institute increased not only their teaching skills but also their knowledge of each others' disciplines. Nursing Outlook, 26 (5), May 1978, 321-324.

2 Batchelor, E.V. The Teaching Centre, Norfolk and Norwich Hospital. (Integration of postgraduate medical and nursing education.) Health and Welfare Libraries Quarterly, 2 (2-4), Jun/Dec 1975, 35-40.

3 Bristow, S. Career opportunities. Shortened statutory courses. (Using the psychiatric nursing course at St. Luke's Woodside Hospital, as an example.) Nursing Times, 72, 10 Jun 1976, 888-889.

4 Buckman, M.J. and Grobe, B. Four years' experience with an evening nursing program. (At Maryville College, St. Louis to enable individuals to train as nurses who would otherwise have found it impossible.) Hospital Progress, 57 (2), Feb 1976, 32-34, 38.

5 CENTRE for Educational Research and Innovation Health, higher education and the community: towards a regional health university. Paris: OECD, 1977.

6 Charrow, K.C. Education of the health professions in the context of the health care system: the Ontario experience. Paris: OECD, 1975.

7 Coventry, M. Experimental training course for graduates. (At Glasgow Northern District College of Nursing and Midwifery.) Nursing Times, 73, 23 Jun 1977, 965-967.

8 Davis, A.J. Undergraduate interdisciplinary educators in the health sciences. Innovative education. (Program at the University of California, San Francisco, for students planning to enter the health professions.) Journal of Nursing Education, 15 (4), Jul 1976, 22-26.

9 Donabedian, D. Teaching clinical public health nursing in a collaborative medical center/ nursing school program. Journal of Nursing Education, 18 (8), Oct 1979, 4-8.

10 Dowling, M.A.C. and others Making educational programmes relevant. WHO Chronicle, 30 (11), Nov 1976, 464-467.

11 Ford, C.W. and Morgan, M.K. editors Teaching in the health professions. St. Louis: Mosby, 1976.

12 Fosdike, H. How to provide a common language and stimulation. Assessment of the South Bank Polytechnic's health education diploma course for health educators.) Health and Social Service Journal, 87, 2 Dec 1977, 1651-1652.

13 Guilbert, J.J. Educational handbook for health personnel. Geneva: WHO, 1977. (WHO offset publication no.35.)

14 Harnar, R. Coordinating nursing with general education. (Multidisciplinary courses for all health workers in India.) Nursing Journal of India, 68 (3), Mar 1977, 81-83.

15 House, V.G. Principles for successful training. (GNC survey based on a comparison of 600 experimental and 1000 traditional course students.) Nursing Times, 73, 20 Jan 1977, 106-107.

16 House, V.G. Survival of the fittest: a summary of an attempt to evaluate experimental schemes of nurse training. (GNC Research Unit Study.) Journal of Advanced Nursing, 2 (2), Mar 1977, 157-170.

17 Jacobs, R.M. editor A flexible design for health professions education: medicine, dentistry, pharmacy, nursing, allied health. New York: Wiley, 1976.

18 Jones, D. Special training for teamwork. (Nursing Mirror Forum 76.) Nursing Mirror, 143, 2 Dec 1976, 52-53.

19 Katz, F.M. Guidelines for evaluating a training programme for health personnel. Geneva: WHO, 1978. (WHO offset publication no.38.)

20 Knopke, H.J. Instructional change in health care education. (Survey of nursing, medical and pharmacy faculties to identify the extent to which recommended changes in their teaching activities had been implemented.) Nursing Research, 25 (4), Jul/Aug 1976, 263-267.

21 Korsak, A. Hospitals have major role in health manpower education. (American Hospital Association survey of training for health occupations including nursing.) Hospitals, 50 (11), 1 Jun 1976, 74-76, 79, 80.

22 Luginbill, C. Nurse-instructors for medical students. (Teaching of clinical skills at the Southern Illinois University School of Medicine.) American Journal of Nursing, 78 (5), May 1978, 868-870.

23 Murray, L. The two-plus-one scheme: has it been successful? (Evaluation of shortened courses of nurse training in six hospitals.) Nursing Times, 73, 10 Feb 1977, 21-24.

24 National League for Nursing Collaboration in health care education. New York: The League, 1976.

25 Nursing Mirror Clinical teamwork—the aim of education. Part 2. Education for teamwork. (Nursing Mirror Forum 76.) Nursing Mirror, 143, 23, 2 Dec 1976, 49-56.

26 Owen, G.M. Curriculum integration in nursing education: a concept or a way of life? A study of six courses integrating basic nursing education and health visiting in a single course.

Journal of Advanced Nursing, 2 (5), Sep 1977, 443-460.

27 Patterson, M. and Hayes, S. Verbal communication between students in multi-disciplinary health teams. (Study among under-graduate students in Australia.) Medical Education, 11 (3), May 1977, 205-209.

28 Pickett, B. Multi-disciplinary education in the health sciences. (Foundation for Multi-Disciplinary Education in Community Health.) Australasian Nurses Journal, 7 (5), Dec 1977, 10-11.

29 Raymond, E.A. Community nursing option: some questions and answers. (With reference to experimental community option based at South Bank Polytechnic.) Nursing Times, 74, 6 Apr 1978, Occ. papers, 37-40.

30 Shephard, R.J. and Ashley, M.J. Attitudes of health science students towards teaching practices, examinations, and other related issues. (Multiple-choice questionnaire used with a group of students (including nurses) in Toronto.) Medical Education, 13 (2), Mar 1979, 111-116.

31 Vuori, H. Approaches to training for co-operation. (Educational experiment at University of Kuopio, Finland.) Public Health, 90 (6), Sep 1976, 281-285.

32 Wieczorek, R.R. and others Interdisciplinary education: a model for the resocialization of faculty. Nursing Forum, 15 (3), 1976, 224-237.

33 World Health Organisation. Division of Health Manpower Development Personnel for health care: case studies of educational programmes, edited by F.M. Katz and T. Fülop. Geneva: WHO, 1978. (Public health papers; 70.)

25 NURSE LEARNERS

a GENERAL

1 Bendall, E.R.D. People who are training to be nurses. (Course, age, sex, marital status, educational qualifications and country of origin, of a sample of 1000 student and pupil nurses indexed with the GNC in January 1976.) Nursing Times, 72 (34), 26 Aug 1976, 1317-1318.

2 Burgess, G. The personal development of the nursing student as a conceptual framework. Nursing Forum, 17 (1), 1978, 96-102.

3 Burgess, G. The self-concept of under-graduate nursing students in relation to clinical performance and selected biographical variables. (Research study.) Journal of Nursing Education, 19 (3), Mar 1980, 37-44.

4 Davis, W.E. ODWIN Expansion program: a study in success. (Study of students with poor academic qualifications who successfully completed nursing training after eight-week preparatory course.) Nursing Research, 27 (4), Jul/Aug 1978, 230-232.

5 De Tornyay, R. Changing student relationships, roles and responsibilities. As a result of social, legal and economic changes. Nursing Outlook, 25 (3), Mar 1977, 188-193.

6 De Tornyay, R. and Russell, M.L. Helping the high-risk student achieve. (Pre-professional programme for minority students at University of Washington to help educationally disadvantaged students.) Nursing Outlook, 26 (9), Sep 1978, 576-580.

7 Durrant, L. The student of nursing needs — the consumer of education. (Strategies to meet needs of students and influence of role models on their behaviour.) Journal of Nursing Education, 17 (6), Jun 1978, 17-19.

8 Gibbs, J.L. Student evaluation of an undergraduate nursing programme. MSc thesis, University of Manchester, Department of Nursing, Oct 1979.

9 Goldstein, J.O. Comparison of graduating AD and baccalaureate nursing students' characteristics. Nursing Research, 29 (1), Jan/Feb 1980, 46-49.

10 Hargreaves, I. A study of the empathic functioning of nurses in training. MSc, Faculty of Medicine, Manchester University, Oct 1976.

11 Ichilov, O. and Dotan, M. Formation of professional images among Israeli student nurses. (Study of the value dimension of the professional socialization process of Israeli student nurses.) International Journal of Nursing Studies, 17 (4), 1980, 247-259.

12 Kakar, D.N. and Dean, M. Nursing students' background, choice of profession and professional satisfaction. (Study at the College of Nursing. Chandigarth.) Nursing Journal of India, 71 (2), Feb 1980, 30-33.

13 Lester, J. Surrey learners benefit from discussion. Value of the student representative meetings in the South-West Surrey district. Nursing Mirror, 142 (24), 10 Jun 1976, 39-40.

14 McKay, S.R. A peer group counseling model in nursing education. Journal of Nursing Education, 19 (3), Mar 1980, 4-10.

15 Malarkey, L. The older student — stress or success on campus. Journal of Nursing Education, 18 (2), Feb 1979, 15-19.

16 Marriner, A. The student's perception of his creativity. (Survey at the New York State University of Plattsburgh.) Nursing Research, 26 (1), Jan-Feb 1977, 57-60.

17 Morris, P.B. and Grassi-Russo, N. Motives of beginning students for choosing nursing school. (Research study.) Journal of Nursing Education, 18 (5), May 1979, 34-40.

18 New Zealand Nursing Journal A survey of role conflict in expectations for student nurses. (Hawkes Bay School of Nursing.) New Zealand Nursing Journal, 70 (2), Feb 1977, 8-10.

19 Nursing Times A day in the life. The pupil nurse. Nursing Times, 73, 20 Jan 1977, 84-85.

20 O'Connor, K. A system to collect information on student nurses. (To be introduced by Nurses Education Board of New South Wales.) Lamp, 35 (12), Dec 1978/Jan 1979, 14-16.

21 Packard, K.L. and others Concerns of final semester baccalaureate nursing students. Nursing Research, 28 (5), Sep/Oct 1979, 302-304.

22 Sayre, J. The role of linguistic style in student learning difficulties. (Problems in writing essays and teaching methods to overcome them.) Journal of Nursing Education, 16 (6), Jun 1977, 16-23.

23 Simpson, I.H. and others From student to nurse: a longitudinal study of socialization. Cambridge: Cambridge University Press, 1979. (American Sociological Association, A. and C. Rose monograph series.)

24 Smoyak, S.A. Teaching as coaching. (Focusing on students' learning history and needs to identify strengths and weaknesses.) Nursing Outlook, 26 (6), Jun 1978, 361-363.

25 Sobol, E.G. Self-actualization and the baccalaureate nursing student's response to stress. Nursing Research, 27 (4), Jul/Aug 1978, 238-244.

26 Tobiason, S.J. A plea to role models. (How learners learn variety of nursing roles from nurse managers.) Supervisor Nurse, 10 (1), Jan 1979, 36-37.

27 Ventura, M.R. Related social behaviors of students in different types of nursing education programs. (Study of 16 American nursing schools comparing associate degree, diploma and baccalaureate degree program students.) International Journal of Nursing Studies, 13 (1), 1976, 3-10.

28 Watson, J. Conceptual systems of undergraduate nursing students as compared with university students at large and practising nurses. (Research study to measure characteristics of abstractness — concreteness.) Nursing Research, 27 (3), May/Jun 1978, 151-155.

29 Webb, M.R. and Herman, A.L. Achieving behaviors in beginning nursing students. (Investigation of achievement-related personality characteristics in new nursing students in the context of nursing's failure to achieve full professional status.) International Journal of Nursing Studies, 15 (2), 1978, 75-82.

30 Webb, M. and Linn, M.W. Open mindedness of first year medical, nursing and social work students. (Study at the University of Miami.) Medical Education, 11 (1), Jan 1977, 4-6.

31 Weinstein, E.L. and others Characteristics of the successful nursing student. (Research study.) Journal of Nursing Education, 19 (3), Mar 1980, 53-59.

32 Wong, S. and Wong, J. Representation of racial minority students in selected Canadian university schools of nursing. Journal of Advanced Nursing, 5 (1), Jan 1980, 83-90.

33 Zorn, J.M. A research profile of today's baccalaureate nursing student. Journal of Continuing Education in Nursing, 11 (2), Mar/Apr 1980, 7-9.

b ATTITUDES

1 Angus, M. Job satisfaction in two schools of nursing. (Study of students in a community college and a hospital in Canada.) Dimensions in Health Service, 56 (8), Aug 1979, 35-37.

2 Auster, D. Sex differences in attitudes toward nursing education. (Survey of male and female students.) Journal of Nursing Education, 18 (6), Jun 1979, 19-28.

3 Claerbaut, D. Expansionist trends in health care and the role of minority students: a challenge for nursing education. (Research study of black nursing students' attitudes.) Journal of Nursing Education, 17 (4), Apr 1978, 42-47.

4 Crout, L. From a learner's point of view. (How present organisation of nurse education inhibits development of questioning attitude in learners.) Nursing Mirror, 151, 3 Jul 1980, 14.

5 Garvin, B.J. Values of male nursing students. (Study at Ohio State University comparing their values with female nursing students and general college students.) Nursing Research, 25 (5), Sep/Oct 1976, 352-357.

6 Gliebe, W.A. Faculty consensus as a socializing agent in professional education. (Study of attitudes of student nurses and tutors.) Nursing Research, 26 (6), Nov/Dec 1977, 428-431.

7 Jones, S.L. Socialization versus selection factors as sources of student definitions of the nurse role (with particular reference to the United States.) International Journal of Nursing Studies, 13 (3), 1976, 135-138.

8 Jones, S.L. and Jones, P.K. Nursing student definitions of the 'real' nurse. (Study of factors influencing their definitions.) Journal of Nursing Education, 16 (4), Apr 1977, 15-21.

9 Kahn, A.M. Modifications in nursing student attitudes as measured by the EPPS: a significant reversal from the past. (Comparison of scores of nursing and non-nursing students on autonomy and deference subtest scales of personality test.) Nursing Research, 29 (1), Jan/Feb 1980, 61-63.

10 Leaf, A.G. and Fraser, B.J. The dimensionality of vocational commitment: an empirical assessment of Ramsay's Three-factor model with trainee nurses. (In New South Wales.) British Journal of Guidance and Counselling, 6 (2), Jul 1978, 191-197.

11 Macdonald, M.R. How do men and women students rate in empathy? (Research study.) American Journal of Nursing, 77 (6), Jun 1977, 998.

12 Minnigerode, F.A. and others Masculinity and femininity in nursing. (Concept of the 'ideal nurse' was rated by male and female nursing students.) Nursing Research, 28 (5), Sep/Oct 1978, 302-304.

13 Mosley, D.Y. Nursing students' perceptions of the urban poor. New York: National League for Nursing, 1977.

14 Nursing Journal of India Students' role in improving the image of a nurse. (Papers from seminar presented by student nurses.) Nursing Journal of India, 67 (1), Jan 1976, 3-5; (2), Feb 1976, 26-28.

15 Parkinson, M.H. Learning the characteristics of helping relationships: nurse-teacher genuineness and student-nurse self-disclosure. Research report. (Into the process whereby nurses learn the characteristics of helping relationships in their basic education.) New Zealand Nursing Journal, 70 (7), Jul 1977, 24-25.

16 Rhodes, B. The instrumental values of nurses. (Study of students in one school of nursing to ascertain the relationship between the values held by several groups of nurses.) Nursing Mirror, 145, 10 Nov 1977, 29-30.

17 Rosswurm, M.A. Changing nursing students' attitudes towards persons with physical disabilities. (Research study.) AORN Journal, 5 (1), Jan/Feb 1980, 12-14.

18 Schwirian, P.M. and Kisker, K.L. Perceptions of health among baccalaureate nursing students. (Research study to examine changes in perception during training.) Journal of Nursing Education, 16 (6), Jun 1977, 2-9.

19 Stoller, E.P. Preconceptions of the nursing role: a case study of an entering class. (Includes a comparison of entering and graduating classes.) Journal of Nursing Education, 17 (6), Jun 1978, 2-14.

20 Stromborg, M.F. Relationship of sex role identity to occupational image of female nursing students. Nursing Research, 25 (5), Sep/Oct 1976, 363-369.

21 Tetreault, A.I. Selected factors associated with professional attitude of baccalaureate nursing students. Nursing Research, 25 (1), Jan-Feb 1976, 49-53.

22 Worsley, A. Exploration of student nurses' stereotypes of patients. (Research study.) International Journal of Nursing Studies, 17 (3), 1980, 163-174.

c EVALUATION OF TEACHERS AND COURSES

1 Brown, D.L. and Hayes, E.R. Evaluation tools: student's assessment of faculty. (Team teaching and clinical teaching.) Nursing Outlook, 27 (12), Dec 1979, 778-781.

2 Elvins, L. and Mackay, L. A preliminary study of nursing students' perceptions of whether a course is achieving its objectives: ongoing evaluation of a College-based programme. (College of Nursing, Australia.) Australian Nurses Journal, 6 (8), Feb 1977, 28-31.

3 Hitchens, E.W. Evaluation: the graffiti technique. (Method of enabling students to evaluate course, teacher and themselves as a group.) Journal of Nursing Education, 18 (3), Mar 1979, 46-47.

4 Jackson, M.O. Instructor and course evaluation based on student-identified criteria. Journal of Nursing Education, 16 (2), Feb 1977, 8-13.

5 Lord, S. Unit assessment from below. (Suggested form for students to complete evaluating performance of trained ward staff and tutors.) Nursing Times, 76, 17 Jul 1980, 1248-1250.

6 Stuebbe, B. Student and faculty perspectives on the role of a nursing instructor. (Research project to examine how students saw the role of nursing instructors and compare this with instructors' own view of their role.) Journal of Nursing Education, 19 (7), Sep 1980, 4-9.

7 Wong, S. Nurse-teacher behaviours in the clinical field: apparent effect on nursing students' learning. (Research study of students' perceptions of teacher behaviours which either facilitate or hinder students' learning.) Journal of Advanced Nursing, 3 (4), Jul 1978, 369-372.

d STUDENT STATUS AND ORGANISATIONS

1 Beckett, C. Time for student status for students. Nursing Mirror, 149, 27 Sep 1979, 14.

2 Cardwell, C. Student or worker? Chris Cardwell reports on his visit to the International Meeting of Student Nurses (European Group.) Nursing Mirror, 143 (19), 4 Nov 1976, 38.

3 Chapman, C. The learner as worker. (Problems in apprenticeship system of nurse education.) Medical Teacher, 2 (5), Sep/Oct 1980, 241-244.

4 Long, R. After the Act. (Controversy over student status for learners and financial costs of educating nurses.) Nursing Times, 75, 1 Nov 1979, 1878-1879.

5 Montag, M.C. Nursing student: learner or worker. Lamp, Dec 1975, 31-34.

6 Nursing Mirror Keep out of party politics warning from European Student Nurses Group. (Conference report.) Nursing Mirror, 145, 13 Oct 1977, 5.

7 Nursing Mirror Wake up to politics student nurses told. (Report of Eighth European Student Nurses Conference.) Nursing Mirror, 145, 29 Sep 1977, 2.

8 Salvage, J. The student nurse of today—the qualified nurse of tomorrow. (Comment on forthcoming conference of European student nurses and nurses' educational needs in the future.) Nursing Mirror, 147, 16 Nov 1978, 19-20.

9 Skyes, P. Politics, yes…party politics, no. (Report of 8th European Student Nurses conference.) Nursing Times, 73, 27 Oct 1977, 1660.

10 South African Nursing Association Student status: the Board's view regarding supernumerary status of student nurses. S.A. Nursing Journal, 44 (9), Sep 1977, 16-17.

11 Young, P. Costing the care-free student. (Student status for learners using comparison with physiotherapy students.) Nursing Times, 74, 7 Dec 1978, 2008.

26 CONTINUING EDUCATION

a GENERAL

1 Burgess, G.R. Self-assessment of continuing education needs. International Nursing Review, 25 (3), May/Jun 1978, 89-92.

2 Castledine, G. Back to school nurse? (Needs of nurses for continuing education.) Nursing Mirror, 151, 4 Sep 1980, 12.

3 Dopson, L. Continuing development. (Report on King's Fund Centre conference on continuing education.) Nursing Times, 76, 19 Jun 1980, 1077.

4 Franklin, V.L. The sabbatical leave. (Need for planning in advance.) Nursing Outlook, 28 (2), Feb 1980, 109-111.

5 Goldiak, S. Continuing education: a 'must' for maintaining competence. International Nursing Review, 24 (6), Nov/Dec 1977, 171, 181.

6 Greaves, F. Learning to learn again. (Advice on study methods for nurses on advanced courses in higher education.) Nursing Mirror, 147, 3 Aug 1978, 38.

7 Ingersoll, D.J. Study leave provisions for nursing staff. (Research study.) Nursing Times, 75, 7 Jun 1979, Occ. papers, 61-64.

8 International Nursing Council ICN policy statement on continuing education for nurses and guidelines. International Nursing Review, 23 (4), Jul/Aug 1976, 102.

9 International Nursing Council Through the eyes of continuing education—the ICN. (Its role generally and statement on continuing education.) Journal of Continuing Education in Nursing, 10 (6), Nov/Dec 1979, 39-41.

10 Royal College of Nursing. Professional Nursing Department Post-basic training opportunities for state enrolled nurses. Rcn, 1976.

11 Studdy, S. and Hunt, C. A computerised survey of learning needs. (Among trained staff at St. Thomas' Hospital, London.) Nursing Times, 76, 19 Jun 1980, 1084-1087.

12 World Health Organization. Regional Office for Europe Continuing education of health personnel: report on a working group, Dublin 18-21 Oct 1976. Copenhagen: WHO, 1977.

13 World Health Organization. Regional Office for Europe Continuing education of health personnel and its evaluation. Copenhagen: WHO, 1980.

b MANDATORY OR VOLUNTARY

1 Adcock, R. Mandatory continuing education: will it raise the standard of nursing practice? Australian Nurses Journal, 9 (10), May 1980, 41-43.

2 American Journal of Nursing The status of continuing education: voluntary and mandatory. (Summary of the position in each State in U.S.) American Journal of Nursing, 77 (3), Mar 1977, 410-416.

3 American Journal of Nursing Survey shows slow but strong movement in States toward mandatory continuing education. American Journal of Nursing, 78 (5), May 1978, 766, 792, 799, 802, 804, 808, 810.

4 Briant, N.J. What every reasonable and prudent nurse should know. (Claims that voluntary systems of continuing education are more effective than mandatory ones.) Canadian Nurse, 73 (6), Jun 1977, 13.

5 Elliott, V. Continuing education for nurses: mandatory or voluntary? (Review of arguments.) Journal of Nursing Care, 13 (5), May 1980, 14-16.

6 Rajabally, M. Continuing education should be mandatory. Dimensions in Health Service, 53 (7), Jul 1976, 22-23.

7 Waddle, F.I. Trends in mandatory continuing education. Journal of Continuing Education in Nursing, 11 (1), Jan/Feb 1980, 39-40.

8 Wolf, D.H. Mandatory CE: it's time to keep up—or get out. (Progress of legislation to introduce compulsory continuing education in the United States.) RN Magazine, 40 (1), Jan 1977, 39-44.

c UNITED STATES

1 Adams, A.E. Continuing education in state

universities. (Survey by questionnaire of financial support.) Nursing Outlook, 24 (5), May 1976, 294-297.

2 American Association of Industrial Nurses AAIN statement on continuing education. New York: the Association, 1975.

3 Barlow, D.J. and Chesney, A.P. Nurses want to keep up to date! (Project to investigate continuing education needs of nurses in Texas.) Journal of Continuing Education in Nursing, 8 (6), Nov/Dec 1977, 15-21.

4 Bell, F. and Rix, P. Attitudes of nurses toward lifelong learning: one hospital examines the issues. (Research study.) Journal of Continuing Education in Nursing, 10 (1), Jan/Feb 1979, 15-20.

5 Bille, D.A. Planning staff development: theory X, or theory Y? (Two theories of motivation—'carrot and stick' or human relations approach.) Journal of Continuing Education in Nursing, 9 (6), Nov/Dec 1978, 10-15.

6 Bille, D.A. Successful educational programming: increasing learner motivation through involvement. (Using patient teaching workshop as example of continuing education.) Journal of Nursing Administration, 9 (5), May 1979, 36-42.

7 Braley, N.L. Programming continuing education activities. Occupational Health Nursing, 25 (3), Mar 1977, 7-15.

8 Brown, S.T. and Lee, B.T. Imogene King's conceptual framework: a proposed model for continuing nursing education. Journal of Advanced Nursing, 5 (5), Sep 1980, 467-473.

9 Butherus, G.C. Where do you stand in… the continuing education picture? (Report of survey by NAPNES of provision by state boards of nursing.) Journal of Practical Nursing, 27 (9), Sep 1977, 14.

10 Cantor, M.M. The roles and responsibilities of continuing education in nursing. Journal of Continuing Education in Nursing, 8 (1), Jan-Feb 1977, 16-24.

11 Chatham, M.A. A continuing education program for nursing aides: communication skills, self concept, and problem solving. Journal of Continuing Education in Nursing, 9 (5), Sep/Oct 1978, 26-29.

12 Chatham, M.A. Discrepancies in learning needs assessments: whose needs are being assessed? (Survey of nursing managers' opinions of their staff's educational needs and those of staff nurses themselves.) Journal of Continuing Education in Nursing, 10 (5), Sep/Oct 1979, 18-22.

13 Conlin, E. How to measure staff development. (Continuing education programme.) Dimensions in Health Service, 55 (9), Sep 1978, 32-33.

14 CONTINUING education philosophy and objectives. AORN Journal, 26 (1), Jul 1977, 174-175.

15 Cooper, S.S. A brief history of continuing education in nursing in the United States. Journal of Continuing Education in Nursing, 4 (3), May-Jun 1973, 5-14.

16 Cooper, S.S. Continuing education—How? (Advice on using libraries, attending

conferences and keeping up-to-date generally.) American Journal of Maternal-Child Nursing, 3 (4), Jul/Aug 1978, 242, 244, 246.

17 Cooper, S.S. Continuing education: yesterday and today. Nurse Educator, 3 (1), Jan/Feb 1978, 25-29.

18 Cooper, S.S. Steps in self-development. Wakefield, Mass.: Contemporary Publishing, 1977. (Contemporary nursing review no.R.3.)

19 Curran, C.L. Factors affecting participation in continuing education activities and identified learning needs of registered nurses. (Research study in Chicago.) Journal of Continuing Education in Nursing, 8 (4), Jul/Aug 1977, 17-22.

20 Curran, C.L. Learning needs of foreign nurses. (Survey in Chicago showing different emphasis placed by foreign educated registered nurses and American nurses on importance of various topics in continuing education.) Supervisor Nurse, 9 (8), Aug 1978, 30-32.

21 Donovan, L. Who's going to pay for all that continuing education? (RN survey of readers about employers' policies.) RN Magazine, 41 (1), Jan 1978, 48-51.

22 Friedrich, R.M. and others Innovations in continuing education: a statewide program for systematic training in interpersonal skills. Journal of Continuing Education in Nursing, 10 (2), Mar/Apr 1979, 29-35.

23 Hauf, B.J. Assuring quality in continuing nursing education. Nursing Leadership, 3 (1), Mar 1980, 7-16.

24 Haymes, H. Running a CE program: administrative strategies. Nursing Outlook, 28 (3), Mar 1980, 183-186.

25 Hicks, B.C. A need oriented approach to staff development. (Assignment of staff development instructor to one clinical area of the hospital.) Journal of Nursing Administration, 7 (7), Sep 1977, 46-47.

26 Jones, M.C. A continuing education dilemma: luring the adult learner. Occupational Health Nursing, 27 (1), Jan 1979, 17-19.

27 Journal of Continuing Education in Nursing Special issue. Selected papers presented at the 1976 National Conference on Continuing Education. Journal of Continuing Education in Nursing, 8 (3), May/Jun 1977, 7-74.

28 Journal of Nursing Administration Staff development: a reader. Wakefield, Mass.: Contemporary Publishing, 1975.

29 Journal of Practical Nursing What LP/VNs think of continuing education. (Results of survey including books and journals read.) Journal of Practical Nursing, 30 (11), Nov/Dec 1980, 31-33, 36-38.

30 Kang, H.S.K. A cybernetics model for continuing education in nursing. Nursing Leadership, 2 (2), Jun 1979, 15-20.

31 Keeling, A.W. and Noriega, L. Continuing education—independently! (Study of the effectiveness of self-instructional modules.) Supervisor Nurse, 9 (4), Apr 1978, 45-46, 50-51.

32 King, P.J. The hospitalwide education department. Journal of Nursing Administration, 7 (4), Apr 1978, 13-19.

33 LaMonica, E.L. and others Empathy training as the major thrust of a staff development program. Nursing Research, 25 (6), Nov-Dec 1976, 447-451. Reprinted in Nursing Mirror, 145, 25 Aug 1977, 22-25.

34 Levine, M.E. Does continuing education improve nursing practice? Hospitals, 52 (21), 1 Nov 1978, 138-140.

35 McGill, C. and Barlow, D. Implementing a regional plan for continuing education in nursing. (Texas.) Journal of Continuing Education in Nursing, 7 (5), Sep/Oct 1976, 30-38.

36 McNally, J.M. A resource model for continuing education in nursing. Journal of Continuing Education in Nursing, 9 (4), Jul/Aug 1978, 33-37.

37 Manuel, B.T. Designing content for CE offering. (Outlines steps in designing educational programme including setting objectives and evaluation.) AORN Journal, 26 (4), Oct 1977, 637-638, 640.

38 Matthews, A.E. and Schumacher, S. A survey of registered nurses' conceptions of and participation factors in professional continuing education. Journal of Continuing Education in Nursing, 10 (1), Jan/Feb 1979, 21-27.

39 Moore, F.I. and Singleton, E.K. A 'temporary systems' approach to nursing education in a health care organization. (Staff development and orientation.) Journal of Nursing Administration, 8 (7), Jul 1978, 7-14.

40 Mote, J.R. Continuing education: enhancing the quality of patient care. Hospitals, 50 (1), 1 Aug 1976, 175-176, 178-180.

41 Murphy, J. Notes on continuing education. The first hour: creating a learning environment. (Organising a day conference.) Journal of Continuing Education in Nursing, 10 (5), Sep/Oct 1979, 42-46.

42 National League for Nursing Implementation of continuing education in nursing. New York: NLN, 1978.

43 Nursing Administration Quarterly Continuing education—who cares? (Issue devoted to this topic.) Nursing Administration Quarterly, 2 (2), Winter 1978, 1-90.

44 O'Connor, A.B. Reasons nurses participate in continuing education. Nursing Research, 28 (6), Nov/Dec 1979, 354-359.

45 Popiel, E.S. editor Nursing and the process of continuing education. 2nd ed. St. Louis: Mosby, 1977.

46 Price, D.J. Continuing education: advancing our basic skills. (Discusses ANA standards, guidelines and criteria for continuing education and current USA practice.) Occupational Health Nursing, 25 (5), May 1977, 7-8.

47 Puetz, B.E. Differences between Indiana registered nurse attenders and nonattenders in continuing education in nursing activities. Journal of Continuing Education in Nursing, 11 (2), Mar/Apr 1980, 19-26.

48 Reilly, D.E. Preparation of objectives for continuing education programs. Occupational Health Nursing, 24 (12), Dec 1976, 30-32.

49 Robinson, V.M. How to initiate change in practice. (Application of knowledge gained through continuing education to nursing practice.) AORN Journal, 26 (1), Jul 1977, 54-61.

50 **Spikes, F.** Planning continuing nursing education programs: a guide to the practitioner. (With model.) Journal of Continuing Education in Nursing, 9 (5), Sep/Oct 1978, 5-10.

51 **Studdy, S.** Continuing education. American attitudes. (Report of study tour.) Nursing Focus, 2 (1), Sep 1980, 9-10.

52 **Tibbles, L.** Theories of adult education: implications for developing a philosophy for continuing education in nursing. Journal of Continuing Education in Nursing, 8 (4), Jul/Aug 1977, 25-28.

53 **Tobin, H.** Quality staff development: a must for change and survival. (Comments on American Nurses Association Standard 9. 'The nursing administration provides programs for orientation and continued learning of nursing personnel.') Journal of Nursing Administration, 6 (4), May 1976, 39-42.

54 **United States Veterans Administration. Department of Medicine and Surgery** Program guide: nursing service. Guidelines for continuing education. Washington: the Administration, 1977.

55 **University of Wisconsin—Extension Department of Nursing** Notes on continuing education. Continuing education: some definitions. Journal of Continuing Education in Nursing, 10 (1), Jan/Feb 1979, 36-38.

56 **University of Wisconsin—Extension Department of Nursing** Notes on continuing education. Journal of Continuing Education in Nursing, 11 (1), Jan/Feb 1980, 46-49.

57 **Van Emden, J.** How can further education help nurses? (Need for nurses to have good academic background including liberal and communication studies.) Journal of Community Nursing, 2 (1), Jul 1978, 10-11.

58 **Wise, P.S.Y.** Curriculum development in continuing education: option or necessity? (Need to base it on conceptual or theoretical framework.) Nursing Outlook, 28 (5), May 1980, 318-320.

d OTHER OVERSEAS COUNTRIES

1 **Bazley, M.** Post basic nursing education in technical institutes. (Letter outlining NZ government proposals for restructuring of post basic courses.) New Zealand Nursing Journal, 71 (8), Aug 1978, 25.

2 **Bergman, R. and others** A practicum—a learning experience in integration and change. (Long term project for students in a post basic baccalaureate nursing course at Tel Aviv University, Israel.) Journal of Advanced Nursing, 1 (3), May 1976, 197-208.

3 **Clark, K.M. and Dickinson, G.** Self-directed and other-directed continuing education: a study of nurses' participation. (Survey of nurses in Vancouver.) Journal of Continuing Education in Nursing, 7 (4), Jul/Aug 1976, 16-24.

4 **Duvillard, M.** Continuing education for nursing personnel in Switzerland. International Nursing Review, 28 (1), Jan/Feb 1980, 18-21.

5 **Hugue, H.** Conceptual aspects of continuing education in nursing. Nursing Journal of India, 46 (11), Nov 1975, 252-253.

6 **Key, L.J. and Heidman, M.** Continuing education: easy steps to conference and seminar planning. Canadian Nurse, 74 (6), Jun 1978, 19-23.

7 **Lamp** Postgraduate courses in nursing education in New South Wales. Lamp, 34 (6), Jun 1977, 28-29.

8 **Love, I.D.** Graduation—the end or the beginning? Australian Nurses Journal, 4 (3), Sep 1974, 38-40.

9 **Mellish, J.M.** Continuing education. (Symposium paper.) S.A. Nursing Journal, 43 (9), Sep 1976, 24-27.

10 **Mussallem, H. and Robertson, M.E.** Through the eyes of continuing education—Canada. Journal of Continuing Education in Nursing, 11 (1), Jan/Feb 1980, 41-45.

11 **NEW Zealand Nurses' Association** Position paper on post-basic nursing education in New Zealand. New Zealand Nursing Journal, 71 (10), Oct 1978, 10-11.

12 **New Zealand Nursing Journal** The history of the New Zealand school of advanced nursing studies (formerly the post-graduate school for nurses). (See also page 2.) New Zealand Nursing Journal, 71 (11), Nov 1978, 16-19.

13 **Ogundeyin, W.M.** Effectiveness of self-instructional units in post-basic nursing education: with special reference to the use of nursing care plans unit. (Research study in Nigeria.) Journal of Advanced Nursing, 5 (2), Mar 1980, 169-178.

14 **Popiel, E.S.** Through the eyes of continuing education—the WHO. (With example of its work in Southeast Asia.) Journal of Continuing Education in Nursing, 11 (3), May/Jun 1980, 66-69.

15 **Pratt, R.** Post-basic nursing education—strategies for the development of clinical skills. Australian Nurses Journal, 8 (2), Aug 1978, 37-41, 61.

16 **Warkentin, W.** Continuing nursing education. Nursing Journal of India, 46 (11), Nov 1975, 247-248.

e INSERVICE EDUCATION

1 **Eldridge, R.M.** The role and function of the in-service training officer. (At Leicester Royal Infirmary south west district personnel department.) Nursing Times, 76, 26 Jun 1980, 1143-1144.

2 **Gardner, O.I.** A study of the opinions and preferences of the staff nurse on in-service education. MSc, University of Manchester, Department of Nursing, Oct 1979.

3 **Gatherer, A.** Time for combined in-service training. (Need for inter-disciplinary inservice education.) Nursing Mirror, 147, 23 Nov 1978, 47-48.

4 **Heath, J.** In-service nurse training in England and Wales. Sheffield: NHS Learning Resources Unit, 1980.

5 **Heath, J.** In-service training. 1. In-service training and all that. (Survey of in-service training officers in England and Wales.) Nursing Times, 76, 19 Jun 1980, 1081-1082.

6 **Hyde White, H.** Do-it-yourself in-service training. Nursing staff of the Guy's health district are organising 'on-site' meetings at which they are able to share their particular clinical expertise. Nursing Times, 74, 21/28 Dec 1978, 2117-2118.

7 **Jackson, G.** In-service training for nurses and other professionals. (With reference to the work of the London Boroughs' Training Committee.) Nursing Times, 76, 19 Jun 1980, 1082-1083.

8 **Kennard, Y.** Continuing education. (Report of in-service training department at Pembury Hospital, Kent. Letter.) Nursing Mirror, 145, 8 Sep 1977, 11.

9 **Parfitt, M.** In-service training. (At The Royal Hospital and Home for Incurables, Putney.) Nursing Mirror, 145, 8 Dec 1977, 19-20.

10 **Pearce, Y.** Meeting the challenge. (In-service training programmes in Nottingham's south district.) Nursing Times, 76, 26 Jun 1980, 1142-1143.

11 **Sparrow, E.** Continuing education—imperative for nurses? Nursing Mirror, 145, 18 Aug 1977, 29-30.

12 **Weetman, S. and Mullin, C.** An approach to in-service education. (Includes clinical and management courses.) Nursing Times, 74, 8 Jun 1978, 968-970.

f INSERVICE EDUCATION: OVERSEAS COUNTRIES

1 **Curran, C.L.** What kind of continuing education? A study of the relationship of employment factors to the learning need, and continuing education activities of registered nurses. (In-service education.) Supervisor Nurse, 8 (7), Jul 1977, 72-75.

2 **Del Bueno, D.J.** Evaluation of a continuing education workshop for inservice educators. Journal of Continuing Education in Nursing, 8 (2), Mar-Apr 1977, 13-16.

3 **Del Bueno, D.J.** No more Wednesday matinees. (Making inservice education effective.) Nursing Outlook, 24 (6), Jun 1976, 359-361.

4 **Del Bueno, D.J.** Organizing and staffing the inservice department. Journal of Nursing Administration, 6 (10), Dec 1976, 12-13.

5 **Del Bueno, D.J.** What can nursing service expect from the inservice department? Journal of Nursing Administration, 6 (7), Sep 1976, 14-15.

6 **Howell, B.K.** Guidelines for presenting an inservice. (Method of presenting teaching project.) AORN Journal, 31 (5), Apr 1980, 839, 842-843, 846-847.

7 **Jensen, D.L.** Challenge: a flexible game for hospital training programs. (Use of gaming as in-service education technique.) Supervisor Nurse, 8 (10), Oct 1977, 34-35.

8 **Kase, S.H. and Swenson, B.** Costs of hospital sponsored orientation and inservice

education for Registered Nurses. USDHEW, 1976.

9 LaMonica, E.L. and Karshmer, J.F. Empathy: educating nurses in professional practice. (Inservice training based on groups.) Journal of Nursing Education, 17 (2), Feb 1978, 3-11.

10 Magner, M.M. Inservice education manual for the nursing department. 2nd ed. St. Louis: Catholic Hospital Association, 1978.

11 O'Leary, M.M. and Holzemer, W.L. Evaluation of an inservice program. (To teach venepuncture.) Journal of Nursing Administration, 10 (3), Mar 1980, 21-23.

12 Personett, J.D. The primary educator. (To act as Liaison Officer between the director of inservice education and nursing personnel.) Journal of Nursing Education, 16 (4), Apr 1977, 38-40.

13 Pierce, S.F. and Thompson, D. Changing practice: by choice rather than chance. (Role of in-service education in implementing change at staff nurse level.) Journal of Nursing Administration, 6 (2), Feb 1976, 33-39.

14 Rinaldi, L.A. and Kelly, B. What to do after the audit is done. (In service education programme.) American Journal of Nursing, 77 (2), Feb 1977, 268-269.

15 Sanford, N.D. Teaching strategies for inservice and staff development educators. Journal of Continuing Education in Nursing, 10 (6), Nov/Dec 1979, 5-10.

16 Tapper, M. Evaluation of inservice programs. AORN Journal, 23 (7), Jun 1976, 1307-1308, 1310, 1312, 1314.

17 Warkentin, F.W. Concept of in-service education. Nursing Journal of India, 47 (9), Sep 1976, 217-218.

g ORIENTATION: FROM STUDENT TO NURSE

1 Alhadeff, G. Anxiety in a new graduate. (Includes chart on treating reality shock.) American Journal of Nursing, 79 (4), Apr 1979, 687.

2 Archbold, C.R. Our nurse-interns are a sound investment. (Programme for newly trained nurses to give them clinical skills.) RN Magazine, 40 (9), Sep 1977, 105, 107, 109-110, 112.

3 Atwood, A.H. The mentor in clinical practice: an experienced clinically expert nurse served as role model and guide to improve both staff development of new graduates and patient care. Nursing Outlook, 27 (11), Nov 1979, 714-717.

4 Bell, E.A. Antidote for 'reality shock'. (Ways of preparing students for leadership of nursing teams and planning patient care.) Journal of Nursing Education, 19 (4), Apr 1980, 4-6.

5 Benner, P. and Benner, R.V. The new nurse's work entry: a troubled sponsorship. New York: Tiresias Press, 1979.

6 Carozza, V. and others An experimental educationally sponsored pilot internship program. (To help newly trained nurse improve clinical skills.) Journal of Nursing Education, 17 (9), Nov 1978, 14-20.

7 Carlson, S.E. Notes on continuing education. What is an orientation? Journal of Continuing Education in Nursing, 10 (4), Jul/Aug 1979, 61-63.

8 Choi-Lao, A.T.H. and Logan, M.S. Bridging the gap between education and service. (Scheme at University of Ottawa whereby second-year nursing students attended inservice programmes organised by hospital and community agencies.) Canadian Nurse, 75 (3), Mar 1979, 34-35.

9 Clarke, L.M. and others Transition: a planned clinical learning experience for associate degree students in nursing. (University of Vermont.) Journal of Nursing Education, 15 (4), Jul 1976, 3-6.

10 Coco, C.D. A report on nurse internship programs. (Structured orientation programs for new graduates.) Supervisor Nurse, 7 (12), Dec 1976, 12-16.

11 Del Bueno, D.J. and Quaife, M.C. Two ways to retain staff. Special orientation units pay off. (Columbia—Presbyterian Medical Center, New York.) American Journal of Nursing, 76 (10), Oct 1976, 1629-1630.

12 Dell, M.S. and Griffith, E. A preceptor program for nurses' clinical orientation. Journal of Nursing Administration, 7 (1), Jan 1977, 37-38.

13 Fraser, D.J. Induction training at the Royal Edinburgh Hospital. (A large psychiatric teaching hospital. For all grades of staff including nurses.) Hospital and Health Service Review, 76 (9), Sep 1980, 293-296.

14 Friesen, L. and Conahan, B.J. A clinical preceptor program strategy for new graduate orientation. Journal of Nursing Administration, 10 (4), Apr 1980, 18-23.

15 Guida, F.K. Orientation and training: treating the orientation overload system. (Orientation manual and case study assignment for new nurse employees.) Supervisor Nurse, 8 (10), Oct 1977, 28-31.

16 Harper, J. Coming out: a confrontation with reality. (Newly trained nurse's reality shock.) Canadian Nurse, 72 (7), Jul 1976, 30-31.

17 Holloran, S. Bicultural training for new graduates. (To help transition from student to staff nurse.) Journal of Nursing Administration, 10 (2), Feb 1980, 17-24.

18 Hulse, A.M. Welcome to our hospital. (Orientation of newly appointed qualified nursing staff.) Nursing Times, 74, 25 May 1978, 883-884.

19 Kaelin, M.S. and Bliss, J.B. Evaluating newly employed nurses' skills. (During orientation, supplemented by self-instruction to improve performance as part of staff development.) Nursing Outlook, 27 (5), May 1979, 334-336.

20 Kaye, N.V. Bushong and Simms, S. Externship: a way to bridge the gap. Hospitals and educational institutions can develop training programs to improve the clinical skills of new graduates. Supervisor Nurse, 10 (6), Jun 1979, 14-16, 19, 22.

21 Kibbee, P. Developing a model for implementation of an evaluation component in an orientation program. Journal of Continuing Education in Nursing, 11 (5), Sep/Oct 1980, 25-29.

22 Kjolberg, G.L. and Glynn, K. Orientation—would it work for you? Part 2. Recruiting for the Far North. (Six month orientation program to attract new graduate nurses.) Canadian Nurse, 71, Nov 1975, 25-26.

23 Kopelke, C.E. The nominal group approach as an evaluation tool. (Orientation programme for recently qualified staff nurses at Johns Hopkins Hospital.) Journal of Nursing Administration, 6 (10), Dec 1976, 32-34.

24 Kramer, M. and Schmalenberg, C. Bicultural training and new graduate role transformation. (Training to ease transition from student to worker.) Nursing Digest, 5 (4), Winter 1977, iii-xii, 1-83.

25 Lewison, D. and Gibbons, L.K. Nursing internships: a comprehensive review of the literature. (Programmes designed to ease transition from student to staff nurse.) Journal of Continuing Education in Nursing, 11 (2), Mar/Apr 1980, 32-38.

26 Leffler, M. A hospital orientation program for agency nurses. Supervisor Nurse, 10 (8), Aug 1979, 46, 49-50.

27 Littlejohn, C.E. From staff nurse to supervisor: a plan of development. (Inservice program in a community health agency.) Nursing Outlook, 24 (10), Oct 1976, 618-621.

28 McGrath, B.J. and Koewing, J.R. A clinical preceptorship for new graduate nurses. (Bridging the gap between student and graduate nurse experience.) Journal of Nursing Administration, 8 (3), Mar 1978, 12-18.

29 Martin, P.O. The graduate nurse transition program. (Orientation programme in Glynn-Brunswick Memorial Hospital, Georgia.) Supervisor Nurse, 7 (12), Dec 1976, 18, 20, 22.

30 Nixon, K. and Russell, M. Orientation—would it work for you? Part 1. Creating a learning environment. (Problems of new graduate nurses.) Canadian Nurse, 71 (11), Nov 1975, 24, 26.

31 Peitchinis, J. Orientation programs and the competent nurse. (Results of research study of three kinds of programmes at Red Deer General Hospital, Calgary.) Dimensions in Health Service, 55 (6), Jun 1978, 12-13.

32 Pohutsky, L. An orientation plan for nurses. Supervisor Nurse, 10 (10), Oct 1979, 23, 25-26.

22 Rantz, M.J. A modular approach to unit orientation. Supervisor Nurse, 11 (6), Jun 1980, 48-51.

34 RN Magazine Reality shock can be handled on the job. (Study of effect of two types of inservice training by M. Kramer, author of 'Reality Shock'.) RN Magazine, 40 (6), Jun 1977, 11.

35 Schmalenberg, C. and Kramer, M. Coping with reality shock: the voices of experience. Wakefield, Mass.: Nursing Resources, 1979.

36 Schmalenberg, C.E. and Kramer, M. Dreams and reality: where do they meet?

(Solutions to the problem of 'reality shock' seen in newly qualified nurses from colleges.) Journal of Nursing Administration, 6 (5), Jun 1976, 35-43.

37 Scipien, G.M. and Pasternack, S.B. Creating more confident baccalaureate graduates. (Course of independent study to aid transition from student to staff nurse.) American Journal of Nursing, 77 (5), May 1977, 818-820.

38 Simpson, I.H. and others From student to nurse: a longitudinal study of socialization. Cambridge: Cambridge University Press, 1979. (American Sociological Association, A. and C. Rose monograph series.)

39 Tobin, H.M. Orientation programs for new nurses: organisation essential for effective performance of new nurses. (General discussion with staff development process model.) AORN Journal, 28 (5), Nov 1978, 952, 954, 958-960, 964, 966.

40 University of Wisconsin—Extension Department of Nursing Notes on continuing education. Individualizing the orientation of staff nurses. Journal of Continuing Education in Nursing, 11 (2), Mar/Apr 1980, 54-59.

41 Weiss, S.J. and Ramsey, E. An interagency internship: a key to transitional adaptation. (Six hospitals share joint project to assist in the role transition from student to graduate nurse.) Journal of Nursing Administration, 7 (8), Oct 1977, 36-42.

42 Wong, J. The inability to transfer classroom learning to clinical nursing practice: a learning problem and its remedial plan. Journal of Advanced Nursing, 4 (2), Mar 1979, 161-168.

h POST-BASIC CLINICAL COURSES

1 Bristow, S. Career opportunities. Joint Board courses. Nursing Times, 72, 10 Jun 1976, 890-891.

2 Brown, A. Beyond a background of basics. (History and current role of Joint Board of Clinical Nursing Studies.) Nursing Mirror, 150, 20 Mar 1980, 7.

3 Committee for Clinical Nursing Studies Report. Edinburgh: The Committee, 1976.

4 Cullinan, J. The approach to postbasic teaching. A workshop for ward nurses. (Account of JBCNS workshop at Westfield College.) Nursing Times, 75, 26 Apr 1979, 693.

5 Darling, V.H. Education—a continuing concern. (Work of Joint Board of Clinical Nursing Studies.) Nursing Focus, 1 (9), Jun 1980, 405-407.

6 Darling, V.H. Through the eyes of continuing education—England and Wales. (Work of Joint Board of Clinical Nursing Studies.) Journal of Continuing Education in Nursing, 10 (5), Sep/Oct 1979, 49-51.

7 Dopson, L. Postbasic development. (Report on recent JBCNS conference on post-basic education.) Nursing Times, 75, 13 Dec 1979, 2148.

8 Dunn, A. Research at the Joint Board. (Work of five researchers at JBCNS.) Nursing Times, 75, 13 Sep 1979, 1562-1563.

9 Edmonds, G. and others The specialist nurse teacher. (New responsibilities for clinical teachers with introduction of JBCNS courses.) Nursing Times, 75, 13 Sep 1979, 1586-1587.

10 European Nurse Researchers Second conference: collaborative research and its implementation in nursing. Copenhagen: Danish Nurses' Organization, 1980.

11 Finn, B. JBCNS short courses. Nursing Times, 72, 29 Apr 1976, 646.

12 Gitterman, G. and Goering, P. Through the looking glass. (Education and practice brought together through nurse tutor updating clinical skills.) Canadian Nurse, 72 (10), Oct 1976, 44-47.

13 Hills, J. and Harris, M. Network analysis for new course planning. (Use of network analysis to plan a course outlined in the Joint Board of Clinical Nursing Studies curriculum no.176 for Operative Department Nursing.) Nursing Times, 72 (20), 20 May 1976, Occ. papers, 73-76.

14 Joint Board of Clinical Nursing Studies Course evaluation package. JBCNS, (1978.) (Occasional publication no.2.)

15 Joint Board of Clinical Nursing Studies Not just observers. The relevance of the Joint Board of Clinical Nursing Studies courses for overseas nurse learners discussed at a weekend workshop organised by the United Kingdom Council for Overseas Student Affairs. Nursing Times, 72, 25 Nov 1976, 1929.

16 Joint Board of Clinical Nursing Studies Notes on the outline curricula published by the Joint Board of Clinical Nursing Studies. The Board, 1978.

17 Joint Board of Clinical Nursing Studies Post-basic/postgraduate courses in specialist aspects of clinical nursing: a guidance document for centres accepting nurses from overseas. JBCNS, 1977.

18 Joint Board of Clinical Nursing Studies Third report. The Board, 1978.

19 Joint Board of Clinical Nursing Studies Review of the work of the Joint Board of Clinical Nursing Studies, 1970-1980. JBCNS, 1980.

20 Young, P. Towards clinical excellence. Day conference held by the Joint Board of Clinical Nursing Studies. Nursing Mirror, 144, 5 May 1977, 39-41.

27 NURSING RESEARCH

a GENERAL AND UNITED KINGDOM

1 Atkinson, F.I. Research summer schools: an evaluation. (Held at Nursing Research Unit, University of Edinburgh.) Nursing Times, 75, 15 Feb 1979, Occ. papers, 17-20; 22 Feb 1979, Occ. papers, 21-24.

2 Brown, M.L. Nursing research; delights and difficulties. (Using a study of procedures carried out in the wards by students at Foresterhill College, Aberdeen, as an example.) Nursing Times, 73, 7 Apr 1977, Occ. papers, 45-48; 14 Apr 1977, Occ. papers, 49-52.

3 Campbell, C. and others Research. (Development of research mindedness in the graduate nurse. Symposium paper.) Nursing Mirror, 144, 10 Feb 1977, 52-53.

4 Cang, S. Janforum. Nursing research: problems of aim, method and content. Journal of Advanced Nursing, 4 (4), Jul 1979, 453-458.

5 Cartwright, A. Professionals as responders: variations in and effects of response rates to questionnaires, 1961-77. (By director of Institute for Social Studies in Medical Care. Includes HVs, district nurses and midwives.) British Medical Journal, 2, 18 Nov 1978, 1419-1421.

6 Cheadle, J. Presenting your research. (Writing journal articles.) Nursing Mirror, 146, 4 May 1978, 26-28.

7 Clark, J. Nursing research in Wales. (Report on Rcn conference in Aberystwyth.) Nursing Mirror, 145, 25 Aug 1977, 7-8.

8 Clark, J.M. and Hockey, L. Research for nursing: a guide for the enquiring nurse. Aylesbury: HM & M Publishers, 1979.

9 Clark, J.M. and Hockey, L. Research for nursing. (Interview by · A. Dunn with Jill MacLeod Clark and Lisbeth Hockey, joint authors of new book on nursing research.) Nursing Times, 75, 6 Sep 1979, 1517-1518.

10 Cormack, D.F.S. Obtaining access to data sources: an exploration of method, problems and possible solutions. (With reference to author's research in Scottish psychiatric hospitals using Flanagan's Critical Incident Technique.) Journal of Advanced Nursing, 5 (4), Jul 1980, 357-370.

11 Cox, C. The Nursing Education Research Unit. The early days. A short history, and summary of the plans for the future. (Chelsea College, University of London.) Nursing Times, 75, 3 May 1979, 747-749.

12 Crow, R. Research into nursing practice. (Interview with Dr Rosemary Crow, director of DHSS Nursing Practice Research Unit at Northwick Park Hospital by C. Kratz.) Nursing Times, 75, 1 Nov 1979, 1875.

13 Davis, A.J. Research as an inactional situation: objectivity in the interview. International Journal of Nursing Studies, 17 (4), 1980, 215-220.

14 DEPARTMENT of Health and Social Security Nursing research fellowships and secondments. (Reprinted from DHSS Report and Handbook of Research and Development 1979.) Nursing Times, 76, 4 Dec 1980, Occ. papers, 127-128.

15 EUROPEAN Nurse Researchers First conference: collaborative research and its implementation in nursing. Utrecht, Netherlands: National Hospital Institute, 1979.

16 EUROPEAN Nurse Researchers Second conference: collaborative research and its implementation in nursing. Copenhagen: Danish Nurses' Organization, 1980.

17 Gott, M. Nursing research: how to plan and implement a project. Nursing Times, 75, 28 Jun 1979, 1089-1092.

18 Hall, D.J. 'What nurse don't see, she don't worry about', or the use of observation in hospital research. Nursing Times, 74, 7 Dec 1978, Occ. papers, 137-140.

19 **Hockey, L.** Clinical research through partnership. (Nursing Mirror Forum 1976.) Nursing Mirror, 142, 1 Apr 1976, 49-57.

20 **Hockey, L.** The Edinburgh University's nursing research unit: the first four years. Journal of Advanced Nursing, 1 (6), Nov 1976, 437-442.

21 **Hockey, L.** Expanding the nursing horizon. (Need to extend knowledge basis of nursing through scientific research and her hopes for change by the year 2000.) Nursing Mirror, 149, 25 Oct 1979, 32-35.

22 **Hoult, B.** Oiling the wheels. (Administrative procedures necessary to get nursing research project organised.) Nursing Mirror, 146, 4 May 1978, 25-26.

23 **House, V.G.** Evaluation research: the need for multiple criteria. (Identification of criteria for evaluating experimental training courses developed by the GNC Research Unit.) Journal of Advanced Nursing, 2 (1), Jan 1977, 15-20.

24 **INTERNATIONAL** Council of Nurses ICN guidelines on nursing research for National Nurses Associations. International Nursing Review, 23 (4), Jul/Aug 1976, 121.

25 **INTERNATIONAL** Council of Nurses ICN statement on nursing research. International Nursing Review, 23 (4), Jul/Aug 1976, 122. Nursing research should be 'socially relevant'. Statement agreed by CNR at Tokyo congress. Nursing Times, 73, 23 Jun 1977, 932. See also Journal of Advanced Nursing, 3 (1), Jan 1978, 88-90.

26 **Journal of Advanced Nursing** Royal College of Nursing Research Society. (Origins and development.) Journal of Advanced Nursing, 2 (5), Sep 1977, 547.

27 **Kilty, J.M.** Can nursing research learn from educational research? International Journal of Nursing Studies, 13 (2), 1976, 96-102.

28 **Lancaster, A.** The nursing research liaison officer scheme. Nursing Times, 73, 10 Nov 1977, 1759-1761.

29 **Lancaster, A.** Towards a research-based profession. (Objectives necessary for research-based teaching and practice.) Nursing Times, 72, 22 Apr 1976, 632-633; 29 Apr 1976, 672-673.

30 **Lelean, S.** Euro research must be for the patient's good. (Report on conference in Netherlands of nurse researchers from 16 European countries.) Nursing Mirror, 148, 3 May 1979, 30-31.

31 **Lelean, S.R.** Research in nursing: an overview of DHSS initiatives in developing research in nursing. (Includes details of the Index of Nursing Research.) Nursing Times, 76, 17 Jan 1980, Occ. papers, 5-8; 24 Jan 1980, Occ. papers, 9-12.

32 **MacDonald, I. and Otto, S.** A way to ensure research is meaningful to the practitioner. (Action research projects with mental handicap nurses and social work agencies.) Health and Social Service Journal, 88, 31 Mar 1978, 366-368.

33 **McFarlane, J.K., Baroness McFarlane of Llandaff** Nursing as a research-based profession. (Work of Manchester University's Department of Nursing Studies to prepare nurses

for research.) Nursing Times, 76, 15 May 1980, Occ. papers, 57-59.

34 **McFarlane, J.K., Baroness** The role of research and the development of nursing theory. Journal of Advanced Nursing, 1 (6), Nov 1976, 443-451.

35 **MacIlwaine, H.** How to get started. (In nursing research: doing a literature search, designing and budgeting.) Nursing Mirror, 146, 4 May 1978, 23.

36 **MANCHESTER** University. Department of Nursing The research process. (Symposium.) Nursing Mirror, 146, 4 May 1978, 23-28.

37 **Mendez, M.A.** Learning about research. (With reference to the remedial professions and links with nursing research interest groups.) British Journal of Occupational Therapy, 42 (6), Jun 1979, 133.

38 **Milne, M.A.** Commencing research—the difficulties. (Personal account.) Health Visitor, 52 (5), May 1979, 180, 182-183, 185.

39 **Milne, M.A.** Research—a learning experience: personal look at the emotions engendered and the qualities which come to the fore when research is undertaken. Nursing Times, 75, 29 Mar 1979, Occ. papers, 40.

40 **Myco, F.** A survey on nursing research in relation to the nursing profession in Northern Ireland. New University of Ulster, 1979. (New University of Ulster nursing studies.)

41 **Norton, D.** Research at work in a region. (Research nurse scheme in SW Thames region with job description of SNO/research.) Nursing Times, 76, 10 Jan 1980, 59-61.

42 **Nursing Research Advisory Group** Report of study day, September 1976. Edinburgh: The Group, 1976.

43 **Nursing Times** Is nursing research-based? (Views of 18 student nurses at Pilgrim Hospital, Boston, who had completed a research appreciation course.) Nursing Times, 76, 11 Dec 1980, 2180.

44 **Nursing Times** Understanding research. (With a list of research interest groups, and information about research appreciation courses.) Nursing Times, 72 (22), 3 Jun 1976, Occ. papers, 77-79.

45 **Richardson, A.M.** Some thoughts on research and the nursing profession. (Examples of research findings which have not been applied in nursing practice.) NATNews, 17 (4), Apr 1980, 10-11.

46 **Roberts, I.** Research and the health visitor. Health Visitor, 49 (11), Nov 1976, 354-357.

47 **Roper, N.** Justification and use of research in nursing. Journal of Advanced Nursing, 2 (4), Jul 1977, 365-371.

48 **Rubin, R. and Erickson, F.** Research in clinical nursing. (Using process recording of patient behaviour as data.) Journal of Advanced Nursing, 3 (2), Mar 1978, 131-144.

49 **SCOTTISH** National Nursing and Midwifery Consultative Committee. Working Group A new concept of nursing 2. Research. (Especially into nursing practice and skills.) Nursing Times, 72 (15), 15 Apr 1976, Occ. papers, 53-56.

50 **Smith, J.P.** Editorial. (On lack of implementation of research in nursing, with reference to Rcn research series.) Journal of Advanced Nursing, 2 (5), Sep 1977, 441-442.

51 **Smith, J.P.** Is the nursing profession really research-based? Journal of Advanced Nursing, 4 (3), May 1979, 319-325.

52 **Trenchard, H.** The research nurse. (Role of research nurse at district level in Wandsworth and East Merton Teaching District.) Nursing Times, 76, 10 Jan 1980, 61-63.

53 **UNIVERSITY** of Edinburgh. Department of Nursing Studies Nursing Research Unit biennial report October 1973-December 1975. The Unit, 1976.

54 **Voss, P.** Matter of fact. (A critique of the Rcn research project 'The study of nursing care.') Nursing Times, 72, 1/8 Jan 1976, 9.

55 **Wilson, K.J.W.** Research and nursing. NATNews, 13 (5), Jul 1976, 18-19.

56 **Young, P.** History of the Department of Nursing Studies at the University of Edinburgh, scene of the Second Nursing Mirror Forum to be held on Friday March 26. Nursing Mirror, 142, 11 Mar 1976, 40.

b UNITED STATES

1 **Abdellah, F.G.** U.S. Public Health Service's contribution to nursing research—past, present, future. Nursing Research, 26 (4), Jul/Aug 1977, 244-249.

2 **Advances in Nursing Science** ANS open forum. (Four contributors' views on current priorities in nursing research.) Advances in Nursing Science, 1 (2), Jan 1979, 79-90.

3 **American Nurses' Association** Reference resources for research and continuing education in nursing: papers presented at a 1976 ANA Convention Program... Kansas City: ANA, 1977.

4 **American Nurses' Association** Research in nursing: towards a science of health care. Kansas City: ANA, 1976.

5 **American Nurses' Association. Commission on Nursing Research** Nursing research: synopses of selected clinical studies. Kansas City: ANA, 1979.

6 **American Nurses' Association. Commission on Nursing Research** Preparation of nurses for participation in research. Kansas City: ANA, 1976.

7 **Bloch, D. and others** The Nursing Research Grants Program of the Division of Nursing, U.S. Public Health Service. Journal of Nursing Administration, 8 (3), Mar 1978, 40-45.

8 **Brand, K.P. and Martinson, I.M.** Evolution of a nursing research center. (University of Minnesota School of Nursing.) Nursing Outlook, 24, Nov 1976, 704-707.

9 **Campos, R.G.** Securing information on funding sources for nursing research (in the United States.) Journal of Nursing Administration, 6 (8), Oct 1976, 16-18.

10 **Carnegie, M.E.** Quo vadis? (Final editorial outlining trends in nursing research as reflected

in the journal over the last five years.) Nursing Research, 27 (5), Sep/Oct 1978, 277-278.

11 De Tornyay, R. Nursing research—the road ahead. (Summary of articles in Nursing Research's anniversary year issue and future directions outlined.) Nursing Research, 26 (6), Nov/Dec 1977, 404-407.

12 Elliott, J.E. and others Update on nursing research in the West. (Work of Western Council of Higher Education in Nursing.) Nursing Research, 29 (3), May/Jun 1980, 184-188.

13 Glass, H.P. Research: an international perspective. (Historical perspectives, current activities and future needs.) Nursing Research, 26 (3), May/Jun 1977, 230-236.

14 Gortner, S.R. Nursing research: out of the past and into the future. Nursing Research, 29 (4), Jul/Aug 1980, 204-207.

15 Gortner, S.R. and Nahm, H. An overview of nursing research in the United States. Nursing Research, 26 (1), Jan-Feb 1977, 10-33.

16 Gramse, C.A. Progress and research in nursing. Journal of Continuing Education in Nursing, 9 (5), Sep/Oct 1978, 30-34.

17 Henderson, V. We've 'come a long way' but what of the direction? (Review of development of nursing research for 25th anniversary issue of Journal.) Nursing Research, 26 (3), May/Jun 1977, 163-164.

18 Hoskins, C.N. Nursing research: its direction and future. Nursing Forum, 18 (2), 1979, 175-186.

19 Hyde, A. The American Nurses' Foundation's contribution to research in nursing. Nursing Research, 26 (3), May/Jun 1977, 225-227.

20 Jacox, A. Strategies to promote nursing research. Nursing Research, 29 (4), Jul/Aug 1980, 213-217.

21 Johnson, W.L. Research programs of the National League for Nursing. Nursing Research, 26 (3), May/Jun 1977, 172-176.

22 Kalisch, P.A. Weavers of scientific patient care. Development of nursing research in the U.S. Armed Forces. Nursing Research, 26 (4), Jul/Aug 1977, 253-271.

23 Kelly, D. What is research in nursing? Editorial. Supervisor Nurse, 8 (4), Apr 1977, 9.

24 Krueger, J.C. and others Nursing research: development, collaboration and utilization. Germantown: Aspen Systems Corporation, 1978.

25 McElmurry, B. Illinois: state-wide council for nursing research. (Expression of the Illinois Nurses' Association research services and activities at the state level.) International Journal of Nursing Studies, 15 (1), 1978, 17-22.

26 Lindeman, C.A. Delphi survey of priorities in clinical nursing research. (A research technique using a series of questionnaires to obtain a consensus of opinion from a group of experts.) Nursing Research, 24 (6), Nov-Dec 1975, 432-441.

27 Lindeman, C.A. and Krueger, J.C. Increasing the quality, quantity and use of nursing research. (Western Interstate Commission for Higher Education (WICHE). Regional programme for Nursing Research Development set up in 1971.) Nursing Outlook, 25 (7), Jul 1977, 450-454.

28 Minckley, B.B. Nursing research and regionalization in the Midwest. Nursing Research, 29 (3), May/Jun 1980, 193-198.

29 Nahm, H. and Gortner, S.R. What has been the impact of the social and biologic sciences and mental health on the development of nursing research? Nursing Research, 26 (1), Jan-Feb 1977, 65-66.

30 Notter, L.E. The case for nursing research. Nursing Outlook, 23 (12), Dec 1975, 760-763.

31 Nursing Research The Editor's report—1976. Nursing Research, 25 (1), Jan-Feb 1976, 3.

32 Nursing Research Not for nurse researchers only. (Development of nursing research conference in U.S.A. from 1957.) Nursing Research, 26 (5), Sep/Oct 1977, 323.

33 Nursing Research Nursing research centers on the rise. (Their development in the USA from 1953.) Nursing Research, 27 (4), Jul/Aug 1978, 211.

34 Perloff, E. A comparative study of authorship and subject matter of articles in Nursing Research. (During its 25-year history.) Nursing Research, 26 (6), Nov/Dec 1977, 471.

35 Schlotfeldt, R.M. Nursing research: reflection of values. (Progress in commitment to research since 1952.) Nursing Research, 26 (1), Jan-Feb 1977, 4-9.

36 See, E.M. The ANA and research in nursing. (ANA's contributions over the last 15 years.) Nursing Research, 26 (3), May/Jun 1977, 165-171.

37 Sills, G.M. Research in the field of psychiatric nursing 1952-1977. Nursing Research, 26 (3), May/Jun 1977, 201-207.

38 Spector, A.E. Regional action and nursing research in the South. (Through the Southern Regional Education Board, Atlanta, Georgia.) Nursing Research, 26 (4), Jul/Aug 1977, 272-276.

39 Wechsler, H. and Kibrick, A.K. editors Explorations in nursing research. New York: Human Sciences Press, 1979.

40 Werley, H.H. Nursing research in perspective. (Review of progress in U.S.A.) International Nursing Review, 24 (3), May/Jun 1977, 75-83.

OTHER COUNTRIES

41 Aggarwal, K.C. Research in nursing—2. It's high time to act now. (Importance of nursing involvement in health care research.) Nursing Journal of India, 67 (12), Dec 1976, 293-294.

42 Aggarwal, K.C. Waiting for a miracle? (Slow progression of nursing research in India due to a reliance on Western ideas.) Nursing Journal of India, 57 (10), Oct 1976, 248-249.

43 Bergman, R. Overview of nursing research in Israel. New Zealand Nursing Journal, 70 (9), Sep 1977, 3-5.

44 Canadian Nurse First national survey identifies nurse researchers in Canada. (In 1976.) Canadian Nurse, 73 (12), Dec 1977, 12.

45 Farrell, M. and Bhaduri, A. What is nursing research? Nursing Journal of India, 68 (5), May 1977, 133-134.

46 Gray, G. Nursing research: is it justified? Australian Nurses Journal, 9 (3), Sep 1979, 41-43, 57.

47 Johnson, M.N. and Okunade, A.O. Roles that nurses in the community can play in nursing research. Nigerian Nurse, 7 (3), Jul-Sep 1975, 28-30.

48 NATIONAL Conference on Nursing Research in Education Bright future predicted for nursing research. (Report.) Canadian Nurse, 72 (1), Jan 1976, 6.

49 Pybus, M. Improving patient care through nursing research. (With list of nursing research studies in New Zealand.) New Zealand Nursing Journal, 71 (11), Nov 1978, 3-4.

50 Storch, J. and others Nurses involved in research. (Study of Canadian nurses in 1976.) Dimensions in Health Service, 56 (1), Jan 1979, 34-35.

51 Storch, J. and others Report on Canadian survey for nurses engaged in research in 1976. Edmonton: University of Alberta, 1977.

52 Williamson, S.B. The meaning and value of research. S.A. Nursing Journal, 44 (12), Dec 1977, 18-21; 45 (1), Jan 1978, 11-14.

c ETHICS

1 Armiger, B. Ethics of nursing research: profile, principles, perspective. Nursing Research, 26 (5), Sep/Oct 1977, 330-341.

2 Bishop, V. Taking a stand on ethics. (Nurse's role in clinical research with reference to the Helsinki Declaration.) Nursing Mirror, 149, 2 Aug 1979, 22-23.

3 Creighton, H. Legal concerns of nursing research. Nursing Research, 26 (5), Sep/Oct 1977, 337-341.

4 Daniel, W.W. Research Q. and A. Q. What are values? How are they calculated? How are they related to levels of significance? Nursing Research, 26 (4), Jul/Aug 1977, 304-306.

5 Farrell, M. and Bhaduri, A. Research orientations in nursing—IX. A question of ethics. Nursing Journal of India, 49 (5), May 1978, 103-104.

6 Faulkner, A. Nursing as a research-based profession—some ethical issues. (Abridged version of prize-winning essay.) Nursing Focus, 1 (12), Aug 1980, 476-479, 481.

7 Kratz, C. The ethics of research. (Symposium on moral dilemmas in nursing.) Nursing Mirror, 145, 21 Jul 1977, 17-20.

8 May, K.A. The nurse as researcher: impediment to informed consent? Nursing Outlook, 27 (1), Jan 1979, 36-39.

9 McShea, M.M. Clinical judgement: an ethical issue. (In relation to psychiatric nursing research and/or practice.) Journal of Psychiatric Nursing and Mental Health Services, 16 (3), Mar 1978, 52-55.

10 Morris, J.J. and others Applying ethical standards to nursing practice. (Letter outlining authors' reasons for not going ahead with planned research study in order to protect patients.) Nursing Research, 27 (2), Mar/Apr 1978, 113.

11 NEW Zealand Nurses' Association Ethics of nursing research. (Prepared by the Steering Committee of the New Zealand Nurses' Association nursing research special interest section.) New Zealand Nursing Journal, 69 (3), Mar 1976, 2.

12 Nursing Research Research Q and A. Q: How is the topic of protection of human subjects taught in undergraduate and graduate nursing research courses? (Rights of patients and ethics of research.) Nursing Research, 27 (5), Sep/Oct 1978, 328-329.

13 Royal College of Nursing Ethics related to research in nursing: guidance for nurses involved in research or any study/project concerning human subjects. Rcn, 1977.

d METHODS

1 AORN Journal Research process is mode of thinking in daily activities. (A comparison of the 'research process' with the 'nursing process.') AORN Journal, 23 (5), Apr 1976, 798-799.

2 Artinian, B.M. and Anderson, N. Guidelines for the identification of researchable problems. Journal of Nursing Education, 19 (4), Apr 1980, 54-58.

3 Batey, M.V. Conceptualization: knowledge and logic guiding empirical research. Nursing Research, 26 (5), Sep/Oct 1977, 324-329.

4 Brand, K.L. and Martinson, I.M. What facilities and equipment are needed for nursing research? How are they identified? Nursing Research, 26 (2), Mar-Apr 1977, 141-143.

5 Brink, P.J. and Wood, M.J. Basic steps in planning nursing research: from question to proposal. North Scituate, Mass.: Duxbury, 1978.

6 Daniel, W.W. and Longest, B.B. Statistical sampling and the nurse researcher. (In relation to survey sampling.) Nursing Forum, 16 (1), 1977, 36-55.

7 Deets, C.A. Methodological concerns in the testing of nursing interventions. Advances in Nursing Science, 2 (2), Jan 1980, 1-11.

8 Diers, D. Research in nursing practice. Philadelphia: Lippincott, 1979.

9 Donaldson, S.K. and Crowley, D.M. The discipline of nursing. (Claim that to qualify as nursing research, studies must be undertaken from a nursing perspective.) Nursing Outlook, 26 (2), Feb 1978, 113-120.

10 Downs, F.S. and Fleming, J.W. Issues in nursing research. New York: Appleton-Century-Crofts, 1979.

11 Downs, F.S. and Newman, M.A. A source book of nursing research. 2nd ed. Philadelphia: Davis, 1977.

12 Farrell, M. and Bhaduri, A. Research orientation in nursing. Nursing Journal of India. 3. Overview of research process. 68 (8), Aug 1977, 208-209, 211.

4. If only I had a problem. . .(Defining a topic for research.) 68 (9), Sep 1977, 220-221.
6. The fundamentals of sampling technique. 68 (11), Nov 1977, 278-279.
8. How to go about data collection. 69 (2), Feb 1977, 37-38.

13 Farrell, M. and Bhaduri, A. The three approaches to research. (Historical, survey and experimental.) Nursing Journal of India, 68 (10), Oct 1977, 245-246.

14 Fawcett, J. The relationship between theory and research: a double helix. Advances in Nursing Science, 1 (1), Oct 1978, 49-62.

15 Felton, G. and McLaughlin, F.E. The collaborative process in generating a nursing research study. Nursing Research, 25 (2), Mar-Apr 1976, 115-120.

16 Field, M. Causal inferences in behavioral research. Advances in Nursing Science, 2 (1), Oct 1979, 81-93.

17 Flaskerud, J.H. Use of vignettes to elicit responses toward broad concepts. (In research. Short, compact descriptions which exemplify the concept.) Nursing Research, 28 (4), Jul/Aug 1979, 210-212.

18 Fox, D.J. Fundamentals of research in nursing. 3rd ed. New York: Appleton-Century-Crofts, 1976.

19 Geden, E.A. and Taylor, S.G. Research Q and A. Q. How do problems encountered in the preliminary stage of research affect a study? Nursing Research, 27 (2), Mar/Apr 1978, 130-132.

20 Gorton, J.V. Parlay those everyday ideas into research dollars. (Writing a research proposal and obtaining funds for research projects.) RN Magazine, 40 (6), 15 Jun 1977, 65, 67-70.

21 Jaspen, N. Research Q and A. (On acceptability of using parametric inferential procedures for analysis of ordinal data.) Nursing Research, 26 (6), Nov/Dec 1977, 470.

22 Lanahan, C.C. Pragmatics of research. Journal of Midwifery, 21 (3), 1976, 14-18.

23 Murphy, J.R. Preparing research data for computerization. American Journal of Nursing, 79 (5), May 1979, 954-956.

24 Notter, L.E. Essentials of nursing research. 2nd ed. Tavistock, 1979.

25 Pavlovich, N. Nursing research: a learning guide. St. Louis: Mosby, 1978.

26 Polit, D.F. and Hungler, B. Nursing research: principles and methods. Philadelphia: Lippincott, 1978.

27 Rains, B. Sounding board: writing a master's thesis. Nursing Outlook, 28 (11), Nov 1980, 685-687.

28 Renoliel, J.Q. The interaction between theory and research. Nursing Outlook, 25 (2), Feb 1977, 108-113.

29 Sweeney, M.A. and Olivieri, P. 'Driving' nurses to research. (Workshop to enable nurses to become comfortable with research.) Nurse Educator, 3 (4), Jul/Aug 1978, 7-13.

30 Verhonick, P.J. editor Nursing research II. Boston: Little, Brown and Co., 1977.

31 Verhonick, P.J. and Seaman, C.C. Research methods for undergraduate students in nursing. New York: Appleton-Century-Crofts, 1978.

32 Warren, M.D. Aide-mémoire for preparing a protocol. (Research proposal.) British Medical Journal, 1, 6 May 1978, 1195-1196.

e EDUCATION

1 Ackerman, W.B. The place of research in the master's program. Nursing Outlook, 24 (12), Dec 1976, 754-758.

2 Birch, J. Nursing should be a research-based profession. (Survey of learners and tutors showed that very few tutors used research findings in teaching.) Nursing Times, 75, 20/27 Dec 1979, Occ. papers, 135-136.

3 Brogan, D.R. An integrated approach to training in research methodology and statistics. (To master's degree students in a U.S.A. university.) International Journal of Nursing Studies, 17 (2), 1980, 101-106.

4 Brownlee, E.B.I. The novelty of research—challenging the post basic student. S.A. Nursing Journal, 44 (3), Mar 1977, 21.

5 Burkhalter, P.K. and Kim, H.T. The honors program approach to undergraduate research in nursing. (University of Hawaii.) Journal of Nursing Education, 15 (1), Jan 1976, 21-25.

6 Cahall, J.B. Research: a vital component throughout the nursing curriculum. (Report of course.) Journal of Nursing Education, 19 (4), Apr 1980, 19-27.

7 Clarke, M. Research in nurse education. (Review of research projects in nurse education over the last two decades.) Nursing Times, 73, 17 Feb 1977, Occ. papers, 25-28.

8 Derwinski, B. and others Fostering the research attitude. (Nursing research course for baccalaureate students at Montana State University.) Journal of Nursing Education, 18 (7), Sep 1979, 23-26.

9 Derwinski, B. and others Research Q. and A. Q: How can research be taught to undergraduate nursing students? Nursing Research, 27 (4), Jul/Aug 1978, 264.

10 Diers, D. The role of continuing education in promoting research in practice. Journal of Continuing Education in Nursing, 8 (3), May/Jun 1977, 54-62.

11 Fawcett, J. Integrating research into the faculty workload. (Nurse teachers in universities.) Nursing Outlook, 27 (4), Apr 1979, 259-262.

12 Fuller, E.O. How does the doctorally prepared nurse develop into a productive researcher? Nursing Research, 25 (2), Mar-Apr 1976, 110-111.

13 Hill, M.S. and others Educational research in nursing—an overview. (Of U.S.A. research.) International Nursing Review, 27 (1), Jan/Feb 1980, 10-17.

14 Hodgman, E.C. Student research in

service agencies. (Problems of providing access to clinical settings for students doing nursing research projects.) Nursing Outlook, 26 (9), Sep 1978, 558-565.

15 Humphrey, P. and Woods, N.F. Involving undergraduate students in faculty research. Journal of Nursing Education, 19 (5), May 1980, 4-6.

16 Joint Board of Clinical Nursing Studies The research objective in Joint Board courses: an introductory guide. JBCNS, 1977. (Occasional publications no.1.)

17 Journal of Advanced Nursing Objectives of undergraduate/baccalaureate nursing education; an international review. Journal of Advanced Nursing, 2 (4), Jul 1977, 405-413.

18 Kilty, J.M. and Potter, F.W. Nursing education research management: establishing priorities and optimizing the use of resources: a methodology. (A research method illustrated by the University of Surrey study of the Midwife Teachers' Diploma.) Journal of Advanced Nursing, 1 (2), Mar 1976, 163-172.

19 King's Fund Centre Research and nursing education (report of a meeting 12th December 1975.) The Centre, 1976, KFC 76/72.

20 Margolius, F.R. and others Research committees in nursing programs. Findings of this survey reveal the scope and direction of faculty and students' activities in conducting research in schools of nursing. Nursing Outlook, 26 (7), Jul 1978, 442-443.

21 Mauger, B.L. and Huggins, K. Developing and implementing collaborative nursing education research in the South. (Project of the Southern Regional Education Board and the Council on Collegiate Education for Nursing.) Nursing Research, 29 (3), May/Jun 1980, 189-192.

22 Noble, M.A. Teaching clinical research: idealism versus realism. Journal of Nursing Education, 19 (2), Feb 1980, 34-37.

23 Nursing Research Research Q. and A. Q: What guidelines should be followed in critically evaluating research reports? Nursing Research, 28 (2), Mar/Apr 1979, 120-126.

24 O'Grady, J. and Haukenes, E. Teaching research methods to undergraduates in nursing — learning by doing. Journal of Nursing Education, 17 (8), Oct 1978, 48-52.

25 Reed, J.C. and Cooley, S. Teaching research by the 'Tell', 'Show' and 'Do' process. Journal of Nursing Education, 15 (1), Jan 1976, 18-20.

26 Rinehart, J.M. One way to learn the research process: when graduate students conduct small studies using each other as subjects. Nursing Outlook, 24 (1), Jan 1976, 38-40.

27 Schare, B.L. An undergraduate research experience. Conducting their own study helps students to recognise the relevance of scientific inquiry to practice. Nursing Outlook, 25 (3), Mar 1977, 178-180.

28 Schlotfeldt, R.M. The professional doctorate: rationale and characteristics. Nursing Outlook, 26 (5), May 1978, 302-311.

29 Sherman, K.M. and Kirsch, A.K. Research

Q. and A. Q: Can nursing educators deal effectively with nursing students' difficulty in critiquing nursing research articles? (Includes guidelines for the critical reading of research publications.) Nursing Research, 27 (1), Jan/Feb 1978, 69-70.

30 Solomons, H.C. and others How faculty members spend their time. (Analysis of workload showed little time devoted to research.) Nursing Outlook, 28 (3), Mar 1980, 160-165.

31 Spector, N.C. and Bleeks, S.L. Strategies to improve students' attitudes to research. Nursing Outlook, 28 (5), May 1980, 300-304.

32 Thomas, B. and Price, M.M. Research preparation in baccalaureate nursing education. Nursing Research, 29 (4), Jul/Aug 1980, 259-261.

33 Treece, E.W. Articulation between courses in nursing research: the need and the process. (Value of a course in nursing research as a part of all educational programmes.) International Nursing Review, 24 (1), Jan/Feb 1977, 11-14.

34 Ward, M.J. and Fetler, M.E. Instruments for use in nursing education research. Boulder, Col.: Western Interstate Commission for Higher Education, 1979.

f RESEARCH AND PRACTICE

1 Baker, V.E. Nursing administration and research. (Need for support by managers for research and utilisation of research findings.) Nursing Leadership, 1 (1), Jun 1978, 5-9.

2 Barnard, K.E. Knowledge for practice: directions for the future. (Target areas for research, with reference to 1974 Delphi Survey of Clinical Research Priorities and ways of disseminating research findings.) Nursing Research, 29 (4), Jul/Aug 1980, 208-212.

3 Chance, H.C. and Hinshaw, A.S. Strategies for initiating a research program. Journal of Nursing Administration, 10 (3), Mar 1980, 32-39.

4 Cogliano, J.F. Clinical research in the nursing home: one viewpoint. Journal of Gerontological Nursing, 5 (6), Nov/Dec 1979, 39-43.

5 COMMISSION on Nursing Research Generating a scientific basis for nursing practice: research priorities for the 1980s. Nursing Research, 29 (4), Jul/Aug 1980, 219.

6 Conway, M.E. Clinical research: instrument for change. (Use of controlled system model to examine how research in clinical settings could become institutionalised.) Journal of Nursing Administration, 8 (12), Dec 1978, 27-32.

7 Conway, M.E. Knowledge generation and transmission: a role for the nurse administrator. (Conference paper on the application and promotion of research with report of group discussion on p.42-44.) Nursing Administration Quarterly, 3 (4), Summer 1979, 29-44.

8 Cruise, R.J. and Cruise, P.D. Research for practicing nurses: an introduction for all nurses who can and should be doing nursing research. Supervisor Nurse, 10 (10), Oct 1979, 52, 54-55.

9 Cuddihy, J.T. Clinical research: translation

into nursing practice. (Small scale study with partial-care paediatric patients to evaluate the quality of nursing care and the effect of the nursing process in relation to patient outcome.) International Journal of Nursing Studies, 16 (1), 1979, 65-72.

10 Dimond, M. and Slothower, L. Research in nursing administration: a neglected issue. Nursing Administration Quarterly, 2 (4), Summer 1978, 1-8.

11 Gortner, S.R. and others Contributions of nursing research to patient care. Journal of Nursing Administration, 6 (3), Mar/Apr 1976, 22-28; Journal of Advanced Nursing, 1 (6), Nov 1976, 507-518.

12 Haller, K.B. and others Developing research-based innovation protocols: process, criteria, and issues. (Process of transferring research-based knowledge into protocols for nursing practice.) Research in Nursing and Health, 2 (2), Jun 1979, 45-51.

13 Hightower, L. and others Putting nursing research to work. (Implementing policy and procedure changes derived from survey described on p.66, 68-69.) Supervisor Nurse, 8 (4), Apr 1977, 18-20.

14 Hodgman, E.C. Closing the gap between research and practice: changing the answers to the 'who', the 'where' and the 'how' of nursing research. International Journal of Nursing Studies, 16 (1), 1979, 105-110.

15 Horsley, J.A. and others Research utilization as an organizational process. (Six phases in applying research findings to nursing practice.) Journal of Nursing Administration, 8 (7), Jul 1978, 4-6.

16 Jacox, A. and Prescott, P. Determining a study's relevance for clinical practice. (Evaluating research.) American Journal of Nursing, 78 (11), Nov 1978, 1882-1889.

17 Johnson, M. and Keslar, A.M. Nursing research and WICHE: impact on patient care. (How authors implemented research findings discovered at WICHE nursing research workshop.) Nursing Administration Quarterly, 2 (4), Summer 1978, 33-37.

18 Jones, L. and Rude, N.V. Research Q. and A. Q. What problems are encountered in using patients' charts as sources of data for research? What impact do these problems have on research? What, if anything, can be done about them? Nursing Research, 27 (3), May/Jun 1978, 195-196.

19 Klein, N. and Johnston, M. Insider-out: the health worker as researcher. (Advantages of inside knowledge of researcher but disadvantage of role ambiguity and conflict.) Nursing Research, 28 (5), Sep/Oct 1979, 312-314.

20 Krueger, J.C. Utilization of nursing research: the planning process. (Application of research findings to nursing practice.) Journal of Nursing Administration, 8 (1), Jan 1978, 6-9.

21 Larson, E. The inquisitive nurse: bringing research to the bedside. (Methods of making clinical nursing research more accessible and relevant to nurses.) Nursing Administration Quarterly, 2 (4), Summer 1978, 9-31.

22 Lindeman, C.A. Implementing nursing research in a critical care setting. (Implementation of Hampe's study of the needs

of grieving spouses published in Nursing Research, 24 (2), 1975, 113-120, at University of California, Los Angeles coronary care unit.) Journal of Nursing Administration, 6 (10), Dec 1976, 14-17.

23 McHugh, N.G. and Johnson, J.E. Clinical nursing research: beyond the methods books. (Report of authors' experience.) Nursing Outlook, 28 (6), Jun 1980, 352-356.

24 Marram, G. Barriers to research in psychiatric-mental health nursing: implications for preparing the nurse researcher. Journal of Psychiatric Nursing and Mental Health Services, 14 (4), Apr 1976, 7-11.

25 Miller, J.R. and Messenger, S.R. Obstacles to applying nursing research findings. (Research study.) American Journal of Nursing, 78 (4), Apr 1978, 632-634.

26 Misner, S.J. Nursing research: key to a locked-in profession. (Gap between research and nursing practice.) Supervisor Nurse, 8 (8), Aug 1977, 37-42.

27 Nursing Administration Quarterly Research: impact on patient care. (Ten articles.) Nursing Administration Quarterly, 2 (4), Summer 1978, 1-114.

28 Padilla, G.V. Incorporating research in a service setting. (Recommends nursing audit as institutional mechanism for implementing and sustaining research activities.) Journal of Nursing Administration, 9 (1), Jan 1979, 44-49.

29 Rubin, R. and Erickson, F. Research in clinical nursing. Maternal-Child Nursing Journal, 6 (3), Fall 1977, 151-164.

30 Smoyak, S.A. Is practice responding to research? (Development of research techniques in the United States.) American Journal of Nursing, 76 (7), Jul 1976, 1146-1150.

31 Stetler, C.B. and Marram, G. Evaluating research findings for applicability in practice. Nursing Outlook, 24 (9), Sep 1976, 559-563.

32 Stevenson, J.S. Developing staff research potential. Journal of Nursing Administration, 8 (5), May 1978, 44-46; (6), Jun 1978, 8-12.

33 Stybel, L.J. Organic research as a planning tool for the nurse administrator. Journal of Nursing Administration, 7 (3), Mar 1977, 28-31.

34 Sylvester, D.C. Nursing administration's responsibilities for research. AORN Journal, 31 (5), Apr 1980, 850, 852, 854-855.

35 United States Department of Health, Education and Welfare. Health Resources Administration Instruments for measuring nursing practice and other health care variables. 2 vols. Hyattsville, Md.: USDHEW, 1978.

36 Western Interstate Commission for Higher Education Communicating nursing research. Vol.8: Nursing research priorities: choice or chance. Boulder, Col.: WICHE, 1977.

37 Western Interstate Commission for Higher Education Communicating nursing research. Vol.9: Nursing research in the bicentennial year. Boulder, Col.: WICHE, 1977.

38 Western Interstate Commission for Higher Education Communicating nursing research. Vol.10: Optimizing environments for health: nursing's unique perspective. Boulder, Col.: WICHE, 1977.

39 Wilcox, R. and others Clinical research in nursing homes. Some practical suggestions on how to avoid problems in conducting nursing care studies on elderly, institutionalized patients. Nursing Outlook, 25 (4), Apr 1977, 255-257.

40 Wooldridge, P.J. and others Methods of clinical experimentation to improve patient care. St. Louis: Mosby, 1978.

HEALTH SERVICES AND HOSPITALS

28 NURSING AND HEALTH OVERSEAS

a WORLD HEALTH AND DEVELOPING COUNTRIES

1 ANALYSIS of health manpower functions: findings in Brazil, Egypt and Hungary: a WHO research programme. WHO Chronicle, 33 (2), Feb 1979, 39-44.

2 **Bridgman, R.F. and others** Health care facilities in developing countries: prevailing concerns and possible solutions. World Hospitals, 16 (1), Feb 1980, 38-43.

3 **Bryant, J.H.** Community health workers: the interface between communities and health care systems. WHO Chronicle, 32 (4), Apr 1978, 144-148.

4 **Feuerstein, M.T.** A comprehensive community approach to rural health problems in developing countries. International Nursing Review, 23 (6), Nov/Dec 1976, 174-182.

5 **Flahault, D.** The relationship between community health workers, the health services, and the community. WHO Chronicle, 32 (4), Apr 1978, 149-153.

6 **Fulop, T.** New approaches to a permanent problem: the integrated development of health services and health manpower. WHO Chronicle, 30 (11), Nov 1976, 433-441.

7 **Gish, O.** Guidelines for health planners: the planning and management of health services in developing countries. Tri-Med Books, 1977.

8 **Hentsch, T.** Community and world health. (International trends in world health.) International Nursing Trends, 23 (4), Jul/Aug 1976, 103-106.

9 **Hornby, P. and others** Guidelines for health manpower planning: a course book. Geneva: WHO, 1980.

10 **Hornby, P. and others** Trends in planning for health manpower. WHO Chronicle, 30 (11), Nov 1976, 447-454.

11 **Kakar, D.N.** Communication and persuasion in health: some guidelines for multipurpose health workers. Nursing Journal of India, 47 (5), May 1976, 103-104.

12 **Kent, P.W. editor** International aspects of the provision of medical care. Oriel Press, 1976.

13 **Kleczkowski, B.M.** Health care facilities in developing countries. (Problems of planning and building with limited resources.) WHO Chronicle, 30 (9), Sep 1976, 363-369.

14 **Kleczkowski, B.M. and Pibouleau, R. editors** Approaches to planning and design of health care facilities in developing areas. Geneva: World Health Organization. (WHO offset publications.) Vol.1, 1976, no.29; Vol.2, 1977, no.37; Vol.3, 1979, no.45.

15 **Kohn, R. and White, K.L.** Health care: an international study. Report of the World Health Organization/International Collaborative Study of Medical Care Utilization. Oxford University Press, 1976.

16 **Levi, G.** Health—an integral part of development. (The relationship between health and environmental conditions seen in a WHO survey.) Nursing Mirror, 143, 5 Aug 1976, 63-66.

17 **Levinson, R.M.** The potentials of cross cultural field study: Emory's comparative health care systems program in London. (Six-week course in London providing comparative study of British and U.S. health care systems.) Journal of Nursing Education, 18 (9), Nov 1979, 46-52.

18 **Llewelyn-Davies, R.** Planning health facilities in developing countries—some case studies and their lessons. World Hospitals, 7 (3), 1976, 159-163.

19 **MacMillan, D.** Demanding an answer to the world's needs. (Need and demand in the planning of health services.) Health and Social Service Journal, 89, 28 Sep 1979, 1238-1240.

20 **Mahler, H.** A social revolution in public health. (New approach to community health problems of developing countries.) WHO Chronicle, 30 (12), Dec 1976, 475-480.

21 **Mejia, A. and Pizurki, H.** World migration of health manpower. WHO Chronicle, 30 (11), Nov 1976, 455-460.

22 **Montacute, C. and Montacute, M.** Administration of health services. Nairobi: Uzima, 1979.

23 **Roemer, M.I.** Health care systems in world perspective. Ann Arbor: Health Administration Press, 1976.

24 **Royal Society** More technologies for rural health: a Royal Society discussion organized by D.A.J. Tyrrell and others held Nov 1-2, 1979. The Society, 1979.

25 **Watson, E.J.** Meeting community health needs: the role of the medical assistant. WHO Chronicle, 30 (3), Mar 1976, 91-96.

26 **White, K.L. and others** Health services: concepts and information for national planning and management. Geneva: WHO, 1977. (Public health papers no.67.)

27 WORLD Health Assembly Demand for a social revolution in community health. (Report of the Thirtieth World Health Assembly in Geneva in May 1977.) WHO Chronicle, 31 (7), Jul 1977, 255-261.

28 **World Health** Issue on village health care. World Health, Jul 1980, 3-29.

29 **World Health** Who's six regions. (Issue on particular health problems of each region.) World Health, Oct 1976, 3-26.

30 **World Health Organization** The long-term future of the International Health Regulations. WHO Chronicle, 32 (11), Nov 1978, 439-447.

31 **World Health Organization** Reference material for health auxiliaries and their teachers. Geneva: WHO, 1976. (WHO offset publication no.28.)

32 **World Health Organization. Regional Office for Europe** Training of senior public health administrators: report of WHO working group Moscow 21-23 June, 1978. Copenhagen: WHO, 1980. (EURO reports and studies; 23.)

33 **World Hospitals** Health care staffing in developing countries. (Four articles on India, Philippines, Guatemala and Bahrain.) World Hospitals, 16 (1), Feb 1980, 25-36.

34 **World Hospitals** Information on planning of health care facilities in developing countries. (A bibliography.) World Hospitals, 13 (1 & 2), 1977, 94-101.

35 **World Hospitals** Three articles on planning health care in developing countries. World Hospitals, 14 (3), Aug 1978, 149-156.

b ENVIRONMENT AND POLLUTION

1 **Archer, A. and Barratt, R.S.** Lead in the environment. Monitoring for lead. Royal Society of Health Journal, 96 (4), Aug 1976, 173-176.

2 **Bean, C.** Lead the age old hazard. Occupational Safety and Health, 10 (12), Dec 1980, 12-14.

3 **Bryce-Smith, D.** Dangers in the air. (With special reference to asbestos, sulphur dioxide and lead.) Nursing Mirror, 146, 1 Jun 1978, 44-46.

4 **Cassidy, M.W.A.** The menace of pollution —fact or fiction? Planning for the control of pollution. Royal Society of Health Journal, 96 (6), Dec 1976, 262-268.

5 Gloag, D. Pollution and people. British Medical Journal. Radiation exposure and the protection of the community. 6 Dec 1980, 1545-1548. Is low-level lead pollution dangerous? 13 Dec 1980, 1622-1625.

6 Healy, M.A. and Aslam, M. The distribution of lead in a roadside environment and its consequences for health. Public Health, 94 (2), Mar 1980, 78-88.

7 Hebel, J.R. and others Mental capability of children exposed to lead pollution. British Journal of Preventive and Social Medicine, 30 (3), Sep 1976, 170-174.

8 Helmsman, A. An acceptable level? The implications of some recent research on lead pollution. Nursing Times, 72, 2 Sep 1976, 1342-1343.

9 Holland, W.W. The menace of pollution— fact or fiction? The assessment of health effects of pollution. Royal Society of Health Journal, 96 (6), Dec 1976, 268-269.

10 Large, J.B. Environmental noise. Methods of assessing community response to environmental noise. Royal Society of Health Journal, 97 (4), Aug 1977, 147-155.

11 Magos, L. Lead, mercury and cadium pollution. Nursing Mirror, 142, 22 Jan 1976, 47-49.

12 Pisharoti, K.A. Guide to the integration of health education in environmental health programmes. Geneva: World Health Organization, 1975. (WHO offset publication no.20.)

13 Reed, S.B. The menace of pollution—fact or fiction? Pollution—myth or menace?— measure it! Royal Society of Health Journal, 96 (6), Dec 1976, 256-262.

14 World Health Water. Issue on water supplies as the key to human health. World Health, Jan 1977, 3-31.

15 World Health Organization Task group on environmental health criteria for noise. Noise. Geneva: WHO, 1980.

16 World Health Organization. Regional Office for Europe Health and the environment. Copenhagen: WHO, 1977. (Public health in Europe no.8.)

17 World Health Organization. Study Group Health hazards from new environmental pollutants. Geneva: WHO, 1976. (Technical report series no.586.)

18 Wynn, M. and Wynn, A. Lead and the unborn. (Comment on Lawther report on lead and health.) New Society, 52, 17 Apr 1980, 104-105.

c WORLD HEALTH ORGANIZATION

1 Corrigan, P. The World Health Organization. Hove: Wayland, 1979.

2 Dorolle, P. Half a century of international health. Royal Society of Health Journal, 95 (1), Feb 1975, 18-19.

3 Mahler, H. The WHO you want: an address to WHO Regional Committees. WHO Chronicle, 34 (1), Jan 1980, 3-8.

4 Mahler, H. Use your WHO. (To achieve WHO's goal of Health for All by the Year 2000.) WHO Chronicle, 34 (12), Dec 1980, 455-460.

5 Nursing Times The nurse's role in WHO. (Account of four-day meeting of European Regional Committee.) Nursing Times, 74, 28 Sep 1978, 1583.

6 Ritchie-Calder, Peter. Baron Ritchie-Calder of Balmashannar Back to the people. (Review of WHO's achievements over the last thirty years. See also editorial on p.3.) World Health, Apr 1978, 4-7.

7 World Health Issue on WHO priorities for the future. World Health, Jul 1976.

8 World Health The Water Decade 1981-1990. (Issue on WHO's resolve to provide clean water for all the world by 1990.) World Health, Jul/Aug 1980, 3-35.

9 World Health Organization Basic documents. 27th ed. Geneva: WHO, 1977; 28th ed. 1978; 29th ed. 1979.

10 World Health Organization Health challenges for 1978-83. WHO Chronicle, 31 (4), Apr 1977, 123-126.

11 World Health Organization Introducing WHO. Geneva: WHO, 1976.

12 World Health Organization The work of WHO: annual report of the Director General. Geneva: WHO, 1976.

13 World Health Organization. Executive Board Formulating strategies for health for all by the year 2000. Geneva: WHO, 1979.

d NURSING: INTERNATIONAL

1 Anstey, O. Goals for ICN. (By the ICN President.) International Nursing Review, 24 (5), Sep/Oct 1977, 153.

2 Anstey, O. Report of the ICN president, 1977-1979. International Nursing Review, 27 (1), Jan/Feb 1980, 22-24.

3 Bristow, S. Career opportunities. Nursing overseas. Nursing Times, 72, 10 Jun 1976, 894-896.

4 COMMONWEALTH Nurses Federation Supplement. The Commonwealth scene. Nursing Times, 72-76.
No.5, 29 Apr 1976, CNF suppl. 33-40.
No.6, 11 Nov 1976, CNF suppl. 41-48.
No.7, 3 Feb 1977, CNF suppl. 49-56.
No.8, 2 Jun 1977, CNF suppl. 57-64.
No.9, 3 Nov 1977, CNF suppl. 65-72.
No.10, 23 Feb 1978, CNF suppl. 73-80.
No.11, 6 Jul 1978, CNF suppl. 81-88.
No.12, 2 Nov 1978, CNF suppl. 89-96.
No.13, 22 Feb 1979, CNF suppl. 97-104.
No.14, 5 Jul 1979, CNF suppl. 105-112.
No.15, 1 Nov 1979, CNF suppl. 113-120.
No.16, 31 Jan 1980, CNF suppl. 121-128.
No.17, 26 Jun 1980, CNF suppl. 129-136.

5 Cornelius, D. Report of the ICN president, 1975-1977. International Nursing Review, 24 (4), Jul/Aug 1977, 116-121.

6 Fawkes, B. Nursing—an international perspective. (With reference to the work of various international organisations.) Australian Nurses Journal, 9 (6), Dec/Jan 1980, 40-42.

7 Forster, M. What ICN means to me. (Student's view.) International Nursing Review, 24 (3), May/Jun 1977, 74.

8 Henkle, J.O. International nursing: a specialty? (Research study of American nurses working overseas and nurses with overseas nursing experience.) International Nursing Review, 26 (6), Nov/Dec 1979, 170-173.

9 Hutchinson, D. Introducing the International Council of Nurses. (Editorial on the scope, objectives, activities and structure of the ICN.) Journal of Continuing Education in Nursing, 8 (1), Jan-Feb 1977, 6-7.

10 International Council of Nurses National reports of member organisations. Revised ed. Geneva: ICN, 1977.

11 International Council of Nurses Policy statements. Geneva: ICN, (1976.)

12 INTERNATIONAL Council of Nurses 16th Quadrennial Congress May 30-June 3, 1977, Tokyo, Japan. Reports. Nursing Mirror, 144, 16 Jun 1977, 7-9; Nursing Times, 73, 23 Jun 1977, 930-935; 7 Jul 1977, 1018-1025; American Journal of Nursing, 77 (8), Aug 1977, 1303-1310.

13 International Nursing Foundation of Japan Nursing in the world: the needs of individual countries and their programmes. Tokyo: the Foundation, 1977.

14 International Nursing Review Special issue on ICN Congress, Tokyo. International Nursing Review, 24 (5), Sep/Oct 1977, 130-154.

15 Joyce, P.M. 'The ambit and orbit of nursing in the 70s.' UNA Nursing Journal, 74 (1), Jan/Feb 1976, 4-6, 8-10.

16 Krebs, D. 'Better conditions for nurses'. The role of the International Council of Nurses in identifying issues crucial to nursing. World of Irish Nursing, 7 (8), Sep 1978 , 1-2; (9), Oct 1978, 5; (11/12), Nov/Dec 1978, 6.

17 Lucas, E. editor Nurses and health care: collected papers from the second King's Fund Transatlantic Seminar of Nurses. King Edward's Hospital Fund, 1976.

18 Manning, M. Problems of Third World nurses. A recent conference 'Third World Workers in the NHS,' organised by Walsall Council for Community Relations. Nursing Mirror, 143, 22 Jul 1976, 39-41.

19 Masson, V. International collaboration in nursing education: the people to people approach. (Project HOPE, American scheme of providing health care assistance overseas.) Journal of Nursing Education, 19 (5), May 1980, 48-54.

20 Masson, V. International nursing: what is it and who does it? (Nurses who work outside their own country.) American Journal of Nursing, 79 (7), Jul 1979, 1242-1245.

21 Masson, V. Nursing for export—let the buyer beware! (Importance of recognising cultural differences when trying to implement ideas in nursing education and practice overseas.) International Nursing Review, 25 (4), Jul/Aug 1978, 113-115.

22 Mooneyhan, E. The professional nurse in developing countries—practice and preparation.

International Nursing Review, 26 (1), Jan/Feb 1979, 17-20, 23.

23 Skeet, M. No nurse is an island. (Need for nurses to be aware of and become involved in international developments in health care.) Nursing Mirror, 151, 18/25 Dec 1980, 35-37.

24 Smith, J. What comes out of a melting pot of the world's nurses? (Report on ICN congress in Tokyo.) Nursing Mirror, 144, 30 Jun 1977, 4-5.

25 World Health Issue devoted to changing aspects of nursing in different parts of the world. World Health, Dec 1978, 2-28.

e EUROPE AND EEC

GENERAL

1 Abel-Smith, B. The cost of health services. (With reference to European health services.) New Society, 49, 12 Jul 1979, 74-76.

2 Abel-Smith, B. and Maynard, A. The organisation, financing and cost of health care in the European Community. Luxembourg: Commission of the European Communities, 1979. (Social Policy series; 36.)

3 Blanpain, J. and Delesie, L. Community health investment: health services research in Belgium, France, Federal German Republic and the Netherlands. Oxford University Press for Nuffield Provincial Hospitals Trust, 1976.

4 Blanpain, J. and others National health insurance and health resources: the European experience. Cambridge, Massachusetts: Harvard University Press, 1978.

5 A CHANCE to break down the European barriers. How the result of the EEC elections will affect nurses. Nursing Mirror, 148, 31 May 1979, 5.

6 Clarke, P. Rcn study tour of the EEC countries, France, Italy, Belgium and Luxembourg 11-23 March 1979. NATNews 16 (9), Sep 1979, 16, 18, 21, 24.

7 Commission of the European Communities National health survey systems in the European Economic Community: proceedings of a conference held in Brussels 6-8 October 1975, edited by P. Armitage. Luxembourg: the Commission, 1977.

8 COUNCIL of the European Communities Council directive 77/453/EEC of 27 Jun 1977 concerning the co-ordination of provisions laid down by law, regulation or administrative action in respect of the activities of nurses responsible for general care. Nursing Times, 73, 29 Sep 1977, Occ. papers, 132; 74, 19 Jan 1978, Occ. papers, 8.

9 Dopson, L. Community spirit. (Effects of EEC directives on nursing in Britain.) Nursing Times, 75, 28 Jun 1979, 1077-1080.

10 Dopson, L. Sheila Quinn—'EEC NO'. (An interview with the president of the standing committee of nurses in Brussels.) Nursing Times, 75, 31 May 1979, 904.

11 EUROPEAN Community Nurse. (Summary of proposals in the two draft directives submitted to the EEC Council.) Queen's Nursing Journal, 19 (10), Jan 1977, 288.

12 EUROPEAN Economic Community. Hospital Committee Hospitals in the EEC: organisation and terminology. Copenhagen: Gyldendal, 1978.

13 Gawn, R.A. The EEC medical directives. Health Trends, 1 (8), Feb 1976, 1-4. Present state of implementation, Feb 1978, 1-4.

14 Hansard Nurses and midwives. EEC Directives. Meetings with organisations involved. 5 Apr 1977, WA 494-
EEC directives agreed 1 Jul 1977, WA 365-366. (Nursing Times, 7 Jul 1977, 1012.)
Implementation, 16 May 1978, WA 155-156; 6 Mar 1979, WA 617-618.
Implications for training, 28 Jul 1978, WA 960-961; 9 Jul 1979, WA 51-52.
Cost of implementation, Lords, 7 Nov 1978, 272-273.
Nursing qualifications (EEC recognition) order 1979. Motion for approval, Lords, 24 Jul 1979, 1843-.

15 Hay, P.R. General nurse training in Denmark, West Germany and the Netherlands. (Report of visit and study of community experience given to nurses.) Health Visitor, 52 (11), Nov 1979, 471, 474.

16 International Nursing Review Nursing and midwifery legislation in Europe requires substantial revision. (Report of WHO meeting in Hamburg.) International Nursing Review, 27 (3), May/Jun 1980, 92-94.

17 Journal of Advanced Nursing Proposals for nurses in the European Economic Community. Journal of Advanced Nursing, 2 (2), Mar 1977, 184-185.

18 Kohn, R. Coordination of health and welfare services in four countries: Austria, Italy, Poland and Sweden: report on a study. Copenhagen: WHO, Regional Office for Europe, 1977. (Public health in Europe; 6.)

19 Kratz, C. WHO launches nursing programme for Europe. (Report of 27th session of WHO Regional Committee for Europe.) Nursing Times, 73, 17 Nov 1977, 1780.

20 LEGISLATION...(E.E.C. nursing directives.) Official Journal of the European Communities, 20, 15 Jul 1977, 1-13.

21 Morris, P. Euro directives will be just another headache. (Cost of implementation.) Nursing Mirror, 148, 28 Jun 1979, 5.

22 Moyle, R. Euro-hiccoughs. (Some of the obstacles facing potential Euronurses.) Nursing Times, 75, 16 Aug 1979, 1385-1386.

23 Nursing Times Nursing Times explains... Nurse education—GNC policy and EEC directives. Nursing Times, 74, 27 Apr 1978, 696. Comment from A. Carr in letter, 25 May 1978, 878-879. GNC for Scotland policy on EEC directives, Nursing Times, 74, 11 May 1978, 780.

24 Paine, L. Eighth conference on hospital services in Europe. World Hospitals, 12 (4), 1976, 238-245.

25 Paine, L.H.W. NHS and EEC—interface and interaction. Hospital and Health Services Review, 72 (4), Apr 1976, 127-129; (5), May 1976, 164-167.

26 Permanent Committee of Nurses in Liaison with the EEC An examination of the working conditions for first level nurses in the public sector in the EEC countries and the four Nordic countries outside the EEC. The Committee, 1975.

27 Permanent Committee of Nurses in Liaison with the EEC Survey of health services and the nursing structure within the health services in the countries affiliated to the EEC. The Committee, 1978.

28 Permanent Committee of Nurses in Liaison with the EEC A survey of post-basic specialties available for nurses in the nine countries affiliated to the EEC. The Committee, 1978.

29 Pyne, R.H. The nursing profession in EEC countries. (Report on the effect of the EEC directives on the regulation of the profession.) Nursing Times, 75, 25 Jan 1979, Occ. papers, 5-12.

30 Quinn, S. The EEC directives: implications for nurse educators. Medical Teacher, 2 (2), Mar/Apr 1980, 88-92.

31 Quinn, S. EEC directives: their implications for the patient in the community. Nursing Mirror, 147, 31 Aug 1978, 38-40.

32 Quinn, S. EEC directives: U.K. makes stand against Belgium. (Problems of the free movement of nurses.) Nursing Times, 72, 1 Jul 1976, 990.

33 Quinn, S. The health professions in Europe. Nursing Focus. 1. EEC directives, 1 (11), Jul 1980, 431-432. 2. Nurses and midwives, 1 (12), Aug 1980, 466-467. 3. Can we control our destiny? 2 (1), Sep 1980, 14-15 .

34 Quinn, S. The implications of the EEC nursing directives. Midwife, Health Visitor and Community Nurse, 14 (2), Feb 1978, 42-43.

35 Quinn, S. Nursing: the EEC dimension. (Royal College of Nursing, Nursing Lecture 1977.) Nursing Times, 74, 5 Jan 1978, Occ. papers, 1-4; 19 Jan 1978, Occ. papers, 5-7 with EEC directive 77/453/EEC reprinted on p.8.

36 Quinn, S.M. Nursing in Europe. (Introduction to series of articles.) Nursing Mirror, 145, 1 Sep 1977, 14-15. Reprinted in International Nursing Review, 26 (1), Jan/Feb 1979, 8-9.

37 Quinn, S. editor Nursing in the European Community. Croom Helm, 1980.

38 Quinn, S.M. Sheila Quinn—Britain's representative on the Permanent Committee of Nurses in Liaison with the EEC talks to Nursing Times about the new EEC directives for general nurses. Nursing Times, 73, 21 Jul 1977, 1102-1103.

39 Royal College of Nursing A background to nursing in the EEC: report of a seminar... 24-28 Jan 1977, King's Fund Centre, London. Rcn, 1977.

40 ROYAL College of Nursing How will Britain meet the problems of implementation? (Report of Rcn conference on the EEC directives, with photograph of Permanent Committee members.) Nursing Mirror, 146, 2 Feb 1978, 4-5.

41 Statutory Instruments 1979 1604. The nursing qualifications (EEC recognition) order 1979.

42 Swaffield, L. Seeking the meaning. European Congress of Catholic Nurses. Nursing Times, 72, 16 Sep 1976, 1422-1423.

43 **Turpin, M.** British nurse takes a look at Scandinavian home health services. Nursing Mirror, 142, 18 Mar 1976, 36.

44 **WHO Chronicle** Health services in Europe. 1. Administration and preventive services. 2. Medical care and health personnel. WHO Chronicle, 30 (10), Oct 1976, 407-412; (12), Dec 1976, 497-500.

45 **WHO Chronicle** Health care management in Europe. (Application of Country Health Programming (CHP) and creation of effective training programmes.) WHO Chronicle, 34 (2), Feb 1980, 53-55.

46 **World Health Organization. Regional Committee for Europe** Medium-term programme in nursing/midwifery in Europe (1976-1983). Copenhagen: WHO, 1977.

47 **World Health Organization. Regional Office for Europe** Nursing services: report on a WHO symposium Stuttgart, 20-23 Nov 1978. Copenhagen: WHO, 1980. (Euro reports and studies; 22.)

48 **World Health Organization. Regional Office for Europe** Relevance of educational planning to health problems: report on a working group. Copenhagen: WHO, 1976.

49 **World Health Organization. Regional Office for Europe** Second liaison meeting with nursing/midwifery associations on WHO's European nursing/midwifery programme, Copenhagen, 21-23 Apr 1976. Copenhagen: WHO, 1976.

50 **World Health Organization. Regional Office for Europe** Third liaison meeting with nursing/midwifery associations on WHO's European nursing/midwifery programme: report...Copenhagen 28 Feb-2 Mar 1978. Copenhagen: WHO, 1978.

51 **World Health Organization. Regional Office for Europe** Use of operational research in European health services: report of a working group, Sofia 7-11 July 1975. Copenhagen: WHO, 1976.

52 **World Health Organization. Regional Office for Europe** Ad Hoc Working Group — International School of Advanced Nursing Education. Report. Copenhagen, 5-6 April 1973. Copenhagen: WHO, 1974.

53 **World of Irish Nursing** The National Florence Nightingale Committee of Ireland. (Functions and objectives.) World of Irish Nursing, 5 (1-2), Jan-Feb 1976, 9.

BELGIUM

54 **Iveson-Iveson, J.** The art of nursing, Belgian style. (Report of visit to Brussels.) Nursing Mirror, 146, 15 Jun 1978, 8-9.

55 **Royal College of Nursing** Nursing in Europe. Belgium. Nursing Mirror, 145, 27 Oct 1977, 24.

DENMARK

56 **Danish Nurses Organisation** Nursing in Europe. Denmark. (Education and conditions of work.) Nursing Mirror, 145, 8 Sep 1977, 16-18.

57 **Iveson-Iveson, J.** Nursing—the Danish way. Nursing Mirror, 146, 4 May 1978, 8-10; 18 May 1978, 8-10.

58 **Paine, L.** Health services in Denmark. World Hospitals, 12 (2), 1976, 106-107.

59 **Paine, L.** Hospital study tour in Denmark. World Hospitals, 12 (4), 1976, 210-223.

EIRE

60 **Ireland. Department of Health** Working Party on General Nursing. Report. Dublin: Stationery Office.

61 **HEALTH** services in the Irish Republic. British Medical Journal, 2, 4 Nov, 1310-1311.

62 **Hensey, B.** The health services of Ireland. 3rd ed. Dublin: Institute of Public Administration, 1979.

63 **Leydon, M.I.** Nursing in Europe. Eire. (Education, conditions of work and the Irish Nurses Organisation.) Nursing Mirror, 145, 15 Sep 1977, 24-26.

64 **Philpot, T.** Will the Irish health service move with the times? Nursing Mirror, 147, 16 Nov, 22-23.

65 **Royal College of Nursing** Notes on Eire. (Education and conditions of work.) Nursing Mirror, 145, 15 Sep 1977, 26.

66 **Taaffe, T.C.** Need for solidarity. (Address by the President of the INO to the AGM.) World of Irish Nursing, 7 (11/12), Nov/Dec 1978, 1-2.

67 **Tierney, B.** Role of the working party. (To examine nursing staff structures in the Irish hospital services.) World of Irish Nursing, 7 (1), Jan 1978, 6.

FRANCE

68 **Alaire, C.** Nursing in Europe. France. (Education.) Nursing Mirror, 145, 6 Oct 1977, 38-40.

69 **Grossman, M.** Here and there: a look at nursing in France. Canadian Nurse, 75 (9), Oct 1979, 30-31.

70 **Ross, T.** When in France. (Use of computer for nursing records, medical records and other aspects of administration at Cannes Hospital, France.) Nursing Mirror, 151, 28 Aug 1980, 22-24.

71 **Royal College of Nursing** Notes on France. (Salary and conditions of work.) Nursing Mirror, 145, 6 Oct 1977, 40.

72 **Williams, J.** All change for France. (Nurse education in France.) Nursing Mirror, 150, 14 Feb 1980, 38.

ITALY

73 **Koelschbach, P.B.** Nursing in Europe. Italy. (Education and salaries.) Nursing Mirror, 145, 22 Sep 1977, 25-26.

74 **Royal College of Nursing** Notes on Italy. (Education and working conditions of nurses.) Nursing Mirror, 145, 22 Sep 1977, 27.

NETHERLANDS

75 **Ashton, K.** British nurses in Holland. (Experiences of two nurses.) Nursing Times, 76, 5 Jun 1980, 1022-1023.

76 **Doeleman, F.** The health care system in the Netherlands. Community Medicine, 2 (1), Feb 1980, 46-56.

77 **Lapre, R.M.** A short outline of health services planning at central level in the Netherlands. World Hospitals, 12 (2), 1976, 114-116.

78 **Levert, A.J.** Nursing in Europe. The Netherlands. (Education and the professional organisation for nurses.) Nursing Mirror, 145, 29 Sep 1977, 29-30.

79 **Royal College of Nursing** Notes on Holland. (Conditions of work.) Nursing Mirror, 145, 29 Sep 1977, 30.

80 **Stolte, J.B.** Democratisation in the hospital: participation in decision making in the Netherlands. Hospital and Health Services Review, 72 (10), Oct 1976, 348-353.

81 **Stoneham, M.W.** The Netherlands experience. (Report of recent visit.) Hospital and Health Services Review, 76 (9), Sep 1980, 297-299.

SWEDEN

82 **Hands, D.** A lesson in Swedish. (Study tour of Swedish health care.) Health and Social Service Journal, 90, 1 Aug 1980, 1006-1009.

83 **HEALTH** services in Sweden. British Medical Journal, 280, 28 Jun 1980, 1640-1641.

84 **Rawlins, T.** Planning a study tour. (Report of visit to Sweden with advice.) Nursing Times, 76, 24 Jul 1980, 1324-1325.

WEST GERMANY

85 **EFFICIENCY** with humanity. (Hospitals in West Germany.) Health and Social Service Journal, 90, 27 Jun 1980, 846-849.

86 **Royal College of Nursing** Notes on West Germany. (Conditions of work.) Nursing Mirror, 145, 20 Oct 1977, 32.

87 **Weinrich, R.** Nursing in Europe. The Federal Republic of Germany. Nursing Mirror, 145, 20 Oct 1977, 31.

USSR

88 **Blenkinsop, D. and others** Bread and circuses. (Report of visit to USSR to study health services there.) Nursing Focus, 1 (7), Mar 1980, 263-264, 266-268.

89 **Easson, G.A.** Professional nursing in the Soviet Union. Journal of Nursing Education, 16 (7), Sep 1977, 23-26.

90 **Hardie, M.** From a Russian notebook. (Health care and nursing.) Nursing Times, 76, 10 Jan 1980, 82-85.

91 **Kaser, Michael** Health care in the Soviet Union and Eastern Europe. Croom Helm, 1976.

92 **Millington, C.** Russia. (Report of visit to operating theatres and intensive care units in Russia.) NATNews, 14 (9), Dec 1977, 18-19.

93 **Ryan, M.** Behind Soviet health curtain. (Medical provision.) Health and Social Service Journal, 88, 20 Jan 1978, 74-76.

94 **Ryan, M.** The organisation of Soviet medical care. Blackwell/Robertson, 1978. (Aspects of social policy series.)

95 **Ryan, M. and Forwell, G.D.** The way forward in the Soviet health service. British Medical Journal, 280, 10 May 1980, 1180-1181.

96 **Weiss, L.D.** Career mobility of mid-level health workers in the USSR. (Includes nurses and feldshers.) Nursing Forum, 18 (3), 1979, 311-316.

OTHER COUNTRIES

97 THE FIGHT for a health service in Poland. Nursing Times, 76, 4 Dec 1980, 2135.

98 FINLAND. National Board of Health. Primary health care in Finland. Health services in Finland. Helsinki: the Ministry, 1978-1979.

99 **Forjaz, Teresa** Interview. Teresa Forjaz. (Nursing Officer (research) at the National Institute of Health in Lisbon, Portugal.) Nursing Times, 14, 30 Mar 1978, 524-525.

100 **Hodkinson, J.M.** Nursing in Finland. (With particular reference to community nursing.) Queen's Nursing Journal, 19 (4), Jul 1976, 100-102.

101 **International Nursing Review** Closer links forged between ICN and Hungarian nurses. (With outline of basic nurse education in Hungary.) International Nursing Review, 27 (4), Jul/Aug 1980, 100-101.

102 **Irving, C.** Franja Bolnica—a partisan hospital (Yugoslavia.) Nursing Times, 73, 3 Mar 1977, 316-317.

103 **Komadina, D.** Integration of consumers and providers of health services. (In Yugoslavia.) World Hospitals, 12 (1), 1976, 40-43.

104 **Llobet, M.A. and Melendez, C.** The professional association, the nurse and the student nurse in Spain. International Nursing Review, 25 (5), Sep/Oct 1978, 136-137.

105 **Paduano, M.A.** Nursing education in Spain. International Nursing Review, 23 (5), Sep-Oct 1976, 150-154.

106 **Richardson, S.A.** The other side of the wall: report on a work study tour to East Germany. Health Visitor, 49 (1), Jan 1976, 2-6.

107 **Robinson, W.** Nursing in Gibraltar. (Health care services.) Nursing Mirror, 145, 22 Sep 1977, 6-9.

108 **Royal College of Nursing** Notes on Luxembourg. Nursing Mirror, 145, 13 Oct 1977, 33.

109 **Schol, D.** Nursing in Europe. Luxembourg. Nursing Mirror, 145, 13 Oct 1977, 31-32.

110 **Skupnjak, B. and Novosel, M.** General practice in Croatia, Yugoslavia. Journal of the Royal College of General Practitioners, 26, Nov 1976, 847-852.

111 **Yorath, A.** A short study in Athens. (Report of visit to Greece and description of nursing and health care there.) Nursing Times, 74, 25 May 1978, 892-893.

f AFRICA

GENERAL

1 **Commonwealth Nurses Federation** Nursing education in West Africa. Nursing Times, 75, 5 July 1979, CNF Supplement, 106.

2 **Jato, M. and others** Adapting nursing textbooks for Africa: a necessity? (Research study in Cameroon.) International Nursing Review, 26 (1), Jan/Feb 1979, 21-23.

3 **Jegede, S.A.** Cultural approach to nursing in Africa. Nigerian Nurse, 7 (3), Jul-Sep 1975, 6-8.

4 **Marshall, R.H.E.** The professional association in Africa: toward the 21st century. International Nursing Review, 26 (1), Jan/Feb 1979, 24-26.

5 **Stranex, R.** Nursing in a remote part of East Africa. S.A. Nursing Journal, 43 (3), Mar 1976, 19-20.

6 **WHO Chronicle** Issue on the health situation in Africa. WHO Chronicle, 30 (1), Jan 1976, 3-37.

KENYA

7 **Ahmed, S.** Potential contribution of primary-school teachers to the health of a developing country. (Kenya.) Lancet, 2, 5 Aug 1978, 307-308.

8 **Ahmed, S.** The primary school and the teacher: new health care roles in developing countries. (With reference to Kenya.) World Hospitals, 16 (1), Feb 1980, 21-23.

9 **Crow, R.** Health care in the Turkana desert. (North-west Kenya.) Nursing Mirror, 144, 31 Mar 1977, 62-65.

10 **National Nurses Association of Kenya** '10 years of nursing in Kenya'. Reports presented at the Seminar hosted by National Nurses Association of Kenya to celebrate. (History from 1946.) Kenya Nursing Journal, 6 (1), Jun 1977, 49-55, 57-58.

11 **National Nurses Association of Kenya** The National Nurses Association of Kenya as the (Professional) Organisation for nurses in Kenya. Kenya Nursing Journal, 5 (3), Dec 1976, 30-38.

12 WHAT role do our nurses play in the health services in Kenya today? Kenya Nursing Journal, 4 (2), Dec 1975, 5, 47.

NIGERIA

13 **Adegoroye, A.** The professional nursing journal in Nigeria: a decade's experience. Nigerian Nurse, 11 (2), Apr/Jun 1979, 4-9.

14 **Adeloye, A.** Nursing in Nigeria. Improvement and the future. Nigerian Nurse, 9 (3), Jul/Sep 1977, 29-31, 51.

15 **Akinsanya, J.** The Nigerian connection. (Nursing in Nigeria.) Nursing Times, 75, 7 Jun 1979, 950-951.

16 **Bailey, A.** Education for the health care providers—a nursing care concept. (Analysis of the problems of nurse education in Nigeria and a proposal for a new training course.) Nigerian Nurse, 8 (1), Jan-Mar 1976, 37-41, 45.

17 **Bailey, A.** The need for nursing textbooks in Nigeria and other developing countries. Nursing Times, 74, 23 Feb 1978, CNF Supplement, 74-75.

18 **Chokreih, A.O. and Adebo, E.O.** Evaluation of nursing knowledge and skills in Nigeria. International Nursing Review, 24 (2), Mar/Apr 1977, 55-60.

19 **Daramola, S.O.** The Nigerian patient: his choice for traditional treatment. Nigerian Nurse, 10 (4), Oct/Dec 1978, 22-23.

20 **Leke, J.** Continuing education for nurses in Nigeria. International Nursing Review, 26 (4), Jul/Aug 1979, 111-112.

21 **Leke, J.T.** Nigerian patients' perception of their nursing care needs. Journal of Advanced Nursing, 3 (2), Mar 1978, 181-187.

22 **Nursing Times** Floating doctor service (Nigeria.) Nursing Times, 72 (45), 11 Nov 1976, CNF Supplement, 43.

23 **Odedere, A.** The need for better conditions of service for the Nigerian nurse. Nigerian Nurse, 8 (4), Oct-Dec 1976, 44-47.

24 **Oyedepo, K.** Development of standards and the evaluation of nurses and nursing services in Nigeria. Nigerian Nurse, 10 (2), Apr/Jun 1978, 23-27.

25 **Oyedepo, K.** Professional responsibility of Nigerian nurses. Nigerian Nurse, 7 (4), Oct-Dec 1975, 36-39.

SOUTH AFRICA

26 **Chamane, J.B.** Cultural factors in nursing education. (The importance of cultural differences on attitudes to health and hygiene with reference to South Africa.) S.A. Nursing Journal, 44 (9), Sep 1977, 26-28.

27 **Donn, M.C.** South Africa 1975. (Study tour of South African Hospitals.) NATNews, 12 (9), Dec 1975, 11-13.

28 **Gilliland, J.** The need for a comprehensive approach to the delivery of health care (in South Africa.) S.A. Nursing Journal, 43 (9), Sep 1976, 8-10.

29 **Jacobson, B.** Apartheid and health care. (In South Africa and Rhodesia.) Nursing Times, 74, 6 Apr 1978, 567.

30 **Lemkus, S.M. and Op't Hof, J.** Genetic training of nurses in South Africa. (Report of survey of nurses' knowledge and attitudes and the development of a training programme.) S.A. Nursing Journal, 44 (11), Nov 1977, 17-18.

31 **Mellish, J.M.** Ethos of nursing: a South African perspective. Durban: Butterworth, 1978.

32 **Mellish, J.M.** Nursing education today. S.A. Nursing Journal, 44 (3), Mar 1977, 6-8.

33 **Muller, O.H. and Smit, J.J.M.** The nursing contributors to health services of the black states. Curationis, 2 (2), Sep 1979, 51-53.

34 **Robson, N.** Reflections on nursing in Owambo. S.A. Nursing Journal, 43 (3), Mar 1976, 18, 17.

35 **Roux, J.P.** The development of health services for Bantu in the R.S.A. with special reference to the development of health services in the Homelands. S.A. Nursing Journal, 43 (10), Oct 1976, 29-30.

36 **S.A. Nursing Journal** Issue on nursing education in South Africa. S.A. Nursing Journal, 44 (3), Mar 1977.

37 **Samson, J.P.** Nursing education and the black nurse...an overview. (With history from 1850.) Curationis, 1 (1), Jun 1978, 47-55.

38 Searle, C. South Africa. Extended role of the nurse in hospital. Part 1. Australasian Nurses Journal, 6 (9), Apr 1977, 9-10.

OTHERS

39 Akita, A. and others Environmental and social change: the effects on nursing practice. (Health problems of developing countries and the effect of technology on nursing, with section on nursing in Ghana.) International Nursing Review, 26 (1), Jan/Feb 1979, 10-16.

40 Bacon, L. Ghana—medical care amid economic problems. Journal of the Royal College of General Practitioners, 30, Jul 1980, 433-436.

41 Bayoumi, A. The history of Sudan health services. Nairobi: Kenya Literature Bureau, 1979.

42 Gish, O. Planning the health sector: the Tanzanian experience. Croom Helm, 1975.

43 Hanrahan, K. Nurse education in Botswana. World of Irish Nursing, 7 (5), Jun 1978, 6-7.

44 Hawes, S. A lesson from the third world. (Work of health volunteers in Yemen including teaching of local birth attendants.) Nursing Times, 76, 13 Mar 1980, Community Outlook, 82.

45 Health and Social Service Journal Two articles on Zambian health services. Health and Social Service Journal, 88, 17 Feb 1978, 194-196.

46 Idriss, A.A. and others The primary health care programme in Sudan. WHO Chronicle, 30 (9), Sep 1976, 370-374.

47 Kaunda, B. Address at the combined Copperbelt Graduation Ceremony. (Outlines government's plans for nursing education in Zambia.) Zambia Nurse, 9 (2), Jul/Aug, 1977, 3-4.

48 Lamb, I. When caring is a challenge. (Nursing and nursing education in Zambia.) Nursing Mirror, 149, 8 Nov 1979, 26-27.

49 Lancet Primary care in Ghana. (Research report.) Lancet, 2, 18 Nov 1978, 1085.

50 Lekgetha, A.N. The comprehensive health care system in Boputhatswana. S.A. Nursing Journal, 43 (8), Aug 1976, 19-20.

51 Lester, J. VSO nurse faces the challenge of Africa. (Alison Gordon, who worked as VSO nurse in Ghana.) Nursing Mirror, 145, 10 Nov 1977, 4-5.

52 Martin-Buss, Y. Health services in Rhodesia. New Zealand Nursing Journal, 71 (7), Jul 1978, 16-17.

53 Mudibany, L. The new emphasis on traditional medicine in Zaire—implications for nursing practice. International Nursing Review, 27 (6), Nov/Dec 1980, 184-186.

54 Smith, P.A. Student nurse rural fieldwork in mainland Tanzania. Journal of Advanced Nursing, 3 (5), Sep 1978, 437-446.

55 Van Eeden, I. The role of the nurse in the Cullinan Refugee Camp. (For Angolans.) S.A. Nursing Journal, 43 (6), Jun 1976, 30-31.

56 Webb, C. A new nursing education programme for independent Mozambique. International Nursing Review, 26 (2), Mar/Apr 1979, 41-48.

g MIDDLE EAST

GENERAL

1 Cox, C. Turkish delights? (Nursing and health care in Turkey and report of visit to discuss establishment of a national centre for research in nursing.) Nursing Mirror, 151, 18/25 Dec 1980, 32-34.

2 Eccles, M.J. A nurse in Lebanon. (Experiences with an Australian medical team there.) Lamp, 35 (6), Jun 1978, 31-33.

3 Mallard, I.Z. The climate is delightful. (Personal account of work in the Middle East with criticisms of conditions.) Nursing Times, 74, 9 Nov 1978, 1864-1867.

4 Meleis, A.I. International issues in nursing education: the case of Kuwait. (Development from 1962.) International Nursing Review, 26 (4), Jul/Aug 1979, 107-110.

5 Meleis, A.I. A model for establishment of educational programmes in developing countries: the nursing paradoxes in Kuwait. Journal of Advanced Nursing, 5 (3), May 1980, 285-300.

6 Meleis, A.I. and Hassan, S.H. Oil rich, nurse poor: the nursing crisis in the Persian Gulf. Improving the image and status of the nurse in these countries will help solve the serious shortage of nurses they are experiencing. Nursing Outlook, 28 (4), Apr 1980, 238-243.

7 Moghadassy, M. and Simozar, M. Progress: baccalaureate nursing in Iran. International Nursing Review, 25 (1), Jan/Feb 1978, 22-24.

8 NURSING services and education develop in Bahrain. International Nursing Review, 25 (6), Nov/Dec 1978, 165.

9 Potts, M. A touch of common sense. (Health service problems in Iran highlighted by a government commission.) World Medicine, 10 (15), 7 May 1975, 45, 47-48.

10 Wallace, D. Medical services in Saudi Arabia. Nursing Mirror, 143, 12 Aug 1976, 45-46.

11 Wren, G.R. The hospitals of Saudi Arabia. World Hospitals, 12 (2), 1976, 120-125.

12 Zeighami, B. and others What's behind the nursing brain drain? A study of the attitudes of Iranian nurses. International Nursing Review, 24 (3), May/Jun 1977, 84-87.

ISRAEL

13 Bergman, R. and others Multi-applications to nursing education programs in Israel—facts and issues. International Journal of Nursing Studies, 15 (2), 1978, 83-90.

14 Bergman, R. and others 'Non-starters' in schools for registered nurses in Israel—1975-1976. International Journal of Nursing Studies, 16 (2), 1979, 151-157.

15 Drummond, G. Health care in Israel. (History of Israel's health care programmes and report of visits to hospital in Jerusalem.) Nursing Mirror, 146, 19 Jan 1978, 21-23.

16 Dunn, A. Israel working holidays. A sense of adventure. (Report on visit to meet volunteers at the Hadassah Medical Centre in Jerusalem.) Nursing Times, 74, 19 Oct 1978, 1707.

17 Margolis, E. Health changes in a changing society. The health services of Israel. Medical Care, 13 (11), Nov 1975, 943-955.

18 Royston, P. and Frost, A. Horizons. Nursing in Israel. Journal of Practical Nursing, 27 (1), Jan 1977, 36.

19 Solly, K. Uneasy peace that opens new frontiers in health and welfare. (Social welfare in Israel.) Health and Social Service Journal, 87, 1 Apr 1977, 580-581.

h ASIA

GENERAL

1 Atteberry, M. and Lewis, L. An international adventure in teaching. (Six week course in advanced clinical nursing for Far East nurses held in Manila.) International Nursing Review, 23 (1), Jan/Feb 1976, 11-14.

2 Commonwealth Nurses Federation Crown colony of Hong Kong. (Health services and nurse training.) Nursing Times, 74, 6 Jul 1978, CNF Supplement, 82.

3 Commonwealth Nurses Federation The Kwun Tong Community Health Project, Hong Kong. Nursing Times, 74, 6 Jul 1978, CNF Supplement, 83.

4 International Nursing Review Nurses association develops in Tonga. (With some information on nurse education.) International Nursing Review, 27 (4), Jul/Aug 1980, 103-104.

5 Kettle, B. At the bamboo roots. (Study tour of the Far East May-July 1974 looking at health services and nurse education.) Nursing Times, 72. 1. General and Singapore, 12 Aug 1976, 1228-1230. 2. Hong Kong, 19 Aug 1976, 1274-1275. 3. Malaysia, 26 Aug 1976, 1311-1313.

6 Maglacas, A.M. and others Nursing education: the changing pattern in Indonesia. WHO Chronicle, 30 (11), Nov 1976, 461-463.

7 NATIONAL survey of nurses and midwives. (Undertaken by the Ministry of Health.) Nursing Journal of Singapore, 17 (1), May 1977, 41-42, 7.

8 Thornton, N.F. Nursing in Nepal. (Report of work in a mission hospital in 1977.) Journal of Practical Nursing, 30 (6), Jun 1980, 32-33.

9 Thornton, N.F. Nursing in Nepal. (Male nurse's experiences in a mission hospital.) Nursing Mirror, 145, 18 Aug 1977, 31.

10 Waldron, E.A. Bangladesh—an unforgettable experience. (Work of a nurse sponsored by TEAR Fund running milk feeding centres and family planning services.) Nursing Times, 73, 10 Mar 1977, ABPN Supplement, 7-8.

CHINA

11 Bissell, C. A glimpse of China in 1977. (Report of study tour.) Health Visitor, 51 (3), Mar 1978, 90-92, 94.

12 Bonsall, M. The health and welfare system in Red China. (Report of study visit.) British Journal of Occupational Therapy, 41 (4), Apr 1978, 135-136.

13 Cathcart, H.R. Chinese health system gets down to basics. (Preventive medicine and primary health care.) Hospitals, 52 (20), 16 Oct 1978, 69-73.

14 Chiang-Wen, W. The barefoot doctors of China's countryside. Nursing Mirror, 146, 30 Mar 1978, 14-16.

15 Garfield, R. China's nurses: redefining roles to improve health. International Journal of Nursing Studies, 15 (3), 1978, 129-134.

16 Garfield, R. Nursing and health care in China. Nursing Forum, 16 (3, 4), 1977, 329-338.

17 Garfield, R. Nursing education in China. Nursing Outlook, 26 (5), May 1978, 312-315.

18 Hicks, C. Caring for the people. (Report of visit to China.) Nursing Times, 75, 11 Jan 1979, 55-59.

19 Hurst, T. The long march to curing the sick man of Asia. (Progress of the Chinese health service since 1949.) Health and Social Service Journal, 89, 18 Jan 1979, 37-39.

20 Klintworth, C. General medical care in China. Australian Nurses Journal, 4 (3), Sep 1974, 33-35.

21 Lubout, J. and others Health and medical care in China. Australian Nurses Journal, 8 (1), Jul 1978, 50-53.

22 Medical Teacher Nurse education in China. (Short report of article in 'China Now'.) Medical Teacher, 1 (2), Mar/Apr 1979, 70.

23 Mitchell, F. The caring revolution. (Observations on health care in China.) Health and Social Service Journal, 86, 24 Sep 1976, 1711-1713.

24 Mitchell, F. Doctor is worker, peasant, soldier and student. (Medicine in China.) Health and Social Service Journal, 86, 1 Oct 1976, 1764-1765.

25 NURSES' study tour of China. New Zealand Nursing Journal, 69 (2), Feb 1976, 17-18; (4), Apr 1976, 12-14.

26 Schorr, T.M. Impressions of China. (Report of study tour, with photographs.) American Journal of Nursing, 78 (3), Mar 1978, 389-394.

27 Sonn, A. Chinese health service. (Study tour report.) Nursing Mirror, 144, 9 Jun 1977, 25-27.

28 Sonn, A. Community participation and self help in China's health service. Midwife, Health Visitor and Community Nurse, 13 (8), Aug 1977, 261-262.

29 Sonn, A. Health care in China in the 70s. (Study tour.) Queen's Nursing Journal, 19 (15), Jun 1977, 426-427, 429.

30 Wen, C.P. and Hays, C.W. Health care planning in China. Medical Care, 14 (3), Mar 1976, 241-254.

31 Varty, B.W. Health care in China. (Impressions of a Canadian hospital admin-istrator.) Hospital Administration in Canada, 18 (11), Nov 1976, 14-16.

32 WHO Chronicle Study tour in China. (On traditional medicine.) WHO Chronicle, 31 (11), Nov 1977, 433-435.

33 World Health Issue on Chinese medicine and acupuncture. World Health, Dec 1979, 2-29.

34 Young, P. Nursing Mirror goes to China. 5 parts. Nursing Mirror, 145, 1 Dec 1977, 6-9; 8 Dec 1977, 7-9; 15 Dec 1977, 6-9; 22 Dec 1977, 6-8; 29 Dec 1977, 4-7.

INDIA

35 Aggarwal, K.C. Some suggested structural changes in nursing education. 2 parts. Nursing Journal of India, 47 (7), Jul 1976, 169, 171; (9), Sep 1976, 220-222.

36 Aggarwal, K.C. There is a difference (between diploma degree and post basic degree courses.) Nursing Journal of India, 46 (12), Dec 1975, 268, 279.

37 Arora, P. Perspectives on Indian nursing. Nursing Journal of India, 47 (8), Sep 1976, 223-224.

38 Chabook, H. Social changes and student nurses. (Address by President of TNAI on nursing in India.) Nursing Journal of India, 70 (12), Dec 1979, 317-319, 324.

39 Chatterjee, M. Gandhiji's interest in nursing, medicine and health. Nursing Journal of India, 66 (10), Oct 1975, 225-238.

40 Cherian, A. Role of nursing in India today. Nursing Journal of India, 67 (11), Nov 1976, 258-259.

41 Crout, E. The sacred cows of east and west. (Development of health services in India.) Nursing Mirror, 151, 18/25 Dec 1980, 27-29.

42 Hailey, M.A. A visit to India. (Report of a study tour.) Health Visitor, 50 (7), Jul 1977, 217-218, 220.

43 Harnar, R.M. A model for nursing education in India. Nursing Journal of India, 47 (1), Jan 1976, 8-11.

44 Harnar, R.M. Societal determinants for nursing education. (National policies for nurse education in India.) Nursing Journal of India, 67 (2), Feb 1976, 39-41.

45 Harnar, R.M. Social forces and factors influencing nursing education in India. Nursing Journal of India, 47 (3), Mar 1976, 54-56.

46 International Nursing Review Indian students celebrate Golden Jubilee. International Nursing Review, 27 (3), May/Jun 1980, 94-95.

47 Kurian, A.P. Education for the change in role of nurses in India. Nursing Journal of India, 70 (11), Nov 1979, 282-284.

48 Nandi, P.K. Cultural constraints on professionalization: the case of nursing in India. International Journal of Nursing Studies, 14 (3), 1977, 125-135.

49 Nursing Journal of India Summary of the main recommendations of the Bhore committee. (Policy on health care in India.) Nursing Journal of India, 70 (10), Oct 1979, 257-260, 263.

50 Pethe, T. Nursing education: new vistas. (New system for four graded courses from nurse's aides to degree students.) Nursing Journal of India, 49 (2), Feb 1978, 33, 35.

51 Philip, R. Association as an agent of change. (Difference between professional association and trade union and role of the Trained Nurses Association of India.) Nursing Journal of India, 68 (9), Sep 1977, 225, 228.

52 Thomas, A. Nurses' place in the health care system. (Government plans.) Nursing Journal of India, 71 (5), May 1980, 121-124, 131.

JAPAN

53 Brown, R.L. Dispelling evil spirits with today's advancing medicine. (Health care in Japan.) Health and Social Service Journal, 86, 4 Feb 1977, 206-207.

54 Inoturan, J.E. Employment and work conditions of nurses in Japan. Philippine Journal of Nursing, 46 (1), Jan/Mar 1977, 13-14.

55 International Council of Nurses An outline of the history of nursing in Japan. Australian Nurses Journal, 6 (12), Jun 1977, 23-26.

56 INTRODUCING the Japanese Nursing Association. (Its function and activities.) International Nursing Review, 24 (4), Jul/Aug 1977, 125-126.

57 Iveson-Iveson, J. A visit to a Japanese hospital. (Report on nursing techniques and organisation seen on visit during trip to Tokyo.) Nursing Mirror, 145, 21 Jul 1977, 8-9.

58 Kratz, C. Some reflections. (On visits to a hospital and school of nursing in Tokyo.) Nursing Times, 73, 7 Jul 1977, 1024.

59 Tokyo Planning Committee. ICN 16th Quadrennial Congress Health services in Japan. International Nursing Review, 24 (2), Mar/Apr 1977, 46-50.

60 Tokyo Planning Committee. ICN 16th Quadrennial Congress Nursing education in Japan. International Nursing Review, 23 (3), May/Jun 1976, 73-79.

61 Tokyo Planning Committee. ICN 16th Quadrenniel Congress Nursing services in Japan. International Nursing Review, 23 (6), Nov/Dec 1976, 169-173.

i AUSTRALASIA

AUSTRALIA

1 Allwright, M. and others Auxiliary nursing in Tasmania: a survey of the role, function and status of the Tasmanian auxiliary nurse. Australian Nurses Journal, 9 (8), Mar 1980, 31-34.

2 Australia. Hospitals and Health Services Commission A report on hospitals in Australia. Canberra: Australian Government Publishing Service, 1974.

3 Australian Nurses Journal The profession. Summary of submission by Australian nursing organisations to the Federal Government Committee of Inquiry into Education and Training. Australian Nurses Journal, 6 (12), Jun 1977, 10, 12, 14, 16.

4 Bates, E.M. A consumer's view of the Australian experience in health insurance. Lancet, 2, 5 Jul 1980, 26-28.

5 Boorer, D. Am I my brother's keeper? An account of the conference 'Innovation through Participation' organised by the New South Wales Nurses' Association and held in Sydney from 15th-19th March 1976. (Speakers included R.W. Revans and Janet Craig.) Lamp, 33 (5), May 1976, 19-22.

6 Boorer, D. Revans over Australia. New South Wales Nurses Association conference 'Innovation through partnership.') Nursing Mirror, 142 (18), 29 Apr 1976, 39-40.

7 Committee of Inquiry into Nurse Education and Training Nurse education and training: report of the Committee of Inquiry into Nurse Education and Training to the Tertiary Education Commission. (Conclusions and recommendations with comments by professional bodies.) Australian Nurses Journal, 8 (7), Feb 1979, 10-14.

8 Curry, G. Educating for nursing professionalism—status or competence? Some recent trends in nursing education in Australia. (Review of article in professional journal and other material.) Lamp, 44 (10), Oct 1977, 5-7.

9 Cuskelly, C. Nurse education—a choice between higher and further education. (Comments on a report by the Nurses' Education Board of New South Wales.) Australian Nurses Journal, 6 (5), Nov 1976, 27-30.

10 Dains, E. The Royal British Nurses Association in Australia. Australasian Nurses Journal, 9 (1), Nov 1979, 20-22.

11 Dickenson, M. and Law, G. Nurses in the national health scheme. (Australia.) Lamp, 33 (3), Mar 1976, 30-36.

12 DIPLOMA in Nursing, College of Nursing, Australia. The beginning of a new era in nursing education in Australia. (Completion of the first college conducted basic nursing course.) Australian Nurses Journal, 6 (6 & 7), Dec 1976-Jan 1977, 7-8, 10, 12.

13 Donaldson, R.J. Personal reflections on a visit to Australia. (Health services.) Community Medicine, 1 (4), Nov 1979, 315-320.

14 Donohue, S. Nursing education conference (on goals for nursing education in Australia). Lamp, 33 (1), Jan 1976, 25, 27-35.

15 Dunlop, M. The role of the CAEs in nurse education. (College of Advanced Education.) Lamp, 34 (3), Mar 1977, 5, 7, 9.

16 Edwards, N.C. A case for first aid? Meeting the challenge of nursing education today in hospital schools of nursing. Australian Nurses Journal, 5 (11), May 1976, 36-37.

17 Fawkes, B. Australian nursing develops on several fronts. (Visit by Barbara Fawkes.) International Nursing Review, 24 (2), Mar/Apr 1977, 39-40.

18 Fischer, L.R. Health dynamics and nursing. (Changes in health care and issues facing nursing.) Australian Nurses Journal, 7 (1), Jul 1977, 44-50.

19 Gehling, M. The Aboriginal connection. (Medical and social problems of Aborigines.) Nursing Mirror, 149, 13 Sep 1979, 28-30.

20 Godfrey, J. Diversification of higher education in Australia. Australian Nurses Journal, 8 (4), Oct 1978, 41-43.

21 Graham, D. The Royal Australian Nursing Federation. A brief consideration of RANF, the representation provided by its governing body, and the role of the organisation in the improvement of standards of nursing care. Australian Nurses Journal, 6 (12), Jun 1977, 38-40.

22 Harte, C. RANF affiliation with ACTU. (Australian Council of Trade Unions.) Australian Nurses Journal, 8 (4), Oct 1978, 24-27.

23 Ibell, B.M. Development of the nursing profession in Australia in Ibell, B.M. Integrated basic theory and practice of nursing. Melbourne: Pitman Medical, 1979.

24 Kelly, B. A background to the history of nursing in Tasmania. Moonah, Tasmania: Davies Brothers, 1977.

25 Lamp First basic course (UG2) students. (Description of new three-year Diploma of Applied Science basic nursing course.) Lamp, 34 (12), Dec 1977, 14-15.

26 Lancet The Royal Flying Doctor Service. (Of Australia. History.) Lancet, 1, 17 Jun 1978, 1303-1304.

27 Kratz, V. Letter from Australia. 6 parts. Nursing Times, 75-76.
1. 4 Oct 1979, 1700-1702.
2. Primary nursing. (Sir Charles Gairdner Hospital, Perth.) 18 Oct 1979, 1790-1791.
3. The Aborigines. 22 Nov 1979, 2042-2043.
4. Linking nursing with education. The Educational Development Unit at the Western Australian Institute of Technology. 24 Jan 1980, 173-174.
5. Enthusiasm and innovation. (District nursing service.) 13 Mar 1980, 478-479.
6. Nurse education. 3 Jul 1980, 1191-1192.

28 Lambert, P. New horizons in nursing. (Implications of the White report on the role of the nurse in Australia and other recent studies of nursing in Australia.) Australian Nurses' Journal, 5 (5), Nov 1975, 31-34, 44.

29 Lawson, J.S. Who will nurse the sick in the eighties? (New educational programmes developed in Tasmania.) Australian Nurses Journal, 9 (4), Oct 1979, 45-46.

30 Maxwell, R.J. The Medical Commons. The keynote address delivered at the National Congress of the Australian Hospital Association at Canberra on 27 October 1977. (Problems faced by developed countries over their health services, with reference to Australia.) Hospital and Health Services Review, 74 (2), Feb 1978, 51-55.

31 Millers, N. and Huntsman, R.W. Nurse education—do we care where we are at? Lamp, 33 (9), Sep 1976, 7, 9, 11; Australian Nurses Journal, 6 (6 & 7), Dec 1976-Jan 1977, 26-27, 35.

32 Murphy, A. Into the bush: a look at life with the Australian Flying Doctor Service. (With facts and figures.) Health Visitor, 53 (1), Jan 1980, 14, 16.

33 Nurses Education Board of New South Wales Nursing resources available in New South Wales training schools. Sydney: The Board, 1976.

34 Parsons, R. Nursing education reform—ten years on. (Institute of Hospital Matrons Report 1967-1969 and NSW government policy 1977.) Lamp, 35 (10), Oct 1978, 9-13.

35 Patten, M.E. The Australian nurse of the 1980s: college-trained for primary care. (Review of developments in nurse education.) Australian Nurses Journal, 9 (2), Aug 1979, 36-38, 52.

36 Quine, S. Nurses' education board of the New South Wales survey findings. (Survey of the educational qualifications of entrants to basic nursing courses.) Lamp, 33 (1), Jan 1976, 19-20; (8), Aug 1976, 5, 7.

37 Richardson, J. Aboriginal health: a vicious circle. Australian Nurses Journal, 6 (2), Aug 1976, 25-26.

38 Royal Australian Nursing Federation The Federation. Highlights from the annual report. (Review of the last six years' activities of the Federation.) Australian Nurses Journal, 6 (10), Apr 1977, 7-8, 10, 11-13, 14, 16.

39 Royal Australian Nursing Federation and others Goals in nursing education. Policy statements of the Royal Australian Nursing Federation, College of Nursing Australia, National Florence Nightingale Committee of Australia, New South Wales College of Nursing. Australian Nurses Journal, 5 (10), Apr 1976, 10-14.

40 Schultz, B. Along the way. (Outline history of the Royal Australian Nurses Federation.) Australian Nurses Journal, 4 (4), Oct 1974, 10-35.

41 Shearman, D.J.C. and Limmer, A.N. A mantle of safety: the 50th year of the Royal Flying Doctor Service. British Medical Journal, 2, 5 Aug 1978, 407-409.

42 Shoebridge, J. Questioning current attitudes in nursing midwifery. (Nursing generally as well as midwifery.) Australian Nurses Journal, 9 (3), Sep 1979, 44-49.

43 Steinitz, B. An I.R.O.'s testament: union support is a clear moral duty. (With reference to Royal Australian Nursing Federation Union of Employees.) Australian Nurses Journal, 9 (4), Oct 1979, 47-48.

44 Thomson, M. Change in nursing education. (Summary of a talk given to visiting nurses explaining New Zealand developments.) New Zealand Nursing Journal, 68 (12), Dec 1975, 22-23.

45 Townsend, J. 'The nurses' among the students. (Experiences of nursing education in a general college of advanced education in Canberra.) Australian Nurses Journal, 5 (9), Mar 1976, 16, 19.

46 Winstanley, J. The practice of nursing. Community and family practice. (Implications of the 'Goals in nursing education' report.) Australian Nurses Journal, 5 (3), Sep 1975, 12-14.

47 Zepps, K. The role of the New South Wales College of Nursing regarding the education and professional development of nursing in New South Wales. Lamp, Dec 1975, 3, 5, 7, 34.

NEW ZEALAND

48 Carroll, M.O. Educating the nurse for the

future. (With reference to New Zealand.) New Zealand Nursing Journal, 70 (11), Nov 1977, 3-6.

49 Carroll, P. Nursing standards and nursing legislation: some considerations. (With history of nursing in New Zealand from 1841.) New Zealand Nursing Journal, 73 (6), Jun 1980, 6-10.

50 CHANGES in nursing education. (Questions and answers on policy of transfer of nursing education from hospital-based schools of nursing to the tertiary education system.) New Zealand Nursing Journal, 73 (3), Mar 1980, 11-13.

51 Crombie, B. Changes in health care delivery which have affected the 'role' and 'status' of health professionals. New Zealand Nursing Journal, 73 (1), Jan 1980, 25-26, 33.

52 Edge, D.P. New Zealand. (Personal experiences of working in New Zealand.) British Medical Journal, 1976, 2, 13 Nov 1976, 1185-1186.

53 Green, D.E. Some factors in nursing recruitment. (With some reference to New Zealand.) New Zealand Nursing Journal, 71 (7), Jul 1978, 11-12.

54 Huddlestone, J. Health manpower in New Zealand. The swinging pendulum. (Health professions generally, with some reference to nursing.) New Zealand Nursing Journal, 70 (12), Dec 1977, 17-19.

55 Hughes, B. The development of nursing as a profession in New Zealand. New Zealand Nursing Journal, 71 (3), Mar 1978, 17-20.

56 Hyland, M.M. The position and role of the enrolled nurse within the nursing structure of New Zealand. New Zealand Nursing Journal, 73 (5), May 1980, 39-41, 43.

57 McGuigan, T. Reorganization of the New Zealand health services. Royal Society of Health Journal, 95 (3), Jun 1975, 159-162.

58 Millers, N. The nurse in contemporary society. (The nursing profession related to status of women in New Zealand.) New Zealand Nursing Journal, 69 (5), May 1976, 23-27.

59 New Zealand Nurses' Association Nurses' Amendment Bill. (Submissions on the Bill.) New Zealand Nursing Journal, 69 (5), May 1976, 12-14.

60 New Zealand Nurses' Association. Nelson Branch Patterns of health care. (Survey by nurses of use of existing NZ health services and ways of extending community nursing services.) New Zealand Nursing Journal, 71 (4), Apr 1978, 6-10.

61 NURSES' Act 1977—what it means for nurses. New Zealand Nursing Journal, 71 (2), Feb 1978, 20-21.

62 Salmon, B. Look toward that mountain. (Paper on past, present and future of nursing in New Zealand.) New Zealand Nursing Journal, 70 (4), Apr 1977, 17-21.

63 Salmond, G.C. New problems—new strategies. (Value of health services research in New Zealand shown by action following community health survey.) World Health, Jan 1980, 14-15, 17.

64 Small, D. The first graduates of technical institute nursing courses: a follow-up. (Evalu-ation of three year full-time course by assessing performance of graduates in employment.) New Zealand Nursing Journal, 70 (11), Nov 1977, 8-14.

65 TECHNICAL Institute nursing programmes. (Details of two basic nursing programmes at Waikato Institute and Southland Polytechnic.) New Zealand Nursing Journal, 71 (8), Aug 1978, 10-12.

66 TRANSFER of nursing education: over 40% complete. (From hospital to technical institute-based programmes.) New Zealand Nursing Journal, 72 (10), Oct 1979, 6-7.

67 Ward, A.R. New Zealand. New method of nurse rostering. Australasian Nurses Journal, 3 (4), Oct 1977, 23-24.

PACIFIC

68 Alimurung, M.M. Nursing and its challenges. Philippine Journal of Nursing, 44 (3), Jul-Sep 1975, 162-165.

69 Commonwealth Nurses Federation Supplement Working group on the collaborative role of WHO in nursing/midwifery in the South Pacific. Nursing Times, 74, 2 Nov 1978 CNF Supplement, 91-92.

70 Metten, A. A day in Dagua. (Catholic Mission Hospital in Papua New Guinea.) Nursing Times, 76, 17 Jul 1980, 1281.

71 RETURN to Tonga. (Interview with Mrs. Akosita Fineanganofo on nursing services in Tonga.) Nursing Times, 72 (45), 11 Nov 1976, 1750-1751.

72 Smith, E.S. Nursing in rural Papua, New Guinea. Nursing Times, 73, 10 Feb 1977, 210-211.

j CENTRAL AND SOUTH AMERICA AND CARIBBEAN

1 Auld, P. Argentina—sense and nonsense. (Health care.) World Medicine, 15 (17), 31 May 1980, 42-43, 45, 47.

2 Borges, M.V. Nursing in primary health care in Brazil. International Nursing Review, 27 (6), Nov/Dec 1980, 173-177, 190.

3 Brosnan, S. Community health in the Guatemalan highlands. Journal of Practical Nursing, 30 (8), Aug 1980, 26-28.

4 Ceeni, H.M. A link with the outside world. (Costa Rica's rural health programme.) World Health, Nov 1976, 24-29.

5 Cuskelly, C. A report submitted to the New South Wales Nurses' Registration Board on a recent visit to Peru. Part 1. Nursing education and practice. Lamp, 34 (7), Jul 1977, 29-31.

6 De Castro, I.B. and others Changes in the image of the nurse in Brazil. International Nursing Review, 23 (2), Mar/Apr 1976, 43-47.

7 Felsted, E. A quarter century of nursing education in Jamaica. Jamaican Nurse, 15 (2), Aug 1975, 15.

8 Feuerstein, M.T. Evaluation—by the people. (Of health services in Honduras, Central America.) International Nursing Review, 25 (5), Sep/Oct 1978, 146-153.

9 Fielding, S. Nursing in Honduras. Journal of Practical Nursing, 27 (2), Feb 1977, 18-19.

10 Gomez, M.P. Nursing in Paraguay. International Nursing Review, 25 (2), Mar/Apr 1978, 48-50.

11 Gonzalez De Alfaro, M.E. Legal and civil responsibilities of nurses. (With special reference to Panama.) International Nursing Review, 24 (6), Nov/Dec 1977, 172-175, 181.

12 Gregory, S. Health care in Haiti. 1. 2. The Tuesday people. (Nutrition clinic for children held on Tuesdays.) Nursing Times, 76, 10 Apr 1980, 660-662; 17 Apr 1980, 707-710.

13 Hampton, S. Expedition nurse. (Author's adventures as nurse to the all woman expedition to the Great Atrato Swamp, Columbia, in South America.) Nursing Mirror, 145, 27 Oct 1977, 7-9.

14 Jones-Hendrickson, S.B. The dynamics of the labour market for nurses from the Commonwealth Caribbean. PhD thesis, Exeter University, Faculty of Social Sciences, 1976.

15 Metcalf, C. Expedition to Ecuador. 2 parts. (Nurse member of medical team describes pre-expedition planning and improvisation in primitive conditions.) Nursing Times, 73, 7 Jul 1977, 1026-1027; 14 Jul 1977, 1087-1091.

16 Seivwright, M.J. The practice of nursing. (Implications of American theories for Jamaica.) Jamaican Nurse, 15 (2), Aug 1975, 20-21.

k NORTH AMERICA

GENERAL

1 Redwood, P.E. North America. (Florence Nightingale scholarship studying paediatric and cardiothoracic nursing.) Nursing Times, 72 (12), 25 Mar 1976, ABPN supplement V-VI.

2 Schlotfeldt, R.M. What's new in nursing practice: North America. Australian Nurses Journal, 7 (2), Aug 1977, 40-43, 54.

3 Speirs, S. A study tour of North America. (Nurse training in Canada and the USA compared with British training.) Nursing Times, 75, 15 Mar 1979, 459-461.

CANADA

4 Alberta Task Force on Nursing Education Report. Edmonton: Department of Advanced Education and Manpower, 1975.

5 Blair, D. and McPhail, E. Future of nursing in Alberta. Dimensions in Health Service, 57 (4), Apr 1980, A14.

6 Brain, M.C. Health care in Ontario. British Medical Journal, 2, 21 Aug 1976, 464-465.

7 Canadian Council on Hospital Accreditation Guide to hospital accreditation. Toronto: The Council, 1977.

8 Canadian Nurse Frankly speaking. (Two articles by nurses on problems presented by economic cuts.) Canadian Nurse, 74 (7), Jul/Aug 1978, 29.

9 Canadian Nurses Association Annual Meeting and Convention, Canadian Nurses' Association, June 20-23 1976, Hotel Nova

Scotian, Halifax. (Report.) Canadian Nurse, 72 (8), Aug 1976, 20-33.

10 **Canadian Nurses Association** CNA intensifies its role as national coordinator. (Programs and decisions of the CNA during the past year.) Canadian Nurse, 71 (12), Dec 1975, 31-33.

11 **Canadian Nurses Association** Index of Canadian nursing studies addendum no.2. Ottawa: the Association, 1976.

12 **Canadian Nurses Association** Putting 'health' into health care: submission to Health Services Review 1979. Ottawa: CNA, 1980.

13 **Gilchrist, J.M.** The continuing challenge for nursing. (With particular reference to nurse education in Canadian universities.) Nursing Papers, 12 (3), Aug 1980, 6-17.

14 **Harvey, K.C. and others** The health care of Canadian Indians in North Western Ontario. (Includes nursing care.) Hospital and Health Service Research, 75 (2), Feb 1979, 43-48; (3), Mar 1979, 80-83.

15 **Hazlett, C.B.** Task analysis of the clinically trained nurse (C.T.N.) (Nurse practising in isolated nursing stations in northern Canada.) Nursing Clinics of North America, 7 (4), Dec 1975, 699-709.

16 **Kelly, N.** Quest for a profession: the history of the Vancouver General Hospital School of Nursing. Vancouver General Hospital, School of Nursing, Alumnae Association, 1973.

17 **Lasor, B. and Elliott, M.R.** Issues in Canadian nursing. Scarborough, Ontario: Prentice-Hall, 1977.

18 **Lee, S.S.** Quebec's health services in a state of dynamic chnage. (Effects of the recommendations of the Royal Commission on Health Services 1964-65.) Hospital Administration in Canada, 19 (1), 1977, 13, 18, 23-24, 47.

19 **Nunes-Vaz, E.** What patterns for Canada's health care? Hospital Administration in Canada, 18 (6), Jun 1976, 58, 60, 62.

20 **Soderstrom, L.** The Canadian health system. Croom Helm, 1978.

21 **Wallace, J.D.** Hospitals and new perspectives in health care. (In Canada.) Hospital Administration in Canada, 18 (3), Mar 1976, 18, 20, 23-24.

22 **Watkin, B.** A lesson from Canada. (Comments on 'A new perspective on the health of Canadians' published in 1974.) Nursing Mirror, 142, 4 Mar 1976, 42.

USA

23 **Abalos, D.T.** Strategies of transformation in the health delivery system. (Historical background to and changes in U.S. health system with reference to changing roles and increased militancy of nurses.) Nursing Forum, 17 (3), 1978, 284-316.

24 **Abdellah, F.G.** Nursing's role in future health care. (As seen by the United States Department of Health, Education and Welfare in forward plan for health 1977-1981.) AORN Journal, 24 (2), Aug 1976, 236-240.

25 **Allen P.** Education changes affect health manpower. (Effect of changes in entry level

requirements.) AORN Journal, 29 (1), Jan 1979, 43-47.

26 **American Journal of Nursing** Can we bring order out of the chaos of nursing education? (Three articles recommending changes in education, by Claire Fagin, Margaret McClure and Rozella Schlotfeldt.) American Journal of Nursing, 76 (1), Jan 1976, 98-107.

27 **American Journal of Nursing** Many nurses active in politics. (Democratic and Republican Conventions.) American Journal of Nursing, 76 (10), Oct 1976, 1542-1543, 1570, 1572-1574.

28 **American Journal of Nursing** A nationwide survey on state action on entry into practice. Special report. American Journal of Nursing, 78 (4), Apr 1978, 535, 566, 568, 570, 572.

29 **American Nurses Association** Nursing: a social policy statement. Kansas City: the Association, 1980.

30 **American Nurses Association** A strategy for change: papers presented at conference in Albuquerque, New Mexico, 9-10 June 1979. Kansas City: ANA, 1979.

31 AMERICAN Nurses' Association Convention '78. (Report.) American Journal of Nursing, 78 (7), Jul 1978, 1231-1246.

32 **Byrne, M.W. and Spatz, A.M.** RNs and LPNs: do they work well together? Journal of Practical Nursing, 30 (11), Nov/Dec 1980, 40-42, 55.

33 **Chopoorian, T. and Craig, M.M.** Nursing and health care delivery. (Features of the Health Planning and Resources Development Act.) American Journal of Nursing, 76 (12), Dec 1976, 1988-1991.

34 CREDENTIALING in nursing: a new approach. Report of the committee for the study of credentialing in nursing. American Journal of Nursing, 79 (4), Apr 1979, 674-683.

35 **Croft, G.D.** American nursing in the Seventies: a summary of trends, problems and progress. Lamp, 36 (1), Feb 1979, 5-8.

36 **DeVries, R.** Future trends in health care in the U.S.A. World Hospitals, 7 (3), 1976, 193-195.

37 **Di Marco, N. and Hilliard, M.** Comparisons of associate, diploma and baccalaureate degree nurses' state board, quality of patient care, competency rating, supervisor rating, subordinates' satisfaction with supervision and self-report job satisfaction scores. International Journal of Nursing Studies, 15 (4), 1978, 163-170.

38 **Draper, J.** Courting the idea of national health. (Current proposals in the USA for a system of health insurance.) Health and Social Service Journal, 90, 22 Feb 1980, 253-255.

39 **Draper, J.** An eye on American welfare. Health and Social Service Journal, 90, 15 Feb 1980, 216-219.

40 **Elliott, C.L. and Kaiser, G.** Patients, not unions, first concern of hospitals. (Labour relations in hospitals in the U.S.) Hospitals, 53 (21), 1 Nov 1979, 76-79.

41 **Flanagan, L. compiler** One strong voice: the story of the American Nurses' Association. Kansas City: ANA, 1976.

42 **Ford, L.C.** U.S. circa 1976: changes and challenges in nursing education and practice. Australian Nurses Journal, 5 (10), Apr 1976, 26-31.

43 **Freidson, E.** The prospects of health services in the United States. (Four models of organisation.) Medical Care, 16 (12), Dec 1978, 971-983.

44 **Haines, S.M.** Health care in the USA: the nursing scene. Nursing Times, 73, 3 Nov 1977, 1723-1724.

45 **Isaacs, M.** Toward a national health policy: a realist's view. American Journal of Nursing, 78 (5), May 1978, 848-851.

46 **Isler, C.** Bicentennial forecast. The promises in your future. (Summary of forecasts of nursing trends.) RN Magazine, 39 (12), Dec 1976, 15-16, 20, 25, 28.

47 **Johnson, W.L.** Educational preparation for nursing—1977. (Statistics from NLN's annual survey of U.S. schools of nursing.) Nursing Outlook, 26 (9), Sep 1978, 568.

48 **Jonas, S. and others** Health care delivery in the United States. New York: Springer, 1977.

49 **Journal of Practical Nursing** Three articles on the 1985 debate. (Proposed change in New York State Law on Licensure in nursing.) Journal of Practical Nursing, 29 (8), Aug 1979, 16-19, 36, 37, 39.

50 **Kalisch, P.A. and Kalisch, B.J.** The advance of American nursing. Boston: Little, Brown and Co., 1978.

51 **Klein, R.** A vision of health in the world's richest nation. (Proposed national health insurance system in the U.S.A.) Health and Social Service Journal, 89, 14 Dec 1979, 1620-1622.

52 **Kniep-Hardy, M. and Burkhardt, M.A.** Nursing the Navajo (American Indians.) American Journal of Nursing, 77 (1), Jan 1977, 95-96.

53 **La Monica, E.L. and Siegel, F.F.** A professional organization that helps all of us. (Need of American Nurses Association to attract more members. Opposite view p.19-21.) Journal of Nursing Administration, 9 (5), May 1979, 16-18.

54 **Landis, L.** Socio-economics of nursing. (Role of the American Nurses Association.) International Nursing Review, 25 (6), Nov/Dec 1978, 182-186.

55 **Lee, A.A.** Mandatory BSN. (Comment on the professional/technical split with the BSN required for 'professional' status.) RN Magazine, 42 (4), Apr 1979, 64-66, 70, 72, 74, 76.

56 **Lee, A.A.** 'There has to be a better way!' Must we have a professional/technical split? Nearly half the respondents to RN's Special Poll offered other alternatives. RN Magazine, 42 (2), Feb 1979, 39-46.

57 **Leininger, M.** Changing foci in American nursing education: primary and transcultural nursing care. (Nursing in primary health care and with people of different cultures and beliefs. ICN congress paper.) Journal of Advanced Nursing, 3 (2), Mar 1978, 155-166.

58 **Lewis, E.P.** Editorial. How it all came

about. (Evolution of American nursing organisations.) Nursing Outlook, 25 (2), Feb 1977, 96-97.

59 Lysaught, J.P. and others Progress in professional service: nurse leaders queried. (Implementation of recommendations of the National Commission for the Study of Nursing and the state of nursing in the U.S.) Hospitals, 52 (10), 16 Aug 1978, 93-94, 96, 98, 120.

60 McMahon, M.B. Health care in the Arctic. (Public health nursing with Eskimos in Alaska.) Nursing Times, 75, 6 Dec 1979, 2107-2110.

61 Moloney, M.M. The integrated baccalaureate curriculum: an opinion survey. Nursing Outlook, 26 (6), Jun 1978, 375-379.

62 National League for Nursing Entry into registered nursing: issues and problems. New York: NLN, 1977.

63 National League for Nursing Health care in the 1980's. Who provides? Who plans? Who pays? New York: NLN, 1979.

64 National League for Nursing NLN Convention Report. Anaheim, California April 24-27. Nursing Outlook, 25 (6), Jun 1977, 378-387.

65 National League for Nursing Nursing service in a specialty, a rural, and an urban hospital. New York: NLN, 1979.

66 National League for Nursing Policies and procedures of accreditation for programs in nursing education. 3rd ed. New York: NLN, 1979.

67 National League for Nursing This is the National League for Nursing. New York: NLN, 1977.

68 National League for Nursing. Council of Diploma Programs Today's issues: tomorrow's achievements: papers presented at the 1976 annual meeting. New York: NLN, 1976.

69 National League for Nursing. Division of Research Nursing data book: statistical information on nursing education and newly licensed nurses. New York: NLN, 1978.

70 Novello, D.J. The National Health Planning and Resources Development Act: what it is and how it works. Nursing Outlook, 24 (6), Jun 1976, 354-361.

71 Nursing Mirror A symposium on nursing in America, how they see themselves and how we see them. Nursing Mirror, 143 (2), 8 Jul 1976, 45-57.

72 Nursing Outlook Outlook on nursing. (Four articles on the past, present and future to commemorate 25 years of Nursing Outlook.) Nursing Outlook, 26 (1), Jan 1978, 28-46.

73 Parker, N.I. and Wain, O. A project for the development of credit examinations for assessing point of entry for diploma graduates into a baccalaureate nursing programme. Journal of Advanced Nursing, 2 (4), Jul 1977, 393-403.

74 Phillips, D.F. American hospitals: a look ahead. Hospitals, 50 (1), 1 Jan 1976, 73-75, 78-79.

75 Powers, E.M. The unification model in nursing. (Integration of service and education in

the United States.) Nursing Outlook, 24 (8), Aug 1976, 482-487.

76 Primeaux, M. Caring for the American Indian patient. American Journal of Nursing, 77 (1), Jan 1977, 91-94.

77 Raheja, K.K. Nursing in transition. (In the U.S.) Nursing Forum, 15 (4), 1976, 413-417.

78 Randall, A. Health care in the USA: an administrator's reactions. Nursing Times, 73, 3 Nov 1977, 1726-1727.

79 Roemer, M.I. Social medicine: the advance of organized health services in America. New York: Springer, 1978. (Springer series on health care and society; 3.)

80 Salvage, J. Jane Salvage in America. (Report of visit to hospitals in Chicago, Minnesota and California.) Nursing Mirror, 150, 10 Jan 1980, 27-29.

81 Siegel, H.J. and Elsberry, N. Master's preparation for joint practice. (New course at University of Wisconsin-Oshkosh.) Nursing Outlook, 27 (1), Jan 1979, 57-60.

82 Soules, M.T. What does a B.S.N. get you? (Survey of hospitals showed that baccalaureate, diploma and associate degree nurses did the same sort of work.) RN Magazine, 41 (6), Jun 1978, 50-51.

83 Spector, A.F. Regional planning for nursing education in the south, 1972-1975: a study in transition. Atlanta: Southern Regional Education Board, 1975.

84 Styles, M.M. and Wilson, H.S. The third resolution. An analysis of the career mobility resolution passed by the 1978 ANA House of Delegates — and a description of a new educational program developed in response. Nursing Outlook, 27 (1), Jan 1979, 44-47.

85 Thompson, D. Health care in the USA: a doctor's impressions. Nursing Times, 73, 3 Nov 1977, 1724-1725.

86 Thompson, J. The ANA in Washington. Kansas City: American Nurses Association, 1972.

87 Tichborne, V. Going to the States? be prepared! (Nurse describes her work in Florida and gives advice to British nurses.) Nursing Times, 76, 7 Feb 1980, 257-258.

88 Torrens, P.R. The American health care system: issues and problems. St. Louis: Mosby, 1978. (Issues and problems in health care series.)

89 Torrens, P.R. Health insurance in the United States: implications for the United Kingdom. Lancet, 1, 5 Jan 1980, 27-31.

90 Trandel-Korenchuk, D.M. and Trandel-Korenchuk, K.M. How state laws recognize advanced nursing practice. Nursing Outlook, 26 (11), Nov 1978, 713-719.

91 TRENDS in nursing and nursing education in the United States and elsewhere. Lamp, 33 (2), Feb 1976, 5, 7, 9, 11, 13-15.

92 Turnbull, A. Nursing in the USA. (American systems of nursing education and nursing care using 'SOAP' nursing care plans.) Nursing Mirror, 146, 27 Apr 1978, 26-28.

93 United States Department of Health,

Education and Welfare. Division of Nursing Redesigning nursing education for public health: report of the conference May 23-25, 1973. The Department, 1975.

94 Wagoner, E.F. The issue of separate licensure enters the nursing arena. (For dependent and independent nursing practice.) Journal of Nursing Education, 16 (1), Jan 1977, 11-13.

95 Walsh, M.E. 25 years of nursing leadership (25th anniversary of the founding of the National League for Nursing.) Nursing Outlook, 25 (4), Apr 1977, 248-249.

96 WHAT future for nursing? (A collection of views of nurses in the United States.) AORN Journal, 24 (2), Aug 1976, 217-235.

97 Williams, S.J. and Torrens, P.R. editors Introduction to health services. New York: Wiley Medical, 1980. (Wiley series in health services.)

98 Wood, J. To have and have not in the land of plenty. (Impressions of the US health service compared with NHS.) Health and Social Service Journal, 89, 13 Apr 1979, 418-419.

99 Youtz, D.J. The Capital City School of Nursing formerly the Washington Training School for Nurses 1877-1972. Alexandria: Capital City School of Nursing Alumnae Association, 1975.

100 Zimmerman, A. AJN interviews the ANA president. (Anne Zimmerman, on the role of the American Nurses' Association.) American Journal of Nursing, 78 (6), Jun 1978, 1018-1021.

UNITED STATES: OVERSEAS NURSES

101 Davitz, L.J. and others Foreign and American nurses: reactions and interactions. (Survey of the attitudes of 95 foreign nurses compared with American attitudes to nursing care and practice.) Nursing Outlook, 24 (4), Apr 1976, 237-242.

102 Dhillon, C.L. Study programs for foreign nurses: special needs of foreign nurses. Nursing Outlook, 24 (1), Jan 1976, 43-44.

103 Drury, R.K. Study programs for foreign nurses: a university based program. (Course at Pace University, New York, to familiarize overseas students with cultural and professional aspects of nursing in USA.) Nursing Outlook, 24 (1), Jan 1976, 41-42.

104 Koehler, C.J. Recruiting abroad: does it pay? (Concludes that recruiting of foreign-educated (including British-trained) nurses is not a feasible method of relieving staff shortages.) American Journal of Nursing, 78 (12), Dec 1978, 2086-2089.

29 NATIONAL HEALTH SERVICE

a GENERAL

1 Atkinson, P. and others, editors Prospects for the National Health. Croom Helm, 1979.

2 Avery Jones, F. Getting the NHS back on course. British Medical Journal, 2, 1 Jul 1978, 5-9.

3 Barnard, K. and Lee, K. Conflicts in the National Health Service. Croom Helm, 1977.

4 Bevan, G. and others Health care priorities and management. Croom Helm, 1980.

5 Black, D. Health care today and tomorrow. (Based on IHSA conference paper.) Hospital and Health Services Review, 74 (9), Sep 1978, 309-312.

6 Black, Sir D. and Thomas, G.P. editors Providing for the health services: proceedings of Section X (General) of the British Association for the Advancement of Science, 1977. Croom Helm, 1978.

7 Bricknell, J.G. The Health Service: reappraisal of priorities. Nursing Mirror, 143, 22 Jul 1976, 69-70.

8 British Medical Journal The next 30 years. (Five working papers and discussion at a BMJ conference, including Prevention or cure? and Home or hospital?) British Medical Journal, 2, 1 Jul 1978, 22-27.

9 Brown, A. NHS: where we lie in the league. (Comparison with other countries.) Nursing Mirror, 149, 2 Aug 1979, 6.

10 Brown, R.G.S. The changing National Health Service. 2nd ed. Routledge and Kegan Paul, 1978.

11 Carstairs, V. and Heasman, M.A. Scotland's health problems and health resources. Hospital and Health Services Review, 75 (5), May 1979, 151-155.

12 CENTRAL Health Services Council. Annual report 1975-1976. HMSO, 1976-1977.

13 Central Office of Information. Reference Division Health services in Britain. 9th ed. HMSO, 1977. (Reference pamphlet no.20.)

14 CIBA Foundation Health care in a changing setting: the U.K. experience. (Symposium held in London, 3-4 December 1975.) Amsterdam, Elsevier, 1976. (Ciba Foundation Symposium 43, new series.)

15 Clode, D. 'Producing health instead of wealth'. (Interview with Dr. Peter Draper, director of the Unit for the Study of Health Policy.) Health and Social Service Journal, 88, 17 Nov 1978, 1308-1310.

16 De Kadt, E. Wrong priorities in health. (Problems of health care provisions in Britain in relation to economics, class and political problems.) New Society, 36, 3 Jun 1976, 525-526.

17 Department of Health and Social Security Annual report 1976-1977. HMSO, 1977-1978.

18 Department of Health and Social Security Health and personal social services in England: DHSS planning guidelines for 1978/79. DHSS, 1978.

19 Department of Health and Social Security Health and personal social services statistics for England, 1976-1979. HMSO, 1976-1979.

20 Department of Health and Social Security Research and development report and handbook 1977. HMSO, 1977.

21 Dixon, E. Crosswinds over the Atlantic. (Comparison of some aspects of health care in Britain and the USA.) Nursing Mirror, 151, 24 Jul 1980, 28-29.

22 Draper, P. and others The NHS in the next 30 years: a new perspective on the health of the British. Unit for the Study of Health Policy, 1978.

23 Ennals, D. The national health service. (Text of speech delivered at IHSA conference 1978 and discussion.) Hospital and Health Services Review, 74 (8), Aug 1978, 265, 268, 275-276.

24 Ennals, D. National Health Service: future of the 'world's best buy'. (Text of a speech made to the Oxford Medical Society, 27 Oct 1976.) Department of Health and Social Security, 1976.

25 Garraway, M. Evaluation in the National Health Service. Health Bulletin, 34 (5), Sep 1976, 256-261.

26 Godber, Sir G. Attainable goals in health. University of Glasgow Press, 1976. (Maurice Bloch lecture no.16.)

27 Godber, Sir G. Problems in the delivery of health care. Community Health, 8 (1), Jul 1976, 2-11.

28 Haugejorden, O. Proposal of a hierarchical classification of health service objectives, activities and resources. Public Health, 93 (6), Nov 1979, 358-362.

29 Hewitt, M. The medical mainliner. (Addiction to health care systems by Western society.) Nursing Times, 73, 22/29 Dec 1977, 1984-1985.

30 HOSPITAL and health services yearbook. 1976-1980. Institute of Health Service Administrators 1976-1980.

31 Jaques, E. editor Health services: their nature and organisation, and the role of patients, doctors, nurses, and the complementary professions. Heinemann, 1978.

32 Jennings, A.M.C. Efficiency in the National Health Service. (Delivering service as and when required.) Lancet, 1, 26 Feb 1977, 474-475.

33 Jones, J.I. The comprehensive approach to health care in Britain: service implications and requirements. (Symposium paper.) S.A. Nursing Journal, 43 (9), Sep 1976, 21-24.

34 Klein, R. Ideology, class and the National Health Service. King's Fund Centre, 1980. (KF project paper: RC4.)

35 McLachlan, G. editor Mixed communications. Oxford: Oxford University Press for Nuffield Provincial Hospitals Trust, 1979. (Problems and progress in medical care: essays on current research; 12th series.)

36 Nelson, A.M. Priorities in health care. (Conference address.) Community Health, 7 (3), Jan 1976, 162-166.

37 Northern Ireland. Department of Health and Social Services Report for period 1 October 1973-31 December 1976. HMSO, 1979.

38 Nuttall, P.D. The British National Health Service. Nursing Outlook, 25 (2), Feb 1977, 98-102.

39 Parston, G. Planners, politics and health services. Croom Helm, 1980.

40 Radical Statistics Health Group In defence of the NHS. The Group, 1977.

41 Roys, P.J. The past—the way ahead. (Presidential address at the annual conference of the Institute of Health Service Administrators.) Hospital and Health Services Review, 73 (7), Jul 1977, 244-250.

42 Scottish Home and Health Department The health service in Scotland: the way ahead. HMSO, 1976.

43 Scottish Home and Health Department Health services in Scotland. Report 1975-1979. HMSO, 1976-1980.

44 Scottish Home and Health Department Structure and management of the NHS in Scotland. Edinburgh: HMSO, 1979.

45 Smith, J. Green fields of learning. (Work of Brunel Institute of Organisation and Social Studies on the structure of the NHS.) Health and Social Service Journal, 89, 1 Feb 1979, 94-96.

46 Stacey, M. People who are affected by the inverse law of care. Some of the variations between medical treatment and health in the different social classes. Health and Social Service Journal, 87, 3 Jun 1977, 898-899, 902.

47 Stacey, M. editor The sociology of the National Health Service. University of Keele, 1976. (Sociological review monograph no.22.)

48 Walters, V. Class inequality and health care: the origins and impact of the National Health Service. Croom Helm, 1980.

49 Welsh Office Health and personal social service statistics for Wales. No.2. 1975-No.6. 1979. HMSO, 1976-1980.

50 Welsh Office The structure and management of the National Health Service in Wales. Cardiff: HMSO, 1980.

51 Widgery, D. Health in danger: the crisis in the National Health Service. Macmillan, 1979. (Crisis points series.)

THIRTIETH ANNIVERSARY

52 Abel-Smith, B. National Health Service: the first thirty years. HMSO, 1978.

53 Abel-Smith, B. Political pendulum swings as clocks chime in the decade. (Review of developments in the health service during 1970s.) Health and Social Service Journal, 90, 4 Jan 1980, 12-15.

54 Briggs, A. The growth of the social services: 1. Making health every citizen's birthright: the road to 1946. New Society, 46, 16 Nov 1978, 383-386.

55 Briggs, A. The growth of the social services: 2. The achievements, failures and aspirations of the NHS. (Developments from 1948 to the present.) New Society, 46, 23 Nov, 1978, 448-451.

56 British Medical Journal Thirty years ago. Six doctors recall the birth of the NHS. British Medical Journal, 2, 1 Jul 1978, 28-33.

57 Castle, B. NHS revisited. Fabian Society, 1976. (Fabian tract 440.)

58 Clark, J. Bevan's masterpiece or Bevan's folly? (Shortened version of her address to 1978 Rcn Congress.) Nursing Mirror, 147, 6 Jul 1978, 16-19.

59 Clark, J. The British National Health Service 1948-1978: should we start again? Journal of Advanced Nursing, 4 (2), Mar 1979, 205-214.

60 Department of Health and Social Security NHS and social services: thirtieth anniversary. DHSS, 1978. (Leaflet NHS 7.)

61 Dunford, J. An old-timer looks back. (At the health services since 1914.) Nursing Mirror, 145, 29 Dec 1977, 18.

62 Harris, J. Beveridge and the Welfare State. Nursing Mirror, 146, 13 Apr 1978, 53, 55.

63 Health and Social Service Journal The thirtieth anniversary. (Events leading up to the NHS and profile of Bevan.) Health and Social Service Journal, 188, 30 Jun 1978, 726-733.

64 Hunter, D. New wine in old bottles? Changes in the NHS since 1948. Health and Social Service Journal, 87, 3 Jun 1977, 890.

65 Lancet The NHS anniversary. Lancet, 2, 15 Jul 1978, 167.

66 Lee, J. Battle for the Health Service. (Interview with Jennie Lee, widow of NHS founder Aneurin Bevan.) Nursing Mirror, 147, 6 Jul 1978, 9-11.

67 Nursing Times 30 years of the NHS. (With reminiscences of 5 July 1948 by some prominent nurses.) Nursing Times, 74, 6 Jul 1978, 1117-1120.

68 Nursing Times 'We must fight for change'. (Report of conference to mark 30 years of the NHS.) Nursing Times, 74, 13 Jul 1978, 1148.

69 Orriss, H.D. Social security and health care since Beveridge. Nursing Times, 72, 11 Mar 1976, 390-391.

70 Ride, T.J. Developments in the post-war health services. Nursing Times, 73, 15 Sep 1977, Occ. papers, 121-124; 22 Sep 1977, Occ. papers, 125-127.

71 Scottish Home and Health Department The National Health Service in Scotland 1948-1978. Edinburgh: SHHD, 1978.

72 Smith, A. How much have we changed? 6. Are we any healthier? (Since NHS established.) New Society, 41, 8 Sep 1977, 485-487.

73 Wakeley, J. NHS is 30 years old. (Comment and comparison with U.S.) Supervisor Nurse, 9 (9), Oct 1978, 66-67.

74 Watkin, B. The National Health Service: the first phase 1948-74 and after. Allen & Unwin, 1978.

75 Yellowlees, H. The National Health Service—thirty years on. Health Trends, 10 (3), Aug 1978, 45-48.

b COMMUNITY HEALTH COUNCILS

1 Ackroyd, E. Health care and the public. (By president of the Patients Association.) Hospital and Health Services Review, 74 (9), Sep 1978, 318-321.

2 Anderson, R. Public awareness and interest in community health councils. (Information from recent national study of general practice.) Health and Social Service Journal, 89, 22 Mar 1979, Centre eight papers C29-C31.

3 Ashworth, W. and Mitchell, G. The CHC and its public. Hospital and Health Services Review, 72 (6), Jun 1976, 204-205.

4 Ball, D. Can the little dog stop the dish running off with the spoon? (Role of CHC in monitoring and influencing change in the City and Hackney Health District (Teaching) against a background of cutbacks.) Health and Social Service Journal, 87, 17 Jun 1977, 920-921.

5 Bochel, D. and MacLaren, M. Local health councils—representatives of the consumer? (Scottish equivalent of CHCs.) Hospital and Health Services Review, 75 (5), May 1979, 164-168.

6 Bradney, D. Watchdogs that give you a say in keeping health services up to scratch. (Functions of CHCs.) Health and Social Service Journal, 89, 5 Jan 1979, 16-17.

7 Clark, C. and Brennan, M. Reflecting local health and care with the right class of person. (Study of two community health councils in Birmingham.) Health and Social Service Journal, 86, 3 Dec 1976, 2154-2155; 10 Dec 1976, 2199.

8 Cox, L.W. CHCs and HCPTs: The Salisbury experience. (Community health councils and health care planning teams.) Hospital and Health Services Review, 72 (8), Aug 1976, 267-269.

9 Cox, L.W. Organising, managing and servicing a community health council. Hospital and Health Services Review, 74 (9), Sep 1978, 305-307.

10 Davidson, N. Opening doors to meet the needs of the people served. (Representatives and influence of CHCs, and views on proposals for electing members to AHAs.) Health and Social Service Journal, 89, 11 May 1979, 566-569.

11 Donald, B.L. Time for a change: finding an identity for the CHC. Hospital and Health Services Review, 72 (1), Jan 1976, 5-7.

12 Farrell, C. and Levitt, R. Consumers, community health councils and the NHS. King's Fund Centre, 1980. (KF project paper; RC4.)

13 Faulkner, R. Involving the consumer. How can community health councils involve consumers in decisions? Health and Social Service Journal, 86, 17 Sep 1976, 1664.

14 Fruin, D. Community health councils: keeping the balance. (In the light of 'Patients first'.) British Medical Journal, 280, 7 Jun 1980, 1385-1386.

15 Gerrard, M. What next?—future perspectives for CHCs. Royal Society of Health Journal, 99 (4), Aug 1979, 169-172, 175.

16 Hallas, J. CHCs in action: a review. Nuffield Provincial Hospitals Trust, 1976.

17 Hallas, J. The Health Service—the patients' eye view. Professionalizing participation. (Role of CHCs in an NHS facing financial problems.) Royal Society of Health Journal, 97 (3), Jun 1977, 119-120.

18 Hallas, J. What CHCs are thinking. A seminar discussion. (At the Nuffield Centre, Leeds.) Hospital and Health Services Review, 74 (8), Aug 1978, 263-264.

19 Ham, C. and Levitt, R. Who speaks for patients? (Survey of age, sex and social class of CHC members attending a training programme.) Hospital and Health Services Review, 75 (10), Oct 1979, 351-352.

20 Harper, A.V. The community health council. Community Health, 8 (1), Jul 1976, 48-52.

21 Hospital and Health Services Review Community health councils. Hospital and Health Services Review, 72 (9), Sep 1976, 298-299.

22 Hospital and Health Services Review Community health councils. (Review of some annual reports.) Hospital and Health Services Review, 72 (1), Jan 1976, 19-20; 72 (2), Feb 1976, 67-68; (3), Mar 1976, 94-95; (11), Nov 1976, 394-396; 73 (1), Jan 1977, 21-22; (5), May 1977, 164-165.

23 Hyde, A. Seeing inside with outside eyes. (Hospital visiting by CHCs.) Health and Social Service Journal, 89, 2 Nov 1979, 1410-1411.

24 Jones, D. As others see us... (Difficulties CHCs face in getting public recognition.) Health and Social Service Journal, 87, 24 Jun 1977, 961.

25 Jones, D.T. Consulting the public: some recent findings. (Consumer participation in the NHS.) British Medical Journal, 2, 22 Oct 1977, 1101-1102.

26 Jones, W.T. Influencing individual and public responses. (Public participation in matters affecting health.) Nursing Mirror, 142, 8 Apr 1976, 65-67.

27 Keywood, O. The NHS and the consumer. Community health councils—1. (Description of functions.) Nursing Times, 74, 2 Feb 1978, 180-181.

28 Klein, R. and Lewis, J. The politics of consumer representation: a study of Community Health Councils. Centre for Studies in Social Policy, 1976.

29 Lanbridge, C. Community health councils—watchdogs or lapdogs? Nursing Mirror, 145, 13 Oct 1977, 42-43.

30 Lancet Representing the patient. (Community health councils.) Lancet, 1976, 1, 17 Apr 1976, 846.

31 Levitt, R. The people's voice in the NHS: community health councils after five years. King Edward's Hospital Fund for London, 1980.

32 Levitt, R. Challenging the apathy of the NHS consumer. (Future of CHCs in the light of 'Patients first'.) Health and Social Service Journal, 90, 18 Apr 1980, 507.

33 Levitt, R. and Ham, C. Gathering new ideas. (Role of CHCs in NHS planning system.) Health and Social Service Journal, 88, 12 May 1978, 544.

34 Levitt, R. An uphill struggle for even the most gregarious CHC. (Difficulties encountered by CHCs in putting forward public's viewpoint.) Health and Social Service Journal, 89, 11 May 1979, 569-570.

35 Lewis, J. The community and health. (The work of community health councils.) Nursing Mirror, 142, 15 Jan 1976, 40-41.

36 McCarthy, S. How a CHC can help with

complaints. Midwife, Health Visitor and Community Nurse, 15 (7), Jul 1979, 276-277, 279.

37 Mackeith, J.S. Community participation in health care—how it has worked out in practice. (In Sunderland, including role of CHC.) Hospital and Health Services Review, 76 (2), Feb 1980, 62-66.

38 Marre, R.M. Community health councils—a personal view. Health Trends, 7 (3), Aug 1975, 45-46.

39 Marre, R.M. Community Health Councils—a personal view. Community Health, 8 (3), Jan 1977, 164-167.

40 Midwife, Health Visitor and Community Nurse Community health councils surveyed. Midwife, Health Visitor and Community Nurse, 12 (2), Feb 1976, 45-46.

41 Mullen, P. Community health councils—planning and health care planning teams. Royal Society of Health Journal, 97 (2), Apr 1977, 85-88.

42 Page, J. Co-ordinating community health. (The advantages and disadvantages of a national body for community health councils.) Health and Social Service Journal, 86, 3 Jul 1976, 1212-1213.

43 Royal Society of Health Journal Consumer satisfaction in the health service: the role of the community health council. (Two articles.) Royal Society of Health Journal, 98 (4), Aug 1978, 173-180, 195.

44 Saunders, M. Would community health councils be missed? (By secretary of Islington CHC who argues that they are valuable.) Nursing Focus, 1 (7), Mar 1980, 278, 280.

45 Skeet, M. Community involvement: ways in which the community health councils can encourage public participation in health care. Nursing Mirror, 143, 14 Oct 1976, 40-41.

46 Stevenson, M.J. The NHS and the consumer. Community health councils—2. (Their development, contribution and relationships to NHS personnel.) Nursing Times, 74, 2 Feb 1978, 181-183.

47 Thomson, W. Local health councils—personal point of view. (Scottish equivalent of community health councils.) Health Bulletin, 36 (4), Jul 1978, 183-186.

c COMPUTERS

1 Alderson, M. A review of the National Health Service's computing policy in the 1970s. British Journal of Preventive and Social Medicine, 30 (1), Mar 1976, 11-16.

2 Iduna, pseud. Computerisation of personal health records. Health Visitor, 51 (6), Jun 1978, 227.

3 Laver, F.J.M. Janforum. The significance of computing. (General assessment of value of computers.) Journal of Advanced Nursing, 4 (5), Sep 1979, 555-558.

4 Linger, T.S. and Davies, J.C. Conversion of the patient master index at Southampton to a computer based system. (All records relating to a patient are integrated.) Health and Social Service

Journal, 88, 24 Mar 1978, Centre eight papers A17-A20.

5 Lucas, R.W. and others Computer interrogation of patients: (to replace routine 'history taking'.) British Medical Journal, 2, 11 Sep 1976, 623-625.

6 Sawicki, F. Use of computers in health services. Copenhagen: World Health Organization, Regional Office for Europe, 1977.

7 Tunnicliffe Wilson, J.C. A review of operational problems tackled by computer simulation in health care facilities. (With extensive bibliography.) Health and Social Service Journal, 90, 18 Jul 1980, Centre eight papers B73-B80.

d FINANCE AND RESOURCES

1 Abel-Smith, B. Value for money in health services: a comparative study. Heinemann, 1976.

2 Acheson, R.M. The definition and identification of need for health care. (With reference to RAWP.) Journal of Epidemiology and Community Health, 32 (1), Mar 1978, 10-15.

3 Age Concern Comments on 'Priorities for health and Personal Social Services in England': DHSS consultative document. Mitcham: Age Concern, 1976.

4 Ashton, J.R. R.A.W.P. and the achievement of equity in the National Health Service. Public Health, 92 (4), Jul 1978, 190-196.

5 Association of Health Service Treasurers Research Committee Internal audit in the National Health Service. The Association, 1977.

6 Avery Jones, F. RAWP, the Royal Commission, and the 'inner cities'. Lancet, 2, 18 Aug 1979, 372-374.

7 Barnard, K. and Ham, C. National Health Service. The reallocation of resources: parallels and past experience. Lancet, 1, 26 Jun 1976, 1399-1400.

8 Barr, A. and Logan, R.F.L. Policy alternatives for resource allocation. (The two reports issued by the RAWP (Resources Allocation Working Party) and future goals.) Lancet, 1, 7 May 1977, 994-996.

9 Bennett, A.E. and Holland, W.W. Rational planning or muddling through? Resource allocation in the NHS. Lancet, 1977, 1, 26 Feb 1977, 464-466.

10 Bosanquet, N. A necessary evil? (Queries need for health service cutbacks.) Nursing Mirror, 150, 12 Jun 1980, 35-36.

11 Bosanquet, N. Spending to best effect. (The implications of the White Paper on public expenditure for the health service.) Nursing Times, 72, 26 Feb 1976, 286-287.

12 Boyd, K.M. editor The ethics of resource allocation in health care. Edinburgh: Edinburgh University Press, 1979.

13 British Medical Journal If I was forced to cut. (Views on ways to save NHS money.) British Medical Journal 2. Community physician, 13 Oct 1979, 905-906; Consultant physician, 20 Oct 1979, 985-986; Consultant pathologist, 27 Oct 1979, 1057-1058.

14 British Medical Journal A policy of despair. (Consultative document on priorities for health and social services.) British Medical Journal, 1976, 1, 3 Apr 1976, 787-788.

15 Clode, D. Health warning on cash policies ...(Report of HVA annual conference.) Health and Social Service Journal, 87, 28 Oct 1977, 1486-1487.

16 Cole, A. Idealism and opportunism. (How RAWP has helped Medway Health District.) Nursing Times, 74, 16 Nov 1978, 1885-1889.

17 Collier, A.J. and Shaw, R.M. Health service priorities in England. 2. The DHSs role in the allocation of financial resources for the NHS. Health Trends, 5 (8), Nov 1976, 81-83.

18 Creese, A.L. and others NHS priorities and RAWP. British Medical Journal, 2, 18 Nov 1978, 1446-1447.

19 Culyer, A.J. and Wright, K.G. editors Economic aspects of health services. Robertson, 1978.

20 Culyer, A.J. Need and the National Health Service: economics and social choice. Martin Robertson, 1976.

21 Davidson, N. The honeymoon is over. (Lack of implementation of RAWP by present government and its effects on Sunderland AHA.) Health and Social Service Journal, 90, 7 Mar 1980, 320-322.

22 Davidson, N. Two and two making five. (Analysis of Government's suggested financial savings which include reductions in divisional nursing officers.) Health and Social Service Journal, 90, 1 Feb 1980, 150-152.

23 Denham, T. How a team finds its way through the budget maze. (Specialty budgeting in East Cumbria.) Health and Social Service Journal, 88, 1 Dec 1978, 1367-1368.

24 Department of Health and Social Security Resource Allocation Working Party. Sharing resources for health in England. HMSO, 1976. (RAWP)

25 Department of Health and Social Security Resource Allocation Working Party. Sharing resources for health in England. HMSO, 1976. (RAWP) Comments on the report. British Medical Journal, 2, 9 Oct 1976, 893-895; Health and Social Service Journal, 86, 1 Oct 1976, 1756-1757; Lancet, 2, 2 Oct 1976, 733-734; Nursing Times, 73, 7 Oct 1976, 1540.

26 Department of Health and Social Security Priorities for health and social services in England: a consultative document. HMSO, 1976.

27 Department of Health and Social Security Priorities in the health and social services: the way forward. Further discussions of the government's national strategy. HMSO, 1977.

28 DIRECT benefit to patient care. (Effect of RAWP on Wigan AHA.) Nursing Times, 75, 15 Mar 1979, 437-440.

29 Dopson, L. The end of a dream? (Comment on recent document 'The Litmus papers' on alternative ways of financing the NHS.) Nursing Times, 76, 11 Dec 1980, 2178.

30 **Draper, P.** Economic policy and health. Unit for the Study of Health Policy, 1976.

31 **Dudley, H.A.F.** Efficiency in the National Health Service. Loosening patient immobility. (Discussion of RAWP.) Lancet, 1, 11 Jun 1977, 1251-1253.

32 **English, M.L.** Budgeting for national health expenditure: the British system. World Hospitals, 7 (3), 1976, 164-170.

33 **Ennals, D.** Better value for money in the N.H.S. Rehabilitation no.100, Jan-Mar 1977, 41-49.

34 **Ennals, D.** Mr. Ennals on closures. (Report of speech at Manchester Business School.) Hospital and Health Services Review, 73 (11), Nov 1977, 397-398.

35 **Ennals, D.** Prospects for 1977. Statement to explain the thinking behind financial allocations for 1977—including the controversial recommendations of the Resource Allocation Working Party. Nursing Times, 73, 6 Jan 1977, 12-13.

36 **Ferrer, H.P. and others** The use of mortality data in the report of the Resource Allocation Working Party. Public Health, 91 (6), Nov 1977, 289-295.

37 **Ferster, G. and Butts, M.** A method for estimating revenue expenditure by specialty in an RHA. Hospital and Health Services Review, 73 (3), Mar 1977, 79-83.

38 **Forsythe, J.M. and Fleming, P.H.J.** Le Health service priorities in England. 4. 'Amid shot and shell': allocation of financial resources for the Area Health Authority. Health Trends, 9 (2), May 1977, 26-29.

39 **Godber, Sir G.** Building on our assets. (Report of an interview on the assets of the present NHS.) British Medical Journal, 1, 13 Mar 1976, 638-640.

40 **Goldacre, M.J. and Harris, R.I.** Mortality, morbidity, resource allocation, and planning: a consideration of disease classification. British Medical Journal, 281, 6 Dec 1980, 1515-1519.

41 **Gravelle, H.S.E. and Williams, A.** Health service finance and resource management. King's Fund Centre, 1980. (KF project paper: RC6.)

42 **Guy's Hospital Medical School. Department of Community Medicine Unit for the Study of Health Policy** Health, money and the National Health Service. The Unit, 1976.

43 **Halpern, S.** 1. All this and RAWP. 2. Where to from here? Health and Social Service Journal, 88, 20 Oct 1978, 1188-1190; 27 Oct 1918, 1212-1214.

44 **Hospital and Health Services Review** Finance in the National Health Service. Hospital and Health Services Review, 73 (3), Mar 1977, 106-109.

45 **Hospital and Health Services Review** Notes for students. Finance in the NHS. Hospital and Health Services Review, 76 (4), Apr 1980, 161-162.

46 **Jeffries, M.** RAWP and the Oxford region. British Medical Journal 1. The impact on medical care of DHSS economics. 18 Feb 1978, 426-427. 2. The hub of the problem. 25 Feb 1978, 495-496.

3. Closures, economies and cuts. 11 Mar 1978, 638-639.

47 **Jenkin, P.** Can we afford a free NHS? (Text of speech and discussion at IHSA conference.) Hospital and Health Services Review, 74 (8), Aug 1978, 269-275.

48 **Journal of Medical Ethics** Who shall die? (Allocation of life-saving resources.) Journal of Medical Ethics, 6 (4), Dec 1980, 171-172.

49 **Klein, R.** The policies of redistribution. (Comments on the report of the Resources Allocation Working Party.) British Medical Journal, 2, 9 Oct 1976, 893-895.

50 **Klein, R.** Resource allocation. (In the NHS.) Hospital and Health Services Review, 73 (8), Aug 1977, 280-283.

51 **Lane, A.J. and Pethybridge, F.** Health service priorities in England. 3. The task of the Regional Health Authority in allocating financial resources and determining priorities. Health Trends, 9 (2), May 1977, 21-25.

52 **Lee, K. editor** Economics and health planning. Croom Helm, 1979.

53 **Marsh, G.N.** Cutting the cost of the National Health Service—a personal view. (General suggestions by a GP.) British Medical Journal, 280, 3 May 1980, 1140-1141.

54 **Maynard, A. and Ludbrook, A.** Applying resource allocation formulae to constituent parts of the U.K. (RAWP formula compared with Scottish, Welsh and Northern Ireland formulae.) Lancet, 1, 12 Jan 1980, 85-87.

55 **Miller, M.** Changed priorities or hidden cuts? (Allocation of health service resources.) New Scientist, 72, 4 Nov 1976, 288-289.

56 **Money-Coutts, D.B.** An alternative method of financing the health services. Community Health, 8 (3), Jan 1977, 168-170.

57 **Morris, P.** Wasting away in the NHS. (Views of nurses on causes and prevention of waste.) Nursing Mirror, 149, 11 Oct 1979, 7.

58 **Muir Gray, J.A.** Choosing priorities. (In health care.) Journal of Medical Ethics, 5 (2), Jun 1979, 73-75.

59 **Nairne, P.** Health service priorities in England. 1. A fair share of national resources? Health Trends, 4 (8), Aug 1976, 61-66.

60 **Nurse, J.** How NHS budgeting has become a bristling form of animal life. (Functional budgeting at district level including providing information on expenditure to nurse managers.) Health and Social Service Journal, 88, 8 Dec 1978, 1391-1392.

61 **Nursing Mirror** Some growth in primary care, geriatric and psychiatric nursing. (Comments on the public expenditure White Paper.) Nursing Mirror, 142, 8, 26 Feb 1976, 34.

62 **Nursing Times** Doing the best we can. (Report of visit to Northumberland AHA, one of the poorest areas in the NHS which is benefiting from RAWP.) Nursing Times, 74, 26 Oct 1978, 1754-1759.

63 **Nursing Times** Nursing Times explains. Resource reallocation. Nursing Times, 74, 23 Nov 1978, 1926-1927.

64 **Office of Health Economics** Scarce resources in health care. OHE, 1979. (Studies of current health problems no.64.)

65 **Owen, D.** Priorities and expenditure. (Interview with Dr. David Owen.) British Medical Journal, 1, 28 Feb 1976, 513-515.

66 **Polytechnic of Central London. Health Services Study Group** Finance in the NHS. Part 1: NHS financial allocations and budgetary control. The Group, 1980.

67 **Radical Statistics Health Group** RAWP deals: a critique of 'sharing resources for health in England'. The Group, 1977.

68 **Rickard, J.H.** Per capita expenditure of the English area health authorities. British Medical Journal, 1, 31 Jan 1976, 299-300.

69 **Rippington, T.** Being on the right side of RAWP after three years. Health and Social Service Journal, 88, 10 Mar 1978, 277-278.

70 **Royal College of Nursing** The effect of financial cutbacks in the National Health Service on standards of care. Rcn, 1977.

71 **Royal College of Nursing** Comments on the consultative document 'Priorities for health and personal social services in England.' Rcn, 1976.

72 **Royal College of Nursing** Priorities for health and social services in England: Rcn initial statement. Rcn, 1976.

73 **Salvage, J.** Crisis of costs? (Effects of cuts on NHS.) Nursing Mirror, 150, 12 Jun 1980, 31-33.

74 **Schrijvers, G.** 'What I miss in England is some sort of devolution to hospitals'. (Interview describing his enquiry into resource allocation in the British and Swedish health services as compared with the Dutch system.) Health and Social Service Journal, 88, 7 Apr 1978, 393-394.

75 **Scottish Health Centre** Health services economics. (Report of conference.) Nursing Mirror, 142, 10 Jun 1976, 63-66; 17 Jun 1976, 55-59.

76 **Smith, A.** The reorganized National Health Service. Priorities for allocation of resources. Royal Society of Health Journal, 96 (2), Apr 1976, 67-69, 85.

77 **Steele, R. and Gray, A.M.** Beyond the programme budget: economics and resource planning in the NHS. Hospital and Health Services Review, 76 (3), Mar 1980, 96-101.

78 **Stone, D.H.** An approach to the analysis of health care needs and resources. (With reference to RAWP and SHARE reports.) Journal of Epidemiology and Community Health, 34 (3), Sep 1980, 208-211.

79 **Thorne, S.** Whose health service is it these days, anyway? (Problems in consultation with the public over cuts in services in the light of recent consultative document.) Health and Social Service Journal, 90, 11 Jan 1980, 57-58.

80 **Trenchard, H.** Cash and care: a question of priorities. Nursing Focus, 1 (9), May 1980, 347-352.

81 **Walker, A.** To the roots of inequality. (The implications of two research reports from the Royal Commission on RAWP and finance.)

Health and Social Service Journal, 88, 18 Aug 1978, 926-927.

82 White, R. Resources. (Comments on the redeployment of resources. Called for in 'Priorities for health and personal social services in England.') Nursing Mirror, 143 (15), 7 Oct 1976, 53.

83 Wilkes, E. Unlimited demand—limited resources: the problem of priorities. Hospital and Health Services Review, 72 (8), Aug 1976, 274-276.

84 Yudkin, J.S. Changing patterns of resource allocation in a London teaching district. (Effects of RAWP in Tower Hamlets.) British Medical Journal, 2, 28 Oct 1978, 1212-1215.

e INFORMATION

1 Barr, A. Information for management and planning in the NHS: proposals for a health care information network. Hospital and Health Services Review, 73 (11), Nov 1977, 387-390.

2 Benjamin, B. editor Medical records. 2nd ed. Heinemann Medical, 1980.

3 Bunch, A.J. Health care administration: an information sourcebook. Capital Planning Information, 1979. (CPI Sourcebooks; 1.)

4 Clode, D. Planning: push-button age. (Some of the methods available nationally for collecting personnel data.) Health and Social Service Journal, 89, 13 Jul 1979, 868-871.

5 Community Health Health information systems. (Three reference papers.) Community Health, 7 (4), Apr 1976, 223-233.

6 Crown, J. Area information services. Health Trends, 10 (2), May 1978, 35-36.

7 Day, P. Private lives on record. (Problems of confidentiality in health information systems.) Health and Social Service Journal, 89, 29 Mar 1979, 312.

8 Fell, P. Ever ready with all the answers. (Information service in Barnsley AHA with special reference to statistics.) Health and Social Service Journal, 88, 8 Sep 1978, 1013.

9 Gandy, R.J. Flexible information profiles for planning. Hospital and Health Services Review, 74 (10), Oct 1978, 346-348.

10 Griffiths, D.A.T. and Wainwright, L. A hospital information room at the Ipswich District General Hospital. (To provide and encourage integrated management approach between medical, nursing and administrative staff.) Hospital and Health Services Review, 75 (4), Apr 1979, 121-126.

11 Griffiths, D.A.T. Evaluating information for management. Hospital and Health Services Review, 74 (8), Aug 1978, 259-263.

12 Hamson, J. The red rag of information. (How cooperation between health and local authorities requires systematic and thorough records.) Health and Social Service Journal, 89, 8 Jun 1979, 702-703.

13 Home Office. Committee on Data Protection Report. HMSO, 1978.

14 McLachlan, G. editor By guess or by what? Information without design in the NHS.

Nuffield Provincial Hospitals Trust/Oxford University Press, 1978. (Problems and progress in medical care essays in current research. 11th series.)

15 McLachlan, G. editor Framework and design for planning: uses of information in the NHS. Nuffield Provincial Hospitals Trust/Oxford University Press, 1977. (Problems and progress in medical care essays in current research. 10th series.)

16 Metcalfe, D.H.H. Toward the definition of the problems to be solved in the medical information system. Medical Record, 17 (2), May 1976, 115-120.

17 National Training Council for the National Health Service Report of a study of information services on training matters in the NHS. NTC, 1979.

18 Nicholson, H.W. and Shepherdson, M. A different approach to information services. The experience within Cleveland AHA. (Description of an information bank on all aspects of the health service.) Hospital and Health Services Review, 73 (7), Jul 1977, 234-235.

19 Prudden, R. and Hall, D. Opening the door to shared services at Redbridge. (Information centre run jointly by the Borough of Redbridge and the East Roding Health District.) Health and Social Service Journal, 86, 28 Aug 1976, 1553.

20 Sutherland, A. Future developments in the provision of health care information. Medical Record, 17 (1), Feb 1976, 89-93.

21 Tyrrell, M. Using numbers for effective health service management. Heinemann, 1975.

22 Vuori, H. Privacy, confidentiality and automated health information systems. Journal of Medical Ethics, 3 (4), Dec 1977, 174-178.

23 Vuori, H. The use of automated health information systems in the management and planning of health services. Public Health, 91 (1), Jan 1977, 33-43.

24 World Health Organization. Regional Office for Europe Information systems for health services, edited by G. McLachlan. Copenhagen: WHO, 1980.

f MANAGEMENT AND STAFFING

1 Association of Chief Administrators of Health Authorities. Wessex Branch The chief administrator in the reorganised health service. 2 parts. Health and Social Service Journal, 87, 12 Aug 1977, 1162-1164; 19 Aug 1977, 1188-1189.

2 Ball, D. Top table. (Report on meeting of regional team of officers, and analysis of NHS management structure generally.) Health and Social Service Journal, 88, 28 Jul 1978, 842-844.

3 Brooks, J. Still a long way to go from limbo to equality. (Survey into discrimination against women managers in the NHS.) Health and Social Service Journal, 89, 19 Oct 1979, 1354-1356.

4 Brown, R.G.S. Accountability and control in the National Health Service. Health and Social Service Journal, 87, 28 Oct 1977, B9-B15.

5 Campey, R. Filling the baskets instead of fulfilling the ideals. (Critical look at

administration in the NHS and the training schemes for administrators.) Health and Social Service Journal, 87, 18 Nov 1977, 1592-1593.

6 Charles-Edwards, D. Personnel priorities for our NHS. Industrial Society, 59, Jul/Aug 1977, 15-16.

7 Chester, D. Can the health service afford to manage like this? (Criticism of functional management in the NHS.) Health and Social Service Journal, 88, 21 Apr 1978, 451-452.

8 Clode, D. 'Plans aren't worth the paper they are written on.' (The relationship between the DHSS and regional administrators.) Health and Social Service Journal, 87, 16 Sep 1977, 1314-1316.

9 Cooper, P. Building the bridges of management. (Administrative structure in the two-district area of Redbridge and Waltham Forest.) Health and Social Service Journal, 86, 14 Aug 1976, 1468-1469.

10 Cuming, M.W. Personnel management in the National Health Service. Heinemann, 1978.

11 Daniels, P. Manpower information—East Anglia's approach. Health and Social Service Journal, 86, 7 Feb 1976, 255-256.

12 Davis, A.C. The rising tide: some aspects of the management of the demand for health care. (Examination of critiques of the NHS provision of care.) Community Health, 9 (2), Nov 1977, 91-100.

13 Dearden, B. How style gives substance to creating real participation. (Participative management in NHS.) Health and Social Service Journal, 87, 7 Oct 1977, 1400-1401.

14 Dennis, A.J. Motivation and the manager in the NHS. Hospital and Health Services Review, 76 (9), Sep 1980, 304-306.

15 Department of Health Management arrangements for the reorganized National Health Service, HMSO, 1972.

16 Donald, B. Towards a more positive manpower policy. (In the N.H.S.) Health Services Manpower Review, 3 (3), Aug 1977, 19-25.

17 Ellis, S. That unspoken prejudice. (Racial prejudice and the NHS.) Nursing Times, 74, 30 Nov 1978, 1964-1965.

18 Flintham, V. The personnel officer and a role. Health and Social Service Journal, 88, 24 Mar 1978, 345-346.

19 Godber, Sir G. Decision making system and structures in the British National Health Service. Hospital Progress, 57 (3), Mar 1976, 82-84, 86, 88, 92, 94, 96.

20 Gooch, S. From the razing of Bristol to the rising of participation. King's Fund Conference on staff participation in management in the NHS. Health and Social Service Journal, 87, 1 Jul 1977, 986-987.

21 Gourley, R. Training for performance review. (Staff development.) Health Services Manpower Review, 4 (2), May 1978, 7-14.

22 Gray, M. From diverse and sometimes even hostile tribes... (Criticism of consensus on management in the NHS.) Health and Social Service Journal, 87, 28 Oct 1977, 1505.

23 Harbridge, E. Where the buck (often) stops... (Work of Brian Smith, Area Administrator for Lincolnshire AHA.) Nursing Mirror, 148, 22 Mar 1979, 22-23.

24 Harris, C. Structures to make the manager creak. (Role of the administrator in NHS.) Health and Social Service Journal, 87, 18 Nov 1977, 1588-1589.

25 Harris, C. and Ball, D. 'Brookwood may well be a warning sign to the DHSS: unless our advice is heeded it could recur throughout the NHS...staff are just fed up'. (Interview with Colin Harris, Chairman of the Association of Health Sector and Unit Administrators concerning decision making in the NHS.) Health and Social Service Journal, 88, 7 Jul 1978, 762-764.

26 Hayton, C. Employee participation—some approaches discussed. Health Services Manpower Review, 4 (3), Aug 1978, 12-14.

27 Hayton, C.R. Management arrangements below district level: a framework for analysis. Hospital and Health Services Review, 76 (5), May 1980, 166-169.

28 Haywood, S.C. More democracy for the NHS? Hospital and Health Services Review, 73 (4), Apr 1977, 123-126.

29 Haywood, S. and Alaszewski, A. Crisis in the health service: the politics of management. Croom Helm, 1980.

30 Heafford, S. and Stokes, R.A. Staff membership of health authorities. Hospital and Health Services Review, 74 (2), Feb 1978, 48-50.

31 Hesmondhalgh, S. Diagnosing management ills in the NHS. (With special reference to personnel management.) Personnel Management, 10 (3), Mar 1978, 37-41.

32 Hill, S.G. NHS management structures past, present and future. British Journal of Occupational Therapy, 40 (9), Sep 1977, 207-209.

33 Hill, S. 'Practices, preferences and attitudes not to mention personalities! (Functional management versus line management.) Health and Social Service Journal, 88, 25 Aug 1978, 963.

34 Institute of Health Service Administrators and others The role of unit and sector administrators in the National Health Service: report of a joint working party. The Institute, 1976.

35 Jarrold, K.W. Health service management below district level. (Institutional coordination, with some reference to the nurse's role.) Hospital and Health Services Review, 74 (10), Oct 1978, 341-343.

36 Kaye, V. The team spirit. (The workings of an interdisciplinary team at the DHSS planning official health policy.) Health and Social Service Journal, 87, 16 Sep 1977, 1317-1319.

37 Klein, R. Accountability in the NHS: whose head on the block? British Medical Journal, 1976, 2, 13 Nov 1976, 1211-1212.

38 Lloyd, T. Democracy, politics and health care. (Need for greater participation in decision-making in the NHS by the public and professionals.) Nursing Mirror, 149, 30 Aug 1979 Supplement ii-iv, vi, viii.

39 McFarlane, J.K. Operational research versus the ubiquitous queue. (Applications in the health service.) Nursing Mirror, 143, 12 Aug 1976, 60-62.

40 McLachlan, G. editor Five years after: a review of health care research management after Rothschild. Nuffield Provincial Hospitals Trust/Oxford University Press, 1978. (Occasional hundreds no.9.)

41 Millard, C. How the Harrow health district works. Health and Social Service Journal, 86, 12 Jun 1976, 1068-1069.

42 Nursing Mirror Participative management recommended by DHSS. Nursing Mirror, 143 (14), 30 Sep 1976, 35. Report of King's Fund Conference, 25 Nov 1976, 36.

43 Owen, D. The organisation and management of the NHS. (HSA annual conference address.) Hospital and Health Services Review, 72 (7), Jul 1976, 239-244.

44 Paine, L. editor The health service administrator: innovator or catalyst? Selected papers from a King's Fund international seminar. King Edward's Hospital Fund for London, 1978.

45 Pantall, J. The role of authority chairmen. Hospital and Health Services Review, 74 (4), Apr 1978, 114-116.

46 Pearce, S.G. Towards an integrated personnel division. Hospital and Health Services Review, 72 (4), Apr 1976, 114-118.

47 Rubin, S.G. Professionals in health service administration. Community Health, 8 (2), Oct 1976, 82-83.

48 Pethybridge, F. Obsessed by structures. (Reply to Brian Watkin who queried the effectiveness of lay members of health authorities.) Health and Social Service Journal, 90, 8 Aug 1980, 1040-1041.

49 Royal College of Nursing Democracy in the National Health Service: election of staff members of authorities. Rcn comments on the consultative paper. Rcn, 1976.

50 Sabel, C. Skeleton in the health service cupboard. (Racial discrimination among health service staff.) Health and Social Service Journal, 86, 15 Oct 1976, 1852-1853.

51 Salvage, J. Democracy stifled in the NHS. (In context of campaign by Tower Hamlets residents and health workers against change of use of Bethnal Green Hospital to provide care for geriatric patients.) Nursing Mirror, 146, 29 Jun 1978, 8-9.

52 Speakman, A.J. Top posts in the National Health Service: report to the Nurses and Midwives, the Administrative and Clerical and the Professional and Technical (B) Whitley Councils. DHSS, 1979.

53 Spencer, J.A. Shaping management in Oxfordshire. (A single district area.) Health and Social Service Journal, 86, 10 Jul 1976, 1254-1255.

54 Spencer, R. and Sirett, K. Establishing a district personnel service you can live with. (Central Birmingham Health District (Teaching).) Health and Social Service Journal, 86, 17 Jan 1976, 110-111; 24 Jan 1976, 167.

55 Stewart, W. Tackling an insidious disease. (Staff counselling as part of health service manager's role.) Health and Social Service Journal, 87, 21 Oct 1977, 1460.

56 Wall, A. Bath health district: management arrangements. Health and Social Service Journal, 86, 15 May 1976, 890-891.

57 Walton, N. The day of small things. A few thoughts about management arrangements for people. (On optimum size of organisations, with particular reference to the NHS.) Hospital and Health Services Review, 73 (6), Jun 1977, 185-187.

58 Walton, M. Just a part of the routine? (How committees work, with some reference to the NHS.) Nursing Mirror, 150, 17 Jan 1980, 32-34.

59 Watkin, B. Health authorities: the time is ripe for a new model. (Problems faced by health authorities as essentially lay bodies.) Health and Social Service Journal, 90, 25 Jan 1980, 116-119.

60 West, C.R. The recruitment and development of administrators. The National Staff Committees consultative document. (Background and comment.) Health Services Manpower Review, 4 (3), Aug 1978, 15-18.

61 Williamson, C. Distribution of knowledge is the distribution of power. (Role of lay members of AHAs.) Health and Social Service Journal, 90, 20 Jun 1980, 804-807.

62 World Health Organization. Expert Committee Application of systems analysis to health management. Geneva: WHO, 1976.

63 Wycherley, G. Don't jump off the fence. (Role of personnel officer in NHS.) Health and Social Service Journal, 87, 15 Jul 1977, 1049.

g MANAGEMENT PLANNING

1 Ball, D. The cost of collaboration. (Functions of the area team of officers in the NHS structure.) Health and Social Service Journal, 88, 21 Jul 1978, 816-818.

2 Ball, D. Probing the heart of the spider's web... (District management team in East Cumbria.) Health and Social Service Journal, 88, 14 Jul 1978, 788-790.

3 Barnard, K. and others NHS planning: an assessment. 2 parts. Hospital and Health Services Review, 76 (8), Aug 1980, 262-265; (9), Sep 1980, 301-303.

4 Boddy, D. Participation in decision-making in the health services. (Report of study of operation of multidisciplinary planning committees in the Greater Glasgow Health Board.) Journal of Advanced Nursing, 3 (4), Jul 1978, 349-358.

5 British Medical Journal District management teams. British Medical Journal, 280, 7 Jun 1980, 1388-1389.

6 Burdett, F. and Battye, G.C. The family way: team management development in the NHS. (The part played by Leicester Polytechnic Health Service Management Unit.) Hospital and Health Services Review, 17 (1), Jan 1976, 17-18.

7 Carr, A. A new rung on the ladder. (Case for corporate team management as opposed to chief executives at each level of the NHS.) Nursing Mirror, 148, 24 May 1979, 20-21.

8 Dearden, R.W. What a district strategy looks like. (Hereford Health District.) Hospital and Health Services Review, 74 (11), Nov 1978, 393-398.

9 Department of Health and Social Security. Regional Planning Division The NHS planning system. The Department, 1976.

10 Diplock, C. and De Vulder, J. Better project management through network planning. Health and Social Service Journal, 89, 22 Jun 1979, Centre eight papers B47-B51.

11 Dunnell, K. editor Health services planning. King Edward's Hospital Fund for London, 1976.

12 Eskin, F. and Nichols, B. Team tactics in Manchester. (Course for management teams wanting to develop team skills.) Health and Social Service Journal, 88, 15 Sep 1978, 1036-1038.

13 Gillott, J. Ivory towers to make one quit, Call for planning to be divorced from day to day issues in health service administration. Health and Social Service Journal, 87, 18 Nov 1977, 1589-1590.

14 Gourlay, J.R. Manpower planning in the NHS—STAMP. (Standard Manpower Planning and Personnel Information System.) Health Services Manpower Review, 4 (3), Aug 1978, 20-22.

15 Green, B. and Simmons, S. The inter-disciplinary health care team. Fact or fiction? (Barriers to effective teamwork.) Nursing Forum, 16 (2), 1977, 165-184.

16 Grun, J. How to smooth the way to better planning. (At local level in the NHS.) Health and Social Service Journal, 88, 6 Oct 1978, 1137-1138.

17 Hansen, R.E.A.S. The district management team: the district community physician and the local government. Community Health, 8 (1), Jul 1976, 45-48.

18 Haywood, S. Team management in the NHS—what is it all about? (Role of teams and analysis of business transacted during meetings.) Health and Social Service Journal, 89, 5 Oct 1979, Centre eight papers B53-B60.

19 Hospital and Health Services Review Notes for students: the NHS planning system: its context and development. Hospital and Health Services Review, 75 (12), Dec 1979, 453-456.

20 Howie, W.B. Problems of area planning (for a Scottish Health Board.) Health Bulletin, 34 (3), May 1976, 145-150.

21 John, H.H. The development and functioning of the area team of officers. Health Trends, 5 (8), Nov 1976, 93-96.

22 Lee, K. and Mills, A. The contribution of economics to health service planning. Health and Social Service Journal, 89, 8 Feb 1979, Centre eight papers C35-C40.

23 Long, A.F. and Mercer, G. NHS manpower planning—towards a positive approach? Health Services Manpower Review, 6 (2), May 1980, 3-6.

24 Malsey, P.W. Talking point. Pulling together. (Comment on recent breakdown of Solihull's area team of officers.) Nursing Times, 73, 4 Aug 1977, 1186.

25 Miles, D.P.B. and Yule, I.G. Health service planning in practice: experience in a new town. (Milton Keynes.) Health Trends, 9 (3), Aug 1977, 63-66.

26 Mills, A. and Reynolds, J. Centre-periphery: can guidelines bridge the gap? (Preparation of planning guidelines from each tier in the NHS for the next level down.) Hospital and Health Services Review, 73 (2), Feb 1977, 50-52.

27 Murray-Sykes, K. Three go in search of England. (Survey of district health care planning teams.) Health and Social Service Journal, 89, 3 Aug 1979, 981-982.

28 Nichol, D. Administrators and management teams in the National Health Service. Manchester: University of Manchester, Health Services Management Unit, 1980. (Working paper no.35.)

29 Overton, P. and Stinson, S.M. Pro-gramme evaluation in health services: the use of experimental designs. Journal of Advanced Nursing, 2 (2), Mar 1977, 137-146.

30 Pethybridge, F. Multi-disciplinary management and decision making in the reorganised National Health Service. Hospital and Health Services Review, 72 (3), Mar 1976, 77-80.

31 Rathwell, T.A. Population and health care planning. Hospital and Health Services Review, 73 (12), Dec 1977, 420-422.

32 Reynolds, M.R.F. The district management team. Community Health, 8 (1), Jul 1976, 43-45.

33 Royal Society of Health Journal The pleasures and perils of joint care planning. (Two articles.) Royal Society of Health Journal, 98 (4), Aug 1978, 165-172, 198.

34 Scott-Samuel, A. Social area analysis in community medicine. (Method of quantifying data to guide health service resource allocation and planning.) British Journal of Preventive and Social Medicine, 31 (3), Sep 1977, 199-204.

35 Smith, G.W. Teamwork in the N.H.S.: myths and models. (Management teams.) Health Services Manpower Review, 5 (1), Feb 1979, 8-13.

36 Thatcher, P.R. Planning progress in West Sussex. Health and Social Service Journal, 86, 7 Aug 1976, 1434-1435.

37 Trace, T. and Tranter, A.W. Health care planning teams: some problems in practice. Health and Social Service Journal, 86, 24 Jan 1976, 158-159.

38 Vincent, E.C. Planning: ensuring the greatest care for the patient. (Analytical approach to health service planning.) Nursing Mirror, 147, 2 Nov 1978, 36-38.

39 Walton, M. and Smith, G. Sense is the key. (How to set up a review of team activity.) Health and Social Service Journal, 90, 15 Feb 1980, 220.

40 Walton, M. and Smith, G. Sharing team expectations. (Importance of clearly setting out team objectives.) Health and Social Service Journal, 90, 11 Jan 1980, 51-53.

41 Watkin, B. Themes in health care planning: a consideration of the NHS interim planning system. University of Manchester, Department of Social Administration, 1976. (Working paper series no.19.)

42 West, R.J. The essentials of planning in the N.H.S. Public Health, 94 (1), Jan 1980, 16-20.

h MANAGEMENT TRAINING

1 Armfield, J. and Jenkin, B. Developing health service managers. (Brooklands Management School course based on acquisition of personal learning skills.) Nursing Times, 73, 20 Oct 1977, Occ. papers, 133-136.

2 Bailey, P. The answer's simple...two plus two makes four. (Training administrators in the NHS.) Health and Social Service Journal, 88, 1 Dec 1978, 1370-1371.

3 Dearden, R.W. and Jones, J.A.G. Learning and management. (Management training project in Hereford Health District.) Hospital and Health Services Review, 73 (12), Dec 1977, 432-436.

4 Edmonstone, J. Leadership in an organ-isational context: an experiential learning design. (Approach developed by Trent RHA OD Unit.) Health Services Manpower Review, 5 (1), Feb 1979, 13-16.

5 Haywood, S. Preparing for 2000 A.D. (Role and training of NHS managers.) Health Services Manpower Review, 6 (4), Nov 1980, 3-8.

6 Hill, J. Management development. (Development of comprehensive management training programme in Brent and Harrow AHA.) Health and Social Service Journal, 89, 22 Mar 1979, Centre eight papers B41-B44.

7 Huczynski, A.A. NHS management courses. Whose responsibility? (A method of evaluating courses.) Nursing Times, 72 (3), 22 Jan 1976, Occ. papers, 9-11.

8 King Edward's Hospital Fund for London The education and training of senior managers in the National Health Service: a contribution to debate. KEHF, 1977.

9 National Staff Committee for Administrative and Clerical Staff The recruitment and career development of administrators: a consultative document. The Committee, 1978.

10 National Training Council for the National Health Service An education and training technology service for the National Health Service. NTC, 1979.

11 National Training Council for the National Health Service Management education and training in the National Health Service. NTC, 1979.

12 Owen, J.W. and Draper, F.W. Manage-ment education, training and development. Hospital and Health Services Review, 72 (9), Sep 1976, 301-303.

13 Paine, L. Thoughts on Thwaites: a commentary on management training in the National Health Service. King Edward's Hospital Fund for London, 1979.

14 **Smith, D.** Training for management: a conspectus of past and present activities in the important field of management education and training in the National Health Service. Health and Social Service Journal, 87, 30 Sep 1977, F1-F4.

15 **Smith, D.** Training in the NHS—administrators. Health and Social Service Journal, 87, 7 Oct 1977, F13-F16.

16 **Stolte, J.B.** On education for health care management. Hospital and Health Services Review, 72 (3), Mar 1976, 83-86.

17 **Toman, J.P.** Health service management training. (Research study to assess and evaluate existing arrangements, philosophies and procedures.) Nursing Times, 73, 7 Jul 1977, 1041-1043.

18 **University of Birmingham. Health Services Management Centre** Management development options in the NHS: a reference manual of alternative methods of management development, and indications for the use of each. Birmingham: The Centre, 1978. (HSMC Occ. paper no.14.)

19 **White, D.K.** The evaluation of middle management training in the National Health Service. PhD thesis, Bath University, 1980.

20 **White, D.K.** New directions in health service management education training and development. Health Services Manpower Review, 2 (3), Oct 1976, 15-20.

i MEDICAL STAFF

1 **Appleyard, J. and Maden, J.G.** Multi-disciplinary teams. (Undermining effect on doctor's clinical independence. See also editorial on p.1245.) British Medical Journal, 2, 17 Nov 1979, 1305-1307.

2 **Armstrong, J.** What's up doc? (Responses to the Merrison Committee report.) Health and Social Service Journal, 86, 3 Dec 1976, 2142-2143.

3 **Bosanquet, N.** Facts of life. (Comments on David Owen's speech on doctors' clinical freedom, Lancet, 1, 8 May 1976, 1006-1009.) Nursing Times, 72, 10 Jun 1976, 880-881.

4 **British Medical Association** The handbook of medical ethics. BMA, 1980.

5 **British Medical Journal** Clinical responsibility. (Papers and discussion on the concept of the multidisciplinary team in hospital care and the effect on the patient.) British Medical Journal, 2, 17 Dec 1977, 1584-1589.

6 **British Medical Journal** London medical education. Flowers Report. (Membership, recommendations and terms of reference. Leading article, p.665-666.) British Medical Journal, 1, 8 Mar 1980, 731-733.

7 **Campbell, A.V.** Establishing ethical priorities in medicine. British Medical Journal, 1, 26 Mar 1977, 818-821.

8 **Committee of Enquiry into Competence to Practice** Report. The Committee, 1976.

9 **Davis, A. and Horobin, G.** Focus: current issues in medical ethics. The problem of priorities. Journal of Medical Ethics, 3 (3), Sep 1977, 107-109.

10 **Denham, M.J. and others** Work of a district ethical committee. British Medical Journal, 2, 27 Oct 1979, 1042-1045.

11 **Duncan, A.** Quality assurance: what now and where next? (Present practices to safeguard quality of medical care and other possible measures.) British Medical Journal, 280, 2 Feb 1980, 300-302.

12 **Duncan, A.S. and others** Dictionary of medical ethics. Darton Longman and Todd, 1977.

13 **General Medical Council. Survey of Basic Medical Education** Basic medical education in the British Isles. 2 vols. Nuffield Provincial Hospitals Trust, 1977.

14 **Health Trends** Functions of the medical staff of the Department of Health and Social Security. Health Trends, 8 (3), Special Issue 1976, 34-60.

15 **Illman, J.** Darker side of a doctor's life. (Suicide attempts, drug dependence and alcoholism in doctors.) Health and Social Service Journal, 88, 24 Nov 1978, 1344-1345.

16 **Joint Working Party of the Conference of Medical Royal Colleges and their Faculties in the UK and the British Medical Association** Discussion document on ethical responsibilities of doctors practising in the National Health Service. British Medical Journal, 1, 15 Jan 1977, 157-159.

17 **King's Fund Centre** The organisation of hospital clerical work: report of a King's Fund Working Party. KFC, 1979.

18 **McCormick, J.** The doctor: father figure or plumber. Croom Helm, 1979.

19 **Martin, A.J.** Duty of care. (The legal basis to the concept of clinical responsibility of doctors.) Nursing Times, 72, 9 Sep 1976, 1379.

20 **Northern Regional Health Authority** Applications for ethical approval: a report by the working group in current medical ethical problems. (Work of ethical committee.) Lancet, 1, 14 Jan 1978, 87-89.

21 **Owen, D.** Clinical freedom and professional freedom. (Preservation of freedom of the medical profession in the National Health Service.) Lancet, 1, 8 May 1976, 1006-1009.

22 **Pappworth, M.H.** Medical ethical committees. A review of their functions. World Medicine, 13, 22 Feb 1978, 19-21, 57, 61, 64, 67-69, 71-72, 74, 76, 78.

23 **Parliament** Medical Act 1978. HMSO, 1978. (Chapter 12.)

24 **Shaw, C.D.** Aspects of audit. British Medical Journal. (Methods of reviewing the quality of medical care.)
1. The background. 24 May 1980, 1256-1258.
2. Audit in British hospitals. 31 May 1980, 1314-1316.
3. Audit in British general practice. 7 Jun 1980, 1361-1363.
4. Acceptability of audit. 14 Jun 1980, 1443-1446.
5. Looking forward to audit. 21 Jun 1980, 1509-1571.

j PATIENTS RIGHTS: UNITED KINGDOM

1 **Ashton, K.** Assessing quality and quantity: Scottish Hospital Advisory Service. Nursing Times, 72 (32), 12 Aug 1976, 1224.

2 **Cooper, P. and others** Who complains? An inconclusive study. Hospital and Health Services Review, 76 (6), Jun 1980, 201-203.

3 **Department of Health and Social Security** Complaints code. (Code of practice issued as a consultative document.) Nursing Mirror, 143, 8 Jul 1976, 38-41; 15 Jul 1976, 39.

4 **Eskin, F. and Newton, P.** Public ignorance of the health service. (Survey by the Department of Community Medicine, Manchester University.) Health and Social Service Journal, 86, 10 Apr 1976, 676-677.

5 **Halpern, S.** Why HAS has no bite may be because it has no teeth. (Ineffectiveness of the Health Advisory Service.) Health and Social Service Journal, 89, 17 Aug 1979, 1038-1041.

6 **Health Advisory Service** Annual report 1976-. HMSO, 1977-.

7 **Health and Social Service Journal** Complaints. (Comments on the hospital complaints procedures.) Health and Social Service Journal, 87, 8 Apr 1977, 620-626.

8 **Health Service Commissioner** Annual report 1975/76-1979/80. HMSO, 1976-1980.

9 **Hospital Advisory Service** Annual report 1976. HMSO, 1976.

10 **International Council of Nurses** ICN statement on the quality of life. (Including rights of individuals to health services.) International Nursing Review, 27 (1), Jan/Feb 1980, 4.

11 **Kelly, L.Y.** The patient's right to know. (Moral and legal aspects.) Nursing Outlook, 24 (1), Jan 1976, 26-32.

12 **Klein, R.** The Health Commissioner: no cause for complaint. British Medical Journal, 1, 22 Jan 1977, 248-249.

13 **Klein, R.** Public opinion and the National Health Service. (Comment on the findings of patient surveys.) British Medical Journal, 1, 12 May 1979, 1296-1297.

14 **Lancet** Commentary from Westminster. Complaints from dissatisfied patients. Lancet, 1, 22 Mar 1980, 663-664.

15 **Marre, A.** Reflections of the Health Service Commissioner. Queen's Nursing Journal, 18 (9), Dec 1975, 241-242, 244-245.

16 **Marre, A.** The role of the ombudsman in Britain. World Hospitals, 12 (4), 1976, 235-237.

17 **Marre, A.** Thoughts and experiences of the first Health Service Commissioner. Royal Society of Health Journal, 96 (4), Aug 1976, 149-151, 195.

18 **Morris, P.** The balance of injustice. (How the scales are tipped against aggrieved patients who wish to make complaints.) Nursing Mirror, 148, 29 Mar 1979, 16-18.

19 **Oliphant, J.** The Scottish Hospital Advisory Service—a nurse looks back. Health Bulletin, 37 (2), Mar 1979, 47-49.

20 Powell, J.E. Human rights. (With comment on the right to medical care, by R.S. Downie.) Journal of Medical Ethics, 3 (4), Dec 1977, 160-162.

21 Pugh, Sir I. The man with the direct line to the patient, by D. Ball. (Interview with Sir Idwal Pugh discussing the role of the Health Commissioner.) Health and Social Service Journal, 87, 8 Apr 1977, 618-619.

22 Rayner, C. Reality and expectation of the British National Health Service consumer. (Analysis of queries received about health care problems and plea for health professionals to give patients more understanding and information.) Journal of Advanced Nursing, 4 (1), Jan 1979, 69-77.

23 Select Committee on the Parliamentary Commissioner for Administration First report session 1977-78: independent review of hospital complaints in the National Health Service. HMSO, 1977.

24 Stimson, G. and Stimson, C. Health rights handbook: a guide to medical care. Dorchester: Prism Press, 1978.

25 Watkin, B. Any complaints? (Survey by a Liverpool CHC.) Nursing Mirror, 145, 24 Nov 1977, 10.

26 Watkin, B. Half a loaf. (Comments on DHSS proposals, for a code of practice for handling patients' complaints.) Nursing Mirror, 142, 11 Mar 1976, 42.

27 Watkin, B. Health Advisory Service. Nursing Mirror, 142, 20 May 1976, 42.

28 Weightman, G. Society at work. Accountable medicine. (Use of hospital complaints procedures.) New Society, 36, 22 Apr 1976, 184-185.

29 Wootton, H. Rights, wrongs and risks of patients' charter campaign. (Resolution at National Consumer Congress.) Health and Social Service Journal, 90, 11 Apr 1980, 470.

k PATIENTS' RIGHTS: OVERSEAS COUNTRIES

1 Australian Nurses Journal Patients' rights. (American, Australian and New Zealand codes.) Australian Nurses Journal, 8 (3), Sep 1978, 12, 14, 16, 18-19.

2 Bandman, E.L. How much dare you tell your patient? (Protecting patients' rights and avoiding malpractice suits.) RN Magazine, 41 (8), Aug 1978, 39-41.

3 Bandman, E.L. and Bandman, B. There is nothing automatic about rights. (Comments on the American Hospital Association's 'Statement on a patient's bill of rights.') American Journal of Nursing, 77 (5), May 1977, 867-872.

4 Breitung, J. The rights of patients. Nursing Care, 9 (9), Sep 1976, 30-32.

5 Laszlo, S.S. and McKenzie, J.L. The use of a simulation game in training hospital staff about patients rights. Journal of Continuing Education in Nursing, 10 (5), Sep/Oct 1979, 30-36.

6 Maher, L. The rights of patients. Lamp, 37 (11), Nov 1980, 11-14.

7 Martin, A. A right to treatment. (American practice of using courts to determine the extent of individual rights.) Nursing Times, 73, 20 Oct 1977, 1620-1621.

8 Sandroff, R. How the 'patient bill of rights' makes honesty easier. (Results of RN survey on the spread of the patient rights movement.) RN Magazine, 41 (8), Aug 1978, 42-47.

9 World Health Health and human rights. World Health, Jan 1976, 3-31.

10 World Health Organization Health aspects of human rights: with special reference to developments in biology and medicine. Geneva: WHO, 1976. Also WHO Chronicle, 30 (9), Sep 1976, 347-359.

l POLITICS

1 Castle, B. The Castle diaries 1974-76. Weidenfeld & Nicolson, 1980.

2 Castle, B. and Bosanquet, N. Talking point. Not crocodile tears. (Achievements of Barbara Castle as Secretary of State for Social Services.) Nursing Times, 72, 29 Apr 1976, 644-645.

3 Clode, D. Smoothing the angles. (DHSS political advisers, appointed by the Secretary of State to brief ministers.) Health and Social Service Journal, 87, 16 Sep 1977, 1319-1320.

4 Draper, P. and Dennis, J. Health at the hustings. Voting for health. Nurses as voters should be aware of the policies of the political parties on economic growth. Nursing Times, 75, 3 May 1979, 736.

5 Ennals, D. David Ennals, the man. (Interview by C. Tomalin.) Health and Social Service Journal, 86, 1 Oct 1976, 1752-1754.

6 Ennals, D. 'I think we have a series of problems—not all on the pay front...' (Interview.) Health and Social Service Journal, 88, 17 Nov 1978, 1304-1306.

7 Ennals, D. The man behind the minister. (Interview by S. Ellis.) Nursing Times, 75, 11 Jan 1979, 60-61.

8 Ennals, D. Six contentious months as Secretary of State. (Interview by D. Wilson.) Social Work Today, 8, 5 Oct 1976, 8-11.

9 Ennals, D. David Ennals—just how much does he care...and does it matter? Social Work Today, 8 (1), 5 Oct 1976, 7.

10 Jenkins, P. The cost of health. (The) chief Conservative social services spokesman looks at new sources of finance for the NHS. Nursing Times, 73, 4 Nov 1977, 1701.

11 Jenkin, P. A freer hand. (The organisation of the NHS and Conservative health policy.) Nursing Times, 73, 1 Dec 1977, 1862.

12 Jenkin, P. Interview with Patrick Jenkin on Tory policy for the health service by C. Tomalin. Health and Social Service Journal, 86, 15 Oct 1976, 1844-1846.

13 Jenkin, P. Patrick Jenkin: the intelligent ingenue. (Critical portrait by H. Macpherson.) World Medicine, 14 (17), 2 Jun 1979, 24-25.

14 Jenkin, P. Standards of care. (Tory policy for the health services.) Nursing Times, 74 (1), 5 Jan 1978, 8-9.

15 Jenkin, P. The NHS: what does the future hold? (Tory policy.) Nursing Times, 74, 2 Feb 1978, 176-178.

16 Klein, R. Parliamentary accountability and the NHS: need for separate committee. British Medical Journal, 1, 3 Jun 1978, 1498, 1499, 1501.

17 Lancet Conservatives and the N.H.S. Lancet, 2, 6 Aug 1977, 292-293.

18 Lewis, S. Promised lands and offers of better times. (Analysis of parties, election manifestos and implications for health services.) Health and Social Service Journal, 89, 27 Apr 1979, 466-467.

19 Liberal Party Our National Health Service: towards a vision for the future. Liberal Publications Department, 1978.

20 Mackenzie, W.J.M. Power and responsibility in health care: the National Health Service as a political institution. Oxford: Oxford University Press for Nuffield Provincial Hospital Trust, 1979.

21 Moyle, R. There is now encouraging concern about the present state of the NHS. (Interview.) Health and Social Service Journal, 89, 11 Mar 1977, 426-428.

22 Nazer, G. Who can control this son of Frankenstein? (Political parties' attitudes towards NHS.) Nursing Mirror, 148, 3 May 1979, 7.

23 Nursing Mirror Election 79. Which way should nurses vote? (Policies of the three parties by David Ennals, Patrick Jenkin and Lord Winstanley.) Nursing Mirror, 148, 3 May 1979, 18-20.

24 Nursing Times Health at the hustings. What's in store for health? By the spokesman for health of each of the three major political parties. Nursing Times, 75, 3 May 1979, 734-735.

25 Owen, D. In sickness and in health: the politics of medicine. Quartet Books, 1976.

26 Owen, D. Looking back. (David Owen's achievements as Minister of State for Health and Social Security.) Nursing Times, 72, 7 Oct 1976, 1548-1549.

27 Powell, J.E. Medicine and politics: 1975 and after. New ed. Pitman, 1976.

28 Ryan, M. Who are the real friends of the NHS? (Examination of myths of impact of Labour and Conservative parties on the NHS in the 1940s and 1950s.) Nursing Mirror, 151, 10 Jul 1980, 14.

29 Smith, C. We need to scrap all the existing systems and start again...streamline our cockeyed service. (Interview with Cyril Smith—Liberal spokesman on health by R. Royston.) Health and Social Service Journal, 86, 5 Nov 1976, 1968-1970.

30 Vaughan, G. Good doctor's cure to quell the service's sea-sickness. (Interview with Gerard Vaughan by D. Clode.) Health and Social Service Journal, 89, 23 Nov 1979, 1518-1521.

31 Vaughan, G. Man at the top. (Interview with Dr. Gerard Vaughan, Minister of Health, on the NHS by A. Brown.) Nursing Mirror, 150, 12 Jun 1980, 26-28.

32 Watkin, B. Politics and the NHS. (Comment on the political nature of the position of AHA chairman.) Nursing Mirror, 145, 27 Oct 1977, 10.

33 Young, Sir G. Turning the wheels on health. (Interview with Sir George Young, Parliamentary Under-Secretary in the DHSS by M. Allen.) Nursing Mirror, 150, 3 Apr 1980, 24-26.

m PRIVATE PRACTICE

1 Association of Independent Hospitals and Kindred Organisations Directory. 8th ed. The Association, 1976.

2 Ball, D. The model and the reality. (Current trends in private medicine.) Health and Social Service Journal, 88, 26 May 1978, 600-604.

3 Ball, D. The state of health of private medicine in Britain. Health and Social Service Journal, 88, 19 May 1978, 572-574.

4 Bolt, D.E. and Grant, K. A vital question of freedom or equality. (Private practice in the NHS.) Health and Social Service Journal, 86, 8 Oct 1976, 1812-1813.

5 British Medical Journal Private medicine. An old chestnut reassessed. (Growth of private practice, its implications and background with statistics.) British Medical Journal, 281, 12 Jul 1980, 123-124. Building a private hospital, 26 Jul 1980, 291-292.

6 British Medical Journal Private practice and NHS. (Outline of key dates 1974-1976.) British Medical Journal, 1, 22 May 1976, 1290.

7 Davidson, N. Long journey to the abolition of pay beds. (The limited powers of the Health Services Board and lukewarm support for it from the Government.) Health and Social Service Journal, 89, 15 Mar 1979, 256-258.

8 Davis, S.E. The N.H.S.—the continuing need for private nursing homes? The contribution of the nursing home. Royal Society of Health Journal, 98 (3), Jun 1978, 132-134.

9 Dennis, K.J. Private practice and nurse training. (Letter suggesting that private hospitals should contribute to a central training board for nurses.) British Medical Journal, 2, 8 Sep 1979, 615.

10 Department of Health and Social Security Health services management: use of NHS facilities by private patients. DHSS, 1978.

11 Drummond, P. Working outside the NHS. A hell of an adventure. (Private sector abroad and in this country.) Health and Social Service Journal, 80, 12 Dec 1980, 1586-1589.

12 Elias, B. Shadowing the NHS to meet the needs of the private patient. (The future of independent hospitals.) Health and Social Service Journal, 86, 4 Mar 1977, 382-383.

13 Fisher, A. Private practice, the NHS, and the unions. An interview with Mr. Alan Fisher. British Medical Journal, 2, 24 Jul 1976, 227-228.

14 Health Services Board Withdrawal of authorisations for the use of NHS hospital accommodation and services by private patients...second proposals. HMSO, 1978.

15 Hoadley, D.M. The N.H.S.—the continuing need for private nursing homes? Interdependence and co-existence. Royal Society of Health Journal, 98 (3), Jun 1978, 130-131.

16 Keller, N.S. The evolution of a successful partnership. (Two nurses run private practice.) Journal of Nursing Administration, 7 (8), Oct 1977, 6-9, 35.

17 Kingman, S. Chief casualty could be the senior service. (Implications of private hospitals and private health insurance for NHS staffing.) Health and Social Service Journal, 89, 31 Aug 1979, 1094-1097.

18 Miller, H.L. and Miller, M.V. Marginal status and role strain in private duty nursing. (Study of 30 nurses by long, focused group interviews.) International Journal of Nursing Studies, 13 (3), 1976, 167-178.

19 Mitchell, B. Private nursing homes: an inquiry into procedures for the registration and inspection of private nursing homes in eleven AHAs. Nursing Times, 75, 22 Nov 1979, 2031-2033.

20 Mollo, S. Causes of the coming boom. (Factors affecting recent expansion of private medicine.) Health and Social Service Journal, 90, 28 Mar 1980, 412-413.

21 Nursing Mirror. Parliamentary Correspondent News from Westminster. Pay beds bill goes to the Lords. Nursing Mirror, 143, 21 Oct 1976, 40; Pay beds bill enters crucial stage, 28 Oct 1976, 39.

22 Nursing Times Pay beds scrapbook. (Diary of events in the phasing out of pay beds.) Nursing Times, 42, 2 Dec 1976, 1866-1867.

23 Poole, A. Pass the hat... (Manpower and cost implications of private hospitals for the NHS nursing service, with statistics.) Nursing Mirror, 150, 28 Feb 1980, 16.

24 Queen's Nursing Journal Private medicine and the patient: does it really help? Queen's Nursing Journal, 19 (12), Mar 1977, 338-339.

25 Smith, J.C. Realities of private medical care. British Medical Journal, 2, 3 Jul 1976, 62-63.

26 Taylor, S., Baron Taylor of Harlow An independent health service. (The case for private practice outside the NHS.) Nursing Mirror, 142, 29 Jan 1976, 40-41.

27 Turner, J. The private hospitals. (With some reference to the shortage of nurses in the NHS.) New Society, 49, 27 Sep 1979, 667-668.

28 Walker, A. Private care: whose freedom to choose? Nursing Mirror, 148, 18 Jan 1979, 14-16.

29 Watkin, B. Does private care provide value for money? Nursing Mirror, 147.
1. Why people prefer to pay for treatment. 30 Nov 1978, 18-20.
2. How much is it going to cost? 7 Dec 1978, 22-24.
3. Why small is beautiful. (Nuffield Nursing Homes Trust). 14 Dec 1978, 24-25.
4. Where morale is high and recruitment no problem. (American Medical (Europe)). 21 Dec 1978, 12-13.

n STAFF AND INDUSTRIAL RELATIONS

1 Agag, pseud. Toward a wider view. The political, health and welfare scene. (Role of trade unions in the health service over the last few years.) British Journal of Occupational Therapy, 44 (1), Jan 1978, 42.

2 Anthony, M.F. Early planning helps hospitals run efficiently during strike. Hospitals, 52 (6), 16 Mar 1978, 105, 108, 110-112.

3 Bosanquet, N. editor Industrial relations in the NHS: the search for a system. King Edward's Hospital Fund for London, 1979.

4 Bosanquet, N. Unions and hospitals: the American case. British Medical Journal, 1, 15 Mar 1980, 806-807.

5 Bosanquet, N. and Healy, G. Is the NHS really torn by strife? (Industrial disputes.) New Society, 48, 10 May 1979, 328-329.

6 Burchill, F. The Advisory Conciliation and Arbitration Service. Health Services Manpower Review, 4 (4), Nov 1978, 18-21.

7 Button, J.H. Industrial action—a learning experience. (The experience of West Glamorgan AHA in dealing with industrial action by ambulance men and ancillary staff.) Hospital and Health Services Review, 75 (6), Jun 1979, 198-201.

8 Button, J. Responses to industrial action. 2. (Review of industrial relations in the NHS in last decade with reference to HC(79)20.) Health Services Manpower Review, 6 (1), Feb 1980, 17-19.

9 Chalmers, J. The ancillary workers' strike—the experience of the Brent Health District. Hospital and Health Services Review, 75 (7), Jul 1979, 234-237.

10 Department of Health and Social Security Health services management: if industrial relations break down. DHSS, 1979. (Health circular: HC(79)20.)

11 Dyson, R. The certification of health service trade unions: the present position. Health Services Manpower Review, 2 (3), Oct 1976, 20-21.

12 Dyson, R. Consultation and negotiation at area and district levels. Health Services Manpower Review, 4 (3), Aug 1978, 3-7.

13 Dyson, R. Industrial action 1979: what can we learn? British Medical Journal, 1, 26 May 1979, 1435-1437.

14 Dyson, R. Industrial relations in the NHS. (Association of Nurse Administrators (AGM lecture.) Queen's Nursing Journal, 19 (9), Dec 1976, 260.

15 Dyson, R. Industrial relations in the NHS. (Review of recent developments including question of Rcn affiliation to TUC.) Midwife, Health Visitor and Community Nurse, 15 (1), Jan 1979, 7-8.

16 Dyson, R. Interunion competition bleeds the NHS. (Reports from Rainhill and Westminster hospitals showing conflict between COHSE and NUPE.) British Medical Journal, 2, 15 Dec 1979, 1606-1608.

17 Dyson, R. A rap over the knuckles from

the professor. (Summary of review of industrial relations problems at Westminster Hospital.) Health and Social Service Journal, 89, 2 Nov 1979, 1404-1405; 9 Nov 1979, 1440-1441.

18 Dyson, R. and Message, M. Industrial relations training for senior management: a new approach. Hospital and Health Services Review, 72 (8), Aug 1976, 269-272.

19 Ellis, N. A panic measure with hidden hazards. (Local disputes procedures in the NHS.) British Medical Journal, 280, 5 Jan 1980, 61-62.

20 Farnham, D. Industrial relations in the National Health Service: an appraisal and some comments. Health Services Manpower Review, 2 (3), Oct 1976, 10-14.

21 Fletcher, S.B. Minimum cost to us, maximum cost to them. (Industrial action in the NHS.) Hospital and Health Services Review, 74 (12), Dec 1978, 429-431.

22 Fox, T.E. Industrial action, the National Health Service and the medical profession. Lancet, 2, 23 Oct 1976, 892-895.

23 Harrison, S.R. Disputes procedure—pathology or panacea? (Comments on proposals on disputes procedure by Secretary of State for Social Services.) Health Services Manpower Review, 5 (2), May 1979, 16-17.

24 Harrison, S. Responses to industrial action. 1. Assumptions and evidence. (Comment on HC(79)20 on the handling of industrial disputes in the health service.) Health Services Manpower Review, 6 (1), Feb 1980, 15-17.

25 Health and Social Service Journal Industrial relations. (Introduction and six articles on aspects of industrial relations in the NHS.) Health and Social Service Journal, 88, 10 Nov 1978, 1272-1289.

26 Hospital and Health Services Review Notes for students. Joint consultation in the NHS. Hospital and Health Services Review, 76 (5), May 1980, 193-194.

27 Lancet Commentary from Westminster. Industrial relations in the N.H.S. Deteriorating relations. Lancet, 1, 18 Mar 1978, 617-618. Comment on proposed disputes procedure. Lancet, 2, 28 Oct 1978, 952-953.

28 Lancet Trades unions and the NHS: a partnership for progress? (Report of a symposium.) Lancet, 2, 23/30 Dec 1978, 1391.

29 McCarthy, Lord Industrial relations in the health service. Hospital and Health Services Review, 73 (8), Aug 1977, 285-287.

30 McGill, I. and Brand, C. An eye on the progress of joint consultation. (Survey of joint consultative machinery used by AHAs.) Health and Social Service Journal, 89, 1 Feb 1979, 97-98.

31 McGill, I. and Brand, C. Joint consultation as a form of joint regulation: a review. Health Services Manpower Review, 5 (1), Feb 1979, 3-8.

32 McGill, I. and Brand, C. Management must take an active role. (In management/staff consultation.) Health and Social Service Journal, 89, 15 Feb 1979, 151-152.

33 McGill, I. and Brand, C. Procedural and substantive issues relating to the joint consultative process. (Research study.) Health

Services Manpower Review, 5 (2), May 1979, 6-13.

34 Mailly, R. The circular on industrial action: in breach of contract? Health Services Manpower Review, 6 (2), May 1980, 9-11.

35 Mallinson, T. Building in industrial relations into the new NHS. Health Services Manpower Review, 5 (4), Nov 1979, 9-11.

36 March, P.J. and Ware, T. Training unions to negotiate—an unusual experience. (For non-affiliated unions in Northamptonshire AHA.) Health Services Manpower Review, 4 (4), Nov 1978, 21-23.

37 Marsh, P.J. Positive approach to a closed shop. How management and unions in Northamptonshire came to an agreement on negotiating union membership agreements or post entry closed shops for employees within the authority. Health and Social Service Journal, 88, 17 Mar 1978, 304-306.

38 Mersey Regional Health Authority Report of a committee of inquiry...to examine the management and deployment of health service resources and the conduct of industrial relations in Liverpool Area Health Authority (Teaching). Liverpool: Mersey RHA, 1978.

39 Open University A suitable case for treatment: a case study of industrial relations in the National Health Service. Milton Keynes: Open University Press, 1976.

40 Rosmann, J. One year under Taft-Hartley. (A high level of union activity has occurred as a result of hospital coverage by Taft-Hartley law.) Hospitals, 49 (24), 16 Dec 1975, 64-68.

41 Royal College of Nursing Rcn stewards handbook. Rcn, 1977.

42 Sisley, B. Joint staff consultation. (Experiences of Camden and Islington Area Joint Consultative Committee.) Health Visitor, 51 (8), Aug 1978, 297-298.

43 Smith, J. Anatomy of industrial action. (Diary of events in Brent Health District Jan-Apr 1979.) Nursing Times, 75, 10 May 1979, 783-789.

44 Spirn, S. Negotiating and coexisting with a union. Hospital Progress, 57 (2), Feb 1976, 54-55.

45 Surrey Area Health Authority Report of the committee of inquiry into industrial relations (in) West Surrey/North East Hampshire Health District Division of Psychiatry. The Authority, 1979.

46 Tibbles, I. How to use that 'low profile' often in industrial relations. Health and Social Service Journal, 89, 25 May 1979, 630-632.

47 Werther, W.B. and Lockhart, C.A. Labor relations in the health professions: the basis of power—the means of change. Boston: Little, Brown and Co., 1976.

30 HEALTH SERVICE REORGANISATION

a GENERAL AND ASSESSMENT

1 Anson, D. The effects of NHS reorganisation upon senior administrators. Health and

Social Service Journal, 28 Apr 1978, Centre eight papers B21-B24.

2 Association of Nurse Administrators 'Big is beautiful' doesn't work. (Conference on the National Health Service.) Nursing Times, 72, 8 Apr 1976, 516.

3 Ball, D. A revolution on the quiet. (Growing commitment towards a single district structure.) Health and Social Service Journal, 88, 3 Mar 1978, 244-246.

4 Bosanquet, N. View from the top. (View of the Association of Chief Administrators of Health Authorities on NHS reorganisation.) Nursing Times, 72 (14), 8 Apr 1976, 522.

5 Brown, R.G.S. Reorganising the National Health Service: a case study in administrative change. Oxford: Blackwell, 1979. (Aspects of social policy series.)

6 Burns, C. NHS reorganisation—an appraisal after two years. Midwife, Health Visitor and Community Nurse, 12 (4), Apr 1976, 114-118.

7 Chairmen of the Regional Health Authorities of the National Health Service Enquiry into the working of the DHSS in relation to regional health authorities. Department of Health and Social Security, 1976.

8 Chester, T.W. and Donald, B.L. Social change and NHS reorganisation. The second anniversary. (Considers objectives for the reorganisation and how far they have been achieved.) Hospital and Health Services Review, 72 (6), Jun 1976, 201-204; (7), Jul 1976, 230-234.

9 Clode, D. 'The area is a godsend to us—it's at least a focal point we can relate to...' (Interview with Wally Herbert, director for Avon Social Services Department on the NHS and social services.) Health and Social Service Journal, 88, 3 Nov 1978, 1242-1244.

10 Donaldson, R.J. The new health service in Britain: its organization outlined. Royal Society of Health, 1977.

11 Emerton, A. Royal Society of Health. Two years of the reorganised service. (Conference report.) Nursing Times, 72, 22 Jan 1976, 83.

12 Eskin, F. and Newton, P. A survey of public knowledge in relation to the National Health Service reorganisation. Community Health, 9 (2), Nov 1977, 114-119.

13 Gammon, M. Fixed rules which govern our human organisations. (Discusses the NHS as a bureaucratic system and suggests that new forms of organisation must be developed.) Health and Social Service Journal, 77, 29 Apr 1977, 742-743.

14 Glorney, M. The autumn look will be lean but far from hungry. (Criticism of existing three-tier administrative structure and Government's likely plans to streamline it.) Health and Social Service Journal, 89, 14 Sep 1979, 1175-1176.

15 Hamburger, S. Self inflicted wounds. (A personal view of present problems facing the NHS.) Nursing Times, 72, 4 Nov 1976, 1704-1705.

16 Haywood, S. Decision making in the new NHS: consensus or constipation? A paper for discussion. King's Fund Centre, 1977. (King's Fund project paper.)

17 Heath, P.J. The likely effects on the National Health Service of devolution to the English regions. Health Trends, 1 (11), Feb 1979, 7-9.

18 Heller, T. Restructuring the health service. Croom Helm, 1978.

19 Hospital and Health Services Review The Health Services Act 1976. Hospital and Health Services Review, 73 (2), Feb 1977, 72-74.

20 Hospital and Health Services Review Notes for students. The shaping of the reorganised NHS. Hospital and Health Services Review, 74 (4), Apr 1978, 145-146; (5), May 1978, 179-180.

21 Hudson, P. The reorganised health service. The first six months and the next ten years. NATNews, 12 (3), Apr 1975, 10-13.

22 Keywood, O. Talking point. Has the NHS really failed? Nursing Times, 73, 24 Mar 1977, 402-403.

23 Klein, R. Examining, diagnosing and treating the health of the service. Health and Social Service Journal, 86, 5 Nov 1976, 1962-1963.

24 Klein, R. Reorganisation: what went wrong? (In health and social services.) New Society, 41, 22 Sep 1977, 592-593.

25 Lancet The coming debate on the National Health Service. Lancet, 2, 6 Nov 1976, 1034.

26 Lessof, M.H. If I were director of the NHS. (Suggested changes in policy and structure.) Lancet, 2, 1 Jul 1978, 27-30.

27 Levitt, R. The reorganised National Health Service. Croom Helm, 1976. 2nd ed. 1977.

28 Lyons, J. NHS reorganisation—has patient care improved? Nursing Mirror, 142, 27 May 1976, 68-70.

29 Maxwell, R.J. Management arrangements—sense or nonsense? (Comments on reorganisation.) Hospital and Health Services Review, 72 (3), Mar 1976, 89-93.

30 Nursing Times NHS in Scotland. A summary of the reorganised structure. Nursing Times, 72, 22 Jul 1976, 1136-1137.

31 Nursing Times The NHS in Wales: a summary of the reorganised structure. Nursing Times, 72, 28 Oct 1976, 1688-1689.

32 Office of Health Economics The reorganised NHS. OHE, 1977. (Studies of current health problems no.58.)

33 Parliament Health services act 1976. HMSO, 1976. (Chapter 83.)

34 Payne, R.W. British changes bring headaches. (Review of NHS by Canadian academic.) Hospital Administration in Canada, 20 (4), Apr 1978, 56-57, 59.

35 Phillips, D. Precedents for establishing district health authorities—RHAs and the establishment of CHCs: a case study. Health and Social Service Journal, 90, 16 May 1980, Centre eight papers B62-B72.

36 Rigden, M.S. What kind of CHA? (Central health authority, which could provide top tier of management of NHS as alternative to DHSS.) Hospital and Health Services Review, 75 (1), Jan 1979, 18-20.

37 Ryan, M. The case for a Health Commission. (A statutory agency to run the NHS in place of direct ministerial control.) Nursing Mirror, 142, 22 Jan 1976, 40-41.

38 Stewart, J.D. The NHS—the structural problem. An edited version of an address at the IHSA Annual Conferece. (With discussion, p.315-316.) Hospital and Health Services Review, 73 (9), Sep 1977, 311-315. Reprinted in Nursing Times, 73, 15 Dec 1977, Occ. papers, 157-160; 22/29 Dec 1977, Occ. papers, 163-164.

39 Strube, G. A critical appraisal of the National Health Service. Hospital Update, 2 (5), May 1976, 269-270, 272.

40 Swaffield, L. Hats off. (Rcn symposium organised by the York and Northallerton centres discussing the reorganised structure.) Nursing Times, 72, 5 Aug 1976, 1188-1189.

41 Teeling-Smith, G. Cost benefit paralysis. (Summary of a conference paper on the reorganised NHS.) Nursing Times, 72, 22 Jan 1976, 88-89.

42 Teeling-Smith, G. The reorganized National Health Service. The cost of ill health. Royal Society of Health Journal, 96 (2), Apr 1976, 62-66.

b ROYAL COMMISSION ON NHS: General and evidence

1 Aylett, M. What I would say to the Royal Commission. Open letter to the chairman. British Medical Journal, 2, 30 Oct 1976, 1064-1065.

2 Bennett, J. Inside the Royal Commission. (Description of how it works.) British Medical Journal, 1, 25 Jun 1977, 1643-1645.

3 British Medical Journal Briefing. The Royal Commission on the N.H.S.: the background. British Medical Journal, 2, 28 Jul 1979, 288-289.

4 Hansard. Royal Commission Hansard references. Statement of appointment. 20 Oct 1975, 35-45; Ords. 20 Oct 1975, 1170-1179.

5 Royal Commission on the National Health Service The task of the Commission: a guide for those who wish to submit evidence. HMSO, 1976.

6 Clode, D. Signs from the mountain as the faithful wait and pray. (Royal Commission on the NHS.) Health and Social Service Journal, 89, 30 Mar 1979, 340-341.

7 Gould, D. Delivering health care wisely and well. (The role of the Royal Commission.) New Scientist, 74, 7 Apr 1977, 15-17.

8 Hospital and Health Services Review The Royal Commission. Hospital and Health Services Review, 72 (6), Jun 1976, 189.

9 Institute of Health Service Administrators NHS structural changes—code of practice and procedure. Hospital and Health Services Review, 74 (4), Apr 1978, 138-139.

10 New Society Health check. (Royal Commission on the National Health Service.) New Society, 36, 13 May 1976, 354-355.

11 Nursing Times First steps to Health Service Commission. Nursing Times, 72, 28 Oct 1976, 1658.

12 Smith, D. Plea to chop the DHSS down to size. (The case which the Royal Commission should consider.) Health and Social Service Journal, 89, 30 Mar 1979, 340-344.

13 White, R. Comment. Re-reorganisation. Nursing Mirror, 143, 16 Dec 1976, 41.

EVIDENCE: GENERAL

14 Ball, D. A quick guide to the published evidence. A cross section of the issues raised in the main written submission to the Royal Commission. (On the NHS.) Health and Social Service Journal, 87, 28 Oct 1977, 1492-1499.

15 Ball, D. Tomorrow's world? (Comment on evidence to the Royal Commission on the NHS from various bodies.) Health and Social Service Journal, 87, 28 Oct 1977, 1490-1491.

16 Beck, J. and others Areas of concern: an examination of evidence to the Royal Commission on the National Health Service. (Extract from project by tutor students at Rcn's IANE.) Nursing Times, 74, 1 Jun 1978, Rcn supplement, 11, 14, 17-19.

17 Brown, A. Everyone agrees: there are far too many bureaucrats. (Evidence to the Royal Commission on the NHS.) Nursing Mirror, 149, 19 Jul 1979, 6.

18 Davies, R. and Farrell, C. Conflict and consensus: an analysis of the evidence submitted to the Royal Commission on the National Health Service 1976-1979. King's Fund Centre, 1980. (KF project paper; RC1.)

19 Lancet Dear Royal Commissioners. Lancet Hospital care for the elderly. 28 Aug 1976, 454-455.
How to set priorities in medicine. 4 Sep 1976, 512-514.
Fair shares in the NHS by Sir G. Godber. 18 Sep 1976, 622-624.
Priorities for health by E.G. Knox. 9 Oct 1976, 790-792.
A bad example of a good idea. (NHS organisation) by L.H.W. Paine, 20 Nov 1976, 1130-1131.

20 Midwives Chronicle Extracts from other evidence. (Selection of evidence by various professional bodies.) Midwives Chronicle, 90 (12), May 1977, 96-99.

21 Occupational Health OH evidence to Royal Commission. (Extracts from evidence of six organisations.) Occupational Health, 29 (5), May 1977, 206-208.

EVIDENCE: INDIVIDUAL (Alphabetically by name)

22 Advisory Conciliation and Arbitration Service Royal Commission on the National Health Service: ACAS evidence. ACAS, 1978. (Report no.12.) For comment see Health and Social Service Journal, 88, 14 Jul 1978, 796.

23 Association of Directors of Social Services Commission 'must not cloak the real problems...' Health and Social Service Journal, 87, 3/10 Jun 1977, 873.

24 British Association of Social Workers The Royal Commission on the National Health

Service: memorandum of evidence. Birmingham: BASW, 1977.

25 British Medical Association Royal Commission on the National Health Service. Report of Council to the Special Representative Meeting, London, 9 Mar 1977. Submission of evidence. British Medical Journal, 1977, 1, 29 Jan 1977, 299-334. For comments on BMA evidence see Lancet, 1, 3 Feb 1977, 293-294.

26 British Medical Association Consultants' tier jerker for the management, by R. McKay. (Comment on the BMA's evidence to the Royal Commission.) Health and Social Service Journal, 89, 27 Apr 1979, 476-480.

27 British Medical Journal What shall I say to the Royal Commission? Compelling needs of our hospitals, by M. Elderkin. British Medical Journal, 2, 9 Oct 1976, 864-865.

28 British Medical Journal What I would say to the Royal Commission. Them and us, by N.B. Sprague. British Medical Journal, 2, 23 Oct 1976, 996-997.

29 British Psychological Society Evidence to the Royal Commission on the National Health Service. Leicester: The Society, 1977.

30 Clode, D. Testing the waters at Bath. (Bath Health District view of what Royal Commission should recommend.) Health and Social Service Journal, 89, 6 Apr 1979, 376-379.

31 Confederation of Health Service Employees Memorandum of evidence to the Royal Commission on the National Health Service. Banstead: COHSE, 1977. Summarised in Nursing Mirror, 144, 12 May 1977, 37.

32 Conservative Medical Society Tory pressure group advocates cash-on-delivery health service. Nursing Times, 73, 4 Aug 1977, 1180.

33 Consumers' Association Managing at home: a report on domiciliary supportive services...including research submitted to the Royal Commission on the National Health Service. The Association, 1978. (A Which? campaign report.)

34 Council for the Education and Training of Health Visitors Summary of evidence presented by the Council to the Royal Commission on the National Health Service. CETHV, 1977.

35 Council for Professions Supplementary to Medicine Submission to the Royal Commission on the National Health Service. The Council, 1976.

36 Davies, T.F. The NHS is dead: long live the NHS. An open letter to Sir Alec Merrison. British Medical Journal, 2, 4 Dec 1976, 1376-1378.

37 Equal Opportunities Commission Evidence to the Royal Commission on the National Health Service. Manchester: The Commission, 1977.

38 Family Planning Association Evidence to the Royal Commission on the National Health Service. FPA, 1977.

39 Harris, R. and Seldon, A. Evidence to the Royal Commission on the National Health Service. Institute of Economic Affairs, 1977.

40 Health Visitors Association Evidence to the Royal Commission on the National Health Service. Health Visitor, 50 (3), Mar 1977, 73-75; Nursing Times, 73, 17 Mar 1977, 361.

41 Hospital and Health Services Review Persuading the Royal Commission. Hospital and Health Services Review, 73 (4), Apr 1977, 111-113.

42 Institute of Health Service Administrators IHSA evidence to the Royal Commission. Hospital and Health Services Review, 73 (5), May 1977, 161.

43 Joint Committee of Professional Nursing and Midwifery Associations The NHS and professionalism. (Memorandum submitted to the Royal Commission on the NHS.) Health Visitor, 51 (1), Jan 1978, 9-10.

44 Joint Committee of Professional Nursing and Midwifery Associations Nurses unite. (Summary of evidence.) Nursing Times, 73, 5 May 1977, 641.

45 Klein, R. Health care, private choice and public provision. (Based on model of health care submitted as evidence by the Institute for Economic Affairs.) British Medical Journal, 1977, 1, 30 Apr 1977, 1170-1171.

46 Labour Party The right to health: the Labour Party's evidence to the Royal Commission on the National Health Service. Labour Party, 1977.

47 MIND Evidence to the Royal Commission on the NHS with regard to services for mentally handicapped people. Mind, 1977.

48 National Association of Theatre Nurses NATN's evidence to the Royal Commission on the NHS. NATNews, 14 (5), Jul 1977, 11-12.

49 National Corporation for the Care of Old People Clear aims for the future in services for the elderly. Edited version of the evidence to the Royal Commission on the NHS. Health and Social Service Journal, 86, 21 Jan 1977, 106-107.

50 National Schizophrenia Fellowship Memorandum to the Royal Commission on the NHS. Surbiton: the Fellowship, 1977. Reported in Nursing Mirror, 145, 25 Aug 1977, 4.

51 Nursing Mirror Nursing Mirror's evidence to the Royal Commission, by Pat Young. Nursing Mirror, 144, 31 Mar 1977, 39-40.

52 Outer Circle Policy Unit Demand to stop structural tinkering by S. Lewis. (Summary of evidence to the Royal Commission on the NHS by the Outer Circle Policy Unit.) Health and Social Service Journal, 89, 25 Jan 1979, 52-53.

53 Regional Librarians' Group Library services in the National Health Service: evidence to the Royal Commission on the National Health Service. The Group, 1976.

54 Royal College of General Practitioners Evidence to the Royal Commission on the NHS. Journal of the Royal College of General Practitioners, 27, Apr 1977, 197-206.

55 Royal College of Midwives The RCM's evidence to the Royal Commission on the NHS. Midwives Chronicle, 90, Apr 1977, 69-75.

56 Royal College of Midwives (Scottish Board) Evidence to the Royal Commission on the NHS. Midwives Chronicle, 90, May 1977, 95-96.

57 Royal College of Nursing Evidence to the Royal Commission on the National Health Service. Rcn, 1977.

58 Royal College of Nursing Royal Commission on the National Health Service: preliminary evidence from the Rcn. Rcn, 1976.

59 Royal College of Nursing Shopping for '76. (Comments on the Rcn proposals for NHS rationalisation.) Nursing Times, 72, 1/8 Jan 1976, 10-11.

60 Society of Chiropodists Royal Commission on the National Health Service. Final evidence submitted by the Society of Chiropodists. Chiropodist, 32 (2), Feb 1977, 39-53.

61 Society of Community Medicine (Formerly Society of Medical Officers of Health) Evidence to the Royal Commission on the NHS. Public Health, 91 (3), May 1977, 151-160.

62 Society of Occupational Medicine Evidence to the Royal Commission on the NHS. Journal of the Society of Occupational Medicine, 27 (3), Jul 1977, 120-121.

63 Trades Union Congress Evidence for submission to the Royal Commission on the National Health Service. TUC, 1977.

c ROYAL COMMISSION: PROPOSALS

1 Royal Commission on the National Health Service Report. Cmnd.7615. HMSO, 1979.

2 Royal Commission on the National Health Service A service for patients: conclusions and recommendations of the Royal Commission's Report, July 1979. HMSO, 1979.

COMMENTS

3 Abbott, M. Report of integrity. (Comment on report of Royal Commission on the NHS.) Nursing Focus, 1 (3), Nov 1979, 118-119.

4 Abel-Smith, B. A critique of the Royal Commission. (Report of lecture.) Hospital and Health Services Review, 76 (1), Jan 1980, 23-24.

5 Andrews, J. The Royal Commission. A geriatrician's view. Lancet, 1, 12 Jan 1980, 87-88.

6 Ashworth, W. CHCs and the Royal Commission. (Comment on report's recommendations.) Hospital and Health Services Review, 75 (12), Dec 1979, 431-432.

7 Bamford, T. Reforming the NHS. (Comment on the findings of the Royal Commission on the NHS.) Social Work Today, 10, 31 Jul 1979, 1.

8 British Medical Journal Royal Commission on the NHS. 'Much to praise, not a little to criticise...' (Comment on report and recommendations.) British Medical Journal, 2, 28 Jul 1979, 227-228, 284-287, 290.

9 British Medical Journal Royal Commission on the NHS. (Four articles commenting on report by J.O. Drife, P.V. Lippiett, G.P. McNicol and R. Klein.) British Medical Journal, 2, 6 Oct 1979, 840-850.

10 Clode, D. Baldly stated ideas on a regional machinery theme. (What a confidential DHSS document said about the role of RHAs in a reorganised NHS structure.) Health and Social Service Journal, 90, 18 Jan 1980, 82-85.

11 Clode, D. The pleading and the bleeding. (Structural change at area tier in the light of possible Royal Commission recommendations.) Health and Social Service Journal, 89, 13 Apr 1979, 410-413.

12 Cole, A. The shape of things to come. (Government proposals for new reorganisation of NHS. See also p.1330.) Nursing Times, 76, 31 Jul 1980, 1335.

13 Deans Weir, R. Towards a simpler organisation. (Comment on some of Royal Commission's recommendations.) Hospital and Health Services Review, 75 (12), Dec 1979, 425-429.

14 Elwood, W. Hold your hatchets and take a close look. (Effects of abolishing the area tier of the NHS on work in community medicine.) Health and Social Service Journal, 88, 28 Jul 1978, 848-849.

15 Ennals, D. Insurance scheme would be disaster. (Comment on report of the Royal Commission on the NHS.) Nursing Mirror, 149, 9 Aug 1979, 17-19.

16 Gruneberg, R.N. The Royal Commission report—a personal view. (Critical comment by a consultant microbiologist.) Nursing Focus, 1 (6), Feb 1980, 227-228, 230.

17 Halpern, S. The dustbin syndrome. (Fate of recent inquiries into the NHS including the report of the Royal Commission.) Health and Social Service Journal, 89, 7 Dec 1979, 1578-1581.

18 Hancock, C. A better service to patients. (Comment on the report of the Royal Commission on the NHS.) Nursing Mirror, 149, 30 Aug 1979, Supplement xii-xv.

19 Health and Social Service Journal Three papers from journal's conference on the report of the Royal Commission on the NHS. Health and Social Service Journal, 89, 5 Oct 1979, 1280-1285.

20 Health and Social Service Journal Five articles on the report of the Royal Commission on the NHS. Health and Social Service Journal, 89, 27 Jul 1979, 930-950.

21 Health and Social Service Journal Ten articles commenting on aspects of the report of the Royal Commission on the NHS. Health and Social Service Journal, 89, 21 Sep 1979, 1194-1214.

22 Health and Social Service Journal Some representations from the black hole. (Comment on proposed Welsh health commission, with reference to Royal Commission on the NHS.) Health and Social Service Journal, 89, 4 May 1979, 512-513.

23 Hospital and Health Services Review The Royal Commission. (Comment on report.) Hospital and Health Services Review, 75 (9), Sep 1979, 301-304.

24 Hunt, P. What the NAHA thinks of the Royal Commission. (National Association of Health Authorities.) Journal of Community Nursing, 3 (3), Sep 1979, 4-5, 34, 38.

25 Jenkin, P. Jenkin set against headlong dash to new Appointed Day. (Interview with

Secretary of State on various aspects of the health service.) Health and Social Service Journal, 89, 29 Jun 1979, 792-795.

26 Lancet Health care in inner city areas. (Views of Royal Commission on the NHS.) Lancet, 2, 4 Aug 1979, 263-264.

27 Lancet Royal Commission on the NHS. (Some of its recommendations.) Lancet, 2, 21 Jul 1979, 142-143.

28 Macara, A.W. Health care or health? (Comment on the report of the Royal Commission.) Royal Society of Health Journal, 99 (6), Dec 1979, 228-234.

29 McFarlane, J.K. Now it's your turn to tell us! (Some of the main recommendations of the Royal Commission.) Nursing Mirror, 149, 26 Jul 1979, 16-18.

30 McFarlane, J.K. and Dopson, L. 'A report to make people think'. (Interview with Jean McFarlane on aspects of the Royal Commission on the NHS report.) Nursing Times, 75, 26 Jul 1979, 1257-1258.

31 Morris, P. First aid is needed—not major surgery. (Summary of report of Royal Commission on the NHS with checklist of the chief recommendations.) Nursing Mirror, 149, 26 Jul 1979, 6-7.

32 Murphy, R. Essential reading for nurse managers. (Comment on report of the Royal Commission on the NHS.) Nursing Focus, 1 (2), Oct 1979, 78-79, 82.

33 Nursing Focus Reorganisation—the government's blueprint. (Summary of proposals.) Nursing Focus, 2 (1), Sep 1980, 5, 7.

34 Pace, D. A treasurer's viewpoint. (On the report of the Royal Commission on the NHS.) Nursing Focus, 1 (5), Jan 1980, 189, 191.

35 Royal College of Nursing Comments on the report of the Royal Commission on the National Health Service. Rcn, 1979.

36 Wells, C.J. The Royal Commission—its task, its work and its report. (By a member of the Commission.) Royal Society of Health Journal, 99 (6), Dec 1979, 225.

37 Wild, D. Teams and plans and misused terms. (Comment on the report of the Royal Commission on the NHS.) Royal Society of Health Journal, 99 (6), Dec 1979, 238, 265.

CONSULTATIVE PAPER: PATIENTS' FIRST

38 Department of Health and Social Security and Welsh Office Patients first: consultative paper on the structure and management of the National Health Service in England and Wales. HMSO, 1979.

39 Bailey, E. Legal notes. NHS organisation and 'Patients First'. Nursing Focus, 1 (8), Apr 1980, 320, 322-323.

40 Bosanquet, N. Patients or doctors first? (Critical comment on 'Patients first'.) New Society, 53, 31 Jul 1980, 220-221.

41 Draper, P. and others The Royal Commission and prevention. (Criticism of aspects of the Commission's views on prevention.) Lancet, 2, 25 Aug 1979, 425-426.

42 Fewtrell, C. Patients first: staff...?

(Report on conference organised by Journal.) Health Services Manpower Review, 6 (1), Feb 1980, 4-6.

43 Hancock, C. 'Patients first'. (Comment.) Nursing Focus, 1 (8), Apr 1980, 303-304.

44 Haywood, S. Remember—structure is a means not an end. (Comment on 'Patients first'.) Health and Social Service Journal, 90, 18 Apr 1980, 518-519.

45 Health and Social Service Journal Reaction and repercussion. (Review of comments on Patients first.) Health and Social Service Journal, 90, 9 May 1980, 608-611.

46 Health Visitor NHS reorganisation. (Summary of circular HC(80)8.) Health Visitor, 53 (9), Sep 1980, 359.

47 Health Visitors Association Comments on 'Patients first'. Health Visitor, 53 (6), Jun 1980, 233, 235.

48 Hospital and Health Services Review Patients first, then structure and management. (Comment on 'Patients first'.) Hospital and Health Services Review, 76 (1), Jan 1980, 2-4.

49 Hospital and Health Services Review Patients first: a day conference of the Institute of Health Service Administrators. Hospital and Health Services Review, 76 (4), Apr 1980, 139-147.

50 Institute of Health Service Administrators On 'Patients first': a summary of the Institute of Health Service Administrators' comments on the consultative paper on the structure and management of the NHS in England and Wales. Hospital and Health Services Review, 76 (5), May 1980, 175-181.

51 Institute of Health Service Administrators Restructuring the NHS: implementation. Appendix 3 of the IHSA comments on 'Patients first'. Hospital and Health Services Review, 76 (6), Jun 1980, 217-219.

52 National Association of Theatre Nurses Comments on 'Patients first'. NATNews, 17 (6), Jun 1980, 16.

53 Ride, T.J. Patients first—a prescription for nursing. (Comment on report's implications for nursing with special reference to need for a clinical career structure.) Nursing Times, 76, 28 Feb 1980, 385-387.

54 Royal College of Midwives Comments on 'Patients first'. Midwives Chronicle, 93, Jun 1980, 204-206, 207.

55 Royal College of Nursing Comments on 'Patients first', March 1980. Rcn, 1980.

56 Royal College of Nursing Patients first. (Report of Rcn conference.) Nursing Times, 76, 6 Mar 1980, 398-399; Health and Social Service Journal, 90, 7 Mar 1980, 306-307.

57 Salvage, J. Prepare to shed a tier. (Comment on 'Patients first'.) Nursing Mirror, 150, 28 Feb 1980, 8-9.

58 Salvage, J. An unhealthy silence? (Progress of the Health Services Bill.) Nursing Mirror, 150, 13 Mar 1980, 7.

59 Scrivens, E. In the light of the last six years. (Comment on consultative document's recommendations for reduction in management tiers.) Health and Social Service Journal, 90, 14 Mar 1980, 350-352.

60 University of Leeds. Nuffield Centre for Health Services Studies 'Patients first'—intentions and consequences: a commentary on the consultative paper on the structure and management of the National Health Service.... Leeds: the Centre, 1980.

RESEARCH PAPER No.1

61 ROYAL Commission on the National Health Service. Research papers. HMSO. No.1. The working of the National Health Service 1978. No.6. Access to primary care 1979.

62 Ball, D. Sorry but there's no easy answer. (Analysis of Royal Commission Research Paper No.1. The working of the National Health Service.) Health and Social Service Journal, 88, 16 Jun 1978, 688-689.

63 Bosanquet, N. Towards a non-political health service? (Comment on research papers published by Royal Commission on the NHS.) New Society, 48, 14 Jun 1979, 644-645.

64 British Medical Journal Royal Commission on the NHS. (Comment on the Royal Commission's Research Paper No.1, The working of the National Health Service.) British Medical Journal, 1, 24 Jun 1978, 1652-1653.

65 Morris, P. Beware the ghost of plans past.... (What the research reports prepared for the Royal Commission said about bureaucracy.) Nursing Mirror, 149, 19 Jul 1979, 7.

d INTEGRATION WITH SOCIAL SERVICES

1 Barnes, C. Machinery that needs more than the occasional facelift. (Joint planning between health and local authorities.) Health and Social Service Journal, 87, 11 Nov 1977, 1561.

2 Booth, T. The swings and roundabouts of sharing out resources: the benefits and drawbacks so far encountered in joint financing schemes between health and social services. Health and Social Service Journal, 87, 25 Nov 1977, 1616-1617.

3 Bosanquet, N. Inside the social services. Nursing Times. History and aims. 73, 24 Feb 1977, 264-265. Organisation and finance. 73, 31 Mar 1977, 452-453. The future of the social services. 74, 5 Jan 1978, 37-38; 26 Jan 1978, 162-163.

4 Brown, M. The dubious advantages of integration. (Of health and social services in Northern Ireland.) Social Work Today, 10, 6 Mar 1979, 21-23.

5 Brown, M. Northern Ireland's marriage troubled by seven-year itch. (Questions value of integration of health and social services.) Health and Social Service Journal, 90, 15 Feb 1980, 222-223.

6 Burningham, S. Making the most creative use of the available resources. (Work of joint planning officer with East Sussex Social Services and AHA.) Health and Social Service Journal, 89, 14 Dec 1979, 1618-1619.

7 Canvin, R. and others Balance of care in Devon: joint strategic planning of health and social services at AHA and county level. Health

and Social Service Journal, 88, 18 Aug 1978, Centre eight papers C17-C20.

8 Clode, D. Setting the seal on the century. (Interview with Lord Seebohm on the effects of his report on reorganisation of the social services.) Health and Social Service Journal, 90, 4 Jan 1980, 20-21.

9 Davies, B.M. Coming to terms with the meaning of partnership. The importance of planning for collaboration between health and personal social services. Health and Social Service Journal, 87, 27 May 1977, 855-858.

10 Department of Health and Social Security Social service teams: the practitioner's view. HMSO, 1978.

11 Department of Health and Social Security Working Party on Manpower and Training for the Social Services Report. HMSO, 1976.

12 Freeman, M. and Hucklesby, D. Beating about the undergrowth. (How Government's proposals for 'organic' change in local government may affect joint planning between health and social services.) Health and Social Service Journal, 89, 15 Mar 1979, 262-263.

13 Hall, P. Reforming the welfare: the politics of change in the personal social services. Heinemann, 1976.

14 Hamson, J. The red rag of information. (How cooperation between health and local authorities requires systematic and thorough records.) Health and Social Service Journal, 89, 8 Jun 1979, 702-703.

15 Harbert, W.B. Moving into overall care. Discusses the potential of joint financing of projects of interest to both the health and social services. Health and Social Service Journal, 77, 29 Apr 1977, 745.

16 Haward, R.A. Five years on—how real is the integration of hospital and community health services. (With two proposals for improving situation.) Public Health, 93 (6), Nov 1979, 377-382.

17 Hospital and Health Services Review Positive discrimination in the health and social services. Hospital and Health Services Review, 76 (6), Jun 1980, 223-226.

18 Institute of Health Service Administrators Collaboration—theory and practice. Open forum at the IHSA annual conference. (Between health and local authorities.) Hospital and Health Services Review, 73 (9), Sep 1977, 317-319.

19 Kahan, B. Co-operation between health and social services: implications for policy. Social Work Service, No.22, Feb 1980, 29-34.

20 Kelly, G. Joint financing: is it greasing the wheel of change or paying Peter to pay Paul? (Report on progress towards co-operation between health and personal social services.) Social Work Today, 9, 1 Aug 1978, 9-11.

21 Keywood, O. The effects of an integrated service on standards of health care. 2 parts. (Baillière Tindall prize winning essay.) Nursing Mirror, 143, 7 Oct 1976, 63-66; 14 Oct 1976, 69-73.

22 Langston, P. Why should health alone pay the piper and call the planning tune? (Joint financing of health and social services.) Health

and Social Service Journal, 88, 28 Jul 1978, 845-846.

23 Lewis, S. Weaving a strategem across boundaries. (Part 1. Joint financing between health service and local government.) Health and Social Service Journal, 89, 6 Apr 1979, 382-383.

24 Lonsdale, S. and others, editors Teamwork in the personal social services and health care: British and American perspectives. Croom Helm, 1980.

25 Morgan, W. and Walker, J.H. The role of the social worker in health care. Community Health, 7 (3), Jan 1976, 122-126.

26 Murray, E.W. State of confusion. The essential differences between the various forms of welfare available in the community from the local authorities and from central government. Nursing Mirror, 146, 12 Jan 1978, 40.

27 Newe, G. Togetherness is the keynote. (Integration of health and personal social services in Northern Ireland.) Health and Social Service Journal, 89, 4 May 1979, 514-515.

28 Owens, J.K. Ten years of social service. Social Service Quarterly, 51 (2), Oct/Dec 1977, 46-48.

29 Personal Social Services Council Collaboration in community care: a discussion document. HMSO, 1978.

30 Price, J.R. The road to Seebohm—or 'How the social services happened.' Midwife, Health Visitor and Community Nurse, 13 (9), Sep 1977, 278, 281, 283-284.

31 Rathwell, T. and Reynolds, J. Conflicts in co-operation. (Barriers to effective joint planning between health and social services.) Health and Social Service Journal, 89, 7 Sep 1979, 1144-1145.

32 Rathwell, T. and Reynolds, J. Keeping up the pioneer spirit. (Suggestions on how joint planning between health and local authorities can be made more effective.) Health and Social Service Journal, 89, 14 Sep 1979, 1172-1173.

33 Rubin, S. and Bradburn, S. Community health officers for new health and social service. (The advantages of integrating health and social services.) Health and Social Service Journal, 86, 12 Nov 1976, 2016-2017.

34 Scottish Home and Health Department Working Party on Relationships between Health Boards and Local Authorities Report. HMSO, 1977.

35 Scottish Education Department. Social Work Services Group and Scottish Home and Health Department Social work services in the Scottish Health Service: report of the working party. HMSO, 1976.

36 Seebohm, F., Baron Seebohm of Hertford The Seebohm reorganisation—what went wrong? Social Work Today, 9 (6), 4 Oct 1977, 10-11.

37 Smith, J. The aspects of collaboration. (Comment on recent DHSS document on collaboration between health and social services.) Health and Social Service Journal, 88, 8 Sep 1978, 1006-1007.

38 Smith, J. Sad mysteries surrounding lack of joint administration. (Comparison of role of members of social service committees with their counterparts in the NHS.) Health and Social Service Journal, 90, 22 Feb 1980, 256-257.

39 Smith, J. Who will now fly the flag of conterminosity? (Sharing of boundaries between health and social services and effect of abolition of AHAs on cooperation between health and social services.) Health and Social Service Journal, 89, 7 Dec 1979, 1584-1585.

40 Willcocks, A. Weakness of consultation. (Criticism of joint consultative committees for health and social service planning.) Health and Social Service Journal, 89, 27 Apr 1979, 481.

41 Wilson, D. Joint financing: where does all the money go? (Some of the projects which have been funded.) Health and Social Service Journal, 88, 28 Apr 1978, 480-481.

e NURSING AND REORGANISATION

1 Allen, P. Great Britain: a common lanuage but an uncommon health care delivery system. (Report of study tour including looking at role of the nurse.) Journal of Nursing Education, 17 (2), Feb 1978, 40-46.

2 Arnold, N. Getting it right—third time around. (Adverse effects of Salmon and NHS reorganisation on nursing management, with some reference to 'Patients first'.) Nursing Mirror, 150, 17 Apr 1980, 36-37.

3 Ashton, K. Caring for a divided land. (Nursing in Ulster. Report of visit.) Nursing Times, 73, 13 Oct 1977, 1580-1585.

4 Auld, M.G. Perfecting the system. (Conference address on health services priorities and resources in relation to nursing.) Nursing Mirror, 146, 30 Mar 1978, 37-38; 6 Apr 1978, 41-42.

5 Baly, M. Professional advisory committee. Nursing Times, 72, 15 Jul 1976, 1074-1077.

6 Carr, A. Let 'adaptable' be the key word. (How new reorganisation could allow nursing management structures to be more flexible.) Nursing Mirror, 151, 24 Jul 1980, 12.

7 Carr, A. Rejig of a rejigged Health Service. (Effects on staff of changes proposed in 'Patients first'.) Nursing Mirror, 150, 17 Jan 1980, 16.

8 Carr, A. A traditional view of the nurse's role. (Comment on Royal Commission on NHS and the author's view that senior nurses should have direct clinical involvement.) Health and Social Service Journal, 89, 5 Oct 1979, 1282-1283.

9 Carr, A. The shape of things to come. (Review of report of Royal Commission on the NHS with reference to nurse manager's role in patient care.) Nursing Times, 75, 18 Oct 1979, 1786-1787.

10 Carr, A. Which way now—area nurse? (Uncertain future due to 'Patients first'.) Nursing Mirror, 150, 21 Feb 1980, 14.

11 Castledine, G. Change for change's sake? (Comment on function and effectiveness of professional nursing and midwifery advisory committees.) Nursing Mirror, 150, 28 Feb 1980, 14.

12 Clark, G. Watching nurses' interests in Parliament. (By parliamentary correspondent from 1955-1977.) Nursing Mirror, 146, 13 Apr 1978, 49, 51.

13 Clark, J. It's all been said before even by Flo Nightingale. (Comment on the Royal Commission's views on nursing.) Health and Social Service Journal, 89, 21 Sep 1979, 1206-1208.

14 Clay, T. The role of nursing and midwifery advisory committees in the reoganised NHS. The author, 1976.

15 Clode, D. Let's bring the present idiotic system to an end. (Views of Sam Richards, Vice-President of Rcn, on needs of staff during coming reorganisation of NHS.) Health and Social Service Journal, 90, 14 Mar 1980, 358.

16 Department of Health and Social Security Nursing 1974-1976. Report of the Chief Nursing Officer. DHSS, 1977. Extracts in Nursing Mirror, 145, 29 Sep 1977, 7-9; 6 Oct 1977, 7-9.

17 Department of Health and Social Security Regional and area nursing and midwifery liaison committees. DHSS, 1976. (HC(76)49.)

18 Dopson, L. and Rowden, R. Devolution. (Effects on nursing if devolution in Scotland and Wales goes ahead.) Nursing Times, 75, 22 Feb 1979, 312-313.

19 Drummond, P. Wessex—changing 'as swiftly and simply as possible'. (Proposals for restructuring to disband 4 AHAs and create 10 'neutral' districts.) Health and Social Service Journal, 90, 8 Aug 1980, 1028-1029.

20 Edwards, E.A. The nursing service in North Lothian. (How unified nursing service was developed to facilitate optimum care for the patient and his family.) Nursing Mirror, 146, 11 May 1978, 21-23.

21 Emerton, A.C. The reorganized National Health Service. Staffing problems in nursing. Royal Society of Health Journal, 96 (2), Apr 1976, 58-62.

22 Ennals, D. The Minister and the NHS. (Interview with David Ennals on nursing and the NHS.) Nursing Mirror, 146, 1 Jun 1978, Supplement 6-7, 9.

23 Friend, P. From where I sit. (Personal impression of the NHS and description of her career by CNO at DHSS.) Nursing Mirror, 147, 6 Jul 1978, 12-14.

24 Frost, W. NHS reorganisation from the point of view of nursing. Midwife, Health Visitor and Community Nurse, 12 (12), Dec 1976, 397-400.

25 Greene, J. Towards a better service. (Defects in nursing organisation in the present NHS structure.) Nursing Mirror, 144, 10 Feb 1977, 41.

26 Hambleton, B. A link in career development. (Functions of National Staff Committee for Nurses and Midwives.) Nursing Focus, 1 (4), Dec 1979, 161.

27 Hospital and Health Services Review Nurses' dilemmas. (Comment on the Rcn's document on the state of nursing in the NHS.) Hospital and Health Services Review, 74 (12), Dec 1978, 421-423.

28 Howell, L.C. Organisation of nursing services. 1. Fine tuning is called for—not a new instrument. (Management structure.) Health and Social Service Journal, 90, 15 Aug 1980, 1066-1068.

29 Jones, D. Perspective on care. (Comment on 'Patients first' and suggestion that patient-oriented non-support clinical services should be under control of nursing management.) Nursing Times, 76, 10 Apr 1980, 627.

30 Knibbs, J. Stemming the stress on senior staff. (Approaches to preventing stress caused by reorganisation.) Health and Social Service Journal, 86, 21 Aug 1976, 1512.

31 Lancet Commentary from Westminster. The strain on nurses. (Comment on Miss Hall's letter to David Ennals.) Lancet, 1, 11 Mar 1978, 566.

32 Lee, M. Professional advisory machinery. (Letter outlining work of National Steering Committee.) Nursing Times, 76, 23 Oct 1980, 1880.

33 Lewis, S. Tough and angry as nurses dissect the state of care. (Summary of and comment on the Rcn's document on the state of nursing in the NHS. See also editorial on p.1231.) Health and Social Service Journal, 88, 3 Nov 1978, 1236-1239.

34 Lloyd, T. Flexibility is the key word. (Suggested structure for nursing management in the new district health authorities.) Health and Social Service Journal, 90, 13 Jun 1980, 780-781.

35 McFarlane, J., Baroness McFarlane of Llandaff Twenty-fifth William Power Memorial Lecture. The implications of the report of the Royal Commission on the National Health Service for nursing and midwifery clinical practice. Midwives Chronicle, 93, Apr 1980, 107-111.

36 Midwives Chronicle Roles and status of professional advisory committee. (Nursing and Midwifery.) Midwives Chronicle, 89, Dec 1976, 293.

37 National Staff Committee for Nurses and Midwives Nursing appointment procedures: a guide to good practice. The Committee, 1980.

38 National Staff Committee for Nurses and Midwives Progress report. A review of the first year's work of the area nursing and midwifery committees. Nursing Times, 72, 29 Jan 1976, 128.

39 The National Staff Committee for Nurses and Midwives Progress report. (Lists achievements and current areas of work. Invites comments and suggestions on future areas to examine.) Nursing Mirror, 144 (17), 28 Apr 1977, 39-40.

40 National Staff Committee for Nurses and Midwives Report to the Secretaries of State.; (1975-1978). HMSO, 1979.

41 Nursing Officer If I was forced to cut. Nursing officer. By a special correspondent. (Including views on nurse staffing.) British Medical Journal, 2, 8 Dec 1979, 1480-1491.

42 Nursing Times Stage set for first area committee elections. (Nursing and midwifery advisory committees.) Nursing Times, 76, 2 Oct 1980, 1726.

43 Nursing Times Nursing secondment to the

DHSS. (Experiences of Grace H. Williams, Judith L. Dickie, Margaret Clarke and M.H. Magowan.) Nursing Times, 73, 28 Apr 1977, Occ. papers, 57-60; 5 May 1977, Occ. papers, 61-62.

44 Paine, R.E. Health and local authority JCCs. (The work of joint consultative committees and their relevance to nurses.) Nursing Times, 73, 17 Feb 1977, 250-251.

45 Pealing, J. If you have tiers to shed shed them for the patient. (Revised nursing management structure implemented in S.E. Staffordshire Health District which omits SNO grade.) Health and Social Service Journal, 90, 22 Feb 1980, 250-252.

46 Poole, A.A.B. Achieving democracy— mark 2. (Revision of electoral procedures in Surrey AHA's nursing and midwifery advisory committee.) Nursing Times, 76, 13 Mar 1980, 470-472.

47 Professional Advisory Machinery Nursing and Midwifery. National Steering Committee The role and status of nursing and midwifery committee. Nursing Mirror, 142, 10 Jun 1976, 40-41.

48 Quinn, S. A nurse's view. (Comment on the report of the Royal Commission on the NHS.) Royal Society of Health Journal, 99 (6), Dec 1979, 234-237.

49 Royal College of Nursing An assessment of the state of nursing in the National Health Service 1978: Rcn submission to the Secretary of State for Social Services. Rcn, 1978.

50 Royal College of Nursing Major issues to be raised with the Secretary of State at the meeting on 19 May 1976. The College, 1976. Summary in Nursing Times, 74, 2 Nov 1978, 1783.

51 Royal College of Nursing Patients first: the implications for nursing. Rcn, 1980.

f REGIONAL REPORTS

1 Cowper-Smith, F. Focus on Colchester—1. (Colchester District health services.) Nursing Mirror, 142, 22 Apr 1976, 47-49.

2 Dopson, L. On location. 1. Nursing at the seaside. (East Dorset health district.) Nursing Times, 76, 3 Jul 1980, 1164-1167.

3 Dopson, L. On location. 2. The challenge of nursing in suburbia. (Visit to Mid-Surrey district.) Nursing Times, 76, 7 Aug 1980, 1382-1386.

4 Dopson, L. On location. 3. Powys: sheep country where integration is complete. Nursing Times, 76, 11 Sep 1980, 1608-1615.

5 Evans, A.M. Three years later—coming to terms with reality. (Work of the South Glamorgan Health Authority (Teaching) since reorganisation.) Hospital and Health Services Review, 73 (3), Mar 1977, 87-92.

6 Halpern, S. How will Wales cope after St. David's Day? (Possible effects of devolution on the health service in Wales.) Health and Social Service Journal, 89, 8 Feb 1979, 122-124.

7 Health and Social Service Journal Ulster— special issue. (Eleven articles on health and social services in Northern Ireland.) Health and Social Service Journal, 86, 24/31 Dec 1976, 2280-2293.

8 Honywood, H. An integrated service— Lichfield. (Hospital—community liaison.) General Practice Team, 54, Jan 1976, 2-4.

9 McKay, R. Questions of dizziness while climbing the peaks of Scottish democracy. (How devolution would affect Scottish health service.) Health and Social Service Journal, 89, 1 Mar 1979, 206-208.

10 Northern Ireland Council for Nurses and Midwives A summary of the work of the Council 1971-1975. Belfast: The Council, (1976.)

11 Nunn, C. Monklands DGH: a case study in devolution. (Monklands and Cumbernauld Health District, Scotland.) Hospital and Health Services Review, 72 (12), Dec 1976, 416-420.

12 Nursing Mirror The nursing services in Scotland. (Ten articles including long term care and care of mentally ill, handicapped and elderly.) Nursing Mirror, 146, 4 May 1978, Supplement i-xvi.

13 Nursing Mirror The nursing services in Wales. (All aspects.) Nursing Mirror, 147, 21 Sep Supplement i-xvi.

14 Nursing Mirror The Ulster scene.
1. (The development of services.)
2. (Special aspects of the service.)
3. Health service planning, manpower and education. Nursing Mirror, 148, 5 Apr 1979, 28-31; 12 Apr 1979, 24-26; 19 Apr 1979, 18-20.

15 Nursing Times Profiles. 72.
Bath Health District. 19 Feb 1976, Profile 5-8.
Blackburn Health District. 19 Aug 1976. Profile 29-32.
Cambridge Health District. 17 Jun 1976. Profile 21-24.
East Birmingham Health District. 18 Nov 1976. Profile 41-44.
Gwynedd Area Health Authority. 28 Oct 1976. Profile 37-40.
Leeds (Western) Health District. 20 May 1976. Profile 17-20.
Leicester: keeping pace with health needs. 18 Mar 1976. Profile 9-12.
Maidstone Health District: integrated care. 22 Jan 1976. Profile 1-4.
Northern Ireland (Western Area). 16 Dec 1976. Profile 45-48.
St. Thomas' Health District (Teaching). 22 Apr 1976. Profile 13-16.
South Derbyshire Health District. 16 Sep 1976. Profile 33-36.
South Lothian. 22 Jul 1976. Profile 25-28.

16 Nursing Times Health services in the Channel Islands. 1. The Bailiwick of Jersey. 2. The Bailiwick of Guernsey. Nursing Times, 75, 19 Apr 1979, Rcn Supplement 3, 5-6, 9-10, 13-14, 16, 19.

17 Ross, T. An oasis north of the border. (The health service in Scotland.) Nursing Mirror, 148, 22 Mar 1979, 18-19.

18 Smith, J. The first 18 months of reorganisation in the Brent Health District. Nursing Mirror, 142, 29 Jan 1976, 60-61.

31 HOSPITALS

a GENERAL

1 Baddeley, S. and others The development of community hospitals. (With G.P. care of patients and control of admissions and dis-

charges.) Community Health, 9 (2), Nov 1977, 60-65.

2 Bennett, A.E. editor Community hospitals: progress in development and evaluation. Oxford Regional Hospital Board, 1974.

3 Billing, A. Concept of the nucleus hospital. 1. Philosophy. 2. Inpatient accommodation. 3. Departments. Nursing Mirror, 144, 26 May 1977, 21-23, 30 Jun 1977, 17-19, 28 Jul 1977, 17-20.

4 Cavenagh, A.J.M. Contribution of general practitioner hospitals in England and Wales. (Survey of one-in-seven sample.) British Medical Journal, 2, 1 Jul 1978, 34-36.

5 Davies, P.M. Medical terminology in hospital practice: a guide for all those engaged in professions allied to medicine. 3rd ed. Heinemann, 1978. (For nurses and others.)

6 Department of Health and Social Security Hospital services: the future pattern of hospital provision in England. DHSS, 1980.

7 Department of Health and Social Security Rationalisation of services: a revised hospital plan for inner London: paper presented…on 30 September 1975. The Department, 1975.

8 Gatherer, A. and others Cornerstone of care for the future health service. (Changing pattern of care in community hospitals with implications for nursing and other staff with special reference to Oxfordshire.) Health and Social Service Journal, 80, 5 Dec 1980, 1562-1563.

9 Halpern, S. Sizing up the size problem. (Comment on new DHSS policy on smaller hospitals.) Health and Social Service Journal, 90, 6 Jun 1980, 730-731.

10 Haynes, R.M. and Bentham, C.E. Community hospitals and rural accessibility. Farnborough: Saxon House, 1979.

11 Hyde, A. A special kind of patient care. (History of and current issues facing the community hospital.) Health and Social Service Journal, 89, 20 Apr 1979, 436-437.

12 Jones, F.A. The London hospitals scene. British Medical Journal, 2, 30 Oct 1976, 1046-1049.

13 Kernick, D.P. and Davies, S.E. The community hospital: a three-year study. (Barry, South Wales.) British Medical Journal, 2, 20 Nov 1976, 1243-1245.

14 Kernick, D.P. and Davies, S. Problems in the development of the community hospital concept. British Medical Journal, 2, 5 Nov 1977, 1238-1239.

15 Kerrane, T. The post-graduate hospital scene in London. (History, present management and future.) Nursing Focus, 1 (3), Nov 1979, 107-110.

16 London Health Planning Consortium Towards a balance: a framework for acute hospital services in London reconciling service with teaching needs. The Consortium, 1980.

17 Marsh, B. Blending old into new. (History and implementation of nucleus hospitals with reference to those at Macclesfield and Chester.) Health and Social Service Journal, 90, 8 Feb 1980, 179-181.

18 Murray, J.F. Improving the hospital service? (Comparison of the Dutch hospital system with the British.) British Medical Journal, 1, 28 Feb 1976, 507-508.

19 Swarbrick, P.J. The first five years: one practice's view of a hospital general practitioner's unit. (Bangour General Hospital, Lothian.) Health Bulletin, 35 (1), Jan 1977, 7-10.

20 Weightman, G. Society at work. Castles to cottages. (The concept of community hospitals using Dike Memorial Hospital, Gloucestershire, as an example.) New Society, 35, 26 Feb 1976, 432-433.

21 While, A.E. The vital role of the cottage-community hospital. Journal of the Royal College of General Practitioners, 28, Aug 1978, 485-491.

22 White, D. Mechanical response. (The image a large hospital presents to its customers.) Health and Social Service Journal, 88, 27 Jan 1978, 97-98.

23 Woodward, J.W. A general practitioner ward in a new district general hospital. (Queen Mary's Hospital, Sidcup.) Journal of the Royal College of General Practitioners, 26, Sep 1976, 660-664.

b BED ALLOCATION AND USE

1 Bridgman, R.F. Hospital utilization: an international study, translated from the French by C.R. Stevenson. Oxford: Oxford University Press for WHO Regional Office for Europe, 1979. (Oxford medical publications.)

2 Davies, T.F. How to prevent cold admissions from freezing. (The reduction of waiting lists and more efficient use of beds.) Lancet, 1977, 1, 29 Jan 1977, 241-242.

3 Hurst, J.W. Saving hospital expenditure by reducing in-patient stay. HMSO, 1977. (Government economic service occasional papers no.14.)

4 Murphy, F.W. Blocked beds. (By social long stay patients especially the elderly.) British Medical Journal, 1, 28 May 1977, 1395-1396.

5 Scott-Samuel, A. Waiting lists and unmet needs. (Factors determining size of waiting lists.) Public Health, 93 (1), Jan 1979, 46-49.

6 Seccombe, C.J.P. Catchment areas—pros and cons. Midwife, Health Visitor and Community Nurse, 13 (5), May 1977, 145-146.

7 Weir, M. Making the most of beds and theatres to shorten the waiting. Health and Social Service Journal, 87, 1 Apr 1977, 564-565.

c DISCHARGE AND CONTINUITY OF CARE

1 Amos, G. Going home. (Work of Continuing Care Project and discussion of needs of elderly on discharge from hospital.) Community View, 5, May 1980, 3-5.

2 Ashley, J.S.A. Community care: continuing or alternative care? (Role of community nurses with patients discharged from hospital or nursed at home instead of being admitted to hospital.) Royal Society of Health Journal, 97 (3), Jun 1977, 127-129, 134.

3 Baxter, M. 'Hospital and community' now.

(Study of patients discharged from the Aberdeen Royal Infirmary in 1972.) Health Bulletin, 34 (3), May 1976, 150-158.

4 Bracken, A. Let's integrate. (Scheme of hospital/community liaison in Northumberland.) Nursing Mirror, 147, 12 Oct 1978, 45.

5 British Association for Service to the Elderly Hospital at home. (Annual conference on the application of the 'hospital at home' scheme started in Paris.) Queen's Nursing Journal, 19 (5), Aug 1976, 146.

6 British Red Cross Society Red Cross gives new look to home nursing. Nursing Times, 72 (1), 1/8 Jan 1976, 3. (See also item nos 152, 154-155.)

7 British Red Cross Society Nursing for the family. (British Red Cross Society national scheme of lectures in home nursing.) Queens Nursing Journal, 18 (10), Jan 1976, 282.

8 Cang, S. An alternative to hospital. (Extension of domiciliary patient care to relieve the burden on hospitals through hospital at home scheme.) Lancet, 1977, 1, 2 Apr 1977, 742-743.

9 Cang, S. Between the devil and the PCT. (Report of talk on Peterborough's Hospital at Home scheme by Stephen Cang.) Nursing Times, 74, 21/28 Dec 1978, 2090.

10 Cass, S. The effects of the referral process on hospital inpatients. (Analysis of the process of referral to other nursing, social work and para-medical agencies in preparation for hospital discharge.) Journal of Advanced Nursing, 3 (6), Nov 1978, 563-569.

11 Cass, S. Homeward bound. (Review of studies on hospital/community liaison and description of her research study into the career of general medical patients and referrals made.) Nursing Mirror, 147, 13 Jul 1978, 26-27.

12 Clarke, F. Hospital caring without walls... (Background to and functioning of Peterborough hospital at home scheme.) Health and Social Service Journal, 89, 29 Mar 1979, 309-310.

13 Clarke, F. Hospital at home. (Letter on concept of full-time and part-time patients with reference to the Peterborough scheme.) Nursing Times, 74, 16 Nov 1978, 1902.

14 Cullinan, J. Continuing care: getting down to working together. (Nursing Times workshop in which draft 'Nurse's guide to effective discharge procedures' was examined.) Nursing Times, 76, 24 Apr 1980, 721-724.

15 Department of Health and Social Security Early discharge from hospital for patients with hernia or varicose veins: report of a randomised controlled trial. HMSO, 1978.

16 Drug and Therapeutics Bulletin The GP and the hospital doctor: sharing care. (Review of research into hospital/community liaison.) Drug and Therapeutics Bulletin, 15 (20), 30 Sep 1977, 77-79.

17 Felstein, I. After care of chronic disease following hospital discharge. Midwife, Health Visitor and Community Nurse, 13 (8), Aug 1977, 257-260.

18 Ferguson, M. Integration between hospital and community. (Patient link project at the Welsh National School of Medicine aimed at a

student's comprehension of the totality of a patient including home background.) Nursing Mirror, 143, 2 Dec 1976, 54-56.

19 Ferguson, M. Patient-link project. (Teaching and learning project at the Department of Advanced Nursing Studies at Welsh National School of Medicine, involving student nurse visiting a patient at home before and after his hospital stay.) Nursing Times, 73, 29 Sep 1977, Occ. papers, 129-131.

20 Furbank, M.E. A nursing referral system: admissions, transfers and discharge to and from hospital. (Research study carried out in the Plymouth Group Hospitals to improve hospital-community liaison.) Nursing Times, 72, 18 Mar 1976, Occ. papers, 41-44.

21 Gabell, A. Nurse could you care more? (Criteria for discharge.) Nursing Times, 76, 1 May 1980, 767.

22 Gay, P. and Pitkeathley, J. The community care of discharge hospital patients. (Research study to discover if there was a role for the volunteer in the care of the discharged patient.) Health and Social Service Journal, 88, 7 Apr 1978, Centre eight papers C9-C16.

23 Gay, P. and Pitkeathley, J. When I went home: a study of patients discharged from hospital. King Edward's Hospital Fund for London, 1979.

24 HOSPITAL at home. (Report on new pilot scheme in Peterborough.) Health and Social Service Journal, 88, 21 Jul 1978, 812.

25 Jasper, M. Catch them early: a project to test the effectiveness of a hospital liaison scheme between the Accident and Emergency Department, paediatric wards and the health visitor. Health Visitor, 52 (4), Apr 1979, 133-134.

26 Kratz, C. Bringing it home. Peterborough's Hospital at Home Scheme. (Correspondence, p.1751.) Nursing Times, 74, 26 Oct 1978, 1748-1751.

27 Kratz, C. Medical nursing? (Comment on 'Hospitals at home' schemes.) Nursing Times, 74, 13 Jul 1978, Community Outlook 179.

28 Lewis, P. and Roberts, V. Discharges planned and unplanned. Health and Social Service Journal, 86, 13 Mar 1976, 490-491.

29 Pritchard, M.A. A concept of continuing care. (Liaison nursing officer in Bury St. Edmunds Health District dealing with all age groups and conditions.) Nursing Times, 76, 24 Jan 1980, 169-172.

30 Rigby, C. The clinical nurse specialist—4. Community liaison. (Royal Marsden Hospital, Sutton.) Nursing Times, 74, 27 Jul 1978, 1246.

31 Roberts, I. The discharged patient—are we doing our best? (Hospital/community liaison.) Nursing Mirror, 145, 22 Sep 1977, 37-39.

32 Robinson, W. Nursing for the family. (Nationwide lecture programme of home nursing organised by the Red Cross.) Nursing Mirror, 142, 8 Jan 1976, 40-42.

33 Shepherd, P. Early discharge from hospital after surgery. (Scheme involving community nursing staff at Bedford General

Hospital.) Midwife, Health Visitor and Community Nurse, 12 (9), Sep 1976, 289-291.

34 Skeet, M. and Stroud, J. Home nursing. (Textbook to accompany British Red Cross scheme of lectures.) Stanley Paul, 1975.

35 Smith, K. Community nursing care study. Liaison in community care. (Liaison between the primary health care team, geriatric hospitals, social services department, and the DHSS.) Nursing Times, 73, 21 Apr 1977, 554-555.

36 Smith, M.A. Nursing care outside the hospital in the integrated health service. Planned early surgical discharge and major out-patient surgery. Queen's Nursing Journal, 19 (3), Jun 1976, 72-73.

37 Watkin, B. Hospitals at home. (Comprehensive domiciliary patient care scheme developed in France.) Nursing Mirror, 146, 2 Feb 1978, 10.

38 Williams, E.V. A successful liaison system (in Walsall). (Correspondence.) Nursing Times, 72 (16), 22 Apr 1976, 625-626.

39 Wood, J. Links in the paper chain: the urgent need for better liaison between GPs and hospitals. Health and Social Service Journal, 87, 15 Jul 1977, 1048.

40 WORKING together. (Review of research showing lack of continuity of care between hospital and community and details of Continuing Care Project.) Nursing Times, 76, 14 Feb 1980, 272-273.

d DISCHARGE AND CONTINUITY OF CARE: OVERSEAS COUNTRIES

1 American Journal of Nursing Making the right moves in discharge planning. (Seven articles.) American Journal of Nursing, 79 (8), Aug 1979, 1439-1454.

2 Ayala, V. and Ross, D.G. Discharge planning. ONA Journal, 6 (10), Oct 1979, 406-408.

3 Barrowclough, F. Hospital at home. (Letter commenting on aspects of the home care scheme in Paris.) Queen's Nursing Journal, 19 (7), Oct 1976, 201-202.

4 Bristow, O. and others Discharge planning for continuity of care, by Opal Bristow, Carol Stickney and Shirley Thompson. New York: National League for Nursing, 1976.

5 Broomfield, S. Involving staff in discharge planning. (Discharge planning committee set up by Quality Assurance coordinator to increase nurse involvement.) Supervisor Nurse, 10 (7), Jul 1979, 35-36.

6 Burkey, S.L. An audit outcome: home going instructions. Supervisor Nurse, 10 (5), May 1979, 21-23, 26-29.

7 Caldera, K. and others Exploration of the effect of educational level on the nurse's attitude toward discharge teaching. (Research study.) Journal of Nursing Education, 19 (8), Oct 1980, 24-32.

8 Capano, K.R. and Brindle, S. Bridging the gaps in discharge planning. (Research study with paediatric nurses and patients.) Paediatric Nursing, 4 (6), Nov/Dec 1978, 53-57.

9 Clarke, F. Home care—an alternative to admission. (Sante-Service-Bayonne 'hospital at home' scheme in France.) Health and Social Service Journal, 86, 21 Feb 1976, 348-349.

10 Cook, R.L. Continuity of care: cliche or viable nursing concept? Nursing Leadership, 2 (4), Dec 1979, 21-25.

11 Dartington, T. Fragmentation and integration in health care: the referral process and social brokerage. (With reference to transfer between hospital and community.) Sociology of Health and Illness, 1 (1), Jun 1979, 12-39.

12 Hicks, A.P. and Ashby, D.J. Teaching discharge planning. (Students act as home health coordinators for a three week block.) Nursing Outlook, 24 (5), May 1976, 306-308.

13 Hushower, G. and others The nursing process in discharge planning. Supervisor Nurse, 9 (9), Sep 1978, 55-58.

14 Lancet Hospitals at home. (Discussion of schemes in France and Switzerland, with reference to care of the elderly.) Lancet, 2, 12 Nov 1977, 1016.

15 Lieber, M. Patient representative is hospital patient liaison. (Ex-administrator guides patients and relatives through hospital system explaining procedures and answering queries.) AORN Journal, 26 (4), Oct 1977, 668-674.

16 McCarthy, E. Comprehensive home care for earlier hospital discharge. (Visiting Nurse Association, Milwaukee.) Nursing Outlook, 24 (10), Oct 1976, 625-630.

17 McKeehan, K.M. Nursing diagnosis in a discharge planning program. Nursing Clinics in North America, 14 (3), Sep 1979, 517-524.

18 McQuire, H.D. Better continuity needed. (Review of 1975 hospital literature on continuity of care.) Hospitals, 50 (7), 1 Apr 1976, 87-89, 90-91.

19 Nerland, E. Patient transfer form provides continuity of care. Hospitals, 52 (19), 1 Oct 1978, 151-152, 154.

20 Peterson, M. A plea for planned discharges for patients. Australian Nurses' Journal, 5 (11), May 1976, 31, 37.

21 Pigache, P. Who goes home? (New 'hospital at home' scheme in France.) World Medicine, 13 (5), 30 Nov 1977, 93-94, 96-97, 99.

22 Previte, V.J. Continuing care in a primary nursing setting: role of a clinical specialist. (Discharge planning at Beth Israel Hospital, Boston, Mass.) International Nursing Review, 26 (2), Mar/Apr 1979, 53-56.

23 Reilly, M.M. Let's set the record straight: preparing the discharge summary and the patient's instruction sheet. Nursing (U.S.), 9 (1), Jan 1979, 56-61.

24 Steagall, B. How to prepare your patient for discharge. (Written plans about diet, medication, etc.) Nursing, 7 (11), Nov 1977, 6-7.

25 Thoms, F.L. and Mott, R. A new role for the RN: discharge coordinator. (RN member of hospital social service staff to improve hospital/community liaison.) Hospital Progress, 39 (2), Feb 1978, 38, 40.

26 Warnock, F.N. and Baszynski, A. Student nurse plus continuity of care equals quality care. (Student nurses visit patients' homes and help in pre-discharge planning.) International Nursing Review, 23 (5), Sep-Oct 1976, 148-149. Slightly extended version in Journal of Nursing Education, 16 (3), Mar 1977, 12-16.

27 Zerr, D. Teaching continuity of care through post-hospital visits by the student nurse. Nursing Papers, 8 (3), Fall 1976, 41-46.

e EQUIPMENT AND FURNITURE

1 Bliss, M.R. The use of ripple beds in hospitals. Hospital and Health Services Review, 74 (6), Jun 1978, 190-193.

2 Buckles, A.M. How should we dispose of our used needles and syringes?: an evaluation of four different types of containers for the disposal of sharps. Nursing Times, 76, 21 Aug 1980, ICNA 5-6, 8, 11.

3 Carr, R. and Sangster, J.A. Equipping health service buildings. Hospital and Health Services Review, 73 (5), May 1977, 154-157.

4 Carr, R. and Sangster, J.A. An introduction to capital equipping (for health service buildings.) Nursing Times, 72, 19 Aug 1976, 1290-1291.

5 Challis, R. Cost and bacteriological implications of replacing tea-towels and dishcloths with paper. Nursing Times, 75, 6 Sep 1979, Contact 5-6, 15.

6 Corner, C. Danger: staff at risk. (Education of staff about disposal of dangerous disposables.) Nursing Mirror, 146, 19 Jan 1978, 32.

7 D'Cruz, D.M. Soleus—a simple foot board device (for maintaining a patient in a sitting position in bed.) Nursing Times, 72, 4 Nov 1976, 1732-1734.

8 Department of Health and Social Security Supply Board Working Group. Report. DHSS, 1978.

9 Dunn, A. Save it. (Inefficiency in supplies departments.) Nursing Times, 75, 29 Nov 1979, 2064.

10 Frost, M. Who's a naughty girl? ('Borrowing' of equipment from the NHS by nurses.) Health and Social Service Journal, 88, 8 Dec 1978, 1394-1395.

11 Galley, J. Equipment research. ('Salisbury Surf bed', an adjustable trolley for patients who have to lie prone.) Health and Social Service Journal, 89, 9 Nov 1979, 1448-1449.

12 Grayson, H. Taking the top off storage. Recent studies at the Medical Architecture Research Unit. Polytechnic of North London and the importance of planning supplies systems for new hospitals. Health and Social Service Journal, 80, 12 Dec 1980, 1590-1591.

13 Green, H. More than just a salesman. (Relationship of medical and nursing staff with commercial representatives.) Nursing Mirror, 142, 10 Jun 1976, 58-59.

14 Hall, E. Agent of change in disposables switch. (Nursing practice committees evaluate products and review and revise procedures.) Hospital Administration in Canada, 19 (11), Nov 1977, 14-15.

15 McGilloway, F.A. A chair is a chair, or is it? (Need for more careful designing of wards and equipment.) Nursing Mirror, 151, 24 Jul 1980, 34-35.

16 Moores, Y. and Pethybridge, F. A supply council for the NHS: some of the initial problems. (By members of the Supply Board Working Group.) Hospital and Health Services Review, 74 (12), Dec 1978, 431-434.

17 Norton, D. Equipment fit for purpose. (The variety of products with the same function purchased within the health service and means of improving their design and selection.) Nursing Times, 74, 6 Jul 1978, Occ. papers, 73-76.

18 Norton, D. Save it! (Development of system in SW Thames region involving product appraisal form to link users of equipment with supplies departments.) Nursing Times, 76, 31 Jan 1980, 188-190.

19 Robertson, C. Life on a Stryker bed. (By patient.) Nursing Times, 74, 4 May 1978, 752.

20 Robertson, J.C. Patient support systems: and so to beds... Nursing Mirror, 148, 24 May 1979, Supplement i-iii, vii, ix, xiii, xvii.

21 Salmon, B.L. Centralisation—good or bad? (Of supplies, based on IHSA conference paper.) Hospital and Health Services Review, 74 (9), Sep 1978, 313-318.

22 Savage, G. Morale sapping bureaucracy. (Support of concept of Common Services Agency in a Scottish context and view of what the Royal Commission should recommend.) Health and Social Service Journal, 89, 4 May 1979, 515-516.

23 Small, C.F. Beds. PhD thesis, University of Strathclyde, 1977.

24 Smith, B. Save it! (Work on evaluation of cost and efficiency of equipment including Kanga and Kylie bed sheets and Flowtron Intermittent Compression System for varicose ulcers.) Nursing Times, 76, 7 Feb 1980, 229-230.

25 Thomas, R. Unidirectional flow vs traditional system. (Friesen system of handling supplies etc.) AORN Journal, 31 (4), Mar 1980, 722, 724, 726, 728, 730, 732-733, 736.

26 Thomson, C.W. and others Fluidised-bead bed in the intensive-therapy unit. Lancet, 1, 15 Mar 1980, 568-570.

27 Thornett, M. Disposal bags in Brent. Report of the nurses' working party. Nursing Times, 73, 24 Feb 1977, ICNA Supplement 45-48.

28 Worthington, L. Things that go BUMP in the night. (Needs and concerns of nurses regarding mechanical equipment such as respirators.) Canadian Nurse, 73 (10), Oct 1977, 18-19.

f FINANCE

1 Coles, J. and others Allocating budgets to wards: an experiment. Hospital and Health Services Review, 72 (9), Sep 1976, 309-312.

2 Hurst, T. Save it! (Suggestions on ways hospitals could save money.) Nursing Times, 75, 6 Dec 1979, 2104-2105.

g FIRE AND ACCIDENTS

1 Australasian Nurses Journal Four articles on safety in hospital, including one on fire and evacuation planning. Australasian Nurses Journal, 8 (1), Sep 1978, 3-19, 22.

2 Bishop, V. It can be lethal in the care unit. (Need to educate nurses to recognise potential dangers of electrical apparatus in hospitals.) Nursing Mirror, 149, 11 Oct 1979, 20-21.

3 Coakley, D. On the dangers of getting out of bed in hospital. (Accidents to patients.) Health Trends, 12 (1), Feb 1980, 5-6.

4 Donn, M. Dangers of faulty and broken equipment. (With reference to the Health and Safety at Work Act.) Nursing Times, 74, 2 Nov 1978, Theatre Nursing 13, 15.

5 Fletcher, J.C. Friday the thirteenth. (How staff at Preston Royal Infirmary coped with a fire there on July 13th, 1979.) Nursing Times, 75, 13 Dec 1979, 2153-2154.

6 Health and Social Service Journal Fire! Fire! Evacuation exercise at Hackney Hospital. (Mainly illustrations.) Health and Social Service Journal, 86, 21 Feb 1976, 354-355.

7 Health and Social Service Journal Fire safety. (In hospitals. Four articles including report of a survey in Scotland, hazards of textiles and automatic alarm systems.) Health and Social Service Journal, 88, 17 Mar 1978, 310-317.

8 Hoenig, S.A. and Scott, D.H. Medical instrumentation and electrical safety: the view from the nursing station. New York: Wiley, 1977.

9 Iacobell, F.P. and Schodowski, L. Fire reaction training that really works. Hospitals, 54 (3), 1 Feb 1980, 64-66.

10 INCIDENT data compiled and compared. (Accidents and injuries to patients.) Hospitals, 53 (22), 16 Nov 1979, 54, 56, 58.

11 Johnson, J. Thoughts on 'cot sides'. (Project at Tolworth Hospital showing that reduction in their use did not increase accidents.) Nursing Focus, 2 (4), Dec 1980, 120-121.

12 Kulikowski, E.S. A study of accidents in a hospital. Supervisor Nurse, 10 (7), Jul 1979, 44-45, 49-50, 52, 55, 58.

13 Leask, E. Electro-medical equipment and patient safety. Health Bulletin, 34 (2), Mar 1976, 98-100.

14 Le Bourdais, E. A Canadian survey. Accidents in hospitals. Dimensions in Health Service, 54 (2), Feb 1977, 25-28.

15 Lynn, F.H. Incidents—need they be accidents? (Accidents to patients on wards.) American Journal of Nursing, 80 (6), Jun 1980, 1098-1101.

16 Lyons, H. Imagining the worst for sake of fire safety. (The case for fire fighting training for hospital staff with reference to a course held at Banstead Hospital, Surrey.) Health and Social Service Journal, 89, 15 Mar 1979, 259-260.

17 McGrath, R. Emergency removal of patients and first aid fire fighting in hospitals. 3rd ed. Chicago: National Safety Council/ American Hospital Association, 1974.

18 McKerral, H. When security is the key issue. (Comparison of security methods used in Chicago hospitals with those used at Charing Cross Hospital.) Health and Social Service Journal, 89, 14 Sep 1979, 1162-1163.

19 Meth, I.M. Electrical safety in the hospital. American Journal of Nursing, 80 (7), Jul 1980, 1344-1348.

20 Morris, C. Problems of creating a sense of security. (Problems of security in hospitals.) Health and Social Service Journal, 90, 18 Apr 1980, 508-509.

21 Morris, P. 'We'll just keep going... (Security at Royal Victoria Hospital, Belfast.) Nursing Mirror, 149, 15 Nov 1979, 7.

22 Nunn, C. There's a fire at DRI. (The efficiency of fire precautions following a fire at Dundee Royal Infirmary.) Hospital and Health Services Review, 70 (6), 1974, 202-207.

23 Nursing Times 55 practices in a year but staff in fire ward unprepared. (Inquiry into fire at Central Middlesex Hospital.) Nursing Times, 72 (6), 12 Feb 1976, 206.

24 Perrin, J. Is your hospital ready for a fire? Dimensions in Health Service, 53 (5), May 1976, 14-16, 17.

25 Shepard, I.M. Hospitals aren't safe enough. (The NIOSH survey of hospital health and safety services.) (National Institute of Occupational Safety and Health.) Hospital Progress, 58 (11), Nov 1977, 85-87.

26 Sklar, C. Hospital hazards and the nurse. (Includes safety of patients.) Canadian Nurse, 74 (7), Jul/Aug 1978, 16-18.

27 Smith, A. An explosive problem. (Hazards of liquid petroleum gas heaters in hospitals and safety guidelines.) Health and Social Service Journal, 90, 26 Sep 1980, 1260-1261.

28 White, D. Learning through experience: how to fight a hospital fire. (Simpson Memorial Maternity Pavilion, Edinburgh.) Health and Social Service Journal, 86, 4 Mar 1977, 376-377.

29 White, D. Our Nordic neighbours. (Council of Europe Fellowship to study the management of safety in hospitals in Denmark and Sweden.) Health and Social Service Journal, 90, 1 Aug 1980, 1010-1111.

30 White, D. and Young, N. Computer lights up gaps in organising the training. (Computer based hospital fire precautions training in Fife.) Health and Social Service Journal, 87, 12 Aug 1977, 1160-1161.

31 Wooliscroft, M. The hospital fire problem—towards a rational approach. Royal Society of Health Journal, 96 (4), Aug 1976, 181-185.

h FOOD AND CATERING

1 EGON Ronay's Lucas guide 1979. Harmondsworth: Penguin, 1978. (Includes survey on food in hospitals.)

2 Evans, E. Special diets in hospital. (Results of recent surveys.) Nursing Times, 73, 26 May 1977, 795-797.

3 Horton, A.R. Food service under stress.

(Food hygiene in hospitals.) Royal Society of Health Journal, 98 (5), Oct 1978, 201-208.

4 Hospitals Food service. (Five articles on cost containment and efficiency.) (19 pages.) Hospitals, 54 (6), 16 Mar 1980, 75-103.

5 Howard, J.P. Hospital dietetics and catering: the science and the art. Royal Society of Health Journal, 99 (1), Feb 1979, 17-22.

6 Janes, E. Hospital food: how well does it go down? Nursing, 11, Mar 1980, 487-489.

7 Konhauser, A. Team provides dietary care in small hospital. (Including nutrition education.) Hospitals, 53 (17), 1 Sep 1979, 99-102.

8 Lancet Food poisoning in hospitals. Lancet, 1, 15 Mar 1980, 576-577.

9 Miller, B. and Balsley, M. JCAH revises dietetic service standards. (Joint Commission on Accreditation of Hospitals.) Hospitals, 54 (21), 1 Nov 1980, 102-105.

10 Thompson, S. Pass the mash. (Poor range of food offered in most hospital canteens.) Nursing Mirror, 150, 17 Apr 1980, 19-20.

i HISTORY

1 Anderson, B. Hospitals: a look at the old and the new. (Stobhill General Hospital and Dumfries and Galloway Infirmary.) Health and Social Service Journal, 86, 22 Oct 1976, 1894.

2 Green, A. The ghosts of Christmas past. (In some British hospitals.) Nursing Mirror, 147, 21 Dec 1978, 16-18.

3 LONDON's hospitals. 250 years of medical care. (Mainly illustrations.) Nursing Times, 72 (18), 6 May 1976, 698-699.

4 Parry Jones, B. Locating and preserving Oxfordshire hospital records. Medical Records, 18 (4), Nov 1977, 328-329.

5 Rhind, N. Royal patronage and the hospital service. (Influence on its development.) Nursing Mirror, 144, 2 Jun 1977, 13-16.

6 A RIGHT royal welcome. (Hospital royal occasions 1953-1976.) Nursing Times, 73, 2 Jun 1977, 812-813.

7 Thompson, J.D. and Goldin, G. The hospital: a social and architectural history. New Haven: Yale University Press, 1975.

8 Winder, J. Royal patronage for village of healing. (The growth of Queen Square and its famous hospitals. Introduction and four articles.) Health and Social Service Journal, 87, 23/30 Dec 1977, 1740-1747.

INDIVIDUAL HOSPITALS

9 Addenbrooke's Hospital—Hyde, A. A contrast in Cambridge. (History of Addenbrooke's Hospital, Cambridge, and new hospital built in 1961.) Health and Social Service Journal, 90, 15 Feb 1980, 210-213.

10 Bethlem Hospital. . .And a look at the past. Nursing Times, 76, 4 Sep 1980, 1560-1562.

11 Bolton Hospital—The Bolton TV 'Hospital' series. 1. How did it happen? (By staff of Bolton AHA.) 2. Were we right to have said 'Yes' to the BBC? Hospital and Health Services Review, 74 (1), Jan 1978, 7-10; (2), Feb 1978, 43-48.

12 Bootham Park Hospital—Sumner, E.C. The first 200 years of Bootham Park Hospital. (York.) Nursing Mirror, 146, 1 Jun 1978, 18-20.

13 Brighton General Hospital—Gooch, J. A brief history of Brighton General Hospital. Phillimore, 1980.

14 Bromley General Hospital—Allen, M. Diary of a hospital. (Report of a week-long educational visit to Bromley General Hospital.) Nursing Mirror, 148, 10 May 1979, 12-15.

15 Chester—Hyde, A. Battling for pastures new. (Nucleus hospital at Chester.) Health and Social Service Journal, 89, 6 Apr 1979, 372-373.

16 Cranleigh Village Hospital—Davidson, N. Cranleigh's loyal army keep its history alive. Health and Social Service Journal, 90, 11 Apr 1980, 476-478.

17 Crumpsall Hospital—Hall, S. and Perry, D.L. Crumpsall Hospital 1876-1976: the story of a hundred years. Crumpsall Hospital, (1977.)

18 Dinorwic Quarry Hospital—Smith, H.B. The quarrymen who built their own hospital. (Dinorwic Quarry Hospital, Llanberis, now a museum.) Occupational Health, 31 (2), Feb 1979, 74-78.

19 Dinorwic Quarry Hospital—Smith, H.B. Quarrymen's hospital. (History of Dinorwic Quarry Hospital, North Wales.) Nursing Mirror, 147, 6 Jul 1978, 26-27.

20 Dreadnought Seamen's Hospital—Goldsmith, E. and McBride, A.G. Dreadnought Seamen's Hospital. British Medical Journal, 1, 19 Jun 1976, 1511-1513.

21 Edgware General—Jennings, G.H. Early memories of the Edgware General 1927-1945. (Includes photograph of the children's ward staff in 1940.) Nursing Mirror, 145, 4 Aug 1977, 25-27.

22 Elizabeth Garrett Anderson Hospital—Manning, M. Last-ditch stand tries the staying power of the EGA. (Elizabeth Garrett Anderson Hospital.) Nursing Mirror, 147, 14 Dec 1978, 8-9.

23 Elizabeth Garrett Anderson Hospital—Meade-King, M. Elizabeth Garrett Anderson—a hospital in jeopardy. Nursing Times, 72, 13 May 1976, 723-726.

24 Great Ormond Street Hospital for Sick Children—Happy birth GOS. (Mainly illustrations.) Nursing Times, 73, 24 Mar 1977, 404-405.

25 Great Ormond Street Hospital for Sick Children—Winder, J. Growth of an extrovert child. (History.) Health and Social Service Journal, 87, 23/30 Dec 1977, 1741-1743.

26 Guy's Hospital—Handler, C.E. editor Guy's Hospital: 250 years. Guy's Hospital Gazette, 1976.

27 Guy's Hospital—Helliwell, P.J. 250 years of Mr. Guy's Hospital. Nursing Mirror, 142, 6 May 1976, 46-50.

28 Hallamshire Hospital—Morris, P. Opening soon. . .the hospital they thought would never open. (Hallamshire Hospital, Sheffield.) Nursing Mirror, 147, 24 Aug 1978, 9.

29 Hamadryad Hospital—Mayberry, J.F. The Hamadryad Hospital ship for seamen, 1866-1905. (Cardiff.) British Medical Journal, 2, 20/27 Dec 1980, 1690-1692.

30 Irvine Memorial Hospital—Irvine, W. A place in the country that is not entirely countrified. (Irvine Memorial Hospital.) Health and Social Service Journal, 90, 22 Aug 1980, 1100-1101.

31 Italian Hospital—A corner for expatriates. Health and Social Service Journal, 87, 23/30 Dec 1977, 1746-1747.

32 Italian Hospital—Turner, J. Hospital, Italian style. New Society, 46, 21/28 Dec 1978, 681-682.

33 King's College Hospital—Iveson-Iveson, J.M. Research at King's. (Report of Open Day at The Voluntary Research Trust of King's College Hospital.) Nursing Mirror, 144, 9 Jun 1977, 7-8.

34 Lincoln County Hospital—Ingham, M.J. County Hospital Lincoln: Sewell Road 1878-1978. Lincoln: Lincolnshire AHA, 1979.

35 Lindenhof Hospital, Berne—Kratz, C.R. New ideas in old institutions. (Nursing care at Lindenhof Hospital, Berne, owned by Swiss Red Cross.) Nursing Times, 73, 6 Oct 1977, 1559-1561.

36 Liverpool Infirmary—McLoughlin, G. A short history of the first Liverpool Infirmary 1749-1824. Chichester: Phillimore, 1978.

37 London Hospital—The London Hospital. (The London Hospital Exhibition to commemorate past royal occasions.) Nursing Times, 73, 2 Jun 1977, 808-809.

38 Lynton Cottage Hospital—Garnham, L. Singing the praises of an unsung gem of the NHS. (Lynton Cottage Hospital in Devon.) Health and Social Service Journal, 90, 2 May 1980, 574-575.

39 Mildmay Mission Hospital—Willcox, Q.E. Mildmay Mission Hospital—100 years old. (History and current role in health service.) Nursing Mirror, 145, 20 Oct 1977, 8-9.

40 Milton Keynes—Hyde, A. The new town's problem child. (New hospital at Milton Keynes.) Health and Social Service Journal, 89, 6 Jul 1979, 828-829.

41 National Hospital for Nervous Diseases Neurological road for horseless carriages. (History of the National Hospital for Nervous Diseases.) Health and Social Service Journal, 87, 23/30 Dec 1977, 1745-1746.

42 New Cross Hospital—Rags to riches: the story of the New Cross Hospital, which this month celebrates its centenary. Nursing Times, 73, 3 Nov 1977, 1698-1699.

43 New Cross Hospital—Kaye, V. Travelling across times remembered. (History of New Cross Hospital and Mildmay Mission Hospital.) Health and Social Service Journal, 87, 25 Nov 1977, 1618-1620.

44 Newcastle Royal Infirmary—Hyde, A. Still set to serve the needy. (Newcastle Royal Infirmary.) Health and Social Service Journal, 90, 7 Mar 1980, 314-315.

45 Queen's Medical Centre, Nottingham. Hospital and Health Services Review, 76 (3), Mar 1980, 108-109.

46 Radcliffe—Gough, M.H. The 'Radcliffe' Hospitals, Oxford. (Past and present.) British Medical Journal, 2, 7 Jul 1979, 33-35.

47 Royal Cornwall Infirmary—Andrews, C.T. The first Cornish hospital. (Royal Cornwall Infirmary.) The author, 1975.

48 Royal Devon and Exeter—Deebie, S. From the days when pigs went squeak in the night. (History of the 200 year old Royal Devon and Exeter Hospital.) Health and Social Service Journal, 86, 1 Oct 1976, 1766-1767.

49 The Royal Free's 150th anniversary. Lancet, 1, 15 Apr 1978, 818.

50 Royal Hospital, Chelsea—Robinson, W. The Royal Hospital, Chelsea. (For Army pensioners.) Nursing Mirror, 145, 22 Dec 1977, 11-13.

51 Royal Infirmary of Edinburgh—Dopson, L. Preserving a hospital's history. (Interview with archivist of Royal Infirmary of Edinburgh.) Nursing Times, 75, 19 Jul 1979, 1239-1240.

52 Royal London Homeopathic Hospital—Winder, J. Facts and faith to beat an epidemic. (History of the Royal London Homeopathic Hospital.) Health and Social Service Journal, 87, 23/30 Dec 1977, 1744.

53 Royal Marsden—Cox, S. Inside the Royal Marsden. Nursing Mirror, 147, 31 Aug 1978, Supplement iii, v, vii.

54 Royal Naval Hospital—Dopson, L. Hospital, the navy way. (RNH Haslar in Gosport.) Nursing Times, 75, 11 Oct 1979, 1748-1752.

55 The Royal Sea Bathing Hospital (Margate). Nursing Times, 73, 10 Mar 1977, Archives 9-12.

56 Royal Sea Bathing Hospital, Margate—Hyde, A. A breath of good sea air. Health and Social Service Journal, 90, 18 Jan 1980, 78-79.

57 Royal South Hants Hospital—Watson, D.M. Proud heritage: a history of the Royal South Hants Hospital 1838-1971. Southampton: G.F. Wilson, 1979.

58 Royal United Hospital, Bath. (Developments.) Hospital and Health Services Review, 72 (5), May 1976, 162-163.

59 Royal Victoria Hospital, Netley. (Its closure in 1978.) QARANC Gazette, 8 (5), 1979, 29-31.

60 Saint Bartholomew's Hospital—Gooddy, J.W. Bart's traditions and treasures. Health and Social Service Journal, 86, 21 Aug 1976, 1510-1512.

61 St. John's Hospital for diseases of the skin—Matron's reports. (Selected extracts 1913-1940.) Nursing Times, 72, 30 Sep 1976, 1506-1509.

62 St. Mary's Hospital, Isles of Scilly—Davidson, N. Beautiful isles with an air of fiction. (St. Mary's Hospital, a cottage hospital in the Isles of Scilly.) Health and Social Service Journal, 90, 20 Jun 1980, 798-799.

63 St. Peter's Hospital for Stone. Nursing Times, 73, 10 Feb 1977, Archive 5-8.

64 St. Stephen's Hospital—Martin, L. Happy birthday, St. Stephen's. (100th anniversary of St. Stephen's Hospital, Chelsea, with photographs.) Nursing Times, 74, 8 Jun 1978, 946-947.

65 St. Thomas's Hospital—Duncum, B. Pay beds a century ago. (Home Hospital Association patients at St. Thomas's.) Hospital and Health Services Review, 72 (5), May 1976, 157-159.

66 St. Thomas's Hospital—Robinson, W. The new St. Thomas' Hospital. Nursing Mirror, 144, 9 Jun 1977, 13-16.

67 St. Thomas's Hospital. The new hospital opened. Hospital and Health Services Review, 73 (2), Feb 1977, 57-59.

68 St. Tydfil's Hospital. (Acute general hospital which was once a workhouse.) Nursing Times, 73, 27 Oct 1977, Archive 29-32.

69 Tarporley Hospital—Davidson, N. Cottage hospitals. Small is beautiful. (Tarporley Hospital, Cheshire.) Health and Social Service Journal, 90, 4 Jul 1980, 869-871.

70 Tenby Cottage Hospital—Davidson, N. The charm has gone but the loyalties remain. (Tenby Cottage Hospital.) Health and Social Service Journal, 80, 5 Dec 1980, 1556-1557.

71 University College Hospital—Merrington, W.R. University College Hospital and its Medical School: a history. Heinemann: 1976.

72 Wallingford Community Hospital—Hyde, A. Mecca and the unbelievers. (Wallingford community hospital.) Health and Social Service Journal, 89, 27 Apr 1979, 472-473.

73 Whitby Hospital—Dopson, L. Whitby Hospital. Integration in practice. (Community hospital.) Nursing Times, 75, 12 Apr 1979, 640-642.

74 Yeatman Cottage Hospital—Davidson, N. An evident future. (Yeatman Cottage Hospital in Sherborne, Dorset.) Health and Social Service Journal, 90, 23 May 1980, 672-674.

75 York—Holroyd, A. and Joy, N. Enthusiasm, nostalgia and a need for real success. Problems in running York's new district hospital. Health and Social Service Journal, 87, 14 Jan 1977, 60-61.

76 York—Stone, P. Building towards new horizons for this historic city. (Construction of a new district hospital at York.) Health and Social Service Journal, 87, 14 Jan 1977, 58-59.

j HOUSEKEEPING

1 Broadley, J. Patients and the profit motive. (The contractor's role in providing hospital domestic and housekeeping services.) Health and Social Service Journal, 90, 27 Jun 1980, 850-851.

2 Burningham, S. Stumbling block for domestic managers. (Need for more staff and adequate recognition of their work.) Health and Social Service Journal, 89, 29 Jun 1979, 804-805.

3 Kaye, V. Stolen linen is put on the line. (Report on International Association for Hospital Security seminar.) Health and Social Service Journal, 90, 2 May 1980, 570-571.

4 Nursing Times Three articles on pest control in hospitals, including report of a DHSS infestation control course and article on cockroaches specifically. Nursing Times, 75, 15 Feb 1979, Contact 4-7.

5 Williams, A. and others Ancillary staff in the hospital service: an investigation. (By the City University Business School at two London hospitals.) Hospital and Health Services Review, 74 (3), Mar 1978, 83-86.

k MANAGEMENT

1 Banyard, R. Skills in close harmony: the working role of the administrator at hospital level. Health and Social Service Journal, 87, 4 Nov 1977, 1579.

2 Deegan, A.X. Management by objectives for hospitals. Germantown, Md.: Aspen Systems Corporation, 1977.

3 Friedman, E. Women CEOs: they're good for the field, but is it good for them? (Women (including nurses) in hospital administration in the U.S.) Hospitals, 54 (3), 1 Feb 1980, 45-48.

4 Griffiths, D.A.T. Information rooms for operational management in general hospitals. (To aid management in decision making.) Hospital and Health Services Review, 74 (4), Apr 1978, 124-127; (5), May 1978, 157-160.

5 Hill, S. Healthy first steps towards harmony in the future. (Northampton General Hospital's experience of introducing system of participative management.) Health and Social Service Journal, 87, 30 Sep 1977, 1370-1371.

6 Hospital and Health Services Review Notes for students. Closures of hospitals: procedures and problems. Hospital and Health Services Review, 76 (2), Feb 1980, 81-82.

7 Hunt, E.J. Participative management—a compromise. The concept of the staff consumer forum in Tameside General Hospital. Hospital and Health Services Review, 73 (2), Feb 1977, 40-44.

8 Kernaghan, S.G. The 'organic approach' to cutting through bureaucracy. Hospital administrator uses democratic principles to improve hospital functioning and patient care. Hospitals, 51, 1 Sep 1977, 71-72, 74.

9 Levesley, R. and Hancock, A. Focal point of identity. (How hospital management teams work in one sector of Leeds Western Health District.) Health and Social Service Journal, 90, 23 May 1980, 665.

10 Marculies, N. Managing change in health care organisations. Medical Care, 15 (8), Aug 1977, 693-704.

11 Marsh, G.V. Hospital administration: the new order—problems of obesity. Royal Society of Health Journal, 97 (2), Apr 1977, 70-73.

12 Nevard, L. The health organisations. (Improving organisational performance by examining individual frustrations and satisfaction.) Hospital and Health Services Review, 73 (1), Jan 1977, 6-9.

13 Rakich, J.S. and Darr, K. editor Hospital organisation and management: text and readings. 2nd ed. New York: Spectrum, 1978.

14 Revans, R.W. Action learning in hospitals: diagnosis and therapy. McGraw-Hill,

1976. (Includes a reprint of 'Standards for morale'.)

15 Rinaldi, L. Managing a hospital audit committee. (With multidisciplinary representation.) Supervisor Nurse, 8 (6), Jun 1977, 60-62.

16 Ryan, J.E. Better style for change: matrix management. (System to recognise and coordinate need to implement radical changes and maintain routine operations.) Hospitals, 54 (22), 16 Nov 1980, 105-106, 108.

17 Shircore, R. and Garrison, T. Deficiencies in efficiency. Technical advances in treating acute illness, particularly cardiac arrest, have outstripped the management capability allowed by the existing administrative structure of acute hospitals. Health and Social Service Journal, 89, 25 May 1979, 626-627.

18 Wild, D. Hospital administration—the new order: the medical administrator's point of view. Royal Society of Health Journal, 96 (5), Oct 1976, 226-229.

19 Wolfson, G. and Dunham, P. Devolution philosophy heads towards a better tomorrow. Health and Social Service Journal, 89, 9 Nov 1979, 1450-1452. Edited version in Nursing Times, 76, 6 Mar 1980, 433-435 under title 'Hospital management for tomorrow'—describes Claybury Hospital's management team.

l NOISE

1 Bentley, S. and others Perceived noise in surgical wards and an intensive care area: an objective analysis. (At St. Mary's Hospital, London.) British Medical Journal, 2, 10 Dec 1977, 1503-1506.

2 Knowland, R. Searching for the golden gift of peace and quiet. (Noise control in hospital design.) Health and Social Service Journal, 86, 22 Oct 1976, 1900-1901.

3 Ogilvie, A.J. Sources and levels of noise on the ward at night. (Research study in two different designs of ward.) Nursing Times, 76, 31 Jul 1980, 1363-1366.

m NURSING HOMES

1 Bowring, D.H. Private nursing homes: the role of these nursing homes and some of the legislation governing them. Nursing Mirror, 146, 12 Jan 1978, 23-24.

2 Davies, R. Alternatives to the NHS. (The Nuffield Nursing Homes Trust.) Midwife, Health Visitor and Community Nurse, 16 (1), Jan 1980, 12, 14-15.

3 Registered Nursing Home Association The register of approved private hospitals and nursing homes. 2nd ed. Exeter: The Association, 1976.

n OUTPATIENTS

1 Beletz, E.E. On creating a nurse clinic. (Superimposed on a traditional hospital outpatient department.) Supervisor Nurse, 7 (9), Sep 1976, 34-35, 38-40.

2 Dorsey, B. and Hussa, R.K. Evaluating ambulatory care: three approaches. (Variations on the methodology of the Joint Commission on

Accreditation of Hospitals.) Journal of Nursing Administration, 9 (1), Jan 1979, 34-43.

3 Felstein, I. Booming into the eighties. (Advantages of the day hospital to both patients and the NHS.) Health and Social Service Journal, 87, 25 Nov 1977, 1628.

4 Goldacre, M.J. and Gatherer, A. Peripheral outpatient clinics: use, costs and benefits. British Journal of Preventive and Social Medicine, 31 (3), Sep 1977, 205-208.

5 Goldacre, M.J. and Gatherer, A. Use of out-patient services: a simple approach to seeking information. (Survey in the Oxfordshire area.) Hospital and Health Services Review, 73 (1), Jan 1977, 14-16.

6 Hanson, S. Ambulatory nursing standards. (Standards compiled by the Outpatient Department, University Hospital, Seattle.) Supervisor Nurse, 6 (12), Dec 1975, 10-15.

7 Ingham, M. Efficiency first but a rethink is the answer. (Zoning of hospital outpatient appointment times in Lincolnshire to improve efficiency of ambulance service.) Health and Social Service Journal, 90, 18 Jan 1980, 91-92.

8 Kirk, R.M. Reducing outpatient attendances. (Using indirect contact by letter and telephone.) British Medical Journal, 1, 19 Jun 1976, 1521-1522.

9 O'Neal, E.A. A framework for ambulatory care evaluation. Journal of Nursing Administration, 8 (7), Jul 1978, 15-20.

10 Raphael, W. and Mandeville, J. Being an outpatient. King Edward's Hospital Fund for London, 1977 (Project paper 15). Summary 'View from the queue', Nursing Times, 73, 9 Jun 1977, 851.

11 Schwartz, M.M. and White, M.A. Motivating clinic patients. (Study to evaluate ways of increasing number of outpatient clinic appointments kept.) Supervisor Nurse, 8 (10), Oct 1977, 48-49.

12 Shrank, A.B. Outpatient suite: a new design. (At Wrekin Hospital, Telford.) British Medical Journal, 2, 7 Oct 1978, 998-999.

13 Singer, M.E. and others Centralized appointment system reduces patients' waiting time (in an out-patient department.) Hospitals, 50 (6), 16 Mar 1976, 151-152, 154, 156, 158.

14 Wilkes, E. and others A different kind of day hospital—for patients with preterminal cancer and chronic disease. (In Sheffield.) British Medical Journal, 2, 14 Oct 1978, 1053-1056.

o PLANNING AND DESIGN

1 Adams, J.F. and Ireland, J.T. An economical multi-purpose ward unit. (To bridge needs of in-patients and outpatients.) Health Bulletin, 38 (2), Mar 1980, 77-79.

2 Allen, D.E. Hospital planning: the development of the 1962 hospital plan: a case study in decision making. Pitman, 1979.

3 Allen, R. and Von Karolyi, I. Hospital planning handbook. New York: Wiley, 1976.

4 Becker, F.D. Employees need role in design of work space. (Staff involvement using workshops and questionnaires resulted in

improved morale.) Hospitals, 54 (22), 16 Nov 1980, 97-98, 101.

5 Besharah, A. CNJ talks to...Gordon Friesen. (Designer of hospitals with no nurses' station and 'Nurserver'—new method of providing each patient's supplies.) Canadian Nurse, 76 (6), Jun 1980, 45.

6 Birren, F. Human response to color and light. (Hospital environment based on studies of their psychological and physiological effect on patients.) Hospitals, 53 (14), 16 Jul 1979, 93-96.

7 Bolton, J. Computers in construction. (Of hospitals.) Health and Social Service Journal, 90, 4 Apr 1980, 441-443.

8 Burrough, E.J.R. A scandalous impromptu. Oxford: Radcliffe Infirmary, 1976. (Critique of the open ward system.)

9 Burrows, J. and Hughes, P. Acute ward planning: an alternative approach. (Y-shaped ward plan.) Nursing Times, 76, 24 Jul 1980, 1322-1323.

10 Canter, D. and Canter, S. editors Designing for therapeutic environments: a review of research. Chichester: John Wiley, 1979.

11 Chartered Institution of Building Services. Lighting Division Hospitals and health care buildings. CIBS, 1979. (CIBS Lighting guide; 12.)

12 Curry, I. How can research assist the nurse in planning capital building projects? North West Thames Nursing Research Bulletin, 2, Autumn 1974, 17-21.

13 Curry, I. Towards a better ward design. (Needs of patient, nurse and doctors.) Nursing Times, 76, 3 Jan 1980, 38-39.

14 Department of Health and Social Security Nucleus hospitals. DHSS, 1976.

15 Dilworth, J.C. The role of the nurse planner. Lamp, 37 (2), Feb 1980, 5-9.

16 Drummond, P. Throwing bricks at design. (Survey of structural defects in new hospitals.) Health and Social Service Journal, 90, 26 Sep 1980, 1256-1259.

17 Edwards, K. The environment inside the hospital. (Importance of colour and furnishings.) Practitioner, 222, Jun 1979, 746-749, 751.

18 Froud, B. Management. Capricode—hospital building procedures explained. Nursing Focus, 1 (3), Nov 1979, 111-113, 115.

19 Gibson, I.R.L. Pitfalls in operational policies. (With some reference to commissioning of new buildings.) Hospital and Health Services Review, 76 (3), Mar 1980, 105-106.

20 Goad, A. Designing your hospitals: requirements of the project team in hospital design. (By a nurse planner.) Royal Society of Health Journal, 99 (2), Apr 1979, 74.

21 Goldstein, J.R. Nursing station design using a social theory model. Journal of Nursing Administration, 9 (4), Apr 1979, 21-24.

22 Green, J.R.B. Ward design. (Letter from architect involved with Greenwich District Hospital.) Nursing Times, 74, 2 Nov 1978, 1809.

23 Grubbs, J. and Short, S.J. Nursing input

to nursing unit design. Journal of Nursing Administration, 9 (5), May 1979, 25-30.

24 Hall, C.L. Designing your hospitals: planning needs. Royal Society of Health Journal, 99 (2), Apr 1979, 70-73.

25 Hardy, O.B. and Lammers, L.P. Hospitals: the planning and design process. Germantown, Md.: Aspen Systems Corporation, 1977.

26 Health and Social Service Journal The painter and the patient. (Brightening the hospital environment at St. Mary's Hospital, Manchester.) Health and Social Service Journal, 86, 10 Jul 1976, 1258-1259.

27 Henderson, M. Planned before the squeeze: the last of the big spenders? (Monklands District General Hospital, Lanarkshire.) Health and Social Service Journal, 86, 19 Nov 1976, 2062-2063.

28 Hoatson, N. The role of the nurse planner. Australian Nurses Journal, 6 (8), Feb 1977, 39-41.

29 Hospitals Design and construction issue. Hospitals, 53 (4), 16 Feb 1979, 82-190.

30 Hospitals Design and construction issue. Hospitals, 54 (4), 16 Feb 1980, 77-147.

31 Howells, S. and Hitchcox, B. Nucleus hospitals. Hospital and Health Services Review, 72 (6), Jun 1976, 206-211.

32 Hyde, A. A phoenix from the ashes. (Design of nucleus hospitals with special reference to the London Borough of Newham.) Health and Social Service Journal, 89, 30 Mar 1979, 336-337.

33 Hyde, A. Your disobedient servant and the Tatton-Brown connection. (Three articles discussing criticism by William Tatton-Brown of DHSS hospital planning system.) Health and Social Service Journal, 89, 4 May 1979, 504-507.

34 Jones, D.T. Hospital rebuilding—where now? (Criticism of the 1962 Hospital Plan and ideas for future policy.) Health and Social Service Journal, 86, 17 Apr 1976, 719-720.

35 Kalisch, P.A. and Kalisch, B.J. Nursing involvement in the health planning process. United States Department of Health, Education and Welfare, 1978. (Nurse planning information series, no.2.)

36 Kaye, V. The Newcastle Hilton. Building and staffing Newcastle's vast new hospital, the Freeman. Health and Social Service Journal, 88, 13 Jan 1978, 34-35.

37 Metcalf, C. Owed to the Nightingale but what about the future? (Reply to recent criticisms of small-cubicled wards with suggestions how

they can form setting for patient allocation.) Nursing Times, 74, 7 Sep 1978, 1476.

38 Miller, J. Starting from scratch. The commissioning of health service buildings. (The William Harvey Hospital, Ashford.) Nursing Times, 73, 16 Jun 1977, 888-890.

39 Moss, R. Boundless scope in space... (Multi-potential theories in hospital planning.) Health and Social Service Journal, 88, 24 Mar 1978, 348-349.

40 Noble, A. and Dixon, R. Ward evaluation, St. Thomas' Hospital: report for the District Management Team. Polytechnic of North London Medical Architecture Research Unit, 1977.

41 Owen, D. Hospital building: Dr. Owen reviews the prospects. Hospital and Health Services Review, 72 (1), Jan 1976, 26-29.

42 Peters, J.P. A guide to strategic planning for hospitals. Chicago, Ill.: American Hospital Association, 1979.

43 Purland, G. From blueprint to bricks and mortar in a legal complex. (Planning of Queen's Medical Centre, Nottingham, including Nottingham School of Nursing.) Health and Social Service Journal, 88, 19 May 1978, 575-576.

44 Pütsep, E. Modern hospital: international planning practices. Lloyd-Luke, 1979.

45 Sears, D. and Auld, R. Evaluation of complex buildings final report supplement 1. Hospital survey: the attitudes of patients, doctors and nurses to aspects of physical environment in hospital wards. University College and London School of Economics. Joint Unit for Planning Research, 1976.

46 Sears, D. and Auld, R. Human valuation of complex environments: a final report on the Evaluation of Complex Buildings Project. University College and London School of Economics, Joint Unit for Planning Research, 1976.

47 Stone, P. editor British hospital and health-care buildings: designs and appraisals. Architectural Press, 1980.

48 Tatton-Brown, W. Owed to the Nightingale. (The advantages of the Nightingale ward by a former chief architect of the DHSS with comment on recent experience as a hospital patient.) Nursing Times, 74, 3 Aug 1978, 1273-1278.

49 Tatton-Brown, W. Owed to the Nightingale—2. Ward evaluation. (Review of three types of ward at St. Thomas' Hospital by PNL Medical Architecture Research Unit. See also editorial on p.1.) Nursing Times, 74, 3 Aug 1978, 1279-1284.

50 Taylor, S., Baron Taylor of Harlow The natural history of windows: a cautionary tale. (With reference to hospital design and their effects on staff and patients.) British Medical Journal, 1, 31 Mar 1979, 870-875.

51 Whitehead, C.A. A management system for hospital commissioning. Hospital and Health Services Review, 72 (11), Nov 1976, 378-382.

52 Zilm, F. The planning process and development of a time line. (Estimating time needed for parts of hospital planning project.) Journal of Nursing Administration, 9 (9), Sep 1979, 40-44.

p RECORDS AND INFORMATION

1 Alderson, M. Hospital activity analysis and health information systems. Health Trends, 4 (8), Aug 1976, 66-68.

2 Anderson, B. Problem-orientated medical records—a critical appraisal. Medical Records, 20 (2), May 1979, 510-515.

3 Butler, E.A. An automated hospital information system. (Computerised system of medical and nursing records at El Camino Hospital, Mountview, California.) Nursing Times, 74, 9 Feb 1978, 245-246.

4 Hill, P.A. Interface. The medical records officer. Nursing Times, 72, 29 Jul 1976, 1162-1163.

5 Martini, C.J.M. and others A study of the validity of the Hospital Activity Analysis information. (Study in Nottinghamshire.) British Journal of Preventive and Social Medicine, 30 (3), Sep 1976, 180-186.

6 Moores, B. Crunching the numbers across the Atlantic. (American system of professional activity study (PAS) for monitoring patient care information compared favourably with British system of hospital activity analysis (HAA).) Health and Social Service Journal, 80, 5 Dec 1980, 1558-1561.

7 Petrie, J.C. and McIntyre, N. editors The problem orientated medical record (POMR): its use in hospitals, general practice and medical education. Edinburgh: Churchill Livingstone, 1979.

8 Revans, R.W. After the decade. An emollient review of the Hospitals' Internal Communications Project (carried out with 10 London hospitals between 1965 and 1968.) Lamp, 33 (7), Jul 1976, 26-31.

9 Yates, D. What we can still learn from the thoughts of Florence... (Florence Nightingale's statistical system for monitoring performance of hospitals.) Health and Social Service Journal, 88, 10 Mar 1978, 281.

COMMUNITY SERVICES

32 COMMUNITY HEALTH

a GENERAL AND PREVENTIVE MEDICINE

1 Arnold, P.J. Physical education and health. (Includes discussion of definitions of health.) Health Education Journal, 38 (1), 1979, 10-17.

2 Ashton, J.R. Poverty and health in Britain today. Public Health, 93 (2), Mar 1979, 89-94.

3 Barefoot, P. and Cunningham, P.J. Community services: the health worker's A-Z. Faber, 1977.

4 Bell, J. and others Patterns of illness and use of services in a new town: a preliminary report. (Survey in new town in Scotland.) Public Health, 93 (6), Nov 1979, 333-343.

5 Black, D. Cui bono? (Medical and social models of health care.) British Medical Journal, 2, 29 Oct 1977, 1109-1114.

6 Bosanquet, N. A missed opportunity. (Comments on 'Prevention and health' everybody's business.) Nursing Times, 72, 29 Apr 1976, 645.

7 Brearley, P. and others The social context of health care. Robertson, 1978. (Aspects of social policy series.)

8 Brotherston, J. The next century of preventive medicine. Prevention. Royal Society of Health Journal, 97 (1), Feb 1977, 4-8.

9 Connolly, P. Definition of health: a key concept in the development of health visiting principles. Health Visitor, 51 (12), Dec 1978, 464-466.

10 Dalzell-Ward, A.J. The new frontier of preventive medicine. Public Health, 90 (3), Mar 1976, 101-109.

11 Davies, J.B.M. Community health and social services. 3rd ed. Hodder and Stoughton, 1977. (Modern nursing series.)

12 Davies, J.B.M. Community health, preventive medicine and social services. 3rd ed. Baillière Tindall, 1975. 4th ed. 1979.

13 Department of Health and Social Security On the state of the public health: the annual report of the Chief Medical Officer of Health. 1974-1976. HMSO, 1976-1977.

14 Department of Health and Social Security and others Prevention and health. HMSO, 1977. Cmnd.7047. Summary of recommendations in Nursing Times, 74, 9 Mar 1978, Community Outlook 71-73, 75, 77.

14 Department of Health and Social Security Prevention and health: everybody's business: reassessment of public and personal health. HMSO, 1976. (Consultative document.)

16 D'Souza, M.F. A general review of current established screening procedures. Health Bulletin, 18 (1), Jan 1976, 54-57.

17 Egbert, E. Concept of wellness. Journal of Psychiatric Nursing, 18 (1), Jan 1980, 9-12.

18 Essex-Cater, A.J. A manual of public health and community medicine. 3rd ed. Bristol: John Wright, 1979.

19 Falconer, T.C. Port health control in the UK. Nursing Times, 74, 21 Sep 1978, 1553-1554.

20 Feuerstein, M.T. Community participation in evaluation: problems and potentials. International Nursing Review, 27 (6), Nov/Dec 1980, 187-190.

21 Fry, J. A new approach to medicine: principles and priorities in health care. Lancaster: MTP, 1978.

22 Gibson, J. Health personal and communal: a short hygiene for nurses. 4th ed. Faber, 1976.

23 Hamilton, M. Benefits of screening. (Royal Society of Health conference session.) Occupational Health, 28 (6), Jun 1976, 296-298.

24 Hannay, D.R. The symptom iceberg: a study of community health. Routledge and Kegan Paul, 1979.

25 Hewitt, M. and Guilfoyle, B. Population statistics—1. Trends in the population level. 2. Indicators of the nation's health care. Nursing Times, 74, 27 Apr 1978, 724-726; 4 May 1978, 766-767.

26 Hobson, W. editor The theory and practice of public health. 5th ed. Oxford: Oxford University Press, 1979.

27 Hunt, S.M. and others A quantitative approach to perceived health status: a validation study. (Tested on four groups of elderly people.) Journal of Epidemiology and Community Health, 34 (4), Dec 1980, 281-286.

28 Hyde, A. Diagnosing new town blues. A sense of adventure. (Health care in Milton Keynes and Peterborough.) Health and Social Service Journal, 88, 18 Aug 1978, 930-932; 25 Aug 1978, 958-960.

29 Illsley, R. Professional or public health? sociology in health and medicine. Nuffield Provincial Hospitals Trust, 1980. (Rock Carling Fellowship 1980.)

30 Jones, J. The community physician: a suitable role for preventive medicine. Health and Social Service Journal, 86, 12 Nov 1976, 2014-2015.

31 Kratz, C. Talking point. (Differences between hospital and community care.) Nursing Times, 73, 11 Aug 1977, Community Outlook 3.

32 Lamb, A.M. Consultative document on prevention. Prevention and health—everybody's business. Health Visitor, 49 (4), Apr 1976, 114-115.

33 Lancet Commentary from Westminster. The new (or not so new) White Paper on prevention. (Critical comment.) Lancet, 2, 24/31 Dec 1977, 1369-1370.

34 Lloyd, O. What is epidemiology? Occupational Health, 32 (11), Nov 1980, 585-588.

35 Long, A. Guide to epidemiology. (Its value in health service planning.) Health and Social Service Journal, 89, 20 Jul 1979, 907-908.

36 Martin, F.M. Social medicine and its contribution to social policy. Lancet, 2, 24/31 Dec 1977, 1336-1338.

37 Melville, J. Coping in the community. (Battersea Action Counselling Centre providing individual, family and group counselling.) New Society, 47, 8 Feb 1979, 300, 302.

38 Morris, J.N. Social inequalities undiminished. (Review of research and discussion of social policy. Reprinted with revisions from Lancet, 1, 13 Jan 1979, 87-90.) Health Visitor, 53 (9), Sep 1980, 361-362, 364-365.

39 Muir Gray, J.A. A case of political medicine. (The political nature of preventive medicine.) Nursing Mirror, 150, 3 Apr 1980, 23.

40 Muir Gray, J.A. The failure of preventive medicine. Lancet, 2, 24/31 Dec 1977, 1338-1339.

41 Muir Gray, J.A. Man against disease: preventive medicine. Oxford: Oxford University Press, 1979.

42 Nursing Times Whatever happened to the red book? (Prevention and health: everybody's business.) Nursing Times, 74, 12 Jan 1978, Community Outlook 19-21.

43 Paine, L.H.W. editor Health care in big cities. Croom Helm, 1978.

44 Parliament. Expenditure Committee First

report, session 1976-77. Preventive medicine: vol.1, report. HMSO, 1977.

45 Priest, M.A. Modern textbook of personal and communal health for nurses: including bacteriology and the principles of asepsis. 5th ed. Heinemann, 1977.

46 Reid, J.J.A. The next century of preventive medicine. The future. Royal Society of Health Journal, 97 (1), Feb 1977, 9-13.

47 Robinson, D. Patients, practitioners and medical care: aspects of medical sociology. 2nd ed. Heinemann, 1978.

48 Rose, G. and Barker, D.J.P. Epidemiology for the uninitiated. Rates. (Prevalence and incidence.) Screening. British Medical Journal, 2, 30 Sep 1978, 941-942; 18 Nov 1978, 1417-1418.

49 Rowe, R.C. Medicine and community medicine: a joint exercise in monitoring. (Epidemiological method of monitoring services to aid planning process.) Health and Social Service Journal, 88, 20 Jan 1978, B16-B19.

50 Royal Society of Health Journal Centenary supplement. Royal Society of Health Journal, 96 (5), Oct 1976, Supplement 1-12.

51 Sreenivasan, B.R. Changing patterns in diseases (during the last 50 years.) Journal of the Royal College of General Practitioners, 26, Nov 1976, 860-862.

52 Stone, D. and others Society at work. Too much screening? New Society, 38, 20 Oct 1976, 192-194.

53 Taylor, S., Baron Taylor of Harlow The natural history of preventive medicine, or breaking the chains of causation. (Changes in social medicine since the 1930s.) British Medical Journal, 281, 27 Sep 1980, 849-853.

54 Topliss, E.P. The arguments for community care. (For the chronic sick, elderly, the handicapped and the mentally ill.) Nursing Times, 74, 13 Apr 1978, Community Outlook 107-108.

55 Totman, R. Social causes of illness. Souvenir Press, 1979.

56 Tuckett, D. editor An introduction to medical sociology. Tavistock Publications, 1976.

57 Tuckett, D. and Kaufert, J.M. editors Basic readings in medical sociology. Tavistock, 1978.

58 West, G.P. Veterinary contributions to human health. Nursing Mirror, 144, 17 Feb 1977, 62-64.

59 White, D. When is a disease not a disease? (Fashions in disease.) New Society, 54, 11 Dec 1980, 506-507.

60 Wilson, J.H.G. Current trends and problems in health screening. (Using phenylketonuria as an example.) Health Bulletin, 18 (1), Jan 1976, 45-53.

61 Wynn, M. and Wynn, A. Are there really diseases of affluence? New Society, 51, 6 Mar 1980, 500-501.

b PRIMARY HEALTH CARE

1 Bodenstein, J.W. Primary health care: its

principles and some of its implications in our South African Development Context. S.A. Nursing Journal, 42 (11), Nov 1975, 20-24.

2 Brayton, M. A first for Africa. (Report of ICN meeting in Nairobi and ICN/WHO workshop on primary health care.) Nursing Times, 75, 25 Oct 1979, 1830-1831.

3 Chapple, M. Is primary care in need of a change? Journal of Community Nursing, 3 (7), Jan 1980, 10, 25.

4 Clark, E.M. and Forbes, J.A. Evaluating primary care: some experiments in quality measurement in an academic unit of primary medical care. Croom Helm, 1979.

5 Cohen, J. and Halpern, A. A practice counsellor. (As member of primary care team in a London practice.) Journal of the Royal College of General Practitioners, 28, Aug 1978, 481-484.

6 Community Outlook The primary health care team—what you told us. (Entries in recent competition.) Nursing Times, 74, 14 Sep 1978 (12p); 12 Oct 1978 (8p); 9 Nov 1978 (6p).

7 Community Outlook Teamwork conference '78. (Communication in the primary care team and schemes for nursing children at home including Gateshead scheme.) Nursing Times, 74, 14 Dec 1978, Community Outlook 368, 371, 375-376, 379-380, 382.

8 Donoso, G. Health care and community action. (WHO's policies regarding primary health care.) WHO Chronicle, 32 (3), Mar 1978, 102-105.

9 Fagin, C.M. Primary care as an academic discipline. Nursing Outlook, 26 (12), Dec 1978, 750-753.

10 Farmer, R.T.D. Primary medical care, where should it go? (Potential and limitations of primary care.) Midwife, Health Visitor and Community Nurse, 15 (11), Nov 1979, 444.

11 Flack, G. Team training to bring the professionals to the people. (The Council for the Education and Training of Health Vistors' viewpoint on multidisciplinary team education in primary health and social care.) Health and Social Service Journal, 86, 10 Dec 1976, 2194-2195.

12 Flahault, D. An integrated and functional team for primary health care. WHO Chronicle, 30 (11), Nov 1976, 442-446.

13 Fry, J. Spotlight on primary health care. (General discussion.) Midwife, Health Visitor and Community Nurse, 13 (12), Dec 1977, 392-393.

14 Heyes, E.N. Aspects of modelling primary health care. MSc thesis, Lancaster University, Department of Operational Research, 1978.

15 Hicks, D. Primary health care: a review. HMSO, 1976.

16 Hicks, D. The way ahead. The future of primary health care. Nursing Mirror, 146, 26 Jan 1978, 39-40.

17 Jameson, J. It takes more than one to make a team. (Multidisciplinary course for primary health care team members at the West London Institute of Higher Education.) Nursing Mirror, 147, 9 Nov 1978, 44-45.

18 Kaprio, L.A. Primary health care in Europe. Copenhagen: WHO, 1979. (Euro reports and studies; 14.)

19 McMahon, R. and others On being in charge: a guide for middle-level management in primary health care. Geneva: World Health Organisation, 1980.

20 Mahler, H. Primary health care. Lecture delivered in Kuala Lumpur on 29 July 1977 at the invitation of the College of General Practitioners Malaysia. (By Director-General of WHO.) New Zealand Nursing Journal, 70 (10), Oct 1977, 3-7.

21 Marshall, S.G. and Eckersley, A.P.R. A primer of primary care. LLoyd-Luke, 1980.

22 Milne, M.A. Student role perception of the primary health care team. 1. Overlap—friend or foe? (Review of functions.) 2. Overlap—guilty or innocent? (Research study.) Nursing Times, 76, 5 Jun 1980, Occ. papers, 61-64; 19 Jun 1980, Occ. papers, 65-68.

23 Milne, M.A. Students' views of the primary health care team. (Research study with trainee GPs, student HVs, district nurses in training and postgraduate social work students.) Nursing Times, 75, 1 Nov 1979, Occ. papers, 113-116.

24 Morgan, M. Lines of communication in rural Wales. (Care based on cottage hospitals and primary care teams.) Nursing Focus, 1 (5), Jan 1980, 198-201.

25 Mullett, L. The role of the surgery. (Work of members of primary care team with case study, by student nurse on community care option.) Nursing Mirror, 146, 5 Jan 1978, 37-39.

26 Nursing Mirror The primary health care team. (Introduction on the team concept and three articles by doctor, HV and district nurse on the care of a fictitious family.) Nursing Mirror, 147, 5 Oct 1978, Supplement i, iii-iv, vii, ix, xi, xv-xvii, xix, xxi-xxiii.

27 Parnell, J.W. Primary health care team seminars (to establish whether specific training is necessary for team members.) Queen's Nursing Journal, 19 (4), Jul 1976, 94-96.

28 Pritchard, P. Manual of primary health care: its nature and organization. Oxford: Oxford University Press, 1978.

29 Rajakumar, M.K. The importance of primary care. (With special reference to the general practitioners.) Journal of the Royal College of General Practitioners, 28 Feb 1978, 91-95.

30 Ross, F. Primary health care in Thamesmead. 2. Nursing Times, 76, 7 Aug 1980, Occ. paper, 85-87.

31 Royal College of Nursing United we stand? (Report of Rcn centre conference on the primary health care team.) Nursing Times, 74, 13 Jul 1978, Community Outlook 187.

32 Royal Commission on the National Health Service Access to primary care. HMSO, 1979. (Research paper no.6.)

33 Saint-Yves, I. The dilemma of primary health care. (Suggests new structure with clinical associate and nursing aid.) Journal of Community Nursing, 4 (2), Aug 1980, 4-5.

34 Saint-Yves, I.F.M. Need general practitioner be patient's first contact with health service? (Suggests new system of continuous comprehensive primary health care staffed by GPs and paramedicals.) Lancet, 2, 13 Sep 1980, 578-580.

35 **Salkind, M.R. and Norell, J.S.** Teaching about the primary care team: an experiment in vocational training. (Multidisciplinary long-term discussion group including HV and practice nurse.) Journal of the Royal College of General Practitioners, 30, Mar 1980, 158-160.

36 **Sartain, B.** Primary health care team—an appraisal. Nursing Mirror, 144, 17 Feb 1977, 67-68.

37 **Skinner, M.** Primary care focus in two communities. (Summary of two surveys, one by the National Consumer Council and one published by the Royal Commission on the NHS.) Health and Social Service Journal, 89, 15 Mar 1979, 252-253.

38 **Stephen, W.J.** An analysis of primary medical care: an international study. Cambridge University Press, 1979.

39 **Turner, V.** How much do you care? (Evaluating care within the primary care team.) Community View, 4, Mar 1980, 3-5.

40 **Weir, S.** Contact before crisis point for those who need care most: primary medical care and the single homeless in Liverpool. Health and Social Service Journal, 86, 25 Feb 1977, 332-333.

41 **World Health Organization** Primary health care in the WHO regions. WHO Chronicle, 32 (11), Nov 1978, 431-438.

42 **World Health Organization** The primary health worker: working guide; guidelines for training; guidelines for adaptation. Geneva: WHO, 1977. Rev. 2nd ed. 1980.

43 **World Health Organization. Regional Office for Europe** The definition of parameters of efficiency in primary care and the role of nursing in primary health care: report on two working groups, Reykjunk 14-18 July 1975. Copenhagen: WHO, 1976.

44 **World Health Organization and United Nations Children's Fund** Primary health care: report of the International conference on primary health care, Alma-Ata USSR, 6-12 Sep 1978. Geneva: WHO, 1978. Reported in Lancet, 2, 11 Nov 1978, 1040-1041, 1061; WHO Chronicle, 32 (11), Nov 1978, 409-430.

45 **Wright-Warren, P. and others** To Russia, for care. (Two articles on trip to Russian conference on primary health care.) Nursing Mirror, 148, 8 Mar 1979, 20-22.

c GENERAL PRACTICE

1 **Adcock, M. and others** Experiment of much binding in the Plumstead marshes. (Report on experiment at Thamesmead to achieve co-operation between GPs, social workers and health visitors.) Health and Social Service Journal, 87, 14 Oct 1977, 1428-1429.

2 **Allsopp, J.** Justice for GPs and patients. (Work of Family Practitioner Committees and the way they deal with complaints against GPs.) Health and Social Service Journal, 90, 25 Jul 1980, 980-982.

3 **Bowling, A.P.** Delegation in general practice—a threat or a panacea? A history of general practice illustrating its problems and a study of the possibilities for their partial resolution by delegation. PhD thesis, University College, Department of Sociology and Anthropology, Swansea, 1979.

4 **Bradshaw-Smith, J.H.** A computer record keeping system for general practice. (Ottery St. Mary health centre, Devon.) British Medical Journal, 1, 5 Jun 1976, 1395-1397.

5 **British Medical Journal** The telephone in general practice. (With review of its uses including nursing.) British Medical Journal, 2, 21 Oct 1978, 1106.

6 **Carr, T.E.A.** Whither general medical practice? (Includes statistics on paramedical staff including nurses.) Health Trends, 4 (11), Nov 1979, 83-88.

7 **Corney, R.H.** Factors affecting the operation and success of social work attachment schemes to general practice. Journal of Royal College of General Practitioners, 30, Mar 1980, 149-150, 154-157.

8 **Corney, R.H. and Bowen, B.A.** Referrals to social workers: a comparative study of a local authority intake team with a general practice attachment scheme. Journal of Royal College of General Practitioners, 30, Mar 1980, 139-142, 144-147.

9 **Corney, R. and Briscoe, M.** Investigation into two different types of attachment schemes. (Research study by the general practice research unit at the Institute of Psychiatry into social worker attachment to general practice.) Social Work Today, 9, 6 Dec 1977, 10-14.

10 **Department of Health and Social Security** The doctor/patient relationship: a study in general practice. HMSO, 1979.

11 **Fry, J. editor** Trends in general practice. 2nd ed. British Medical Journal for Royal College of General Practitioners, 1979.

12 **Gerrard, J.** Working in a group practice. (Attachment of social worker to two practices in Edgware, London.) Social Work Today, 10, 24 Oct 1978, 16-17.

13 **Gilchrist, I.C. and others** Social work in general practice. (Survey of working arrangements and problems encountered.) Journal of the Royal College of General Practitioners, 28, Nov 1978, 673-675, 680-686.

14 **Gunton, G.F.** Conflict or co-operation? (Between doctors, social workers and health visitors in general practice.) Practice Team, 53, Oct 1975, 10.

15 **Lycett, C.D.L. and others** The need for health care—a pilot survey with general practice. (Survey involving health visitors.) Journal of Royal College of General Practitioners, 29, Aug 1979, 489-493.

16 **Mackichan, N.D.** The GP and the primary health care team: a handbook for those employed in, attached to, and working with a family practice. Pitman, 1976.

17 **Marsh, G.N.** 'Curing' minor illness in general practice. (Campaign to encourage self care among patients including nurse care of minor illness.) British Medical Journal, 2, 12 Nov 1977, 1267-1269.

18 **Marsh, G.N.** The practice brochure: a patient's guide to team care. British Medical Journal, 281, 13 Sep 1980, 730-732.

19 **Marsh, G. and Kaim-Caudle, P.** Team care in general practice. Croom Helm, 1976.

20 **Murray, T.S. and Mackay, J.** Managing the practice: ancillary staff. (Includes practice nurse.) Practitioner, 221, Nov 1978, 663-665.

21 **Reedy, B.L.E.C. and others** Attachment of a physician's assistant to an English general practice. British Medical Journal, 281, 6 Sep 1980, 664-666.

22 **Reilly, P.M. and others** Communications between doctors and social workers in a general practice. Journal of the Royal College of General Practitioners, 27 (178), May 1977, 289-293.

23 **Royal College of General Practitioners. Birmingham Research Unit** Self evaluation in general practice (of quality of medical care.) Journal of the Royal College of General Practitioners, 27 (178), May 1977, 265-270.

24 **Sloan, R.E.G. and others** Records in general practice—4. The cost and advantages of establishing an age-sex register. (See also editorial 515-516.) Journal of the Royal College of General Practitioners, 27, Sep 1977, 532-533.

25 **Stevens, J.L.** Quality of care in general practice: can it be assessed? Journal of the Royal College of General Practitioners, 27, Aug 1977, 455-466.

26 **Westcott, R.** The length of consultations in general practice. (Related to sex, diagnosis, age, and social class of patient.) Journal of the Royal College of General Practitioners, 27, Sep 1977, 552-555.

27 **Williams, W.O. and Dajda, R.** General practitioners and their staff. (Survey of GPs about their ancillary staff including nurses, with special reference to qualities looked for in a receptionist.) Journal of the Royal College of General Practitioners, 29, Mar 1979, 145-149.

28 **Wright, J.** The practice...and perfection. (Scheme of attachment of social worker to general practice in Warwick.) Health and Social Service Journal, 88, 13 Oct 1978, 1160-1162.

d HEALTH CENTRES

1 **Ashton, J.** The Peckham Pioneer Health Centre: a reappraisal. Community Health, 8 (3), Jan 1977, 132-138.

2 **Baker, G. and Bevan, J.** The management and administration of health centres—a study of the effects of the 1974 reorganisation of the National Health Service. Canterbury: Health Services Research Unit, 1978. (Report no.33.)

3 **Beales, J.G.** Dawson Report. The centres of discontent. Health and Social Service Journal, 80, 16 May 1980, 638-641.

4 **Beales, G.** Sick health centres: and how to make them better. Pitman, 1978.

5 **Follis, P.** Conference special. If you have a hive beware the queen bee and her drones. (Report of a conference on health centre design organised by the Association of Health Centre and Practice Administrators.) Health and Social Service Journal, 87, 24 Jun 1977, 952-953.

6 **Gordon, H. and Bennett, R.A.** Health

centre apparent in Bookham. (Planning of centre with plan showing layout.) British Medical Journal, 2, 29 Sep 1979, 811-812.

7 **Gordon, J.** Why not keep community clinics? (Brief report of two surveys which suggest that the public like using clinics.) Journal of the Royal College of General Practitioners, 30, Sep 1980, 546.

8 **Hannay, D.R.** The use and perception of a health centre. (Woodside Health Centre, Glasgow.) Practitioner, 218, Feb 1977, 260-266.

9 **Health and Social Service Journal** Dawson Report. (Six articles on health centres with reference to 1920 report advocating service based on primary and secondary health centres and teaching hospitals.) Health and Social Service Journal, 90, 16 May 1980, 638-650.

10 **Ivory, J. and others** Does small mean success? (Successful health centre in Northumberland refutes Dr. J.G. Beales' article of 16 May 1980, 638-641, in which he casts doubt on their value.) Health and Social Service Journal, 80, 5 Dec 1980, 1564.

11 **Lewis, S.** The greening of the Meadows. (Social work team in health centre in South Nottingham.) Health and Social Service Journal, 89, 20 Jul 1979, 909-911.

12 **McCreadie, D.W.A. and MacGregor, I.M.** Aspects of health centre provision in Scotland. Hospital and Health Services Review, 75 (5), May 1979, 160-164.

13 **MacGregor, I.M. and others** Health centre practice in Scotland. (Includes review of function of nurses in the primary health care team.) Health Bulletin, 37 (6), Nov 1979, 240-254; 38 (1), Jan 1980, 5-22.

14 **Rowley, A.** Numerical filing of health centre records. Hospital and Health Services Review, 73 (7), Jul 1977, 236-240.

15 **Silverstone, R. and Salkind, M.R.** Doctors' attitudes to health centres. (Results of interviews with GPs in Inner London.) Journal of the Royal College of General Practitioners, 30, Dec 1980, 748-750.

e HEALTH EDUCATION

1 **Aldridge, W.G. and others** Joint approach to health education. (Campaign to prevent salmonellosis by a health co-ordinating committee in North Staffordshire.) Health and Social Service Journal, 86, 7 Aug 1976, 1428-1429.

2 **Anderson, W.A.** Teaching old dogs new tricks—changing attitudes to health education at work. Occupational Health, 30 (11), Nov 1978, 538-541.

3 **Barnett, J.W.** A unique opportunity to participate in health education. (Health education by pharmacists.) Health and Social Service Journal, 90, 11 Apr 1980, 479-480.

4 **Burkitt, A.** What is health education? Nursing Times, 73, 23 Jun 1977, Health Education 3, 5, 7.

5 **Burningham, S.** Why the art of health education is more than a pretty poster. (History and functions of the Health Education Council.) Health and Social Service Journal, 88, 1 Sep 1978, 984-986.

6 **Butterfield, W.J.H.** Health education—changing concepts of health knowledge and self care. Royal Society of Health Journal, 96 (4), Aug 1976, 152-155.

7 **Chisholm, M.** 'Cosh, con, or conscience?' (Ways in which the public can be induced to follow advice on health education.) Nursing Times, 72, 13 May 1976, 722.

8 **Clarke, W.D. and others** Health education in the doctor's waiting room. (Use of audio-tapes transmitted by telephone in a group practice in South East London.) Health Education Journal, 35 (1), 1976, 135-141.

9 **Clarke, W.D. and others** Health education, with a display machine, in the surgery. Health Education Journal, 36 (4), 1977, 100-103, 113.

10 **Cole, R.** The understanding of medical terminology used in printed health education materials. (Research study with general practice patients and polytechnic students.) Health Education Journal, 38 (4), 1979, 111-121.

11 **Cowley, J.C.P.** In-service education of professionals as health educators: it's not the same as just running courses. Health Education Journal, 39 (2), 1980, 35-44.

12 **Cust, G.** The Health Education Council and its work. Health Trends, 3 (11), Aug 1979, 57-59.

13 **Cust, G.** The implications for health education. (With people travelling abroad.) Royal Society of Health Journal, 97 (5), Oct 1977, 214.

14 **Davies, R. and Evans, D.** New strategy for spreading the message of health. (Improving health education.) Health and Social Service Journal, 86, 24 Sep 1976, 1714-1715.

15 **Dodds, J.** Taking a positive approach to society's negative attitudes. (Factors which limit effectiveness of health education.) Health and Social Service Journal, 87, 26 Aug 1977, 1220-1221.

16 **Draper, P.** Accident and illness promotion. The challenge to prevention. Nursing Times, 74, 12 Jan 1978, Community Outlook 14-16, 18.

17 **Draper, P. and others** Health and wealth. (Conflict between the production of wealth in society and the promotion of health, eg cigarette and alcohol production.) Royal Society of Health Journal, 97 (3), Jun 1977, 121-126.

18 **Draper, P. and others** Three types of health education. (With discussion of type 3, about the wider environment within which health choices are made.) British Medical Journal, 281, 16 Aug 1980, 493-495.

19 **Elliston, L.** Points of view. (Developments in health education in the U.K. over the last 25 years.) Health Education Journal, 36 (2), 1977, 46-48.

20 **Fisher, D.W.** Adult education theory necessary in health education practice. International Journal of Health Education, 14 (2), 1976, 129-135.

21 **Gardner, M.D.** Health education presenters—an experiment in health education. (Job creation scheme to train and employ teachers to teach health education.) Health Bulletin, 36 (2), Mar 1978, 72-78.

22 **Gatherer, A. and others** Is health education effective?: abstracts, bibliography and overview of evaluated studies. Health Education Council, 1979. (Monograph series; 2.)

23 **Graham, J.L.** Message and medium. (Scottish research project in health education involving AV material.) Health and Social Service Journal, 90, 11 Jul 1980, 911-912; 18 Jul, 1980, 948-949.

24 **Gunaratne, V.T.H.** Health for all by the year 2000: the role of health education. International Journal of Health Education, 23 (1), 1980, Supplement 1-11.

25 **Hall, C.P.** Group health education by health visitors. MPhil thesis, Surrey University, Department of Biological Sciences, 1977.

26 **Harte, J.D.** The role of the general practitioner in health education. Community Health, 7 (3), Jan 1976, 144-148.

27 **Hazeltine, K.** Delivering goods in a depressed market. (Aims and functions of health education officers.) Health and Social Service Journal, 88, 1 Sep 1978, 987-988.

28 **Health Education Council** Health education in the workplace: a report of a workshop…Feb 1980. The Council, 1980.

29 **Health Education Journal** Research and the Health Education Council. Health Education Journal, 37 (4), 1978, 242-243.

30 **Hobbs, P. and others** Health education with patients in hospital. Health Education Journal, 36 (2), 1977, 35-41.

31 **Horner, J.S.** Health education and public policy in the United Kingdom. Community Medicine, 2 (3), Aug 1980, 229-235.

32 **Hospital and Health Services Review** Notes for students. Health education in the National Health Service. Hospital and Health Services Review, 74 (3), Mar 1978, 110.

33 **Jacob, A.** Help yourself to health—an evaluation. (Study to assess effectiveness of health education booklet, involving questionnaire distributed by health visitors.) Health Bulletin, 37 (4), Jul 1979, 154-157.

34 **Jones, L.** The health education unit. (South Glamorgan Health Authority mobile unit.) Nursing Mirror, 143, 9 Sep 1976, 64-65.

35 **Ley, P. and others** Effects of source, context of communication and difficulty level on the success of health educational communications concerning contraception and the menopause. (Survey in general practice of the effectiveness of booklets when received from doctor, nurse or receptionist.) Health Education Journal, 38 (2), 1979, 47-52.

36 **Mackie, A.** Communication problems in health education in the consumer society. Royal Society of Health Journal, 95 (3), Jun 1975, 133-135.

37 **Macqueen, I.A.G.** The guardian—health promotion or crisis intervention. (Expansion of preventive health services, with particular reference to the health visitor, as the best way of improving the nation's health.) Health Visitor, 50 (3), Mar 1977, 66-69.

38 **Moyle, R.** The promotion of health. (1976

conference paper.) Royal Society of Health Journal, 96 (6), Dec 1976, 240-242.

39 Myer, E.M. Help yourself to good health? (Value of health education.) Journal of Medical Ethics, 5 (1), Mar 1979, 4-8.

40 Nicklin, L. Towards a plan for environmental health education. Health Education Journal, 35 (1), 1976, 153-158.

41 Nursing Times Health education. (Five articles in special supplement.) Nursing Times, 73, 23 Jun 1977, Health Education 1, 3, 5, 7-8, 11-12, 14, 17-18, 20, 22, 24.

42 Parrish, R. The cost benefit debate in evaluating health education. (Methods of evaluation.) Health and Social Service Journal, 89, 20 Apr 1979, 442-444.

43 Raikes, A. Points of view. Health education. (The need for clarification of the aims, content and direction of health education.) Public Health, 90 (2), Jan 1976, 79-81.

44 Randell, J. Health education. (With special reference to the role of the nurse and several definitions of health.) Nursing, 16, Aug 1980, 714-716.

45 Randell, J. and Sutherland, I. British health education—some long term aims. (Work of Health Education Council.) International Journal of Health Education, 21 (4), 1978, 232-248.

46 Randell, J. Health education without tears. (Need to define objectives.) Midwife, Health Visitor and Community Nurse, 16 (6), Jun 1980, 248, 250-251.

47 Randell, J. and Farmer, D. A survey of students on Certificate in Health Education courses in England and Wales. (To investigate the effect of courses in the performance and development of the individual.) Health Education Journal, 35 (4), 1976, 238-246.

48 Richards, N.D. Towards a redefinition of health education: the role of the social sciences. Community Health, 7 (3), Jan 1976, 135-143.

49 Runswick, H. and Davis, C.C. Health education: practical teaching techniques. Aylesbury: HM&M Publishers, 1976. (Topics in community health series.)

50 Scottish Home and Health Department. Scottish Health Education Unit Annotated bibliography of health education research completed in Britain from 1948-1978. Edinburgh: the Unit, 1979.

51 Sheiham, A. Evaluating health education programmes. Health Education Journal, 37 (1), 1978, 127-131.

52 Stone, D.H. An approach to planning for prevention. Public Health, 94 (2), Mar 1980, 95-102.

53 Sutherland, I. editor Health education: perspectives and choices. Allen & Unwin, 1979.

54 Tennant, B.T.J. Self help in community health education. MEduc thesis, Manchester University, Department of Adult Education, 1980.

55 Thomas, J. Health education research—a UK venture. (Evaluation of national publicity

campaign.) International Journal of Health Education, 21 (4), 1978, 245-248.

56 Thomas, S. A recipe for health. (Role of health education officer.) Nursing Mirror, 150, 3 Apr 1980, 30-31.

57 Thomson, W. Health education. Nursing Times, 74.
1. The problem. 14 Sep 1978, 1517-1518.
2. How do we communicate? 21 Sep 1978, 1561-1562.
3. Using the media. 28 Sep 1978, 1614-1615.
4. Whom do we educate? 5 Oct 1978, 1652-1653.

58 Tones, K. Teaching about health: education or medicine? (Reprinted from Health Education News for Teachers, 4, Autumn 1975.) Health Visitor, 49 (1), Jan 1976, 15, 17.

59 Vuori, H. The medical model and the objectives of health education. International Journal of Health Education, 23 (1), 1980, 12-19.

60 Wallace, J.M. Health education and the control of stress. Health Education Journal, 35 (3), 1976, 199-207.

61 Watson, L. Prescription for health education. Health Bulletin, 18 (1), Jan 1976, 9-11.

62 Wolfson, J. and Bailey, L. A community education approach to health: the Open University. International Journal of Health Education, 21 (4), 1978, 249-252.

63 Yarrow, A. Representative body? (Role of the community health council in health education.) Nursing Times, 72, 18 Nov 1976, 1788.

f HEALTH EDUCATION: OVERSEAS COUNTRIES

1 Bennett, B.E. A model for teaching health education skills to primary care practitioners. (Developed at Johns Hopkins University School of Health Services.) International Journal of Health Education, 20 (4), 1977, 232-239.

2 Chacko, A. In the realm of health education. (Role of nurses in health education in India.) Australasian Nurses Journal, 6 (9), Apr 1977, 8-9.

3 Chacko, A. The role of a nurse in health education as practised in and around Church of South India Hospital, Bangalore, India. International Journal of Nursing Studies, 14 (3), 1977, 121-123.

4 Curtin, B. Health Hazard Appraisal. (Summary of research study on effectiveness of a tool designed to influence behavioral changes in health habits.) Nurse Practitioner, 5 (2), Mar/Apr 1980, 67.

5 Graham, B. and Gleir, C. Health education: are nurses really prepared? Journal of Nursing Education, 19 (8), Oct 1980, 4-6.

6 Hellman, S. The health educator—a resource for nurses. Supervisor Nurse, 7 (9), Sep 1976, 18, 21-22.

7 Hibbs, G. Believing is seeing. (How health education can be carried out by all health staff illustrated by outline of strategy for promoting protection of the eyes.) Occupational Health, 31 (11), Nov 1979, 512-518.

8 Jinadu, M.K. The role of community health

nurses in family health education at home in a southern province of Iran (Fars). (With emphasis on reduction of child mortality and excessive fertility.) International Journal of Nursing Studies, 17 (1), 1980, 47-53.

9 Krawczyk, R.M. Well persons: their importance to nursing education and practice. (Course to prepare nursing students for the role of maintaining health and preventing ill-health.) Nursing Forum, 18 (3), 1979, 220-230.

10 Lazes, P.M. Health education project guides outpatients to active self care. (Martland Hospital, Newark, N.J.) Hospitals, 51, 16 Feb 1977, 81-82, 84, 86.

11 Logan, K. National agency to be health education troubleshooter. (National Center for Health Education, New York.) Hospitals, 50 (9), 1 May 1976, 69-71.

12 McGrath, B.J. Nursing in area health education centers. (North Carolina.) American Journal of Nursing, 76 (10), Oct 1976, 1605-1607.

13 McMurray, A.E. The body shop: marketing a healthy lifestyle. (A Canadian nurse working in Australia in a community health project using advertising techniques.) Canadian Nurse, 76 (4), Apr 1980, 46-48.

14 Minett, N. Health education in the bush. (In Sierra Leone.) International Nursing Review, 27 (6), Nov/Dec 1980, 165-168.

15 National League for Nursing Community involvement in health-related programs. New York: NLN, 1978.

16 Sheffield, R. Community health education: beyond fad to commitment. (Courses run by New England Memorial Hospital, Stoneham, Ma. for local community.) Hospitals, 51, 1 Sep 1977, 99-102.

17 Somers, A.R. Consumer health education—to know or to die. (Role of the hospital.) Hospitals, 50 (9), 1 May 1976, 52-56.

18 Tubesing, D.A. and others The wholistic health center project: an action-research model for providing preventive, whole-person health care at the primary level. Medical Care, 15 (3), Mar 1977, 217-227.

19 WHO Chronicle Development of health education services (in the African region.) WHO Chronicle, 30 (1), Jan 1976, 35-37.

20 WHO Chronicle Global health learning materials programme. (For auxiliary health workers.) WHO Chronicle, 34 (12), Dec 1980, 461-464.

21 Wilson, D. How the Finns are tackling their CHD problem. (Health education programme involving community nurses.) Journal of Community Nursing, 1 (7), Jan 1978, 13, 25.

22 Woodward, V. The ward sister as a health educator. Curationis, 3 (1), Jun 1980, 9.

23 World Health Who will care for health? Issue on health education in developing countries. World Health, Apr 1977, 3-29.

g PATIENT PARTICIPATION AND SELF-HELP

1 Anderson, J.A.D. and others Users and

non-users of doctors—implications for self-care. (Comparison between 60 pairs of patients.) Journal of the Royal College of General Practitioners, 27, Mar 1977, 155-159.

2 **Bennet, G.** Patients and their doctors: the journey through medical care. Baillière Tindall, 1979.

3 **Bennett, A.E. editor** Communication between doctors and patients. Oxford University Press for Nuffield Provincial Hospitals Trust, 1976.

4 **Bradshaw, J.S.** British barefoot doctors? (Review of studies of self-management of illness.) Royal Society of Health Journal, 97 (4), Aug 1977, 159-164.

5 **British Medical Journal** Patient participation groups. (For modification of Central Ethical Committee's guidelines see BMJ, 10 Nov 1979, 1235.) British Medical Journal, 2, 3 Nov 1979, 1160-1161.

6 **Browne, K. and Freeling, P.** The doctor-patient relationship. 2nd ed. Edinburgh: Churchill Livingstone, 1976.

7 **Burnington, S.** Providing a platform for patients. (Kentish Town Health Centre's patient participation group.) Health and Social Service Journal, 89, 15 Feb 1979, 148-150.

8 **Bury, J.** Some thoughts on the doctor/patient relationship. (Suggested change in approach involving encouraging more self-care.) Midwife, Health Visitor and Community Nurse, 13 (7), Jul 1977, 202, 205, 207.

9 **Dakin, A. and Milligan, J.** Patient participation. (Description by two patients of the formation and organisation of Practice Association in Bristol.) Journal of the Royal College of General Practitioners, 30, Mar 1980, 133-135.

10 **Davis, A. editor** Relationships between doctors and patients. Farnborough: Saxon House, 1978.

11 **Dopson, L.** Patient power? (Report of conference at Royal College of General Practitioners on patient participation groups.) Nursing Times, 76, 31 Jan 1980, 185.

12 **Dunn, S. and Moss, T.** Groupwork: a vehicle to self help. (Two self help organisations for haemodialysis and mastectomy patients set up by social workers.) Social Work Today, 10, 28 Nov 1978, 16-17.

13 **Felstein, I.** Never mind the dirt! (Types of self-help group.) Nursing Mirror, 150, 19 Jun 1980, 38-39.

14 **Graffy, J.P.** Patient participation in primary health care. (Study to investigate the background, organisation and activities of six patient participation groups.) Journal of the Royal College of General Practitioners, 30, Sep 1980, 542-545.

15 **Henry, S.** Sometimes the best medicine is hardest to swallow: the range and aims of self help groups. Health and Social Service Journal, 87, 3 Jun 1977, 892-893.

16 **Heywood Jones, I.** Sharing in caring. (Value of self-help groups and details of Self-help Clearing House to register groups and give advice.) Nursing Times, 75, 18 Oct 1979, 1816-1817.

17 **Jankowski, R.F. and others** Patients' expectations of health care: fulfilled and unfulfilled. (Survey in general practice of patients with rheumatoid arthritis.) Practitioner, 224, Apr 1980, 351-353.

18 **Journal of the Royal College of General Practitioners** Patient participation in general practice. (Review of literature from 1974.) Journal of the Royal College of General Practitioners, 30, Mar 1980, 132.

19 **Klein, J.** Self-help groups. (Social psychology of groups and examples of self-help groups in nurses' working situations.) Nursing Mirror, 145, 29 Dec 1977, 33-34.

20 **McKenna, S.P. and others** Looking at health from the consumers' point of view. (Development of the Nottingham Health Profile, a socio-medical indicator of health.) Occupational Health, 32 (7), Jul 1980, 350-355.

21 **Robinson, D.** Self-help in relation to health care. (Role of self-help groups.) Midwife, Health Visitor and Community Nurse, 14 (8), Aug 1978, 265-267.

22 **Robinson, D.** Self-help in health care. (How self-help groups work and their value and limitations.) Journal of Medical Ethics, 6 (1), Mar 1980, 4-6.

23 **Robinson, D. and Henry, S.** Self-help and health: mutual aid for modern problems. Robertson, 1977.

24 **Shaw, I.** General practice and the consumer. (Patient participation groups.) Hospital and Health Services Review, 76 (2), Feb 1980, 47-49.

25 **Thompson, T.** An ordinal evaluation of the consumer participation process in community health programs. Nursing Research, 29 (1), Jan/Feb 1980, 50-54.

26 **Tomalin, C.** Patient power in Wales. (Patients Committee, Aberdare.) Health and Social Service Journal, 86, 22 May 1976, 930.

27 **Turton, P.** Patience for progress. (Report on meeting of the National Association for Patient Participation in General Practice.) Nursing Times, 74, 9 Nov 1978, 1834.

28 **Williamson, J.D. and Danaher, K.** Self-care in health. Croom Helm, 1978.

29 **Wilson, A.T.M.** A new kind of health service. An address given at the annual meeting of the Association of Welsh health authorities. (Includes description of elected patients' committee at Aberdare Health Centre.) Hospital and Health Services Review, 74 (3), Mar 1978, 91-93, 95.

30 **Wilson, A.T.M.** Patients' participation in a primary care unit. (Patients' Committee at Aberdare Health Centre.) British Medical Journal, 1, 5 Feb 1977, 398.

31 **Wilson, A.T.M.** Why we must try to utilise this great, untapped wealth. (Progress in Aberdare towards a democratic patient-orientated health service.) Health and Social Service Journal, 88, 20 Jan 1978, 66-67.

32 **Wood, J. and Metcalfe, D.H.H.** Professional attitudes to patient participation groups: an exploratory study. (Interviews with GPs from ten practices.) Journal of the Royal

College of General Practitioners, 30, Sep 1980, 538-541.

h VOLUNTEERS

1 **Bamford, T.** Volunteers: the future direction. (Comment on the Good Neighbour Campaign and the Wolfenden report on Voluntary Organisations.) Social Work Today, 9, 22 Nov 1977, 1.

2 **Chamberlain, J.** Community spirit is there—it can happen everywhere. (Coordination of voluntary and statutory health and social service agencies in Bracknell.) Health and Social Service Journal, 90, 11 Jan 1980, 54-55.

3 **Crouch, A.F.** Voluntary service in a health district. Queen's Nursing Journal, 19 (8), Nov 1976, 225-226.

4 **Garvock, S.L. and Jabes, J.** Rewarding hospital volunteers. Dimensions in Health Service, 57 (2), Feb 1980, 26-27.

5 **Moss, J.** Volunteers in the primary care team. (Pilot scheme in Kent involving British Red Cross Society volunteers.) Midwife, Health Visitor and Community Nurse, 16 (7), Jul 1980, 287, 290, 292.

6 **Nelson, J.** Doing it for love? The motives of the voluntary workers in our hospitals. Nursing Mirror, 143, 30 Dec 1976, 47.

7 **Royal Society of Health Journal** The role of the volunteer in the Welfare State. (Five articles referring to the health service with one on the role of CHCs.) Royal Society of Health Journal, 98 (5), Oct 1978, 216-230, 237.

8 **Skeet, M. and Crout, E.** Health needs help: results of a study into the role and preparation of volunteers working within the reorganised National Health Service. Blackwell, 1977.

9 **Skeet, M.** Health needs help. (Role of volunteer in health care.) Nursing Mirror, 146, 16 Mar 1978, 40-42.

10 **Skeet, M.** Tapping voluntary resources in the Welfare State: the practical problems. Royal Society of Health Journal, 99 (1), Feb 1979, 23-27.

11 **Skeet, M.** Voluntary services and the NHS. Midwife, Health Visitor and Community Nurse, 13 (11), Nov 1977, 360-362.

12 **Smith, J.P.** Health needs help. The role and preparation of volunteers in the NHS. (King's Fund conference.) Nursing Mirror, 144, 10 Feb 1977, 39-40.

13 **Smith, J. and Hinton, N.** The voluntary sector: a debate. (The case against, by Jef Smith and the case for by Nicholas Hinton.) Social Work Today, 9, 22 Nov 1977, 8-10.

14 **Volunteer Centre** Volunteer involvement in the National Health Service...evidence to the Royal Commission on the National Health Service. Berkhamsted: The Centre, 1976.

33 COMMUNITY HEALTH NURSING

a GENERAL

1 **Ashton, K.** Community nurses in

Scotland—the facts... (Comments on the Scottish Home and Health Department reports—'A profile of qualified nurses'...and 'Nurse staffing (community) survey book of tables.') Nursing Times, 73, 27 Jan 1977, 118-119.

2 Benson, E.R. and McDevitt, J.Q. Community health and nursing practice. Englewood Cliffs: Prentice-Hall, 1976.

3 Bolton, G. Community nursing in the United Kingdom: personal research project for the N.S.W. Nurses' Registration Board. The Author, 1980.

4 Braden, C.J. and Price, J.L. Encouraging client self-discovery. (Four facets of community health nursing behavior help clients to develop their self-reliance.) American Journal of Nursing, 76 (3), Mar 1976, 444-446.

5 Bristow, S. Career opportunities. Community care. Nursing Times, 72, 10 Jun 1976, 893-894.

6 Community Outlook Specialists in the community. (Report of first Nursing Times Community Outlook Conference.) Nursing Times, 74, 21 Sep 1978, 1546.

7 Community Outlook Telephone talk. (Sheffield's community nurses' involvement with local radio phone-in and Salop midwives' 24-hour telephone advice service.) Nursing Times, 75, 12 Jul 1979, Community Outlook 199.

8 Dalton, J.M. Nursing diagnosis in a community health setting. Nursing Clinics of North America, 14 (3), Sep 1979, 525-531.

9 Edinburgh University. Nursing Research Unit Lots of questions. (Report of conference on evaluation and assessment of nursing care in the community.) Nursing Times, 75, 14 Jun 1979 Community Outlook 163-164, 166, 168.

10 Ellis, M.A. In the community. (Adaptation of nursing skills in hospital to meet community needs. Symposium on the graduate nurse.) Nursing Mirror, 144, 10 Feb 1977, 53-55.

11 Flack, G. Looking for dividends from the co-operative movement. (Multidisciplinary seminar for teachers of district nursing, health visiting, general practice and social work.) Health and Social Service Journal, 86, 11 Mar 1977, 432-435.

12 Fromer, M.J. Community health care and the nursing process. St. Louis: Mosby, 1979.

13 George, V.M. Twenty-five years on. (Changes in community nursing since 1952.) Queen's Nursing Journal, 19 (15), 424-425.

14 Going, M. Should community nurses be informed? (With list of basic information sources compiled by M. Going and K. Carter on p.160-161.) Nursing Times, 75, 14 Jun 1979 Community Outlook 157-158.

15 Hughes, J. and Roberts, J.A. Problems in the development of London's community nursing services. London School of Hygiene and Tropical Medicine, Dept. of Community Health, 1980.

16 Illing, M. Community nursing. A forum for ideas. (Miss Illing, consultant adviser to the supplement 'Community Nursing' states her hopes for it.) Nursing Mirror, 144, 30 Jun 1977, 46.

17 Kasteler, J.M. The community nurse as a resource in the patient's ability to cope with illness. International Nursing Review, 24 (3), May/Jun 1977, 88-92.

18 Keywood, O. Nursing in the community. Baillière Tindall, 1977.

19 Kretzer, V. and Morgan, Z. The community nursing services in McCarthy, M. and Millard, P.H. editors Management of chronic illness... King Edward's Hospital Fund for London, 1979.

20 McKeown, P. Nursing care outside hospital in the integrated health service. Developments in care (in Tayside). Queen's Nursing Journal, 19 (3), Jun 1976, 70-71, 73.

21 Meggitt, C. The future of community nursing. A district nurse who qualified this year looks forward. Queen's Nursing Journal, 19 (15), Jun 1977, 432, 434.

22 Mitchell, A.M. Nursing services in the community. (Experience of three-month secondment from the hospital service.) Nursing Mirror, 73, 24 Mar 1977 Health Centre iv, vii, ix.

23 Muir Gray, J.A. A difficult decade: a look at the future of community nursing. Nursing Mirror, 145, 15 Sep 1977, 36-37.

24 O'Connor, A.B. compiler Nursing in community health settings. New York: American Journal of Nursing, 1978. (Contemporary nursing series, 18.)

25 Poole, A.A.B. 'Patients first' and its impact on the community nursing services. Nursing Times, 76, 20 Mar 1980, 523-524.

26 Price, J.C. Integrated client centering in community health nursing. (Focusing on the patient rather than the nursing problem.) Health Visitor, 49 (10), Oct 1976, 320-324.

27 Scottish Home and Health Department A profile of qualified nurses working in the Scottish community nursing service in 1973. Edinburgh: The Department, 1976. (Nursing manpower planning report no.7.)

28 Society of Chief Nursing Officers (Public Health) (Report) 1969-1975. The Society, 1979.

29 Tinkham, C.W. and Voorhies, E.F. Community health nursing: evolution and process. 2nd ed. New York: Appleton-Century-Crofts, 1977.

30 Trangmar, J.A. Urban change. (And the role of the community nurse.) Nursing Mirror, 146, 23 Mar 1978, 40-42.

31 Volante, R.S. and Winn, R.L.N. Humanizing the teaching of community nursing. International Nursing Review, 24 (2), Mar/Apr 1977, 51-54.

32 Walker, H.B. Snags, safeguards, and satisfactions. (Discussion of the extended role of the nurse, with reference to community nursing and call for clearly defined agreements between the medical and nursing professions.) Nursing Mirror, 146, 25 May 1978, 37-38.

33 Walton, M. Integration—fact or friction? (With reference to community nursing.) Health Visitor, 53 (4), Apr 1980, 122-124.

34 Williams, C.A. Community health nursing—what is it? (Argues that it's a matter of focus on group health problems, in contrast to individual, clinically-oriented care.) Nursing Outlook, 25 (4), Apr 1977, 250-254.

b MANAGEMENT AND STAFFING

1 Bergman, R. Evaluation of community health nursing. (Areas of examination and methods.) New Zealand Nursing Journal, 71 (3), Mar 1978, 23-26.

2 Bernal, H. Levels of practice in a community health agency: a three-tier system for classifying staff nurses. (Visiting Nurse Association.) Nursing Outlook, 26 (6), Jun 1978, 364-369.

3 Brown, B.I. Realistic workloads for community health nurses: an analysis of time studies. Nursing Outlook, 28 (4), Apr 1980, 233-237.

4 Cearlock, H.A. The development and implementation of nursing audit in a community health agency. Journal of Nursing Education, 19 (8), Oct 1980, 18-23.

5 Chapple, M. The Barnsley dispute: its importance nationally. (The question of geographical allocation of caseloads.) Journal of Community Nursing, 4 (1), Jul 1980, 14-15.

6 Decker, F. and others Using patient outcomes to evaluate community health nursing. (Scheme in Minnesota.) Nursing Outlook, 27 (4), Apr 1979, 278-282.

7 Eccles, T. Community nurses and the computer. (For record keeping and management information.) Queen's Nursing Journal, 19 (14), May 1977, 391-392.

8 Engle, J. and Barkauskas, V. The evolution of a public health nursing performance evaluation tool. Journal of Nursing Administration, 9 (4), Apr 1979, 8-16.

9 Flynn, B.C. and Ray, D.W. Quality assurance in community health nursing. (Evaluating effectiveness of services.) Nursing Outlook, 27 (10), Oct 1979, 650-653.

10 Gatherer, A. Are you being well served? (Assistance for community nurses in the form of secretarial help, statistical support and auxiliaries.) Nursing Mirror, 148, 15 Mar 1979, 26.

11 Hughes, J. and others Nurses in the community: a manpower study. (Survey in inner London of health visitors and district nurses to provide data base for planning future manpower needs of service.) Journal of Epidemiology and Community Health, 33 (4), Dec 1979, 262-269.

12 Irish Nurses Organisation Survey of workload of public health nurses. (Memorandum.) World of Irish Nursing, 5 (5), May 1976, 4-5.

13 Jacox, A.K. and Norris, C.M. editors Organising for independent nursing practice. New York: Appleton-Century-Crofts, 1977.

14 Kelly, M.E. and Rossler, L.M. Development of interdisciplinary problem oriented recording in a public health nursing agency. Journal of Nursing Administration, 6 (10), Dec 1976, 24-31.

15 Lamp Quality assurance in community nursing workshop papers. (Three short articles with one on audit of nursing records.) Lamp, 36 (11), Dec 1979, 5-10.

16 Lohmann, G. A statewide system of record audit. (In primary care programs in Iowa.) Nursing Outlook, 25 (5), May 1977, 330-332.

17 Morris, P. Primarily semi-detached. (Reorganisation of community nursing services in Barnsley AHA to provide part GP attachment, part geographical allocation.) Nursing Mirror, 149, 1 Nov 1979, 7.

18 Nimmo, A.W. and Wilkes, J.S. An approach to planning staff levels in community nursing: case study in the Peterhead area. Aberdeen: Grampian Health Services Information Unit, 1978.

19 Risk, M.M. The community clinical nurse specialist: a two-year perspective. Nursing Clinics of North America, 7 (4), Dec 1975, 761-769.

20 Roberts, J.A. Recruitment. 12. Staffing community nursing services in London. (With reference to the community Nursing Manpower Study in 1977 and 1978.) Nursing Times, 76, 4 Dec 1980, 2164-2166.

21 Saint-Yves, I.F.M. Point of view: nurses hold the key. (Suggests new structure in community nursing services with nursing aid, community nurse and clinical associate.) Journal of Community Nursing, 2 (10), Apr 1979, 7, 14.

22 Shelton, W. Sorting out the communications problem. (Nursing and Midwifery Request Unit, set up by two Notts health districts to channel requests for nursing service to appropriate nurse or clinic.) Journal of Community Nursing, 2 (4), Oct 1978, 21-22.

23 Thomson, C. Staffing structure. (Review and recommendations for domiciliary midwives and district nurses in Leek and Cheadle.) Queen's Nursing Journal, 18 (10), Jan 1976, 270-272; (11), Feb 1976, 299-300.

24 Werner, J.R. Effective community health nursing: a framework for actualizing standards of practice. Nursing Forum, 15 (3), 1976, 265-276.

25 Wilkes, J.S. and Nimmo, A.W. An analysis of work patterns in community nursing. 2 parts. (Surveys of health visitors and district nurses in 3 Aberdeenshire health centres to produce a formula for staffing.) Nursing Times, 72, 29 Jan 1976, Occ. papers, 13-16; 5 Feb 1976, Occ. papers, 17-18.

26 Wiseman, J. Hidden messages. (Value of community nursing statistics for nurse managers.) Nursing Mirror, 150, 19 Jun 1980, 40-41.

27 Wray, J.G. Problem oriented recording in community nursing—a new experience in education. (Adaptation at Queen's University, Kingston, Ontario.) International Journal of Nursing Studies, 13 (4), 1976, 243-250; International Nursing Review, 24 (4), Jul/Aug 1977, 114-115; Journal of Nursing Education, 16 (9), Nov 1977, 12-15.

c OVERSEAS COUNTRIES

1 Adams, R. Origins of public health nursing in Israel. Curationis, 1 (2), Sep 1978, 43-46.

2 Adebo, E.O. Integration of community health nursing concepts into the basic nursing curriculum. (In Nigeria.) Nigerian Nurse, 7 (4), Oct-Dec 1975, 9-11, 17.

3 Aggarwal, K.C. A wider role for our nurses. (In the community, with reference to India.) Nursing Journal of India, 68 (7), Jul 1977, 184-186.

4 Archer, S.E. A descriptive study of community health nursing in Australia 1975-1976. Brisbane: Royal Australian Nursing Federation, 1977.

5 Archer, S.E. Selected issues confronting community health nursing. Australian Nurses Journal, 5 (10), Apr 1976, 15-17; 5 (11), May 1976, 14-17.

6 Batley, N. and Kratz, C. Two-way process. (Report of Tokyo workshop on community nursing at which British practice was described.) Nursing Times, 73, 28 Jul 1977, 1172-1173.

7 Brann, J. A Churchill Fellow sees for herself. (Study of community nursing in the United States, Canada, England and Malaya.) Australian Nurses Journal, 6 (2), Aug 1976, 31-35.

8 Brofman, J.L. An evening home visiting program. (Met patients' needs and proved cost-effective and safe.) Nursing Outlook, 27 (10), Oct 1979, 657-661.

9 Burgess, M. Community health nursing at Wellington Polytechnic: points and progress. New Zealand Nursing Journal, 70 (10), 9-11.

10 Burrett, B.A. The nurse and community care in East Bhutan. (Setting up of community health programme in Assam.) Nursing Mirror, 145, 1 Dec 1977, 22-23.

11 Canadian Public Health Association A statement of functions and qualifications for the practice of public health nursing in Canada. Canadian Journal of Public Health, 159, May 1968, 204.

12 Chapple, M. Is America ripe for prevention? (Report of her visit to and lecture at symposium of Primary Care Nurse Practitioners in Colorado.) Journal of Community Nursing, 1 (7), Jan 1978, 18-19.

13 Clark, J.H. and Ansett, M. The supervisor-shared home visit. (As a means of observing and evaluating knowledge and skills of district nurse and assisting her.) Nursing Outlook, 27 (1), Jan 1979, 54-56.

14 Dickie, C. Community health nursing. (A review of New Zealand services.) New Zealand Nursing Journal, 69 (2), Feb 1976, 12-14.

15 Erasmus, C.A. The future of community health nursing. (In South Africa.) Curationis, 2 (2), Sep 1979, 10-15.

16 Essex, N. Supportive staff and services for all registered nurse practice. (Description of generalist community nursing in the Western Metropolitan Health Region.) Lamp, 35 (10), Oct 1978, 52-54.

17 Ferguson, M. The Canadian way: primary care nursing in Canada. Nursing Times, 74, 13 Jul 1978, 195-196, 198.

18 Fonseca, J.D. The community health

nurse: a profile. Nursing Outlook, 25 (10), Oct 1977, 627.

19 Harnish, Y. Patient care guides: practical information for public health nurses. New York: National League for Nursing, 1976.

20 Highriter, M.E. The status of community health nursing research. (Review of articles 1972-1976.) Nursing Research, 26 (3), May/Jun 1977, 183-192.

21 Karafiath, D.D. Home care makes sense today. (The advantages and barriers to home care.) Journal of Nursing Administration, 6 (5), Jun 1976, 31-34.

22 Keith, P.M. and Castles, M. Community health nurses' preferences for systems of protection. (Preferences for escort protection in dangerous areas.) Nursing Research, 25 (4), Jul/Aug 1976, 252-255.

23 Kinlein, M.L. Independent nursing practice with clients. Philadelphia: Lippincott, 1977.

24 Knox, J. We did it. You can too. (Development of philosophy, objectives and standards of community nursing in Alberta.) Canadian Nurse, 74 (11), Dec 1978, 24-26.

25 Koltz, C.J. Private practice in nursing: development and management. Germantown, Md.: Aspen Systems, 1979.

26 Kratz, C. Our day in Hong Kong. (Description of community nursing service.) Nursing Times, 73, 7 Jul 1977, 1025.

27 Kratz, C. The sun rises for community nurses? The ICN congress in Tokyo and its significance for community nurses. Nursing Times, 73, 11 Aug 1977, Community Outlook 7.

28 Lowe, G.G. Community health nursing lectures. (Inservice training in Geelong.) UNA Nursing Journal, 73 (7), Nov-Dec 1975, 8-9.

29 Martin, E.M. Transition without trauma—the community nurse. (Merging of the domiciliary and community nurse into the generalist community nurse at Manning River Region, New South Wales.) Lamp, 33 (8), Aug 1976, 28-31.

30 Mellish, J.M. The extended role of the nurse in the community. (Symposium report.) S.A. Nursing Journal, 43 (9), Sep 1976, 30-32, 38.

31 Miles, J. Community health nursing. Definition of community health nursing. S.A. Nursing Journal, 43 (8), Aug 1976, 7-9.

32 Morris, J. Mufakose Clinic. (Primary care clinic in Rhodesia.) Rhodesian Nurse, 8 (4), Dec 1975, 6-8.

33 New South Wales Council of Community Nursing Patients cared for at home—their dependency. (Results of survey.) Lamp, 35 (7), Jul 1978, 34-37; Australian Nurses Journal, 8 (3), Sep 1978, 45-47.

34 New Zealand Nursing Journal The educational preparation of the practice nurse. (In New Zealand—notes on a paper at a study day on the place of the practice nurse in the community.) New Zealand Nursing Journal, 70 (12), Dec 1977, 7-8.

35 Nursing Clinics of North America Symposium on community nursing in Canada. Nursing Clinics of North America, 7 (4), Dec 1975, 687-778.

36 Pakshong, D.I. The role of the nurse in community health. Nursing Journal of Singapore, 17 (1), May 1977, 25-27.

37 Queen's Nursing Journal Community nursing in Hong Kong. Queen's Nursing Journal, 19 (12), Mar 1977, 337, 339.

38 Rees, R. Independent of the institutionalised practice of nursing. (The development of Australian community health services in relation to nursing practice.) Australian Nurses Journal, 8 (1), Jul 1978, 31-33.

39 Rice, V. The Diploma in Community Health Nursing, Cumberland College of Health Sciences. A report on four years of development. Lamp, 35 (3), Mar 1978, 6-9, 11-13.

40 Shillington, P. A nurse in the camp. (TB nursing and public health education in Kampuchea.) Community View, 6, Aug 1980, 3-5.

41 Shreeve, G. Dai care. (Role of traditional mothers and women (dais) in India's primary health care.) Nursing Times, 73, 24 Feb 1977, 260.

42 Simpson, J.M. Community services in Norway. (District and public health nursing services.) Queen's Nursing Journal, 19 (3), Jun 1976, 77-78.

43 Spanton, V. The nurse retraining programme in Yogyakarta, Indonesia. (To prepare community oriented nurses capable of developing primary care.) New Zealand Nursing Journal, 73 (1), Jan 1980, 20-24.

44 Tulloch, E. Preparation for nursing leadership in tropical community health care teams. (The Master's degree in International Community Health at Liverpool University, which six nurses are currently taking alongside doctors.) Nursing Times, 73, 3 Nov 1977; Commonwealth Nurses Federation Supplement, 67-68.

45 Tully, M. Nursing with a research unit in Africa. (Community health nursing with a nutrition research unit in Sierra Leone.) Nursing Times, 74, 9 Mar 1978, 401-405.

46 United States Department of Health, Education and Welfare. Division of Nursing Surveys of public health nursing 1968-1972. The Department, 1976.

47 Warner, A.R. editor Innovations in community health nursing: health care delivery in shortage areas. St. Louis: Mosby, 1978.

48 Yew, D. A decade of private nursing service to the community. Nursing Journal of Singapore, 19 (2), Dec 1979, 86-87.

d INTERPROFESSIONAL RELATIONSHIPS

1 Council for the Education and Training of Health Visitors Interprofessional co-operation: multidisciplinary seminar Sep 1976. A report by the planning group. CETHV, 1977. (Occasional paper.)

2 Hirshson, R. Nurses and social workers—

we can learn from each other. American Journal of Nursing, 76 (12), Dec 1976, 1972-1973.

3 Kendall, P. The role relationship dilemma of health visitor and social worker. Health Visitor, 50 (8), Aug 1977, 261-262, 264.

4 Nursing Mirror Better communications for HVs. (Liaison scheme between health visitors and midwives in the City and Hackney Health District.) Nursing Mirror, 142 (10), 4 Mar 1976, 36.

5 Payne, L. Interdisciplinary experiment: an account of the Southampton study group. (Study groups consisting of GPs, health visitors and social workers to discuss mutual problems of training and professional role.) Social Work Today, 6 (22), 5 Feb 1976, 691-693.

6 Sullivan, J.A. Comparison of manifest needs of nurses and physicians in primary care practice. (Results suggest an emerging assertiveness in nurses compared with earlier studies showing need for order, deference and endurance.) Nursing Research, 27 (4), Jul/Aug 1978, 255-259.

7 Swailes, S.S. Establishing good communications. (Experiences of a community charge nurse in establishing contact with other health professionals.) Queen's Nursing Journal, 18 (11), Feb 1976, 307-308.

34 FAMILY CARE

a GENERAL PRACTICE NURSING

1 Acheson, H.W.K. Making better use of our nurses. (Letter on expanding role of nurse in general practice.) British Medical Journal, 2, 23 Jul 1977, 265.

2 Allen, V.P. The practice nurse. (Author describes her work.) Nursing Mirror, 146, 23 Mar 1978, 10.

3 Barber, J.H. and others Urgency and risk in first contact decisions in general practice. (Survey at Woodside Health Centre, Glasgow, using a nurse to make initial home calls and estimate the urgency of each case.) Health Bulletin, 18 (1), Jan 1976, 21-29.

4 Bowling, A.P. To do or not to do? (Research study of general practitioners' and nurses' attitudes towards the delegation of medical tasks.) Nursing Mirror, 151, 17 Jul 1980, 30-32.

5 Bowling, A. Nurses in the primary care team. (Letter giving results of a survey of nurses and GPs showing doctors' opposition to delegation.) Lancet, 2, 13 Sep 1980, 590.

6 Brash, J.S. and West, S.R. Education for practice nurses. (Research study in Auckland.) New Zealand Nurses Journal, 72 (11), Nov 1979, 26-29.

7 Dawar, A. Who deals with it now? 3. The nurse in McCarthy, M. and others Management of minor illness... King Edward's Hospital Fund for London, 1979, 45-58.

8 Griffin, A.M. and Steel, R. The general practitioner and the community nurse. Practitioner, 224, Dec 1980, 1231-1233.

9 Jacka, S.M. The need for training. (Nursing

in general practice.) General Practice Team, 57, Oct/Nov 1976, 2.

10 Josse, S.E. Employment of practice nurses. (Letter outlining position regarding contracts and pension rights.) Journal of the Royal College of General Practitioners, 28, Apr 1978, 239-240.

11 Keywood, O. Attachment scheme or geographical patch? (Suggests small teams of HVs, district nurses and midwives led by nurse with all three qualifications.) Nursing Mirror, 147, 10 Aug 1978, 35.

12 Mackichan, N.D. The nurse in the primary health care team. Contained in: Mackichan, N.D. The G.P. and the primary health care team. Pitman, 1976. (Chapter 12, 212-224.)

13 Marsh, G.N. Further nursing care in general practice. (Work of nurses at Norton Medical Centre, Stockton on Tees in family planning and well woman screening.) British Medical Journal, 2, 11 Sep 1976, 626-627.

14 Miller, D.S. and Backett, E.M. A new member of the team? Extending the role of the nurse in British primary care. (Results of a questionnaire to GPs showing two-thirds were in favour of the nurse's extended role.) Lancet, 2, 16 Aug 1980, 358-361; Letter from J.M. Bevan, Lancet, 2, 6 Sep 1980, 541.

15 Mourin, K. A practice nurses' course— content and evaluation. (At Norwich City College.) Journal of the Royal College of General Practitioners, 30, Feb 1980, 78-82, 84.

16 Mourin, K. The role of the practice nurse. (Objectives of course developed by author at Norwich City College.) Journal of the Royal College of General Practitioners, 30, Feb 1980, 75-77.

17 Nisbet, E. Assessing the urgency of home visits. (Research project in which nurse visited and assessed GP's patients requesting house calls.) Nursing Times, 73, 22 Sep 1977, 1472-1474.

18 Reedy, B.L.E.C. and others A comparison of the activities and opinions of attached and employed nurses in general practice. Journal of the Royal College of General Practitioners, 30, Aug 1980, 483-489.

19 Reedy, B.L.E.C. and others Nurses and nursing in primary medical care in England. (Survey of the nursing reception and administrative duties of qualified nurses in general practice by the Medical Care Research Unit, University of Newcastle upon Tyne.) British Medical Journal, 2, 27 Nov 1976, 1304-1306.

20 Reedy, B.L.E.C. and others The social and occupational characteristics of attached and employed nurses in general practice. Journal of the Royal College of General Practitioners, 30, Aug 1980, 477-482.

21 Ruthven, H. Attachment of local authority nurses to general practice prior to reorganisation (in Scotland.) Health Bulletin, 18 (1), Jan 1976, 29-35.

22 Sachs, H. The practice nurse—a practical asset. (Survey of two group practices by Bedford College which outlines four-fold role: to assist, supplement and complement the doctor and provide alternative source of care.) Nursing Mirror, 147, 26 Oct 1978, 60-62.

23 Salmond, G. The contribution of the practice nurse. (Report of inter-disciplinary study day.) New Zealand Nursing Journal, 70 (12), Dec 1977, 3-8.

24 Saltman, B.M. Group practice nurse. (Gatley Health Centre.) Nursing Times, 73, 24 Mar 1977 Health Centre xvi, xviii, xx.

25 Waters, W.H.R. and others A four-year prospective study of the work of the practice nurse in the treatment room of a South Yorkshire practice. (Including extended role.) (See also letter 26 Jan 1980, 255.) British Medical Journal, 280, 12 Jan 1980, 87-89.

26 Wilson, D. The practice nurse—an entity at last. Journal of Community Nursing, 3 (11), May 1980, 22, 29.

b PRIMARY HEALTH CARE NURSING

1 Aiken, L.H. Primary care: the challenge for nursing. (In the American health care system.) American Journal of Nursing, 77 (11), Nov 1977, 1828-1832.

2 Alford, D.M. and Jensen, J.M. Primary health care. Reflections on private practice. American Journal of Nursing, 76 (12), Dec 1976, 1966-1968.

3 Batley, N. Education and training for primary care as seen by a health visitor. Nursing Times, 76, 17 Apr 1980, Occ. papers, 41-43.

4 Bergman, R. Extending health care through the utilization of nursing/midwifery personnel. (Primary health care, with reference to ICN and WHO recommendations.) International Nursing Review, 27 (2), Mar/Apr 1980, 53-58.

5 Chen, S-P. C. and others Patient encounters by primary care nurse students. (Analysis of health problems.) Research in Nursing and Health, 1 (1), Apr 1978, 18-28.

6 Colliere, M.F. Development of primary health care. (Role of nurse.) International Nursing Review, 27 (6), Nov/Dec 1980, 169-172.

7 Commonwealth Nurses Federation Supplement Nurse education for primary health care for rural populations. (Report of workshop in Bangladesh, India and Sri Lanka.) Nursing Times, 74, 2 Nov 1978 CNF Supplement 90-91.

8 Craven, R.F. Primary health care. Practice in a nursing home. American Journal of Nursing, 76 (12), Dec 1976, 1958-1960.

9 Department of Health Primary health care nursing services in inner city areas. A DHSS discussion document. Nursing Mirror, 145, 18 Aug 1977, 38.

10 Friend, P. Nursing in primary health care. CNO(77)8. (A paper recently distributed to regional areas, and district nursing officers to aid them in future planning.) Nursing Mirror, 145, 14 Jul 1977, 41-42.

11 Hart, C. The independent contractor and the primary care team. (Letter suggesting extending independent practitioner status to all nurses in primary care teams.) Journal of the Royal College of General Practitioners, 27, Jun 1977, 377.

12 Jones, J.I. The extended role of the nurse in the community (in primary care teams in Britain.) S.A. Nursing Journal, 43 (10), Oct 1976, 18, 21.

13 Jones, P.E. Nurses in Canadian primary health care settings: a review of recent literature. Toronto: University of Toronto, 1980.

14 Jones, P.E. A program in continuing education for primary health care. Nursing Clinics of North America, 7 (4), Dec 1975, 691-695.

15 Kratz, G. A measure of care. (Report of WHO working groups on measuring the efficiency of primary care and deciding on the role of the nurse.) Nursing Times, 72, 16 Dec 1976, 1952.

16 Kratz, C. Talking point. (Comment on DHSS circular Nursing in primary health care.) Nursing Times, 73, 13 Oct 1977 Community Outlook 67.

17 Lamb, A.M. Primary health nursing: a description of the work of health visitors, district nurses, domiciliary midwives and school nurses. Baillière Tindall, 1977.

18 Lee, M.K.S. Nursing in primary health care. Philippines Journal of Nursing, 48 (3), Jul/Sep 1978, 64-68.

19 Lindars, M.E. Primary health care: influencing change. (Comment on recent circular CNO (77) 8 on the primary health care team.) Nursing Mirror, 145, 22 Dec 1977, 31.

20 Morton, P. Developments in the organisation of primary health care nursing services (1900-1977). MPhil thesis in Applied Social Science, Nottingham University, 1978.

21 PRIMARY care nursing: a manual of clinical skills. Philadelphia: Davis, 1977.

22 Quesada, M.L.M. The primary health care project of the Philippine Nurses Association. Philippines Journal of Nursing, 48 (3), Jul/Sep 1978, 69-76.

23 Reedy, B.L.E.C. and others Nurses and nursing in primary medical care in England. University of Newcastle upon Tyne Medical Care Research Unit, (1976.)

24 Royal College of Nursing Primary health care nursing. (Report of the inaugural meeting of the Rcn Society of Primary Health Care.) Queen's Nursing Journal, 19 (4), Jul 1976, 96.

25 Royal College of Nursing. Society of Primary Health Care Nursing Primary health care nursing: a team approach. Rcn, 1980.

26 Schwartz, D. Interview—Doris Schwartz. (Associate professor of nursing, Cornell University, New York, and nurse director of the Primex programme which trains community nurses for a wider role in primary care.) Nursing Times, 72 (25), 24 Jun 1976, 963-965.

27 World Health Organisation WHO resolution. The role of nursing/midwifery personnel in primary health care teams. International Nursing Review, 24 (6), Nov/Dec 1977, 184.

28 World Health Organisation. Regional Office for Europe The definition of parameters of efficiency in primary care and the role of nursing in primary health care: report on two working groups, Reykjavik, 14-18 Jul 1975. Copenhagen: WHO, 1976.

c FAMILY CARE AND NURSE PRACTITIONER

1 Archer, S.E. Community nurse practitioner: another assessment. (Second report of a study of these nurses' activities and characteristics. For Part 1—see Nursing Outlook, 23, Jun 1975, 358-364.) Nursing Outlook, 24 (8), Aug 1976, 499-503.

2 Blake, R.A. and others A method of integrating family nursing in an undergraduate curriculum. (Texas Women's University College of Nursing, Houston.) Journal of Nursing Education, 15 (6), Nov 1976, 22-25.

3 Bowling, A. A nurse practitioner in Britain? (With some reference to author's research with treatment room nurses and district nurses.) Nursing Times, 76, 4 Dec 1980, 2157-2158.

4 Chafetz, L. and Gaillard, J. The impact of a therapeutic nurse-family relationship on post graduate public health nursing students. International Journal of Nursing Studies, 15 (1), 1978, 37-49.

5 Chambers, L. and others A controlled trial of the impact of the family practice nurse on volume, quality, and cost of rural health services. (Family nurse practitioner.) Medical Care, 15 (12), Dec 1977, 971-981.

6 Flynn, B.C. Predictors of family nurse practitioner program success. (Survey in Indiana.) Nurse Practitioner, 3 (1), Jan-Feb 1978, 32-33.

7 Geary, M.C. Supporting family coping. Supervisor Nurse, 10 (3), Mar 1979, 52-53, 57-59.

8 Gibson, K.W. If you've ever thought of being a nurse practitioner. (Two nurses run primary health care clinic.) RN Magazine, 40 (5), May 1977, 38-41.

9 Grandall, S.C. Primary health care. How an FNP won over the bureaucracy. (Family nurse practitioner in a community health centre.) American Journal of Nursing, 76 (12), Dec 1976, 1962-1964.

10 Hoole, A.J. and others, editors Patient care guidelines for family nurse practitioners. Boston: Little, Brown and Co., 1976.

11 Hunnings, V. If you've ever thought of being a nurse practitioner...I'm finally fulfilling my potential. (Nurse runs primary health care clinic in rural town and does home visits.) RN Magazine, 40 (5), May 1977, 35-38.

12 Lewis, C.E. and Cheyovich, T.K. Who is a nurse practitioner? Processes of care and patients' and physicians' perceptions. (Study at the University of Kansas of two different styles of care provided by nurse practitioners.) Medical Care, 14 (4), Apr 1976, 365-371.

13 Lewis, H.L. Nurse practitioners in prevention and health education. (Family nurse practitioners.) Hospital Progress, 59 (1), Jan 1978, 80-83.

14 Lewis, M.A. and Lewis, C.E. Protocols for the nurse practitioner: uses and problems. American Journal of Nursing, 76 (8), Aug 1976, 1312-1313.

15 Linn, L.S. Patient acceptance of the family nurse practitioner. (Research study in Southern

California.) Medical Care, 14 (4), Apr 1976, 357-364.

16 Porter, L.S. Health care workers' role conceptions and orientation to family-centered child care. Nursing Research, 28 (6), Nov/Dec 1979, 330-337.

17 Reedy, B.L.E.C. Family nurse practitioners. (Letter commenting on the bias of The Lancet against nurse practitioners.) Lancet, 1, 12 Mar 1977, 607.

18 Ross, H.K. and Ross, M.S. A new nursing role within the neighbourhood family context: the nurse as a member of the family. (Identification of needs of elderly, follow up and organisation of well-adult health programme for the elderly in Florida.) Community Health, 9 (4), May 1978, 195-200.

19 Rothwell, M.G. A patient centered group practice. (The problem oriented system as the philosophic base for a group practice in which the nurse is full partner. Nursing Outlook, 24 (12), Dec 1976, 745-748.

20 Shaw, D. and others Multiple impact therapy. (An intensive two-day meeting of a family and a multidisciplinary professional team.) American Journal of Nursing, 77 (2), Feb 1977, 246-248.

21 Stewart, B. Counselling. Hidden conflicts: a case study of the Fisher family—2. (Counselling by nurse.) Occupational Health, 32 (1), Jan 1980, 22-29; (2), Feb 1980, 76-83.

22 Thomas, P. The nurse's role. (In the care of fictitious family by the primary care team.) Nursing Mirror, 147, 5 Oct 1978 Supplement xvii, xix.

23 Thorpe, E. A woman's place... (Socialisation of children with reference to health visitor's possible radical role with mothers.) Nursing Times, 75, 1 Mar 1979, 348-349.

24 Vacek, P. and Ashikaga, T. Educational program evaluation: the University of Vermont family nurse practitioner program. Nursing Research, 27 (1), Jan/Feb 1978, 36-41.

25 Ward, M.J. Family nurse practitioners: perceived competencies and recommendations. (Mail questionnaire throughout USA.) Nursing Research, 28 (6), Nov/Dec 1979, 343-347.

26 White, M. Inside family life: an arena for health education. Nursing Forum, 18 (3), 1979, 246-252.

27 Wiseman, J. Family care study. Coping with a mentally handicapped son and a physically disabled grandmother. Nursing Times, 73, 8 Dec 1977, 1907-1909.

28 Woolf, M. and Pegden, S. Families five years on: a survey. HMSO, 1976.

29 Wright, E. Family nurse clinicians: physicians' perspective. (A survey by questionnaire to physicians to determine factors which would help or hinder primary care nurses trained in an expanded role.) Nursing Outlook, 23 (12), Dec 1975, 771-773.

30 Wright, E. Registered nurses' opinions on an extended role concept. (Survey of the opinions of 800 nurses from Texas on the family nurse clinician.) Nursing Research, 25 (2), Mar-Apr 1976, 112-114.

d ETHNIC MINORITIES

1 Abrahams, A. Can the strong arm of the law smash racial inequalities? (Work of the Community Relations Commission and the Race Relations Board during the last 8 years.) Health and Social Service Journal, 86, 28 Jan 1977, 158-161.

2 Ahmed, S. Asian girls and culture conflict. Social Work Today, 9, 8 Aug 1978, 14-16.

3 Anwar, M. Young Asians between two cultures. New Society, 38, 16 Dec 1976, 563-565.

4 Barchard, B. Caring for immigrant children. (Health problems.) New Zealand Nursing Journal, 72 (5), May 1979, 9-14.

5 Bentham, I.A. My friend Kashmir Kaur. (Health visitor's experience of teaching an Indian English.) Nursing Times, 72, 29 Apr 1976, 665-666.

6 Community Relations Commission Aspects of mental health in a multi-racial society: notes for the guidance of doctors and social workers. The Commission, 1976. (Reference series, no.10.)

7 Community Relations Commission Between two cultures: a study of relationships between generations in the Asian community in Britain. The Commission, 1976.

8 Community Relations Commission. Reference and Technical Services Division Caring for under-fives in a multi-racial society. The Commission, 1977.

9 Coombe, V. Health and social services and minority ethnic groups. Royal Society of Health Journal, 96 (1), Feb 1976, 34-38.

10 Davis, S.S. and Aslam, M. Eastern treatment for Eastern health? (Study in Nottingham of Asians' compliance with medication instructions.) Journal of Community Nursing, 2 (11), May 1979, 16-18, 20.

11 Fitzgerald, M.J. and MacLachlan, I.D. Immigrants: do we understand them enough to help them? Nursing Mirror, 147.
1. Identifying the problem. 27 Jul 1978, 35-36.
2. Background. 3 Aug 1978, 40-42.
3. Foreground. 10 Aug 1978, 37-38.
4. Communication. 17 Aug 1978, 34.

12 Fosdike, H. Assessing the needs of an ethnic community. (Project with the Moroccan community in North Kensington.) Midwife, Health Visitor and Community Nurse, 16 (4), Apr 1980, 148, 150, 152, 154.

13 Furlong, E. Training course for staff working with Asians. (Brent Health District.) Nursing Times, 73, 24 Mar 1977, 428-429.

14 Goel, K.M. Diseases of immigrant children. Nursing Mirror, 142, 15 Apr 1976, 55-57.

15 Gray, J. Health education for Asians. Cultural bridge building. (Scheme in Blackburn.) Health and Social Service Journal, 90, 8 Aug 1980, 1042-1043.

16 Health and Social Service Journal Cultural shock. (News item on CHC report on health care of Asian women by local maternity services.) Health and Social Service Journal, 88, 1 Sep 1978, 978-979.

17 Health and Social Service Journal Ethnic policy. (Community Health Project for Ethnic Minorities, new group to help them and health professionals involved with them.) Health and Social Service Journal, 88, 15 Dec 1978, 1406-1407.

18 Hill, R. When the boat comes in: the anatomy of a refugee camp. (Preparations by Lincolnshire AHA for arrival and medical treatment of Vietnamese boat people.) Health and Social Service Journal, 89, 2 Nov 1979, 1414-1417.

19 Hollingsworth, A.O. and others The refugees and childbearing: what to expect. (Indochinese in America.) RN Magazine, 43 (11), Nov 1980, 45-49.

20 Houston, A.H. Sopley: medical services for refugees. (From Vietnam.) British Medical Journal, 2, 10 Nov 1979, 1191-1192.

21 Judge, S. Some social aspects of illness among Italian migrants. Australian Nurses Journal, 6 (12), Jun 1977, 41-43.

22 Kallarackal, A.M. and Hertbert, M. The happiness of Indian immigrant children. (A study showing the importance of the family.) New Society, 35, 26 Feb 1976, 422-424.

23 Khan, V.S. editor Minority families in Britain: support and stress. Macmillan, 1979. (Studies in ethnicity.)

24 Knight, L. Eastern promise in the East End? (Bengali nurse whose primary task is health education with Bengali immigrants in Tower Hamlets, East London.) Nursing Mirror, 149, 25 Oct 1979, 35-37.

25 Lam, E. Health visiting Vietnamese refugees in Britain. Health Visitor, 53 (7), Jul 1980, 254-255.

26 Learmonth, A. Asians' literacy in their mother tongue and English. (Survey by health education officer of Bengalis and Pakistanis attending clinics or community groups in Oldham.) Nursing Times, 76, 28 Feb 1980, Occ. papers, 27-28.

27 Littlewood, R. and Cross, S. Ethnic minorities and psychiatric services. Sociology of Health and Illness, 2 (2), Jul 1980, 194-201.

28 Lobo, E. de H. Children of immigrants in Britain: their health and social problems. Hodder and Stoughton, 1978.

29 Loynes, A.P. Working with families from Bangladesh. (Role of HV.) Midwife, Health Visitor and Community Nurse, 15 (12), Dec 1979, 501, 504, 505.

30 McKay, R. Spreading the right words. (Barriers to communication with the Asian community and measures to overcome them.) Health and Social Service Journal, 88, 8 Dec 1978, 1388-1390.

31 Malgarinou, M. The changing Greek family structure: influence upon the psychosocial development of children. (Includes nurse's role.) International Nursing Review, 26 (5), Sep/Oct 1979, 157-158.

32 New Society Society at work. A guide to the race act. (Race Relations Act 1976.) New Society, 39, 3 Feb 1977, 230-233.

33 Philpot, T. Asians and the NHS.

(Comment on recent report by Wandsworth Council for Community Relations published by the Commission for Racial Equality.) Nursing Mirror, 147, 13 Jul 1978, 9.

34 Pushkin, I. Prejudice among ethnic groups. Midwife, Health Visitor and Community Nurse, 14 (11), Nov 1978, 391-393.

35 Ronalds, C. and others Asian mothers' use of general practitioner and maternal/child welfare services. Journal of the Royal College of General Practitioners, 27 (178), May 1977, 281-284.

36 Royal Society of Health The needs of immigrant families. (Papers presented at a conference, 20 November 1975.) The Society, 1976. Report by A. Kirby in Health and Social Service Journal, 85, 20/27 Dec 1975, 2794.

37 Santopietro, M.C.S. and Lynch, B.A. What's behind the 'inscrutable' mask? (Mental health and other problems of Indochinese refugees in America and nursing implications.) RN Magazine, 43 (10), Oct 1980, 55-62.

38 Slack, P.A. Minority report. (Role of HV with minority groups.) Nursing Times, 74, 13 Jul 1978 Community Outlook 190.

39 Smith, D.J. The facts of racial disadvantage: a national survey. PEP, 1976.

40 Social Work Today Social work for a multi-racial society. (Six articles. See also editorial on p.1.) Social Work Today, 10, 20 Feb 1979, 15-31.

41 Tauber, I.J. and others Preliminary results of a picture recognition study amongst Bangladeshi women. (With reference to health education materials.) Health Visitor, 53 (7), Jul 1980, 251-253.

42 Thornton, P. Family planning and immigrants. Nursing, 16, Aug 1980, 704, 707-708.

43 Watson, J.L. editor Between two cultures: migrants and minorities in Britain. Blackwell, 1977.

44 Wilson, A. Finding a voice: Asian women in Britain. Virago, 1978.

e ONE-PARENT FAMILIES

1 Armstrong, J. and West, J. The unsupported mother. (Description of students' project illustrated by cartoons of sources of help.) Midwives Chronicle, 90 (1073), Jun 1977, 144-146.

2 Bailey, D.J. and others The problems of one-parent families. (Survey by medical students from Charing Cross Hospital.) Midwife, Health Visitor and Community Nurse, 16 (3), Mar 1980, 102, 104, 108.

3 Corney, R.H. Group work with single parents—the consumer's viewpoint: participants' impressions. (Research study.) Health and Social Service Journal, 88, 22 Sep 1978, Centre eight papers D30-D32.

4 Ferri, E. and Robinson, H. Coping alone. NFER Publishing Co. for National Children's Bureau, 1976. (A National Children's Bureau report.)

5 Ferri, E. Growing up in a one-parent family—a long-term study of child development.

NFER Publishing Co., 1976. (A National Children's Bureau report.)

6 Green, M. Goodbye father. Routledge and Kegan Paul, 1976.

7 Mack, J. Children half alone. (The effect of one-parent life on children.) New Society, 38, 7 Oct 1976, 6-8.

8 Poole, C.J. Adolescent mothers: can they be helped? Paediatric Nursing, 2 (2), Mar/Apr 1976, 7-11.

9 Ritson, S. Gill—a mother at 15 years. (Family study by student HV of single mother and her baby.) Health Visitor, 52 (2), Feb 1979, 36-37, 43.

10 Rushton, A. and Winny, J. Group work with single parents—a single and separated parents' group. (Organised by social workers attached to a health centre.) Health and Social Service Journal, 88, 22 Sep 1978, Centre eight papers D27-D29.

11 Turner, J. The Gingerbread women. (Activities of Keighley Gingerbread.) New Society, 51, 14 Feb 1980, 339-340.

12 Turner, J. One-parent families: the undeserving poor? New Society, 45, 6 Jul 1978, 11-12.

13 Webb, D. compiler Finer report: action and inaction. The Government's record on implementing the Finer report. 2nd ed. National Council for One Parent Families, 1978. (Facts series no.1.)

f PROBLEM FAMILIES AND BATTERED WIVES

1 American Journal of Nursing The battered wife. (Two articles.) American Journal of Nursing, 78 (4), Apr 1978, 650-656.

2 Borland, M. editor Violence in the family. Manchester University Press, 1976.

3 Brandon, S. Violence in the family. Royal Society of Health Journal, 97 (5), Oct 1977, 201-205.

4 Cade, B. Family violence: an interactional view. Social Work Today, 9, 28 Feb 1978, 15-17.

5 Coote, A. and Gill, T. Battered women and the new law. Rev.ed. Inter-Action Inprint; National Council for Civil Liberties, 1979. (Inter-action guide; 1.)

6 Coward, A.M. Community nursing care study. A family at war. Nursing Times, 72, 9 Dec 1976, 1914-1916.

7 Daniels, R. Battered women—the role of Women's Aid refuges. Social Work Today, 9, 15 Nov 1977, 10-13.

8 Davies, J. Violence in the home. (The role of the nurse and health visitor in relation to child abuse, marital violence and granny-bashing.) Nursing Mirror, 146, 22 Jun 1978, 26-27.

9 Dobash, R. and Dobash, R. Wife beating—still a common form of violence. Social Work Today, 9, 15 Nov 1977, 14-16.

10 Fisher, E. Homeless families: a scheme of notification to ensure effective care. (Survey in

Kensington involving HVs as a result of which new system of notification evolved.) Nursing Times, 76, 3 Jul 1980, Occ. papers, 77-80.

11 Freeman, M.D.A. Violence in the home: a socio-legal study. Farnborough: Gower, 1979.

12 Gayford, J.J. Battered wives one hundred years ago. (History from 1521 to the present.) Practitioner, 219, Jul 1977, 122-128.

13 Harrisson, S.P. Families in stress: a study of the long-term medical treatment of children and parental stress. Royal College of Nursing, 1977. (Research series.)

14 Hartie, M. An eviction. (Community nursing care study of a 'problem family'.) Nursing Times, 72, 21 Oct 1976, 1635-1637.

15 Marcovitch, A. Refuges for battered women. (Work of Acton Women's Aid.) Social Work Today, 7, 15 Apr 1976, 34-35.

16 Martin, J.P. Violence and the family. Chichester: Wiley, 1978.

17 Mitchell, A.R.K. Violence in the family. Hove: Wayland, 1978.

18 National Women's Aid Federation The existing research into battered women. The Federation, 1976.

19 Open University The battered wife. (Excerpt from course on conflict in the family.) Nursing Times, 76, 11 Sep 1980, Community Outlook 264.

20 Pahl, J. A refuge for battered women: a study of the role of a women's centre. HMSO, 1978.

21 Parker, B. Communicating with battered wives. Topics in Clinical Nursing, 1 (3), Oct 1979, 49-53.

22 Renvoize, J. Web of violence: a study of family violence. Routledge and Kegan Paul, 1978.

23 Richards, I.D. and others A hundred vulnerable families. (Study of medical and social needs of families in Glasgow.) Public Health, 93 (1), Jan 1979, 16-24.

24 Robb, G and Moore, J.G. The yo-yo syndrome and the community. (Study of the effects on children in 23 violent matrimonial cases.) Community Health, 8 (2), Oct 1976, 79-81.

25 Royal Society of Health 'Disorganisation can kill.' (Symposium on violence in the home.) Nursing Times, 72, 4 Mar 1976, 319.

26 Select Committee on Violence in the Family First report: session 1975-76. Battered wives. First report: session 1976-1977. Violence to children. Vol.1 Report. Vol.2 Evidence. Vol.3 Appendices. Second report: session 1976-77. Battered wives. HMSO, 1976-1977. Summary of first report 1976-77 in Nursing Mirror, 144, 23 Jun 1977, 5.

27 Select Committee on Violence in the Family Minutes of evidence 18 May 1976: Health Visitors Association, Royal College of Nursing, Association of British Paediatric Nurses. HMSO, 1976.

28 Smith, J. Antidote to violence. (Analysis of report of the Select Committee on Violence in the Family.) Health and Social Service Journal, 87, 2 Sep 1977, 1239.

29 WIFE batterers. (Men's Aid—set up by Chiswick Women's Aid for helping husbands.) New Society, 37, 19 Aug 1976, 400-401.

g WOMEN'S ROLE AND THE FAMILY

1 Beresford, S.A.A. Why do women consult doctors? Social factors and the use of the general practitioner. British Journal of Preventive and Social Medicine, 31 (4), Dec 1977, 220-226.

2 Blair, P. Are women's hospitals necessary? Health and Social Service Journal, 85, 20/27 Dec 1975, 2790-2791.

3 Evans, M. and Morgan, D. Work on women: a guide to the literature. Tavistock, 1979. (Social science paperbacks.)

4 Kitzinger, S. Women as mothers. Oxford: Martin Robertson, 1978.

5 Klein, R. Removing the veils that surround women's health. (Growing concern among women about discrimination in health service provision.) Health and Social Service Journal, 89, 27 Apr 1979, 484-485.

6 Kush-Goldberg, C. The health self help group as an alternative source of health care for women. (Research study including seeking members' attitudes towards nurse involvement in groups.) International Journal of Nursing Studies, 16 (3), Aug 1979, 283-294.

7 New Society Women and their role: articles from 'New Society'. New Society, 1976.

8 New Society Woman's place. New Society, 46, 9 Nov 1978 Society Today i-iv.

9 New Society Woman's role. New Society, 46, 23 Nov 1978 Society Today i-iv.

10 Splane, V.H. World Conference on International Women's Year. (An official ICN observer's report.) International Nursing Review, 23 (2), Mar/Apr 1976, 57-59.

11 Stacey, M. editor Health and the division of labour. Croom Helm, 1977. (Explorations in sociology series, no.10.)

12 Thoms, P. The role of women over three centuries. Australian Nurses Journal, 6 (3), Sep 1976, 30-33.

13 World Health Issue on a decade for women 1976-1985. World Health, Aug-Sep 1976, 3-43.

14 World Health Women, health and development. (Eight articles.) World Health, Jun 1980, 3-29.

35 DISTRICT NURSING

a GENERAL

1 Aish, A. Not all patients need hospitals. (Description of British district nursing service by a Canadian nurse who worked here during sabbatical leave.) Canadian Nurse, 75 (3), Mar 1979, 23-25.

2 Ashton, K. Community nursing in Scotland

...the reality. (Comments on Scottish Health Service Studies No.37. Work study of district nursing staff.) Nursing Times, 73, 27 Jan 1977, 119.

3 Carroll, S.J. District v ward: a comparison of nurses in both environments. (By a student nurse.) Nursing Mirror, 146, 27 Apr 1978, 41.

4 Dancer, M. Developments in district nursing. (Evaluation of programme of nursing in Hampshire, Wiltshire, Dorset and the Isle of Wight.) Nursing Times, 73, 5 May 1977, 666-668.

5 Frost, D. The district nurse. Nursing Times, 72, 27 May 1976 Community Care Supplement v, vii, viii.

6 Gee, J.L. and Gee, R.C. Handbook of community nursing (district nursing.) The authors, 1980.

7 General Practice Team District nurse or nurse practitioner? General Practice Team, 57, Oct/Nov 1976, 14.

8 Greaves, R. and Dodd, P.A. In praise of geographical working. (District nursing service in Barnsley.) Journal of Community Nursing, 3 (12), Jun 1980, 22-23.

9 Hicks, D. Home nurses and home nursing. Contained in Hicks, D. Primary health care: a review. HMSO, 1976. Chapter xi, 299-359.

10 Hockey, L. District nursing today—the obstacles and opportunities. (Based on lecture, with reference to SHHD report on district nursing in Scotland.) Nursing Mirror, 147, 16 Nov 1978, 58-60.

11 Hockey, L. A study of district nursing: the development and progression of a long-term research programme. PhD thesis, City University, Dept. of Social Science and Humanities, Mar 1979.

12 Hopson, B. Queer individual moves on. (Personal experiences of a district nurse.) Nursing Mirror, 142, 29 Jan 1976, 65-66.

13 Howell, J.F. and Bottoms, D. Case load—with a difference. (Development in East Surrey Health District of district nurses' bag to carry CSSD equipment.) Nursing Mirror, 146, 29 Jun 1978, 39-40.

14 Jordan, P. District nurse. Weidenfeld and Nicolson, 1977.

15 Keywood, O. Extension of nurse duties. (Suggests district nurse could do some chiropody and physiotherapy.) Nursing Mirror, 146, 5 Jan 1978, 40.

16 Kratz, C. Letter from Australia. 5. Enthusiasm and innovation. (District nursing services.) Nursing Times, 76, 13 Mar 1980, 478-479.

17 Kratz, C. Out in the cold. (Recent publications with worrying implications for district nurses—DHSS circular on aspects of Briggs, the Court report and the report of the Working Party on District Nurse Training.) Nursing Times, 73, 10 Feb 1977, 186.

18 Kratz, C. Towards district nursing. (Comment on SHHD's report on district nursing in Scotland.) Nursing Times, 74, 11 May 1978 Community Outlook 125.

19 Lake, T. SOS...patients in distress.

(Three groups of patients with emotional problems with whom the district nurse may have contact.) Nursing Mirror, 151, 11 Sep 1980 Supplement xi-xiv.

20 Lamb, A. Changing patterns of community care must be firmly founded on teamwork. (Report of district nurse tutors' conference.) Nursing Times, 74, 23 Mar 1978, 480.

21 Lightowlers, J. Men under the microscope. (Interviews with two male district nurses.) Journal of Community Nursing, 1 (6), Dec 1977, 25.

22 Martin, A. The nurse and the law. The unacceptable patient. (The district nurse and heavy or helpless patients.) Journal of Community Nursing, 4 (1), Jul 1980, 7.

23 O'Hare, E. The gingerbread man. (Use of pictorial tool by district nurses for assessment of patient.) Nursing Times, 76, 21 Feb 1980, 318-320.

24 Potter, D. and Hockey, L. The work of district nurses in England. University of Edinburgh Nursing Research Unit, 1976.

25 Queen's Nursing Institute Nursing in the community. Rev.ed. The Institute, 1976.

26 Queen's Nursing Institute Nursing in the community. (The work of the district nurse.) Nursing Mirror, 144, 14 Apr 1977, Supplement i-iii, v, vii, ix.

27 QUEEN'S Nursing Institute—pattern for the future. (Five items on the functions of the QNI.) Queen's Nursing Journal, 19 (6), Sep 1976, 158-162.

28 Robbottom, B.M. District nursing in the 1980s. Nursing Focus, 2 (4), Dec 1980, 118-119.

29 Royal College of Nursing. Society of Primary Health Care Nursing 'The Rcn and the district nurse': a precis of Rcn comments 1977. Rcn, 1977.

30 Scottish Home and Health Department District nursing in Scotland. Edinburgh: HMSO, 1978. Summary in Nursing Times, 74, 23 Mar 1978, 478.

31 Spicer, J. The district nurse as a life-saver. Nursing, 15, Jul 1980, 644-646.

32 Spicer, J. Practice in squalor. (The application of aseptic technique in poor home conditions.) Community View, 5, May 1980, 8-9.

33 White, C.M. A study of some of the factors influencing the district nurse's decision to discharge patients from her care. MSc thesis, Manchester University, Department of Nursing, 1979.

34 Yarnold, M.W. and Billings, J.E. A new district nursing case. (A case designed by district nurses at Macclesfield.) Queen's Nursing Journal, 19 (2), May 1976, 48.

b EDUCATION AND TRAINING

1 Batley, N. Miss Batley sets the record straight on district nurses. (Full text of letter from Director of CETHV on its position on district nurse education.) Nursing Times, 73, 8 Dec 1977, 1894.

2 Brooks, R. District nurses want action. (Report on meeting in Glasgow about campaign for statutory committee and speech by Charlotte Kratz.) Nursing Mirror, 145, 20 Oct 1977, 7.

3 Carr, A. Beyond the brief. (Conference paper on the Panel of Assessors' report on education and training of district nurses.) Nursing Times, 73, 10 Mar 1977, 328-329.

4 Carr, A.J. District nurse training in the 1980s. Address given at the Annual Open Meeting of the Queen's Nursing Institute. Nursing Mirror, 145, 3 Nov 1977, 45-47; Journal of Community Nursing, 1 (6), Dec 1977, 4-6.

5 Carr, A.J. DNs' training. (Letter from chairman of Working Party on the Education and Training of District Nurses welcoming DHSS' acceptance of new curriculum.) Nursing Times, 74, 26 Oct 1978, 1767.

6 Cawdell, A.E. and Swyer, C. The experiment that failed. (Educational exercise for hospital medical staff who accompanied district nurses to learn about poor home conditions of geriatric patients.) Journal of Community Nursing, 1 (7), Jan 1978, 22-23.

7 Chapple, M. An act for the future. (National District Nursing Campaign during passage of Nurses, Midwives, and Health Visitors Bill.) Community View, Sep 1979, 2-3.

8 Community Outlook Special report outlining the main events shaping district nurse training over the past 30 years. Nursing Times, 73, 15 Sep 1977, 1420-1421.

9 Crichton, M.S. and Walsh, A. There's a big wide world outside nursing. (Description by two district nurse practical work teachers of the City and Guilds 730 Further Education Certificate.) Journal of Community Nursing, 2 (3), Sep 1978, 7-8, 26.

10 Cottrell, M.T. Recent Briggs' proposals and the district nurse. (Letter.) Queen's Nursing Journal, 19 (5), Aug 1975, 138.

11 Damant, M. District nurse training. Prospecting for the future. (A new training syllabus.) Nursing Times, 75, 12 Apr 1979 Community Outlook 100, 102.

12 Dancer, M. The practical work teacher—role and preparation. Nursing Mirror, 145, 8 Sep 1977, 43-44.

13 Dancer, M. Teaching in the practical situation—1. Selection and preparation for practical work teaching. Queen's Nursing Journal, 19 (11), Feb 1977, 307.

14 Dancer, M. and Rumbold, G. Education and the district nurse. 4. Selection of district nurses: the tutor's role. Journal of Community Nursing, 4 (6), Dec 1980, 8, 10, 13.

15 Department of Health and Social Security Panel of Assessors for District Nurse Training. Curriculum in district nursing for state registered nurses and registered general nurses. DHSS, 1978.

16 Department of Health and Social Security. Panel of Assessors for District Nurse Training Report on the education and training of district nurses. DHSS, 1976. Comment in Nursing Times, 72, 16 Dec 1976, 1944.

17 Elliott, A. and others District nurse training. (History and outline curriculum of new training course.) Journal of the Royal College of General Practitioners, 30, Feb 1980, 69-70, 74.

18 Elliott, A. District nurses: new training proposals. (Comment by a GP and brief history of district nurse training.) British Medical Journal, 2, 4 Nov 1978, 1316.

19 Friend, P. CNO clarifies position on training. (Full text of letter on DHSS position on training and qualification of district nurses.) Nursing Times, 73, 3 Nov 1977, 1695.

20 Gastrell, P. Teaching in the practical situation—2. Preparation of field staff for teaching responsibilities. Queen's Nursing Journal, 19 (12), Mar 1977, 333-334.

21 Gibson, S. A critique of the 'objectives model of curriculum design' applied to the education and training of district nurses. Journal of Advanced Nursing, 5 (2), Mar 1980, 161-167.

22 Gibson, S. and Jarvis, P. Training for practice. (Outline of the University of Surrey's education and training for district nursing.) Nursing Times, 74, 10 Aug 1978 Community Outlook 233, 235, 237.

23 Green, J. The role of the nursing officer in district nurse training. Nursing Times, 75, 12 Apr 1979 Community Outlook 102, 104, 106.

24 Hall, C.M. 'Concern'. (Full text of letter from Catherine Hall to Roland Moyle, re the refusal to set up statutory committee on district nursing training.) Nursing Mirror, 145, 25 Aug 1977, 41; Extracts in Nursing Times, 73, 18 Aug 1977, 1260.

25 Hall, C.M. Breakthrough. (Full text of second letter to Roland Moyle re district nurses' campaign and correspondence.) Nursing Times, 73, 29 Sep 1977, 1496-1497; Nursing Mirror, 145, 6 Oct 1977, 49.

26 Hansard District nurses training.
Possible statutory qualifications. 5 Jul 1977, WA 477.
Briggs Co-ordinating Committee. Terms of reference. 22 Nov 1977, WA 663.
Statutory recognition. 11 Nov 1977, WA 282; 14 Nov 1977, WA 54-55; 15 Nov 1977, WA 122; 22 Nov 1977, WA 658-659; 5 Dec 1977, WA 517; 13 Dec 1977, WA 151-152.

27 Harstedt, L. and Jemmott, A. Direct entrants to district nurse training in Kent. Queen's Nursing Journal, 19 (9), Dec 1976, 249-250.

28 Harstedt, L. Kent's blueprint for the 1980s. (Pilot scheme of district nurse training in Kent.) Nursing Mirror, 149, 5 Jul 1979, 26-29.

29 Illing, M. Introduction to a series on education. (Of district nurses, aimed at potential teachers.) Nursing Mirror, 145, 1 Sep 1977, 35-36.

30 Illing, M. A small ray of hope. (Response to refusal of Minister of Health to set up a Statutory Committee for district nurses.) Nursing Mirror, 145, 4 Aug 1977, 33.

31 Jarvis, P. Assessment as a teaching tool. (Assessment by practical work teachers of district nurse students.) Journal of Community Nursing, 2 (10), Apr 1979, 13-14.

32 Jarvis, P. District nurse examiners—how do they score? (Data from marking workshop during a study day for district nurse examiners.) Nursing Times, 74, 9 Mar 1978 Community Outlook 68-69.

33 Journal of Community Nursing Round up. Just keep on rocking the boat. (District nurses' campaign for statutory committee.) Journal of Community Nursing, 1 (4), Oct 1977, 7, 12.

34 Kratz, C. District nurses' campaign. (Letter explaining events at the June 8 meeting of the District Nursing Action Campaign Committee.) Nursing Times, 74, 29 Jun 1978, 1091.

35 Kratz, C. Same again. The background to the current controversy on district nurse training. Nursing Times, 74, 8 Sep 1977 Community Outlook 52-53.

36 Lightowlers, J. The report that is still top secret. (Report of the working party to the Panel of Assessors for District Nurse Training.) Journal of Community Nursing, 1 (1), Jul 1977, 20.

37 Lovett, R.M. Assessment: a many headed process. (Of district nurse students.) Nursing Mirror, 146, 15 Jun 1978, 41-42.

38 MacKenzie, A. Monitoring practical experience in district nurse training. (Record book for students used in Essex AHA.) Nursing Times, 76, 31 Jan 1980, 210-212.

39 McKerrow, E. editor The education and training of district nurses. Bolton College of Education (Technical), 1977.

40 Miller, P. A sign of the times. (New curriculum for and definitions of role of district nurses developed by Panel of Assessors' Working Party.) Nursing Mirror, 151, 11 Sep 1980 Supplement i-ii.

41 Mills, A.R. Before the door is closed... the case for a statutory committee. (By Div NO who gave oral evidence to Briggs Working Group 4.) Journal of Community Nursing, 1 (12), Jun 1978, 16-17.

42 Moyle, R. Lagging legislation—recent releases from the statutory saga. (Letters from Roland Moyle and Chairman of the Panel of Assessors for District Nurse Training on the Briggs Bill.) Nursing Mirror, 146, 1 Jun 1978, 43.

43 Moyle, R. Thumbs down on DN statutory committee in Briggs structure: 'Intolerably rigid' Minister tells panel. (Includes full text of letters from Roland Moyle.) Nursing Mirror, 145, 28 Jul 1977, 35.

44 Nursing Mirror District nurses must not be left behind. (Summaries of evidence submitted by QNI and DNA to Briggs Coordinating Committee—Working Group 4.) Nursing Mirror, 146, 9 Feb 1978, 41-42.

45 Nursing Mirror Nurses declare war on Moyle's decision. (Report of Rcn open meeting of district nurses. Editorial comment on p.1. Report of delegation.) Nursing Mirror, 145, 15 Sep 1977, 2; 20 Oct 1977, 2.

46 Nursing Times DN training. (Correspondence on proposed statutory body.) Nursing Times, 73, 4 Aug 1977, 1199-1200.

47 Nursing Times Save district nursing. (Report of Campaign for Statutory Committee.) Nursing Times, 73, 6 Oct 1977, 1534-1535.

48 Price, I. A key role for the practical work

teacher. Nursing Mirror, 145, 10 Nov 1977, 43-46.

49 Price, I. Practical work teachers courses 1975: a subjective review. Queen's Nursing Journal, 19 (5), Aug 1976, 141-142.

50 Prince, J. The proposed new district nurse education and training. (Guide to the Report from the Panel of Assessors for District Nurse Training.) Midwife, Health Visitor and Community Nurse, 14 (1), Jan 1978, 18-19.

51 Prince, J. Psychology for district nurses. (Significance in district nurse training.) Queen's Nursing Journal, 18 (11), Feb 1976, 301-302.

52 Queen's Nursing Institute Statutory training committee. (Full text of statement by QNI on Minister's refusal to appoint Statutory Committee for district nurses.) Nursing Mirror, 145, 18 Aug 1977, 37.

53 Queen's Nursing Journal Reflections on district nurse training. A layman looks at developments during the past thirty years. Queen's Nursing Journal, 19 (15), Jun 1977, 426-427.

54 Robottom, B. The district nursing voice on Briggs, by D. Wilson. (Interview with Barbara Robottom, the only district nurse on the Briggs Cooordinating Committees.) Journal of Community Nursing, 1 (2), Aug 1977, 23.

55 Robottom, B. From conception to birth— a long labour. (Background to development of new syllabus for district nurse training, with outline curriculum.) Journal of Community Nursing, 4 (3), Sep 1980, 4-6, 30.

56 Robottom, B.M. Integration of theory and practice. (In curricula for district nurse education and training.) Nursing Mirror, 145, 1 Sep 1977, 36-38.

57 Ruddick-Bracken, H. Advanced training for the district nurse? (Implications of six-month training.) Nursing Mirror, 147, 9 Nov 1978, 46.

58 Ruddick-Bracken, H. New course, new scope, new prestige. (Comment on new subjects in curriculum for district nurse training.) Nursing Mirror, 151, 11 Sep 1980 Supplement xxvii-xxviii.

59 Rumbold, G. Teaching in the practical situation—3. The tutor's role in developing the skills of the PWT. Queen's Nursing Journal, 19 (13), Apr 1977, 369.

60 Sharman, R.L. District nurse tutors— selection and preparation. Nursing Mirror, 145, 29 Sep 1977, 43-44.

61 Waddison, P.E. From report to reality. (Problems associated with implementing the Panel of Assessors' report on district nurse training.) Nursing Times, 73, 17 Mar 1977, 366-367.

62 Wilson, D. District nurses go to college. (Plans for district nursing courses reported to the annual meeting of district nurse tutors.) Journal of Community Nursing, 3 (11), May 1980, 13, 25.

63 Young, E.J. The teaching process. (With reference to the role of the district nurse tutor.) Nursing Times, 76, 3 Apr 1980, 605-606.

c MANAGEMENT AND STAFFING

1 Goldstone, L.A. and Worrall, J. The problems of variations in work patterns of district nurses. (With reference to authors' study in Wigan.) Nursing Times, 76, 24 Apr 1980, Occ. papers, 45-51.

2 Harris, E. and Jones, R.V.H. District nurses: how many in AD 2000? (Research study to discover the amount of home nursing needed by different age groups.) Nursing Mirror, 145, 11 Aug 1977, 35-36.

3 Keywood, O. Where duties overlap. (Need for guidance on where district nurse's duties end and others, eg home help and relative—begin.) Nursing Mirror, 146, 9 Mar 1978, 43.

4 McIntosh, J.B. Decision making on the district. (Based on time and observation study of registered and enrolled district nurses.) Nursing Times, 75, 19 Jul 1979, Occ. papers, 77-80.

5 McIntosh, J.B. Making the best use of time. (Work of district nurse and practice nurse in treatment room.) Nursing Mirror, 149, 9 Aug 1979, 32-33.

6 McIntosh, J.B. and Richardson, I.M. Work study of district nursing staff. Scottish Home and Health Department, 1976. (Scottish health service studies no.37.)

7 McIntosh, J.B. Community nursing. Record keeping—a boon or a bind? (District nurses' records.) Nursing Mirror, 147.
1. Record content. 6 Jul 1978, 43-44.
2. Nurses'. views. 13 Jul 1978, 39-40.
3. The way forward. 20 Jul 1978, 36-37.

8 Mills, A.R. Management of the home nursing service. Nursing Mirror, 145, 20 Oct 1977, 43-44.

9 Nimmo, A.W. Treatment room work: an analysis. (Survey of how district nurses used their time in three treatment rooms with discussion of the findings' implications for staffing.) Nursing Times, 74, 28 Sep 1978, Occ. papers, 109-112; 5 Oct 1978, Occ. papers, 113-116.

10 Ross, F. Primary health care in Thamesmead. (Research study of district nurse's work in homes and at the health centre.) Nursing Times, 76, 24 Jul 1980, Occ. papers, 81-84; 7 Aug 1980, Occ. papers, 85-87.

11 Sartain, B. Community (home) nurse workload monitoring. (In Southampton.) Health Services Manpower Review, 3 (4), Nov 1977, 21-23.

12 Watts, D.E. District nurses in East Birmingham health district: a study of their work. (A survey of one week's activities of 42 nurses.) Nursing Times, 72, 11 Nov 1976, Occ. papers, 157-160; 18 Nov 1976, Occ. papers, 161-164.

13 Whitaker, M.S.R. A district nurse work analysis: a method of measuring work and staff levels. (Scheme tested in Mid-Oxon Sector.) Nursing Times, 73, 21 Jul 1977, Occ. papers, 97-100.

14 Williams, A. and Anderson, R. Provision of district nurse services at minimum cost contained in Williams, A. and Anderson, R. Efficiency in the social services. Blackwell, 1975. Chapter 2, 9-16.

15 Worrall, J. A general study of district nursing in Wigan. (Work study based on completed diary sheets to develop management information system for service planning.) Nursing Times, 76, 28 Feb 1980, Occ. papers, 21-26.

d NIGHT NURSING SERVICE

1 Bracken, A. In the small dark hours. (Setting-up of a community night nursing service in Northumberland AHA.) Nursing Mirror, 148, 1 Mar 1979, 43.

2 Hornby, A. 24 hour community nursing—a pilot scheme in the Lancaster area. Nursing Times, 72, 18 Mar 1976, 428-429.

3 Hubbard, P. The battle of Hastings. (Description of Hastings Health District night nursing service, with SNO's views by Carrie Paxton.) Journal of Community Nursing, 4 (1), Jul 1980, 4-6.

4 Jack, M. A home night nursing service. (Aberdeen.) Nursing Times, 72, 23 Sep 1976, Occ. papers, 140.

5 McBeath, C.M. Small is beautiful—and it works! (Setting up of night sitter service in North Lothian District.) Journal of Community Nursing, 3 (1), Jul 1979, 13-14.

6 NURSING at night. (Enfield's district night nursing service.) Community View, 7, Sep 1980, 11-12.

36 HEALTH VISITING

a GENERAL

1 Batley, N. Prevention and health. (Letter on drop in health visitor recruitment and need for shift of emphasis by Government towards preventive medicine.) British Medical Journal, 2, 20 Aug 1977, 522.

2 Beech, C. Health visiting in a changing society. Nursing, 15, Jul 1980, 639-641.

3 Bolton, G. Prevention: an exploratory study of health visiting in England, Wales and Scotland. Health Visitor, 53 (6), Jun 1980, 203-206.

4 British Medical Journal Health visitors of the future. (Summary and comment on the CETHV's 'An investigation into the principles of health visiting'.) British Medical Journal, 2, 29 Jul 1978, 308-309.

5 Castle, A.J. Towards an educational model of health visiting. (How HVs can use problem-solving approach in helping clients.) Health Visitor, 53 (1), Jan 1980, 9-10.

6 Chapel, L.M. Yet another definition of health. (With reference to the aims of health visiting.) Health Visitor, 52 (3), Mar 1979, 79-82.

7 Chapel, L.M. Health visiting: where do we go from here? (With reference to the CETHV's report.) Nursing Mirror, 147, 24 Aug 1978, 36-38.

8 Clark, J. The role of the health visitor: a study conducted in Berkshire, England. Journal of Advanced Nursing, 1 (1), Jan 1976, 25-36.

9 Clode, D. In search of an identity. (Reprint of extracts from an earlier article on problems health visitors face.) Health and Social Service Journal, 88, 27 Oct 1978, 1220-1221.

10 **Clode, D.** Of primary concern... (Professional identity crisis in health visiting.) Health and Social Service Journal, 88, 12 May 1978, 538-540.

11 **Community Outlook** HVs—question or challenge? (Need for HVs to demonstrate their effectiveness and evaluate visits.) Nursing Times, 75, 12 Jul 1979 Community Outlook 201.

12 **Community Outlook** HVs—starting research. (Problems experienced as discussed at South Bank Polytechnic workshop.) Nursing Times, 75, 12 Jul 1979 Community Outlook 203.

13 **Cotton, L.** The health visitor's contribution. (To the care of a fictitious family by the primary care team.) Nursing Mirror, 147, 5 Oct 1978 Supplement xi, xv-xvi.

14 **Council for the Education and Training of Health Visitors** An investigation into the principles of health visiting. The Council, 1977. Summary in Nursing Times Community Outlook, 74, 11 May 1978, 127-129.

15 **Council for the Education and Training of Health Visitors** Report of workshop on the principles and practice of health visiting, Nottingham University, 21-24 March 1976. CETHV, 1976.

16 **Court, D.** Dual role for HVs in Court report. Nursing Mirror, 143, 23 Dec 1976, 19.

17 **Cowell, A.** Health visiting objectives in Havering. Health Visitor, 53 (3), Mar 1980, 86, 88.

18 **Cowper-Smith, F.** Changes in health visiting. (History, discussion with polytechnic students and a day at a clinic in North London.) Nursing Times, 75, 12 Apr 1979, 615-618; 19 Apr 1979, 660-663.

19 **Davis, J.** How nice to see you, do come in. (Role of health visitor in supporting and listening to clients.) Health Visitor, 50 (6), Jun 1977, 182-183.

20 **Dawtry, E.** The health visitor in primary care: a general study of health visitors in two health centres and a detailed survey of their contrasting work patterns in one centre. MPhil thesis, CNAA (Polytechnic of North London, Medical Architecture Research Unit), 1976.

21 **Dingwall, R.** What future for health visiting? Evidence to the Royal Commission on the NHS. (Personal views based on research.) Nursing Times, 73, 2 Jun 1977, Occ. papers, 77-79.

22 **Dingwall, R. and Watson, P.** Pausing before a rush to change. (Need for evaluation before change to geographically-based health visiting from practice attachment.) Health and Social Service Journal, 90, 6 Jun 1980, 749-750.

23 **Dopson, L.** A case for courage. (Health visiting and school nursing aspects of the Lester Chapman case.) Nursing Times, 75, 1 Nov 1979, 1874.

24 **Farnese, M.** 'Belonging' in suburbia... (Formation of social group by HVs which became focus for community activities.) Nursing Mirror, 149, 20 Sep 1979, 38.

25 **Farnese, M.** The HV—an adviser on

grants? (Recent Ombudsman's ruling that health visitor is not obliged to advise on the attendance allowance.) Nursing Mirror, 148, 22 Mar 1979, 28.

26 **Fraser, M.** Health Visitors' Association annual study conference. 'Five formative years'—a new era for health visitors? Nursing Mirror, 143, 28 Oct 1976, 36-37.

27 **Goodwin, S.A.** Health visitors and the TUC. (HVA's affiliation with TUC.) Health Visitor, 51 (6), Jun 1978, 229.

28 **Hall, M.** Opportunity in health visiting. (Letter advocating a separate profession with direct entry.) British Medical Journal, 2, 9 Dec 1978, 1646.

29 **Harrison, S.P.** Compliance or non-compliance with treatment? (The role of the health visitor in influencing patients to comply with treatment illustrated by the cases of children with cystic fibrosis.) Health Visitor, 49 (3), Mar 1976, 78.

30 **Hawkins, V.C.** Health visiting in the Forces. (Work with Soldiers', Sailors' and Airmen's Families Association (SSAFA) in Germany.) Health Visitor, 52 (10), Oct 1979, 422, 426, 429.

31 **Health Visitors Association** Annual Conference. Report. Health Visitor, 50 (11), Nov 1977, 358-360, 362, 364, 367-368, 370-371, 373-374, 376; 51 (11), Nov 1978, 418-429.

32 **Health Visitors Association** Annual report. Health Visitor.
1975. 49 (7), Jul 1976, 229-240.
1976. 50 (7), Jul 1977, 226, 228, 232-240.
1977. 51 (7), Jul 1978, 257-264, 267, 269-272.
1978. 52 (8), Aug 1979, 330-339.
1979. 53 (7), Jul 1980, 274-279.

33 **Henderson, J.C.** Health visiting in Hampshire: a descriptive study of the day to day work of health visitors in Hampshire Area Health Authority and of the clientele served. MSc thesis in Educational Research, Surrey University, 1977.

34 **Hendry, J.** Lady from 'the welfare'. (A health visitor in Hackney describes her work.) New Society, 42, 22/29 Dec 1977, 622-624.

35 **Hicks, D.** Health visitors and health visiting. Contained in Hicks, D. Primary health care: a review. HMSO, 1976. Chapter X, 245-298.

36 **Hudson, R.** Jack of all trades? (Role of HV in general and with the elderly in particular.) Health and Social Service Journal, 88, 3 Mar 1978, 251.

37 **Jack, S.** An investigation into the principles of health visiting. (Comment on reactions to the report by chairman of the working party.) Health Visitor, 51 (12), Dec 1978, 463.

38 **Kendall, P.** The health visitor in court. Health Visitor, 51 (4), Apr 1978, 126-128.

39 **Keywood, O.** High rise problems. (Suggests having health visitors based in tower blocks.) Nursing Mirror, 146, 5 Jan 1978, 39.

40 **Kornreich, R.** The relevance of sociology to health visiting—which type of sociology? Which type of health visiting? Health Visitor, 50 (8), Aug 1977, 264-265.

41 **Kratz, C.** Talkingpoint. (On the CETHV's claims for health visiting's separate training and status.) Nursing Times, 73, 8 Dec 1977 Community Outlook 123.

42 **Luker, K.A.** Adjusting to being a health visitor. Nursing Times, 72 (39), 30 Sep 1976, HV Supplement, 22, 24, 26.

43 **Luker, K.A.** Goal attainment: a possible model for assessing the role of the health visitor. Nursing Times, 74, 27 Jul 1978, 1257-1259.

44 **McClymont, M.** Some quandaries facing the health visitor in these times of change. Contained in CIBA Foundation Health care in a changing setting: the UK experience. Amsterdam: Elsevier, 1976, 75-95.

45 **Mead, A.M.** The health visitor. Nursing Times, 72 (21), 27 May 1976 Community Care Supplement xi-xvii.

46 **Midwife, Health Visitor and Community Nurse** Help for health visitors. (Five letters describing clerical assistance.) Midwife, Health Visitor and Community Nurse, 13 (10), Oct 1977, 326-327.

47 **Morrow, M.** The HV—a professional friend. (General description of her work.) Nursing Mirror, 148, 28 Jun 1979, 28-29.

48 **Orr, J.** Health visiting in focus: a consumer view of health visiting in Northern Ireland. Rcn, 1980. (Rcn research series.) Based on 'Consumer perceptions of health visiting'. MSc thesis, University of Manchester, Department of Nursing, 1978.

49 **Owen, G.M. editor** Health visiting. Baillière Tindall, 1977.

50 **Ranson, B.H.A.** Health visiting: the personal touch or the professional image—which is more important? (The role and identity of the HV.) Health Visitor, 50 (8), Aug 1977, 258-261.

51 **Scott, C.S.** The relevance of sociology to health visitors. Health Visitor, 53 (6), Jun 1980, 212, 215.

52 **SCOTTISH HVA.** (Report on annual conference.) Nursing Times, 73, 11 Aug 1977 Community Outlook 5.

53 **Simpson, K.** The health visitor in court. (Letter describing experiences and calling for more legal advice for health visitors.) Health Visitor, 53 (6), Jun 1980, 223, 227.

54 **Spicer, F.** A support group for health visitors. (At London Youth Advisory Centre.) Health Visitor, 53 (9), Sep 1980, 377, 379.

55 **Swaffield, L.** Changing sides? (Report of HVA annual study conference.) Nursing Times, 73, 3 Nov 1977, 1700-1701.

56 **Swaffield, L.** So much to do... Some issues raised at the Health Visitors' Association Study Conference. Nursing Times, 72, 28 Oct 1976, 1662-1663.

57 **Thompson, J.** From conception to the grave. (Preventive role of the health visitor.) Nursing Mirror, 150, 3 Apr 1980, 28-29.

58 **Tucker, P.** Why not 'penalise' the health visitor? The health visitor has an enormous amount to offer in any community orientation of penal policy. Midwife, Health Visitor and Community Nurse, 14 (3), Mar 1978, 77-78.

59 Turner, M. A new look at health visiting. Nursing Times, 72, 1 Jul 1976, 1022-1023.

60 Turner, V. 'Health' visitors? (Definitions of health and the HV's role.) Health Visitor, 51 (3), Mar 1978, 82-83.

61 Venvell, D. The health visitor as a link between home and education. (With reference to links with educational home visitor schemes.) Health Visitor, 51 (6), Jun 1978, 215-216.

62 Walsworth-Bell, J.P. Patch-work: a study of the effect of geographical organisation, compared with attachment to a primary care team, on three aspects of health visitors' work. MSc thesis in Social Medicine, London University, 1978.

63 While, A.E. On becoming a health visitor. MSc dissert., CNAA, Polytechnic of the South Bank, 1980.

64 Whincup, M. Law report—duties of a health visitor. (The case of a health visitor dismissed for incompetence, especially poor record keeping.) Health Services Manpower Review, 6 (4), Nov 1980, 21-22.

65 Wightman, F. Health visiting in Belfast. Nursing Times, 72, 16 Dec 1976, 1964-1965.

b BRIGGS REPORT AND LEGISLATION

1 Batley, N. Big is beautiful. The director of the CETHV puts forward her personal views on a Briggs Bill. Nursing Times, 74, 9 Mar 1978, 389.

2 Batley, N. In company with the big battalions. (Problems of health visitor organisation following NHS reorganisation and the Briggs proposals.) Nursing Times, 72, 30 Sep 1976, 1502-1503.

c EDUCATION AND TRAINING

1 Anderson, A. Sociology in the health visitor's training. Health Visitor, 52 (5), May 1979, 185-187.

2 Batley, N. An alternative view. (Why the CETHV does not approve inclusion of HV tutor students on new Diploma in Nursing Education.) Nursing Times, 76, 25 Sep 1980, 1719-1720.

3 Batley, N. HV education and training. (Letter describing context of recent critical NFER report.) Nursing Mirror, 145, 7 Jul 1977, 8.

4 Chapman, V.A. The fieldwork teacher: an exploratory case study of the role of the fieldwork teacher. MSc thesis, Surrey University, 1979.

5 Chevannes-Reeves, M. Health visiting and health visiting courses: a health visitor looks at three sociologists' accounts. Health Visitor, 51 (2), Feb 1978, 40-41.

6 Council for the Education and Training of Health Visitors Issues in health visiting training. Nursing Times, 72, 30 Sep 1976 HV Supplement, 1.

7 Council for the Education and Training of Health Visitors Report of the working group on a revised curriculum for a certificate in fieldwork teaching. CETHV, 1977.

8 Davenport, J. Problems of a student health visitor. Nursing Times, 72, 30 Sep 1976 HV Supplement, 16, 18, 20, 22.

9 Dellar, C.J. The selection of students for a health visitors' training course: an interim investigation of the relationships between predictors in the selection procedure and performance on the course. MSc thesis, University of Aston in Birmingham, 1978.

10 Dingwall, R. The social organisation of health visitor training. Nursing Times, 72, 19 Feb 1976, Occ. papers, 25-28; 26 Feb 1976, Occ. papers, 29-32; 4 Mar 1976, Occ. papers, 33-36; 11 Mar 1976, Occ. papers, 37-40.

11 Dingwall, R. The social organisation of health visitor training. Croom Helm, 1977.

12 Fader, W. Qualifying procedures for health visitors. Windsor: NFER Publishing Co., 1976.

13 Hasler, J.C. and Klinger, M. Common ground in general practitioner and health visitor training—an experimental course. (Course organised by the Oxford Regional Health Authority at Milton Keynes College of Education to modify attitudes and increase knowledge of each other's work.) Journal of the Royal College of General Practitioners, 26, Apr 1976, 266-276.

14 Hindle, L. The fieldwork teacher. (Description of her work.) Nursing Times, 75, 13 Dec 1979 Community Outlook, 390-391.

15 Llewellyn, E.M. Student units—a new concept of health visitor training. Midwife, Health Visitor and Community Nurse, 12 (6), Jun 1976, 192-194.

16 Magill, E. A further education course for health visitors. (In psychiatric care for senior members of Greater Glasgow Health Board's staff.) Health Visitor, 53 (6), Jun 1980, 209, 211.

17 McClymont, M.E. Grouping field work teachers. (Health visiting course at Stevenage College of Further Education.) Nursing Times, 72, 30 Sep 1976, HV Supplement, 13-16.

18 McClymont, M.E. A study of selected health visitor schools to identify how they perceive their role in the preparation of health visitors for practice. MSc thesis, University of Manchester, Department of Nursing, Oct 1978.

19 O'Connell, P. Health visitor education at university: a developmental study of community nurse education at Southampton University 1948-1974. Royal College of Nursing, 1978. (Research series.)

20 O'Connell, P.E. The professional education of health visitors and their role in health care in Black, Sir D. and Thomas, G.P. editors Providing for the health services... Croom Helm, 1978, 47-57.

21 O'Sullivan, S.R. Thoughts on the course for health visitors. Nursing Times, 72 (47), 25 Nov 1976, Occ. papers, 165-168.

22 Scott, C. Teaching sociology to health visitor students. Health Visitor, 49 (12), Dec 1976, 399-400.

23 SURVEY into 'no access' visits by health visitors 1978. (Research study by students on HV fieldwork teachers course.) Health Visitor, 51 (10), Oct 1978, 404-405.

24 Tittmar, H.-G. and others Health visitor training. The moulding of health visitors. The evolved role played by mini-training. Health Visitor, 51 (4), Apr 1978, 130, 132-134.

25 Walters, M.J. A post registration course in health visitor training. Nursing Times, 72, 30 Sep 1976, HV Supplement, 7, 9, 11.

d MANAGEMENT AND STAFFING

1 Henderson, J. What do health visitors do? (Research study into the day-to-day work of the health visitor based on diary sheets.) Nursing Mirror, 147, 14 Sep 1978, 30-32.

2 McIlwain, A. Health visitor bank. (Letter describing the setting up of a bank in Bromley.) Health Visitor, 49 (1), Jan 1976, 12-13.

3 Mulholland, R.C. A performance appraisal scheme for health visitors. Nursing Times, 72, 22 Jul 1976, Occ. papers, 101-104.

4 Public Health How best can we deploy our health visitors? Public Health, 89 (6), Sep 1975, 243-246.

5 Robinson, J.A. Appraisal of health visitors. Nursing Times, 72, 30 Sep 1976, 1521.

6 Strehlow, M.S. Recruitments to health visiting. (Surveys of how students received information on health visiting carried out by the Council for the Education and Training of Health Visitors.) Nursing Times, 72, 30 Sep 1976, HV Supplement, 3, 5, 7.

7 Wiseman, J. Health visiting: the allocation problem. A research study to determine an approach for an allocation plan. MSc thesis, University of Lancaster, 1979.

37 SCHOOL HEALTH

a GENERAL

1 Bosanquet, N. End of term report. (Comments on the school health service 1908-1974, by the Department of Education and Science.) Nursing Times, 72, 25 Mar 1976, 440.

2 Brower, E.W. and Nash, C.L. Evaluating growth and posture in school-age children. (With photographs.) Nursing (U.S.), 9 (4), Apr 1979, 58-63.

3 Canadian Nurse A school screening program that works. (Early detection of adolescent idiopathic scoliosis.) Canadian Nurse, 73 (12), Dec 1977, 24-29.

4 Department of Education and Science Safety at school: general advice. 2nd ed. HMSO, 1979. (DES safety series; 6.)

5 Edwards, L. and Kelly, E. A three-level school health program. Nursing Outlook, 25 (6), Jun 1977, 388-391.

6 Gordon, R.R. 'All they ever do is measure them' (Importance of measuring school children's height to detect abnormally small stature.) Health Visitor, 52 (5), May 1979, 178-179.

7 Hardy, S.M. School health 1896-1921. (History of school in Suffolk from headmaster's log-book.) Health Visitor, 52 (9), Sep 1979, 362-363.

8 Hill, F. After-school care of children in first school. (Research study by HVs.) Health Visitor, 52 (11), Nov 1979, 463-465.

9 Iduna Schools and health. Health Visitor, 49 (4), Apr 1976, 118.

10 Jeanneret, O. and Raymond, L. Health statistics on children of school age. WHO Chronicle, 30 (3), Mar 1976, 101-107.

11 Lynch, G.W. The hungry child and his school performance. (Analysis of a national survey by the social nutrition unit, Queen Elizabeth College.) Health and Social Service Journal, 86, 24 Apr 1976, 761-762.

12 Morris, J.B. and Hird, M.D. Employment of local general practitioners in the school health service. (Pilot study in primary schools in Brechin City, Tayside.) Health Bulletin, 35 (3), May 1977, 119-128.

13 Morris, J.B. and Hird, M.D. School health service: review of 11 year old's screening programme. (In Angus District, Tayside Health Board.) Health Bulletin, 38 (4), Jul 1980, 153-159.

14 Orton, C. The child with a medical problem in the ordinary school. Home + School Council Public., 1979.

15 Radway, J. Trends in school health. Midwife, Health Visitor and Community Nurse, 16 (3), Mar 1980, 110, 112.

16 Rona, R.J. The National Study of Health and Growth (NSHG): surveillance on nutritional status of primary schoolchildren. Health Visitor, 53 (8), Aug 1980, 309, 311-312.

17 Thurmott, P. A history of the school health service. Nursing Times, 74, 12 Oct 1978, 1666-1667.

18 Tyrrell, S. Thoughts on the 'new look' school medical officer. (Role of the doctor in the school health team.) Public Health, 90 (3), Mar 1976, 127-130.

19 WHO Chronicle Problems of younger children of school age. WHO Chronicle, 30 (6), Jun 1976, 253-254.

20 World Health Organization Summary report of a working group on problems of children at school age III (14-18 years). (Seventeen conclusions and recommendations.) Journal of Advanced Nursing, 3 (2), Mar 1978, 215-217.

b HEALTH AND SEX EDUCATION

1 Bacon, C. and Doran, K. An experiment in health education in a Newcastle primary school. Health Education Journal, 39 (2), 1980, 58-59.

2 Bevis, R. The keep fit club. (Run by health visitor/school nurse with infant school children on healthy living.) Nursing Times, 75, 8 Nov 1979 Community Outlook, 361, 363.

3 Brunel University. Educational Studies Unit The role of the health visiting team in relation to secondary schools: Hillingdon Area Health Authority. Uxbridge: Brunel University, 1977.

4 Community Outlook Teenage health education. (Two articles on health education with fourth-formers.) Nursing Times, 76, 11 Dec 1980 Community Outlook, 375-377.

5 Department of Education and Science Health education in schools. HMSO, 1977.

6 Edelman, S.K. Sex and life education in a rural school. (Details of health education course by school nurse.) American Journal of Maternal-Child Nursing, 2 (4), Jul/Aug 1977, 234-239.

7 Engel, E. Health education in schools—a philosophical dilemma. Health Education Journal, 37 (4), 1978, 231-233.

8 Evans, M.W Background notes for the health visitor involved in school health education. Health Visitor, 50 (1), Jan 1977, 2-3.

9 Evans, M.W. Sex education—a co-operative venture. (Report of programme by health education officers based on junior school and involving parents.) Health Visitor, 51 (10), Oct 1978, 378.

10 Felstein, I. A consummation devoutly to be wished. (Nurses' role in sex education.) Midwife, Health Visitor and Community Nurse, 12 (4), Apr 1976, 127-128.

11 Guy, C.J. Health education in schools. Health Education Journal, 35 (3), 1976, 214-220.

12 Hiskins, G. Community help in health education. (Role of the health visitor in health education in schools.) Midwife, Health Visitor and Community Nurse, 14 (5), May 1978, 144-146.

13 Hiskins, G. Health education in schools and the community. Health Visitor, 49 (4), Apr 1976, 115-117.

14 Hubbard, K. Time—scheduled health: critique. (Problems of teaching health education to school children.) Health Education Journal, 35 (3), 1976, 208-211.

15 Langmaid, W.O. Health education in North Yorkshire Junior Schools. (Survey to investigate the extent of health education and the possible assistance of a Health Education Service.) Health Education Journal, 34 (4), 1975, 121-127.

16 McGuffin, S.J. Health knowledge and behaviour of fifth-formers. Health Education Journal, 38 (4), 1979, 107-110.

17 Pearson, R. and Lambert, L. Sex education, preparation for parenthood and the adolescent. (Data from National Child Development Study showing scope of sex education in schools.) Community Health, 9 (2), Nov 1977, 84-90.

18 Reid, D. What's new in schools? (In health education.) Nursing Times, 73, 23 Jun 1977, Health Education, 14, 17-18, 20.

19 Richardson, J. The health visitor, schools and teaching. Midwife, Health Visitor and Community Nurse, 16 (5), May 1980, 198, 201-202, 204.

20 Schools Council Health education at school—the future. (Schools Council project into health education for 13-18 age group.) Nursing Times, 75, 10 May 1979, Community Outlook, 141.

21 Schools Council. Working Party on Health Education Health education in secondary schools: an account of current practice. Evans/Methuen Educational, 1976. (Schools Council working paper 57.)

22 Silman, A.J. A survey of attitudes to health among school leavers. Health Education Journal, 38 (3), 1979, 88-91.

23 Thomas, S. 'Our baby' is growing nicely. (Health education class at a junior school including observation of babies and visits from health professionals.) Nursing Mirror, 150, 13 Mar 1980, 20-22.

24 Thomson, W. Health education—5. Let's start at school. Nursing Times, 74, 12 Oct 1978, 1692-1693.

25 Thorpe, W.R. Health education and the schoolchild. Midwife, Health Visitor and Community Nurse, 12 (11), Nov 1976, 359-560.

26 Toluhi, J.O. A guide to health education for primary teachers. Evans Brothers, 1976.

27 Walshe-Brennan, K.S. The role of the health visitor in sexual development. Health Visitor, 49 (12), Dec 1976, 392-394.

c NURSING

1 Bromelow, I. Strangest job in the NHS? (Area nurse, child health/school health.) Nursing Times, 72, 5 Feb 1976, 196.

2 Brown, M. Secondary school nursing: a changing focus. Canadian Nurse, 73 (10), Oct 1977, 42-45.

3 Community Outlook School nurses. (Five articles including history and current role.) Nursing Times, 74, 12 Oct 1978, Community Outlook, 289, 291, 293, 295, 297-298, 300-301, 303-304.

4 Conrad, J. The high school nurse as a pediatric nurse practitioner. Pediatric Nursing, 1 (6), Nov/Dec 1975, 15-17.

5 Davis, A. and others A school health teaching elective. (One month clinical experience for nursing students.) Nursing Outlook, 25 (10), Oct 1977, 637-639.

6 Gastrell, P. Training scheme for school nurses. (Experimental course organised by Hampshire AHA.) Nursing Mirror, 146, 20 Apr 1978, 37-38.

7 Health Visitor The school nurse. (Editorial.) Health Visitor, 50 (9), Sep 1977, 287.

8 Holt, S.J. and Robinson, T.M. The school nurse's 'Family Assessment Tool'. (Developed in Boulder, Colorado and based on home visit.) American Journal of Nursing, 79 (5), May 1979, 950-953.

9 McAtee, P.R. New directions in school health: school nurse practitioners. Pediatrics, 4 (2), Mar/Apr 1978, 29-31.

10 Nash, W.E. School nurses. (Letter on duties and salary.) Health Visitor, 50 (8), Aug 1977, 267-268.

11 Pendle, A. Long term relationships: the work of the community staff nurse. (With school children in catchment area of health clinic, with special reference to audiology.) Nursing Times, 73, 15 Dec 1977, 1971-1972.

12 Quin, P. Nursing in a girls' school. Nursing Mirror, 142, 27 May 1976, 71.

13 Riches, B. School nursing—a personal

view. (History and current role.) Nursing Times, 76, 11 Sep 1980, Community Outlook, 250, 252, 255.

14 Slack, P.A. School nursing: a basic introduction to nursing in primary and secondary education. Baillière Tindall, 1978.

15 Slack, P. School nursing in the USA. Nursing Times, 76.
1. An American approach to school health. 28 Feb 1980, 365-366.
2. The nurse practitioner in the schools. 6 Mar 1980, 420-421.
3. Aspects of clinical practice and management. 13 Mar 1980, 468-469.
4. Special education. 20 Mar 1980, 521-522.
5. Lessons we can learn. 27 Mar 1980, 557-558.

16 Smiley, O.R. Public health nurses and teachers in school health programmes: a problem in communication. International Nursing Review, 23 (5), Sep-Oct 1976, 141-143.

17 Society of Area Nurses. Child Health. Working Party on the School Nursing Service Review of the school nursing service, May 1980. Newcastle upon Tyne: Newcastle Health Authority, 1980.

18 Thurmott, P. Health and the school: an exploratory survey of the school nursing service in an English county. Royal College of Nursing, 1976. Rcn Research Society summary in Nursing Times, 74, 26 Jan 1978, Occ. papers, 12.

d HEAD INFESTATION

1 British Medical Journal Oust the louse. (Current treatment procedures.) British Medical Journal, 2, 22 Oct 1977, 1043-1044.

2 Community Outlook What happened at Humberside. A review of Humberside AHA's pilot scheme of 1976. (For eradication of head lice, organised by Health Education Council.) Nursing Times, 73, 8 Sep 1977, Community Outlook, 50-51.

3 Donaldson, R.J. The head louse in England: prevalence amongst schoolchildren. Royal Society of Health Journal, 96 (2), Apr 1976, 55-57.

4 Donaldson, R.J. Head infestation. Nursing Mirror, 144, 20 Jan 1977, 56-57.

5 Donaldson, R.J. Head infestation—a persistent problem. Health Visitor, 51 (9), Sep 1978, 336-337.

6 England, P.M. A health education campaign against the head louse. (In Humberside AHA.) Health Education Journal, 36 (2), 1977, 42-45.

7 Health Education Council Head infestation fact sheet. (Produced in context of Health Education Council's campaign.) Nursing Times, 73, 8 Sep 1977, Community Outlook, 48-49.

8 Horridge, D. The louse war. (The role of the community nurse in health education and prevention.) Nursing Mirror, 144, 20 Jan 1977, 56-59.

9 Krushner, J.A. Farewell to lice. (Methods of treatment.) Journal of Community Nursing, 1 (2), Aug 1977, 26.

10 Krushner, J.A. Head lice—a growing

problem. Queen's Nursing Journal, 18 (12), Mar 1976, 325.

11 Preston, S. and Fry, L. Malathion lotion and shampoo: a comparative trial in the treatment of head lice. (In City and Hackney Health District, involving school nurses.) Royal Society of Health Journal, 97 (6), Dec 1977, 291.

12 Priddy, R.F. Head lice infestation—a practical approach. Queen's Nursing Journal, 19 (11), Feb 1977, 308-309, 316.

13 Slack, P. Head infestation. Nursing Times, 72, 12 Feb 1976, 225-227.

38 SOCIAL PROBLEMS

a GENERAL

1 Bosanquet, N. Inside the social services. Young offenders. Nursing Times, 73, 29 Sep 1977, 1528-1529.

2 Darnborough, D. and Gilrea, D. The caring crypt. (Medical care of homeless men at St. George's Crypt, Leeds.) Nursing Mirror, 147, 30 Nov 1978, 56-57.

3 Fidler, J. Loneliness—the problems of the elderly and retired. Royal Society of Health Journal, 96 (1), Feb 1976, 39-41, 44.

4 Fogg, N. Vagrancy in London. Midwife, Health Visitor and Community Nurse, 12 (10), Oct 1976, 326-328, 330.

5 Foster, J. Loneliness: the group solution to isolation. The success of two groups set up three years ago for lonely people in Hampshire. Nursing Mirror, 147, 12 Oct 1978, 28-29.

6 Francis, G.M. Loneliness: measuring the abstract. International Journal of Nursing Studies, 13 (3), 1976, 153-160; 17 (2), 1980, 127-130.

7 Gunn, J. Aggression—is it avoidable? Midwife, Health Visitor and Community Nurse, 12 (9), Sep 1976, 280-283.

8 Hill, J. The psychological impact of unemployment. New Society, 43, 19 Jan 1978, 118-120.

9 Jones, B. Social isolation: how can we help? (Social skills training for the lonely and isolated.) Nursing Times, 76, 31 Jan 1980, 208-209.

10 Kelly, E. Homeless young people in cities. Midwife, Health Visitor and Community Nurse, 14 (10), Oct 1978, 357-358.

11 Kelvin, P. 'If you can't find any work to do, you have the feeling you're not human, you're out of place.' Social Work Today, 12, 2 Dec 1980, 8-11.

12 Knight, L. An alternative way of caring. (Great Chapel Street Medical Center for young homeless people in Soho.) Nursing Mirror, 150, 24 Jan 1980, 16-18.

13 Kosidlak, J.G. Improving health care for troubled youths. (Survey of the health problems of 296 youths carried out by a public health nurse in a detention centre.) American Journal of Nursing, 76 (1), Jan 1976, 95-97.

14 McLaughlin, B. When daddy loses his job.

(Effect of unemployment on families with young children and HV's role.) Nursing Mirror, 149, 18 Oct 1979, 25-27.

15 Maclean, U. and Naumann, L. Primary medical care for the single homeless: the Edinburgh experiment. (Includes discussion of role of HV and district nurse.) Health Bulletin, 37 (1), Jan 1979, 6-10.

16 Martin, I.C.A. Clinical parable. The English malady. (Loneliness.) Nursing Times, 74, 4 May 1978, 768-769; 18 May 1978, 843-844.

17 Martin, I.C.A. Clinical parable. The gates of the day. (Loneliness and the importance of interpersonal relationships.) Nursing Times, 74, 30 Mar 1978, 553-554.

18 Moran, E. When gambling becomes a problem. Midwife, Health Visitor and Community Nurse, 14 (7), Jul 1978, 213, 215.

19 National Association for the Care and Resettlement of Offenders General practitioners, health visitors and the prevention of crime: proceedings of a day conference, 14 May 1975. Barry Rose (Publishers), 1976.

20 Norman, K. Caring for down and outs in the East End. (Primary medical care unit for homeless men and women in Cable Street, Stepney.) Nursing Mirror, 147, 21 Sep 1978, 44-46.

21 Payne, M. Defining an assistant: the achievements and failings of Shelter and changes needed for its future success. Health and Social Service Journal, 87, 1 Jul 1977, 989-991.

22 Quantrill, D. Pop come the health problems. (Health and hygiene problems of open air pop festivals.) Nursing Mirror, 147, 13 Jul 1978, 13-15.

23 Royal Society of Health Journal Juvenile crime. (Four articles.) Royal Society of Health Journal, 96 (1), Feb 1976, 6-9, 18.

24 Rumney, S. Capital Radio's special helpline. (HV describes her experience of answering questions.) Health Visitor, 53 (3), Mar 1980, 98.

25 Skeet, M. Poverty—the disease the world must cure. Nursing Mirror, 145, 29 Sep 1977, 24-28.

26 Skillern, K.D. Sin or sickness?—Stealing, vandalism and violence. 'Ours but to reason why.' Royal Society of Health Journal, 96 (5), Oct 1976, 220-223.

27 Thomas, T. Where the last laugh may go to the villain of the piece. (Treatment of vagrants by the health and social services.) Health and Social Service Journal, 88, 8 Sep 1978, 1016-1017.

28 Tredgold, R.F. The psychology of violence. Community Health, 8 (1), Jul 1976, 20-23.

29 Venvell, D. Health education and the delinquent youngster. Health Visitor, 51 (8), Aug 1978, 296-297.

30 Wai-On, P. The medical aspect of high-rise and high-density living. (Review of studies from various countries, including Britain.) Nursing Journal of Singapore, 15 (2), Nov 1975, 69-75.

31 Walshe-Brennan, K.S. Community roots of delinquency. Community Health, 8 (2), Oct 1976, 74-78.

32 Walshe-Brennan, K.S. The roots of child crime. Nursing Mirror, 143, 26 Aug 1976, 66-68.

33 Wassner, A. Social and racial effects. (Social isolation in urban societies.) New Zealand Nursing Journal, 68 (11), Nov 1975, 14-16.

34 Zeitlin, H. Breeding adult 'belly achers' from an ineffective system. (The increasing problem of juvenile delinquency.) Health and Social Service Journal, 86, 4 Feb 1977, 200-201.

b PRISON NURSING

1 Alexander-Rodriguez, T. Could prison nursing be the specialty for you? Nursing, 8 (3), Mar 1978, 80-81.

2 Blackburn, T. We need recognition. (Letter on role of forensic psychiatric nurse in prison medical departments.) Nursing Mirror, 144, 23 Jun 1977, 11-12.

3 Broster, J. 'Prison just seems to turn you into a zombie'. (Exclusive view from the inside of medical care and the use of drugs in a women's prison in England.) Mind Out, 36, Sep/Oct 1979, 3-4.

4 Cowper-Smith, F. Caring for women in prison. (Problems confronting the prison authorities and report of visits to Holloway and Askham Grange women's open prison near York.) Nursing Times, 75, 1 Feb 1979, 186-192.

5 Ellis, M.J.L. Doctors, prisoners and state: a conflict of interest? (By a prison doctor.) Midwife, Health Visitor and Community Nurse, 16 (2), Feb 1980, 52, 54, 56.

6 Nursing Times Prison reform leaves nurses second best. (Reorganisation of prison service.) Nursing Times, 76, 8 May 1980, 804.

7 Phillips, M. Nursing in a forensic unit. Dimensions in Health Service, 56 (2), Feb 1979, 28, 30-31.

8 Smith, L. A review of forensic psychiatry. (With some reference to Canadian practice.) Canadian Journal of Psychiatric Nursing, 17 (6), Nov/Dec 1976, 12-14.

9 Strank, R.A. Nursing within American prison systems. Home Office, n.d.

10 Warden, J. Caring for the forensic patient: a supportive approach to individuals in conflict with society. (Forensic Inpatient Unit, Clarke Institute of Psychiatry, Toronto.) Canadian Nurse, 73 (1), Jan 1977, 21-22.

c ALCOHOLISM

1 Advisory Committee on Alcoholism Report on education and training: for professional staff and voluntary workers in the field. DHSS and Welsh Office, 1979.

2 Advisory Committee on Alcoholism Report on prevention. DHSS, 1977.

3 Al-Anon Alcoholism *is* a family disease. (Function of Al-Anon Family Groups.) Nursing Mirror, 144, 23 Jun 1977, 23.

4 Al-Anon Public Information Committee Help for families of problem drinkers. Health Trends, 12 (1), Feb 1980, 8.

5 Archard, P. The bottle won't leave you: a study of homeless alcoholics and their guardians. Alcoholics Recovery Project, 1976.

6 Arroyave, F. and others The role of detoxification in alcoholism: three years' results from the Oxford Unit. Health Trends, 12 (2), May 1980, 36-38.

7 Ashton, K. Help for alcoholics. (Alcohol treatment unit, Withington Hospital, Manchester.) Nursing Times, 72, 19 Feb 1976, 248.

8 Baird, K. Special unit treats problems of teenagers. (Adolescent alcoholism unit.) Hospitals, 54 (3), 1 Feb 1980, 50-53.

9 Booth, P.G. and Darragh, P.P. What happens to alcoholics? (Report of progress of first 50 inpatient clients of Windsor Clinic one year after discharge.) Nursing Times, 76, 28 Feb 1980, 380-382.

10 Booth, P.G. and others The Windsor Clinic. (Alcoholism treatment unit serving North Merseyside.) Nursing Times, 75, 29 Mar 1979, 547-551.

11 Bragg, T.L. Teen-age alcohol abuse. Journal of Psychiatric Nursing and Mental Health Services, 14 (12), Dec 1976, 10-18.

12 Brewer, C. Alcohol and the brain. Nursing Times, 72, 23/30 Dec 1976, 2018-2019.

13 British Medical Journal Homes for tuberculous homeless alcoholics. (Home in East London with visits from doctor, social worker and nurse from local chest clinic.) British Medical Journal, 2, 21 Oct 1978, 1107-1108.

14 Camberwell Council on Alcoholism *and* **Campaign for the Homeless and Rootless** Out of sight, out of mind: a report on women in trouble with drink and the law. CHAR, 1976.

15 Caruana, S. and O'Hagan, M. Social aspects of alcohol and alcoholism. Edsall, 1976.

16 Coleman, J.W. The Spitalfields Crypt. The care and rehabilitation of vagrant methylated spirit drinkers in London's East End. Nursing Mirror, 143, 30 Dec 1976, 45-46.

17 Cowper-Smith, F. I thought excess gave me credit until... (Report of day conference on alcoholism.) Nursing Times, 74, 20 Jul 1978, 1191-1193.

18 Craig, W.G. Day programme to help alcoholics. (Organised by Southern General Hospital, Glasgow.) Nursing Times, 75, 4 Oct 1979, 1727-1729.

19 Davies, D.L. Preventing alcoholism. Royal Society of Health Journal, 99 (5), Oct 1979, 196-198.

20 Ditzler, J. Alcoholism: a family illness. (Work of Broadway Lodge in Weston-super-Mare, a non-profit making charitable foundation.) Nursing Times, 76, 19 Jun 1980, 1103-1105.

21 Durrant, L.K. The alcohol problem from an historical perspective. Royal Society of Health Journal, 96 (1), Feb 1976, 42-44.

22 Edwards, G. and Grant, M. editors Alco-holism: new knowledge and new responses. Croom Helm, 1977.

23 Freed, E.X. Some barriers to effective alcoholism research. Journal of Psychiatric Nursing and Mental Health Services, 14 (12), Dec 1976, 7-9.

24 Gayford, J.J. Alcoholic illness—who cares? Tomorrow's alcoholics. Royal Society of Health Journal, 96 (4), Aug 1976, 186-188.

25 Gayford, J.J. 6. Alcoholism. Nursing Mirror, 143 (20), 11 Nov 1976, Nursing care supplement series 3, i-iv.

26 Gibson, D.E. Reminiscence, self-esteem and self-other satisfaction in adult male alcoholics. (Research study.) Journal of Psychiatric Nursing, 18 (3), Mar 1980, 7-11.

27 Glatt, M.M. Alcohol misuse and alcoholism among the young. Midwife, Health Visitor and Community Nurse, 13 (3), Mar 1977, 77-79.

28 Glatt, M.M. The future of regional alcoholic units. (Effect of Advisory Committee on Alcoholism's recommendations.) Lancet, 1, 14 Apr 1979, 814-816.

29 Glatt, M.M. Motivation in alcoholics and drug addicts. (Problems for the team of therapists caused by patients' lack of motivation with particular mention of the role of the physiotherapists.) Nursing Mirror, 142, 15 Jan 1976, 59-61.

30 Grant, M. and Gwinner, P. Alcoholism in perspective. Croom Helm, 1979.

31 Hamilton, J.R. Helping the drunken offender. Health and Social Service Journal, 86, 28 Aug 1976, 1550-1551.

32 Hamilton, J.R. and others The Chief Scientist reports... A detoxification unit for habitual drunken offenders. (At the Royal Edinburgh Hospital. See also editorial on p.110-111.) Health Bulletin, 35 (3), May 1977, 146-154.

33 Hamilton, J.R. and others Detoxification of habitual drunken offenders. Edinburgh: Scottish Home and Health Department, 1978. (Scottish health service studies no.39.)

34 Hebblethwaite, D. Alcoholic illness—who cares? Reflections on healing alcohol abuse. Royal Society of Health Journal, 96 (4), Aug 1976, 189-192.

35 Helping Hand Organisation Aspects of female alcoholism. The Organisation, 1976.

36 Helping Hand Organisation Drugs, suburbia and subway: the pattern of addiction in the seventies. The Organisation, 1978.

37 Henry, S. and Robinson, D. Self help. Talking out of alcoholism: results from a survey of Alcoholics Anonymous in England and Wales. Journal of the Royal College of General Practitioners, 28, Jul 1978, 414-419.

38 Henry, S. and Robinson, D. Understanding alcoholics anonymous. Results from a survey in England and Wales. Lancet, 1, 18 Feb 1978, 372-375.

39 John, H.H. Primary medical care at hostels for alcoholics: a report of two surveys. Health Trends, 3 (12), Aug 1980, 61-64.

40 **MacIntyre, D.** Alcohol-related problems among male patients admitted to a general medical ward—their identification and follow-up. Health Bulletin, 37 (5), Sep 1979, 213-217.

41 **Mead, J. and others** Control yourself—and enjoy a drink. (Programme of controlled drinking for alcoholics at West Midlands Regional Drug and Alcohol Addiction Treatment Unit, with case study.) Nursing Mirror, 149, 4 Oct 1979, 20-24.

42 **Merry, J.** An alcoholism service. (Unit in the psychiatric department of an Epsom District Hospital.) British Medical Journal, 1, 21 Jan 1978, 161-162.

43 **National Council of Women. Working Party on Alcohol Problems of Women and Young People** Report. The Council, 1976. (Chairman: May W. Holland.)

44 **Page, A.R.** An integrated approach to problem drinkers. (Work of multidisciplinary team at Windsor Clinic, Rainhill Hospital.) British Journal of Occupational Therapy, 43 (3), Mar 1980, 84-87.

45 **Plant, M.A. and others** Evaluation of the Scottish Health Education Unit's 1976 campaign on alcoholism. Edinburgh: Medical Research Council Unit for Epidemiological Studies in Psychiatry, 1978.

46 **Rix, K.J.B. and Rix, E.M.L.** The alcohol withdrawal states: clinical features and treatment. Nursing Times, 74, 6 Apr 1978, 578-580.

47 **Robinson, D.** Talking out of alcoholism: the self-help process of Alcoholics Anonymous. Croom Helm, 1979.

48 **Rose, M.W.** Society at work. Who wants to be sober? (Specialist alcoholic unit at Harvey House, Lancaster Moor Hospital.) New Society, 37, 16 Sep 1976, 600-601.

49 **Royal College of Psychiatrists** Alcohol and alcoholism: the report of a special committee of the Royal College of Psychiatrists. Tavistock, 1979.

50 **Royal Society of Health Journal** Juvenile drinking. (Four articles.) Royal Society of Health Journal, 97 (1), Feb 1977, 14-28.

51 **Simnett, I.** Towards an alternative life. (Guidelines for counselling young alcoholics.) Health and Social Service Journal, 87, 19 Aug 1977, 1191.

52 **Toshney, J.** An alcoholism and detoxification centre. (At Withington Hospital, Manchester.) Nursing Times, 74, 6 Apr 1978, 573-576.

53 **Trethowan, W.H.** Alcoholism: the possibilities for prevention. (By chairman of the Advisory Committee on Alcoholism's sub-group on prevention.) Health Education Journal, 36 (4), 1977, 95-99.

54 **Valentine, N.M.** Women and alcoholism: a bibliography. Journal of Psychiatric Nursing and Mental Health Nursing, 14 (12), Dec 1976, 23-27.

d ALCOHOLISM: NURSING

1 **Arthur, H.** Women in distress. (Alcoholics, with reference to treatment regime in a New Zealand Hospital.) Health Visitor, 51 (10), Oct 1978, 380, 382, 385.

2 **Beaton, W.** Community psychiatry nursing. An alcoholic patient. (A case study.) Nursing Times, 72, 4 Nov 1976, 1710-1711.

3 **Calton, E.** Nursing care study: alcoholism. (Man who died at age of 39.) Nursing Mirror, 147, 16 Nov 1978, 39-40.

4 **Carbury, L.J.** When your patient is an alcoholic. Nursing Care, 9 (2), Feb 1976, 24-28.

5 **Cornish, R.D. and Miller, M.V.** Attitudes of registered nurses toward the alcoholic. (Study at the Veterans Administration Hospital, Iowa City, Iowa.) Journal of Psychiatric Nursing and Mental Health Services, 14 (12), Dec 1976, 19-22.

6 **Cote, W. and Roche, M.** The alcoholism nurse specialist. (Programme at Newport Hospital in Rhode Island.) Supervisor Nurse, 9 (12), Dec 1978, 24-31.

7 **Crowshaw, T.** As others see you. (Description of hospital treatment for alcoholism by former patient.) Nursing Times, 74, 6 Apr 1978, 576-577.

8 **Estes, N.J. and others** Nursing diagnosis of the alcoholic person. St. Louis: Mosby, 1980.

9 **Ferrario, E.A.** Community nursing care study. Seeking oblivion. (An elderly alcoholic.) Nursing Times, 73, 14 Apr 1977, 527.

10 **Floyd, T.** Alcoholism addiction: rewards hasten the cure. (Token economy system used at Addiction Treatment Unit, All Saints Hospital, Birmingham.) Nursing Mirror, 149, 6 Sep 1979, 53-54.

11 **Forton, M.L.** Detoxification, then what? A community nursing course in alcoholism. American Journal of Nursing, 80 (1), Jan 1980, 113-114.

12 **Freddy, C.** Alcoholism—the friendly foe. (Personal experiences of alcoholism.) Nursing Mirror, 144, 10 Mar 1977, 71-72.

13 **Gareri, E.A.** Assertiveness training for alcoholics. Journal of Psychiatric Nursing, 17 (1), Jan 1979, 31-36.

14 **Goodman, L.M.** OR nursing intervention for the alcoholic. AORN Journal, 24 (5), Nov 1976, 867-874.

15 **Gurel, M.** An alcoholism training program: its effect on trainees and faculty. (University of Washington, School of Nursing.) Nursing Research, 25 (2), Mar-Apr 1976, 127-132.

16 **Hardin, K.** Treating intoxicated patients in the emergency department. (Drug addiction and alcohol abuse.) Journal of Education in Nursing, 5 (1), Jan/Feb 1979, 11-14.

17 **Harlow, P.E. and Goby, M.J.** Changing nursing students' attitudes toward alcoholic patients: examining effects of a clinical practicum. Nursing Research, 29 (1), Jan/Feb 1980, 59-60.

18 **Hartie, M.** Nursing care study. Alcoholism. The sins of the father... (By health visitor.) Nursing Mirror, 151, 14 Aug 1980, 38-41.

19 **Heinemann, E. and Estes, N.** Assessing alcoholic patients. (Interview guide developed at the University of Washington School of Nursing.) American Journal of Nursing, 76 (5), May 1976, 785-789.

20 **Hewitt, M.** Nursing care study. The one who got away. (Failure of psychiatric services to treat uncooperative alcoholic patient.) Nursing Times, 73, 24 Nov 1977, 1839-1840.

21 **Holt, S. and others** Alcohol and the emergency service patient. (Results of survey.) British Medical Journal, 281, 6 Sep 1980, 638-640.

22 **Janosik, E.** Reachable and teachable: report on a prison alcoholism group. (Group therapy led by psychiatric nurse.) Journal of Psychiatric Nursing and Mental Health Services, 15 (4), Apr 1977, 24-28.

23 **Jenkins, J.** Stephen is sick...but how sick? (Description of poor nursing care received by her brother who was in hospital with alcoholic poisoning.) Nursing Mirror, 149, 22 Nov 1979, 23-25.

24 **Leins, J.A.** Merging the treatment of alcoholism into an existing drug sustained program for addicts. (Nanaimo Chemical Dependency Centre.) Canadian Journal of Psychiatric Nursing, 18 (2), Mar-Apr 1977, 10-11.

25 **Lewin, D.C.** Care of the dependent patient. (Nursing care and general management of alcoholism.) Nursing Times, 74, 6 Apr 1978, 570-573.

26 **McGee, A.** Nursing the alcoholic patient. (In a treatment centre.) Canadian Nurse, 73 (6), Jun 1977, 30-33.

27 **Madden, J.S.** A guide to alcohol and drug dependence. Bristol: Wright, 1979. (For nurses and others.)

28 **Marks, V.L.** Health teaching for recovering alcoholic patients. American Journal of Nursing, 80 (11), Nov 1980, 2058-2061.

29 **Meyer, M.L.** Counselling families of alcoholics. Health Visitor, 50 (5), May 1977, 136-142.

30 **Meyer, M.L.** Counselling families of alcoholics: a guideline for the helping profession. London Council on Alcoholism, 1978. (By a nurse.)

31 **Nursing Clinics of North America** Symposium on alcoholism and drug addiction. Nursing Clinics of North America, 11 (3), Sep 1976, 481-563.

32 **Nyapadi, T.J.** Alcoholism—restoring the personality. Nursing Times, 72, 19 Aug 1976, 1279-1280.

33 **Pormorski, M.E.** The alcoholic as a surgical patient. AORN Journal, 24 (5), Nov 1976, 875-886.

34 **Rix, K.J.B. and Rix, E.M.L.** The alcohol withdrawal states: nursing care. Nursing Times, 74, 6 Apr 1978, 581-583.

35 **Rodman, M.J.** Treating alcoholics: which drugs work best when? RN Magazine, 40 (9), Sep 1977, 95-96, 99, 101, 103.

36 **Rotherham, F.** Nurses and alcohol-related problems. (Survey of knowledge and attitudes of some male psychiatric nurses in a Glasgow

hospital.) Nursing Times, 76, 11 Dec 1980, 2197-2198.

37 Schwerdtfeger, T.H. Developing a nursing staff in an alcoholism center: an effective, therapeutic team approach. Supervisor Nurse, 11 (2), Feb 1980, 43-45.

38 Segal, M. and others Alcoholism: practical aspects of management. (By staff at the Halifax Hospital Group, West Yorkshire, with review of methods available.) Nursing Times, 74, 19 Jan 1978, 98-102.

39 Skelt, A.D. The alcoholic patient in casualty. (Referral to social service agencies.) Nursing Times, 74, 6 Apr 1978, 583.

40 Sorgen, L.M. Student learning following an educational experience at an Alcohol Rehabilitation Centre in Saskatoon, Saskatchewan, Canada. (Research study to assess students' increased knowledge of and attitude towards alcoholism.) International Journal of Nursing Studies, 16 (1), 1979, 41-50.

41 Starkey, P.J. Nurses' attitudes toward alcoholism. AORN Journal, 31 (5), Apr 1980, 819, 822-823, 826, 828.

42 Turton, B. A new experience. (Description of work of sub panel of the JBCNS planning a short course on alcoholism.) Nursing Times, 76, 24 Jul 1980, 1293-1294.

43 Ufer, L. How to recognize and care for the alcoholic patient. Nursing, 7 (10), Oct 1977, 37-38.

44 Wiley, L. Confronting alcoholism—how one medical/surgical unit faced the problem. (Panel give tips on caring for hospitalised alcoholics.) Nursing, 77, 7 (5), May 1977, 56-61.

45 Wilson, A. Treatment of chronic alcoholism according to a three-process model. Psychiatric Nursing, 17 (1), Jan-Feb 1976, 10-11.

e ALCOHOLISM: WORK SETTING

1 Bissell, L.C. Alcoholism. Occupational Health Nursing, 24 (8), Aug 1976, 20-23.

2 Durkin, W.G. Recovery from alcoholism—only the first hurdle. (Research study into firms' attitudes and practices towards recovered alcoholics.) Occupational Health Nursing, 26 (9), Sep 1978, 22-25.

3 Gillespie, J.M. Chemical dependency—a practical personnel policy. (Policy for the alcoholic or drug dependent employee devised by the Greater Glasgow Health Board, Eastern District.) Hospital and Health Services Review, 72 (4), Apr 1976, 112-113.

4 Guida, M. The occupational health nurse's role in the corporate alcoholism program. Occupational Health Nursing, 24 (3), Mar 1976, 22-24.

5 Hamilton, M. Treatment of working alcoholics. (Out-patient clinic, Central Middlesex Hospital.) Occupational Health, 28 (8), Aug 1976, 398-399.

6 Heyman, M.M. Alcoholism programs in industry: the patient's view. New Brunswick, N.J.: Rutgers Center of Alcohol Studies, 1978. (Monograph; 12.)

7 Madden, J.S. The problem and management of alcoholism in industry. Journal of the Society of Occupational Medicine, 26 (2), Apr 1976, 61-64.

8 National Council on Alcoholism Report of the working party on alcohol and work. The Council, (1977.) (Chairman: Sir Bernard Braine.)

9 Tennent, G. Alcoholism in industry. Occupational Health, 30 (4), Apr 1978, 164-166.

10 Thomas, M. The nurse's role in the detection and treatment of alcoholism. Occupational Health Nursing, 24 (5), May 1976, 17-19.

11 Whyte, E.L. Coping with alcoholism in industry. Occupational Health Nursing, 25 (7), Jul 1977, 9-11.

f DRUG ADDICTION

1 Boyd, P. Drug addiction. Midwife, Health Visitor and Community Nurse, 12 (12), Dec 1976, 390-394.

2 Clarke, A. A follow-up of drug clinic attenders. (Research study at St. George's Drug Clinic.) Nursing Times, 74, 31 Aug 1978, Occ. papers, 98-100.

3 Davidson, N. Placard gives rise to the fears of Phoenix. (Alpha House, a drug rehabilitation unit in Hampshire.) Health and Social Service Journal, 88, 7 Apr 1978, 400-401.

4 Dell, D.D. and Snyder, J.A. Marijuana: pro and con. (Review of evidence.) American Journal of Nursing, 77 (4), Apr 1977, 630-635.

5 Donn, N. and Thompson, A. Decision making skills: a possible goal for 'drug education.' Health Education Journal, 35 (4), 1976, 248-257.

6 Dorn, N. and Thompson, A. Evaluation of drug education in the longer term is not an 'optional extra.' (Survey by the Institute for the Study of Drug Dependence.) Community Health, 7 (3), Jan 1976, 154-161.

7 Ghodse, A.H. Casualty departments and the monitoring of drug dependence. (Their potential role in research.) British Medical Journal, 1, 28 May 1977, 1381-1382.

8 Glatt, M.M. editor Drug dependence: current problems and issues. Lancaster: MTP, 1977.

9 Hickey, P. From heroin to new hope... (New policies in the treatment for withdrawal from drugs at the Addiction Clinic, Welwyn Garden City.) Nursing Mirror, 149, 15 Nov 1979, 25-27.

10 Imlah, N. and Akhter, M. Bitter-sweet success. (Work of multidisciplinary team at addiction unit at All Saints' Hospital, Birmingham, for alcoholics and drug addicts.) Nursing Mirror, 148, 1 Feb 1978, 18-20.

11 Iveson-Iveson, J. Behind the smokescreen. (Cannabis.) Nursing Mirror, 151, 28 Aug 1980, 30-31.

12 Lane, D.A. Predictors of drug use. (The value of studying personality and motivation in predicting drug dependence.) Community Health, 8 (1), Jul 1976, 12-15.

13 Mitcheson, M. Government health warning for cannabis? (Assessment of its dangers.) Midwife, Health Visitor and Community Nurse, 15 (4), Apr 1979, 142-143, 146.

14 Rose, B. City Roads: a signpost to the future. (Report on new short-stay unit for drug abusers.) Nursing Times, 74, 25 May 1978, 865.

15 Warner, J. The main line to Europe. (Problems of maintaining effective drug enforcement programmes.) Nursing Mirror, 148, 1 Feb 1979, 13-16.

16 WHO Chronicle Control of drug abuse in developing countries. WHO Chronicle, 34 (2), Feb 1980, 56-59.

g DRUG ADDICTION: NURSING

1 Gossop, M. Drug dependence—1. The pattern of drug abuse. 2. Treatment and nursing care. Nursing Times, 74, 15 Jan 1978, 996-998; 22 Jun 1978, 1060-1061.

2 Detzer, E. and others Detoxifying barbiturate addicts: hints for psychiatric staff. American Journal of Nursing, 76 (8), Aug 1976, 1306-1307.

3 Fultz, J.M. and others When a narcotic addict is hospitalized. American Journal of Nursing, 80 (3), Mar 1980, 478-481.

4 Greenblatt, D.J. and Shader, R.I. Treating the drug abuser in the ED. RN Magazine, 38 (5), May 1975, OR 1, 5, 8, 10.

5 Johnson, E. and Klotkowski, D. Turning an addicted patient on to turning drugs off. RN Magazine, 41 (5), May 1978, 90-92, 94, 96, 98.

6 Lewin, D.C. Care of the drug-dependent patient. Nursing Times, 74, 13 Apr 1978, 621-624.

7 Love, R. Nursing care study. Brian—heroin addict. Nursing Mirror, 143, 15 Jul 1976, 50-52.

8 Nursing Times A stop on the path to destruction. (Care of drug abusers in Middlesex Hospital casualty department.) Nursing Times, 74, 25 May 1978, 862-864.

9 Stevens, P.F. Kate and Paul. (Case history of two drug addicts.) Nursing Times, 72, 1 Jul 1976, 1024-1025.

10 Wiley, L. Managing a hospitalized drug addict. (Multidisciplinary panel of experts discuss a case.) Nursing, 77, 7 (6), Jun 1977, 47-51.

11 Yowell, S. and Brose, C. Working with drug abuse patients in the ER. American Journal of Nursing, 77 (1), Jan 1977, 82-85.

h SMOKING

1 Action on Smoking and Health Mothers who smoke and their children. (Report of committee.) Practitioner, 224, Jul 1980, 735-740.

2 Ashton, W.D. Cigarette smoking and associated disease. (Undergraduate medical student project consisting of questionnaire survey to assess level of public knowledge about harmful effects of smoking.) Journal of the Royal College of General Practitioners, 29, Apr 1979, 229-233.

3 Atkinson, A.B. and Townsend, J.L. Economic aspects of reduced smoking. (Effects of economic measures and health publicity programmes on use of health services and Government revenue.) Lancet, 2, 3 Sep 1977, 492-494.

4 Baric, L. Health education and the smoking habit. Health Education Journal, 37 (1), 1978, 132-137.

5 Baric, L. and others Acquisition of the smoking habit. (Research study.) Health Education Journal, 38 (3), 1979, 71-76.

6 Baric, L. Non-smokers, smokers, ex-smokers: three separate problems for health education. International Journal of Health Education, 22 (1), 1979 Supplement 1-20.

7 Bewley, B.R. and Bland, M. The child's image of a young smoker. (Research study of children's self-images compared with their image of young person who smokes.) Health Education Journal, 37 (4), 1978, 236-241.

8 Bewley, B.R. and others Teachers' smoking. (Influence on children's smoking.) Journal of Epidemiology and Community Health, 33 (3), Sep 1979, 219-222.

9 Bewley, B.R. and others Trend in children's smoking. (Survey among Derbyshire children aged 11-15 years between 1974 and 1977.) Community Medicine, 2 (3), Aug 1980, 186-189.

10 Bostock, Y. and Davies, J.K. Recent changes in the prevalence of cigarette smoking in Scotland compared with trends in England and Wales. (Reproduced with minor changes from Health Bulletin, Nov 1979.) Health Trends, 12 (2), May 1980, 41-44.

11 Capell, P.J. Trends in cigarette smoking in the United Kingdom. (With statistics.) Health Trends, 10 (3), Aug 1978, 49-54; Health Bulletin, 36 (6), Nov 1978, 286-294.

12 Dale, J.J. An evaluation of a programme of school health education on smoking. Health Education Journal, 37 (1), 1978, 142-144.

13 Department of Health and Social Security Smoking and professional people. DHSS, 1977.

14 Doll, R. Smoking and disease: prospects for control. Royal Society of Health Journal, 97 (4), Aug 1977, 167-176.

15 Fee, W. Searching for the simple answer to cure the smoking habit. (Research at the anti-smoking clinic operated by the Tayside Health Board.) Health and Social Service Journal, 86, 18 Feb 1977, 292-293.

16 Haines, A.P. and others Psychoneurotic profiles of smokers and non-smokers. (Self-rating inventory, the Middlesex Hospital Questionnaire, administered to participants in the Northwick Park Heart Study.) British Medical Journal, 280, 14 Jun 1980, 1422.

17 Horn, D. Smoking and disease—what must be done. WHO Chronicle, 31 (9), Sep 1977, 355-361.

18 Jarvis, M.J. and Russell, M.A.H Comment on the Hunter Committee's second report. (Independent Scientific Committee on Smoking and Health.) British Medical Journal, 280, 5 Apr 1980, 994-995.

19 Khosla, T. Ineffectiveness of health warning in cigarette smoking related diseases. Health Education Journal, 38 (2), 1979, 58-62.

20 Maryon-Davis, A. Change is in the air. (Advice on giving up smoking.) Nursing Mirror, 150, 10 Apr 1980, 23-25.

21 Melrose, D. The promotion of an epidemic. (Increase in smoking in the Third World.) Nursing Mirror, 151, 17 Jul 1980, 26-27.

22 Muir Gray, J.A. Warning: cigarettes may do you good. (The positive aspects of smoking in dealing with stress, with some reference to doctors and nurses.) Nursing Mirror, 150, 10 Apr 1980, 21-23.

23 Olsen, N. A case of not-so-gentle persuasion. (Need for health personnel to promote health with reference to smoking.) Nursing Mirror, 150, 26 Jun 1980, 18-20.

24 Royal College of Physicians Smoking or health. Pitman, 1977.

25 Schurer, M. Smoking—and the consequences. Nursing Times, 76, 3 Apr 1980, 585-588.

26 Thomson, W. Health education—6. Smoking is awful. Nursing Times, 74, 19 Oct 1978, 1728-1729.

27 Townsend, J. Smoking and class. (Current trends and morbidity and mortality rates.) New Society, 43, 30 Mar 1978, 709-710.

28 WHO Expert Committee on Smoking Control New recommendations. (Summary.) British Medical Journal, 1, 26 May 1979, 1379.

29 Willard, N. Smoking—a man-made dragon. (History and current trends.) World Health, Jun 1979, 5, 7-9.

30 World Health Issue on smoking or health, with reference to developing countries. World Health, Mar 1980, 3-39.

31 WORLD Health Day 1980. Smoking or health, the choice is yours. (Director-General's message and background paper.) WHO Chronicle, 34, Apr 1980, 127-130.

32 World Health Organization. Expert Committee on Smoking Control Controlling the smoking epidemic. Geneva: WHO, 1979. (Technical report series no.636.)

i SMOKING IN HOSPITALS

1 Ball, K. and Stevenson, A. Hospital action on smoking. (Report of action taken by Central Middlesex Hospital.) British Medical Journal, 2, 29 Sep 1979, 777-778.

2 Campbell, D. Smoking policies in hospitals. Dimensions in Health Service, 53 (12), Dec 1976, 20-23.

3 Crofton, E.C. The sale of cigarettes in Scottish hospitals: an ASH enquiry. (Results of a questionnaire.) Health Bulletin, 35 (1), Jan 1977, 36-39.

4 Crofton, E.C. The sale of cigarettes in general and maternity hospitals in Scotland: an ASH enquiry. Health Bulletin, 38 (4), Jul 1980, 150-153.

5 Crofton, E.C. Smoking as a fire risk in Scottish hospitals: an ASH enquiry. Health Bulletin, 35 (1), Jan 1977, 39-43.

6 Daube, M. No smoke without fire. (ASH survey of smoking among hospital personnel.) Nursing Times, 73, 10 Mar 1977, 330-331.

7 Fewtrell, C. An experiment in banning smoking. (Bristol Royal Infirmary.) Hospital and Health Services Review, 74 (7), Jul 1978, 219-220.

8 Garratt, D.J. and others Smoking in hospital: a survey of attitudes of staff, patients and visitors. Journal of Epidemiology and Community Health, 32 (3), Sep 1978, 226-228.

9 Jacobson, B. Showing an example. (Evaluation of success of non-smoking policy at the Central Middlesex Hospital.) Nursing Times, 74, 16 Nov 1978, 1877.

10 Laycock, E. No smoking in patient rooms—please. (Policy at a Toronto hospital.) Hospital Administration in Canada, 17 (10), Oct 1975, 45-46.

11 Nursing Times No smoking—by arrangement with the management. (Report on Survey on Smoking in Scottish Hospitals sponsored by ASH.) Nursing Times, 74, 16 Feb 1978, 262-263.

12 Wilkinson, P. Smoking in hospitals. (Analysis of results of survey into smoking policy in Leeds' hospitals.) Health and Social Service Journal, 88, 27 Oct 1978, 1215-1216.

13 Zimmerman, M.W. No smoking, please! (Establishment of No-Smoking patient unit is popular with patients.) Hospitals, 52 (15), Aug 1978, 183-184, 186.

j SOLVENT ABUSE

1 Campbell, D. and Watson, J.M. A comparative study of 18 glue sniffers. Community Health, 9 (4), May 1978, 207-210.

2 Masterton, G. and Sclare, A.B. Solvent abuse. (Survey of cases referred to a Glasgow psychiatric unit.) Health Bulletin, 36 (6), Nov 1978, 305-309.

3 Thorpe, W.H. Sniffing and inhalation of aerosols, glue, paint and petrol. (Techniques, effects and prevention.) Midwife, Health Visitor and Community Nurse, 13 (7), Jul 1977, 221-222.

4 Watson, J.M. Glue sniffing: a community dilemma. (Survey in Lanarkshire.) Community Health, 8 (3), Jan 1977, 160-163.

5 Watson, J.M. 'Glue-sniffing' in profile. (Survey in Scotland.) Practitioner, 218, Feb 1977, 255-259.

6 Watson, J.M. The dangers of glue sniffing. Nursing Mirror, 143, 28 Oct 1976, 40-41.

7 Watson, J.M. Glue sniffing. Nursing Times, 72, 28 Oct 1976, 1690-1691.

8 Watson, J.M. The growing problem of glue sniffing. (Study of solvent abuse in Lanarkshire.) Social Work Today, 8 (3), 19 Oct 1976, 10-11.

9 Watson, J. The problem nobody wanted. (Prevention of solvent sniffing carried out in Lanarkshire.) Health and Social Service Journal, 86, 17 Sep 1976, 1666-1667.

MATERNITY SERVICES

39 MIDWIFERY AND MATERNITY SERVICES

a MATERNITY SERVICES

1 Alberman, E. Prevention and health—are we positive enough? (Paper given at a National Association for Maternal and Child Welfare conference.) Queen's Nursing Journal, 19 (10), Jan 1977, 281-283.

2 Baird, D. The perinatal mortality rate as a measure of the efficiency of the maternity services. Health Bulletin, 35 (5), Sep 1977, 234-242.

3 Beard, R.W. What I would say to the Royal Commission. Maternal and neonatal health—a priority. British Medical Journal, 2, 18 Sep 1976, 679-680.

4 Blair, E.M. and others Instrument development: measuring quality outcomes in ambulatory maternal-child nursing. Nursing Administration Quarterly, 2 (4), Summer 1978, 87-93.

5 Bull, M.J.V. Ten years' experience in a general practice obstetric unit. Journal of the Royal College of General Practitioners, 30, Apr 1980, 208-212, 214-215.

6 Chamberlain, G. Dear Royal Commissioners. The maternity services. Lancet, 2, 27 Nov 1976, 1188-1189.

7 THE CINDERELLA of the service? (Critical review by a midwife of average postnatal care given in maternity units.) Midwife, Health Visitor and Community Nurse, 14 (11), Nov 1978, 389.

8 Clare, A.W. Treatment or torture? (Conflict in psychiatry and current obstetrics and gynaecology compared.) Midwife, Health Visitor and Community Nurse, 14 (7), Jul 1978, 205-206.

9 Cudby, H.E. Large and small maternity units. Some comparisons. Midwives Chronicle, 91, Feb 1978, 37.

10 Fergusson, I.L.C. and Watson, J.M. Assessment of the obstetric flying squad in an urban area. (Review of one year's services in South London found few calls were justifiable.) British Medical Journal, 1, 21 Feb 1976, 446-448.

11 International Federation of Gynaecology and Obstetrics *and* **International Confederation of Midwives. Joint Study Group** Maternity care in the world: international survey of midwifery practice and training. 2nd ed. Southampton: Worthy Publications, 1976.

12 James, D.K. Obstetric flying squad service —a defence. (Review of calls made by the flying squad in West Berkshire to patient's homes and G.P. units.) British Medical Journal, 1, 22 Jan 1977, 217-219.

13 King, A.E.M. Changing patterns in maternity care in the 1970s. Nursing Mirror, 144, 9 Jun 1977, 19-22.

14 Lewis, B.V. and others Changing patterns in a general practitioner obstetric unit. British Medical Journal, 1, 25 Feb 1978, 484-485.

15 Littlepage, B.N.C. General practitioner maternity units. (A study of the type of information available in the South-Western Regional Hospital Board for monitoring obstetric care.) Journal of the Royal College of General Practitioners, 26, Apr 1976, 263-265.

16 McCarthy, M. and McCarthy, T.G. Current trends in obstetric services. Public Health, 89 (5), Jul 1975, 191-197.

17 Munro, H.D.R. Livingston: an integrated medical service for women. 1. Obstetrics. Health Bulletin, 35 (5), Sep 1977, 253-259.

18 Pharoah, P.O.D. Obstetrics and neonatal care related to outcome. A comparison of two maternity hospitals. (Follow-up study of infants born in two district hospitals until six years.) British Journal of Preventive and Social Medicine, 30 (4), Dec 1976, 257-261.

19 Rishworth, C.M. Staffing maternity units. (With statistics on aspects of maternity care.) Nursing Times, 76, 24 Apr 1980, 731-733.

20 Sangster, J.A. Some aspects of equipping for midwives. Midwives Chronicle, 90, Jul 1977, 164-165.

21 Savage, W. Have Dr. Ballantyne's aims been achieved? Part 2. (Ways of improving quality of care.) Midwife, Health Visitor and Community Nurse, 16 (6), Jun 1980, 238, 240, 242.

22 Scambler, A. Midwifery care within the 'new obstetrics'. Midwife, Health Visitor and Community Nurse, 15 (5), May 1979, 174-177.

23 Scott-Samuel, A. Why don't they want our health services? (Non-users of maternal and child health services.) Lancet, 1, 23 Feb 1980, 412-413.

24 Shapland, D.E. Extended role for general practitioners in obstetrics? A medical audit. (Study of four GP obstetric units in isolated areas.) British Medical Journal, 1, 5 May 1979, 1199-1200.

25 Tacchi, D. Changing attitudes to maternity. (Women's and staff attitudes and patient management.) Midwives Chronicle, 92, Jan 1979, 4-7.

26 Taylor, A. With grateful thanks... (Problems of maternity care discussed by the Secretary of the Association for improvements in Maternity Services.) Midwife, Health Visitor and Community Nurse, 12 (3), Mar 1976, 83-84.

27 Taylor, G.W. GP maternity units: implications of closure. British Medical Journal, 1, 16 Apr 1977, 1015-1044.

28 Taylor, G.W. and others How safe is general practitioner obstetrics? (Comparative study showing the general practitioner unit to be as safe as a consultant unit for low-risk women.) Lancet, 2, 13 Dec 1980, 1287-1289.

29 Tew, M. Obstetric hospitals and general-practitioner maternity units—the statistical record. Journal of the Royal College of General Practitioners, 27, Nov 1977, 689-694.

30 Waterhouse, I. Dial a midwife—the extension of postnatal care. (Integrated service of West Berkshire.) Midwives Chronicle, 90, Jul 1977, 159-160.

31 WHO Chronicle Something for all and more for those in greater need. A 'risk approach' for integrated maternal and child health care. WHO Chronicle, 31 (4), Apr 1977, 150-151.

32 World Health Organization Risk approach for maternal and child health care. Geneva: WHO, 1978. (WHO offset publication no.39.)

33 World Health Organization Towards a better future: maternal and child health. Geneva: WHO, 1980.

34 World Health Organization. Expert Committee on Maternal and Child Health New trends and approaches in the delivery of maternal and child care in health services: 6th report of the Committee. Geneva: WHO, 1976. (Technical report series no.600.)

b TEXTBOOKS

1 Bailey, R.E. Mayes' midwifery: a textbook for midwives. 9th ed. Baillière Tindall, 1976.

2 BAILLIÈRE's midwives dictionary; edited by Vera de Cruz and Margaret Adams. 6th ed. Baillière Tindall, 1976.

3 Bethea, D.C. Introductory maternity nursing. 3rd ed. Philadelphia: Lippincott, 1979.

4 Bleier, I.J. Bedside maternity nursing. 4th ed. Philadelphia: W.B. Saunders, 1979.

5 Burnett, C.W.F. The anatomy and physiology of obstetrics: a short textbook for students and midwives. Revised by Mary M. Anderson. 6th ed. Faber and Faber, 1979.

6 Clark, A.L. and others Childbearing: a nursing perspective. 2nd ed. Philadelphia: F.A. Davies, 1979.

7 Clyne, D.G.W. A concise textbook for midwives. 5th ed. Faber, 1980.

8 Fream, W.C. Notes on obstetrics. Churchill Livingstone, 1977.

9 Friesner, A. and Raff, B. Maternity nursing. 2nd ed. Flushing: Medical Examination Publishing Co., 1977.

10 Green, J. Review of maternal/child nursing. New York: McGraw-Hill, 1979. (Multiple choice questions.)

11 Hallum, J.L. Midwifery. 2nd ed. Hodder and Stoughton, 1976.

12 Hamilton, P.M. Basic maternity nursing. 4th ed. St. Louis: Mosby, 1979.

13 Hector, W. Modern gynaecology with obstetrics for nurses. 6th ed. Heinemann Medical, 1980.

14 Hickman, M.A. An introduction to midwifery. Blackwell, 1978.

15 Hope, A. and others Sample standard nursing care plans for patients in obstetrical units. Vancouver: Registered Nurses' Association of British Columbia, 1977.

16 Jensen, M.D. and others Maternity care: the nurse and the family. St. Louis: Mosby, 1977.

17 Lerch, C. and Bliss, V.J. Maternity nursing. 3rd ed. St. Louis: Mosby, 1978.

18 McNall, L.K. and Galeener, J.T. editors Current practice in obstetric and gynaecologic nursing. St. Louis: Mosby, 1976.

19 Malo-Juvera, D. and others Obstetrical nursing, continuing education review. 2nd ed. New York: Medical Examination Publishing Co., 1979. (Essay questions and referenced answers.)

20 Quixley, J.M.E. and Cameron, M.D. Obstetrics and gynaecology. 4th ed. Hodder and Stoughton, 1979. (Modern nursing series.)

21 Roch, S.E.G. Midwifery revision: objective and other tests for students of midwifery and obstetrics. Edinburgh: Churchill Livingstone, 1980.

22 Sweet, B.R. and Cape, I.F. Obstetric care. Aylesbury: HM & M, 1976. (Nursing modules series.)

23 Towler, J. and Butler-Manuel, R. Modern obstetrics for student midwives. 2nd ed. Lloyd-Luke, 1980.

24 Varney, H. Nurse-midwifery. Boston; Oxford: Blackwell Scientific, 1980.

c PROFESSIONAL ASPECTS

1 Ashton, R. The quiet secretary. (Interview with Ruth Ashton, General Secretary of RCM),

by C. Dopson. Nursing Times, 76, 17 Jul 1980, Midwifery supplement 3-4.

2 Auld, M.G. Midwifery standards. Midwives Chronicle, 93, Jan 1980, 5-11.

3 Bamfield, T. The Association of Radical Midwives. (Issues for concern in midwifery and role of ARM.) Midwife, Health Visitor and Community Nurse, 15 (9), Sep 1979, 342, 344-345.

4 Barnett, Z.H. The changing pattern of maternity care and the future role of the midwife. Midwives Chronicle, 92, Nov 1979, 381-384.

5 Barnett, Z.H. Communications between doctors, midwives and patients. Midwives Chronicle, 89, Oct 1976, 240.

6 Beak, J.A. Should the RCM set up an English board? (For discussion of matters which are solely the concern of midwives working in England.) Midwives Chronicle, 91, Nov 1978, 320-321.

7 Bent, E.A. The future role of the midwife: the midwives' viewpoint. (With reference to CNO (76) 20.) Midwives Chronicle, 91, Mar 1978, 51-54.

8 Bonnar, J. Ethical problems in obstetrics and gynaecology. World of Irish Nursing, 6 (4), Apr 1977, 1.

9 Bristow, S. Career opportunities. Midwifery. Nursing Times, 72, 10 Jun 1976, 892-893.

10 Central Midwives Board Annual report for year ended March 31, 1976. The Board, 1976.

11 Cowper-Smith, F. The midwife and human prosperity. (Report of International Confederation of Midwives congress.) Nursing Times, 74, 28 Sep 1978, 1589-1593.

12 Cronk, M. Getting back into practice. (Dissatisfaction with present state of midwifery and her reasons for joining Association of Radical Midwives.) Nursing Mirror, 149, 25 Oct 1979, 38-39.

13 Dening, F.C. The 5th International Congress of Psychosomatic Obstetrics and Gynecology. (Report.) Midwives Chronicle, 91, Feb 1978, 25-26.

14 Dingwall, R. Improving labour planning. (Health service administration and the future of midwifery.) Nursing Times, 73, 1 Sep 1977, 1346-1347.

15 Donnison, J. The role of the midwife. Midwife, Health Visitor and Community Nurse, 15 (7), Jul 1979, 265, 267-268, 270.

16 Farrer, M.I. 'You stay in midwifery'... and she did. (Wendy Robinson interviews Margaret Farrer, recently retired Hon. Treasurer of the Royal College of Midwives.) Nursing Mirror, 143 (9), 26 Aug 1976, 36-37.

17 International Confederation of Midwives Report of the 18th international congress for midwives in Jerusalem, 3-8 Sept, 1978. ICM, 1978.

18 Iveson-Iveson, J. The midwife—a key to human prosperity. (Report on 18th Congress of the International Confederation of Midwives.) Nursing Mirror, 147, 21 Sep 1978, 7-9.

19 Karpf, A. Giving birth to the revolution. (The Association of Radical Midwives and its concerns about the current role of midwives.) Health and Social Service Journal, 88, 13 Oct 1978, 1166-1167.

20 Klein, R. An antidote for apathy. (The Association of Radical Midwives.) Nursing Mirror, 148, 15 Mar 1979, 18-19.

21 Lightowlers, J. Midwifery under scrutiny. (New research project to be undertaken at Chelsea College Nursing Education Research Unit.) Journal of Community Nursing, 2 (1), Jul 1978, 18.

22 Lobban, M. The organisation of midwifery services. (In Scotland.) Nursing Mirror, 146, 4 May 1978, Supplement v-viii.

23 Mee, B.D. Midwives and industrial relations. Midwife, Health Visitor and Community Nurse, 13 (3), Mar 1977, 66-69.

24 Midwives Chronicle The Briggs controversy. (Letters and comment on aspects of the Briggs bill affecting midwives.) Midwives Chronicle, Dec 1978, 368-369.

25 Midwives Chronicle The legal position of the midwife. Midwives Chronicle, 91, Feb 1978, 23.

26 Midwives Chronicle TUC affiliation. (Advantages and disadvantages with reference to the RCM.) Midwives Chronicle, 92, Mar 1979, 73-74.

27 Moores, B. Some notes stemming from an investigation into how various quantitative concepts could aid in devising a manpower planning strategy for midwives. Manchester: UMIST, Dept of Management Sciences, 1978.

28 Moores, B. Towards rational midwifery service planning. Journal of Advanced Nursing, 5 (3), May 1980, 301-311.

29 Newstead, M.W. Midwives, management and legislation—a discussion of some recent Acts and Bills. Midwives Chronicle, 89, Jun 1976, 151.

30 Robinson, S. Are there enough midwives? (Report of findings from pilot study of research project at Chelsea College.) Nursing Times, 76, 24 Apr 1980, 726-730.

31 Roch, S.E.G. Midwives at the crossroads. Midwives Chronicle, 89, Oct 1976, 244.

32 Ross, T. Through the looking glass. (Research project at Chelsea College on the role of the midwife.) Nursing Mirror, 151, 10 Jul 1980, Supplement i-iii.

33 Royal College of Midwives Annual general meeting.
95th. Midwives Chronicle, 90, Sep 1977, 203-205; Nursing Mirror, 145, 21 Jul 1977, 4-5.
96th. Midwives Chronicle, 91, Sep 1978, 239-241; Nursing Times, 74, 3 Aug 1978, 1270-1271.
98th. Midwives Chronicle, 93, Sep 1980, 314-318.

34 Royal College of Midwives Comments on proposals on aspects of the Briggs report on nursing. Midwives Chronicle, 89, Nov 1976, 262-263.

35 Royal College of Midwives The future role of the midwife in the maternity services.

(Comments to the DHSS.) Midwives Chronicle, 89, Sep 1976, 222-224.

36 Royal College of Midwives Midwives decide it's time to take the union plunge. Nursing Mirror, 143, 22 Jul 1976, 35-36; Nursing Times, 72, 14 Oct 1976, 1580.

37 Royal College of Midwives Supervision of midwifery. RCM symposium report. Midwives Chronicle, 89, Jan 1976, 10-11.

38 Thomson, A.M. Planned or unplanned? Are midwives ready for the 1980s? Midwives Chronicle, 93, Mar 1980, 68-72.

39 Walker, J.F. Improving maternity care by midwifery research. Nursing Times, 73, 22 Sep 1977, 1489-1491.

40 Walker, J.F. Midwife or obstetric nurse? Some perceptions of midwives and obstetricians of the role of the midwife. (A small exploratory study of the relationship between midwives and the medical profession.) Journal of Advanced Nursing, 1 (2), Mar 1976, 129-138.

41 Walker, J.F. Practitioners in their own right: a study of some aspects of the role of the midwife. MSc(Econ) thesis, University of Wales, University College, Cardiff, 1978.

42 Ward, J.P. Nursing research in obstetrics and gynaecology. (Work of the nursing officer (research) Department of Obstetrics and Gynaecology, University of Liverpool.) Nursing Times, 72, 11 Nov 1976, 1778-1779.

d EUROPE AND THE EEC

1 Beaufils, F. and Bouet, A. (Better perinatal health) France. Lancet, 2, 22/29 Dec 1979, 1352-1353.

2 Bent, E.A. The EEC Midwives Directives. The current position—what is it? Midwives Chronicle, 91, Sep 1978, 246-248.

3 Friend, P. U.K. midwifery services under pressure from Europe. Nursing Mirror, 143, 16 Dec 1976, 36.

4 Garside, D. Midwifery in Scandinavia. (Report of a study tour.) Nursing Times, 72, 6 May 1976, 702-704.

5 Gillies, E. A visit to Sweden. (Brief report of visit to look at maternal and child care.) Health Visitor, 53 (8), Aug 1980, 334, 336.

6 Lepper, E. Midwifery services in Holland. (Report of study tour with emphasis on postnatal care.) Nursing Times, 75, 29 Nov 1979, 2084-2086.

7 Lord, A.P. The health of the mother and child. (Report of course at International Childrens Centre in Paris and study tour to Bulgaria.) Nursing Times, 73, 8 Sep 1977, ABPN Supplement 6-7.

8 McEwen, J. Study visit to Finland. (Maternal and child health services.) Health Visitor, 51 (2), Feb 1978, 41-43.

9 Magill-Gueriden, J. Not such a 'Common Market' for midwives. (Study tour of midwifery training in Holland, Germany and Finland.) Midwives Chronicle, 90, Apr 1977, 76-78.

10 Mee, B.D. Midwives and the EEC. Midwives Chronicle, 89, Jun 1976, 152-153.

11 Mee, B. Negotiating the EEC Midwives' Directives. Nursing Mirror, 142, 3 Jun 1976, 39-41.

12 Romilly, V.P. E.E.C. permanent committee of midwives. (Report of a meeting in London, Feb 1976.) World of Irish Nursing, 5 (10), Oct 1976, 7.

13 Ross, T. The Dutch stay-at-homes. (Dutch midwives.) Nursing Mirror, 148, 10 May 1979, 16-18.

14 Ross, T. The Finnish success story. (Maternity services and primary health care in Finland.) Nursing Mirror, 148, 17 May 1979, 16-19.

15 Ross, T. A simple Swedish recipe. (Maternity services and midwifery in Sweden.) Nursing Mirror, 148, 24 May 1979, 18-19.

e OTHER OVERSEAS COUNTRIES

1 Ansell, C. Health care in the Yemen. (Maternal and child health.) Midwife, Health Visitor and Community Nurse, 14 (12), Dec 1978, 425-426, 428-429.

2 Baskett, T.F. Obstetric care in the central Canadian Arctic. (Among the Eskimos, involving nurse practitioners and medical staff.) British Medical Journal, 2, 7 Oct 1978, 1001-1004.

3 Beischer, N.A. Projected developments in midwifery. (In Australia.) Australian Nurses Journal, 8 (2), Aug 1978, 52-56, 61.

4 Bland, J. A better midwife. (Traditional midwives in Peru.) World Health, Jul 1978, 24, 26-27.

5 Burst, H.V. The American College of Nurse-Midwives: a professional organisation. Journal of Nurse-Midwifery, 25 (1), Jan/Feb 1980, 4-6.

6 Corbould, C. Medical care in rural Bangladesh. (By nurse who worked in family planning and maternal and child health project.) Nursing Mirror, 146, 16 Mar 1978, 25-27.

7 Dean, M. Nurse-midwife—a 'multipurpose worker'. Nursing Journal of India, 47 (4), Apr 1976, 91-92.

8 Etzel, R.A. Liberian obstetrics. The birth and development of midwifery (in Liberia.) Part 1. Journal of Nurse-Midwifery, 21 (4), Winter 1976, 24-37.

9 Field, P.A. Countdown on O.B. nurses. (Three research studies of obstetric nursing practice and education.) Canadian Nurse, 75 (9), Oct 1979, 18-20.

10 Gordon, A.C.M. Health work the Western African way. (Report of midwife's work in Ghana as member of VSO with antenatal patients and children under 5.) Health Visitor, 50 (12), Dec 1977, 420.

11 Gupta, K. Qualified personnel or traditional midwives? Women's choice in rural India. International Nursing Review, 25 (6), Nov/Dec 1978, 175-181.

12 Kamalamma, A. and others Trends in utilisation of maternal care services in a rural community. (Research study.) Nursing Journal of India, 70 (6), Jun 1979, 162-164.

13 Kimbro, C.D. The relationship between nurses and nurse-midwives. (With history of development of nurse-midwifery in USA.) Journal of Nurse-Midwifery, 22 (4), Winter 1977, 29-31.

14 Klein, R. Unqualified and outside the law. (Position of non-nurse midwives in America.) Nursing Mirror, 150, 7 Feb 1980, 30.

15 Larsen, J.V. and others The midwifery nursing associate: an experiment in a rural obstetric unit. (African homelands.) S.A. Nursing Journal, 53 (11), Nov 1976, 7-8.

16 Lawson, J.S. and Savage, N. From haemorrhage to harmony in the labour ward. (Survey of midwifery practices in Sydney.) Australian Nurses Journal, 9 (7), Feb 1980, 31-32.

17 Levine, N.H. A conceptual model for obstetric nursing. The need for and purpose of a more comprehensive theoretical basis for nursing practice, research and education. Journal of Obstetric, Gynecologic and Neonatal Nursing, 5 (2), Mar/Apr 1976, 9-15.

18 Lumley, J. Better perinatal health. Australia. Lancet, 1, 12 Jan 1980, 79-81.

19 Macleod, J. Ten months in East Africa. (As midwife.) Midwives Chronicle, 91, Mar 1978, 62-63.

20 Mulligan, J.E. Professional transition: nurse to nurse-midwife. Nursing Outlook, 24 (4), Apr 1976, 228-233.

21 Powis, J. Nurse-midwifery: are we missing the boat? (Position in the U.S.A., education programmes in Canada and C.N.A. Statement on the nurse-midwife.) Canadian Nurse, 75 (9), Oct 1979, 21-23.

22 Reches, R. Midwifery and professional training of the midwife in Israel. Midwives Chronicle, 91, Jul 1978, 167-169.

23 Reedy, N.J. Nurse-midwife in complicated obstetrics: trend or treason? Journal of Nurse-Midwifery, 24 (1), Jan/Feb 1979, 11-17.

24 Reese, M.C. Meeting maternal and child health care needs in Tanzania. (Using barefoot doctors.) International Nursing Review, 25 (1), Jan/Feb 1978, 10-13.

25 Rooks, J.B. American nurse-midwifery: are we making an impact? Journal of Nurse-Midwifery, 23, Fall 1978, 15-19.

26 Runnerstrom, L. and others The nurse midwife in the obstetric health team. (Expanding role in the United States.) Nursing Forum, 15 (1), 1976, 59-68.

27 Salmond, G.C. Inequality of health care. (Consumer study of maternity and infant health services in Wellington.) New Zealand Nursing Journal, 69 (1), Jan 1976, 23-28.

28 Simpson, Sister Mary Stella Sister Stella's babies: days in the practice of a nurse-midwife. New York: American Journal of Nursing Co., 1978.

29 Spiegelman, J.M. The midwife in the Third World. Midwives Chronicle, 89, Aug 1976, 200-201.

30 Thompson, H.O. and Beebe, J.E. 'Nurse-midwifery and ethics...a beginning.' Journal of Nurse-Midwifery, 21 (4), Winter 1976, 7-11.

31 Turner, Sister M. Nursing care study. Obstetrics in a health sub-centre. (Montfort Catholic Mission, Papua, New Guinea.) Nursing Mirror, 146, 12 Jan 1978, 19-20.

32 Whaley, P. Two home births: a Melbourne midwife reports on the growing trend towards childbirth in the home. Australian Nurses Journal, 8 (1), Jul 1978, 41-44, 47.

33 WHO Chronicle Training traditional birth attendants. (Conference in Brazzaville.) WHO Chronicle, 30 (5), May 1976, 204.

34 Wohlert, H. NAACOG—the first 10 years. (Nurses Association of The American College of Obstetricians and Gynecologists.) Journal of Obstetric, Gynecologic and Neonatal Nursing, 8 (1), Jan/Feb 1979, 9-22.

f DOMICILIARY MIDWIFERY

1 Ashton, K. A home delivery in Holland. (Author describes her experience of care by Dutch domiciliary midwifery service.) Nursing Times, 76, 14 Aug 1980, 1442-1446.

2 Burfitt, M.D. The cost of a community midwifery service. (Description of service in Hounslow district.) Midwives Chronicle, 90, Nov 1977, 264-265.

3 Cox, C.A. and others Critical appraisal of domiciliary obstetric and neonatal practice. (A study of home confinements in the catchment area of the West Middlesex Hospital.) British Medical Journal, 1, 10 Jan 1976, 84-86.

4 Flint, C. A continuing labour of love. (Scheme in South London where three midwives cooperate in providing continuity of care for patients.) Nursing Mirror, 149, 15 Nov 1979, 16-18.

5 Fotheringham, M.R. Night rota system for community midwives. (Havering District of the Barking and Havering A.H.A.) Queen's Nursing Journal, 19 (10), Jan 1977, 270-272.

6 Grove, G. The community midwife. Nursing Times, 72, 27 May 1976, Community Care Supplement viii,x.

7 Hosford, E. Alternative patterns of nurse-midwifery care. The home birth movement (in the U.S.). Journal of Nurse-Midwifery, 21 (3), 1976, 27-30.

8 Huygen, F.J. Home deliveries in Holland: Dutch maternity care and home confinements. Journal of the Royal College of General Practitioners, 26, Apr 1976, 244-248.

9 Kolle, R. The midwife and the family unit. (ICM Congress paper.) Midwives Chronicle, 92, May 1979, 140-141.

10 O'Dwyer, I. The role of the midwife in family life. World of Irish Nursing, 5 (6), Jun 1976, 7.

11 Page, N.E. Community experience in an integrated area. (In Telford, Shropshire.) Midwives Chronicle, 91, Apr 1978, 81.

12 Willmott, J.A.D. Less at risk than some: the work of the Islington community midwife. Midwives Chronicle, 89, Oct 1976, 236-238.

13 Willmott, J.A.D. A matter of choice: the case for domiciliary midwifery. Nursing Mirror, 133, 12 May 1977, 39-41.

14 Willmott, J.A.D. The midwife's place: is it at the mother's home or in the hospital? (Role of community midwife.) Nursing Mirror, 148, 8 Feb 1979, 8.

15 Willmott, J.A.D. Specialists in birth. (Changing role of community midwives, with statistics of Islington Community Midwives service.) Nursing Mirror, 151, 17 Jul 1980, 34-36.

g EDUCATION AND TRAINING

1 Allis, P.A. Outline of curriculum development for midwifery training. (Based on report of working party of Sheffield District Midwives Teachers Group.) Midwives Chronicle, 91, Feb 1978, 23.

2 Balch, B. and Kilty, J.M. The Midwife Teachers' Diploma Course at the Royal College of Midwives and the University of Surrey. Midwives Chronicle, 89, Sep 1976, 214-216.

3 Bent, E.A. and Kilty, J.M. Teachers' page. 18. Theory and practice. Midwives Chronicle, 89, Nov 1976, 269-272.

4 Bent, E.A. and others Educating the midwife for her changing role. Midwives Chronicle, 89, Jul 1976, 174-176.

5 Bent, E.A. and others Preparing today's midwife educator and instructor. Midwives Chronicle, 89, May 1976, 111-113.

6 Bry, B.H. and Marsico, T. Personality characteristics associated with success in learning and practicing nurse-midwifery. (Research study.) Journal of Nurse-Midwifery, 25 (3), May/Jun 1980, 11-15.

7 Central Midwives Board Notices. (Programme for obstetric module to comply with EEC directives.) Midwives Chronicle, 91, Jul 1978, 173.

8 Da Cruz, V. C.M.B. questions and how to answer them. 5th ed. Faber, 1977.

9 Golden, J. Midwifery training: the view of newly qualified midwives. (Survey by Chelsea College of Nursing Education Research Unit.) Midwives Chronicle, 93, Jun 1980, 190-194.

10 Grenu, M. Midwifery training and practice. (ICM Congress Paper.) Midwives Chronicle, 92, Jun 1979, 167-168.

11 Kitson, L.M. Midwifery education in the 1980s. Midwives Chronicle, 93, Feb 1980, 37-40.

12 Matson, T.J. Teaching tomorrow's midwives. (With history from 1788.) Australian Nurses Journal, 7 (6), Dec/Jan 1978, 41-44.

13 Morgan, J.A. A traumatic experience. (Criticism of proposals to reduce period of obstetric experience for student nurses.) Midwives Chronicle, 91, Dec 1978, 359.

14 Newson, K. A thought for the future. (Suggests new type of training based on direct entry.) Midwives Chronicle, 92, May 1979, 142.

15 Newson, K. and Hallworth, C. Time for a change? (Need for change in current system of training midwives.) Nursing Mirror, 151, 10 Jul 1980 Supplement iii-vi, x.

16 Rankin, S. Midwives first—nurses second? (The case for direct entry to midwifery i.e. without nursing qualifications.) Nursing Mirror, 151, 11 Dec 1980, 22-23.

17 Royal College of Midwives Case studies for examination purposes. Results of a questionnaire set by the RCM Yorkshire Group of Midwife Teachers. Midwives Chronicle, 89, Aug 1976, 196-197.

18 Shaw, M.E. A course to aid midwives in clinical teaching. (Plymouth maternity unit.) Midwives Chronicle, 90, Mar 1977, 54-56.

19 Ward, M.E. and Adams, M.E. A masters degree in midwifery. (Proposal.) Midwives Chronicle, 92, Feb 1979, 37-38.

20 Warpinski, D.H. and Adams, C.J. Characteristics of applicants to nurse-midwifery educational program. (Research study.) Journal of Nurse-Midwifery, 24 (4), Jul/Aug 1979, 5-9.

21 Williams, S.M.K. Student nurses' attitudes towards midwifery. (Questionnaire survey of 65 learners.) Nursing Times, 75, 5 Apr 1979, Occ. papers, 41-43.

h HISTORY

1 Arthure, H. Changes in obstetric practice between 1952 and 1977. Midwife, Health Visitor and Community Nurse, 13 (10), Oct 1977, 322-325.

2 Arthure, H. Princess Charlotte of Wales—a Royal tragedy. (Death in childbirth.) Midwife, Health Visitor and Community Nurse, 13 (5), May 1977, 147-149.

3 Blackman, J. Lessons from the history of maternal care and childbirth. Midwives Chronicle, 90, Mar 1977, 46-49.

4 Bowler, V.M. Midwifery notes from the past. (Notes from 'Lectures to Midwives' by F.R. Humphreys, 1899.) Nursing Mirror, 143 (24), 9 Dec 1976, 69-70.

5 Brian, V.A. The deepest cut of all. (History of the Caesarean section.) Nursing Mirror, 143, 30 Sep 1976, 68-69.

6 Carswell, G.W. and Hamilton, A.R. William Smellie—master of British obstetrics. Midwife, Health Visitor and Community Nurse, 12 (4), Apr 1976, 122-123.

7 Carter, M. The royal midwives. (In the 15th-17th centuries.) Midwives Chronicle, 90, Dec 1977, 300-301.

8 Chaney, J.A. Birthing in early America. Journal of Nurse-Midwifery, 25 (2), Mar/Apr 1980, 5-13.

9 Clark, L. Portrait of an Edwardian midwife. (Ester Roberts.) Midwives Chronicle, 91, May 1978, 111-113.

10 Copcutt, D.I. Midwifery in the Nineteenth Century. S.A. Nursing Journal, 43 (4), Apr 1976, 22-24; (8), Aug 1976, 15-17.

11 Donegan, J.B. Women and men midwives: medicine, morality and misogyny in early America. Westport, Conn.: Greenwood Press, 1978. (Contributions in medical history; 2.)

12 Donnison, J. Midwives and medical men:

a history of inter-professional rivalries and women's rights. Heinemann, 1977.

13 Ezrati, J.B. Midwifery in the media. (In USA. Historical account from 1925.) Journal of Nurse-Midwifery, 22 (2), Summer 1977, 35-38.

14 Gordon, J.E. Pioneers of British nursing. Midwifery pioneers. Nursing Mirror, 144, 14 Apr 1977, 67.

15 Kobrin, F.E. The American midwife controversy: a crisis of professionalization. *In* Leavitt, J.W. and Numbers, R.L. editors Sickness and health in America... Madison: University of Wisconsin Press, 1978. (Chapter 16, 217-225.)

16 Liebermann, J.J. Childbirth practices: from darkness into light. (Childbirth in the Middle Ages.) Journal of Obstetric, Gynecologic and Neonatal Nursing, 5 (3), May/Jun 1976, 41-45.

17 Rouch, R.E. The development of midwifery—male and female, yesterday and today. (Including Greek and Roman eras, Renaissance and the U.S.A.) Journal of Nurse-Midwifery, 24 (3), May/Jun 1979, 27-37.

18 Tom, S.A. Rose McNaught: American nurse-midwifery's own 'sister tutor'. (First teacher of nurse-midwifery in USA.) Journal of Nurse-Midwifery, 24 (2), Mar/Apr 1979, 3-8.

19 Withers, M. Agnodike: the first midwife/obstetrician. (In Athens in third century BC.) Journal of Nurse-Midwifery, 24 (3), May/Jun 1979, 4.

i MALE MIDWIVES

1 American Journal of Nursing First certified male midwife practices in New Haven. American Journal of Nursing, 78 (4), Apr 1978, 689-690.

2 Beilby, B.G. A place for the male midwife. (Report of obstetric nurse training at the Royal Sussex County Hospital, Brighton.) Midwives Chronicle, 90, Dec 1977, 295-297.

3 Chalmers, K. Introduction to obstetrics for male nurses. (Experiences of a student at the Royal Free Hospital during obstetric allocation.) Midwives Chronicle, 90, Jan 1977, 3-4.

4 Chalmers, K. A male nurse practises obstetrics. (Experiences of a second year student at the Royal Free Hospital School of Nursing.) Nursing Times, 72, 16 Dec 1976, 1980.

5 Darby, C. Where now for male midwives? (DHSS evaluation of consumer reaction to experiment.) Nursing Mirror, 147, 20 Jul 1978, 13-15.

6 Dicker, K. Toward sexual equality. (Male midwives.) Nursing Mirror, 144, 19 May 1977, 31.

7 Hall, M. Unforgettable experience. (A male nurse on an eight week obstetric appreciation course at Newcastle Polytechnic.) Midwives Chronicle, 90, Jan 1977, 4-5.

8 Lindsay, G.P. Centuries of controversy. But the male midwife is no new species... (Evidence from eighteenth century parish records in Somerset.) Nursing Mirror, 147, 20 Jul 1978, 15.

9 SEX Discrimination Act brings 'equality' for

men. (Issue of male midwives.) Nursing Mirror, 142, 1 Jan 1976, 34.

40 PREGNANCY

a ANTENATAL PREPARATION

1 Backhouse, J. The National Childbirth Trust teacher. (With details of training for antenatal education.) Nursing Times, 76, 17 Jul 1980 Midwifery supplement 15.

2 Billung-Meyer, J. The single mother: can we help? (Special programme of antenatal classes for teenage expectant mothers in Massachusetts.) Canadian Nurse, 75 (10), Nov 1979, 26-28.

3 Boother, B. Antenatal defaulters. Midwives Chronicle, 89, Jul 1976, 170-171.

4 Brant, H.A. Improving the quality of antenatal care. Text of an address to last month's RCM Annual Conference. Nursing Mirror, 147, 10 Aug 1978, 7-9.

5 Brant, H.A. The quality of prenatal care. (With reference to the prevention of handicap.) Midwives Chronicle, 91, Nov 1978, 315-318.

6 Browne, J.C.M. and Dixon, G. Antenatal care. 11th ed. Churchill Livingstone, 1978.

7 Chalmers, J.A. Modern antenatal care—an appraisal. Midwife, Health Visitor and Community Nurse, 12 (1), Jan 1976, 9-12; (2), Feb 1976, 50-52.

8 Chamberlain, G. The prepregnancy clinic. (At Queen Charlotte's Hospital for women worried about possible problems.) British Medical Journal, 281, 5 Jul 1980, 29-30.

9 Chamberlain, G. and Chave, S. Antenatal education. (Programme at Queen Charlotte's Hospital and survey of expectant mothers' sources of information.) Community Health, 9 (1), Aug 1977, 11-16.

10 Clode, D. Action now could save paying later. (Antenatal care and perinatal mortality rates.) Health and Social Service Journal, 89, 5 Jan 1979, 6-8.

11 Copeland, D.Z. Unwed adolescent primigravidas identify subject matter for prenatal classes. (Research study.) Journal of Obstetric, Gynecologic and Neonatal Nursing, 8 (4), Jul/Aug 1979, 248-253.

12 Davies, M. Antenatal teaching. (Work of the National Childbirth Trust, which celebrates its 21st anniversary this year.) Nursing Times, 73, 20 Oct 1977, 1646-1647.

13 Davis, L. and Katz, B.M. Knowledge and attitude toward nurse-midwifery among women taking childbirth education classes. (Research study.) Journal of Nurse-Midwifery, 24 (4), Jul/Aug 1979, 18-26.

14 Dennis, K.J. Antenatal paediatrics. Nursing Mirror, 142, 19 Feb 1976, 63-65.

15 Department of Health and Social Security Prevention and health: reducing the risk. Safer pregnancy and childbirth: a discussion paper. HMSO, 1977.

16 Drummond, G. Community nursing care study. Preparing for Lisa. (Ante- and postnatal care.) Nursing Times, 73, 19 May 1977, 734-736.

17 Gerken, A. Microbiology and midwifery. Antenatal clinics arrange an important series of microbiological tests. Midwife, Health Visitor and Community Nurse, 13 (5), May 1977, 140-142.

18 Gillett, J.R. Helping those who have not been to preparation for childbirth classes. Midwives Chronicle, 90, Feb 1977, 32-34.

19 Gillett, J.R. A report on the survey on preparation for childbirth within the catchment area of Copthorne Maternity Unit Shrewsbury: December 1972-June 1973. International Journal of Nursing Studies, 13 (1), 1976, 25-46.

20 Gillett, J.R. Teacher training through the National Childbirth Trust. Midwife, Health Visitor and Community Nurse, 16 (9), Sep 1980, 380-381.

21 Hall, M. and others Is routine antenatal care worthwhile? (Analysis of case records in Aberdeen.) Lancet, 2, 12 Jul 1980, 78-80.

22 Heward, J.A. and Clarke, M. Communications to an antenatal clinic. (Survey of information provided by general practitioners for the Royal Infirmary Maternity Unit, Leicester.) British Medical Journal, 1, 15 May 1976, 1203-1204.

23 Heywood Jones, I. Antenatal care...or coercion? (Possible role of financial incentives in encouraging pregnant women to attend antenatal clinics.) Nursing Times, 75, 15 Nov 1979, 1964.

24 Hibbard, B.M. and others The effectiveness of antenatal education. (Survey in Cardiff.) Health Education Journal, 38 (2), 1979, 39-46.

25 Kennedy, I. and Stephens, B. A novel antenatal record to help midwives. (Developed in Botswana.) Practitioner, 223, Jul 1979, 18-24.

26 Kitzinger, S. Challenges in antenatal education. 1. Immigrant women in childbirth—an anthropologist's view. 2. Giving support in labour. 3. A fresh look at the second stage. Nursing Mirror, 144, 23 Jun 1977, 19-22; 30 Jun 1977, 20-22; 7 Jul 1977, 17-20.

27 Liffers, T. A survey on preparation for childbirth. (Review of the survey at Copthorne Maternity Unit, Shrewsbury.) Midwife, Health Visitor and Community Nurse, 13 (2), Feb 1977, 50-51.

28 Merkur, H. Normal and abnormal antenatal cardiographic patterns. (With report of study of 900 traces.) Midwives Chronicle, 92, May 1979, 132-135.

29 Moore, D.S. Prepared childbirth: the pregnant couple and their marriage. (Effect of childbirth education and presence of husband on women's birth experience.) Journal of Nurse-Midwifery, 22 (2), Summer 1977, 18-26.

30 Mowat, S. Ante-natal care—some thoughts on the role of the health visitor. Health Visitor, 52 (3), Mar 1979, 78-79.

31 Oakley, A. and MacFarlane, A. A poor birthright. (Antenatal care and the report of the Select Committee on Perinatal and Neonatal Mortality.) New Society, 53, 24 Jul 1980, 172-173.

32 Roberts, J.E. Priorities in prenatal education. Journal of Obstetric, Gynecologic and Neonatal Nursing, 5 (3), May/Jun 1976, 17-20.

33 Rothenstein, L. Prepared childbirth. (Psychoprophylaxis.) Journal of Practical Nursing, 27 (4), Apr 1977, 20-25.

34 Sasmor, J.L. Childbirth education: a nursing perspective. New York: John Wiley, 1979.

35 Savage, W. Antenatal care: have Dr. Ballantyne's aims been achieved? Part 1. Midwife, Health Visitor and Community Nurse, 16 (5), May 1980, 190, 192, 194.

36 Simpson, H. and Walker, G. When do pregnant women attend for antenatal care? (Study of sample in N.E. Thames region.) British Medical Journal, 281, 12 Jul 1980, 104-107.

37 Soep, M. The consumer's view of pregnancy — a reply. (An example of pre-natal preparation organised by health visitors and midwives.) Nursing Times, 72, 8 Apr 1976, 549.

38 Timm, M.M. Prenatal education evaluation. (Survey of relationship between amount of medication used by women during labour and the birth weight of their infants following participation in prenatal classes.) Nursing Research, 28 (6), Nov/Dec 1979, 338-342.

39 Turnbull, A.C. and Woodford, F.P. joint editors Prevention of handicap through antenatal care. Associated Scientific Publishers, 1976. (IRMMH review of research and practice no.18.)

40 Whitley, N. A comparison of prepared childbirth couples and conventional prenatal class couples. (Research study.) Journal of Obstetric, Gynecologic and Neonatal Nursing, 8 (2), Mar/Apr 1979, 109-111.

41 Wynn, M. and Wynn, A. Prevention of handicap and the health of women. Routledge and Kegan Paul, 1979. (Inequality in society series.)

42 Wynn, M. and Wynn, A. Prevention of handicap of perinatal origin: an introduction to French policy and legislation. Foundation for Education and Research in Child-Bearing, 1976.

43 Wynn, M. and Wynn, A. The prevention of preterm birth: an introduction to some European developments aimed at the prevention of handicap. Foundation for Education and Research in Child-Bearing, 1977.

b PREGNANCY

1 British Medical Journal School pregnancies. British Medical Journal, 280, 19 Apr 1980, 1061-1062.

2 British Pregnancy Advisory Service School-girl pregnancies. Wootton-Wawen: BPAS, (1978.)

3 Chao, Y-M. An habitual aborter's self-concept during the course of a successful pregnancy. Maternal-Child Nursing Journal, 6 (3), Fall 1977, 165-175.

4 Chiota, B.J. and others Effects of separation from spouse on pregnancy, labor and delivery and the postpartum period. Journal of Obstetric, Gynecologic and Neonatal Nursing, 5 (1), Jan/Feb 1976, 21-23.

5 Curtin, L.L. and Petrick, J.A. Reproductive manipulation: technical advances, options, and ethical ramifications. ('Test tube babies'.) Nursing Forum, 16 (1), 1977, 6-25.

6 Fawcett, J. Body image and the pregnant couple. (Research study with husbands and wives.) American Journal of Maternal-Child Nursing, 3 (4), Jul/Aug 1978, 227-233.

7 Fawcett, J. The relationship between identification and patterns of change in spouses' body images during and after pregnancy. International Journal of Nursing Studies, 14 (4), 1977, 199-213.

8 Harris, M. Louise: the test-tube miracle. (Procedures for first in-vitro fertilisation and Caesarian section.) Nursing Mirror, 147, 2 Nov 1978 Supplement xv-xvi, xix.

9 Kitzinger, S. Pregnancy and childbirth. Joseph, 1980.

10 Kuczynski, H.J. Sexual relations in pregnancy. Midwives Chronicle, 92, Jul 1979, 215-217.

11 Lederman, R.P. and others Relationship of psychological factors in pregnancy to progress in labor. Nursing Research, 28 (2), Mar/Apr 1979, 94-97.

12 Leslie, J. Nutrition and diet in pregnancy. Part 1. (Written for community nurses.) Nursing Mirror, 144, 16 Jun 1977, 18-20.

13 Malinowski, J.S. Sex during pregnancy: what can you say? (Includes advice on postpartum sex.) RN Magazine, 41 (11), Nov 1978, 48-51.

14 Mantle, M.J. and others Backache in pregnancy. (Survey of 180 women delivered in The London Hospital.) Rheumatology and Rehabilitation, 16 (2), May 1977, 95-101.

15 Moore, D.S. The body image in pregnancy. (Research study.) Journal of Nurse-Midwifery, 22 (4), Winter 1977, 17-27.

16 Munday, D. The price of advice. (Finances of charitable pregnancy advisory bureaux.) Nursing Times, 73, 1 Sep 1977, 1344-1345.

17 O'Donovan, M. Nursing care study. Twin pregnancy following artificial insemination. Nursing Mirror, 142, 20 May 1976, 47-49.

18 Philipp, E. Pregnancy in prison. (Nursing and medical care.) Midwife, Health Visitor and Community Nurse, 14 (2), Feb 1978, 36, 38, 41.

19 Porter, L.S. and Demeuth, B.R. The impact of marital adjustment on pregnancy acceptance. (Research study.) American Journal of Maternal-Child Nursing, 8 (2), Summer 1979, 103-113.

20 Rothwell, H. Pregnancy — a state of ignorance. (The author looks back on her pregnancy and asks for more education, more information, and some changes in health service policy.) Midwives Chronicle, 91, Feb 1978, 28-30.

21 Snehendu, B.K. and others Pregnancy risk-taking among young unmarried women: an analysis of its determinants and prevention. Patient Counseling and Health Education, 1 (4), Summer/Fall 1979, 151-163.

22 Symonds, E.M. Care of the pregnant woman. (Review of obstetric practice.) Midwife, Health Visitor and Community Nurse, 16 (3), Mar 1980, 94, 96, 99.

23 Warnyca, J. and others Healthiest babies possible. The Vancouver Perinatal Health Project. (Multidisciplinary team approach during pregnancy and six months postpartum.) Canadian Nurse, 75 (10), Nov 1979, 18-21.

24 Wasley, G.D. Laboratory pregnancy testing. (Methods.) Nursing Times, 74, 5 Jan 1978, 25-27.

25 WHO Chronicle Pregnancy and the unmarried girl. WHO Chronicle, 30 (3), Mar 1976, 108-110.

c COMPLICATIONS

1 Ademowore, A.S. and Myers, E. Use of problem-oriented medical record by nurses caring for high risk antepartum patients. Journal of Obstetric, Gynecologic and Neonatal Nursing, 6 (1), Jan/Feb 1977, 17-22.

2 Arthure, H. Uncommon accidents in obstetric practice. Midwife, Health Visitor and Community Nurse, 15 (1), Jan 1979, 14-16; (2), Feb 1979, 52-53.

3 Auber, E.S. Case study: obstetric patient 'at risk' with a gynaecological complication. Midwives Chronicle, 89, Sep 1976, 217-219.

4 Austin, M.A. Intra-uterine blood transfusion. (In cases of Rhesus iso-immunisation.) Nursing Times, 74, 11 May 1978, 806-809.

5 Bascom, L. Women who refuse to believe: persistent denial of pregnancy. American Journal of Maternal-Child Nursing, 2 (3), May/Jun 1977, 174-177.

6 Beilin, L.J. Hypertension during pregnancy. Nursing Mirror, 142, 20 May 1976, 57-58.

7 Bowyer-Kearns, S. Ectopic gestation. (Care study.) Nursing Times, 76, 11 Sep 1980, 1621-1623.

8 Brown, A.K. Peripartal cardiomyopathy. (Heart failure in the puerperium or later stages of pregnancy.) Nursing Times, 73, 3 Feb 1977, 165.

9 Caldicott, J.A. Nursing care study. Cardiac disease in pregnancy. Nursing Mirror, 142, 3 Jun 1976, 46-48.

10 Cooper, F. Thrombosis and embolism in obstetrics. Nursing Mirror, 142, 11 Mar 1976, 65-67.

11 Duru, H. Nursing care study. Double uterus. Nursing Mirror, 142, 24 Jun 1976, 50-51.

12 Eagle, M. Nursing care study. Septicaemia proceeding to disseminated intravascular coagulation. (Puerperal septicaemia with endotoxic shock.) Nursing Times, 74 (1), 5 Jan 1978, 17-21.

13 Goggin, M.J. Urinary tract and renal consequences of pregnancy. Nursing Mirror, 145, 22 Sep 1977, 22-24.

14 Guthrie, T.E. Case study: successful outcome of abdominal pregnancy. Midwives Chronicle, 91, May 1978, 107-109.

15 Harder, G.M. Nursing decisions. Experiences in clinical problem solving: complications in a young primigravida. RN Magazine, 39 (1), Jan 1976, 47-50.

16 Hewitt, S.R. Ectopic pregnancy. Nursing Times, 72, 26 Aug 1976, 1308-1310.

17 Hurley, R. Viral infections in pregnancy. Midwife, Health Visitor and Community Nurse, 13 (4), Apr 1977, 117-119.

18 Lewis, K. Nursing care study. Management of phaeochromocytoma in pregnancy. Nursing Times, 72, 1 Apr 1976, 492-493.

19 Norris, L. Nursing care study. Abdominal pregnancy. Nursing Times, 73, 14 Jul 1977, 1084-1085.

20 Oakley, C.M. Heart disease in pregnancy. Nursing Times, 72, 9 Dec 1976, 1923-1924.

21 Oliver, S. Nursing care study. Fulminating eclampsia. (In hospital in the Yemen Arab Republic.) Nursing Mirror, 147, 9 Nov 1978, 28-29.

22 Peckham, C. Cytomegalovirus infection in pregnancy. Midwife, Health Visitor and Community Nurse, 14 (9), Sep 1978, 297, 299.

23 Redman, C.W.G. The management of severe pre-eclampsia. Midwife, Health Visitor and Community Nurse, 12 (10), Oct 1976, 322-325.

d DRUGS

1 Cooper, P. Progress in therapeutics. Drug hazards during pregnancy. Part 2. Midwife, Health Visitor and Community Nurse, 12 (4), Apr 1976, 129.

2 DiPalma, J.R. Drug therapy today. The ubiquitous anaerobe: cause for concern in OBG. RN Magazine, 38 (12), Dec 1975, 61-62, 64, 65.

3 Fraser, A.C. Drug addiction in pregnancy. Lancet, 2, 23 Oct 1976, 896-899.

4 Fraser, A.C. Pregnancy and drug addiction. Midwife, Health Visitor and Community Nurse, 14 (5), May 1978, 132, 135.

5 Lewis, P. Drugs: the bitter pill in pregnancy. The possible adverse effects of drugs given in pregnancy on the developing brain. Nursing Mirror, 147, 5 Oct 1978, 38-39.

6 Richards, M.P.M. Obstetric analgesics and the development of children. (Effect of drugs on infant development.) Midwife, Health Visitor and Community Nurse, 12 (2), Feb 1976, 37-40.

e FETUS

1 American Journal of Nursing Fetal and maternal monitoring. (Home study feature for continuing education accreditation.) American Journal of Nursing, 78 (12), Dec 1978, 2097-2120.

2 Applegate, J. and others Electronic fetal monitoring: implications for obstetrical nursing. Nursing Research, 28 (6), Nov/Dec 1979, 369-371.

3 Beard, R.W. and Rivers, R.P.A. Better perinatal health. Fetal asphyxia in labour. Lancet, 2, 24 Nov 1979, 1117-1119.

4 Beazley, J.M. Assessment of life 'in utero'. Nursing Times, 76, 8 May 1980, 825-828.

5 Beazley, J. and Kurjak, A. Fetal progress:

why palpate a pregnant abdomen? (With value of ultrasonic screening.) Nursing Mirror, 149, 9 Aug 1979, 35-37.

6 Boyce, E.S. and others Doppler ultrasound method for detecting human fetal breathing in utero. British Medical Journal, 2, 3 Jul 1976, 17-18.

7 Bruce, S. Implications for amniocentesis. (By pupil midwife.) Midwives Chronicle, 92, Nov 1979, 389-391.

8 Davies, B.L. and Boniface, W.J. Prenatal testing for birth defects and nursing practice. (Includes parental reactions to stresses encountered.) Journal of Advanced Nursing, 4 (5), Sep 1979, 485-491.

9 Dunlop, C. Fitting into the routine. (Use of ultrasound by midwives in antenatal clinic to confirm presence of live foetus and assess gestational age.) Nursing Mirror, 151, 21 Aug 1980, 36-37.

10 Fox, A. Fetal heart rate monitoring. Lamp, 37 (11), Nov 1980, 15-24.

11 Gordon, A.D.G. Bicarbonate for a boy, vinegar for a girl. (Techniques to assist pre-selection of the sex of children.) Nursing Times, 74, 4 May 1978, 764-765.

12 Higginbottom, J. and others Ultrasound monitoring of fetal movements. A method of assessing fetal development? Lancet, 1, 3 Apr 1976, 719-721.

13 Hodnett, E. Fetal monitoring—why bother? Canadian Nurse, 73 (3), Mar 1977, 44-47.

14 Hudson, C.A. Antenatal determination of fetal sex. Nursing Mirror, 143, 23 Dec 1976, 34-35.

15 Iveson-Iveson, J. The use of ultrasound in midwifery. (History of its development and current use.) Nursing Mirror, 145, 21 Jul 1977, 7-8.

16 Kohn, C.L. and others Gravidas' responses to realtime ultrasound fetal image. (How perceptions of the fetus change.) Journal of Obstetric, Gynecologic and Neonatal Nursing, 9 (2), Mar/Apr 1980, 77-80.

17 Lancet Commentary from Westminster. Prenatal screening for spina bifida. Lancet, 1, 21 Jan 1978, 164-165.

18 Lancet Who's for amniocentesis? (Use and value of this procedure.) Lancet, 1, 7 May 1977, 986-987.

19 Lynaugh, K.H. The effects of early elective amniotomy on the length of labor and the condition of the fetus. (Research study.) Journal of Nurse-Midwifery, 25 (4), Jul/Aug 1980, 3-9.

20 Milford Ward, A. Alpha fetoprotein—an advance in antenatal diagnosis. (Of anencephaly and open spina bifida.) Nursing Mirror, 146, 25 May 1978, 23-25.

21 Muir, V.Y. Concept of the fetus as a transplant. (How nature has resolved the problem of rejecting transplants in the case of pregnancy.) Nursing Mirror, 146, 9 Jan 1978, 25-28.

22 Parer, J.T. and Dulock, H.L. Intrapartum

evaluation of the fetus. Journal of Obstetric, Gynecologic and Neonatal Nursing, 5 (5), Sep/Oct 1976, Supplement 1-80.

23 Pearson, J.F. Fetal monitoring in labour. Midwife, Health Visitor and Community Nurse, 14 (6), Jun 1978, 179-182.

24 Pearson, J.F. Fetal movements: a new approach to antenatal care. Nursing Mirror, 144, 21 Apr 1977, 49-51.

25 Roberts, A.B. Fetal movement and breathing. (As prognostic sign.) Midwife, Health Visitor and Community Nurse, 14 (8), Aug 1978, 256, 259.

26 Rodeck, C.H. Fetoscopy in prenatal diagnosis. (Inspection of uterine contents and fetal blood sampling.) Midwife, Health Visitor and Community Nurse, 14 (12), Dec 1978, 421-423.

27 Seller, M.J. The value of alpha fetoprotein measurements in pregnancy. Midwife, Health Visitor and Community Nurse, 14 (4), Apr 1978, 108, 112.

28 Stott, D.H. Children in the womb: the effects of stress. Detailed research (in Glasgow and Lanarkshire) seems to back up the importance of 'prenatal experience'. New Society, 40, 19 May 1977, 329-331.

29 Valman, H.B. and Pearson, J.F. The first year of life. What the fetus feels. British Medical Journal, 280, 26 Jan 1980, 233-234.

30 Yannes, M.O. Reducing infant mortality. Fetal monitoring. Journal of Practical Nursing, 27 (4), Apr 1977, 26, 27, 34.

f FETAL ABNORMALITIES

1 Clarren, S.K. and Smith, D.W. The fetal alcohol syndrome. Lamp, 35 (10), Oct 1978, 4-7.

2 Cowie, V. Antenatal diagnosis of genetic abnormalities. Nursing Mirror, 142, 22 Jan 1976, 61-62.

3 Crandon, A.J. Antenatal diagnosis of fetal abnormality. (Reprinted from Medical News.) Midwife, Health Visitor and Community Nurse, 16 (2), Feb 1980, 46, 48-49, 51.

4 Kessel, N. The fetal alcohol syndrome from the public health standpoint. Health Trends, 4 (9), Nov 1977, 86-89.

5 Lewis, J. A case of fetal hibernation? Midwives Chronicle, 89, Apr 1976, 88-89.

6 Luke, B. Maternal alcoholism and fetal alcohol syndrome. American Journal of Nursing, 77 (12), Dec 1977, 1924-1926.

7 Powledge, T. Prenatal diagnosis—now the problems. (Medical and ethical problems of abortion after genetic defects are revealed by amniocentesis.) New Scientist, 69, 12 Feb 1976, 332-334.

8 Slater, M.J. Congenital abnormalities and selective abortion. Journal of Medical Ethics, 2 (3), Sep 1976, 138-141.

9 Wallis, S. and Harvey, D. Intrauterine infection of the fetus. Nursing Times, 74, 1 Jun 1978, 912-916.

10 Watt, M. Management of patients at risk

of fetal malformation. (Western General Hospital, Edinburgh.) Nursing Mirror, 142, 6 May 1976, 61-63.

g PLACENTA

1 **Heys, R.F.** Understanding the placenta. Nursing Mirror, 145, 29 Sep 1977, 16-17; 6 Oct 1977, 33-35; 13 Oct 1977, 27-29.

2 **Pickles, B.G.** Abruptio placentae. (Bleeding due to placental detachment.) Nursing Times, 75, 1 Mar 1979, 356-357.

3 **Symonds, E.M.** Management of patients with placenta praevia. Nursing Times, 74, 16 Mar 1978, 453-455.

h SMOKING IN PREGNANCY

1 **Baric, L. and others** A study of health education aspects of smoking in pregnancy. (A study at Bolton District General Hospital to examine factors affecting women who stop smoking.) International Journal of Health Education, 14 (2), 1976 Supplement 1-16.

2 **Davies, D.P. and others** Cigarette smoking in pregnancy: associations with maternal weight gain and fetal growth. Lancet, 1, 21 Feb 1976, 385-387.

3 **Donovan, J.W.** Randomised controlled trial of anti-smoking advice in pregnancy. British Journal of Preventive and Social Medicine, 31 (1), Mar 1977, 6-12.

4 **Evans, D.R. and others** Maternal smoking habits and congenital malformations: a population study. British Medical Journal, 2, 21 Jul 1979, 171-173.

5 **Goldstein, H.** Smoking in pregnancy: some notes on the statistical controversy. British Journal of Preventive and Social Medicine, 31 (1), Mar 1977, 13-17.

6 **Lewis, P.** Smoking and pregnancy. (Its effect on the fetus, and smoking habits of pregnant women.) Midwife, Health Visitor and Community Nurse, 13 (6), Jun 1977, 167, 169-170, 173.

i PREGNANCY AND WORK

1 **Beckett, C.** Ante-natal care in industry. (John Player and Sons.) Physiotherapy, 64 (8), Aug 1978, 233-234.

2 **Greenberg, J.** Implications for primary care providers of occupational health hazards on pregnant women and their infants. Journal of Nurse-Midwifery, 25 (4), Jul/Aug 1980, 21-30.

3 **Johnston, E.E.** A pregnancy committee in industry. (Procedure to protect pregnant employees.) Occupational Health Nursing, 25 (4), Apr 1977, 12-13.

4 **Lerner, S.** Pre-employment examination and job placement of the pregnant woman. Occupational Health Nursing, 24 (9), Sep 1976, 15-18.

5 **Stasiewicz, J.H.** Pregnancy in the workplace. (Advice on maternity policy with list of toxic agents.) Occupational Health Nursing, 28 (5), May 1980, 13-17.

6 **United States Department of Health, Education and Welfare. National Institute for Occupational Safety and Health** Guidelines on pregnancy and work. Rockville, Md.: USDHEW, 1977.

41 CHILDBIRTH

a GENERAL AND PATIENTS' VIEWS

1 **Andersen, J.** A clarification of the Lamaze method. (Of education for childbirth.) Journal of Obstetric, Gynecologic and Neonatal Nursing, 6 (2), Mar/Apr 1977, 53-54.

2 **Barron, L.** Home or hospital delivery? Midwife, Health Visitor and Community Nurse, 15 (3), Mar 1979, 94-95.

3 **Barry, C.N.** Home versus hospital confinement. (Review of research.) Journal of the Royal College of General Practitioners, 30, Feb 1980, 102-107.

4 **Beard, R.W.** Future developments in obstetrics. Part 1. Hospital versus home. (Delivery—advantages and disadvantages of each.) Midwife, Health Visitor and Community Nurse, 13 (8), Aug 1977, 240, 243, 245, 247-248.

5 **Becker, C.** The postpartum period what is reality? Canadian Nurse, 76 (11), Dec 1980, 24-27.

6 **Berezin, N.** The gentle birth book: a practical guide to Leboyer family-centred delivery. Murray, 1980.

7 **Blackwell, J.** Husband in the labour ward. (Account of birth of author's second child and attitudes of staff.) Midwives Chronicle, 90, Nov 1977, 270-272. Reprinted under title 'Labour pains' in Nursing Mirror, 146, 2 Feb 1978, 26-29.

8 **Bond, S.** Shave it...or save it? (Review of research on perineovulval shaving before childbirth.) Nursing Times, 76, 28 Feb 1980, 362-363.

9 **Brewer, C.** Risks in being born. (Comparison between home and hospital delivery as shown in two studies.) (See correspondence 15 Nov 1979, 389-390, 22 Nov 1979, 452.) New Society, 50, 1 Nov 1979, 250-257.

10 **British Medical Journal** Home or hospital confinement? (Review of research.) British Medical Journal, 2, 1 Oct 1977, 845-846.

11 **British Medical Journal** A place to be born. (Hospital v home confinement.) British Medical Journal, 1, 10 Jan 1976, 55-56.

12 **Butani, P. and Hodnett, E.** Mothers' perceptions of their labour experiences. (Research study.) American Journal of Maternal-Child Nursing, 9 (2), Summer 1980, 73-82.

13 **Carlson, B. and Sumner, P.** Hospital 'at home' delivery: a celebration. (Providing a home-like atmosphere in hospital using the Lamaze technique.) Journal of Obstetric, Gynecologic and Neonatal Nursing, 5 (2), Mar/Apr 1976, 21-27.

14 **Chalmers, I.** Perinatal epidemiology. (Statistics including Caesarian section rates and discussion of research by midwives.) Midwife, Health Visitor and Community Nurse, 14 (11), Nov 1978, 380-382.

15 **Chamberlain, G. and others** British births 1970: a survey...Vol.2: obstetric care. Heinemann, 1978.

16 **Champagnie, M.L.** Nursing care study. And a baby was born. (Treatment of burns and delivery of pregnant woman.) Nursing Mirror, 145, 10 Nov 1977, 16-17.

17 **Clark, A.L.** Labor and birth: expectations and outcomes. (Interview with 24 expectant mothers.) Nursing Forum, 14 (4), 1975, 413-428.

18 **Close, S.** Birth report: extracts from over 4000 personal experiences. Windsor: National Foundation for Educational Research, 1980.

19 **Crowe, V.J.** Great expectations! (Comments by the Midwife Teachers' Groups Representatives of RCM on National Childbirth Trust's 'Expectations of a Pregnant Woman in Relation to her Treatment'.) Midwives Chronicle, 91, Aug 1978, 210-211.

20 **Cutts, D.E.** Home or hospital? A survey looks at the attitudes of birthing couples. Australian Nurses Journal, 9 (5), Nov 1979, 35-37.

21 **Davies, R. and others** A sensitive approach to childbirth. (Based on Leboyer's ideas, by mothers who experienced it and two midwives who have used this approach.) Nursing Times, 74, 9 Feb 1978, 222-223.

22 **Dooher, M.E.** Lamaze method of childbirth. (Research study of its effect on marital adjustment and crisis experienced during postpartum period.) Nursing Research, 29 (4), Jul/Aug 1980, 220-224.

23 **Dunn, P.M.** Obstetric delivery today: for better or for worse? Lancet, 1, 10 Apr 1976, 790-793.

24 **Dutton, A.** Excesses of modern obstetrics: the mother's dilemma. (Epidural analgesia, institutionalisation, bottle feeding and induction are discussed.) Nursing Mirror, 146, 26 Jan 1978, 28-29.

25 **Elliman, A.M.** A paediatrician's view of planned early transfer following childbirth. Midwife, Health Visitor and Community Nurse, 13 (11), Nov 1977, 352-354.

26 **Faxel, A.M.H. and Kieffer, M.J.** The birthing room concept at Phoenix Memorial Hospital. 1. Development and eighteen months' statistics. 2. Consumer satisfaction during one year. Journal of Obstetric, Gynecologic and Neonatal Nursing, 9 (3), May/Jun 1980, 151-159.

27 **Gillett, J.** Childbirth. (Visit to Maternity Unit at Pithiviers in France where natural childbirth methods are used.) International Journal of Nursing Studies, 17 (4), 1980, 271-274.

28 **Gillett, J.** Childbirth in Pithiviers, France. (Report of visit to Dr. Michel Odent's maternity unit with use of 'birth room' and freedom of mother to adopt any position she finds comfortable.) Lancet, 2, 27 Oct 1979, 894-896.

29 **Goodlin, R.C.** Low-risk obstetric care for low-risk mothers. (Complication rates in an alternative birth centre compared with labour and delivery rooms.) Lancet, 1, 10 May 1980, 1017-1019.

30 **Gough, L.N.** Case study: home confinement. Midwives Chronicle, 90, Apr 1977, 67-68.

31 **Grossman, M.** The Leboyer method: what does it mean now? Canadian Nurse, 75 (9), Oct 1979, 28-30.

32 **Hardy, C.T. and Ekbladh, L.** Hospital meets patient demand for 'home-style' childbirth. ('Home-style' delivery room at North Carolina Memorial Hospital.) Hospitals, 52 (5), Mar 1978, 73-74, 79-80.

33 **Henschel, D.** 'Tranquil delivery' at King's College Hospital. (Pilot study into Leboyer method of delivery.) Midwives Chronicle, 92, Jun 1979, 170-172.

34 **Hott, J.R.** Best laid plans: pre- and postpartum comparison of self and spouse in primiparous Lamaze couples who share delivery and those who do not. Nursing Research, 29 (1), Jan/Feb 1980, 20-27.

35 **Huprich, P.A.** Assisting the couple through a Lamaze labor and delivery. American Journal of Maternal-Child Nursing, 2 (4), Jul/Aug 1977, 245-253.

36 **Iveson-Iveson, J.** Birth—a family affair? (Report of National Childbirth Trust's 21st Birthday Conference.) Nursing Mirror, 145, 24 Nov 1977, 8.

37 **Jackson, M.** Case study—quadruplets. Midwives Chronicle, 89, May 1976, 121-123.

38 **Kitzinger, S.** Birth at home. Oxford University Press, 1979.

39 **Kitzinger, S.** Education and counselling for childbirth. Baillière Tindall, 1977.

40 **Kitzinger, S.** The good birth guide. Croom Helm, 1979.

41 **Kitzinger, S. and Davis, J.A.** The place of birth: a study of the environment in which birth takes place with special reference to home confinements. Oxford University Press, 1978.

42 **Lancet** Whose baby is it anyway? (New attitudes to childbirth and evaluation of Leboyer method.) Lancet, 1, 14 Jun 1980, 1284-1285.

43 **Landry, K.E. and Kilpatrick, D.M.** Why shave a mother before she gives birth? (Advantages and disadvantages of perineal shaving.) American Journal of Maternal-Child Nursing, 2 (3), May/Jun 1977, 189-190.

44 **Leboyer, F.** Birth without violence. Wildwood House, 1975.

45 **Lubic, R.W.** The impact of technology on health care—the childbearing center: a case for technology's appropriate use. (With emphasis on psychological aspects of childbearing.) Journal of Nurse-Midwifery, 24 (1), Jan/Feb 1979, 6-10.

46 **Lubic, R.W. and Ernst, E.K.M.** The childbearing center: an alternative to conventional care. (Unit in New York offering comprehensive care in homelike atmosphere.) Nursing Outlook, 26 (12), Dec 1978, 754-760.

47 **McIlwaine, G.** Perinatal audit and surveillance. (Report of RCOG multidisciplinary study group.) Community Medicine, 2 (3), Aug 1980, 225-228.

48 **Marut, J.S. and Mercer, R.T.** Comparison of primiparas' perceptions of vaginal and caesarian births. Nursing Research, 28 (5), Sep/Oct 1979, 259.

49 **Meyer, B.J.** Childbirth at home—a family-centred affair. (Personal experience of planned home delivery.) Journal of Obstetric, Gynecologic and Neonatal Nursing, 5 (2), Mar/Apr 1976, 20, 28-31.

50 **Midwife, Health Visitor and Community Nurse** Editorial. Leboyer and all that. (Comment on 'Childbirth without violence.') Midwife, Health Visitor and Community Nurse, 13 (7), Jul 1977, 199.

51 **National Childbirth Trust** Expectations of a pregnant woman in relation to her treatment. (Ten statements.) Midwife, Health Visitor and Community Nurse, 14 (1), Jan 1978, 5. Discussion by Lady Micklethwait, Professor Richard Beard, Kathleen Shaw, DNO, and Tony Smith. British Medical Journal, 2, 15 Jul 1978, 188-191.

52 **Nazer, G.** Hospital or home? (Report of survey into risk factors of home confinements and views of doctors and RCM spokesman.) Nursing Mirror, 147, 9 Nov 1978, 9.

53 **Norr, K.L. and others** The second time around: parity and birth experience. (Attitudes and physical and psychological experiences of multiparas.) Journal of Obstetric, Gynecologic and Neonatal Nursing, 9 (1), Jan/Feb 1980, 30-36.

54 **Oakley, A.** Becoming a mother. Oxford: Robertson, 1979.

55 **Oakley, A.** Women confined: towards a sociology of childbirth. Oxford: Martin Robertson, 1980.

56 **O'Brien, M.** Home and hospital: a comparison of the experiences of mothers having home and hospital confinements. Journal of the Royal College of General Practitioners, 28, Aug 1978, 460-466.

57 **Oliver, C.M. and Oliver, G.M.** Gentle birth: its safety and its effect on neonatal behavior. (Research study of deliveries based on modification of Leboyer method.) Journal of Obstetric, Gynecologic and Neonatal Nursing, 7 (5), Sep/Oct 1978, 35-40.

58 **Rosen, E.L.** Implementation alternative: the birth room. (Combined labour/delivery room with home-like atmosphere.) Canadian Nurse, 76 (3), Mar 1980, 30-32.

59 **Salter, A.** Birth without violence: a medical controversy. (Research study of the Leboyer method of childbirth.) Nursing Research, 27 (2), Mar/Apr 1978, 84-88.

60 **Sayle, D.** Midwifery care study. The normal delivery of a baby in hospital. Nursing Times, 72, 13 May 1976, 732-735.

61 **Seymour, A.** Labour report. An account by a father of his wife's confinement and the birth of their first baby. Midwife, Health Visitor and Community Nurse, 12 (5), May 1976, 157-158.

62 **Shields, D.** Nursing care in labor and patient satisfaction: a descriptive study. (Subjective needs of patients based on interviews in postpartum wards.) Journal of Advanced Nursing, 3 (6), Nov 1978, 535-550.

63 **Smeaton, V.** Happy childbirth. (Letter describing author's experience of Leboyer-style delivery at the West London Hospital.) Nursing Times, 74, 23 Feb 1978, 326.

64 **Smith, W.E.** What risk a home confinement? (Care study of first baby delivered at home, with accounts by parents.) Nursing Times, 76, 17 Jul 1980, Midwifery supplement 7, 9-12, 14.

65 **Stephenson, F.A.** Interdisciplinary co-operation and preparation for childbirth. Physiotherapy, 64 (8), Aug 1978, 231-233.

66 **Tew, M.** Society at work. Where to be born? (A comparison of birth and stillbirth rates at home and hospital.) New Society, 39, 20 Jan 1977, 120-121.

67 **Tricker, I.** Community nursing care study. Painless childbirth. (Normal delivery at home.) Nursing Times, 74, 9 Feb 1978, 225-228.

68 **Willmuth, R. and others** Satisfaction with prepared childbirth and locus of control. (Test of sense of personal control over life events.) Journal of Obstetric, Gynecologic and Neonatal Nursing, 7 (3), May/Jun 1978, 33-37.

b ANAESTHESIA AND ANALGESIA

1 **Beazley, J.M. and Ward, J.P.** Perineal pain after epidural analgesia in labour. (Research study.) Midwives Chronicle, 91, Aug 1978, 204-206.

2 **Crawford, J.S.** Use of anaesthesia. Anaesthetists in the obstetric department. British Medical Journal, 281, 12 Jul 1980, 119-120.

3 **Drug and Therapeutics Bulletin** Epidural anaesthesia in obstetrics. Drug and Therapeutics Bulletin, 14 (3), 30 Jan 1976, 9-11.

4 **Jones, D.H.** Epidural analgesia in obstetrics. Midwives Chronicle, 88, Nov 1975, 367-369.

5 **Kitzinger, S.** Pain in childbirth. Journal of Medical Ethics, 4 (3), Sep 1978, 119-121.

6 **McAllister, R.G.** Obstetric anaesthesia—a two-way street. Journal of Obstetric, Gynecologic and Neonatal Nursing, 5 (1), Jan/Feb 1976, 9-13.

7 **McDonald, S.M.** Thoughts on epidurals. (Role of epidural analgesia in labour.) Midwives Chronicle, 91, Aug 1978, 206-208.

8 **McKenna, J.** Antenatal preparation and epidural anaesthesia. Midwife, Health Visitor and Community Nurse, 12 (3), Mar 1976, 78-81.

9 **Nicholson, C.J.** Who administers obstetrical anaesthesia? American Association of Nurse Anesthetists Journal, 45 (5), Oct 1976, 485-489.

10 **O'Driscoll, K.** An obstetrician's view of pain. Inverse ratio between the need for analgesia and the quality of care in a delivery unit. Midwife, Health Visitor and Community Nurse, 12 (7), Jul 1976, 213, 215, 217-221.

11 **Ryan, D.** Taking the pain out of labour. (Review of methods of analgesia including lumbar epidural analgesia.) Nursing Mirror, 146, 8 Jun 1978, 33-36.

12 **Taylor, A.B.W. and others** Lumbar epidural analgesia in labour: a 24-hour service provided by obstetricians. (In which midwives managed the analgesia.) British Medical Journal, 2, 6 Aug 1977, 370-372.

c LABOUR

1 Bekhit, S.M. Active management of labour. Nursing Times, 72, 29 Apr 1976, 655-658.

2 Bell, M.L. The first stage of labour—how long? (Research study.) Midwives Chronicle, 91, Apr 1978, 84-88.

3 Browne, M.J. The complications of difficult forceps. Midwife, Health Visitor and Community Nurse, 16 (9), Sep 1980, 358, 360-361, 364.

4 Burke, M.F. and Buck, P. Forceps delivery. Nursing Times, 73, 31 Dec 1977, 454-456.

5 Chou Liu, Y. Position during labour and delivery: history and perspective. (Review of research.) Journal of Nurse-Midwifery, 24 (3), May/Jun 1979, 23-26.

6 Crawford, J.W. and Henry, M.J. Computer assisted monitoring of labour and the fetus. Health Bulletin, 34 (3), May 1976, 177-179.

7 Duncan, G. The partogram: a graphic guide to the progress of normal and abnormal labour. Nursing Mirror, 144, 24 Mar 1977, 63-65.

8 Elias, J.A. The quality of intrapartum care. (With reference to the prevention of handicap.) Midwives Chronicle, 91, Dec 1978, 353-354.

9 Flynn, A.M. and others Ambulation in labour. (Its benefits.) British Medical Journal, 2, 26 Aug 1978, 591-593.

10 Fullman, P.M. Disordered action of the uterus in labour. (Value of graphic representation of labour in its detection.) Nursing Times, 74, 27 Apr 1978, 706-707.

11 Harrison, E. Nursing care study. Hydatidiform mole: Sharon's 'miniature' labour. Nursing Mirror, 148, 29 Mar 1979, 43-46.

12 Larsen, J.V. and Muller, E.J. The management of high risk labours by midwives with advanced training. (Research study.) Curationis, 2 (4), Mar 1980, 43-44.

13 McManus, T.J. and Calder, A.A. Upright posture and the efficiency of labour. (Survey in Glasgow.) Lancet, 1, 14 Jan 1978, 72-74.

14 Malinowski, J.S. and others Nursing care of the labor patient. Philadelphia: Davis, 1978.

15 Milrea, L. and others Specialised care. 7. Complicated labour. (Mainly historical account.) Nursing Mirror, 145, 27 Oct 1977 Nursing care supplement series 6, i-iv.

16 Pavlou, C. Conduct of labour. (Modern management) Midwife, Health Visitor and Community Nurse, 13 (6), Jun 1977, 179-181; 13 (12), Dec 1977, 394-398.

17 Roberts, J. Alternative positions for childbirth. Part 1. First stage of labor. (Includes review of research findings.) Journal of Nurse-Midwifery, 25 (4), Jul/Aug 1980, 11-18.

18 Roberts, J.E. Maternal positions for childbirth: a historical review of nursing care practices. Journal of Obstetric, Gynecologic and Neonatal Nursing, 8 (1), Jan/Feb 1979, 24-32.

19 Stewart, C.R. A revised partogram for use in labour wards. (Method of recording progress of labour graphically. Devised for use at Jessop Hospital, Sheffield.) Midwives Chronicle, 90, Jun 1977, 124-126.

20 Whitley, N. and Mack, E. Are enemas justified for women in labour? (Research study.) American Journal of Nursing, 80 (7), Jul 1980, 1339.

d INDUCTION

1 Ball, H.G. Revolutionary methods in childbirth. (Study of labour induction at Derby City Hospital.) Midwives Chronicle, 89, Jun 1976, 146-148.

2 Beard, R.W. Future developments in obstetrics. Part 2: Modern techniques. Induction of labour and the use of oxytocin. Midwife, Health Visitor and Community Nurse, 13 (10), Oct 1977, 315.

3 British Medical Journal Induction of labour. (Editorial.) British Medical Journal, 1, 27 Mar 1976, 729-730.

4 Cartwright, A. The dignity of labour? A study of childbearing and induction. Tavistock, 1979.

5 Cartwright, A. Mothers' experience of induction. (Research study.) British Medical Journal, 2, 17 Sep 1977, 745-749.

6 Cartwright, A. and Simms, M. Midwives and induction. (Survey of midwives' attitudes.) Midwife, Health Visitor and Community Nurse, 15 (3), Mar 1979, 86-88.

7 Chaloner, J. Prostaglandins. (Study of the use of prostaglandin E2 given orally for the induction of labour.) Midwives Chronicle, 90, Feb 1977, 29.

8 Craft, I. Induction of labour. Midwife, Health Visitor and Community Nurse, 12 (2), Feb 1976, 42-44.

9 Fedrick, J. and Yudkin, P. Obstetric practice in the Oxford record linkage study area 1965-1972. (Trends in induction.) British Medical Journal, 1, 27 Mar 1976, 738-740.

10 Howie, P. Induction of labour—does it save babies? (Review of research studies.) Nursing Mirror, 146, 30 Mar 1978, 21-24.

11 Kitzinger, S. Effects of induction on the mother baby relationship. (National Childbirth Trust study.) Practitioner, 217, Aug 1976, 263-267.

12 Kitzinger, S. Happy inductions. (A study based on National Childbirth Trust records to compare 35 happy experiences of induction with 35 unfavourable ones.) Nursing Mirror, 142 (6), 12 Feb 1976, 41-42.

13 MacKenzie, I.Z. Prostaglandins in modern obstetric practice. (Use in the induction of labour.) Midwife, Health Visitor and Community Nurse, 15 (12), Dec 1979, 494, 496-497.

14 Midwife, Health Visitor and Community Nurse Editorial. Induction of labour. Midwife, Health Visitor and Community Nurse, 12 (3), Mar 1976, 69.

15 O'Driscoll, K. and others Selective induction of labour. (Survey of 1000 patients in the National Maternity Hospital, Dublin.) British Medical Journal, 1975, 4, 27 Dec 1975, 727-729.

16 Stewart, P. Patients' attitudes to induction and labour. (Research study.) British Medical Journal, 2, 17 Sep 1977, 749-752.

17 Taylor, R.W. Induction of labour. Nursing Mirror, 143, 23 Sep 1976, 58-59.

18 West, W.E.G. Inducing labour with the Cardiff Infusion System. (Pump to control IV administration of oxytocin and monitor.) Nursing Mirror, 147, 7 Sep 1978, 27-30.

19 Whittaker, B.A. A history of induction. (Pupil midwife's project.) Midwives Chronicle, 92, Apr 1979, 108-110.

20 Williams, S.M.K. Effect of planned deliveries on labour ward staffing. Midwife, Health Visitor and Community Nurse, 12 (12), Dec 1976, 387-389.

21 York, R. A comparative study of the physiological and psychological needs of the labours of inducted and spontaneous parturients. (Summary of paper read at research seminar in 1977.) Journal of Advanced Nursing, 3 (1), Jan 1978, 80-83.

e SURGICAL PROCEDURES

1 AORN Journal Should fathers attend cesarean section deliveries? (Views of parents, physicians and nurses.) AORN Journal, 28 (3), Sep 1978, 434-435, 438-439, 442-443, 446-447, 450-451, 454.

2 Bekhit, S.M. The use of episiotomy. Nursing Times, 72, 12 Aug 1976, 1231-1233.

3 Buchan, P.C. and Nicholls, J.A.J. Pain after episiotomy—a comparison of two methods of repair. (Suturing with black silk or 'Dexon'.) Journal of the Royal College of General Practitioners, 30, May 1980, 297-300.

4 Conklin, M.M. Discussion groups as preparation for cesarean section. Journal of Obstetric, Gynecologic and Neonatal Nursing, 6 (4), Jul/Aug 1977, 52-54.

5 Donovan, B. The Cesarean birth experience: a practical, comprehensive, and reassuring guide for parents and professionals. Boston: Beacon Press, 1977.

6 Donovan, B. and Allen, R.M. The Cesarean birth method. (Comprehensive approach with antenatal classes designed specifically for elective and repeat Cesarean births.) Journal of Obstetric, Gynecologic and Neonatal Nursing, 6 (6), Nov/Dec 1977, 37-48.

7 Fischer, S.R. Factors associated with the occurrence of perineal lacerations. (Review of literature and research study.) Journal of Nurse-Midwifery, 24 (1), Jan/Feb 1979, 18-26.

8 Fox, J.S. Episiotomy. (Incision and repair.) Midwives Chronicle, 92, Oct 1979, 337-340.

9 Kitzinger, S. Episiotomy. Midwife, Health Visitor and Community Nurse, 15 (6), Jun 1979, 233-234.

10 Limb, D.G. and Thelwall-Jones, H. Perineal repair. Midwives Chronicle, 88, Apr 1975, 116.

11 Loach, G.A. Pregnancy with dwarfism.

(Antenatal care and care during Caesarian section of achondroplastic mother with care of infant in SCBU. By nurse on JBCNS theatre nursing course.) Nursing Times, 76, 21 Feb 1980, 336-339.

12 Schlosser, S. The emergency C-section patient: why she needs help...what you can do. (Resentment and anger at being deprived of birth experience.) RN Magazine, 41 (9), Sep 1978, 53-57.

13 Stichler, J.F. and others Cesarean birth. (Three articles including women's reactions and father's presence.) American Journal of Nursing, 80 (3), Mar 1980, 466-472.

14 Trudinger, B.J. Caesarean section in modern obstetrics. Midwife, Health Visitor and Community Nurse, 13 (7), Jul 1977, 213, 216-217, 218-219.

15 Wright, J.D. Caesarean section. Nursing Mirror, 144, 27 Jan 1977, 51-53.

f PSYCHOLOGICAL ASPECTS

1 Beattie, J. Observations on post-natal depression, and a suggestion for its prevention. (Discussions and therapy during antenatal period.) International Journal of Social Psychiatry, 24 (4), Winter 1978, 247-249.

2 Burns, A. With a lot of help from my friends. (Author describes her experience of postnatal depression.) Nursing Mirror, 146, 18 May 1978, 22.

3 Ferguson, I. A psychological approach to pregnancy and childbirth: some of the aspects which should concern midwives. Midwives Chronicle, 90, Aug 1977, 187-188.

4 Hatrick, J.A. Puerperal mental illness. Nursing Times, 72, 8 Apr 1976, 533-534.

5 Journal of the Royal College of General Practitioners Family medicine. (With reference to causes and effects of depression in young mothers.) Journal of the Royal College of General Practitioners, 29, Feb 1979, 67-68.

6 Kirgie, C.A. and others Predicting infant Apgar scores. (Study to identify psychological and sociological factors affecting women during pregnancy which contribute to poor neonatal outcome.) Nursing Research, 26 (6), Nov/Dec 1977, 439-442.

7 Macfarlane, A. The psychology of childbirth. Open Books, 1977. (The developing child series.)

8 Marks, J. Maternal depression—who is at risk? (Research study and discussion of role of HV.) Health Visitor, 53 (1), Jan 1980, 7-9.

9 Measey, L.G. Psychiatric problems in obstetrics. Practitioner, 220, Jan 1978, 120-122.

10 Oakley, A. The baby blues. (Postnatal depression.) New Society, 48, 5 Apr 1979, 11-12.

11 Pitt, B. Psychological aspects of pregnancy. (Risk of having a psychiatric breakdown.) Midwife, Health Visitor and Community Nurse, 13 (5), May 1977, 137-139.

12 POSTNATAL depression: does no one care? (By the husband of a sufferer.) British Medical Journal, 2, 8 Dec 1979, 1487-1488.

13 Prince, J. and Adams, M.E. Minds, mothers and midwives: the psychology of childbirth. Churchill Livingstone, 1978.

14 Sayers, S. Nursing care study. Puerperal psychosis. Nursing Times, 72, 20 May 1976, 774-776.

15 Welburn, V. Postnatal depression. Manchester: Manchester University Press, 1980.

g MATERNAL DEATHS

1 Cowper-Smith, F. One maternal death is one too many. (Summary of and comment on report on confidential inquiries into maternal deaths in England and Wales (1973-1975).) Nursing Times, 76, 7 Feb 1980, 225-226.

2 Department of Health and Social Security Report on confidential enquiries into maternal deaths in England and Wales 1964-1966. HMSO, 1979. (Report on health and social subjects; 14.)

3 Steigrad, S.J. Address given by N.S.W. College of Nursing on avoidable factors in maternal morbidity. Lamp, 33 (1), Jan 1976, 13-16.

42 FAMILY PLANNING

a GENERAL AND SERVICES

1 Barnett, M. Socio-economic factors affecting contraception. Nursing Times, 72, 25 Nov 1976, 1842-1843.

2 Bone, M. The family planning services: changes and effects. HMSO, 1978.

3 Bone, M.R. Trends in contraceptive practice among married couples. Health Trends, 12 (4), Nov 1980, 87-90.

4 Cartwright, A. How many children? Routledge and Kegan Paul, 1976.

5 Cartwright, A. Recent trends in family building and contraception. HMSO, 1978. (Studies on medical and population subjects no.34.)

6 Chamberlain, A. Mothers of large families and birth control education. (Survey in Leeds of mothers' knowledge and attitudes.) Health Education Journal, 37 (4), 1978, 219-230.

7 Diggory, P. and McEwan, J. Planning or prevention?: the new face of 'family planning'. Marion Boyars, 1976. (Ideas in progress series.)

8 Hannay, D.R. Family planning in Glasgow. (Survey of symptoms, referral patterns and sociographic data of patients at Woodside Health Centre.) Royal Society of Health Journal, 96 (4), Aug 1976, 193-195.

9 Jones, M. Family planning—is it working in the NHS? (Criticism of effects of health service cuts by FPA spokesman.) Midwife, Health Visitor and Community Nurse, 16 (2), Feb 1980, 58, 62.

10 Leathard, A. The fight for family planning: the development of family planning services in Britain 1921-74. Macmillan, 1980.

11 Leathard, A. Keep the official flag flying over birth control services. (History and current

problems of the Family Planning Association.) Health and Social Service Journal, 90, 30 May 1980, 704-707.

12 Sai, F.T. Some ethical issues in family planning. International Planned Parenthood Federation, 1976. (Occasional essay no.1.)

13 Sikes, O.J. Education in family planning: what route to take? What difference does it make? International Journal of Health Education, 22 (4), 1979, 206-210.

14 Stewart, M. Crossing the community barrier in family planning. (Co-ordination of medical advisers in community clinics, general practice, and hospitals in Cleveland to form a comprehensive service.) Health and Social Service Journal, 86, 12 Nov 1976, 2018-2019.

15 Stott, P.C. Contraceptive behaviour and fertility patterns in an Inner London group practice. (Involving the giving of questionnaires by nurses.) Journal of the Royal College of General Practitioners, 30, Jun 1980, 340-346.

16 Thornton, P. Family planning and immigrants. Nursing, 16, Aug 1980, 704, 707-708.

b OVERSEAS COUNTRIES

1 Andrews, S.W. A college contraceptive clinic. American Journal of Nursing, 76 (4), Apr 1976, 592-593.

2 Bachu, A. Family planning services in India. Nursing Mirror, 142, 24 Jun 1976, 60-62.

3 Calder, J. Tubal ligation in Bangladesh. ('Mini-Lap' method described, as performed by 'barefoot doctors.') Nursing Mirror, 145, 15 Dec 1977, 32-33.

4 Hewitt, P. Developments in family planning overseas. Australian Nurses Journal, 7 (10), May 1978, 32-35; (11), Jun 1978, 34-37.

5 International Children's Centre and World Health Organization. Regional Office for Europe Family health and family planning. Paris: International Children's Centre, 1979.

6 Martin, J.F. Family planning and family health. (With reference to the Third World.) International Nursing Review, 25 (6), Nov/Dec 1978, 172-174.

7 Rangnekar, M.V. Accent on family planning. Nursing practice in the community. Nursing Journal of India, 47 (9), Sep 1976, 219-220.

8 United Nations. Department of Economic and Social Affairs Social welfare and family planning. New York: UNO, 1976.

9 World Health Issue on family planning. World Health, Aug/Sep 1978, 2-37.

c NURSE, MIDWIFE AND HEALTH VISITOR

1 Abcede, J. Midwives among the chocolate hills. (Bohel Province Family Planning Project in the Philippines.) World Health, Apr 1976, 24-27.

2 Bachu, A. The nurse's role in family planning services in India. International Nursing Review, 23 (1), Jan/Feb 1976, 25-28.

3 **Belanger, C.F. and others** The nurses' health study. (Research study of health effects of various contraceptive methods, using nurses as study participants.) American Journal of Nursing, 78 (6), Jun 1978, 1039-1040.

4 **Bibb, B.N.** The effectiveness of non-physicians as providers of family planning services. (Review of research with recommendations on future role of nurses.) Journal of Obstetric, Gynecologic and Neonatal Nursing, 8 (3), May/Jun 1979, 137-143.

5 **Chamberlain, A.** Birth control motivation —what does it mean? (With reference to the health visitor's role.) Health Visitor, 51 (10), Oct 1978, 374-377.

6 **Chisholm, N.** Prescribing and family planning. (Letter suggesting that Rcn has misinterpreted part of the Medicines Act regarding nurse's role with oral contraceptives.) British Medical Journal, 2, 21 Oct 1978, 1167-1168.

7 **Clark, J.** Note of dissent. (Criticism of Rcn objections to the recommendations of the Joint Working Group on Oral Contraceptives.) Nursing Times, 73, 20 Jan 1977, 80-81.

8 **Clark J.** Using skills. (Rcn family planning symposium.) Nursing Mirror, 142, 27 May 1976, 51-53.

9 **Clark, S.M.** Family planning in the practice of midwifery in England and Wales. (Historical review.) Journal of Nurse-Midwifery, 24 (3), May/Jun 1979, 11-16.

10 **Crabbe, P.** Teenagers at risk. (Nurse's role with teenage girls seeking contraceptive advice.) Nursing Times, 73, 11 Aug 1977, 1229.

11 **Dusitin, N. and others** Post-partum tubal ligation by nurse-midwives and doctors in Thailand. Lancet, 1, 22 Mar 1980, 638-639.

12 **Elder, R.G.** Orientation of senior nursing students toward access to contraceptives. (Survey of 264 students' attitudes towards freely available contraceptives.) Nursing Research, 25 (5), Sep/Oct 1976, 338-345.

13 **Fairweather, D.V.I. and Law, B.** Multidisciplinary training in family planning. (Three years' experience of fourteen courses attended by the medical, nursing, education and social work professions.) Medical Education, 12 (3), May 1978, 205-208.

14 **Family Planning Association** Nurses 'should be able to prescribe the pill' with training and back-up. (Family Planning Association conference.) Nursing Times, 72, 1 Apr 1976, 476.

15 **Flynn, M.** The contribution of nurse practitioners to service delivery in family planning. Lamp, 35 (10), Oct 1978, 14-16.

16 **Flynn, M.** The family planning nurse practitioner: suggested guidelines for role expansion and utilisation. Lamp, 34 (6), Jun 1977, 30-31.

17 **Foley, M.** The nurse and family planning. Queen's Nursing Journal, 19 (12), Mar 1977, 330-331.

18 **General Practice Team** The team approach to family planning. (Three talks on recent enquiries—the Bone report, the Runcorn survey and the role of nurse midwife, and health visitor.) General Practice Team, 55, Mar 1976, 5-10.

19 **Guimei, M.K.** Effectiveness of a programmed instruction module on oral contraceptives. (On increase of knowledge in student nurses during obstetric experience.) Nursing Research, 26 (6), Nov/Dec 1977, 452-455.

20 **Holroyd, M.S.** Prevention in primary health care—everybody's business. (Role of nurse in domiciliary family planning service.) Journal of Community Nursing, 3 (4), Oct 1979, 36, 39-40, 42.

21 **Irish Nurses Organisation** Policy document on family planning. World of Irish Nursing, 7 (5), May 1978, 7.

22 **JOINT** Board of Clinical Nursing Studies. 9. Family planning. Nursing Mirror, 143 (13), 23 Sep 1976 Nursing care supplement series 2, i-iv.

23 **Kamal, I.** Role of the nurse and the midwife in MCH/family planning programme. Pakistan Nursing and Health Review, 6 (1), 1975, 6-15.

24 **McWeeney, E.** JBCNS Family Planning Course 900—a student's impression. Midwives Chronicle, 90, Jan 1977, 11.

25 **Manisoff, M.** Impact of family planning nurse practitioners. (Survey of family planning clinics.) Journal of Obstetric, Gynecologic and Neonatal Nursing, 8 (2), Mar/Apr 1979, 73-77.

26 **Nazer, G.** Chaos for 'illegal' family planners. (Legal problems for students on course at King's College Hospital which is designed to train nurses to provide full range of family planning services.) Nursing Mirror, 147, 26 Oct 1978, 2.

27 **Newton, J.** A nurse-practitioner clinic. (Family planning clinic at King's College Hospital.) General Practice Team, 55, Mar 1976, 10-11.

28 **Newton, J. and others** Nurse specialist work in family planning. (Report of pilot study at King's College Hospital, London.) Midwives Chronicle, 90, Dec 1977, 290-291.

29 **Newton, J. and others** Nurse specialists in family planning. (Training programme and the results of a year's work in an experimental clinic at King's College Hospital.) British Medical Journal, 1, 17 Apr 1976, 950-952.

30 **Oates, D.M.** A new venture in Norwich: Joint Board of Clinical Nursing Studies Course 900. (Family Planning.) Midwives Chronicle, 90, Jan 1977, 10.

31 **Peach, E.H.** Counseling sexually active very young adolescent girls. American Journal of Maternal-Child Nursing, 5 (3), May/Jun 1980, 191-195.

32 **Royal College of Nursing** Family planning. (Rcn symposium on the use of nursing skills in family planning.) Nursing Mirror, 142, 27 May 1976, 47-53.

33 **Royal College of Nursing** Family Planning Nurses Forum. Working Party on Nurse Prescribers of Oral Contraceptives for the Well Woman. Nurse prescribers of oral contraceptives for the well woman. Rcn, 1980.

34 **Shevas, A.** Pill power for nurses? (Views of nurses and the BMA on Rcn Family Planning Nurses' Forum's proposals.) Nursing Mirror, 150, 28 Feb 1980, 9.

35 **Thompson, S.** Why it is right for family planning nurses to prescribe the pill... (Problems of legal and insurance cover for nurses.) Nursing Mirror, 147, 19 Oct 1978, 9.

36 **Tyrer, L.B. and Hunt, R.** Counseling the patient on fertility control. 1. The Pill. 2. Intrauterine devices. Journal of Practical Nursing, 26 (11), Nov 1976, 14-17, 31, 36; (12), Dec 1976, 20-22, 32.

37 **White, T.G.E.** Nurse specialists in family planning. (Letters stating a doctor's view of using nurses as substitutes for doctors.) British Medical Journal, 1, 22 May 1976, 1275-1276.

38 **Wiltshire, J.** Extending skills. (Psycho-sexual seminar training described at an Rcn family planning symposium.) Nursing Mirror, 142, 27 May 1976, 49-51.

39 **Woodside, M.** Family planning. (The role of the nurse and health visitor in promoting family planning.) Nursing Times, 73, 24 Mar 1977, 430-431.

40 **Zabarenko, M.R. and Bednarz, P.K.** A selected annotated bibliography on midwives and family planning. Part 1. (Includes British literature.) Journal of Nurse-Midwifery, 22 (2), Summer 1977, 39-46.

d METHODS

1 **Barnes, J.** Essentials of family planning. Blackwell, 1976.

2 **Berlin, L.E. and others** Increase in diaphragm use in a university population. (Between 1973 and 1976.) Journal of Obstetric, Gynecologic and Neonatal Nursing, 8 (5), Sep/Oct 1979, 280-282.

3 **Committee on the Safety of Medicines** Oral contraceptives: CSM statement. (On two recent studies of mortality associated with the pill.) British Medical Journal, 2, 8 Oct 1977, 965.

4 **Deibel, P.** Natural family planning: different methods. American Journal of Maternal-Child Nursing, 3 (3), May/Jun 1978, 144-152.

5 **Elder, M.G.** Contraception—a review of methods and their effectiveness. Midwife, Health Visitor and Community Nurse, 12 (2), Feb 1976, 47-49.

6 **Family Planning Association** The pill...on or off prescription? A conference organised by the Family Planning Association at the Royal Commonwealth Society, London, 23 Mar 1976. The Association, 1976.

7 **Gibbons, C.** Natural family planning: a detailed survey of previous studies, combined with the author's personal research. (With history.) Nursing Times, 76, 14 Aug 1980, 1454-1456.

8 **Gorline, L.L.** Teaching successful use of the diaphragm. (For suggested improved technique of diaphragm removal see Mar 1980, 411.) American Journal of Nursing, 79 (10), Oct 1979, 1732-1735.

9 **Gray, R.H. and others** Manual for the provision of intrauterine devices (IUDs). Geneva: WHO, 1980.

10 **Gunn, A.** The 'pill' for men—fact or

fantasy. Journal of Community Nursing, 3 (10), Apr 1980, 4-5.

11 Hamilton, D. and Hamilton, C. Candidates for the pill. (Uses and abuses of three main groups of oral contraceptives.) Nursing Mirror, 150, 28 Feb 1980, 43-45.

12 Howard, G. Injectable contraception. (Includes a report of a clinical trial of Norigest at Charing Cross Hospital.) Nursing Mirror, 144, 3 Mar 1977, 59-62.

13 Joint Working Group on Oral Contraceptives Report. HMSO, 1976.

14 Kay, C.R. The happiness pill? (Development of the oral contraceptive pill from the 1930s.) Journal of the Royal College of General Practitioners, 30, Jan 1980, 8-13, 16-19.

15 Kessler, A. and Standley, C.C. Fertility regulating methods. Recent progress in the WHO programme in human reproduction. WHO Chronicle, 31 (5), May 1977, 182-193.

16 Klaus, H. Fertility awareness as a method of conception control. (Natural family planning.) Nursing Times, 74, 12 Jan 1978, 63-64.

17 Louden, N.B. Contraception for teenagers. (Review of methods.) Midwife, Health Visitor and Community Nurse, 15 (9), Sep 1979, 356, 358, 362.

18 Loudon, N.B. and others Acceptability of an oral contraceptive that reduces the frequency of menstruation: the tri-cycle pill regimen. British Medical Journal, 2, 20 Aug 1977, 487-490.

19 Morris, P. Injecting into a controversy... (Depo-Provera, an injectable contraceptive.) Nursing Mirror, 149, 13 Dec 1979, 6.

20 Norris, C. Natural family planning. (Based on monitoring the production of mucus as predictor of ovulation.) Nursing Mirror, 145, 27 Oct 1977, 29-30.

21 Pauncefort, Z. Methods of contraception: a guide to current methods of fertility regulation and their significance. Queen's Nursing Journal, 19 (14), May 1977, 394-396.

22 Seed, M. and Houston, S. The pill and its effects—metabolic research at St. Mary's. (Day ward at present investigating the biochemical effects of the pill on non-European women.) Nursing Times, 72, 1 Apr 1976, 509-510.

23 Smith, A. Ancient and modern—a brief history of contraception. Nursing Mirror, 142, 26 Feb 1976, 55-56.

24 Swenson, I. Oral contraceptives: a review of the literature. Journal of Nurse-Midwifery, 20 (1), Spring 1975, 7-14.

25 Thomas, A.K. Ovarian hormones. (Physiology, pathology and use in contraception.) Nursing Times, 73, 9 Jun 1977, 867-870.

26 Timby, B.K. Ovulation method of birth control. American Journal of Nursing, 76 (6), Jun 1976, 928-929.

27 Vessey, M.P. Contraceptive methods: risks and benefits. British Medical Journal, 2, 9 Sep 1978, 721-722.

28 Vessey, M.P. and others Fertility after stopping different methods of contraception.

(Survey.) British Medical Journal, 1, 4 Feb 1978, 365-367.

29 Vessey, M.P. and others Mortality among women participating in the Oxford/Family Planning Association contraceptive study. (See also editorial on page 747-748 and RCGP and RCOG recommendations on page 757.) Lancet, 2, 8 Oct 1977, 731-733.

30 Royal College of General Practitioners Research Unit Mortality among oral-contraceptive users. (See also editorial on page 747-748 and RCGP and RCOG recommendations on page 757.) Lancet, 2, 8 Oct 1977, 727-731.

31 Whitehead, S. New trends in contraception. Nursing Times, 72, 25 Nov 1976, 1841-1842.

e STERILISATION, MALE AND FEMALE

1 Arthure, H. Puerperal sterilisation. Midwife, Health Visitor and Community Nurse, 12 (7), Jul 1976, 225-226.

2 Bennett, A. Nursing care study. Surgical female sterilisation. It's all done with tubes and clips. (By student nurse who describes her own experience as a patient.) Nursing Mirror, 148, 8 Mar 1979, 42-44.

3 Bledin, K.D. and others Recent trends in sterilization in women. Health Trends, 4 (10), Nov 1978, 84-87.

4 Howard, G. Motivation for vasectomy. Lancet, 1, 11 Mar 1978, 546-548.

5 Teper, S. Sterilisation: the Aberdeen experience, and some broader complications. Journal of Medical Ethics, 4 (1), Mar 1978, 18-24.

6 Whitelaw, R. 10-year survey of 485 sterilisations. 1. Sterilisation or hysterectomy. 2. Patients' views on their sterilisation. British Medical Journal, 1, 6 Jan 1979, 32-35.

7 Winston, R.M.L. Why 103 women asked for reversal of sterilisation. British Medical Journal, 2, 30 Jul 1977, 305-307.

43 TERMINATION OF PREGNANCY

a GENERAL

1 Adamkiewicz, V.W. What are the bonds between the fetus and the uterus. (Viewpoint on abortion.) Canadian Nurse, 72 (2), Feb 1976, 27-28.

2 Ashton, J.R. and others The Wessex Abortion Studies. 1. Interdistrict variation in provision of abortion services. 2. Attitudes of consultant gynaecologists to provision of abortion services. Lancet, 1, 12 Jan 1980, 82-85; 19 Jan 1980, 140-142.

3 Atkinson, J. editor Abortion reconsidered: the Methodist statement and its background. Methodist Publishing House, 1977.

4 Birth Control Trust Abortion: the NHS and the charities. Papers presented at a symposium... The Trust, 1977.

5 Burningham, S. Research, preparation and not having to turn them away. (Day care abortion clinic at the South London Hospital for Women.) Health and Social Service Journal, 89, 9 Nov 1979, 1456-1457.

6 Catford, J.C. and Fowkes, F.G.R. Economic benefits of day care abortion. Community Medicine, 1 (2), May 1979, 115-122.

7 Fowkes, F.G.R. and others Abortion and the NHS: the first decade. British Medical Journal, 1, 27 Jan 1979, 217-219.

8 Francome, C. Abortion and opinion. (Report of recent poll.) New Society, 47, 22 Mar 1979, 678.

9 Francome, C. and Brewer, C. Abortion. 1. The fall. (Reasons for the recent statistical changes in abortion.) 2. The risk. New Society, 39, 3 Feb 1977, 234-235; 10 Feb 1977, 281-282.

10 Gardner, R.F.R. The ethics of abortion. Practitioner, 223, Aug 1979, 244-248.

11 Goldthorp, W.G. Ten-minute abortions. (Report on service in a district general hospital using menstrual aspiration.) British Medical Journal, 2, 27 Aug 1977, 562-564.

12 International Planned Parenthood Foundation The human problem of abortion: medical and legal dimensions. IPPF, 1979.

13 Lafitte, F. Recent and possible future trends in abortion. Journal of Medical Ethics, 4 (1), Mar 1978, 25-29.

14 Nursing Times NHS is 'punitive and judgemental' towards women seeking abortion. (Symposium organised by Coordinating Committee in Defence of the 1967 Abortion Act.) Nursing Times, 73 (23), 9 Jun 1977, 846.

15 Office of Population Censuses and Surveys Abortion statistics 1974: England and Wales. HMSO, 1977.

16 Potts, M. and others Abortion. Cambridge University Press, 1977.

17 Ross, T. Facing up to reality. (British Pregnancy Advisory Service's Birmingham centre.) Nursing Mirror, 150, 21 Feb 1980, 40-41.

18 Tietze, C. and Lewit, S. Legal abortion. (Abortion practices in different countries.) Scientific American, 236 (1), Jan 1977, 21-27.

19 Tomalin, C. Day-care abortion: facts and fantasies. Health and Social Service Journal, 86, 21 Feb 1976, 353.

20 Turner, J. The battle of abortion. New Society, 35, 11 May 1976, 541-542.

21 White, D. The wider context of abortion. (Legal position throughout the world.) New Society, 51, 7 Feb 1980, 280-281.

22 Whitehead, S. Abortion practice: could drugs replace doctors? Nursing Times, 72, 15 Apr 1976, 564-565.

b LEGISLATION

1 British Pregnancy Advisory Service Abortion committee is biased, says British Pregnancy Advisory Service. Nursing Times, 72, 11 Nov 1976, 1745.

2 British Pregnancy Advisory Service A charitable rejoinder to the Select Committee: memorandum. . .on the First Report of the Select Committee on Abortion Session 1975-76. Wootton Wawen: The Association, 1976.

3 Darby, C. The Abortion Act: right or wrong? (Interview with William Benyon, MP and Helene Hayman, MP.) Nursing Mirror, 144, 17 Mar 1977, 35.

4 Kingman, S. Throwing out baby with legislation? (Background to Corrie bill.) Health and Social Service Journal, 89, 3 Aug 1979, 962-963.

5 Lancet Commentary from Westminster. The Braine Bill. (On abortion.) Lancet, 1, 4 Mar 1978, 511-512.

6 Select Committee on Abortion First report, together with the proceedings of the Committee and appendices. Session 1975-76. HMSO, 1976.

c COUNSELLING

1 Anders, R.L. Program consultation by a clinical specialist. (Development of abortion counselling programme by psychiatric nurse clinical specialist.) Journal of Nursing Administration, 8 (11), Nov 1978, 34-38.

2 Brewer, C. Incidence of post abortion psychosis: a prospective study. (In the West Midlands comparing it with the incidence of puerperal psychosis.) British Medical Journal, 1, 19 Feb 1977, 476-477.

3 Burkle, F.M. A developmental approach to post-abortion depression. Practitioner, 218, Feb 1977, 217-225.

4 Cheetham, Juliet Unwanted pregnancy and counselling. Routledge and Kegan Paul, 1977.

5 Devore, N.E. The relationship between previous elective abortions and postpartum depressive reactions. Journal of Obstetric, Gynecologic and Neonatal Nursing, 8 (4), Jul/Aug 1979, 237-240.

6 Kay, B.J. and Thompson, C.W.N. An outcome evaluation of counselling services provided by abortion clinics. (In Chicago.) Medical Care, 15 (10), Oct 1977, 858-868.

7 Marcus, R.J. Evaluating abortion counselling. (Survey in Vancouver.) Dimensions in Health Services, 56 (8), Aug 1979, 16-18.

8 Shane, F. Therapeutic abortion—some psychiatric aspects. Canadian Journal of Psychiatric Nursing, 17 (2), Mar/Apr 1976, 11-13.

9 Simms, M. Report on non-medical abortion counselling. Revised ed. Birth Control Trust, 1977.

d NURSING

1 Aby-Nielsen, K. Physical sensations during stressful hospital procedures: a preliminary study of saline abortion patients. (With reference to preparing patients for such experiences.) Journal of Obstetric, Gynecologic and Neonatal Nursing, 8 (2), Mar/Apr 1979, 105-106.

2 Allen, D.V. and others Two measures of nurses' attitudes toward abortion as modified by experience. (Research in Michigan and New York.) Medical Care, 15 (10), Oct 1977, 849-857.

3 Anderson, C. and Hassanein, R. Psychoprophylaxis in midtrimester abortions. (Study of responses to nursing care received by 15 abortion patients who had been taught a modified form of the Lamaze relaxation technique.) Journal of Obstetric, Gynecologic and Neonatal Nursing, 5 (6), Nov/Dec 1976, 29-33.

4 Berger, J.M. The relationship of age to nurses' attitudes toward abortion. (Research study.) Journal of Obstetric, Gynecologic and Neonatal Nursing, 8 (4), Jul/Aug 1979, 231-233.

5 British Medical Journal Medicolegal. Nurses' role in abortion. (Report of Rcn v DHSS case.) British Medical Journal, 281, 13 Sep 1980, 750.

6 De Tornyay, R. Nursing decisions. Experiences in clinical problem solving. Series 2, number 8. Joyce H. An elective abortion patient. RN Magazine, 40 (6), 15 Jun 1977, 55-61.

7 Department of Health and Social Security Termination of pregnancy by medical induction: the role of the nurse or midwife and others who are not registered medical practitioners. DHSS, 1980 (CMO(80)2, CNO(80)2), Reprinted in Midwives Chronicle, 93, Apr 1980, 112-113.

8 Dewhurst, J.E. and Weeks, A.R.L. Occult manifestations of septic abortion. (Two case studies.) Nursing Mirror, 142, 29 Apr 1976, 62-63.

9 Donachie, E. Dilemmas and pressures. Part 2. On patients and nurses—Abortion legislation. (Position of Catholic nurses regarding abortion.) World of Irish Nursing, 6 (6), Jun 1977, 1-2.

10 Heath, M. Nurses for LIFE. (Pressure group of nurses who are anti-abortion and its position on the Corrie bill.) Nursing Times, 75, 13 Dec 1979, 2145-2146.

11 Hurwitz, A. and Eadie, R.F. Psychologic impact on nursing students of participation in abortion. (A study of dreams which compared the abortion experience with other stressful experiences.) Nursing Research, 26 (2), Mar-Apr 1977, 112-120.

12 McQueen, A. Nursing care study. Termination of pregnancy using extra-amniotic prostaglandin. Nursing Mirror, 142, 17 Jun 1976, 45-47.

13 Martin, A. A question of balance. (Comment on dispute between Rcn and DHSS over nurse's role in medical abortion.) Nursing Mirror, 151, 18 Sep 1980, 9.

14 Nursing Times Nurse could you care more? (Account by a nurse who aborted who reports lack of compassion and good nursing care.) Nursing Times, 75, 5 Apr 1979, 569.

15 Nuttall, P. PPS. (Comment on DHSS circular on nurses' position on termination of pregnancy by medical induction.) Nursing Times, 76, 27 Mar 1980, 569.

16 Olson, M. Helping staff nurses care for women seeking saline abortions. (With nursing care plan for abortion patients.) Journal of Obstetric, Gynecologic and Neonatal Nursing, 9 (3), May/Jun 1980, 170-174.

17 Royal College of Nursing College gives the OK on abortion. (Rcn advice on nurse's role in medical induction.) Nursing Times, 76, 7 Aug 1980, 1376.

18 Sandroff, R. Is it right? (Results of survey of nurses' attitudes to abortion, sterilization and birth control.) RN Magazine, 43 (10), Oct 1980, 25-30.

19 Simms, M. Abortion: why I don't believe Mr. Rye. (Criticises Rcn's judgement on proceedings with abortion dispute.) Nursing Mirror, 151, 4 Dec 1980, 10.

CHILD HEALTH

44 CHILD HEALTH SERVICES

a GENERAL

1 Alberman, E.D. and others After Court. (Critical review of Court report and suggested alternative ways of providing care.) Lancet, 2, 20 Aug 1977, 393-396.

2 Association of British Paediatric Nurses Fit for the future. Comments on the report of the Committee on Child Health Services. (The Court Report.) Nursing Times, 73, 8 Sep 1977 ABPN Supplement, 2-4.

3 Bacon, C.J. and others Individual response from a teaching area to 'Fit for the Future.' Report of an independent working group in Newcastle upon Tyne. (Based on survey and discussions with health professionals.) British Medical Journal, 2, 24 Sep 1977, 811-813.

4 Bain, D.J.G. Child care in the new towns in the UK. (General practice orientated review.) Journal of the Royal College of General Practitioners, 27, Sep 1977, 556-557.

5 Bray, P. Forty years of paediatrics. An address to the Wales and South West Branch of the ABPN. Nursing Times, 73, 8 Sep 1977 ABPN Supplement, 4-5.

6 Brian, V.A. Infant welfare in the Bible. Nursing Times, 76, 18/25 Dec 1980, 2230-2231.

7 Brimblecombe, F. and Barltrop, D. Children in health and disease. Baillière Tindall, 1978.

8 British Medical Association. Board of Science and Education Our children's health: report of the Working Party on our children's health, 1979. BMA, 1979.

9 British Medical Journal Problems of childhood: articles published in the 'British Medical Journal.' British Medical Association, 1976.

10 British Paediatric Association. Working Party on Ethics of Research in Children Guidelines to aid ethical committees considering research involving children. British Medical Journal, 280, 26 Jan 1980, 229-231.

11 Butler, N. Child health and education in the seventies: some results on the 5-year follow up of the 1970 British Births cohort. Health Visitor, 53 (3), Mar 1980, 81-82.

12 Chamberlain, R. British births 1970: a survey...Vol.I: the first week of life. Heinemann, 1975. (National Birthday Trust Fund) Reprinted in Midwives Chronicle, 89, May 1976, 116-117.

13 Children's Committee Out-of-hours social and health care: report of a working group of the Children's Committee. (With some reference to community nursing.) Health and Social Service Journal, 90, 13 Jun 1980, 776-778.

14 Children's Committee Services for adolescents: an issues paper. The Committee, 1979.

15 Clark, J. A good job with one exception. (Role of proposed grade of child health visitor as proposed in Court Report.) Nursing Times, 73, 23 Jun 1977, 936-937.

16 Clark, J. In defence of Court. (The Court report on child health services.) Journal of Community Nursing, 1 (1), Jul 1977, 8-9.

17 Clark, J. Thoughts on Court. Nursing Mirror, 144, 17 Feb 1977, 39-41.

18 Committee on Child Health Services Fit for the future: report of the Committee. HMSO, 1976. 2 vols. (Chairman S.D.M. Court. Cmnd 6684.)

19 Committee on Child Health Services Fit for the future. Comments and summaries. Health Visitor, 50 (2), Feb 1977, 44-45, 48; 51 (1), Jan 1978, 10-12. Hospital and Health Services Review, 73 (2), Feb 1977. Editorial 37-38, Summary 66-68. Lancet, 1, 8 Jan 1977, 79-80. Nursing Mirror, 143, 23 Dec 1976, 19. Nursing Times, 72, 23/30 Dec 1976, 1985. Queen's Nursing Journal, 19 (12), Mar 1977, 328-329.

20 Commonwealth Nurses Federation International Year of the Child. Nursing Times, 75, 22 Feb 1979 CNF Supplement, 98-99.

21 Court, S.D.M. Has the Court Report been misunderstood? An interview with Professor Donald Court. British Medical Journal, 1, 11 Jun 1977, 1522-1525.

22 Court, S.D.M. A less drab response from Court. (Comment on Government proposals from the former chairman of the Committee on Child Health Services.) Lancet, 1, 25 Mar 1978, 653-654.

23 Department of Health and Social Security Advisory and counselling services for young people. HMSO, 1978. (Research report no.1.)

24 Fogelman, K. editor Britain's sixteen-year-olds: preliminary findings from the third follow-up of the National Child Development Study (1958 cohort.) National Children's Bureau, 1976.

25 Ford, L.R. A child health service or a child health system? (Pros and cons of computerised child health records.) Public Health, 92 (4), Jul 1978, 177-180.

26 Franklin, A.W. Widening horizons of child health: a study of the medical health needs of children in England and Wales. Lancaster: MTP Press, 1976.

27 General Medical Services Council Court Report on child health services. (Report of GMSC working party studying its implications.) British Medical Journal, 1, 11 Jun 1977, 1552-1553.

28 Graham, H. Women's attitudes to the child health services. (Survey of attitudes to health visitor and child health clinic.) Health Visitor, 52 (5), May 1979, 175-178.

29 Gray, F.D. The Court report reviewed. Midwife, Health Visitor and Community Nurse, 13 (5), May 1977, 143-144.

30 Green, L.W. and others Guidelines for health education in maternal and child health. International Journal of Health Education, 21 (3), Jul/Sep 1978, 1-32.

31 Harker, P. Taking the child health services into the arena of Court. Health and Social Service Journal, 86, 24/31 Dec 1976, 2272-2273.

32 Haynes, M.V. and others Why mothers attend child health clinics. (Research project of five health visitor students.) Health Visitor, 50 (6), Jun 1977, 184, 186.

33 Hine, D. Afterthoughts on Court: philosophy into practice. (How the Court report's recommendations could be implemented.) Royal Society of Health Journal, 98 (4), Aug 1978, 161-164.

34 Hunter, M. Integration of the child health nursing services in Scotland. Nursing Times, 72 (43), 28 Oct 1976, ABPN Supplement, 4-5.

35 Illingworth, R.S. Some experience in an area health authority child health clinic. (With some reference to the training of health visitors.) British Medical Journal, 1, 31 Mar 1979, 866-869.

36 International Council of Nurses ICN statement on the rights of children. International Nursing Review, 27 (1), Jan/Feb 1980, 5.

37 INTERNATIONAL Year of the Child. Children in Britain and children overseas. Nursing Times, 75, 31 May 1979 IYC Supplement, 2-22.

38 Jackson, J. Paediatric primary care in Inner London. (Survey of children attending family doctors or hospital A and E departments.) Journal of the Royal College of General Practitioners, 30, Sep 1980, 520-528.

39 **Jenkins, G.C.** Developmental and paediatric care of the pre school child. (Survey of opinion and provision in the United Kingdom undertaken on a travelling fellowship.) Journal of the Royal College of General Practitioners, 26, Nov 1976, 795-801.

40 **Jepson, A.M.** Child health services today — aims and objectives. Midwife, Health Visitor and Community Nurse, 13 (1), Jan 1977, 19-21.

41 **Jones, R.H.T.** Integration of hospital and community child health services. (In South Wales.) Health Trends, 1 (11), Feb 1979, 10-13.

42 **Journal of the Royal College of General Practitioners** International Year of the Child. (Six articles on child care in general practice.) Journal of the Royal College of General Practitioners, 29, Nov 1979, 641-665.

43 **King, M. and others** Primary child care: a manual for health workers. Oxford University Press, 1978.

44 **Komrower, G.M.** The role of the hospital in primary care for the child in the community. British Medical Journal, 2, 24 Sep 1977, 787-789.

45 **Lancet** Born in Britain 1970. (Survey of the first week of life.) Lancet, 1976, 1, 3 Apr 1976, 729-730.

46 **Laurence, B.M. and Lawrie, B.** Health and nutrition education unit in a children's hospital. (Queen Elizabeth Hospital for Children, London.) British Medical Journal, 2, 25 Nov 1978, 1469-1471.

47 **Lucas, S.** Some aspects of child health care: contacts between children, general practitioners and school doctors. (With reference to Court report's recommendations.) Community Medicine, 2 (3), Aug 1980, 209-218.

48 **Lupton, G.** The International Year of the Child — 1979. (Gives outline of organisation and activities.) Social Work Service, 19, Mar 1979, 1-3.

49 **Mactaggart, J.M.** The place of preventive medicine in the community care of babies and young children. Nursing Mirror, 144, 6 Jan 1977, 30-31.

50 **Madeley, R.J.** Relating child health services to needs by the use of simple epidemiology. (Scoring system for high risk babies based on indices of social deprivation to facilitate intensive follow-up by health visitors.) Public Health, 92 (5), Sep 1978, 224-230.

51 **Meadow, R.** Paediatric advances: the struggle for child survival. Nursing Mirror, 149, 27 Sep 1979, 34-35.

52 **Mitchell, R.G. editor** Child health in the community: a handbook of social and community paediatrics. Edinburgh: Churchill Livingstone, 1977. 2nd ed. 1980.

53 **Morrell, D.C. and others** Management of minor illness. (Study to measure the effect of a booklet describing common symptoms in childhood, how to treat them and when to call the doctor on the pattern of demand on a group practice in Lambeth.) British Medical Journal, 1, 15 Mar 1980, 769-771.

54 **Morton, E.J.** Health visitors and child health. (Letter on Court Report.) British Medical Journal, 2, 23 Jul 1977, 265-266.

55 **National Children's Bureau** At your service. (Activities and services of the National Children's Bureau.) Nursing Times, 73, 8 Dec 1977 Community Outlook, 140-142.

56 **Nursing Times** Views on Court. (Six articles by nurses involved in various aspects of child health.) Nursing Times, 73, 23 Jun 1977, 936-947.

57 **Office of Population Censuses and Surveys** Child health: a collection of studies. HMSO, 1976. (Studies on medical and population subjects no.31.)

58 **Owen, C.M.** Bridging the information gap. (Between parents and professions in child health.) Nursing Mirror, 148, 24 May 1979, 24-25.

59 **Owen, C.M.** Child health record booklet. (To record child's progress and containing information, produced by the Society of Area Nurses (Child Health).) Midwife, Health Visitor and Community Nurse, 16 (4), Apr 1980, 156, 158, 162.

60 **Owen, C.M.** Health surveillance programme for children. 0-5 years. (In Surrey AHA.) Health Visitor, 53 (3), Mar 1980, 88.

61 **Peckham, C. and Pearson, R.** Preliminary findings at the age of 16 years on children in the National Child Development Study (1958 Cohort.) Public Health, 90 (6), Sep 1976, 271-280.

62 **Pike, L.A.** Teaching parents about child health using a practice booklet. Journal of the Royal College of General Practitioners, 30, Sep 1980, 517-519.

63 **Rogers, B.** Stronger links for the under-fives. (Recent circular from DHSS and DES recommending better coordination of services.) Nursing Mirror, 146, 16 Feb 1978, 47-48.

64 **Royal College of Midwives** Comments on 'Fit for the Future.' Report of the Committee on Child Health Services. Midwives Chronicle, 90, Aug 1977, 191-192; Nursing Times, 73, 14 Jul 1977, 1056.

65 **Royal College of Nursing** Comments on the Court report. Rcn, 1977.

66 **Royal College of Nursing** Fit for the future: the Court report. Summary of main recommendations. Rcn, 1976.

67 **Slack, P.** Prevention in the child health services. (Summary of and comment on new DHSS paper.) Nursing Times, 76, 3 Apr 1980, 581-582.

68 **Smith, C.S.** Child health: what of the future. Public Health, 91 (6), Nov 1977, 305-311.

69 **Smith, J.** Not with an axe but a scythe. (Work of Children's Committee.) Health and Social Service Journal, 90, 18 Jan 1980, 90.

70 **Society of Area Nurses (Child Health)** Child health record. Edsall, 1979.

71 **Society of Community Medicine** Implications of Court. (Discussion by London and Home Counties Branch of the Society of Community Medicine.) Public Health, 91 (5), Sep 1977, 266-268.

72 **Steiner, H.** An evaluation of child health clinic services in Newcastle upon Tyne during 1972-1974. British Journal of Preventive and Social Medicine, 31 (1), Mar 1977, 1-5.

73 **Valman, H.B. and others** Child health in an integrated health service. Health Trends, 9 (2), May 1977, 30-32.

74 **Valman, H.B.** The first year of life. Health services for children. British Medical Journal, 280, 28 Jun 1980, 1588-1591.

75 **West, R.R. and Lowe, C.R.** Regional variations in need for and provision and use of child health services in England and Wales. British Medical Journal, 2, 9 Oct 1976, 843-846.

76 **Wickstead, P. and others** The integration of child health services for pre-school children: a working model. (Scheme involving HV, social worker, GP and clinical medical officer at health clinic and Charing Cross Hospital.) Practitioner, 224, Sep 1980, 875-878.

77 **World Health** Special issue to mark International Year of the Child. World Health, Feb/Mar 1979, 2-36.

78 **Yale, R.** Closing gaps in the care of under fives. (Reasons behind low uptake of preventive services in inner city area.) Health and Social Service Journal, 89, 4 May 1979, 518-519.

b OVERSEAS COUNTRIES

1 **Adams, R.** Development of maternal and child health services in Israel. International Nursing Review, 27 (4), Jul/Aug 1980, 112-113.

2 **Arthur, J.** 'Namaste didi.' (Mother and child health clinic in Nepal.) Nursing Mirror, 143, 15 Jul 1976, 66-67.

3 **Association of British Paediatric Nurses** Spotlight on children: child care in other countries. (Seven articles including care in the Middle East, Bangladesh and Nepal.) Nursing Times, 75, 8 Nov 1979 ABPN, 1-8.

4 **Bates, S.M.** Scandinavia. (Florence Nightingale scholarship studying child care.) Nursing Times, 72 (12), 25 Mar 1976 ABPN supplement, VII-VIII.

5 **Betts, D.** Nursing round the world with Save the Children. (Experiences of twenty years work with the Fund.) Nursing Mirror, 144, 20 Jan 1977, 36-37.

6 **Curnock, D.A.** The 'road to health' — child health in developing countries. (With reference to Nigeria.) Midwife, Health Visitor and Community Nurse, 15 (9), Sep 1979, 350, 352, 354.

7 **Deakin, B.** History of child health services in Victoria. Australian Nurses Journal, 8 (6), Dec/Jan 1978/1979, 29-33, 59.

8 **De Maio, D.** The born-again nurse. (Nurse's expanded role in child health services in Newark, New Jersey during early 20th century.) Nursing Outlook, 27 (4), Apr 1979, 272-273.

9 **Dourado, H.G. and Coelho, C.P.** Nursing and child health in Brazil. (With brief historical review.) International Nursing Review, 27 (3), May/Jun 1980, 70-75.

10 **Ebrahim, G.J.** Child care in the tropics. Macmillan, 1978. (Macmillan tropical community health manuals.)

11 **Ebrahim, G.J.** A handbook of tropical paediatrics. Macmillan, 1978. (Macmillan tropical community health manuals.)

12 **Jolly, J.D.** Child care in North America — 1. Round-the-clock home care. (Home care unit at Montreal Children's Hospital.) Nursing Times, 73, 24 Nov 1977, 1843-1844.

13 **Kum, E. and Uyer, G.** Child health and health and nursing services for children in Turkey. International Nursing Review, 26 (5), Sep/Oct 1979, 147-149.

14 **Lindstrom, C.J.** No shows: a problem in health care. (A study of 30 Mexican-American families to find out the characteristics of mothers who attended a child health clinic regularly compared with those who failed to keep appointments.) Nursing Outlook, 23 (12), Dec 1975, 755-759.

15 **Mendelievich, E. editor** Children at work. Geneva: ILO, 1979.

16 **Munoz, N. and others** Health care for children in Argentina. (Including role of nurse.) International Nursing Review, 26 (5), Sep/Oct 1979, 150-152.

17 **Nash, E.** Paediatric work in the developing countries. (The work of Miss Margaret Woodland, MBE, SRN, SCM, HV.) Nursing Times, 72, 9 Sep 1976, 1408-1409.

18 **Okunade, A.O.** Screening for handicaps in children: are Nigerian nurses equipped? (Survey of community nurses and health centres.) International Journal of Nursing Studies, 17 (3), 1980, 181-187.

19 **Oyediran, M.A. and others** A scoring system for sick children. (To provide an easy means of identifying need for medical treatment in child welfare clinics in developing countries.) British Journal of Preventive and Social Medicine, 31 (2), Jun 1977, 127-130.

20 **Robinson, M.J. and Lee, E.L. editors** Paediatric problems in tropical countries. Churchill Livingstone, 1978.

21 **Sandall, A.** Child health care in France. Health Visitor, 50 (4), Apr 1977, 96-99.

22 **WHO Chronicle** Health of the world's children. WHO Chronicle, 33 (4), Apr 1979, 120-124.

23 **Wynn, M. and Wynn, A.** Some developments in child health care in Europe. Royal Society of Health Journal, 99 (6), Dec 1979, 259-264.

c CHILD DEVELOPMENT AND PSYCHOLOGY

1 **Aves, B.** Stycar. (Game to teach student health visitors and nursery nurses about stages of child development.) Nursing Times, 75, 13 Dec 1979 Community Outlook 378, 380-381, 383, 385.

2 **Bain, D.J.G.** Methods used by general practitioners in developmental screening of preschool children. (Study in Livingston, Scotland of examinations by GPs and HVs.) British Medical Journal, 2, 6 Aug 1977, 363-365.

3 **Baker, P.** Social development during the first two years of life. Nursing Mirror, 142, 10 Jun 1976, 70-71.

4 **Barber, J.H. and others** A new visual chart for pre-school developmental screening. (Developed at Woodside Health Centre, Glasgow.) Health Bulletin, 34 (2), Mar 1976, 80-91.

5 **Berman, C.M.** Significance of animal play. (With reference to children's play.) Nursing Mirror, 145, 29 Dec 1977, 10-13.

6 **Brain, J.** Child's play. (Its importance in child development.) Midwife, Health Visitor and Community Nurse, 13 (6), Jun 1977, 182-185.

7 **Bryant, G.M.** Use of the Denver Developmental Screening Test for health visitors. (Screening test for neuro-developmental disorders used routinely by HV in South Glamorgan AHA.) Health Visitor, 53 (1), Jan 1980, 2-5.

8 **Colyer, M.** Assessment in the community. (Of child development, by health visitor.) Nursing Mirror, 145, 8 Dec 1977 Supplement v, vii.

9 **Curtis Jenkins, G.H. and others** Developmental surveillance in general practice. (Two-year study which showed that routine surveillance on the lines proposed by the Court Committee is worthwhile.) British Medical Journal, 1, 10 Jun 1978, 1537-1540.

10 **Dinnage, R.** Growing up with the Newsons. (Profile of Prof. John and Dr. Elizabeth Newson and their work at University of Nottingham's Child Development Research Unit.) New Society, 52, 10 Apr 1980, 55-57.

11 **Downs, F.S. and Fitzpatrick, J.J.** Preliminary investigation of the reliability and validity of a tool for the assessment of body position and motor activity. (To evaluate health status of 14 children.) Nursing Research, 25 (6), Nov-Dec 1976, 404-408.

12 **Elliman, A.M.** Developmental assessment of the infant and young child. Midwife, Health Visitor and Community Nurse, 15 (8), Aug 1979, 312, 314, 318.

13 **Fergusson, J.H.** Late psychologic effects of a serious illness in childhood. (Report of a study in Philadelphia.) Nursing Clinics of North America, 11 (1), Mar 1976, 83-93.

14 **Fieldhouse, P.** Health interests of children. (Survey of 450 children in four schools.) Health Visitor, 53 (8), Aug 1980, 313, 315.

15 **Freer, C.B. and Ogunmuyiwa, T.A.** Pre-school development screening in a health centre—the problem of non-attendance. Journal of the Royal College of General Practitioners, 27, Jul 1977, 428-430.

16 **Health Visitors Association** New baby's first three years. Edsall/Health Visitor's Association, 1976.

17 **Hutchings, J.** Community nursing and psychology. 16. More about the ABC. (Advice on advising mothers on toilet training.) Journal of Community Nursing, 4 (2), Aug 1980, 6, 16.

18 **Illingworth, R.S.** The development of the infant and young child normal and abnormal. Edinburgh: Churchill Livingstone, 1980.

19 **Illingworth, R.S.** The normal child: some problems of the early years and their treatment. 7th ed. Edinburgh: Churchill Livingstone, 1979.

20 **Illingworth, R.S. and Illingworth, C.** Babies and young children: a guide for parents. 6th ed. Churchill Livingstone, 1977.

21 **Jacobs, R. and Hall, C.J.** Periodic developmental assessment of pre-school children in Newham. Public Health, 90 (4), May 1976, 179-186.

22 **Krajickek, M.J. and Tearney, A.I. editors** Detection of developmental problems in children: a reference guide for community nurses and other health care professionals. Baltimore: University Park Press, 1977.

23 **Lawrence, W.C.M. and Sklaroff, S.A.** Who should carry out developmental screening examinations? (Study in Scotland using GPs, HVs and health authority doctors.) Health Bulletin, 36 (1), Jan 1978, 25-33.

24 **Lobascher, M.E. and Cavanagh, N.P.C.** The other handicap: brightness. (With four case reports.) British Medical Journal, 2, 12 Nov 1977, 1269-1271.

25 **Mann, S.** Recognising and understanding gifted children. Midwife, Health Visitor and Community Nurse, 14 (1), Jan 1978, 16-17.

26 **Milligan, N.** The gifted child. Health Visitor, 52 (11), Nov 1979, 474, 478, 482.

27 **Mitchell, N.** The gifted child. Nursing Mirror, 146, 9 Feb 1978, 14-16.

28 **Montague, J.** Teaching teenagers about child development. (Scheme in Norfolk whereby teenage girls visit playgroups and do child studies.) Midwife, Health Visitor and Community Nurse, 15 (4), Apr 1979, 150-151.

29 **Morris, D.** The hazards in toilet training. Nursing Mirror, 147, 14 Sep 1978, 26-27.

30 **Newsom, J. and Newsom, E.** Joys and playthings in development and remediation. Allen and Unwin, 1979.

31 **Nursing Mirror** Child development. (Supplement of five articles, four of them by staff at Wolfson Centre, London.) Nursing Mirror, 145, 8 Dec 1977 Supplement, i, iii, v, vii, ix, xi, xiii, xv.

32 **O'Brien, R.A.** Relationship of parent-child communication to child's exploratory behavior and self-differentiation. Nursing Research, 29 (3), May/Jun 1980, 150-156.

33 **Ounsted, M.** The first-born child: patterns of development and problems. (Research study of 209 mothers.) Health Visitor, 53 (3), Mar 1980, 78-80.

34 **Pidgeon, V.A.** Characteristics of children's thinking and implications for health teaching. Maternal Child Nursing Journal, 6 (1), Spring, 1-8.

35 **Pringle, M.K.** How early is early? (Demonstration of individual differences in behaviour.) Midwives Chronicle, 90, Oct 1977, 239-241.

36 **Pringle, M.K.** The needs of children: a personal perspective. 2nd ed. Hutchinson, 1980.

37 **Quiggin, V.** Beginning research. Children's knowledge of their internal body parts. (Information useful for health educators.) Nursing Times, 73, 28 Jul 1977, 1146-1151.

38 Reid, R. My children, my children: life before and after birth. An account of some recent developments. British Broadcasting Corporation, 1977.

39 Rendle-Short, J. The child: a guide for the paediatric team. 2nd ed. Bristol: Wright, 1977.

40 Robson, P. Screening for children. Developmental paediatrics. Royal Society of Health Journal, 98 (5), Oct 1978, 231-237.

41 Routledge, L. Children's drawings. British Journal of Occupational Therapy, 39 (9), Sep 1976, 219-221.

42 Shaffer, D. and Dunn, J. editors The first year of life: psychological and medical implications of early experience. Chichester: John Wiley, 1979.

43 Smith, E.C. and others Re-establishing a child's body image (after a disfiguring injury.) American Journal of Nursing, 77 (3), Mar 1977, 445-447.

44 Smith, P.K. Play is only one way to learn. (Its role in child development and education.) New Society, 45, 27 Jul 1978, 180-182.

45 Stallibrass, A. The self-respecting child: a study of children's play and development. Rev. ed. Harmondsworth: Penguin, 1977.

46 Starte, G.D. Results from a developmental screening clinic in general practice. Practitioner, 216, Mar 1976, 311-316.

47 Taylor, S.C. The effect of chronic childhood illnesses upon well siblings. (Research study.) Maternal-Child Nursing Journal, 9 (2), Summer 1980, 109-116.

48 Valman, H.B. and others Rocking horse paediatric weighing machine. Lancet, 2, 25 Dec 1976, 1389.

49 Walshe-Brennan, K.S. The role of games in personality development. Nursing Mirror, 142, 19 Feb 1976, 66-67.

50 Williams, P.D. A comparison of Philippine and American children's concepts of body organs and illness in relation to five variables. International Journal of Nursing Studies, 15 (4), 1978, 193-202.

51 World Health Organization. Expert Committee Child mental health and psychosocial development. Geneva: WHO, 1977. (Technical report series no.613.)

d CHILD PSYCHIATRY

1 Armstrong, A.A. A closer look at children with neurotic and conduct disorders. British Journal of Occupational Therapy, 41 (12), Dec 1978, 391-393.

2 Barcroft, J. Depression in childhood. Journal of Community Nursing, 4 (3), Sep 1980, 18-19, 21.

3 Barker, P. Basic child psychiatry. 2nd ed. Crosby Lockwood Staples, 1976.

4 Benians, R. In defence of child psychiatry. Mind Out, 38, Jan/Feb 1980, 20.

5 Bentovim, A. Problems of childhood. Disobedience and violent behaviour in children: family pathology and family treatment. British Medical Journal, 1, 17 Apr 1976, 947-949; 24 Apr 1976, 1004-1006.

6 Bhaduri, R. Managing agressive children. (Description of group work with children and their parents in a paediatric ward.) Nursing Times, 75, 13 Dec 1979, 2159.

7 Bhoyrub, J.P. School phobia: in-patient treatment. (Includes case study of 13 year old boy.) Nursing Times, 73, 8 Sep 1977, 1388-1392.

8 Blair, C. Hyperactivity in children: viewed within the framework of synergistic man. (Man seen as a whole.) Nursing Forum, 18 (3), 1979, 293-303.

9 Clark, D.A. and Long, K.A. Nurses as health educators with emotionally disturbed children. (Programme at University of Maryland Hospital.) Perspectives in Psychiatric Care, 17 (4), Jul/Aug 1979, 167-173.

10 Colley, M. Another kind of handicap. (Problems of maladjusted children.) New Society, 35, 12 Feb 1976, 327-328.

11 Connell, H.M. Essentials of child psychiatry. Oxford: Blackwell Scientific, 1979.

12 Cormier, P.P. Identification of typologies derived from child behaviors in the hospital as predictors of psychological upset. (Research study.) Journal of Psychiatric Nursing, 17 (6), Jun 1979, 28-35.

13 Cottingham, B. Nursing care study. Stuart—a child with behaviour problems. Nursing Mirror, 144, 20 Jan 1977, 49-52.

14 Dawson-Butterworth, K. Head banging in young children. Practitioner, 222, May 1979, 676-677, 679.

15 Edgcumbe, R. Development of aggressiveness in children. Nursing Times, 72 (13), 1 Apr 1976, Rcn Supplement, vii, ix-x, xii, xv.

16 Fergus, F.M. and Buchanan, K. The use of activity groups as an integral part of OT in child psychiatry. British Journal of Occupational Therapy, 40 (4), Apr 1977, 82-83.

17 Field, M. and Bhoyrub, P. A limit to a child's aggression. (Limit setting, a method of treatment of children with conduct disorders.) Nursing Mirror, 149, 6 Dec 1979, 36-37.

18 Field, M. and Bhoyrub, P. When illness is a refuge. (Treatment of children whose physical illness may point to psychological disorder.) Nursing Mirror, 149, 15 Nov 1979, 34-35.

19 Furneaux, B. and Roberts, B. compilers Autistic children: teaching, community and research approaches. Routledge and Kegan Paul, 1977. (Special needs in education series.)

20 Gilliam, J.E. and others The status of nurses' knowledge and beliefs about autism. (Research study.) International Journal of Nursing Studies, 17 (3), 1980, 189-195.

21 Gordon, N. Hyperkinesis: the overactive child makes the whole family suffer. Nursing Mirror, 147, 12 Oct 1978, 35-36.

22 Graham, P. Causes of aggressive behaviour. (In children.) Nursing Times, 75, 4 Oct 1979, 1703-1704.

23 Green, D.E. Aspects of infantile autism. New Zealand Nursing Journal, 72 (1), Jan 1979, 18-22.

24 Greenfield, M. Child psychiatric day centres. (At the Children's Hospital, Sunderland AHA.) Nursing Times, 76, 12 Jun 1980, 1064-1065.

25 Gross, D. Helping children deal with loss in a psychiatric setting. Journal of Psychiatric Nursing, 17 (1), Jan 1979, 17-20.

26 Hamilton, W.B. Disturbed children. Children at odds with the world. Nursing Mirror, 147, 19 Oct 1978, 32-36.

27 Hamilton, W.B. Role of the nurse in child psychiatry. Nursing Mirror, 144, 26 May 1977, 29-32.

28 Hamilton, W.B. 'The whining schoolboy . . . creeping like a snail unwillingly to school'. (School phobia.) Nursing Mirror, 146, 25 May 1978, 12-17.

29 Harris, M. Understanding the autistic child. American Journal of Nursing, 78 (10), Oct 1978, 1682-1685.

30 Hegadoren, K. 'Problem children' aren't problems any more. (Role of nurse as paediatric psychiatric nursing coordinator with children in general children's ward needing psychiatric help.) Canadian Nurse, 75 (1), Jan 1979, 31-33.

31 Herbert, M. and Iwaniec, D. Children who are hard to love. (Problems of hyperactive children.) New Society, 40, 21 Apr 1977, 111-112.

32 Hersov, L.A. Emotional disorders in childhood. Anxiety states, depression, obsessional disorders, hysterical 'conversion' reactions and hypochondriasis. Nursing Times, 73, 9 Jun 1977, 864-866.

33 Higgins, B. Building play skills. (Work with two children in child psychiatry unit.) Nursing Times, 76, 24 Jul 1980, 1317-1318.

34 Holland, C.J. and others The student nurse as therapeutic consultant. (Research study of Directive Parental Counselling by student nurses with families having a child with behaviour problems.) International Journal of Nursing Studies, 15 (3), 1978, 153-157.

35 Horne, A.M. Autism and the psychiatric nurse. Canadian Journal of Psychiatric Nursing, 15 (3), May/Jun 1974, 6-7, 16.

36 Howlin, P. Autistic children. (Problems faced by autistic children and their parents.) Health and Social Service Journal, 88, 24 Feb 1978, 228.

37 Hutchens, C. Subtracting additives. (Diet modification in care of severely handicapped child.) (Hyperkinetic children and the Feingold diet, 15-16.) Journal of Practical Nursing, 29 (7), Jul 1979, 13-14, 38.

38 Hutchings, J. Community nursing and psychology. 11. A resource for nurses. 13. Learning the wrong lesson. 15. As easy as ABC? (Behaviour disorders in children.) Journal of Community Nursing, 3 (2), Aug 1979, 26-27; (5), Nov 1979, 28, 30; (9), Mar 1980, 26, 29.

39 HYPERACTIVE Children's Support Group. (Details of aims and activities.) Health Visitor, 53 (1), Jan 1980, 10, 12.

40 Jones, L. Paediatric psychiatry. 9. The role of the hospital nurse in the therapeutic team. Nursing Mirror, 143, 8 Jul 1976, 66-67.

41 Knight, L. No labels at Larchwood. (Residential psychiatric unit for children in the grounds of St. Francis Hospital, Haywards Heath.) Mind Out, 37, Nov/Dec 1979, 14-15.

42 Lancet Integrating child psychiatry. (Comments on the recommendations of the Court Committee for psychiatric services.) Lancet, 1, 9 Apr 1977, 789-790.

43 Lancet What is childhood autism? Lancet, 2, 2 Oct 1976, 723-724.

44 Lask, B. Emotional and behaviour problems in childhood. Midwife, Health Visitor and Community Nurse.
1. Enuresis and faecal soiling. 13 (11), Nov 1977, 363-365.
2. Sleep and feeding disorders. 13 (12), Dec 1977, 384, 387, 389.
3. The management of temper tantrums and problems of speech as well as the most common phobias. 14 (2), Feb 1978, 44-46.

45 Liebermann, S. With rigour. (Report on opening of new special secure unit at Aycliff School, County Durham, for disturbed children.) Health and Social Service Journal, 88, 6 Oct 1978, 1130.

46 Meyer, A. 'This stranger, our son'. (Behaviour disorder in 11-year-old boy.) Nursing Times, 74, 30 Nov 1978, 1975-1977.

47 Miller, S.R. Children's fears: a review of the literature with implications for nursing research and practice. Nursing Research, 28 (4), Jul/Aug 1979, 217-223.

48 Pinkerton, P. Paediatric psychiatry. Nursing Mirror, 142.
4. Stress outside the family structure. 12 Feb 1976, 52-54.
5. Childhood neurosis reconsidered. 11 Mar 1976, 58-61.
6. Childhood psychosis reconsidered. 15 Apr 1976, 52-54.
7. Conduct disorder reconsidered. 13 May 1976, 63-65.
8. Emerging outlines for paediatric nursing. 10 Jun 1976, 60-61.

49 Quinn, D. The conduct-disordered child—a psychiatric nursing approach. Nursing Times, 73, 24 Mar 1977, 426-427.

50 Ross, T. Searching for the X-factor in the child under stress. (Report of international conference.) Nursing Mirror, 147, 30 Nov 1978, 21-23.

51 Rouslin, S. Developmental aggression and its consequences. Perspectives in Psychiatric Care, 8 (4), Oct/Dec 1975, 170-175.

52 Stewart, B. Finding feelings behind the words. (Case study of counselling a family over child's stealing and threatening behaviour.) Nursing Mirror, 151, 18 Sep 1980, 43-51.

53 Tomalin, C. Forging the missing link in care of disturbed children. (Day hospital giving intensive therapy to children attached to the Westminster Hospital.) Health and Social Service Journal, 86, 21 Jan 1977, 112-113.

54 Tuckwell, P. Autistic children swim with the tide of normal school. (Unit in an ordinary junior school which aims to cope with special

needs.) Health and Social Service Journal, 86, 3 Dec 1976, 2152-2153.

55 Walshe-Brennan, K.S. Role of the nurse in child guidance. Nursing Mirror, 144, 27 Jan 1977, 66-67.

56 Weir, K. The state of psychiatry. 3. Is child psychiatry growing up? Mind Out, 37, Nov/Dec 1979, 12-13.

57 Wong, S.C. Child psychiatric care. Nursing Times, 73, 16 Jun 1977, 918-919.

e ADOLESCENT PSYCHIATRY

1 Community Outlook Teenagers today. (Physical health, home life and need for sex education.) Nursing Times, 75, 10 May 1979 Community Outlook, 132, 135-136.

2 Corry, L. Youth counselling in a health authority. (Contraception advice and counselling for emotional problems.) Public Health, 93 (1), Jan 1979, 39-41.

3 Crabbe, P. Adolescents in present day society. (Work of Brook Advisory Centres.) Midwife, Health Visitor and Community Nurse, 14 (8), Aug 1978, 253-254.

4 Davis, J. School phobia in adolescence. (Reasons for and treatment given in the Adolescent Unit, Bethlem Royal Hospital.) Nursing Mirror, 144 (77), 28 Apr 1977, 61.

5 Duffey, M. Factors contributing to the development of a cohesive adolescent psychotherapy group. Journal of Psychiatric Nursing, 17 (1), Jan 1979, 21-24.

6 Hanlon, S. Social skills: training with disturbed adolescents. (Unit at Hollymoor Hospital.) British Journal of Occupational Therapy, 40 (11), Nov 1977, 271-272.

7 Henry, W.D. Psychiatric problems of late adolescence. Nursing Mirror, 142, 22 Apr 1976, 57-60.

8 Herry, S.M.J. Nursing care study. A diagnostic dilemma. (A severely emotionally disturbed adolescent at High Trees Adolescent Unit, Foxhall Hospital, Ipswich.) Nursing Mirror, 144, 6 Jan 1977, 43-45.

9 Lambert, L. Measuring the gap in teenagers' knowledge of sex and parenthood. (Survey of 16-year-olds in the third follow up of the National Child Development Study in 1974.) Health and Social Service Journal, 87, 15 Apr 1977, 668-669.

10 Lobet, P. Community care of disturbed adolescents. (Community psychiatric nurse working with out-patient adolescents and their families.) Nursing, 15, Jul 1980, 642-643.

11 Meyer, A. School phobia. Care in the community. (Case study of 15-year-old boy.) Nursing Times, 73, 8 Sep 1977, 1393-1394.

12 O'Hagan, M. Simmons House: an adolescent unit. (At St. Luke's, Woodside Hospital, London.) Nursing Focus, 1 (8), Apr 1980, 314, 316-317.

13 Sands, D. Nursing care study. Acute psychotic disturbance and regression in an adolescent girl. Nursing Times, 74, 14 Dec 1978, 2055.

14 Seymour, R.M. An experimental group for parents of adolescents. Midwife, Health Visitor and Community Nurse, 12 (3), Mar 1976, 88-90.

15 Spicer, F. Aggression in the home. (Psychology of adolescence.) Nursing Mirror, 145, 15 Dec 1977, 45-46.

16 World Health Issue on adolescence. World Health, Dec 1976, 3-29.

17 World Health Organization. Expert Committee Health needs of adolescents. Geneva: WHO, 1977. (Technical report series no.609.)

f MOTHER CHILD BONDING

1 Allan, J.A.B. The identification and treatment of 'difficult' babies. Early signs of disruption in parent-infant attachment bonds. (Role of community nurse in preventing problems.) Canadian Nurse, 72 (12), Dec 1976, 11-16.

2 Avant, K. Nursing diagnosis: maternal attachment. (Research study to validate model of maternal attachment for use in nursing diagnosis.) Advances in Nursing Science, 2 (1), Oct 1979, 45-55.

3 Bardon, D. A mother and baby unit in a psychiatric hospital. (Their history, description of unit at Shenley Hospital, and recent research on mother/child bonding.) Nursing Mirror, 145, 8 Dec 1977, 30-33.

4 Barnard, K.E. and Neal, M.V. Maternal-child nursing research: review of the past and strategies for the future. Nursing Research, 26 (3), May/Jun 1977, 193-200.

5 Barrie, H. Personal opinion: of human bondage. (The dangers of over-emphasizing mother-child bonding.) Midwife, Health Visitor and Community Nurse, 12 (6), Jun 1976, 182-186.

6 Bowlby, J. Attachment and loss. Volume 3: loss sadness and depression. Hogarth Press; Institute of Psychoanalysis, 1980. (International psycho-analytical library; 109.)

7 Bowlby, J. The making and breaking of affectional bonds. Tavistock, 1979.

8 British Medical Journal Helping mothers to love their babies. (Review of studies on mother/child bonding and suggested changes in maternity unit practice.) British Medical Journal, 2, 3 Sep 1977, 595-596.

9 Britton, G.R. Early mother-infant and infant temperature stabilization. (The results indicate that separating normal newborns from their mothers for the purpose of stabilising temperature may not be necessary.) Journal of Obstetric, Gynecologic and Neonatal Nursing, 9 (2), Mar/Apr 1980, 84-86.

10 Cannon, R.B. The development of maternal touch during early mother-infant interaction. Journal of Obstetric, Gynecologic and Neonatal Nursing, 6 (2), Mar/Apr 1977, 28-33.

11 Crow, R. Sensory deprivation. 1. In children. (Development of attachment and effects of maternal deprivation.) Nursing Times, 75, 8 Feb 1979, 229-233.

12 Dunbar, J. First encounters of mothers

with their infants. Maternal-Child Nursing Journal, 5 (1), Spring 1976, 1-4.

13 Funke-Furber, J. and Roemer, C. Failure to thrive. (With chart to assess mother/infant interaction.) Canadian Nurse, 74 (11), Dec 1978, 30-34.

14 Goodwin, A. Snap-happy parents. (Providing photograph of baby in special care unit for separated mother. Letter.) British Medical Journal, 1, 25 Mar 1978, 787.

15 Graham, H. and McKee, L. The first months of motherhood: summary report of a survey of women's experiences of pregnancy, childbirth, and the first six months after birth. Health Education Council, 1980. (Health Education Council's monograph series; 3.)

16 Harris, J. When babies cry. (Research study into mothers' feelings, actions and responce to their babies' cries one month after delivery.) Canadian Nurse, 75(2), Feb 1979, 32-34.

17 Harrison, L. A jaundiced view. (Problems of a mother with a newborn baby in a special care unit.) Nursing Times, 72, 22 Jul 1976, 1110-1111.

18 Herbert, P. Getting to know baby straight away. (Advantage of 'rooming-in' where newborn baby stays with mother in maternity ward rather than being placed in central nursery.) Nursing Mirror, 149, 13 Dec 1979, 32-33.

19 Hill, S.T. and Shronk, L.K. The effect of early parent-infant contact on newborn body temperature. (Research study.) Journal of Obstetric, Gynecologic and Neonatal Nursing, 8 (5), Sep/Oct 1979, 287-290.

20 Jolly, H. The importance of 'bonding' for newborn baby, mother...and father. Nursing Mirror, 147, 31 Aug 1978, 19-21.

21 Law, M.M. Mother-baby-nurse relationship. (Project undertaken while on SCBU course.) Midwives Chronicle, 91, Jun 1978, 148-151; Jul 1978, 182-188.

22 Ludington-Hoe, S.M. Postpartum: development of maternicity. The motherhood role can be divided into two components; emotional factors (maternicity) and physical caretaking (mothering). American Journal of Nursing, 77 (7), Jul 1977, 1171-1174.

23 Mercer, R.T. Postpartum: illness and acquaintance-attachment process. (Effect of delay in mother-infant interaction.) American Journal of Nursing, 77 (7), Jul 1977, 1174-1178.

24 Mercer, R.T. Teenage motherhood: the first year. 1. The teenage mother's views and responses. 2. How the infants fared. Journal of Obstetric, Gynecologic and Neonatal Nursing, 9 (1), Jan/Feb 1980, 16-27.

25 Murphy, N.J. Helping a family and their premature baby grow together. (Nurse's role in neonatal unit in fostering mother-child bonding.) Canadian Nurse, 93 (9), Sep 1977, 42-45.

26 Peddie, B. The nurse's role in the promotion of mental health in obstetrics. (Importance of bonding.) New Zealand Nursing Journal, 71 (2), Feb 1978, 14-16.

27 Rees, B.L. Measuring identification with the mothering role. Research in Nursing and Health, 3 (2), Jun 1980, 49-56.

28 Reynolds, D. Mum's the word for babies in hospital. (Encouragement of close contact between mothers and babies in the special care baby unit at Wycombe General Hospital, Buckinghamshire.) Nursing Mirror, 148, 29 Mar 1979, 20-22.

29 Riesch, S. Enhancement of mother-infant social interaction. (Interviews with mothers to determine their perceptions of the social behavioural potential of their babies.) Journal of Obstetric, Gynecologic and Neonatal Nursing, 8 (4), Jul/Aug 1979, 242-246.

30 Rubin, R. Binding-in in the postpartum period. (Process of relationship-forming between mother and child.) Maternal Child Nursing Journal, 6 (2), Summer 1977, 67-75.

31 Rubin, R. Maternal tasks in pregnancy. (Ensuring the safety and acceptance of the unborn child and developing the maternal role and relationship.) Journal of Advanced Nursing, 1 (5), Sep 1976, 367-376.

32 Schaffer, H.R. editor Studies in mother-infant interaction: proceedings of the Loch Lomond symposium, University of Strathclyde, September 1975. Academic Press, 1977.

33 Sills, J.A. and Handley, J.L. Snap-happy parents. (Scheme at Bangour General Hospital of taking photos of babies in special care nursery for mothers to encourage bonding. Letter.) British Medical Journal, 1, 11 Feb 1978, 368.

34 SPOTLIGHT on children 'I didn't know what 'SBCU' was...'. (Study by two JBCNS course students of communication between parents and staff and SCBU staff and postnatal staff, with reference to the promotion of bonding.) Nursing Times, 76, 18 Sep 1980 ABPN 5-APBN 7.

35 Stern, D. The first relationship: infant and mother. Open Books, 1977. (The developing child series.)

36 Swanson, J. Nursing intervention to facilitate maternal-infant attachment. Journal of Obstetric, Gynecologic and Neonatal Nursing, 7 (2), Mar/Apr 1978, 35-38.

37 Toase, M. Bonding. (Bibliography of items in RCM library.) Midwives Chronicle, 93, Aug 1980, 282.

38 Valman, H.B. The first year of life. Mother-infant bonding. British Medical Journal, 280, 2 Feb 1980, 308-310.

39 Weir, K. New ideas in early development. (Including the newborn's development of the concept of bonding and attachment, with temperamental characteristics.) Health Visitor, 53 (2), Feb 1980, 38-39.

40 Yu Chao, Y-M. Cognitive operations during maternal role enactment. (Research study into how eleven mothers formed concepts about the baby and themselves as mothers.) Maternal-Child Nursing Journal, 8 (4), Winter 1979, 211-274.

g PARENTHOOD AND FATHER'S ROLE

1 Adams, M.E. Providing a service. (Parentcraft teaching.) Nursing Mirror, 145, 29 Sep 1977, xii-xiii.

2 Ashton, R.M. The parentcraft teacher. (Advice on planning a course and teaching methods.) Nursing Mirror, 145, 29 Sep 1977, xv.

3 Ashton, R.M. and Crowe, V.J. Development of programmes to prepare the midwife for education of parents for childbirth and parenthood. Midwives Chronicle, 92, Aug 1979, 248-250.

4 Barlow, U. Personally speaking: maternal deprivation. (Comment on how research can be used in teaching and as a mother.) Midwife, Health Visitor and Community Nurse, 16 (1), Jan 1980, 9, 11.

5 Bassett, W.J. and Bain, D.J.G. The use of multiple choice questionnaire in measuring maternal child health knowledge. (A sample of mothers at developmental screening clinics at Craighill Health Centre, Livingston.) Health Bulletin, 34 (6), Nov 1976, 335-343.

6 Birch, K. and Chambers, M. Preparation for parenthood. (Small-scale pilot study in Calderdale AHA by HV and health education officer.) Health Visitor, 52 (12), Dec 1979, 507, 510.

7 Bishop, B. A guide to assessing parenting capabilities. (By a clinical specialist.) American Journal of Nursing, 76 (11), Nov 1976, 1784-1787.

8 Boswell, J. Are classes 4 and 5 paying attention? (Research study into social characteristics of primipara and their attendance and non-attendance at parentcraft classes.) Nursing Mirror, 148, 22 Mar 1979, 24-25.

9 Brown, H. Fathers and childbirth: changing attitudes and expectations. Midwife, Health Visitor and Community Nurse, 15 (10), Oct 1979, 398, 400.

10 Brown, I. Attitudes of men towards labour and delivery. (Survey of twenty-one men.) Midwife, Health Visitor and Community Nurse, 16 (7), Jul 1980, 278, 280-281.

11 Clulow, C. Love's labour and loss. (Preparation for parenthood and the stress and loss experienced by new parents.) Health Visitor, 52 (3), Mar 1979, 74-76.

12 Cogan, R. and Edmunds, E.P. Pronominalization: a linguistic facet of the maternal-parental sensitive period. (Use of neuter pronoun by parents to describe newborn infant.) Nursing Research, 29 (4), Jul/Aug 1980, 225-227.

13 Cronenwett, L.R. Elements and outcomes of a postpartum support group program. (Result of questionnaire.) Research in Nursing Health, 3 (1), Mar 1980, 33-41.

14 Danyiger, K. Not today, thank you. (Role of women as mothers and the problems this presents.) Nursing Times, 74, 2 Nov 1978, 1788-1789.

15 Donnelly, G.F. and Conroy, N. Parent-neonate communication in the care-giving system. Topics in Clinical Nursing, 1 (3), Oct 1979, 1-9.

16 Elfert, H. Helping preschool children learn to be safe. (Role of nurse with families.) Canadian Nurse, 75 (11), Dec 1979, 26-29.

17 Fiddes, S.A. ...faith as a grain of mustard seed...' (Progress of parentcraft classes at Frank Swire Health Centre, Halifax.) Midwives Chronicle, 93, Apr 1980, 121-123.

18 Fiddes, S.A. Not for the want of trying: some reflections on parentcraft teaching. (Changes in services following surveys of deliveries which showed low level of response to parentcraft teaching.) Midwives Chronicle, 90, Sep 1977, 214-215.

19 Field, C. A venture into in-service training for health visitors. (On preparation for parenthood, by Milton Keynes College of Education.) Nursing Times, 75, 11 Oct 1979, 1771-1772.

20 Freeman, K. A postpartum program that really works. (In-hospital classes, telephone check, new infant classes and home visit.) Canadian Nurse, 76 (3), Mar 1980, 40-42.

21 Friend-Nash, W. and Phillips, L. A venture in community care. A social group work scheme operating at local health centres, involved with young mothers suffering from depression. (By two social workers.) Health Visitor, 51 (7), Jul 1978, 248-251.

22 Gath, A. Emotional needs in a new family. (The importance of screening for problem parents during antenatal care.) Nursing Mirror, 144, 6 Jan 1977, 52-54.

23 Gillies, E. The mothers' club. 1. (HV describes setting-up and success of post-natal support group.) Nursing Times, 76, 10 Apr 1980 Community Outlook, 99-100.

24 Gordon, V.C. Teaching concepts of good parenting. International Nursing Review, 26 (5), Sep/Oct 1979, 137-138.

25 Guerden, J.H.M. Parentcraft education in Holland, Germany and Finland. Nursing Mirror, 142, 12 Feb 1976, 63-64.

26 Haggerty, L. and Kidzma, E.C. Expectant parents' classes: an alternative environment for learning health maintenance. Journal of Nursing Education, 29 (2), Feb 1980, 13-19.

27 Harris, B.G. Learning about parenting. (Course for nursing and other university students.) Nursing Outlook, 25 (7), Jul 1977, 457-459.

28 Hennessy, D. and others With a little help from my friends. (Experimental group counselling scheme in Hampshire for mothers of pre-school children run by three health visitors.) Nursing Times, 74, 13 Apr 1978 Community Outlook, 103-106.

29 Hill, P. The mothers' club. 2. (How mother's club on council housing estate did not succeed.) Nursing Times, 76, 10 Apr 1980 Community Outlook, 100, 102.

30 Hiskins, G. Group help for young mothers. (Self-help groups to provide support.) Midwife, Health Visitor and Community Nurse, 14 (7), Jul 1978, 216, 218, 219.

31 Hiskins, G. How mothers help themselves: a study of post-natal support groups 1978-1979. The author, 1980.

32 Hospitals Parents help children learn and play in public health clinics and hospital-based school. (Parents as Resources (PAR) Scheme to help parents become aware of their role in their child's early years.) Hospitals, 53 (5), 1 Mar 1979, 14-15.

33 Hott, J.R. The crisis of expectant fatherhood. American Journal of Nursing, 76 (9), Sep 1976, 1436-1440.

34 Hutchings, J. Community nursing and psychology. 14. Good morning! (Ways in which parents can change children's behaviour.) Journal of Community Nursing, 3 (7), Jan 1980, 12, 25.

35 Hutchins, P. The father's role. (In child care and need for parentcraft education.) Nursing Mirror, 145, 29 Sep 1977, v-vi, xi.

36 Hutchins, P. New fathers. (Care by health professionals.) Midwife, Health Visitor and Community Nurse, 15 (1), Jan 1979, 10-11.

37 Johnston, M. and others Putting more PEP in parenting. (Using experienced mothers as teachers on post-natal wards.) American Journal of Nursing, 77 (6), Jun 1977, 994-995.

38 Jones, L.D. Starting a mother and toddler group. (Description of club in Swansea started by health visitor.) Health Visitor, 52 (10), Oct 1979, 419, 421.

39 Lambert, L. and Hart, S. Who needs a father? (National Child Development Study assessing the father's part in bringing up children carried out by a questionnaire to mothers.) New Society, 37, 8 Jul 1976, 80.

40 Leonard, L. The father's side. (Study of the reactions of 20 fathers to labour, delivery and nursing care.) Canadian Nurse, 73 (2), Feb 1977, 16-20.

41 Linde, B.S. and Engelhardt, K.F. What do parents know about infant development? (Research study.) Pediatric Nursing, 5 (1), Jan/Feb 1979, 32-36.

42 Linney, J. The emotional and social aspects of having twins. (By HV who is mother of twins.) Nursing Times, 76, 14 Feb 1980, 276-279.

43 Lipkin, G.B. Parent-child nursing: psychosocial aspects. 2nd ed. St. Louis: Mosby, 1978.

44 McKee, L. Fathers and childbirth: 'just hold my hand'. (Research study of fathers' intentions, expectations and knowledge concerning labour and delivery.) Health Visitor, 53 (9), Sep 1980, 368, 371-372.

45 MacLaughlin, S. First-time fathers' childbirth experience. Journal of Nurse-Midwifery, 25 (3), May/Jun 1980, 17-21.

46 Meleis, A.I. and Swendsen, L.A. Role supplementation: an empirical test of a nursing intervention. (Use of the reference group, role modelling and role rehearsal with families facing the birth of their first child.) Nursing Research, 27 (1), Jan/Feb 1978, 11-18.

47 Midwives Chronicle Husband at the delivery. (Selection of readers' letters.) Midwives Chronicle, 91, Jan 1978, 9-11.

48 Murphy, N. Training professionals to support and increase the competence of young parents. (Programme with first year paediatric nursing students.) Journal of Nursing Education, 17 (7), Sep 1978, 41-49.

49 Nash, W.F. and Phillips, L. A venture in community care. (Group for depressed young mothers run by social workers.) Midwife, Health Visitor and Community Nurse, 15 (1), Jan 1979, 12-13.

50 National Childbirth Trust Pregnancy and parenthood, edited by Anne Loader. Oxford: Oxford University Press, 1980.

51 National Children's Bureau Preparation for parenthood: some current initiatives and thinking. The Bureau, 1980.

52 Nursing Clinics of North America Symposium of parenting. (Includes the psychology of and education for parenthood.) Nursing Clinics of North America, 12 (3), Sep 1977, 447-533.

53 Nursing Mirror A supplement on parentcraft. Nursing Mirror, 145, 29 Sep 1977, i, iii, v-vi, xi-xiii, xv.

54 Orbzut, L.A.J. Expectant fathers' perception of fathering. (Interviews with 20 fathers.) American Journal of Nursing, 76 (9), Sep 1976, 1440-1442.

55 Palermo, E. Remarriage: parental perceptions of steprelations with children and adolescents. Journal of Psychiatric Nursing and Mental Health Services, 18 (4), Apr 1980, 9-13.

56 Perkins, E.R. Education for childbirth and parenthood. Croom Helm, 1980.

57 Pinkerton, P. Paediatric psychiatry. 3. The pathology of parent/child interaction. Nursing Mirror, 142, 15 Jan 1976, 56-58.

58 Pitcairn, L. Parents of the future. (Work of National Association for Maternal and Child Welfare Education Department.) Midwife, Health Visitor and Community Nurse, 14 (11), Nov 1978, 386, 388.

59 Smith, D. and Smith, H.L. Towards improvements in parenting: a description of prenatal and postpartum classes with teaching guide. Journal of Obstetric, Gynecologic and Neonatal Nursing, 7 (6), Nov/Dec 1978, 22-27.

60 Stranik, M.K. and Hogberg, B.L.L. Transition into parenthood. (Support group for new parents at University of Minnesota Hospital.) American Journal of Nursing, 79 (1), Jan 1979, 90-93.

61 Sweeny, S.L. and Davis, F.B. Transition to parenthood: a group experience. (Group for husbands and wives before and after birth of their child, led by psychiatrist and psychiatric nurse.) Maternal-Child Nursing Journal, 8 (1), Spring 1979, 59-64.

62 Tankson, E.A. The adolescent parent: one approach to teaching child care and giving support. (Project of maternal-child health care, education and day-care facilities in Minnesota.) Journal of Obstetric, Gynecologic and Neonatal Nursing, 5 (3), May/Jun 1976, 9-15.

63 Thistleton, A.S. The abusive and neglectful parent: treatment through parent education. Nursing Clinics of North America, 12 (3), Sep 1977, 513-524.

64 Toase, M. Father's role. (Bibliography of items in RCM Library.) Midwives Chronicle, 93, Mar 1980, 79.

65 Wheeler, L.A. A concept of maternity care. (Family centred care emphasising continuity of care and the family's role in decision making.) Journal of Obstetric,

Gynecologic and Neonatal Nursing, 5 (1), Jan/Feb 1976, 15-17.

66 Whitehouse, J. Mothers go to college. (A description of mothercraft classes run by the Social Services Department at Warwickshire.) Social Work Service, 5, Dec 1974, 23-26.

67 Young, C. The need for parentcraft. (Education.) Nursing Mirror, 145, 29 Sep 1977, i, iii.

45 INFANTS AND NEWBORN

a GENERAL AND NURSING

1 Aikens, R.M. Hats and lamps in the prevention of neonatal hypothermia. Nursing Mirror, 144, 21 Apr 1977, 65-66.

2 Alberman, E. Better perinatal health. Prospects for better perinatal health. (Concluding article.) Lancet, 1, 26 Jan 1980, 189-192.

3 Bacon, C. and others Heatstroke in well-wrapped infants. Lancet, 1, 24 Feb 1979, 422-425.

4 Baird, S.F. and Dzik, R.S. Nursing roles. Emotional crisis and maternal-child nursing. (Two articles on crisis intervention.) Journal of Obstetric, Gynecologic and Neonatal Nursing, 5 (1), Jan/Feb 1976, 30-39.

5 Binzley, V. State: overlooked factor in newborn nursing. (Level of arousal or consciousness.) American Journal of Nursing, 77 (1), Jan 1977, 102-103.

6 Boccuzzi, N.K. A systematic approach to neonatal nursing management. (Patient classification system to predict staffing needs in neonatal intensive care unit.) American Journal of Maternal-Child Nursing, 3 (6), Nov/Dec 1978, 333-335, 381.

7 Chamberlain, G. Better perinatal health. Background to perinatal health. Lancet, 2, 17 Nov 1979, 1061-1063.

8 Duxbury, M.L. and Thiessen, V. Staff nurse turnover in neonatal intensive care units. (Survey in U.S.A.) Journal of Advanced Nursing, 4 (6), Nov 1979, 591-602.

9 Ebrahim, G.J. Care of the newborn in developing countries. Macmillan, 1979. (Macmillan tropical community health manuals.)

10 Erickson, M.P. Trends in assessng the newborn and his parents. American Journal of Maternal-Child Nursing, 3 (2), Mar/Apr 1978, 99-103.

11 Fardig, J.A. A comparison of skin-to-skin contact and radiant heaters in promoting neonatal thermoregulation. (Research study.) Journal of Nurse-Midwifery, 25 (1), Jan/Feb 1980, 19-28.

12 Friedemann, M.L. and Emrich, K.A. Emergence of infant sleep-wake patterns in the first three months after birth. International Journal of Nursing Studies, 15 (1), 1978, 5-16.

13 Gardner, S. The mother as incubator—after delivery. Decreases in body temperature of 10 nude babies who were held next to their mothers' bodies were compared with the decreases in temperatures of 9 babies who were kept in heated beds. Journal of Obstetric, Gynecologic and Neonatal Nursing, 8 (3), May/Jun 1979, 174-176.

14 Hiley, R. and others Communication in a neonatal unit. (Research study by JBCNS students to examine parent/staff, parent/baby and staff/staff communication.) Nursing Times, 74, 26 Oct 1978, 1771-1772.

15 Hill, A. Neonatal care. Good teamwork: a key to saving the ill newborn baby. (Current approaches to neonatal care and importance of clinical team.) Nursing Mirror, 147, 7 Dec 1978, 44-46.

16 Iles, J.P. and McCrary, M. Cuddle bathing can be fun. (Research into infant bathing routines leading to a new procedure called the 'Cuddle bath'.) Canadian Nurse, 73 (5), May 1977, 24-27.

17 Johnson, M. and Gash, J. Transport of neonates a matter of prevention. (Nursing care before and during journey.) Canadian Nurse, 72 (5), May 1976, 19.

18 Keay, A.J. and Morgan, D.M. Craig's care of the newly born infant. 6th ed. Churchill Livingstone, 1978.

19 Konefal, M.M. Continuing education pays off in the care of high risk infants. Journal of Continuing Education in Nursing, 8 (2), Mar-Apr 1977, 22-25.

20 Lancet The newborn in hospital. (Review of studies recommending improvements in services.) Lancet, 1, 20 May 1978, 1081.

21 Laryea, M.G.G. The midwives' role in the post-natal care of primiparae and their infants in the first 28 days following childbirth. MPhil thesis, CNAA (Newcastle upon Tyne Polytechnic, Department of Health Studies), 1980.

22 Marcil, V. Physical assessment of the newborn. (Detailed guide.) Canadian Nurse, 72 (3), Mar 1976, 21-24.

23 Milliken, D. Changing patterns in staffing of neonatal units. Australian Nurses Journal, 7 (1), Jul 1977, 33-34.

24 Normand, I.C.S. Dilemmas in neonatal care. (Based on lecture.) Midwives Chronicle, 91, Oct 1978, 285-288.

25 Nursing Clinics of North America Symposium on neonatal care. Nursing Clinics of North America, 13 (1), Mar 1978, 1-84.

26 Nursing Mirror The neonate. (Supplement of three articles with historical survey.) Nursing Mirror, 148, 11 Jan 1979 Supplement, i-ii, iv, vi-vii, x-xii, xiv-xv.

27 O'Doherty, N. Characteristics of the normal infant at term. Midwives Chronicle, 90, Jun 1977, 110-123.

28 Ostrea, E.M. and Schuman, H. The role of the pediatric nurse practitioner in a neonatal unit. (Reprinted from Journal of Pediatrics, 86 (4), Apr 1975, 628-631.) Nursing Digest, 4 (2), Mar/Apr 1976, 8-9.

29 Pillitteri, A. Nursing care of the growing family: a maternal-newborn text. Boston: Little, Brown and Co., 1976.

30 Porth, C.M. and Kaylor, L.E. Temperature regulation in the newborn. American Journal of Nursing, 78 (10), Oct 1978, 1691-1693.

31 Pugh, R.E. Perinatal care. Major hazards ahead—unless... (Neonatal care and problems still facing doctors.) Nursing Mirror, 147, 26 Oct 1978, 18-22.

32 Purdy, C.J. and others Retrospective audit of the pediatric nurse practitioner in the normal newborn nursery. Pediatric Nursing, 5 (6), Nov/Dec 1979, 55-57.

33 Rhodes, H. Health visiting study. A first baby. (Based on the nursing process.) Nursing Mirror, 147, 19 Oct 1978, 27-30.

34 Roberts, F.B. Perinatal nursing: care of newborns and their families. New York: McGraw-Hill, 1977.

35 Stevens, S. and Whitfield, M.F. How accurate is clinical test weighing of the newborn? Midwives Chronicle, 93, May 1980, 148-149.

36 Tyne, M.D. The nurse and nursery planning. Pediatric Nursing, 1 (3), May/Jun 1976, 14-17.

37 Valman, H.B. and others The first year of life. British Medical Association, 1980. (Articles published in the British Medical Journal.)

38 Valman, H.B. The first year of life. Routine examination of the newborn. British Medical Journal, 280, 12 Jan 1980, 91-94.

39 Vulliamy, D.G. The newborn child. 4th ed. Churchill Livingstone, 1977.

40 Whiteside, D. Proper use of radiant warmers. American Journal of Nursing, 78 (10), Oct 1978, 1694-1696.

41 WHO Chronicle Attempts to improve the prospects of survival of newborn infants. WHO Chronicle, 31 (2), Feb 1977, 66-71.

42 Wibberley, J. Voluntary work in Oxford's well baby clinics. Midwives Chronicle, 89, Feb 1976, 29.

b ABNORMALITIES AND AT RISK

1 Ashton, K. Detecting birth defects. Nursing Times, 72, 17 Jun 1976, 924-925.

2 Barrie, H. Resuscitation and the midwife. Midwives Chronicle, 89, Apr 1976, 78-79.

3 Bellman, M.H. National Childhood Encephalopathy Study—a progress report. Health Visitor, 51 (9), Sep 1978, 338.

4 Betts, G.A. A frame for the management of babies with Pierre Robin syndrome. (Mandibular hypoplasia.) Nursing Times, 73, 18 Aug 1977, 1295.

5 Boxall, J. Eye mask for phototherapy. (Advantages of an easily removable eye mask for the infant needing treatment for jaundice and psychological benefit to the mother.) Nursing Mirror, 142 (3), 15 Jan 1976, 65-66.

6 Brimacombe, J. Nursing care study. Congenital choanal atresia. (Obstruction to airway between nose and pharynx in newborn baby.) Nursing Mirror, 147, 30 Nov 1978, 43-46.

7 Campbell, A.G.M. and Duff, R.S. Deciding the care of severely malformed or dying infants. Journal of Medical Ethics, 5 (2), Jun 1979, 65-67.

8 **Carruthers, J.** Nursing care study. Lobectomy for congenital unilobar emphysema. (In six-week-old baby.) Nursing Times, 74, 19 Jan 1978, 94-97.

9 **Charles, M.B.** Nursing care study. Left herniotomy in a baby with multiple congenital abnormalities. Nursing Times, 73, 28 Apr 1977, 600-603.

10 **Clarke, K.** Resuscitation of the newborn and mother. Nursing Mirror, 142, 18 Mar 1976, 61-63.

11 **Community Outlook** Need it happen? (Report on Spastics Society campaign to reduce the number of handicapped children born.) Nursing Times, 74, 13 Jul 1978 Community Outlook, 189.

12 **Curnock, D.A.** The breath of life—resuscitation of the newborn. (Outline scheme.) Midwife, Health Visitor and Community Nurse, 13 (9), Sep 1977, 286-291.

13 **Farrell, H.M.** Crisis intervention following the birth of a handicapped infant. Journal of Psychiatric Nursing and Mental Health Services, 15 (3), Mar 1977, 32-36.

14 **Freeman, N.V.** Pyloric stenosis. (Congenital abnormality.) Nursing Times, 72, 7 Oct 1976, 1553-1555.

15 **Guy's Hospital Medical School. Prince Philip Research Laboratories Paediatric Research Unit** Research on birth defects. Spastics Society, 1976.

16 **Harbin, R.E.** Death, euthanasia and parental consent. (Infants with severe congenital defects.) Pediatric Nursing, 2 (4), Jul/Aug 1976, 26-28.

17 **Hill, P.E.** Southall abnormal births survey. (Survey by HVs in a district of Southall.) Health Visitor, 53 (2), Feb 1980, 47-48.

18 **Komrower, G.M. and others** The Manchester regional screening programme: a 10-year exercise in patient and family care. (Work of Willink Biochemical Genetics Unit at Royal Manchester Children's Hospital which screens and treats babies for metabolic abnormalities including phenylketonuria.) British Medical Journal, 2, 15 Sep 1979, 635-638.

19 **Lancaster, V.A.** Preparing the infant with a major surgical congenital abnormality for discharge home. Nursing Times, 76, 18 Sep 1980, ABPN 2-ABPN 5.

20 **Lancet** Non-treatment of defective newborn babies. (By a consultant paediatrician.) Lancet, 2, 24 Nov 1979, 1123-1124.

21 **Littlewood, J.M.** Neonatal screening: the present position. Midwives Chronicle, 90 (12), May 1977, 91-93.

22 **Lobo, E. and Marshall, W.C.** The problem of congenital cytomegalovirus infections. (Virus infection of mother affecting newborn baby.) Nursing Times, 75, 27 Sep 1979, 1666.

23 **McCarthy, J. and others** Congenital malformations. Nursing Mirror, 142 (26), 24 Jun 1976, Nursing care supplement, 6, i-iv.

24 **McDonagh, M.** Nursing care study.

Posterior urethral valves: a sick baby makes a fresh start. (Three-week old baby with congenital abnormality of the bladder and kidney damage and septicaemia due to infected right kidney. By Diploma in Nursing student.) Nursing Mirror, 150, 3 Jan 1980, 34-36.

25 **McElroy, C.** Caring for the untreated infant. (After the decision to withhold active treatment has been made.) Canadian Nurse, 71 (12), Dec 1975, 26-27, 30.

26 **Madeley, R.J. and Latham, A.** Management aspects of high risk strategies in child health. (Scheme in Nottingham involving follow up of high risk babies by HVs.) Community Medicine, 1 (1), Feb 1979, 36-39.

27 **Marshall, W.** Congenital cytomegalovirus infection. Nursing Mirror, 142, 3 Jun 1976, 49-50.

28 **Miller, D.L. and Ross, E.M.** National Childhood Encephalopathy Study: an interim report. British Medical Journal, 2, 7 Oct 1978, 992-993.

29 **Roberts, C.S.** Ethical issues in the treatment of neonates with severe anomalies. Nursing Forum, 18 (4), 1979, 352-365.

30 **Stern, H.** Cytomegalovirus infection. (A cause of congenital abnormality.) Nursing Times, 73, 10 Feb 1977, 190-192.

31 **Swinyard, C.A. editor** Decision making and the defective newborn: proceedings of a conference on spina bifida and ethics. Illinois: Thomas, 1978.

32 **Thieme, R.** Crisis: a baby is born with a defect. (Role of nurse in counselling family.) Nursing, 7 (11), Nov 1977, 45-47.

33 **Thompson, O.** Resuscitation of the depressed newborn. American Association of Nurse Anesthetists Journal, 44 (2), Apr 1976, 174-179.

34 **Tuck, F.** Nursing care study. Pierre Robin syndrome. Nursing Mirror, 143, 23 Sep 1976, 49-52.

35 **Valman, H.B.** The first year of life. Some congenital abnormalities. British Medical Journal, 280, 5 Jan 1980, 24-26.

36 **Waechter, E.H.** Bonding problems of infants with congenital anomalies. Nursing Forum, 16 (3, 4), 1977, 298-318.

37 **World Health Organization. Regional Office for Europe** Early detection of handicap in children: report on a WHO working group 15-18 May 1979. Copenhagen: WHO, 1980.

38 **Youmans, P.M.** Helping babies with developmental disabilities: the developmental pediatric nurse practitioner. Nursing (U.S.), 9 (11), Nov 1979, 13-15.

39 **Young, R.K.** Chronic sorrow: parents' response to the birth of a child with a defect. American Journal of Maternal Child Nursing, 2 (1), Jan/Feb 1977, 38-42.

c DISEASES AND DISORDERS

1 **Boylan, P.** Oxytocin and neonatal jaundice. (Study of the effects of induced labour.) British Medical Journal, 1976, 2, 4 Sep 1976, 564-565.

2 **Brown, R.** The blue baby. (Cyanosis in the newborn.) Nursing Times, 73, 13 Oct 1977, 1596-1597.

3 **Castellette, P.** A baby with oesophageal atresia. Nursing, 7, Nov 1979, 330-332, 335.

4 **Chalmers, I.** Neonatal jaundice—cause not known. Nursing Times, 72 (28), 15 Jul 1976, 1084-1086.

5 **Clark, H.** Nursing care study. Haemophilus influenzae meningitis. Nursing Times, 73, 20 Jan 1977, 89-91.

6 **Coles, H.M.T.** Croup. Nursing Times, 73, 20 Oct 1977, 1634-1635.

7 **Collins, J.E.** Cardiac responses during mechanical ventilation of neonates with respiratory distress syndrome. (Summary of paper read at research seminar in 1977.) Journal of Advanced Nursing, 3 (1), Jan 1978, 73-77.

8 **Crawford, A.M.** Nursing care study. A baby with enterogenous cyst. Nursing Times, 73, 7 Apr 1977, 486-490.

9 **Devlin, J.** Nursing care study. Hyaline membrane disease: born with a fighting chance. (Respiratory distress syndrome of the newborn, treated with artificial ventilation and parenteral nutrition.) Nursing Mirror, 148, 28 Jun 1979, 38-39.

10 **Dodge, J.A.** Infantile hypertrophic pyloric stenosis. Nursing Times, 73, 26 May 1977, 780-782.

11 **Drummond, G.** Nursing care study. Meconium aspiration. (Airway obstruction resulting from fetal distress caused by intra-uterine hypoxia.) Nursing Mirror, 147, 17 Aug 1978, 24-27.

12 **Ennis, S. and Harris, T.R.** Positioning infants with hyaline membrane disease. (Study with nine infants.) American Journal of Nursing, 78 (3), Mar 1978, 398-401.

13 **Fleming, P.J.** Neonatal respiratory distress. Practitioner, 224, Dec 1980, 1239, 1241-1244.

14 **Goad, D.M.** Superficial neonatal infection. (Trial of cord powder and detergent solution for bathing which both contained chlorhexidine.) Nursing Times, 75, 7 Jun 1979, 965-966.

15 **Graham, H. and Kenwright, M.** ABO haemolytic disease of the newborn. Nursing Mirror, 144, 31 Mar 1977, 48-50.

16 **Grover, M.** The tale of the tube. (A mother's account of her child's treatment for tracheal-oesophageal fistula.) Nursing Times, 73, 30 Jun 1977, 1008-1009.

17 **Hudson, M.J.** Fetal or maternal blood? (Techniques used in the prevention of haemolytic disease of the new born.) Midwives Chronicle, 90, Aug 1977, 183-184.

18 **Ironside, A.G.** Infectious diseases. Gastroenteritis of infancy. Nursing Mirror, 142, 19 Feb 1976, 55-56.

19 **Kelnar, C.J.H. and Harvey, D.R.** Hyaline membrane disease. (Respiratory distress syndrome of the newborn.) Nursing Mirror, 145, 17 Nov 1977, 20-23.

20 **Lander, A.J.** Nursing care study. Oesophageal atresia with tracheo-oesophageal fistula associated with hydramnios. Nursing Times, 72, 2 Sep 1976, 1351-1353.

21 **McCrae, W.M.** Kernicterus in the newborn. Nursing Times, 72, 15 Jul 1976, 1086-1088.

22 **Midgley, C.** Neonatal and perinatal infections. (Report of symposium.) Midwives Chronicle, 91, Sep 1978, 251-252.

23 **Minns, H.** Nursing care study. A baby with trisomy E or 18. Nursing Times, 72, 16 Sep 1976, 1430-1433.

24 **Nalepka, C.D.** The oxygen hood for newborns in respiratory distress. American Journal of Nursing, 75 (12), Dec 1975, 2185-2187.

25 **Neligan, G.** The quality of the survivors. (Results of the Newcastle Study of Child Development, and a survey focusing on survivors of adverse neonatal factors born at Princess Mary Maternity Hospital.) Midwives Chronicle, 89, Jan 1976, 6-8.

26 **Oddy, R.Z.** Nursing care study. Collodion baby. Nursing Mirror, 143, 23 Dec 1976, 29-30.

27 **Robinson, L.A. and Brown, A.L.** Colic: pharmaceutic and medical intervention. Pediatric Nursing, 5 (6), Nov/Dec 1979, 61-64.

28 **Rutter, N. and Metcalfe, D.H.** Febrile convulsions—what do parents do? (Survey of medical and parental management.) British Medical Journal, 2, 11 Nov 1978, 1345-1346.

29 **Siddall, J. and others** Breathless babies who can't complain. (Anaemia in newborn babies.) Nursing Mirror, 150, 31 Jan 1980, 20-22.

30 **Speidel, B.D.** Iatrogenic problems of the newborn. Midwife, Health Visitor and Community Nurse, 16 (1), Jan 1980, 6-8.

31 **Umphenour, J.H.** Bacterial colonization in neonates with sibling visitation. Journal of Obstetric, Gynecologic and Neonatal Nursing, 9 (2), Mar/Apr 1980, 73-75.

32 **Valman, H.B.** The first year of life. Bacterial infection in the newborn. British Medical Journal, 1, 15 Mar 1980, 772-775.

33 **Valman, H.B.** The first year of life. Convulsions in the newborn. British Medical Journal, 1, 22 Mar 1980, 839-841.

34 **Valman, H.B.** The first year of life. Convulsions in the older infant. British Medical Journal, 280, 26 Apr 1980, 1113-1114.

d INTENSIVE CARE

1 **Alberman, E. and others** Arrangements for special and intensive care of the newborn. (Census of infants, staffing and facilities in three Thames health regions.) British Medical Journal, 2, 22 Oct 1977, 1045-1047.

2 **American Journal of Nursing** Care of the critically ill newborn. (Four articles on intensive care of the newborn.) American Journal of Nursing, 76 (4), Apr 1976, 566-581.

3 **Baldridge, A.E.** Crisis intervention: in a neonatal intensive care unit. Journal of Practical Nursing, 26 (6), Jun 1976, 22-23, 38.

4 **Barnes, C.M.** Levels of consciousness indicated by responses of children to phenomena in the intensive care unit. Maternal-Child Nursing Journal, 4 (4), Winter 1975, 215-285.

5 **Baylis, J.M.** Trafford community special care baby service. Midwives Chronicle, 91, Jan 1978, 3-5.

6 **Blake, A.M. and others** Referral of mothers and infants for intensive care. (Survey at University College Hospital and discussion of implications for the organisation of perinatal care.) British Medical Journal, 2, 18 Aug 1979, 414-416.

7 **Boxall, J.** North America. (Report of a Winston Churchill Memorial Trust scholarship visiting paediatric intensive care units.) Nursing Times, 72 (12), 25 Mar 1976, ABPN supplement V.

8 **Boxall, J. and Gendle, N.** Intensive care of the newborn—6. Measuring and passing a duodenal/jejunal feeding tube. Nursing Times, 75, 23 Aug 1979, 1459-1460.

9 **Brimblecombe, F.S.W. and others** Separation and special-care baby units. Heinemann, 1978. (Clinics in developmental medicine, no.68.)

10 **Brown, J.E. and Johnson, W.L.** A fetal intensive care nursing program. (School of Medicine, State University of New York at Buffalo.) Journal of Obstetric, Gynecologic and Neonatal Nursing, 5 (3), May/Jun 1976, 23-25.

11 **Bucher, R.M.** Creative nursing saved this infant's life. (Care in ITU of postcardiac surgery child with bilateral phrenic nerve paralysis, based on giving him the will to live.) RN Magazine, 41 (11), Nov 1978, 38, 40-43.

12 **Carpenter, R.G. and Gardner, A.** Identification of some infants at immediate risk of dying unexpectedly and justifying intensive study. (Score based on data collected at birth and by HVs at one month.) Lancet, 2, 18 Aug 1979, 343.

13 **Consolvo, C.A.** Nurse turnover in the newborn intensive care unit. (Definition of stress factors and management methods introduced over three year period during which turnover decreased.) Journal of Obstetric, Gynecologic and Neonatal Nursing, 8 (4), Jul/Aug 1979, 201-204.

14 **Conway, A. and Williams, T.** Care of the critically ill newborn. Parental alimentation. Administration of fat emulsions in addition to alimentation fluids. American Journal of Nursing, 76 (4), Apr 1976, 574-577.

15 **Cowper-Smith, F.** Improving special care for babies. 1. Developing relationships in special care units. 2. The clinical aspects. (Report of two conferences.) Nursing Times, 75, 17 May 1979, 816-818; 24 May 1979, 858-860.

16 **Derbyshire, F.M. and Davies, D.P.** Special care of babies in the community. (Scheme at Leicester Royal Infirmary Maternity Hospital involving health visitors.) Midwives Chronicle, 92, May 1979, 138.

17 **Douek, E. and others** Effects of incubator noise on the cochlea of the newborn. Lancet, 2, 20 Nov 1976, 1110-1113.

18 **Ferrara, A. and Harin, A.** Emergency transfer of the high-risk neonate: a working manual for medical, nursing and administrative personnel. St. Louis: Mosby, 1980.

19 **Fuller, R.A.** Quality assurance in the special care nursery. (Research study of nurses' knowledge of and attitudes to the quality assurance programme.) Supervisor Nurse, 10 (10), Oct 1979, 16-19.

20 **Hyde, D.J.** Special care of babies in the community: How can we improve our service? (Manchester's special care baby service.) Midwives Chronicle, 92, Feb 1979, 42-44.

21 **Jacobson, S.F.** An insider's guide to field research. (As opposed to laboratory experiments. Report of author's experiences of field study of nurses' stress in neonatal intensive care units.) Nursing Outlook, 26 (6), Jun 1978, 371-374.

22 **Jacobson, S.P.** Stressful situations for neonatal intensive care nurses. (Research study, with commentary on its implications for practice by Holly Weeks.) American Maternal-Child Nursing Journal, 3 (3), May/Jun 1978, 144-152.

23 **Jay, S.S.** Paediatric intensive care: involving parents in the care of their child. Maternal-Child Nursing Journal, 6 (3), Fall 1977, 195-204, Reprinted in Canadian Nurse, 74 (5), May 1978, 28-31.

24 **Joint Board of Clinical Nursing Studies** 5. Special and intensive care of the newborn. Nursing Mirror, 143 (9), 26 Aug 1976, Nursing care supplement series, 2, i-iv.

25 **Kinston, M.** Care of the unwell neonate. (Formation of nursing staff group in ITU to help nurses facilitate mother/child bonding.) Nursing Mirror, 147, 17 Aug 1978, 22-23.

26 **Korones, S.B.** High-risk newborn infants: the basis for intensive nursing care. 2nd ed. St. Louis: Mosby, 1976.

27 **Layton-Jones, M.E.A.** Special and intensive nursing care of the newborn—the work of the Joint Board of Clinical Nursing Studies. Midwives Chronicle, 89, Mar 1976, 52-54.

28 **Levin, D.L. editor** A practical guide to pediatric intensive care. St. Louis: Mosby, 1979.

29 **Lewandowski, L.A. and Kramer, M.** Role transformation of special care unit nurses: a comparative study. (With reference to job satisfaction and stresses experienced.) Nursing Research, 29 (3), May/Jun 1980, 170-179.

30 **Mangurten, H.H. and others** Parent-parent support in the care of high-risk newborns. (Value of parents' group.) Journal of Obstetric, Gynecologic and Neonatal Nursing, 8 (5), Sep/Oct 1979, 275-277.

31 **Maternal-Child Nursing Journal** Neonatal intensive care. (Four articles on primary nursing, support for parents and fostering parent-child bonds.) Maternal-Child Nursing Journal, 2 (5), Sep/Oct 1977, 286-297.

32 **Meier, P.P.** A crisis group for parents of high-risk infants. (Report of pilot study by nurse in special care nursery.) Maternal-Child Nursing Journal, 7 (1), Spring 1978, 21-30.

33 **Michie, M.M.** The quality of neonatal care in special and intensive care baby units. (With reference to the prevention of handicap.) Midwives Chronicle, 92, Jan 1979, 13-15.

34 Nethercott, S.G. and Price, J.F. Management of chronically ventilated infants. (The respiratory intensive care unit at Great Ormond Street.) Nursing Times, 74, 6 Jul 1978, 1130-1131).

35 Norman, A.P. Intensive care of the new born. Chest, Heart and Stroke Journal, 2 (2), Summer 1977, 3-7.

36 Nursing Times Intensive care of the newborn. Macmillan, 1980.

37 Opirhory, G.J. Counseling the parents of a critically ill newborn. (Advice to nurses.) Journal of Obstetric, Gynecologic and Neonatal Nursing, 8 (3), May/Jun 1979, 179-182.

38 Roberton, C. Which babies should be admitted to Special Care Units? (Claims that unnecessary admissions deprive mothers of contact in the vital first few days.) Midwife, Health Visitor and Community Nurse, 14 (7), Jul 1978, 208-209, 211.

39 Spikes, J. and Bowen, T. Nursing care plans for the special care nursery. (With example.) Supervisor Nurse, 10 (1), Jan 1979, 23-26.

40 Strong, G. When a baby can't go home. (Criteria for admission to the Special Care Baby Unit.) Nursing Mirror, 148, 11 Jan 1979 Supplement, vii, x-xii, xiv.

41 Todd, R.M. Intensive care of the newborn. Nursing Mirror, 142, 1 Jan 1976, 52-54.

42 Whaley, P.A. and others Relieving parental anxiety: a booklet for parents of an infant in NICU. (With text of booklet.) Journal of Obstetric, Gynecologic and Neonatal Nursing, 8 (1), Jan/Feb 1979, 49-55.

43 Zaslow, S. New touches in caring for preemies. (Sensory stimulation programme for babies in intensive care involving the parents.) RN Magazine, 39 (2), Feb 1976, 31-36.

e PREMATURE AND LOW BIRTH WEIGHT

1 Beaney, A. Case study: a premature baby with Cri-du-Chat syndrome. Midwives Chronicle, 89, Jun 1976, 158-160.

2 Berger, H. The nutritional consequences of premature birth. (Feeding of premature babies.) Midwife, Health Visitor and Community Nurse, 15 (2), Feb 1979, 54-58.

3 British Medical Journal Caring for babies of very low birth weight. (Need for separate neonatal intensive care and special-care baby units.) British Medical Journal, 2, 21 Oct 1978, 1105-1106.

4 Brown, R. The low birth-weight infant. Nursing Times, 74, 2 Nov 1978, 1805-1807.

5 Burroughs, A.K. and others The effect of nonnutritive sucking on transcutaneous oxygen tension in noncrying, preterm neonates. Research in Nursing Health, 1 (2), Jul 1978, 69-75.

6 Chapman, J.S. The effect of pre-term infants' decreasing mortalilty on their future morbidity: preliminary examination of long-term outcomes of stimulation programs for pre-term infants. (Research study.) Nursing Papers, 10 (2), Summer 1978, 31-54.

7 Christensen, A.Z. Coping with the crisis of a premature birth—one couple's story. American Journal of Maternal-Child Nursing, 2 (1), Jan/Feb 1977, 33-37.

8 Cockburn, F. and Taylor, M.L. Feeding the preterm infant. Nursing Mirror, 145, 18 Aug 1977, 19-23.

9 Connolly, A. Nursing care study. Survival against the odds. (Twenty week old premature baby.) Nursing Mirror, 142, 13 May 1976, 59-60.

10 Davies, D.P. and others When should preterm babies be sent home from neonatal units? Lancet, 1, 28 Apr 1979, 914-915.

11 Fancourt, R. and others Follow up study of small for dates babies. (Showing that slow growth and development continued after birth.) British Medical Journal, 1, 12 Jun 1976, 1435-1437.

12 Fiddes, S.A. Low birth weight babies in Calderdale. (Analysis of social and obstetric factors.) Midwives Chronicle, 93, Jul 1980, 245-246.

13 Greer, M. Nursing care study. Pre-term baby. An inheritance of a different kind. (Including adverse reactions to drugs which his mother took during pregnancy.) Nursing Mirror, 149, 6 Dec 1979, 42-44.

14 Harper, H.G. Nursing care study. Special baby care. (Twin born prematurely.) Nursing Times, 73, 29 Sep 1977, 1511-1513.

15 Heredia-Perez, J.A. Nursing care study. A special care baby. (Premature baby.) Nursing Times, 76, 1 May 1980, 778-782.

16 Jeffcoate, J.J. Caring for parents of low birthweight babies. Midwife, Health Visitor and Community Nurse, 16 (3), Mar 1980, 122, 124.

17 Jeffcoate, J.J. Looking at the need for support for families of low birth-weight babies. (Research study.) Health Trends, 12 (2), May 1980, 29-31.

18 Lancet The fate of the baby under 1501g at birth. (Review of research.) Lancet, 1, 1 Mar 1980, 461-463.

19 Measel, C.P. and Anderson, G.C. Non-nutritive sucking during tube feedings: effect on clinical course in premature babies. (Value of sucking on dummy.) Journal of Obstetric, Gynecologic and Neonatal Nursing, 8 (5), Sep/Oct 1979, 265-272.

20 Priestley, B.L. Low birth weight: born too early or too small. (The management and prognosis of premature and small-for-dates infants.) Nursing Mirror, 148, 29 Mar 1979, 38-40.

21 Rothfeder, B. and Tiedman, M. Feeding the low birth-weight neonate. Nursing, 7 (10), Oct 1977, 58-59.

22 Sadler, C. Intravenous feeding of the newborn and small baby. Nursing Mirror, 143, 30 Dec 1976, 42-44.

23 Shosenberg, N. Self-help groups for parents of premature infants. Canadian Nurse, 76 (7), Jul/Aug 1980, 30-34.

24 Speidel, B.D. Adverse effects of routine procedures on preterm infants. (In neonatal intensive care units.) Lancet, 1, 22 Apr 1978, 864-866.

f INFANT DEATH AND STILLBIRTH

1 Battye, J. and Deakin, M. Surveillance reduces baby deaths. (Survey in Sheffield, which showed increased surveillance by health visitors can help to prevent unnecessary deaths, and which has been used as a basis for new visiting programmes.) Nursing Mirror, 148, 26 Apr 1979, 38-40.

2 Beard, R.W. and others Help for parents after stillbirth. (Letter with leaflet of notes for parents. For letters commenting on leaflet see British Medical Journal, 4 Feb, 298 and 18 Feb, 439-440.) British Medical Journal, 1, 21 Jan 1978, 172.

3 Bluglass, K. Psychiatric morbidity after cot death. Practitioner, 224, May 1980, 533, 535, 537, 539.

4 Bourne, S. Coping with perinatal death. Part 1. After effects and theory. (Mourning after stillbirth.) 2. Management problems and strategies. Midwife, Health Visitor and Community Nurse, 15 (2), Feb 1979, 59, 62; (3), Mar 1979, 89, 91-92.

5 Bourne, S. Stillbirth, grief and medical education. (Letter on the danger of families bypassing grief after a stillbirth, with a bibliography of 15 articles.) British Medical Journal, 1977, 1, 30 Apr 1977, 1157.

6 British Medical Journal Grief and stillbirth. British Medical Journal, 1977, 1, 15 Jan 1977, 126.

7 British Medical Journal Help for parents after stillbirth. (Letters commenting on recent leaflet and its limited value.) British Medical Journal, 1, 4 Feb 1978, 298; 18 Feb 1978, 439-440.

8 Carr, A. The first line of defence. (With reference to perinatal mortality rates and value of primary health care team.) Nursing Times, 75, 19 Jul 1979, 1209-1210; 26 Jul 1979, 1259-1260.

9 Clapp, L. and Price, J.H. A review of sudden infant death syndrome. Journal of Nursing Care, 13 (3), Mar 1980, 13-17, 24.

10 Clarke, M. and Williams, A.J. Depression in women after perinatal death. Lancet, 1, 28 Apr 1979, 916-917.

11 Cooper, J. 'End this conspiracy of silence'. (Survey of reactions of 17 couples who experienced a stillbirth.) Nursing Mirror, 149, 6 Dec 1979, 31-33.

12 Deal, A.W. and Bordeaux, B.R. The phenomenon of SIDS. (Sudden Infant Death Syndrome.) Pediatric Nursing, 5 (1), Jan/Feb 1980, 48-50.

13 Department of Health and Social Security Working Party on the Prevention of Early Neonatal Mortality and Morbidity Report. The Department, 1974. (Chairman T.E. Oppé.) (Attached to HC(76)40.)

14 Devlin, R. From both sides now. (Government response to Short report on perinatal and neonatal mortality with comment by Association of Radical Midwives.) Nursing Mirror, 151, 18/25 Dec 1980, 8.

15 **Dunlop, J.L.** Bereavement reaction following stillbirth. Practitioner, 222, Jan 1979, 115-118.

16 **Favorito, J. and others** Apnea monitoring to prevents SIDS. (Sudden Infant Death Syndrome.) American Journal of Nursing, 79 (1), Jan 1979, 101-104.

17 **Foundation for the Study of Infant Deaths** Sudden death in infancy. (Papers given at a Society of Community Medicine conference describing a pilot project in Inner North London boroughs.) Public Health, 89 (4), May 1975, 143-163.

18 **Foundation for the Study of Infant Deaths** Towards a better understanding of cot death. A summary compiled with the guidance of the Scientific Advisory Committee of the Foundation for the Study of Infant Deaths. Health Visitor, 49 (6), Jun 1976, 182-184.

19 **Francis, G.M.** Guidance on symptoms of illness in babies: a further service from the FSID. (Green card giving guidance to mothers from Foundation for the Study of Infant Deaths.) Health Visitor, 52 (10), Oct 1979, 430-432.

20 **Goldstein, H. and Butler, N.R.** Definition of perinatal mortality. Lancet, 1, 11 Jun 1977, 1254-1255.

21 **Grubb, C.A.** Body image concerns of a multipara in the situation of intrauterine fetal death. Maternal Child Nursing Journal, 5 (2), Summer 1976, 93-116.

22 **Gunther, M.H.D.** The relation of infant feeding to cot death. Nutrition, 26 (5), Oct 1972, 290-292.

23 **Health Education Journal** From the editor. (Methods of reducing perinatal mortality.) Health Education Journal, 38 (4), 1979, 106, 136.

24 **Journal of Nurse-Midwifery** The perinatal bereavement crisis. (Three articles.) Journal of Nurse-Midwifery, 24 (5), Sep/Oct 1979, 13-21.

25 **Knox, E.G. and others** Social and health care determinants of area variations in perinatal mortality. Community Medicine, 2 (4), Nov 1980, 282-290.

26 **Kowalski, K. and Osborn, M.R.** Helping mothers of stillborn infants to grieve. American Journal of Maternal Child Nursing, 2 (1), Jan/Feb 1977, 29-32.

27 **Lancet** The abhorrence of stillbirth. (Emotional effects and need for counselling.) Lancet, 1, 4 Jun 1977, 1188-1190.

28 **Lewis, E.** The management of stillbirth: coping with an unreality. Lancet, 2, 18 Sep 1976, 619-620.

29 **Lewis, H.** Nothing was said sympathy wise. (Areas which cause distress to parents following a stillbirth and how these are related to the mourning process.) Social Work Today, 10, 24 Jul 1979, 12-13.

30 **Limerick, S., Countess of Limerick and Downham, M.A.P.S.** Cot deaths—the bereaved parents' need for support. Midwives Chronicle, 90, Oct 1977, 231-234.

31 **Limerick, S., Countess of Limerick and Downham, M.A.P.S.** Counselling after a cot death. Health Visitor, 49 (8), Aug 1976, 256-257.

32 **Limerick, S.R.P., Countess of Limerick and Downham, M.A.P.S.** The mystery of cot deaths. Social Service Quarterly, 50 (3), Jan-March 1977, 250-253.

33 **Limerick, S., Countess of Limerick and Downham, M.A.P.S.** Support for families bereaved by cot death: joint voluntary and professional view. (Lady Limerick is chairman of the welfare and information committee of the Foundation for the Study of Infant Deaths.) British Medical Journal, 1, 10 Jun 1978, 1527-1529.

34 **Lister, R.** The urgent need to reduce baby deaths. (With statistics showing AHAs with high perinatal and infant mortality rates.) New Society, 46, 16 Nov 1978, 392-393.

35 **McElroy, E. and others** Sudden infant death syndrome: a framework for preventive mental health. (Psychosocial aspects of SIDS and programme developed by nurse to help families after SIDS.) Nursing Clinics of North America, 14 (3), Sep 1979, 391-403.

36 **MacNaughton, M.C.** Perinatal mortality surveys. What value are they? (Survey in Scotland.) Midwife, Health Visitor and Community Nurse, 16 (8), Aug 1980, 322-323.

37 **McNay, M.B. and others** Perinatal deaths: analysis by clinical cause to assess value of induction of labour. (Study at Glasgow Royal Maternity Hospital.) British Medical Journal, 1, 5 Feb 1977, 347-350.

38 **Mason, J.K. and others** Cot deaths in Edinburgh: infant feeding and socioeconomic factors. Journal of Epidemiology and Community Health, 34 (1), Mar 1980, 35-41.

39 **Midwives Chronicle** Two letters on the midwife's role in counselling parents after a stillbirth. Midwives Chronicle, 91, Jun 1978, 142-143.

40 **Miles, M.S.** SIDS: parents are the patients. (Counselling parents after death of child from Sudden Infant Death Syndrome.) Journal of Emergency Nursing, 3 (2), Mar/Apr 1977, 29-32.

41 **Moore, A.** The cot death syndrome. Midwife, Health Visitor and Community Nurse, 12 (5), May 1976, 154-156.

42 **Morris, D. and others** A leaflet for parents whose child was stillborn. Midwives Chronicle, 91, Mar 1978, 57-58.

43 **Nakushan, J.M.** Restoring parents' equilibrium after sudden infant death. A public health nurse describes family reactions and what nurses do during their follow up visits. American Journal of Nursing, 76 (10), Oct 1976, 1600-1604.

44 **Newson, K.** It's not just a question of cash. (Ways in which perinatal mortality rate can be improved.) Nursing Mirror, 151, 31 Jul 1980, 11.

45 **Nightingale, S.** Loss of a child—a personal account of mourning. Social Work Today, 9, 13 Jun 1978, 14-16.

46 **Oakley, J.R. and others** Possibly avoidable deaths in hospital in the age-group one week to two years. Lancet, 1, 10 Apr 1976, 770-772.

47 **Palmer, S.R. and others** Infant deaths in Inner London: a health care planning team study. Community Medicine, 2 (2), May 1980, 102-108.

48 **Parliament. House of Commons Social Services Committee** Perinatal and neonatal mortality: second report from the Social Services Committee session 1979-80. Vol.1. HMSO, 1980. Chairman Renée Short.

49 **Parrish, S.** Letting go: new dimensions in assisting bereaved parents. (After stillbirth or perinatal death.) Canadian Nurse, 76 (3), Mar 1980, 34-37.

50 **Ross, T.** Stillbirth—a new approach. (Interview with Hugh Jolly who recommends that mothers should be allowed to see their babies in order to mourn and express their grief.) Nursing Mirror, 143, 7 Oct 1976, 40-41.

51 **Russell, W.** Minister's discouraging response to perinatal report. British Medical Journal, 281, 13 Dec 1980, 1653.

52 **Savage, W.** Perinatal loss and the medical team. (Reactions of doctors and dilemmas they face with advice on management of stillbirth.) Midwife, Health Visitor and Community Nurse, 14 (9), Sep 1978, 292, 295; (10), Oct 1978, 348-349, 351.

53 **Saylor, D.E.** Nursing response to mothers of stillborn infants. Journal of Obstetric, Gynecologic and Neonatal Nursing, 6 (4), Jul/Aug 1977, 39-42.

54 **Scott, D.J. and others** Respiratory viruses and cot death. British Medical Journal, 2, 1 Jul 1978, 12-13.

55 **Slack, P.** Bricks without mortar. (Summary of and comment on House of Commons report on perinatal and neonatal mortality.) Nursing Times, 76, 31 Jul 1980, 1336-1337.

56 **Southall, D.** Studying the unknown. (New British Heart Foundation research project into causes of sudden infant death syndrome.) Nursing Mirror, 151, 11 Sep 1980, 38-40.

57 **Speck, P.** Easing the pain and grief of stillbirth. Nursing Mirror, 146, 1 Jun 1978, 38-41.

58 **Stanton, A.N. and others** Terminal symptoms in children dying suddenly and unexpectedly at home: preliminary report of the DHSS multicentre study of postneonatal mortality. British Medical Journal, 2, 4 Nov 1978, 1249-1251.

59 **The STILLBIRTH and Perinatal Death Association.** Health Visitor, 53 (5), May 1980, 165-166.

60 **Sylva, K. and Bryce, A.** Coping with stillbirth. Midwives Chronicle, 92, Feb 1979, 35-36.

61 **Tew, M.** Facts, not assertions of belief. (Criticism of the House of Commons Social Services Committee report on neonatal and perinatal mortality.) Health and Social Service Journal, 90, 12 Sep 1980, 1194-1197.

62 **Tew, M.** Perinatal mortality: is home a safer place? (Suggests that it is, with reference to statistical study.) Health and Social Service Journal, 90, 30 May 1980, 702-705.

63 **Toase, M.** Stillbirth and perinatal death.

(Bibliography of items held in RCM Trust Library.) Midwives Chronicle, 93, Feb 1980, 33.

64 Turner, J. Saving babies. (Report on the save-a-baby campaign and perinatal mortality rates.) New Society, 44, 27 Apr 1978, 200, 202-203.

65 Worlow, D. What do you say when the baby is stillborn? RN Magazine, 41 (7), Jul 1978, 74.

46 INFANT FEEDING

a GENERAL

1 Addy, D.P. Problems of childhood. Infant feeding: a current view. British Medical Journal, 1, 22 May 1976, 1268-1271.

2 Ansell, C.J. Milk for babies. (A guide to artificial milk products.) Midwife, Health Visitor and Community Nurse, 12 (8), Aug 1976, 153-156.

3 Ayliffe, G.A.J. Contamination of infant feeds in hospital. (Survey of preparation methods and treatment of equipment in 37 hospitals.) Midwife, Health Visitor and Community Nurse, 12 (1), Jan 1976, 18-20.

4 Bacon, C.J. and Wylie, J.M. Mothers' attitudes in infant feeding at Newcastle General Hospital in summer 1975. (A survey of attitudes, influences, personal and social backgrounds of 200 mothers.) British Medical Journal, 1, 7 Feb 1976, 308-309.

5 Barnes, D. and Barnes, P. Infant feeding. A survey of mothers' practices and attitudes. (Study of mothers attending antenatal classes organised by the National Childbirth Trust in the Nottingham area.) Nursing Times, 72, 5 Aug 1976, 1210-1211; 12 Aug 1976, 1250-1253.

6 Brooke, O.G. Infant feeding: the perennial problem. Practitioner, 221, Sep 1978, 314-319.

7 Brown, M.S. and Grunfeld, C.C. Taste preferences of infants for sweetened or unsweetened foods. Research in Nursing and Health, 3 (1), Mar 1980, 11-17.

8 Chute, D. Creating a learning environment. (For mothers and mothers-to-be regarding infant feeding. Review of educational methods.) Canadian Nurse, 74 (1), Jan 1978, 48-51.

9 Clark, J. The baby-milk controversy. Nursing Mirror, 142, 26 Feb 1976, 39-40.

10 Crow, R.A. An ethological study of the development of infant feeding. Journal of Advanced Nursing, 2 (2), Mar 1977, 99-109.

11 Crow, R. and Wright, P. The development of feeding behaviour in early infancy. (Nursing Mirror Forum 1976.) Nursing Mirror, 142, 1 Apr 1976, 57-59.

12 Department of Health and Social Security Committee on Medical Aspects of Food Policy. Working Party on the Composition of Foods for Infants and Young Children Artifical feeds for the young infant. HMSO, 1980. (Reports on health and social subjects; 18.)

13 Department of Health and Social Security Committee on Medical Aspects of Food Policy. Working Party on the Composition of Foods for Infants and Young Children The composition of mature human milk. HMSO, 1977. (Chairman T. E. Oppé.) (Report on health and social subjects, no.12.)

14 Department of Health and Social Security Committee on Medical Aspects of Food Policy. Panel on Child Nutrition. Working Party on Infant Feeding Present day practice in infant feeding. HMSO, 1980. (Reports on health and social subjects, no.20.)

15 De Swiet, M. and others Effect of feeding habit on weight in infancy. Lancet, 1, 23 Apr 1977, 892-894.

16 Gatherer, A. A review of standards of infant hygiene in the home. (Research study involving health visitors of mothers' sterilising of bottle feeding equipment.) Nursing Times, 74, 12 Oct 1978, 1684-1685.

17 Gunn, S. The bottlefeeding mother needs your help too. RN Magazine, 42 (2), Feb 1979, 53.

18 Harker, P. Infant feeding confusion. (Report of research study involving health visitor.) Nursing Times, 75, 11 Jan 1979 Community Outlook, 17-18.

19 Holly, D. and Cullen, D. A comparison of weight gain in breast fed and bottle fed babies. Public Health, 91 (3), May 1977, 113-116.

20 Jones, R.A.K. and Belsey, E.M. Common mistakes in infant feeding: survey from a London borough. British Medical Journal, 1, 8 Jul 1978, 112-114.

21 Jones, R.A.K. and Davies, P.A. Infant feeding. Midwife, Health Visitor and Community Nurse, 15 (11), Nov 1979, 438, 440, 443.

22 Kirk, T.R. Appraisal of the effectiveness of nutrition education in the context of infant feeding. (In the light of the DHSS 1974 recommendations.) Journal of Human Nutrition, 34 (6), Dec 1980, 429-438.

23 Laurance, B. and others Feeding babies in the 70s. A feeding policy document approved by the paediatricians of the North East Thames Regional Health Authority. (Based on the DHSS report 'Present day practice in infant feeding'.) Nursing Times, 73, 3 Mar 1977 Supplement, i-iv.

24 Leslie, J. Nutrition and diet. Part 2. Care of the infant. Nursing Mirror, 144, 30 Jun 1977, 28-31.

25 Lindley, P. Vitamin D—too much of a good thing? Health Visitor, 53 (8), Aug 1980, 318-319.

26 Lyall, R. and Skipworth, G.E. Baby milk dispensing. (Survey in Middlesbrough involving HVs on mothers' inaccuracy in making up feeds.) Health Visitor, 53 (2), Feb 1980, 46.

27 Mackieth, R. and Wood, C. Infant feeding and feeding difficulties. 5th ed. Churchill Livingstone, 1977.

28 Maclean, G.D. An appraisal of the concepts of infant feeding and their application in practice. (Survey in the Swansea District of the West Glamorgan Area Health Authority.) Journal of Advanced Nursing, 2 (2), Mar 1977, 111-126.

29 Maclean, G.D. Whoever told you that. 1. 'To feed, but how to feed? That is the question!' Midwives Chronicle, 90 (12), May 1977, 101-104.

30 Maclean, G.D. Whoever told you that. 3. 'Measure for measure.' (Artificial feeding recommendations.) Midwives Chronicle, 80, Jul 1977, 167-169.

31 Martin, J. Infant feeding 1975: attitudes and practice in England and Wales. HMSO, 1978.

32 Ounsted, M. Infant feeding. (Study at John Radcliffe Hospital, Oxford of milk intake and weight gain.) Nursing Times, 72, 6 May 1976, 700-701.

33 Parnell, G.P. Mothers' attitudes to pre-packed feeds. (Survey at St. Mary's Hospital, Kettering, Northants.) Midwives Chronicle, 89, Nov 1976, 267-268.

34 Poskitt, E.M.E. Is it bad to be 'bonny'? (Health problems of overweight infants.) Health Visitor, 51 (6), Jun 1978, 208-210.

35 Poskitt, E.M.E. and Cole, T.J. Do fat babies stay fat? (Study of feeding practices of weight in infancy reviewed 5 years later.) British Medical Journal, 1, 1 Jan 1977, 7-9.

36 Schwarz, V. Malnutrition in our society. 3. Milk: where to go wrong from the beginning. Health Visitor, 49 (9), Sep 1976, 292-293.

37 Smith, B.A.M. Dangers in artificial feeding. Midwives Chronicle, 89, Feb 1976, 24-25.

38 Valman, H.B. The first year of life. Feeding and feeding problems. British Medical Journal, 280, 16 Feb 1980, 457-460.

39 Waller, J. Patterns of infant feeding. An evaluation of a survey on infant feeding patterns in Port Lincoln, South Australia. Australian Nurses Journal, 5 (11), May 1976, 32-34.

40 Wharton, B.A. and Berger, H.M. Problems of childhood. Bottle feeding. British Medical Journal, 1, 29 May 1976, 1326-1331.

41 White, M. Infant feeding. (Three month survey by health visitors to discover current practice.) Nursing Mirror, 46, 19 Jan 1978, 42-44.

42 Wills, B.B. Food becomes fun for children. (Nutrition education for mothers. Includes Denver Developmental Screening Test of child development.) American Journal of Nursing, 78 (12), Dec 1978, 2082-2085.

43 Winckler, I. How well fed are our children? (Factors mitigating against balanced nutrition.) Nursing Times, 74, 30 Mar 1978, Supplement, iii, v-vi, viii.

44 World Health Organization Infant feeding. Code of marketing practice. (WHO resolution.) Lancet, 1, 7 Jun 1980, 1239-1240.

45 Wrangham, M.R. Deep freezing specialised formula baby foods. Nursing Times, 76, 12 Jun 1980, 1056-1060.

46 WHO/UNICEF meeting on infant and young child feeding. (With recommendations of meeting on p.437-443.) WHO Chronicle, 33 (12), Dec 1979, 435-443; Lancet, 2, 20 Oct 1979, 841-843, Editorial, 833.

b BREAST FEEDING

1 Atkinson, L.D. Prenatal nipple conditioning for breastfeeding. (Study showed that regime reduced amount of nipple pain experienced during first few days of breast feeding.) Nursing Research, 28 (5), Sep/Oct 1979, 267-271.

2 Auerbach, K.G. The role of the nurse in support of breast feeding. Journal of Advanced Nursing, 4 (3), May 1979, 263-285.

3 BREAST feeding: an up to date review of the help available to nursing mothers in the Blackburn Health District. (Survey by midwifery students.) Nursing Mirror, 143, 2 Sep 1976, 39-41.

4 Brimblecombe, F.S.W. and Cullen, D. Influences on a mother's choice of method of infant feeding. (Survey to assess effect of professional advice and other influences.) Public Health, 91 (3), May 1977, 117-126.

5 Brown, M.S. and Hurlock, J.T. Preparation of the breast for breastfeeding. (To evaluate effectiveness of three commonly suggested methods, nipple rolling, application of cream and expression of colostrum.) Nursing Research, 24 (6), Nov-Dec 1975, 448-451.

6 Campbell, R. Characteristics and attitudes of mothers who choose to breast feed their babies. (Study of 60 mothers in Nottingham.) Midwives Chronicle, 89, Apr 1976, 82-84.

7 Canadian Nurse A practical guide to successful breast-feeding. (Information for nurses giving support to mothers.) Canadian Nurse, 72 (3), Mar 1976, 25-35.

8 CIBA Foundation Breast-feeding and the mother. Amsterdam: Elsevier, 1976. (CIBA Foundation symposium 4J (new series).)

9 Clayton, S. and others Response and initiative: breast feeding in the community. (Ways in which HVs and midwives can promote breast feeding.) Midwives Chronicle, 93, Aug 1980, 272-275.

10 Coles, E.C. and others Increasing prevalence of breast-feeding. (Survey in 1975 and 1977.) British Medical Journal, 2, 21 Oct 1978, 1122.

11 Community Outlook Weaning. (Fact sheet and three articles, one on vegetarian babies.) Nursing Times, 76, 12 Jun 1980 Community Outlook, 165-173.

12 Coombes, S. Breastfeeding—a problem conquered. (How author, a health visitor, improved her own knowledge and was able to teach breast feeding more effectively at parentcraft classes.) Nursing Times, 75, 13 Dec 1979 Community Outlook, 387-389.

13 Croucher, M. Midwives can make it. (Description of making of film on breast-feeding.) Midwives Chronicle, 92, Apr 1979, 100-103.

14 Culley, P. and others Are breast-fed babies still getting a raw deal in hospital? (Results of survey and recommendation that early and more frequent feeding should be practised.) British Medical Journal, 2, 13 Oct 1979, 891-893.

15 Davies, D.P. Is inadequate breast-feeding an important cause of failure to thrive? Lancet, 1, 10 Mar 1979, 541-542.

16 Davies, M. Breast feeding. (By Chairman of Breast-Feeding Promotion Group of the National Childbirth Trust.) Nursing Times, 73, 27 Oct 1977, 1678-1679.

17 Deacon, S. Weaning the normal baby. Nursing Times, 73, 3 Feb 1977, 166-167.

18 Department of Health and Social Security Breast feeding: based on a one-day conference 14 Jul 1975. Newman Scientific, 1976. (Report of conference in Journal of Human Nutrition, 30 (4), Aug 1976, 223-280.)

19 Eastham, E. and others Further decline of breast feeding. (A survey into reasons for choice of breast or bottle feeding at Princess Mary Maternity Hospital, Newcastle upon Tyne.) British Medical Journal, 1, 7 Feb 1976, 305-307.

20 Ellison, S.L. and others Sucking in the newborn infant during the first hour of life. (Research study.) Journal of Nurse-Midwifery, 24 (6), Nov/Dec 1979, 18-25.

21 Frantz, K.B. and Kalmen, B.A. Breast-feeding works for cesareans, too...and here is precisely how you can help the mother do it. (With chart showing effect of various drugs on breastfeeding.) RN Magazine, 42 (12), Dec 1979, 39-47.

22 Freedman, G.R. Breast feeding—a year's experience of one group practice. (Survey of ante natal and post partum advice on breast feeding in a Newcastle practice carried out by interviews with a health visitor.) Journal of the Royal College of General Practitioners, 26, Jul 1976, 507-513.

23 Gomm, R. Breast—best or bestial? Midwife, Health Visitor and Community Nurse, 12 (10), Oct 1976, 317-318.

24 Greenbank, G.E. and Hafez, S. Factors influencing breastfeeding. (Research study to establish whether age, formal education and prenatal education and experience influenced the decision to breastfeed.) Journal of Nursing Care, 12 (8), Aug 1979, 6-9.

25 Hahn, M.J. and Hurst, J.E. Hormonal influences in lactation. Nursing Times, 76, 28 Aug 1980, 1522-1523.

26 Hall, J.M. Influencing breastfeeding success. (Report of research study and details of nursing support used with experimental group.) Journal of Obstetric, Gynecologic and Neonatal Nursing, 7 (6), Nov/Dec 1978, 28-32.

27 Herbert, P. Putting a case for the breast. (Breast feeding's value with review of research.) Nursing Mirror, 149, 19 Jul 1979, 19-21.

28 Houston, M.J. and others The contraceptive effects of lactation. (Research study in Edinburgh.) Nursing Times, 76, 10 Jul 1980, 1231-1232.

29 Howie, P.W. and McNeilly, A.S. The initiation of lactation. Midwife, Health Visitor and Community Nurse, 16 (4), Apr 1980, 142, 144, 147.

30 Jeffs, J. Why do mothers breast feed? (Survey of mothers' feeding method during the first postnatal week.) Nursing Times, 73, 16 Jun 1977, 911-914. Comment by J F Walker, 21 Jul 1977, 1126-1127.

31 Jelliffe, D.B. and Jelliffe, E.F.P. Human milk in the modern world: psychosocial, nutri-

tional and economic significance. Oxford University Press, 1978.

32 Jolly, H. Why breast feeding is good for mother and baby. (Reprinted from 'The Times.') Midwives Chronicle, 88, Nov 1975, 374-375.

33 Kitzinger, S. The experience of breast-feeding. Harmondsworth: Penguin, 1979.

34 Kitzinger, S. 'When im seem bellyful im burps and stops.' Breastfeeding contrasts. (A comparison of breast feeding habits of Jamaican mothers, West Indian immigrants and English mothers.) Health Visitor, 49 (2), Feb 1976, 34-36.

35 Knafl, K.A. Research and studies. Negotiating hospital care: La Leche League Members and Hospital Personnel. (Survey of attitudes to breast feeding amongst hospital staff.) Journal of Obstetric, Gynecologic and Neonatal Nursing, 5 (4), Jul/Aug 1976, 47-51.

36 Krishna, L.M. Attitudes to breast feeding by mothers in Newham health district. Public Health, 93 (6), Nov 1979, 383-386.

37 Krishna, L.M. Breast feeding and development. (Small research study of differences in aspects of behaviour between breast fed and bottle fed infants and children.) Public Health, 94 (1), Jan 1980, 21-24.

38 LA LECHE League International and The National Childbirth Trust. (Their role in promoting breastfeeding.) Health Visitor, 52 (6), Jun 1979, 214-216.

39 Lancet Breast is best. Lancet, 2, 21 Aug 1976, 412-413.

40 Llewellyn-Jones, J.D. Breast feeding and sexuality. Australasian Nurses Journal, 8 (2), Oct 1978, 22-24.

41 Lucas, A. and others Pattern of milk flow in breast-fed infants. Lancet, 2, 14 Jul 1979, 57-58.

42 Maclean, G.D. Whoever told you that. 1. 'The milk of human kind.' (Recommendations on breast feeding made by Working Party on Infant Feeding.) Midwives Chronicle, 90, Jun 1977, 129-132.

43 Messenger, M. Breast feeding. (General discussion by chairman of NCT Breastfeeding Promotion Group.) Health Visitor, 52 (6), Jun 1979, 227, 229.

44 Moore, A. Weaning—fact and fashion. Nursing Times, 75, 30 Aug 1979, 1481-1483.

45 Morgan, P. Breast feeding: the mystic maternal cult. New Society, 36, 20 May 1976, 413-414.

46 Nursing Mirror Breast-feeding: the natural way. (Three articles on ways to promote it with reference to research.) Nursing Mirror, 148, 31 May 1979, 14-20.

47 O'Connell, P.E. Promoting breast feeding: the contribution of the health visitor. Journal of Human Nutrition, 30 (4), Aug 1976, 266-268.

48 Ragheb, S. and Smith, E.W. Beliefs and customs regarding breast feeding among Egyptian women in Alexandria. (Research study.) International Journal of Nursing Studies, 16 (1), 1979, 73-83.

49 Richards, M.P.M. Support for breast

feeding. Midwife, Health Visitor and Community Nurse, 12 (3), Mar 1976, 85-87.

50 Roberts, A. Body fluids 12. Breast milk. Nursing Times, 74, 18 May 1978 Body fluids, 45-48.

51 Sacks, S.H. and others To breast feed or not to breast feed. A survey of primiparae. (Southmead Hospital, Bristol.) Practitioner, 216, Feb 1976, 183-186, 188-191.

52 Salariya, E.M. and others Duration of breast-feeding after early initiation and frequent feeding. (Survey showing that duration was increased.) Lancet, 2, 25 Nov 1978, 1141-1143.

53 Savage, R.L. Drugs and breast milk. Adverse Drug Reaction Bulletin, 61, Dec 1976, 212-215.

54 Savage, R.L. Let's not poison the breast milk! Why certain drugs are contra-indicated during lactation. Nursing Mirror, 146, 29 Jun 1978, 24-26.

55 Simpson Memorial Maternity Pavilion 'Breast feeding your baby': a leaflet distributed to mothers attending the Simpson Memorial Maternity Pavilion, Edinburgh. (With introductory note by parentcraft sister.) Midwives Chronicle, 91, Aug 1978, 215-216.

56 Stables, J. Breastfeeding twins. (Personal experience.) Nursing Times, 76, 21 Aug 1980, 1493-1494.

57 Stanway, P. and Stanway, A. Breast is best: a common sense approach to breast feeding. Pan, 1978.

58 Stanway, P. and Stanway, A. Successful breast feeding. Midwife, Health Visitor and Community Nurse, 14 (9), Sep 1978, 304-306.

59 Valman, H.B. The first year of life. Weaning. British Medical Journal, 1, 29 Mar 1980, 913-915.

60 Whichelow, M.J. Breast feeding in Cambridge, England: factors affecting the mother's milk supply. (Research study.) Journal of Advanced Nursing, 4 (3), May 1979, 253-261.

61 Whichelow, M. and Greenfield, M. Coping with colic in the breast fed baby. (Advice on milk-free diet.) Health Visitor, 53 (1), Jan 1980, 6-7.

62 Whitelaw, A. The new wonder ingredients in breast milk. (Recent advances in understanding breast milk and its advantages for low birthweight babies.) Midwife, Health Visitor and Community Nurse, 14 (7), Jul 1978, 220-221.

63 Whitley, N. Preparation for breastfeeding: a one-year follow-up of 34 nursing mothers. (Research study.) Journal of Obstetric, Gynecologic and Neonatal Nursing, 7 (3), May/Jun 1978, 44-48.

64 Wilkinson, P.W. and Davies, D.P. When and why are babies weaned? (Prospective study of weaning practices of 50 mothers.) British Medical Journal, 1, 24 Jun 1978, 1682-1683.

65 World Health Organization. Maternal and Child Health Unit Breast feeding. Geneva: WHO, 1979.

c MILK BANKS

1 Baum, D. Development of human milk banks. Midwife, Health Visitor and Community Nurse, 15 (4), Apr 1979, 126, 128, 131.

2 Birmingham, J.M. A method for pasteurising human milk. Nursing Times, 74, 7 Dec 1978 Contact, 5-6.

3 Bjorksten, B. and others Collecting and banking human milk: to heat or not to heat? British Medical Journal, 281, 20 Sep 1980, 765-769.

4 Choi, M.W. Breast milk for infants who can't breast feed. American Journal of Nursing, 78 (5), May 1978, 852-855.

5 Heywood Jones, I. The milk run. The National Childbirth Trust has organised the collection of excess breast milk from mothers at home for the use of babies in hospital. Nursing Times, 76, 12 Jun 1980, 1055-1056.

6 Lucas, A. and Roberts, C.D. Bacteriological quality control in human milk-banking. British Medical Journal, 1, 13 Jan 1979, 80-82.

7 McEnery, G. and Chattopadhyay, B. Human milk bank in a district general hospital. British Medical Journal, 2, 16 Sep 1978, 794-796. Leading article 'The special care of human milk', 781-782.

d SPECIAL DIETS

1 Baxter, S. Coping with special diets (for babies.) Nursing Mirror, 143, 30 Sep 1976, 63-64.

2 Buchan, J. The 'Bottle Baby' syndrome. (Increasing use of bottled milk substitutes instead of breast feeding in underdeveloped countries.) International Nursing Review, 26 (5), Sep/Oct 1979, 141-144, 152.

3 Goel, K.M. and others Infant-feeding practices among immigrants in Glasgow. (Survey of Asian, African, Chinese and Scottish children.) British Medical Journal, 2, 28 Oct 1978, 1181-1183.

4 Hide, D.W. Isle of Wight infant feeding survey. (Research involving HVs plus case history of a cow's milk allergy baby.) Health Visitor, 53 (2), Feb 1980, 43.

5 Hongladarom, C.C. and Russell, M. An ethnic difference—lactose intolerance. Nursing Outlook, 24 (12), Dec 1976, 764-765.

6 Lipscomb, P. Nursing care study. No milk today. (Dietary care and tests carried out on a small baby who developed cow's milk protein intolerance following gastroenteritis.) Nursing Mirror, 151, 18 Sep 1980, 37-38.

7 Marks, J. Infant feeding across cultures. Health Visitor, 52 (7), Jul 1979, 271-274, 276.

8 Poh Tann, S. and Wheeler, E.F. Food intakes and growth of young Chinese children in London. (With recommendations to health personnel regarding infant feeding advice.) Community Medicine, 2 (1), Feb 1980, 20-24.

9 Roberts, I.F. and others Malnutrition in infants receiving cult diets: a form of child abuse. (Vegetarian and macrobiotic diets.) British Medical Journal, 1, 3 Feb 1979, 296-298.

10 Rosenberg, F.H. Lactose intolerance. American Journal of Nursing, 77 (5), May 1977, 823-824.

11 Smith, T.C.G. That villain milk: the problem of milk intolerance in babies. Nursing Mirror, 142, 22 Apr 1976, 67-68.

12 West, M.J. Nursing care study. A baby with a feeding problem. (In a paediatric ward.) Nursing Times, 74, 12 Jan 1978, 65-68.

e HISTORY

1 Fildes, V. It's a wonder babies ever survived. (History of infant feeding.) Nursing Mirror, 149, 12 Jul 1979 Supplement, viii, x-xi, xiii-xiv.

2 Fildes, V. On the bottle again. (Diseases of weaning during the period 1600-1800.) Nursing Mirror, 151, 11 Dec 1980, 18-21.

3 Fildes, V. Putting mum in the picture. (Infant feeding between 1500 and 1800.) Nursing Mirror, 149, 19 Jul 1979, 22-24.

4 Fildes, V. Weaning the Elizabethan child. Nursing Times, 76, 31 Jul 1980, 1357-1359; 7 Aug 1980, 1402-1403.

5 Fildes, V. The Elizabethan wet nurse. Nursing Times, 74, 16 Mar 1978, 472-473.

6 Griffiths, C. Bottleless babies. (History of infant feeding with illustrations of methods and early bottles.) Nursing Mirror, 151, 10 Jul 1980 Supplement, xi-xii, xiv-xvi.

7 Nursing Times Pap boats and bubby pots. (Cow and Gate Collection of vessels used for artificial infant feeding.) Nursing Times, 72, 11 Nov 1976, 1748-1749.

8 Prince, J. Infant feeding through the ages. Midwives Chronicle, 89, Dec 1976, 283-285.

47 PAEDIATRIC NURSING

a TEXTBOOKS

1 Alexander, M.M. and Brown, M.S. Pediatric history taking and physical diagnosis for nurses. 2nd ed. New York: McGraw-Hill, 1979.

2 Bates, S.M. Practical paediatric nursing. 2nd ed. Blackwell Scientific, 1979.

3 Brandt, P.A. and others, editors Current practice in pediatric nursing. St. Louis: Mosby, 1976. (Mosby's current practice and perspectives in nursing series.)

4 Decastro, F.J. and others The pediatric nurse practitioner: guidelines for practice. 2nd ed. St. Louis: Mosby, 1976.

5 Duncombe, M. and Weller, B.F. Paediatric nursing. 5th ed. Baillière Tindall, 1979. (Nurses' aids series.)

6 Franklin, A.W. Pastoral paediatrics. Pitman, 1976.

7 Hamilton, P.M. Basic pediatric nursing. 3rd ed. St. Louis: Mosby, 1978.

8 Hospital for Sick Children, Toronto, Canada. Department of Nursing Manual of pediatric nursing care plans edited by U.F. Matthews. Boston: Little, Brown & Co., 1979.

9 Jolly, H. Diseases of children. 3rd ed. Blackwell, 1976.

10 Kessel, I. The essentials of paediatrics for nurses. 5th ed. Edinburgh: Churchill Livingstone, 1976.

11 Latham, H.C. and others Pediatric nursing. 3rd ed. St. Louis: Mosby, 1977.

12 Leifer, G. Principles and techniques in pediatric nursing. 3rd ed. Philadelphia: Saunders, 1977.

13 Liverpool Area Health Authority (Teaching) Alder Hey book of children's doses. 3rd ed. Liverpool AHA, 1979.

14 Marlow, D.R. Textbook of pediatric nursing. 5th ed. Philadelphia: Saunders, 1977.

15 Roberts, F.B. Review of pediatric nursing. 2nd ed. St. Louis: Mosby, 1978. (Mosby's review series.)

16 Scipien, G.M. and others Comprehensive pediatric nursing. 2nd ed. New York: McGraw-Hill, 1979.

17 Steele, S. editor Nursing care of the child with long-term illness. 2nd ed. New York: Appleton-Century-Crofts, 1977.

18 Waechter, E.H. and Blake, F.G. Nursing care of children. 9th ed. Philadelphia: Lippincott, 1976.

19 Whaley, L.F. and Wong, D.L. Nursing care of infants and children. St. Louis: Mosby, 1979.

b GENERAL

1 Association of British Paediatric Nurses Newsletter. Nursing Times, 72, 28 Oct 1976, ABPN Supplement, 1-8; 73, 10 Mar 1977, ABPN Supplement, 1-8.

2 Association of British Paediatric Nurses Paediatric News. Nursing Times, 73, 8 Sep 1977, ABPN Supplement, 1-8; 74, 16 Mar 1978, PN, 1-8; 14 Sep 1978, PN, 1-8; 75, 15 Mar 1979, PN, 1-8; 13 Sep 1979, PN, 1-8.

3 Association of British Paediatric Nurses Spotlight on children. Nursing Times, 76, 6 Mar 1980, ABPN, 1-8; 18 Sep 1980, ABPN, 1-8.

4 Baird, I.A. Patient assignment nursing in a psychopaedic unit. (For physically and mentally handicapped children.) New Zealand Nursing Journal, 70 (10), Oct 1977, 17.

5 Barsteiner, J.H. Bicentennial forecast. Pediatric nursing. RN Magazine, 39 (11), Nov 1976, 21, 24, 28-29, 31-32.

6 Bernard, P. and Schachtel, M.D. The pediatric nurse practitioner: origins and challenges. Medical Care, 16 (12), Dec 1978, 1019-1026.

7 Bollinger, E. The role of the pediatric nurse associate. (Wyler Children's Hospital, University of Chicago.) Hospital Topics, 54 (3), May/Jun 1976, 38-39.

8 Breslau, N. The role of the nurse-practitioner in a pediatric team: patient definitions. (Survey in Cleveland, Ohio.) Medical Care, 15 (12), Dec 1977, 1014-1023.

9 Bullough, B. and others Pediatric nurse practitioners in the work setting. A follow up study of the graduates of a short term training program. Pediatric Nursing, 3 (6), Nov/Dec 1977, 13-18.

10 Burns, B.J. and others Personality profile of pediatric nurse practitioners associated with role change. Nursing Research, 27 (5), Sep/Oct 1978, 286-290.

11 Butt, J.M. Paediatric nurses of the future. Australasian Nurses Journal, 4 (10), Apr 1976, 49-51.

12 Cleary, J. The distribution of nursing attention in a children's ward. (Research study shows how nursing attention was distributed over time and gives samples of the way this distribution affected individual children and events.) Nursing Times, 73, 14 Jul 1977, Occ. papers, 95-96.

13 Coffey, H. and Koch, C.N. Psycho-social care of the paralyzed child. A technique in intensive care nursing. Pediatric Nursing, 1 (5), Sep/Oct 1975, 21-23.

14 Czamiecki, L. The integration of sex education in pediatric nursing practice. Pediatric Nursing, 2 (2), Mar/Apr 1976, 12-16.

15 Dening, F.C. Paediatric nurses fight for survival. (Report of ABPN conference.) Nursing Mirror, 146, 27 Apr 1978, 7-9.

16 Evans, J. Nursing care study. Fallot's tetralogy. (In six-year-old boy.) Nursing Times, 74, 1 Jun 1978, 917-920.

17 General Nursing Council for England and Wales Report of the working party on the changing role of the Registered Sick Children's Nurse and the implications for training. GNC, 1979. (Chairman Miss Thompson.) (Enclosed with circular 79/11.)

18 George, A.M. The critical hour in pediatric recovery. AORN Journal, 26 (6), Dec 1977, 1042-1047.

19 Goodman, H.C. and Perrin, E.C. Evening telephone call management by nurse practitioners and physicians. History-taking, disposition, and telephone communication skills of pediatric nurse practitioners, pediatric house officers, and practicing pediatricians were assessed and compared. Nursing Research, 27 (4), Jul/Aug 1978, 233-237.

20 Hohman, J. Nurse mentor system cuts costs, boosts quality of patient care. (Team leader for total patient care system at Children's Hospital of San Francisco.) Hospitals, 53 (1), 1 Jan 1979, 93-94, 101.

21 Holmes, D. The nursing role in paediatric haematology and oncology. Australian Nurses Journal, 9 (3), Sep 1979, 37-40.

22 Hunter, M.H.S. Making effective use of scarce paediatric nursing resources. Nursing Times, 75, 15 Mar 1979, PN, 5-7.

23 Hymovich, D.P. The effects of primary nursing care on childrens', parents' and nurses' perceptions of the pediatric nursing role. (Summary of findings.) Nursing Research Report, 12 (2), May 1977, 6-7, 11.

24 Hymovich, D.P. How children, mothers, and nurses view primary and team nursing. (Small exploratory study.) American Journal of Nursing, 80 (11), Nov 1980, 2041-2045.

25 Ireland, J.D. and Power, D.J. The pae-diatric primary care clinical nurse in South Africa — at the crossroads of progress. Curationis, 2 (2), Sep 1979, 33-39.

26 Iveson-Iveson, J. Problems of Midland children. Report on the autumn conference of the British Association of Paediatric Nurses in Birmingham. Including necrotising enterocolitis and problems associated with intravenous feeding. Nursing Mirror, 146, 12 Jan 1978, 13-14.

27 Iveson-Iveson, J. Students' forum. Pae-diatrics. (With multiple choice and long answer questions.) Nursing Mirror, 150, 3 Apr 1980, 40-43.

28 Jones, P.F. Acute abdominal pain in childhood. Nursing Mirror, 144, 28 Apr 1977, 51-54.

29 Jurk, I. Objective — optimal nursing care. (A charge sister's viewpoint.) (Haematology ward in Royal Children's Hospital, Melbourne.) Australian Nurses Journal, 8 (3), Sep 1978, 48-50.

30 King, C. and others The PNP in a university hospital pediatric group practice. (University of Colorado Medical Center.) Pediatric Nursing, 3 (1), Jan/Feb 1977, 29, 32-33.

31 Lawrie, B. Education in child health and nutrition. (Clinical nurse consultant at Queen Elizabeth Hospital for Children, East London, who works both in the hospital and in the community.) Nursing Times, 73, 10 Nov 1977, 1741-1744.

32 McBride, M.M. Assessing children with pain. Can you tell me where it hurts? Pediatric Nursing, 3 (4), Jul/Aug 1977, 7-8.

33 McCain, G.C. Children speak out on the role of the nurse. (Research study of 36 sick and well school age children's perceptions.) Pediatric Nursing, 4 (3), May/Jun 1978, 47-50.

34 Parfit, J. They're all different. (Problems of assessing the type of handling each child needs illustrated by several research studies.) Nursing Times, 72, 29 Jan 1976, 156-157.

35 Podratz, R. The nursing management of pediatric nursing therapy. Pediatric Nursing, 2 (1), Jan/Feb 1976, 13-15.

36 Richards, C. Nursing care study. A child in need. (Child with an unstable home background who had peritonitis.) Nursing Times, 72, 20 May 1976, 781-784.

37 Rumfelt, J.J.M. How five year old children perceive the role of the nurse. (Research study.) Maternal-Child Nursing Journal, 9 (1), Spring 1980, 13-24.

38 Spitz, P. Kids in crisis. 1. Bedside assessment — special considerations. (Differences in physiology between adults and children.) Nursing, 8 (3), Mar 1978, 70-72, 74, 76-79.

39 Storms, P.D. Just what to do as a pediatric nurse practitioner? Pediatric Nursing, 2 (3), May/Jun 1976, 42-43.

40 Tingey, L. An English nurse in a 'new world' in a Tokyo hospital. (Experiences of working in the paediatric ward of a cardiac unit in a Japanese hospital.) Nursing Mirror, 147, 24 Aug 1978, 22-25.

41 Thorp, R.J. The use of the pediatric nurse

practitioner in comprehensive health care. Pediatric Nursing, 1 (3), May/Jun 1975, 33-35.

42 Wadsworth, Y. Child health nursing in 1984: generalist, specialist or extinct species? Australian Nurses Journal, 8 (6), Dec/Jan 1978/1979, 34-35, 59-60.

43 Watson, J. Research and literature on children's responses to injections. Some general nursing implications. Pediatric Nursing, 2 (1), Jan/Feb 1976, 7-8.

44 Whitelaw, A. and Valman, B. Procedures in practice. Taking blood and putting up a drip in young children. British Medical Journal, 281, 30 Aug 1980, 602-604.

45 Wirth, P. and others An analysis of the fifty graduates of the Washington University pediatric nurse practitioner program. Part 1: Scope of practice and professional responsibility. (Research study.) Nurse Practitioner, 2 (6), Jul/Aug 1977, 18-23.

c EDUCATION AND TRAINING

1 Burr, S.M. Parent participation in paediatric nurse education. (At the Royal Alexandra Hospital for Sick Children, Brighton, mothers with congenitally handicapped babies demonstrate their experiences to nursing staff.) Nursing Times, 72, 15 Jan 1976, 76-77.

2 Hellings, P. and others Education of the PNP—present and future. Pediatric Nursing, 2 (6), Nov/Dec 1976, 6-9.

3 Jolly, J.D. We need more RSCNs. (Implications of Court report for training of paediatric nurses.) Nursing Times, 73, 23 Jun 1977, 937-938.

4 Kahn, L. and Wirth, P. An analysis of 50 graduates of the Washington University pediatric nursing program. 4. Perceptions and expectations of physician supervisors. Nurse Practitioner, 3 (1), Jan-Feb 1978, 27-31.

5 Murphy, N. A broader perspective on teaching pediatric nursing: graduate students' reactions. Journal of Nursing Education, 19 (2), Feb 1980, 54-59.

6 Spees, E. and others The making of a PNA. (Establishment of a pediatric nurse associate program at Los Angeles County Hospital.) Pediatric Nursing, 1 (2), Mar/Apr 1975, 7-15.

7 Telfer, H. Neonatal nursing education. Australian Nurses Journal, 7 (1), Jul 1977, 34, 50-51.

8 Thompson, M. Reference to RSCN training. (Survey of available training.) Nursing Times, 72, 28 Oct 1976 ABPN Supplement, 6.

9 Tomita, H. Japan. (Paediatric nurse education.) Nursing Times, 72, 25 Mar 1976 ABPN Supplement VII-VIII.

10 Williams, H. Guidelines for learners in paediatrics. Nursing Times, 75, 5 Apr 1979, 598.

d COMMUNITY NURSING

1 Armitage, B.E. The role of the nurse in the primary health care of children: bibliography 1960—mid-1976. South East Thames Regional Health Authority, 1976. (Bibliography series no.1.)

2 Campbell, D. Nurses at work: follow-up and follow-through. (Work of the Visiting Nursing Service of Princess Margaret Hospital for Children, Perth.) Australian Nurses Journal, 6 (5), Nov 1976, 12-14.

3 Farr, K.S. Communication pitfalls in routine counseling. (With reference to routine visiting of parents by community nurse.) Pediatric Nursing, 5 (1), Jan/Feb 1979, 55-57.

4 Gow, M.A. Domiciliary paediatric care in Southampton. Queen's Nursing Journal, 19 (7), Oct 1976, 192, 205.

5 Hally, M.R. and others Paediatric home nursing scheme for Gateshead. (Using specially trained district nurses.) British Medical Journal, 1, 19 Mar 1977, 762-764.

6 Hunter, M.H.S. Paediatric hospital and home care. 1. Integrated programmes. (Home care programmes in Paddington, Birmingham, Edinburgh, Southampton and Gateshead.) Nursing Times, 73, 10 Mar 1977, Occ. papers, 33-36.

7 Kehoe, K. The nurse in child health services: some aspects. (In Australia.) Australian Nurses Journal, 6 (12), Jun 1977, 33-34, 37.

8 Morrow, H. and Amoako, D. An expanded role for nurses as paediatric health care providers in Ghana. (Paediatric nurse practitioners.) International Nursing Review, 27 (3), May/Jun 1980, 76-78.

9 Nursing They all call Linda. (Paediatric nurse practitioner who works in one of five nurse/doctor teams in an outpatient clinic.) Nursing, 7 (12), Dec 1977, 11-14.

10 Parkinson, M.W. The role of the area nurse child health. Nursing Times, 73, 27 Oct 1977, 1684-1685.

11 Reedy, B.L.E.C. and others A study of paediatric community nursing in a northern town. University of Newcastle upon Tyne Medical Care Research Unit, 1978.

12 Smith, J.P. Brent's integrated paediatric nursing unit. (Planning and development of integrated services.) Nursing Mirror, 145, 4 Aug 1977, 22-24.

13 Thiraudeau, M.F. and Reidy, M.M. Nursing makes a difference. A comparative study of the health behavior of mothers in three primary care agencies. (Their knowledge of the child's illness and care, and compliance with recommended care.) International Journal of Nursing Studies, 14 (2), 1977, 97-101.

14 Thomas, E. Paediatric liaison. (Attachment of a health visitor to a hospital paediatric department in Mid-Glamorgan.) Health Visitor, 49 (2), Feb 1976, 38.

15 Valman, H.B. The potential of paediatric day care. (To reduce hospital admission and perform outpatient clinic procedures in more relaxed atmosphere. Description of unit at Northwick Park Hospital.) Health Trends, 11 (2), May 1979, 34-35.

e SURGERY

1 Fochtman, D. and Raffensperger, J.G. editors Principles of nursing care for the pediatric surgery patient. 2nd ed. Boston: Little, Brown and Co., 1976.

2 Gatch, G. Intraoperative nursing care of pediatric patients. (Care of children in the operating theatre.) AORN Journal, 25 (5), Apr 1977, 873-877.

3 Ringrose, M. Nursing care in neonatal surgery. Nursing Mirror, 145, 6 Oct 1977, 19-21.

4 Smith, V.M. Seafield warm air contact mattress. (The development of a hot air mattress to prevent hypothermia during neonatal anaesthesia and surgery.) Nursing Times, 73, 10 Mar 1977 ABPN Supplement, 3-5.

5 Wagget, J. Advances in neonatal surgery. Nursing Mirror, 145, 1 Dec 1977, 13-17.

6 Waggoner, S.K. Nursing care of the infant in surgery. AORN Journal, 28 (5), Nov 1978, 827-839.

7 Young, D.G. and Weller, B.F. Baby surgery: nursing management and care. 2nd ed. Aylesbury: HM & M, 1979.

48 CHILD IN HOSPITAL

a GENERAL

1 Alcock, D. Hey, what about the kids? (Survey of practices regarding hospitalization of children in Ontario.) Canadian Nurse, 73 (11), Nov 1977, 38-41.

2 Alderson, P. compiler What is a children's ward: a summary of Department of Health and Social Security reports and recommendations. 2nd ed. National Association for the Welfare of Children in Hospital, 1980.

3 Association of British Paediatric Nurses Spotlight on children. (Issue on children in hospital.) Nursing Times, 76, 4 Dec 1980 ABPN1-ABPN8.

4 Australasian Nurses Journal Special issue on the Adelaide Children's Hospital, including its history. Australasian Nurses Journal, 4 (10), Apr 1976, 1-21.

5 Brennan, M. and Stoten, B. Children, poverty and illness. (Study of admissions to children's wards in Coventry which showed a relationship between parental unemployment and child hospitalisation.) New Society, 36, 24 Jun 1976, 681-682.

6 Castledine, G. Make it the year of the child. (Nursing care and psychological needs of children in hospital.) Nursing Mirror, 148, 8 Feb 1979, 12.

7 Consumers' Association Children in hospital: a report on the extent to which hospitals have implemented DHSS recommendations since the Platt Report. The Association, 1980.

8 Dartington, T. and others The psychological welfare of young children making long stays in hospital: an action research study Apr 1971-Jun 1975. Tavistock Institute of Human Relations, 1976.

9 Duberley, J. Sick children in hospital. (Implications of the Court report.) Nursing Times, 73, 23 Jun 1977, 942-944.

10 Freeman, A. A day in the life of a child in hospital. (An experiment in patient oriented nursing when a student nurse devotes a day to caring for only one child.) Nursing Times, 72, 16 Dec 1976, 1974-1976.

11   Gibb, A.   Stress in children's wards. (Based on a discussion with Anne Gibb.) Nursing, 10, Feb 1980, 444-446.

12   Gohsman, B.   Parents and staff: 'trying on' the problem. (Educating staff about the needs of the hospitalized child at St. Vincent's Hospital, Billings, Montana.) Pediatric Nursing, 3 (1), Jan/Feb 1977, 14-17.

13   Gruppo, P.A.   Helping the hospitalized child. 1. (Interviewing parents and reducing fear through play.) 2. The older child. Journal of Practical Nursing, 27 (5), May 1977, 14-17; (6), Jun 1977, 24-26.

14   Hall, D.J.   Bedside blues: the impact of social research on the hospital treatment of sick children. Journal of Advanced Nursing, 3 (1), Jan 1978, 25-37.

15   Hall, D.J. and Stacey, M. editors   Beyond separation: further studies of children in hospital. Routledge and Kegan Paul, 1979. (Routledge social science series.)

16   Halpern, S.   A pat on the back for a unique family hospital. (Stannington Children's Hospital in Northumberland which treats chronically ill children with social and emotional problems.) Health and Social Service Journal, 89, 23 Nov 1979, 1524-1525.

17   Hyde, A.   The kindly kidnappers. (Report on work of NAWCH and Children in Hospital Week.) Health and Social Service Journal, 89, 15 Jun 1979, 722-723.

18   Jolly, J.D.   Child care in North America — 2. How to be in hospital without being frightened. Nursing Times, 73, 1 Dec 1977, 1887-1888.

19   Jolly, J.D.   Child care in North America — 3. For those to whom hospitals must be home. (Children living in institutions.) Nursing Times, 73, 8 Dec 1977, 1930-1931.

20   Klinzing, D.R. and Klinzing, D.G.   The hospitalized child: communication techniques for health personnel. Englewood Cliffs, N.J.: Prentice-Hall, 1977.

21   Lyth, I.M.   Young children in long-stay hospitals. Midwife, Health Visitor and Community Nurse, 14 (9), Sep 1978, 308-310.

22   Lyttle, C.P.   'Business as usual' in Belfast's Falls Road. The past, present and future of the Royal Belfast Hospital for Sick Children. Nursing Mirror, 146, 29 Jun 1978, 13-14.

23   MacCarthy, D.   In the year of the child 1979: a report on the emotional well-being of children aged 0-5 years in hospital. National Association for the Welfare of Children in Hospital, 1979.

24   MacCormack, D.M.   The Sheffield Children's Hospital. A century of growth. (Three articles on the historical development, emotional needs of children and nurse education.) Nursing Mirror, 143, 1 Jul 1976, 45-47.

25   Medenwald, N.A.   Children's liberation — in a hospital! (With two pediatric bills of rights.) American Journal of Maternal-Child Nursing, 5 (4), Jul/Aug 1980, 231-232, 234.

26   Oswin, M.   Children in long-stay hospitals. Heinemann/Spastics International Medical Publications, 1978. (S.I.M.P. research monograph, no.5.)

27   Oswin, M.   The nurses. Contained in Oswin, M. Children in long-stay hospitals. Heinemann, 1978. Chapter 6, 76-99.

28   Paediatric News   Maintaining a paediatric environment within a general hospital. (Three short articles on intensive care, overcoming traumatic anaesthesia and the struggle to establish child medicine.) Nursing Times, 74, 14 Sep 1978 PN, 4-5.

29   Petrillo, M. and Sanger, S.   Emotional care of hospitalised children: an environmental approach. Philadelphia: Lippincott. 2nd ed. 1980.

30   Reekie, P.   One-hundred-year testimony to the care of children. (Centenary of the Royal Aberdeen Children's Hospital.) Health and Social Service Journal, 87, 9 Sep 1977, 1269-1271.

31   Reynolds, D.   When a granny fills in for Mum. (Mothering-type care of children in hospital through granny schemes.) Nursing Mirror, 148, 15 Feb 1979, 20-22.

32   Roberts, J.   Freedom from pain and fear — a nursing viewpoint. (Of children's reactions, especially in hospital.) Australasian Nurses Journal, 8 (9), Jul 1979, 19, 23-24.

33   Robinson, G.C. and Clarke, H.F.   The hospital care of children: a review of contemporary issues. Oxford University Press, 1980.

34   Sail, T. and Sail, L.   Children in hospital. Gloucester: Thornhill Press, 1976. (Thornhill Guide, no.2.)

35   Savage, J.H.   Anti-climbing hospital — cot attachment. (Description and details of construction.) Nursing Mirror, 144, 12 May 1977, 68-69.

36   Savage, J.H.   Mattress-tilting devices. (For cots.) Nursing Mirror, 144, 2 Jun 1977, 32-34.

37   Shumaker Al Ageel, M.C.   Reactions of a hospitalized school-age child to separation and restricted mobility. (Nursing intervention to overcome health crisis.) Maternal-Child Nursing Journal, 7 (3), Fall 1978, 163-173.

38   Travis, G.   Chronic illness in children: its impact on child and family. Stanford University Press, 1976.

39   Wessex Regional Library and Information Service   Children in hospital. Southampton: Wessex Regional Library and Information Service, 1977. (Communication series.)

40   Woodward, J.   Has your child been in hospital? National Association for the Welfare of Children in Hospital, 1978.

41   Wynne, J. and Hull, D.   Why are children admitted to hospital? (Analysis of 399 admissions to Nottingham Children's Hospital.) British Medical Journal, 2, 29 Oct 1977, 1140-1142.

42   Young, M.   Children in hospital. Caring for the needs of the child and the family. Careful preparation before admission, and individualised care during their stay. Nursing Times, 75, 3 May 1979, 740-741.

43   Younger, N.R.   Children in hospital. (Review of studies and current trends.) Nursing Times, 74, 16 Mar 1978, Paediatric News, 5-8.

b ADOLESCENTS

1   Bamford, F.N. and others   An adolescent ward. (At St. Mary's Hospital, Manchester.) British Medical Journal, 2, 20 Aug 1977, 503-506.

2   Freeberg, S. and others   Nursing care in a combined adolescent medical-psychiatric unit. Journal of Psychiatric Nursing and Mental Health Services, 14 (11), Nov 1976, 13-15.

3   Hofmann, A.D. and others   The hospitalized adolescent: a guide to managing the ill and injured youth. Collier Macmillan, 1976.

4   Jelneck, L.J.   The special needs of the adolescent with chronic illness. American Journal of Maternal Child Nursing, 2 (1), Jan/Feb 1977, 57-61.

5   Lincoln, L.   Effects of illness and hospital procedures on body image in adolescence: a review of the literature. Maternal Child Nursing Journal, 7 (2), Summer 1978, 55-60.

6   Macherski, H.   Nursing care study. A teenage homosexual. (In the Adolescent Unit, Bethlem Hospital.) Nursing Mirror, 147, 5 Oct 1978, 29-32.

7   Parker, G. and Gibson, C.   Development of the hospitalized adolescent anxiety tool. (Self-appraisal questionnaire for nurses to use in assessing adolescent patients' anxieties.) Journal of Psychiatric Nursing and Mental Health Services, 15 (12), Dec 1977, 21-24.

8   Turner, J.   Nursing in the adolescent service. (Role of nurse in Young People's Unit, Macclesfield.) Nursing Times, 74, 14 Dec 1978, 2049-2051.

c FAMILY

1   Bakare, P.O.   Attitudes towards mothers' participation in nursing activities: nursing research. (Survey of the role of the parent in caring for the hospitalized child.) Nigerian Nurse, 8 (2), Apr/Jun 1976, 6-14.

2   Chadwick, B.J. and others   Maintaining the hospitalized child's home ties. American Journal of Nursing, 78 (8), Aug 1978, 1361-1362.

3   Dew, T.A. and others   Parents in pediatric R.R. (Visiting by parents in recovery room.) AORN Journal, 26 (2), Aug 1977, 266-273.

4   Fagin, C. and Nusbaum, J.G.   Parental visiting privileges in pediatric units: a survey. (Of selected US hospitals.) Journal of Nursing Administration, 8 (3), Mar 1978, 24-27.

5   Goyea, H.S.   Parents-staff communication in a children's ward and parents' knowledge of their children's illnesses. (Survey in Nigeria.) Community Health, 9 (1), Aug 1977, 44-48.

6   Hennessey, J.A.   Hospitalized toddlers' responses to mothers' tape recordings during brief separations. Maternal Child Nursing Journal, 5 (2), Summer 1976, 69-91.

7   Hymovich, D.P.   Parents of sick children, their needs and tasks. Pediatric Nursing, 2 (5), Sep/Oct 1976, 9-13.

8 Jolly, J.D. Child care in North America — 4. Parental involvement: how far will it go? (Policy of children's hospitals.) Nursing Times, 73, 15 Dec 1977, 1969-1970.

9 McNeur, R. Parents in the paediatric ward. New Zealand Nursing Journal, 68 (11), Nov 1975, 20-21.

10 Oberlander, R. Parent care units bring home to the hospital. (Hospital units designed to treat whole child rather than just the illness.) Hospitals, 54 (21), 1 Nov 1980, 81-85.

11 Pederson, C.J. and Anderson, J.M. Factors that impact data collection from children. (Importance of establishing rapport with child and parent and their psychosocial needs.) Cancer Nursing, 3 (6), Dec 1980, 439-444.

12 Purcal, K.M. Towards understanding the hospitalised child and his visiting mother from a single-parent family. Australasian Nurses Journal, 5 (8), Mar 1977, 15-19, 22, 24.

13 Reynolds, D. Parents on the wards: when the child goes into hospital, let the mother go in, too. (Report on current progress towards implementation of the Platt report's recommendations.) Nursing Mirror, 147, 2 Nov 1978, 15-18.

14 Tibble, J. Family receptionist in a paediatric unit. (Mother who looks after needs of parents visiting children at Northwick Park Hospital. Includes guidance notes given to parents.) Nursing Times, 75, 1 Feb 1979, 211-212.

15 Veitch, A. Victims of after thoughts. (On barriers to unrestricted visiting by parents of their children in hospital.) Guardian, 22 Dec 1977, 9.

d PATIENT TEACHING AND ANXIETY

1 Astin, E.W. Self reported fears of hospitalised and non-hospitalised children aged ten to twelve. Maternal Child Nursing Journal, 6 (1), Spring 1977, 17-24.

2 Australasian Nurses Journal 'I'm to have my tonsils out'. (Disc of song and dialogue to tell parents and children about hospitalisation.) Australasian Nurses Journal, 3 (4), Oct 1977, 28.

3 Burke, D. and others Health helpers. (Student nurses teach nursery school children about hospitalisation.) Canadian Nurse, 72 (12), Dec 1976, 17.

4 Canadian Nurse A child life program in action. (At the Children's Hospital, Eastern Ontario, with aim of minimising trauma of hospitalization.) Canadian Nurse, 73 (11), Nov 1977, 42-45.

5 Cox, N.C. Psychological effects of surgery on children. AORN Journal, 24 (3), Sep 1976, 425-432.

6 Davis, J.L. Preoperative program prepares children for surgery. (Pre-admission tours.) AORN Journal, 26 (2), Aug 1977, 249-256.

7 Ferguson, F. and others Learning about the hospital at home. (Scheme at Alberta Children's Hospital involving pre-admission visits by hospital nurse to patient's home.) Canadian Nurse, 75 (1), Jan 1979, 44-48.

8 Ferguson, U. What Danny didn't know. (14 year-old's fear of a tracheostomy and the importance of patient teaching.) Nursing (U.S.), 10 (11), Nov 1980, 31.

9 Gohsman, B. and Yunck, M. Dealing with the threats of hospitalization. Pediatric Nursing, 5 (5), Sep/Oct 1979, 32-35.

10 Grant, D. VIP treatment proves this hospital really cares. (Hospital visits for well children in Nova Scotia.) Canadian Nurse, 72 (7), Jul 1976, 24-27.

11 Jolly, J.D. Preparing children for hospital. (Study tour of innovative centres in North America.) Nursing Times, 72, 30 Sep 1976, 1532-1533.

12 Klinzing, D.R. and Klinzing, D.G. Improving the communication between a nursing staff and hospitalized children. Journal of Continuing Education in Nursing, 11 (5), Sep/Oct 1980, 16-19.

13 Lukanivk, C. and others Nurses in tabards. (In Bristol Ward, Charing Cross Hospital, to gain children's confidence.) Nursing Times, 76, 31 Jul 1980, 1346-1347.

14 McCann, B. Tell me about your picture. (Encouraging hospitalised children to express feelings as part of nursing care plan.) Canadian Nurse, 72 (9), Sep 1976, 50-51.

15 Meng, A.L. Parents' and childrens' reactions toward impending hospitalization for surgery. (Research study.) Maternal-Child Nursing Journal, 9 (2), Summer 1980, 83-98.

16 Pidgeon, V.A. Child thought and counselling implications in the hospital. Patient Counseling and Health Education, 1 (1), Spring 1978, 4-7.

17 Rasmussen, M. Hospital admission through a child's eyes. Pediatric Nursing, 3 (3), May/Jun 1977, 43-46.

18 Ritchie, J.A. Preparation of toddlers and preschool children for hospital procedures. Canadian Nurse, 75 (11), Dec 1979, 30-32.

19 Roskies, R. and others Emergency hospitalization of young children: some neglected psychological considerations. Medical Care, 8 (7), Jul 1975, 570-581.

20 Schrader, S. Hospital tours for well children help them to cope. (In University of Colorado Medical Center.) AORN Journal, 26 (1), Jul 1977, 13-14.

21 Schrader, E.S. Preparation play helps children in hospitals. (To reduce anxiety and help prepare them for surgery.) AORN Journal, 30 (2), Aug 1979, 336, 340-341.

22 Schrader, E.S. Preparing children for surgery. (Reprinted from AORN Journal.) NATNews, 17 (6), Jun 1980, 11, 13-14.

23 Smith, E.C. Are you really communicating? A test of what pre-school hospitalized children really gleaned from explanations of their bodies and their illnesses yielded some surprises. American Journal of Nursing, 77 (12), Dec 1977, 1966-1968.

24 Snell, B. and McLellan, C. Whetting hospitalized preschoolers' appetites. Nurses use knowledge of child development and information from parents to encourage eating in the hospital. American Journal of Nursing, 76 (3), Mar 1976, 413-415.

25 Suran, B.G. and Hatcher, H.P. The psychological treatment of hospitalized children with failure to thrive. Pediatric Nursing, 1 (5), Sep/Oct 1975, 10-17.

26 Visintainer, M. The effects of pre-admission psychological preparation on children's stress responses and adjustment during and following hospitalization for minor surgery. (Synopsis of final report.) Nursing Research Report, 12 (2), May 1977, 3-5.

27 Williams, P.D. Preparation of school-age children for surgery: a program in preventive pediatrics — Philippines. (Research study.) International Journal of Nursing Studies, 17 (2), 1980, 107-119.

e PLAY

1 Australasian Nurses Journal Special issue on play in hospitals. Australasian Nurses Journal, 5 (4), Oct 1976, 2-63.

2 Burr, S. Play for children in hospital. (Comments on the report of the 'Expert Group on Play in Hospital' issued with DHSS Health Circular (76) 5.) Nursing Times, 73, 10 Mar 1977, ABPN Supplement, 5-6.

3 Butler, A. and others Child's play in therapy. (The pre-school child in hospital.) Canadian Nurse, 71 (12), Dec 1975, 35-37.

4 Cook, A. Play schemes for children in hospital. Midwife, Health Visitor and Community Nurse, 14 (3), Mar 1978, 82-83.

5 Department of Health and Social Security Report of the expert group on play for children in hospital. (DHSS, 1976.) Summarised in Journal of Advanced Nursing, 1 (5), Sep 1976, 425-428. Comment in Health and Social Service Journal, 86, 6 Jun 1976, 1020.

6 Goldman, M. and others A play program in a community hospital? (Scheme in Michigan using nursing students.) Maternal Child Nursing Journal, 3 (1), Jan/Feb 1978, 42-45.

7 Hall, D.J. Social relations and innovation: changing the state of play in hospitals. Routledge and Kegan Paul, 1977. (Medicine, illness and society series.)

8 Harding, V. The importance of play for children in hospital (and the role of the play specialist). Nursing Mirror, 144, 20 Jan 1977, 46-48.

9 Harvey, S. Hospital play schemes. Health and Social Service Journal, 86, 5 Jun 1976, 1026-1027.

10 Harvey, S. Only jungle-trained mechanics with nerves of steel need apply. (Provision of play for children in acute and psychiatric hospitals.) Health and Social Service Journal, 86, 10 Dec 1976, 2200-2201.

11 Hunter, M.H.S. Planning play for children in hospital. (In Scotland.) Nursing Mirror, 146, 4 May 1978, Supplement, viii-ix.

12 Jolly, H. Why children must be able to play in hospital. Times, 21 Apr 1976, 19.

13 Knudsen, K. Play therapy. Preparing the

young child for surgery. Nursing Clinics of North America, 7 (4), Dec 1975, 679-686.

14 Latimer, E. Play is everybody's business in the children's ward. (Need for all staff to join in this aspect of care and the role of the playleader and play coordinator.) Nursing Mirror, 147, 14 Sep 1978, 21-24.

15 Maxwell, G.I. A school for children in hospital. (At Guy's Hospital.) Nursing Times, 76, 4 Dec 1980, ABPN 2-ABPN 3.

16 National Union of Teachers Hospital schools: a challenge for education? NUT, 1978.

17 Shufer, S. Communicating with young children. Teaching via the play-discussion group. (In hospital.) American Journal of Nursing, 77 (12), Dec 1977, 1960-1962.

18 Taylor, M.M. and Williams, H.A. Use of therapeutic play in the ambulatory pediatric hematology clinic. Cancer Nursing, 3 (6), Dec 1980, 433-437.

19 Welch, C. The nurse's role in play. Nursing Care, 10 (1), Jan 1977, 14-15.

20 Weller, B.F. Helping sick children play. Baillière Tindall, 1980.

21 Young, M. Children in hospital. The growth and organisation of playgroups: play seminars for student nurses. Nursing Times, 75, 3 May 1979, 738-739.

f TERMINAL CARE AND DEATH

1 Association of British Paediatric Nurses Spotlight on children. (Issue on the dying child and his family.) Nursing Times, 76, 19 Jun 1980, ABPN 1-8.

2 Ball, M. Nurse or mortician? (Problems nurses face in caring for children on life-support systems who have suffered total cerebral death.) Journal of Neurosurgical Nursing, 10 (2), Jun 1978, 66-67.

3 Bhaduri, R. Care of the terminal patient—4. A family's sorrow. (Death of a child of a family from Bangladesh.) Nursing Times, 75, 12 Apr 1979, 638-639.

4 Bluebond-Langner, M. The private worlds of dying children. Princeton: Princeton University Press, 1978.

5 Chapman, J.A. and Goodall, J. Dying children need help too. (Neglect of control of symptoms in dying children illustrated by two case studies of children with cystic fibrosis.) British Medical Journal, 1, 3 Mar 1979, 593-594.

6 Chapman, J.A. and Goodall, J. Helping a child to live whilst dying. (Case-history of child with cancer over three-year period.) Lancet, 1, 5 Apr 1980, 753-756.

7 Codden, P. The meaning of death for parents and the child. Maternal Child Nursing Journal, 6 (1), Spring 1977, 9-16.

8 Coplestone, J. Nursing care study. Brain tumour: a child dies—and ward staff give support in the home. Nursing Mirror, 148, 18 Jan 1979, 20-23.

9 Gyulay, J.E. Care of the dying child. Nursing Clinics of North America, 11 (1), Mar 1976, 95-107.

10 Gyulay, J.E. The dying child. New York: McGraw-Hill, 1978.

11 Leyn, R.M. Terminally ill children and their families: a study of the variety of responses to fatal illness. Maternal Child Nursing Journal, 5 (3), Fall 1976, 179-188.

12 Martinson, I.M. Caring for the dying child. (Nursing care of children, predominantly children dying of cancer.) Nursing Clinics of North America, 14 (3), Sep 1979, 467-474.

13 Martinson, I.M. Dying children at home. (Research project and development of model of care involving comfort-orientated care provided by family with assistance of a home care nurse and doctor.) Nursing Times, 76, 18/25 Dec 1980, Occ. papers, 129-132.

14 Martinson, I.M. editor Home care for the dying child: professional and family perspectives. New York: Appleton-Century-Crofts, 1976.

15 Martinson, I.M. Why don't we let them home to die? (Nurse's experiences of caring for dying children at home.) RN Magazine, 39 (1), Jan 1976, 58-65.

16 Martinson, I.M. and others Death and dying: selected attitudes of Minnesota's registered nurses. (Regarding home care for dying children.) Nursing Research, 27 (4), Jul/Aug 1978, 226-229.

17 Martinson, I.M. and others When the patient is dying. Home care for the child. (Research project in Minneapolis to evaluate its benefits and costs.) American Journal of Nursing, 77 (11), Nov 1977, 1815-1817.

18 Mills, G.C. Books to help children understand death. American Journal of Nursing, 79 (2), Feb 1979, 291-295.

19 Moldow, D.G. and Martinson, I.M. From research to reality—home care for the dying child. (Pilot project and evaluation of programmes in Minnesota.) Maternal Child Nursing Journal, 5 (3), May/Jun 1980, 159-160, 162, 166.

20 Renshaw, D.C. The nurse's role with parents of the dying child. Journal of Nursing Education, 18 (1), Jan 1979, 17-20.

21 SPOTLIGHT on children. Death, the child and his family. (Editorial and four articles including role of hospital chaplain.) Nursing Times, 76, 6 Mar 1980, ABPN 1-ABPN 8.

22 Vidovich, M. Caring for kids—death in the I.C.U. (Psychological aspects of care.) Australian Nurses Journal, 9 (6), Dec/Jan 1980, 43-44.

23 Zach, H. Children and death. Social Work Today, 9, 13 Jun 1978, 12-13.

49 HANDICAPPED CHILDREN

a GENERAL

1 Apley, J. editor Care of the handicapped child: a festschrift for Ronald MacKeith. Heinemann, 1978. (Clinics in developmental medicine, no.67.)

2 Baker, J. and others A specialized service for handicapped children. (In Leicester.) Health Visitor, 53 (5), May 1980, 164-165.

3 Brooks, B.G.B. Psychiatric aspects of chronic physical handicap in adolescents. Community Health, 8 (3), Jan 1977, 170-174.

4 Darbyshire, P. Nursing care study. A severely mentally and physically handicapped child. (Child with cerebral palsy and epilepsy. By staff nurse.) Nursing Times, 76, 10 Jan 1980, 64-68.

5 Dawson, J. The severely disabled. (Role of specialist HV in survey of young dependent disabled and formation of register.) Health Visitor, 52 (7), Jul 1979, 262-264.

6 Disabled Living Foundation The specialised health visitor for the handicapped baby, young child and schoolchild: a report. Disabled Living Foundation, 1979.

7 Egan, D. The young handicapped child—a true concern. Public Health, 90 (3), Mar 1976, 93-99.

8 Elliott, P. The garden and the handicapped child. Disabled Living Foundation, 1978.

9 Gruppo, P.A. Helping the handicapped child. (Includes section on nursing considerations for the hospitalised handicapped child.) Journal of Practical Nursing, 28 (9), Sep 1978, 30-32, 36-37.

10 Gunn, A.D.G. The physically handicapped adolescent. Journal of Community Nursing, 1 (11), May 1978, 14-15.

11 Last, M. and others Community nursing and psychology—4: Toilet training; 2: Children with special needs. (Handicapped children.) Journal of Community Nursing, 2 (4), Oct 1978, 16-17.

12 A NEW place in the world. (Problems of designing furniture for severely disabled children.) Nursing Times, 72, 34, 26 Aug 1976, Key Clinical, 25-28.

13 Nursing Mirror The management of gross handicaps. (Catheterisation of the terminally ill, in spina bifida and hydrocephalus, congenital abnormalities of the kidney and intermittent non-sterile catheterisation of children.) Nursing Mirror, 146, 6 Apr 1978, Supplement, i, iii, v, vii, ix, xi, xiii, xv.

14 Peckham, C. and Pearson, R. The prevalence and nature of ascertained handicap in the National Child Developmental Study (1958 Cohort). Public Health, 90 (3), Mar 1976, 111-121.

15 Riley, P.M. The occupational therapist's role with the younger disabled. British Journal of Occupational Therapy, 43 (1), Jan 1980, 10-12.

16 Robinson, W. Language of love. (Bliss symbols: a new system of communication for severely handicapped children.) Nursing Mirror, 144, 12 May 1977, 64-67.

17 Russell, P. The wheelchair child. Souvenir Press, 1978. (Human horizons series.)

18 Ryan, M. Feeding a handicapped child. (Problems and their solution.) Health and Social Service Journal, 87, 9 Sep 1977, 1278.

19 Scrutton, D.R. The physical management

of children with hemiplegia. Physiotherapy, 62 (9), Sep 1976, 285-293.

20 Shearer, A. Children in residence: provision for handicapped children. (Mentally and physically handicapped.) Social Work Today, 10, 3 Apr 1979, 14-19.

21 Skellern, J. The self concept of children and adolescents and the effects of physical disability. Australian Nurses Journal, 8 (6), Dec/Jan 1978/1979, 36-38.

22 Slack, P.A. N.O. news. (Nursing Officer for the district handicap team recommended in the Court report.) Nursing Times, 74, 13 Apr 1978, Community Outlook, 98.

23 Stacey, M. Charisma, power and altruism: a discussion of research in a child development centre. (Staff's and parents' attitudes in a multidisciplinary assessment centre for pre-school handicapped children.) Sociology of Health and Illness, 2 (1), Mar 1980, 64-90. 64-90.

24 Stephens, M.K.J. Handicapped children in Denmark. (Council of Europe Medical Fellowship study tour.) Queen's Nursing Journal, 19 (7), Oct 1976, 193, 196.

25 Sunday Times Suffer the children: the story of thalidomide. André Deutsch, 1979.

26 Treharne, D.A. Management of feeding difficulties. (In physically and mentally handicapped children.) Nursing Times, 75, 18 Jan 1979, 108-109.

27 Webb, Y. Feeding and nutrition problems of physically and mentally handicapped children in Britain: a report. (Based on visits to institutions.) Journal of Human Nutrition, 34 (4), Aug 1980, 281-285.

28 Weller, S.D.V. Points of view. Co-operation in the care of handicapped children. Public Health, 90 (4), May 1976, 187-190.

29 Wightman, F. Community nursing care study. A handicapped child. Nursing Times, 72, 16 Dec 1976, 1966-1967.

30 Wisbeach, A. The treatment of a young handicapped child. (Programme designed by physiotherapist and occupational therapist.) Nursing Mirror, 145, 8 Dec 1977, Supplement, xi, xiii, xv.

31 Wisbeach, A. and Holt, K.S. Children in wheelchairs. (Survey of problems of using wheelchairs and need for guidance and advice for parents.) British Medical Journal, 281, 19 Jul 1980, 199-201.

b EDUCATION

1 Beresford, P. and Tuckwell, P. Schools for all. (The case for integrated education for severely mentally handicapped children.) Nursing Times, 74, 19 Oct 1978, 1708-1709.

2 Beresford, P. and Tuckwell, P. Schools for all: education of severely mentally handicapped children. Mind/Campaign for the Mentally Handicapped, 1978.

3 Bowley, A.H. and Gardner, L. The handicapped child: educational and psychological guidance for the organically handicapped. 4th ed. Edinburgh: Churchill Livingstone, 1980.

4 Brown, A. Too young to be left on the shelf. (Comment on Warnock report and reactions to it.) Nursing Mirror, 150, 3 Apr 1980, 8.

5 Browning, E. Speech impairment. (Management and education of the speech impaired child.) Health and Social Service Journal, 88, 6 Jan 1978, 18.

6 Clark, J. Special educational needs of the young handicapped. After Court comes Warnock. Summary of and comments on the Warnock Report and its implications for nurses. Nursing Mirror, 147, 27 Jul 1978, 7-9.

7 Committee of Enquiry into the Education of Handicapped Children and Young People Special educational needs: report of the Committee. HMSO, 1978. (Cmnd 7212. Chairman Mrs H.M. Warnock.)

8 Critchley, M. and Critchley, E.A. Dyslexia defined. Heinemann, 1978.

9 Darbyshire, P. Play and profoundly handicapped children. Nursing Times, 76, 28 Aug 1980, 1538-1543.

10 Dasari, B.D. The role of recreation for the handicapped child. British Journal of Occupational Therapy, 40 (2), Feb 1977, 40-42.

11 Department of Education and Science The education of children in hospitals for the mentally handicapped. HMSO, 1978. (HMI Series: matters for discussion; 7.)

12 Duffen, W.W. Reading before talking: a father's programme of home teaching. National Society for Mentally Handicapped Children, 1978.

13 Elias, B. 499 reasons to think twice. (Effect of 1976 Education Act on special schools, and reasons why they should not be abolished.) Health and Social Service Journal, 87, 5 May 1978, 510-511.

14 Franklin, A.W. Understanding dyslexia. Nursing Mirror, 146, 5 Jan 1978, 12-14.

15 Freeman, P. Tactile learning methods: the education of deaf/blind children. Health and Social Service Journal, 88, 13 Jan 1978, 48.

16 Hales, A. The children of Skylark Ward: teaching severely handicapped children. Cambridge University Press, 1978.

17 Hickey, K. Teaching dyslexic children. Nursing Mirror, 146, 5 Jan 1978, 15-17.

18 Higgs, C.J. Entry into special schools: new assessment procedures and their impact. Royal Society of Health Journal, 99 (1), Feb 1979, 32-33.

19 John, E. The Warnock report. (On the education of handicapped children.) Midwife, Health Visitor and Community Nurse, 15 (2), Feb 1979, 47-48, 50.

20 Josefowicz, A. Preparing the young handicapped child for school. British Journal of Occupational Therapy, 43 (7), Jul 1980, 230-232.

21 Lancet Commentary for Westminster. Children with special educational needs. (Comment on the Warnock report.) Lancet, 1, 3 Jun 1978, 1218-1219.

22 Lear, R. Play helps: toys and activities for handicapped children. Heinemann, 1977.

23 Leyland, S.J. Special playgroups in an assessment centre. (Wilfrid Sheldon Paediatric Assessment Centre, Belgrave Hospital for Children—part of King's College Hospital.) Nursing Times, 72, 18 Nov 1976, 1815-1817.

24 Marais, E. Children safely at play. (Made-to-order play apparatus for severely physically handicapped children.) Nursing Mirror, 150, 7 Feb 1980, 26-27.

25 Marfleet, J. Educational subnormality. (Factors influencing the decision to send a child to a special school.) Nursing Times, 72, 13 May 1976, 747-749.

26 Miller, L. Education of pre-school handicapped children. (Role of Advisory Service for Pre-School Handicapped Children in Hertfordshire.) Midwife, Health Visitor and Community Nurse, 16 (8), Aug 1980, 334-385.

27 Moreland, L. Toy libraries. Health and Social Service Journal, 86, 5 Jun 1976, 1024-1025.

28 Newell, P. Strategies for education. (Debate over integration of mentally handicapped children into 'normal' education system.) Mind Out, 28, May/Jun 1978, 9-12.

29 Nusson, F.A. When a woman's place is not in the home. (Florence Treloar School in Hampshire for physically handicapped girls.) British Medical Journal, 1, 30 Apr 1977, 1141-1142.

30 Pavlidis, G.T. Dyslexia: why the eyes have it. The main characteristics and functional significance of the four oculomotor sub-systems, and the different kinds of eye movements found in different visual tasks. Nursing Mirror, 150, 24 Jan 1980, 24-27.

31 Pavlidis, G.T. Eye movements in reading and beyond. (Dyslexia.) How to catch his eye. Nursing Mirror, 150, 17 Jan 1980, 22-26; 31 Jan 1980, 24-27.

32 Pearson, R. and Peckham, C. Handicapped children in second schools from The National Child Development Study (1958 Cohort.) Public Health, 91 (6), Nov 1977, 296-304.

33 Penney, A.O. and Bignell, S.G.L. The provision of nursing care in special schools. Department of Health and Social Security, 1977.

34 Pre-School Playgroups Association Guidelines for playgroups with a handicapped child. PPA, 1979.

35 Rapp, D. When production lines can help develop the mentally handicapped... (Scheme at Meldreth Manor School for ESN cerebral palsy children in which the children make and market electronic behaviour modification devices.) Health and Social Service Journal, 88, 27 Oct 1978, 1222-1223.

36 Robinson, W. Ingfield Manor. Spastics Society's special school where young multi-handicapped children are being educated by a revolutionary new system. Nursing Mirror, 143, 16 Dec 1976, 65-67.

37 Robinson, W. Westoning Manor. (A MacIntyre School for the mentally handicapped in Bedfordshire.) Nursing Mirror, 143, 28 Oct 1976, 64-65.

38 **Rogers, M.** Early identification and intervention of children with learning problems. (Assessment at the Children's Hospital, Columbus, Ohio.) Pediatric Nursing, 2 (1), Jan/Feb 1976, 21-26.

39 **Ross, T.** Betwixt and between... (Problems of dyslexic children.) Nursing Mirror, 148, 1 Mar 1979, 14-16.

40 **Sloss, J.** Play therapy for maladjusted children. Social Work Today, 9, 1 Aug 1978, 14-15.

41 **Smith, L.F.** An experiment with play therapy. (Psychotherapy with nine-year-old boy.) American Journal of Nursing, 77 (12), Dec 1977, 1963-1965.

42 **Stafford, S.F.** Play and toy library. (For handicapped children.) Physiotherapy, 64 (3), Mar 1978, 68-69.

43 **Stevens, M.** The educational and social needs of children with severe handicap. 2nd ed. Arnold, 1976.

44 **Stevens, M.** Observe, then teach: an observational approach to teaching mentally handicapped children. 2nd ed. Arnold, 1978.

45 **Swaffield, L.** Then there were toys. (Report of visit to Toy Libraries Association, with details of publications on p.204-205, and useful organisations on p.208.) Nursing Times, 76, 10 Jul 1980, Community Outlook, 203-205, 207-208.

46 **Waddon, A.** Understanding dyslexia. (Diagnosis, characteristics, causes and remedial teaching.) Nursing Mirror, 144, 5 May 1977, 53-54.

47 **Warnock, M.** Children with special needs: the Warnock Report. British Medical Journal, 1, 10 Mar 1979, 667-668.

48 **Wertheimer, A.** Warnock: another forgotten report? (Issues in and problems in implementation of the Warnock report.) Mind Out, 37, Nov/Dec 1979, 16-17.

49 **Wroe, B.** Organising a toy library: a description of the IMS toy library service. Kidderminster: Institute of Mental Subnormality, 1979.

c FAMILY

1 **Australian Nurses Journal** The extended role for the nurse—involvement with the family. (Two articles on the role of Appliance Centre, Royal Children's Hospital, Melbourne, in providing support for the handicapped child and their family.) Australian Nurses' Journal, 5 (8), Feb 1976, 33-36.

2 **Ballard, R.** Sharing the pain—help for parents with a handicapped child. Health Visitor, 49 (12), Dec 1976, 395-396.

3 **Bradshaw, J.** Services that miss their mark and leave families in need. (Families of handicapped children.) Health and Social Service Journal, 87, 15 Apr 1977, 664-665.

4 **Brown, M.S.** The Gordons needed all the help they could get. (Case study of family with

deaf-blind child, by paediatric nurse practitioner, with bibliography.) Nursing, 7 (10), Oct 1977, 40-43.

5 **Crout, E.** Parents who need care too. (Role of nurses including HVs with parents of handicapped children.) Nursing Mirror, 149, 18 Oct 1979, 33-35.

6 **Ford, J.D.** An interpersonal-effectiveness approach to consumer health education. (Workshops for parents of handicapped children.) Medical Care, 17 (10), Oct 1979, 1061-1067.

7 **Gordeuk, A.** Motherhood and a less than perfect child: a literary review. (Motivation for motherhood and the effects of a handicapped child on the maternal role.) Maternal Child Nursing Journal, 5 (2), Summer 1976, 57-68.

8 **Gregory, D.** Family assessment and intervention plan: (for parents with a handicapped or impaired child.) Pediatric Nursing, 1 (4), Jul/Aug 1975, 23-29.

9 **Haus, B.F. and Thompson, S.** The effect of nursing intervention on a program of behavior modification by parents in the home (of nine neurological impaired children.) Journal of Psychiatric Nursing and Mental Health Services, 14 (8), Aug 1976, 9-16.

10 **Hyde, A.** A view from the hill top of problems in the real world. (Honeylands Family Support Unit, Exeter, for local families with handicapped child which offers day and short-term residential care.) Health and Social Service Journal, 89, 14 Dec 1979, 1612-1615.

11 **Institute for Research into Mental and Multiple Handicap. Library and Information Service** Books for parents of a handicapped child: an annotated reading list. The Institute, 1976.

12 **Jacobs, J.** Improving communications between health service professionals and parents of handicapped children: a case study. (Survey in Brighton of parents' knowledge of sources of help including health visitors.) British Journal of Mental Subnormality, 23 (2), Dec 1977, 54-60.

13 **Kirakowska, W.** Counselling for special need. The birth of a handicapped child puts a great strain on a marriage relationship. New Psychiatry, 3 (9), 29 Apr 1976, 14-15.

14 **Miller, M.** Childhood disability—group-work with mothers. Social Work Today, 7 (1), 1 Apr 1976, 15-16.

15 **Miller, M.** The family and the handicapped child: disinherited marriage. (How three couples have coped with a handicapped child.) Midwife, Health Visitor and Community Nurse, 12 (1), Jan 1976, 13-14.

16 **Nettles, O.** Counselling parents of children wtih handicap. Crawley: Tappenden Print Co., 1978.

17 **Porter, S.F.** Family-centered conferences for better trauma care. (Rehabilitation of paraplegic teenager.) Nursing, 8 (10), Oct 1978, 70-77.

18 **Pugh, G. and Russell, P.** Shared care: support services for families with handicapped children. National Children's Bureau, 1977.

19 **Robinson, T.** Self-help parents' groups.

(Parents of handicapped children.) Social Service Quarterly, 50 (4), Apr/Jun 1977, 291-294.

20 **Rocheleau, S.W.** I've got the greatest 24-hour-a-day job in the world. (Respite care, where nurse provides short-term care for handicapped children in her home to relieve parents.) RN Magazine, 40 (10), Oct 1977, 54-58.

21 **Webster, E.J.** Counseling with parents of handicapped children: guidelines for improving communication. New York: Grune and Stratton, 1977.

22 **Wilkin, D.** Responsibility that becomes a prison for mothers. (Study by interview with 120 mothers of severely handicapped children.) Health and Social Service Journal, 86, 28 Jan 1977, 152-153.

d HOSPITALS AND UNITS

1 **ALISON House** Home from home in London. (Alison House, which opened on January 4, is the first short-stay home for mentally and physically handicapped young people in central London.) Nursing Times, 73, 3 Mar 1977, 290-291.

2 **ASHBY Ward**: a new unit for the disabled. (First purpose-built unit for the younger disabled.) Nursing Mirror, 142, 22 Jan 1976, 71.

3 **Bailey, M.** Centre for young handicapped. (Facilities available at the new Ryegate Centre for handicapped children at the Children's Hospital, Sheffield.) Nursing Mirror, 146, 12 Jan 1978, 8-9.

4 **Bailey, M.** Home from home. (Ryegate Centre at the Children's Hospital, Sheffield, for handicapped children.) Nursing Times, 74 (2), 12 Jan 1977, 53.

5 **Benson, T.B. and Williams, E.** The younger disabled unit at Fazakerley Hospital. British Medical Journal, 2, 11 Aug 1979, 369-371.

6 **Brown, H.J. and Sutcliffe, R.L.G.** Favell House: a young disabled unit. Practitioner, 217, Nov 1976, 773-776, 779-782.

7 **Green, R. and Hisley, T.** Orchestrating all the strings. (Work of the Ormskirk Child Development Centre for physically and mentally handicapped children.) Health and Social Service Journal, 89, 6 Apr 1979, 381.

8 **Honeylands Unit** Family unit. (Royal Devon and Exeter Hospital. Honeylands unit to support families of handicapped children.) Nursing Times, 72 (42), 21 Oct 1976, 1625.

9 **Kuosma, C.** Rehabilitation of the handicapped child. (Neurological ward in a Helsinki hospital.) International Nursing Review, 26 (5), Sep/Oct 1979, 139-140.

10 **Pellatt, D.J.R.** Caring for the younger disabled. (Orchard View, Ham Green Hospital, Bristol.) Nursing Mirror, 142, 3 Jun 1976, 57-59.

11 **Pill, R.** The long-stay child patient: the problems. (Survey at the Medical Sociology Research Centre, Swansea, of physically impaired children.) Nursing Times, 73, 7 Jul 1977, Occ. papers, 89-92.

12 **Sheahan, J.** Caring for handicapped children at the Leon Gillis Unit. (At Queen Mary's Hospital, Roehampton.) Nursing Mirror, 147, 21 Sep 1978, 32-34.

13 Urie, N.A. Care of the young disabled. (British Red Cross centre for work, recreation, treatment, and training at Largs, Ayrshire.) Health and Social Service Journal, 86, 29 May 1976, 974-975.

14 WAKERLEY Lodge (Eight articles describing a unit for the young disabled in the grounds of Leicester Hospital, including description of nursing care by L.M. Murray, p.694-695.) Nursing Times, 73, 12 May 1977, 688-699.

15 Wedgwood, J. Accommodation for the young disabled. (The Royal Hospital and Home for Incurables, Putney.) Nursing Mirror, 145, 8 Dec 1977, 13-14.

e CYSTIC FIBROSIS

1 Anderson, C.M. and Goodchild, M.C. Cystic fibrosis: manual of diagnosis and management. Blackwell, 1976.

2 Buchanan, M. Paediatric hospital and home care. 2. Easing parents' problems. (Special needs of children with cystic fibrosis.) Nursing Times, 73, 17 Mar 1977, Occ. papers, 39-40.

3 Clement, M. and others Prone immersion physical exercise therapy in three children with cystic fibrosis: a pilot study. Nursing Research, 28 (6), Nov/Dec 1979, 325-328.

4 Dodge, J.A. and others Effectiveness of counselling in cystic fibrosis. Patient Counseling and Health Education, 1 (1), Spring 1978, 8-12.

5 Duberley, J.D. The nurse-teacher and carer for mother and child. (With cystic fibrosis.) Nursing Mirror, 147, 24 Aug 1978, 15-18.

6 Flower, K.A. and others New mechanical aid to physiotherapy in cystic fibrosis. (Percussor to enable adolescents and adults to treat themselves.) British Medical Journal, 2, 15 Sep 1979, 630-631.

7 Harrisson, S.P. Dysfunctional aspects of a supportive group. (The Cystic Fibrosis Research Trust with reference to author's research with fibrocystic children.) Community Health, 9 (1), Aug 1977, 17-19.

8 Holzel, A. Malabsorption. (In infancy and childhood, including coeliac disease and cystic fibrosis.) Midwife, Health Visitor and Community Nurse, 14 (3), Mar 1978, 79-81.

9 Iveson-Iveson, J. Cystic fibrosis. A disease of unknown causes. (Gives details of Cystic Fibrosis Research Trust.) Nursing Mirror, 148, 24 May 1979, 40.

10 Mallinson, B.M. Seven rules for physiotherapy. (In cystic fibrosis.) Nursing Mirror, 147, 24 Aug 1978, 18-19.

11 Norman, A.P. Cystic fibrosis. Nursing Times, 72, 18 Nov 1976, 1804-1806.

12 Nursing Mirror Cystic fibrosis. (Three articles on research and management, nursing care of relatives and physiotherapy.) Nursing Mirror, 147, 24 Aug 1978, 13-19.

13 Phillips, B.M. Cystic fibrosis. The challenge in research and management. Nursing Mirror, 147, 24 Aug 1978, 13-15.

14 Practitioner Special report. Cystic fibrosis. (Four articles with one on psychological and social aspects.) Practitioner, 224, Mar 1980, 291-295, 297-299, 301-303, 305-307.

15 Russell, G. Cystic fibrosis—1. Clinical aspects. 2. Genetic and social aspects. Nursing Times, 74, 23 Mar 1978, 486-489; 30 Mar 1978, 538-541.

16 Sams, C.A. One breath at a time: a family teaching program for children with cystic fibrosis. Canadian Nurse, 75, (8), Sep 1979, 20-23.

17 Selekman, J. Cystic fibrosis: what is involved in the home treatment program for these children, adolescents and young adults? Pediatric Nursing, 3 (2), Mar/Apr 1977, 32-35.

18 Williams, R.F. Fight the good fight. (Cystic fibrosis.) Journal of Community Nursing, 4 (6), Dec 1980, 18-19, 26.

19 Williams, R.F. Infection of the respiratory tract and lungs in cystic fibrosis. Nursing Times, 76, 20 Mar 1980, 517-520.

f SPINA BIFIDA AND HYDRO-CEPHALUS

1 Anderson, E.M. and Spain, B. The child with spina bifida. Methuen, 1977.

2 Armour, C. A patient's view of spina bifida. Physiotherapy, 63 (7), Jul 1977, 221-222.

3 Bernardo, M.L. When your caseload includes a hydrocephalic child. Pediatric Nursing, 5 (3), May/Jun 1979, 27-29.

4 Brown, G. Care study. Sharon—total care. (Community care of child with hydrocephalus due to acute meningitis.) Nursing Times, 73, 13 Oct 1977, 91-94.

5 Childs, V. Physiotherapy for spina bifida. Physiotherapy, 63 (7), Jul 1977, 218-221.

6 Clarke, C.A. Anencephaly and spina bifida: two unsolved problems. (Epidemiology and theories of causation.) Nursing Mirror, 144, 2 Jun 1977, 22-24.

7 Corcoran, R. Patterns of the imperfect. (The risks of spina bifida and anencephaly.) Midwives Chronicle, 89, Jun 1976, 142-144.

8 Cowie, V. Spina bifida: peace of mind from antenatal diagnosis. (Causes, effects and antenatal diagnosis.) Nursing Mirror, 147, 9 Nov 1978, 34-35.

9 Davies, J.B. and Lucas, D. The Salop skate. (Aid to walking for the spina bifida child.) Physiotherapy, 63 (4), Apr 1977, 115-116.

10 Dromgoole, D. Nursing care study. Spina bifida cystica. Nursing Times, 73, 24 Mar 1977, 406-408.

11 Durham Smith, E. and others The care of an ileal conduit and urinary appliances in children: a practical guide. Association for Spina Bifida and Hydrocelphalus, 1976.

12 Eagles, J.D. Intensive care of the newborn —5. Deborah: a spina bifida baby. Nursing Times, 75, 16 Aug 1979, 1410-1412.

13 Floyd, C.C. A defective child is born: a study of mothers of newborns with spina bifida and hydrocephalus. Journal of Obstetric, Gynecologic and Neonatal Nursing, 6 (4), Jul/Aug 1977, 56-62.

14 Geddes, N. Intermittent catheterization for patients with spina bifida. (Special reference to children and young adults.) Canadian Nurse, 74 (6), Jun 1978, 34-36.

15 Henderson, M.L. and Synhorst, D.M. Bladder and bowel management in the child with myelomeningocele. 1. Roots: source of understanding. (Spina bifida. Advice on teaching parents and child.) Pediatric Nursing, 3 (5), Sep/Oct 1977, 24-31.

16 Hendry, J.M. Peter: an infant with a myelomeningocele. Canadian Nurse, 73 (1), Jan 1977, 15-18.

17 Hendry, J. and Geddes, N. Living with a congenital anomaly: how nurses can help the parents of children born with spina bifida to develop lasting patterns of creative caring. Canadian Nurse, 74 (6), Jun 1978, 29-33.

18 Higgon, G.J. The child with spina bifida in the special school. Physiotherapy, 63 (7), Jul 1977, 216-218.

19 Iveson-Iveson, J. Spina bifida. Report on a Day Conference held at the Post Graduate Centre, Morriston Hospital, Swansea. Nursing Mirror, 146, 16 Feb 1978, 8-9.

20 Lancet Neural-tube defects. (Recent controversy over treatment and need for screening.) Lancet, 1, 11 Feb 1978, 312-313.

21 Lorber, J. Ethical problems in the management of myelomeningocele and hydrocephalus. Nursing Times, 72, 26 Feb 1976, Key Clinical, 5-8; 72, 25 Mar 1976, Key Clinical, 9-11.

22 Nursing Mirror Spina bifida: to treat or not to treat? (Differing views on selective treatment by two paediatricians.) Nursing Mirror, 147, 14 Sep 1978, 13-19.

23 Paterson, D.A. Nursing care study. A child who developed hydrocephalus due to listeria meningitis. Nursing Times, 72, 1 Jul 1976, 1006-1008.

24 Physiotherapy Four articles on spina bifida. Physiotherapy, 63 (6), Jun 1977, 182-192.

25 Platt, G.L. Nursing care study. A child with an infected Spitz-Holter valve. (Child with spina bifida and associated hydrocephalus.) Nursing Times, 76, 10 Jul 1980, 1219-1223.

26 Pouw, R.M. An easily applied and comprehensive assessment of pre-school abilities—based on spina bifida children. (Queen Mary's Hospital, Roehampton.) British Journal of Occupational Therapy, 40 (3), Mar 1977, 61-64.

27 Sandford, T. Nursing care study. Hydrocephalus and blocked shunt: and Mother came too. (Care of six-year-old boy and parents.) Nursing Mirror, 148, 4 Jan 1979, 22-25.

28 Seller, M. Spina bifida. (Research into the mechanisms of neural tube development.) Midwives Chronicle, 93, Jul 1980, 234-235.

29 Stark, G.D. Spina bifida: problems and management. Blackwell, 1977.

30 Tindale, S. Urinary management of spina bifida and hydrocephalus. Nursing Mirror, 146, 6 Apr 1978, Supplement, v, vii.

31 Vigliarolo, D. Managing bowel incontinence in children with meningomyelocele. American Journal of Nursing, 80 (1), Jan 1980, 105-107.

32 Watt, M.S. Towards the prevention of CNS malformations. Congenital abnormalities are a significant cause of infant mortality and malformations of the CNS form a particularly large percentage of these conditions. (Spina bifida and anencaphaly.) Midwife, Health Visitor and Community Nurse, 13 (6), Jun 1977, 174-175, 177, 178.

33 Zachary, R.B. Life with spina bifida. (Includes discussion of 'no treatment' methods and criteria for operation.) British Medical Journal, 2, 3 Dec 1977, 1460-1462.

50 MENTALLY HANDI-CAPPED CHILDREN

a GENERAL AND NURSING

1 Alcott, M. Achieving full potential. (Work of British Institute for the Achievement of Human Potential which organises 'patterning' sessions for mentally handicapped children.) Nursing Times, 74, 10 Aug 1978, 1348-1349.

2 Barker, P. and others Living and learning: a nurse administered token economy programme involving mentally handicapped schoolboys. (In Dundee.) International Journal of Nursing Studies, 15 (2), 1978, 91-102.

3 Benicki, A. and Cull, A. The toy library. (Establishment of library in Gogarburn Hospital, Edinburgh, for the mentally handicapped and report of two surveys of nursing staff's reactions.) Nursing Times, 76, 6 Mar 1980, Occ. papers, 29-32.

4 Berry, R. and others Behavioural principles. A multi-disciplinary approach to the management of severely mentally handicapped children. (Staff training and implementation of programme at Lea Castle Hospital, Worcs.) Nursing Times, 74, 10 Aug 1978, 1327-1330.

5 Campion, J. The children's ward annexe, Mayday Hospital. (Children suffering from developmental retardation.) Nursing Times, 76, 1 May 1980, 769-776.

6 Candy, A. A long way to manhood. National Society for Mentally Handicapped Children, 1976.

7 Cash, J. Symposium on ascertainment of national needs. 1. Child development centres and registers of mental handicap. (Compilation of a register in Warwickshire.) British Journal of Mental Subnormality, 22 (2), Dec 1976, 58-69.

8 Cass, H. and others Take six children: account of a...project...by...volunteers, designed to help severely handicapped children in a subnormality hospital. National Society for Mentally Handicapped Children, 1978.

9 Comley, R. Self-injurious behaviour in a retarded child. (Based on a case study.) Nursing Mirror, 142, 18 Mar 1976, 66-68.

10 Cowie, V.A. Subnormality in children. (Detection, assessment and treatment.) Midwife, Health Visitor and Community Nurse, 14 (7), Jul 1978, 226-228.

11 Dixon, G. Pictures in nursing. Helping mentally handicapped children to eat. Nursing, 11, Mar 1980, 479-483.

12 Dunham, M. and others The physical environment of the mentally handicapped. XI. Children's units in hospitals for the mentally handicapped. Some findings relating to architectural briefing. British Journal of Mental Subnormality, 22 (1), Jun 1976, 47-53.

13 Dyer, B. Children left in hospitals. (Mentally handicapped children in long-stay hospitals.) New Society, 46, 7 Dec 1978, 580-581.

14 Fairbrother, P. Love and affection. (Sexual needs of mentally handicapped children.) Health and Social Service Journal, 87, 2 Dec 1977, 1684.

15 Godfrey, M. Nursing care study. Happy puppet syndrome. (Case study at St. Francis Home for Mentally Handicapped Children, Bulawayo, Rhodesia.) Nursing Mirror, 143, 30 Sep 1976, 45-46.

16 Gorman, V. Improving life for children in mental handicap hospitals. Nursing Mirror, 147, 21 Sep 1978, 24-25.

17 Gray, M. It's O.K. to cry: feeling outlets for mentally retarded children. Journal of Psychiatric Nursing, 18 (3), Mar 1980, 22-24, 29-31.

18 Gunzburg, A.L. The physical environment of the mentally handicapped. 12. An operational philosophy of enrichment applied to the design of a children's family unit. British Journal of Mental Subnormality, 22 (2), Dec 1976, 112-117.

19 Harding, J.T. Nursing care study. Severely handicapped adolescent girl. (Care in mental subnormality hospital.) Nursing Times, 74, 2 Feb 1978, 188-189.

20 Hendry, M. and Rathey, S. Austrian antics. (Skiing holiday for mentally handicapped children.) Nursing Times, 72, 4 Mar 1976, 342-343.

21 Heywood Jones, I. The National Society for Mentally Handicapped Children. (Description of activities.) Nursing Times, 75, 15 Nov 1979, 1991-1992.

22 Hong, C.S. and Cockerill, H. Working with the profoundly handicapped child. (Approach at Chase Village, a purpose-built unit for the care of mentally handicapped children and adults at Enfield.) British Journal of Occupational Therapy, 42 (10), Oct 1979, 235-239.

23 Hulland, F. Coping with a mentally handicapped child. (Sources of information and help.) Mind Out, 38, Jan/Feb 1980, 21.

24 Jackson, D. and Morrison, C. Wednesday's children. (The authors' work as ward sisters who get great satisfaction out of working with mentally handicapped children at Gogarburn Hospital, Edinburgh.) Nursing Mirror, 147, 20 Jul 1978, 32.

25 Kinnell, H.G. Self-mutilation in the retarded child. Nursing Times, 75, 22 Nov 1979, 2023-2024.

26 Klein, R. Pathway to independence. Scheme pioneered by the National Society for Mentally Handicapped Children. Health and Social Service Journal, 90, 15 Aug 1980, 1071-1073.

27 Lees, A.J. Nursing care study. De Lange's syndrome. (Long-term care of twelve-year-old boy of severely subnormal intelligence.) Nursing Times, 74, 3 Aug 1978, 1296-1298.

28 Lock, J. Eight men in a boat. (Adventure course on the Thames for four mentally handicapped children from Normansfield Hospital.) Nursing Mirror, 146, 5 Jan 1978, 25-27.

29 McNab, P. Importance of early intervention in mental handicap. (Includes assessment of child and support to parents.) Nursing Mirror, 145, 24 Nov 1977, 38-40; 1 Dec 1977, 41-42.

30 Males, J. The mentally handicapped child: a plan for action. Royal Society of Health Journal, 99 (2), Apr 1979, 79-81.

31 Marais, E. Learning while living in hospital. (The Kevill-Davies School at Little Plumstead Hospital for mentally handicapped children.) Nursing Times, 74, 13 Jul 1978, 1156-1157.

32 Morris, D. A problem of growth. (Development of mentally handicapped children.) Health and Social Service Journal, 87, 21 Oct 1977, 1466-1467.

33 National Development Group for the Mentally Handicapped Mentally handicapped children: a plan for action. The Group, 1977. (Pamphlet no.2.)

34 National Society for Mentally Handicapped Children Evidence to the Jay Committee (on mental handicap nursing and care.) NSMHC, 1977.

35 National Society for Mentally Handicapped Children Mental handicap A-Z: your questions answered. 14th ed. NSMHC, 1978. (Parents information bulletin, no.4.)

36 Orton, D. Behavioural treatment of hyperactivity in a mentally handicapped child. (Behaviour Modification Unit at Glenfrith Hospital, Leicester.) Nursing Times, 75, 3 May 1979, 758-760.

37 Peer, B. Our special children: caring for the retarded child in an acute care setting. Canadian Nurse, 75 (1), Jan 1979, 34-35.

38 Pickstock, J. and Taylor, J. Behaviour modification in a severely subnormal child. Nursing Mirror, 142, 26 Feb 1976, 47-49.

39 Ray, R. The mentally handicapped child's reaction to bereavement. Health Visitor, 51 (9), Sep 1978, 333-334.

40 Roberts, M.J. and Canfield, M. Behaviour modification with a mentally retarded child. American Journal of Nursing, 80 (4), Apr 1980, 679.

41 Robinson, W. St. Blazey hospital unit for handicapped children. (Behaviour modification project.) Nursing Mirror, 142, 11 Mar 1976, 62-64.

42 Scott, J. Nursing care study. Multiple handicap: stimulating Stanley—one small step at a time. (Severely subnormal boy with mild spastic quadraplegia.) Nursing Mirror, 148, 11 Jan 1979, 34-36.

43 Siantz, M.L. de L. editor The nurse and the developmentally disabled adolescent. Baltimore: University Park Press, 1977.

44 Smith, C.S. and others Aetological factors in mental handicap in relation to possible preventive measures. (Survey of mentally handicapped children under 6.) Public Health, 92 (1), Jan 1978, 30-37.

45 Stoner, R. Nursing care study. Philip: a severely subnormal child. Nursing Mirror, 142, 19 Feb 1976, 53-54.

46 Thomas, D.A. and others Consulting the consumers. (Evaluation of short stay care for mentally handicapped children in Northumberland AHA.) Health and Social Service Journal, 90, 15 Feb 1980, 225-226.

47 Whitney, R.P. I dared to seek surgery for my retarded daughter. (Hysterectomy for a child unable to cope with menstruation.) RN Magazine, 39 (12), Dec 1976, 39-45.

48 Wilkin, D. Caring for the mentally handicapped child. Croom Helm, 1979.

49 Worsley, N. Faith—a case study. (A subnormal and autistic child.) Social Work Today, 8, 18 Jan 1977, 9-11.

b FAMILY

1 Bentley, J. Group therapy for parents of mentally handicapped children. (Southend Hospital.) Nursing Mirror, 142, 6 May 1976, 53.

2 Bromley, D. and Lister, T. What the parents want. (Survey in North Tyneside of parents' attitudes towards short-term relief and holiday breaks.) Health and Social Service Journal, 90, 8 Feb 1980, 191-193.

3 Chesham, I. Helping to keep the mentally handicapped child at home. Public Health, 90 (3), Mar 1976, 135-138.

4 Cunningham, C. and Sloper, P. Helping your handicapped baby. Souvenir Press, 1978. (Human horizons series.)

5 Hencher, J.H. A family with a handicapped child. (Role of HV with a family with a mentally handicapped child where the mother resisted her interventions.) Nursing Times, 76, 24 Jan 1980, 157-158.

6 Hoyle, A. Community nursing care study. A family tragedy. (Two children with microcephaly.) Nursing Times, 72, 28 Oct 1976, 1669-1671.

7 Jones, C. The 'Portage' system in Gwent. (Education of the handicapped pre-school child, with training and counselling in the home involving the whole family and health visitor.) Health Visitor, 53 (2), Feb 1980, 42.

8 Jones, M.E.O. Teaching the parents to help the child. (Hospital-based family support services for mentally handicapped children in Clwyd in teaching basic skills and treating severe problem behaviours.) Nursing Mirror, 148, 24 May 1979, 26-28.

9 Kaines, I. A model for teaching skills to parents of retarded children—philosophy, implementation, future developments. (Behaviour shaping skills.) Australasian Nurses Journal, 8 (1), Sep 1978, 22-23, 30.

10 King's Fund Centre and Association of Professions for the Mentally Handicapped Collaboration between parents and professionals. KEHF, 1976. (Mental handicap papers, no.9.)

11 Larcombe, E.J. A handicapped child means a handicapped family. (Case history of 16-year-old mentally handicapped girl.) Journal of the Royal College of General Practitioners, 30, Sep 1980, 533-534, 536-537.

12 McCormack, M. A mentally handicapped child in the family. Constable, 1978.

13 Mather, J. Make the most of your baby. National Society for Mentally Handicapped Children, 1976.

14 Mellor, M. Healing the deep hurt and living for today. (Development of self-help groups for parents of mentally handicapped children.) Health and Social Service Journal, 89, 16 Nov 1979, 1492.

15 Nursing Mirror Family participation at new children's unit. (Turner Village, Colchester, for the mentally handicapped.) Nursing Mirror, 142, 5 Feb 1976, 69.

16 Rhodes, H. Ismail's world. (Health visiting care study of Pakistani family with 3-year-old mentally handicapped child, based on the nursing process.) Nursing Times, 76, 8 May 1980, Community Outlook, 139-140, 145, 147, 150.

17 Ross, J. When support is needed. (National Society for Mentally Handicapped Children service of voluntary welfare visitors to help parents.) Social Service Quarterly, 49 (2), Oct-Dec 1975, 53, 55.

18 Shearer, A. The Barnardo Chorley project. (Project involving toy library and social work visits to families with mentally handicapped children.) Social Work Today, 10, 10 Oct 1978, 10-11.

19 Wallace, E. Mental handicap: meeting the real needs of families. (Caring for children at home.) Social Work Today, 9, 25 Apr 1978, 21-23.

c DOWNS SYNDROME

1 Baker, M.H. When the Down's syndrome baby is yours. (Mother's experiences.) RN Magazine, 40 (7), Jul 1977, 67-70.

2 Banning, J. The nurse in the community: infant stimulation. (Programme for Down's syndrome children in Ottawa.) Canadian Nurse, 75 (10), Nov 1979, 36-37.

3 Barker, P. and Hunter, M.H. Minor self mutilation. (Case study using behaviour therapy techniques in a boy with Down's syndrome.) Nursing Times, 73, 7 Apr 1977, 500-502.

4 Beare, S. Children with Down's syndrome: a look at some of the current ideas on management. Health Visitor, 52 (7), Jul 1979, 266-268.

5 Brinkworth, R. The challenge that society must accept. (Help available for Down's children.) Health and Social Service Journal, 88, 17 Feb 1978, 200.

6 Cameron, S. O.B. staff alert. (Mother's account of her feelings after the birth of her Down's syndrome baby, with advice for nurses.) Canadian Nurse, 75 (10), Nov 1979, 30-32.

7 Community Outlook Issue on Down's Syndrome, with reference to role of HV, projects in Leeds and Manchester, toys and the National Society for Mentally Handicapped Children. Nursing Times, 74, 8 Jun 1978, Community Outlook, 153, 155, 157-158, 160-161, 163, 167, 169, 171, 173.

8 Cranston, J.A. Nursing care study. A Down's baby. (Hospital care during his 20 weeks of life, by second-year student nurse.) Nursing Times, 75, 18 Oct 1979, 1792-1794.

9 Cunningham, C.C. and Sloper, P. Down's syndrome infants: a positive approach to parent and professional collaboration. (Study of the problems faced by parents in the first year of life.) Health Visitor, 50 (2), Feb 1977, 32-37.

10 Docherty, P. Operant conditioning: success is sweet as John speaks up. (Teaching Down's syndrome boy to communicate in normal voice.) Nursing Mirror, 147, 16 Nov 1978, 45-48.

11 Gath, A. Down's syndrome and the family: the early years. Academic Press, 1978.

12 Johnson-Allen, B. A little help and understanding. (Work of National Society for Mentally Handicapped Children.) Midwife, Health Visitor and Community Nurse, 14 (8), Aug 1978, 260, 263-264.

13 Kromberg, J.G.R. Responses of parents to the birth of a baby with Down's syndrome. S.A. Nursing Journal, 44 (11), Nov 1977, 33-35.

14 Long, A. Health visiting care study. Down's syndrome. Nursing Times, 76, 8 May 1980, 814-819.

15 Lowenstein, L.F. Down's syndrome: a short account of the condition known as mongolism. National Society for Mentally Handicapped Children, 1978.

16 Neumann, D. Down's syndrome—crisis intervention and nursing education. Australian Nurses Journal, 8 (5), Jan 1979, 34-35.

17 Nurse, I. The functions and operation of workshops for mothers of young Down's syndrome children. S.A. Nursing Journal, 44 (11), Nov 1977, 24-26.

18 Physiotherapy Issue on Down's Syndrome. Physiotherapy, 62 (1), Jan 1976, 2-26.

19 Smith, W.W. Teaching a Down's child: an analytical approach. East Grinstead and District Society for Mentally Handicapped Children, 1977.

20 Smithson, M. Lesley: the child we chose. Foster care of a mongol baby. National Society for Mentally Handicapped Children, 1977.

d PHENYLKETONURIA

1 Wyatt, D.S. Phenylketonuria: the problems vary during different developmental stages. American Maternal-Child Nursing Journal, 3 (5), Sep/Oct 1978, 296-302.

51 CHILD WELFARE

a DEPRIVATION

1 Bosanquet, N. Inside the social services. Services for children. Nursing Times, 73, 28 Jul 1977, 1168-1169.

2 Bosanquet, N. The right to care. (The Children's Act.) Nursing Times, 72, 18 Nov 1976, 1790-1791.

3 Bowder, B. Who is deprived? (Cycle of deprivation.) Nursing Mirror, 146, 23 Feb 1978, 38-40.

4 Cowper-Smith, F. Give the kids a break. (Kids—a holiday centre for deprived and handicapped children.) Nursing Times, 72, 9 Dec 1976, 1912-1913.

5 Ellmers, J. The story of Pauline. (Case study of child who suffered maternal deprivation in first three months.) Midwife, Health Visitor and Community Nurse, 13 (10), Oct 1977, 328-329.

6 Ford, L.R. The community's unmet child health needs. (A comparison of 3-year-old non-attenders and attenders at clinics in Glasgow to isolate factors of children 'at risk.') Public Health, 90 (2), Jan 1976, 59-64.

7 Greenwood, G. A cry in the night—and help is immediate. (Huddersfield's Crying Baby Advisory/Relief Service involving health visitors.) Nursing Mirror, 148, 11 Jan 1979, 24-27.

8 Hart, T. Love is all we have. (Problems of children arriving at the Cumberlow Regional Assessment Centre, South London.) Nursing Times, 73, 24 Mar 1977, 424-425.

9 Hughes, J. A cycle of deprivation. (A research project to design a method of intervention in the cycle—Maws' Scholarship 1974.) Health Visitor, 49 (8), Aug 1976, 266-267.

10 Jackson, B. A minister for children? (To protect the only large minority without a political spokesman.) New Society, 35, 15 Jan 1976, 94-96.

11 Nangle, D. Emotional deprivation and neglect in child patients. (Role of the therapist.) Physiotherapy, 62 (9), Sep 1976, 297-298.

12 Parliament Child care act 1980. HMSO, 1980.

13 Pilling, D. A destiny shaped before the child is born. (Health and learning handicaps of socially disadvantaged children.) Health and Social Service Journal, 88, 4 Aug 1978, 879.

14 Rutter, M. and Madge, N. Cycles of disadvantage: a review of research. Heinemann, 1976.

15 Turner, J. Charities for children. New Society, 48, 17 May 1979, 381-383.

16 Wilson, H. Babies in a poverty trap. (Behaviour patterns in deprived families.) New Society, 42, 6 Oct 1977, 14-15.

b FOSTERING AND ADOPTION

1 Bosanquet, N. Inside the social services.

Fostering and adoption. Nursing Times, 73, 1 Sep 1977, 1374-1375.

2 Cowper-Smith, F. Wanted—parents for children. (Work of a new adoption agency finding homes for difficult to place children.) Nursing Times, 73, 14 Apr 1977, 514-515.

3 Department of Health and Social Security and others. Working Party on Fostering Practice Guide to fostering practice. HMSO, 1976. (Chairman Mrs J. Thomas.)

3 Dudley, A. Foster grandparents. American fostering scheme with a difference for mentally handicapped and deprived children. Nursing Mirror, 143 (21), 18 Nov 1976, 75.

4 Halpin, H. Adoption in the seventies. Midwife, Health Visitor and Community Nurse, 12 (3), Mar 1976, 72-74.

5 Hammons, C. The adoptive family. (Stresses of adoption for child and family.) American Journal of Nursing, 76 (2), Feb 1976, 251-257.

6 Holmes, J. Discovering one's identity. (Author describes how she traced her natural parents.) Midwife, Health Visitor and Community Nurse, 14 (4), 113-114.

7 Kornitzer, M. New adoption legislation and the health visitor. Health Visitor, 51 (1), Jan 1978, 4-7.

8 Lafferty, M. Operation orphan. (Treating Vietnamese orphans at Fairfield Hospital, Melbourne.) Australian Nurses Journal, 5 (5), Nov 1975, 24-30.

9 Mattingly, R. Adoption and the Children Act. 1. Progress in implementing the Act and the right of adopted people to obtain their birth certificate. 2. Further provisions that have recently become law and the parts of the Act still not implemented. Nursing Mirror, 144, 28 Apr 1977, 63-64; 5 May 1977, 65-66.

10 Morris, M. Fostering and adoption of black children. Report on a seminar, held by the Medical Group of the Association of British Adoption and Fostering Agencies. Health Visitor, 53 (7), Jul 1980, 284.

11 Parliament Adoption act 1976. HMSO, 1976. (Chapter 36.)

11 Robinson, W. Problems and joys of adoption. (Experiences of a couple adopting children of mixed racial origins.) Nursing Mirror, 142, 19 Feb 1976, 71-73.

13 Royston, R. Money buys more than love as care moves on with the times. (Dr. Barnardo's.) Health and Social Service Journal, 87, 13 May 1977, 802-804.

14 Selman, P. Patterns of adoption in England and Wales since 1959. Social Work Today, 7 (7), 24 Jun 1976, 194-197.

15 Social Work Today Children in residence: the voluntary agencies. (Dr. Barnardo's and the National Children's Home.) Social Work Today, 10, 3 Apr 1979, 20-27.

16 Stroud, J. Adoption counselling and the new Children's Act 1975. Midwife, Health Visitor and Community Nurse, 13 (10), Oct 1977, 308, 311-312, 314.

17 Stroud, J. At the rainbow's end. (Reunion

of adopted people with natural parents.) Health and Social Service Journal, 87, 12 Aug 1977, 1165.

18 Stroud, J. Rewinding the umbilical cord. (Prescribed procedure for adopted people to trace their natural parents.) Health and Social Service Journal, 87, 5 Aug 1977, 1139.

19 Tizard, B. Adoption: a second chance. Open Books, 1977.

20 Tolfree, D. Problems of inter-country adoption. (e.g. of Vietnamese children.) Social Work Today, 10, 21 Nov 1978, 16-18.

21 Tucker, P. Adoption problems stimulate public interest. (Comment on the 1975 Children's Act.) Midwife, Health Visitor and Community Nurse, 14 (1), Jan 1978, 14-15.

22 Walker, L.O. A survey of the needs of adoptive parents. (Research study.) Pediatrics, 4 (2), Mar/Apr 1978, 29-31.

c NON-ACCIDENTAL INJURY

1 Apley, J. Whose sickness? (Causes and management of child abuse cases.) British Medical Journal, 1, 25 Mar 1978, 774-775.

2 Arthur, L.J.H. and others Non accidental injury in children: what we do in Derby. (Team care including doctors, policemen and social workers.) British Medical Journal, 1, 5 Jun 1976, 1363-1366.

3 Barrie, H. Personal opinion—on case conferences. (In cases of child abuse.) Midwife, Health Visitor and Community Nurse, 15 (5), May 1979, 188, 190, 192.

4 Bayne, R. Children at risk—a cause for concern. The circumstances surrounding child abuse. (By student while on RNMS community option.) Nursing Mirror, 146, 2 Feb 1978, 42-44.

5 Black, J.A. and Hughes, F. Legal aspects of child injury or neglect. British Medical Journal, 2, 13 Oct 1979, 910-912.

6 Bosanquet, N. Who is really to blame? (In the case of battered baby, Stephen Meurs.) Nursing Times, 72, 29 Jan 1976, 126-127.

7 British Association of Social Workers The central child abuse register: a BASW working party report. Birmingham: BASW, 1978. (Chairman David N. Jones.)

8 British Medical Journal Non-accidental immersion in bath water: another aspect of child abuse. British Medical Journal, 1, 29 Jan 1977, 271-272.

9 Carter, J. Co-ordination and child abuse. Social Work Service, 9, Apr 1976, 22-28.

10 Carver, V. editor Child abuse: a study text. Milton Keynes: Open University Press, 1978.

11 Creighton, S.J. and Owtram, P.J. Child victims of physical abuse: a report on the findings of NSPCC Special Units' registers. NSPCC, 1977.

12 Department of Health and Social Security and others Violence to children: a response to the First Report from the Select Committee on Violence in the Family (Session 1976-77). HMSO, 1978. (Cmnd.7123)

13 **Desborough, C. and Stevenson, O.** Case conferences: interprofessional communication concerning children at risk. (Paper based on small DHSS sponsored research project.) Health and Social Service Journal, 88, 24 Mar 1978, Centre eight papers, C5-C8.

14 **Doyle, C.** Effective methods for tackling child abuse. Social Work Today, 12, 9 Dec 1980, 13-14.

15 **Elliman, A.** Battered babies. (General discussion.) Midwife, Health Visitor and Community Nurse, 14 (11), Nov 1978, 383-385.

16 **Figgins, P.** Child abuse—associated factors. Nursing Mirror, 145, 22 Sep 1977, 20-21.

17 **Fosson, A.R. and Kaak, H.O.** Child abuse and neglect case studies. Kimpton, 1977.

18 **Francis, J. and Sutton, A.** Two views on non-accidental injury. 2. The battered child and his parents: can we help? Social Work Today, 8, 4 Jan 1977, 16-18.

19 **Franklin, A.W.** The challenge of child abuse: proceedings of a conference sponsored by the Royal Society of Medicine, 2-4 Jun 1976. Academic Press, 1977.

20 **Franklin, A.W. editor** Child abuse: prediction, prevention and follow-up: papers presented by the Tunbridge Wells Study Group... Churchill Livingstone, 1977.

21 **Gallwey, P.** Paedophilia. Midwife, Health Visitor and Community Nurse, 14 (3), Mar 1978, 68, 71.

22 **Guedj, N.** Battered children in the paediatric ward and the role of the psychologist. International Child Welfare Review, 44, Mar 1980, 50-56.

23 **Guirguis, W.R.** Child abuse: the child's view. (Diagnostic tools used by occupational therapists.) British Journal of Occupational Therapy, 43 (3), Mar 1980, 88-89.

24 **Hilton, J.E.** Battered babies. (By police surgeon, with illustrations.) Practitioner, 221, Oct 1978, 607-614.

25 **Holder, V.** The battered child at school. (Research into educational problems.) Health and Social Service Journal, 86, 10 Jan 1976, 71-72.

26 **Howells, J.G.** Death and disorganization. (The effects of disorganization in social services as seen by the child abuse cases of Maria Colwell and Stephen Meurs.) Royal Society of Health Journal, 96 (3), Jun 1976, 98-99, 128.

27 **Hutchinson, F.P.** The probation service and child abuse. Health Visitor, 52 (4), Apr 1979, 130, 133.

28 **Jolly, J.D.** Child care in North America— 5. Child abuse: can it be prevented? Nursing Times, 73, 22/29 Dec 1977, 1994-1995.

29 **Jones, C.O.** Children at risk. Meeting the needs of abused children. (Psychotherapy and placement in care.) Social Work Today, 9, 28 Feb 1978, 9-14.

30 **Kempe, C.H. and Helfer, R.E. editors** The battered child. Chicago: University of Chicago Press. 3rd ed. 1980.

31 **Kempe, R.S. and Kempe, C.H.** Child abuse. Fontana/Open Books, 1978. (The developing child series.)

32 **Lahiff, M.** Softly, softly... Police involvement in case conferences on child abuse could create more problems than it solves. Nursing Times, 72, 16 Dec 1976, 1950-1951.

33 **Lancet** No not non-accidental injury! Lancet, 2, 9 Oct 1976, 775-776.

34 **Landriau, M.** Studies in child abuse. (Work of the NSPCC in research and assistance to families.) Social Service Quarterly, 50 (1), Jul-Sep 1976, 175-178.

35 **Lee, C.M. editor** Child abuse: a reader and sourcebook. Milton Keynes: Open University Press, 1978. Extracts in Nursing Times, 74, 9 Feb 1978, Community Outlook, 37-44.

36 **Lee, C.M.** The Open University. (Preparation of a course in child abuse in a joint project between Newcastle Polytechnic and the Open University.) Nursing Times, 72, 9 Sep 1976, 1386-1388.

37 **Mirza, M.R.** Disturbing new trends in parental violence against children. Social Work Today, 11, 26 Feb 1980, 18.

38 **National Center on Child Abuse and Neglect** Child abuse and neglect: the problem and its management. 3 vols. U.S. Government Printing Office, 1976.

39 **National Society for the Prevention of Cruelty to Children. Battered Child Research Department** At risk: an account of the work of the...department; by E. Baker and others. Routledge and Kegan Paul, 1976.

40 **Nobel, M. and Mason, J.K.** Incest. Journal of Medical Ethics, 4 (2), Jun 1978, 64-70.

41 **Olson, R.J.** Index of suspicion: screening for child abuses. American Journal of Nursing, 76 (1), Jan 1976, 108-110.

42 **Parton, N.** Recording concern—the case against child abuse registers. Social Work Today, 11, 26 Feb 1980, 12-14.

43 **Pickett, J. and Maton, A.** Children at risk (3). (Description of the NSPCC's non-accidental injury special unit in Manchester.) Social Work Today, 9, 14 Mar 1978, 10-18.

44 **Pietroni, R.G.** The battered baby and the GP. Midwife, Health Visitor and Community Nurse, 12 (8), Aug 1976, 145-147.

45 **Roberts, J. and others** Postneonatal mortality in children from abusing families. (Results of study.) British Medical Journal, 281, 12 Jul 1980, 102-104.

46 **Rodriguez, A.** Handbook of child abuse and neglect. Kimpton, 1977.

47 **Royal College of General Practitioners** Ill treated children. (Evidence to the Select Committee on Violence in the Family.) Journal of the Royal College of General Practitioners, 26, Nov 1976, 804-805.

48 **Schmitt, B.D. editor** The child protection team handbook: a multidisciplinary approach to managing child abuse and neglect. New York: Garland STPM, 1978.

49 **Slack, P.** Extending the register. (Comment on new DHSS circular on child abuse registers.) Nursing Times, 76, 4 Sep 1980, 1556.

50 **Smith, S.M. editor** The maltreatment of children. Lancaster: MTP, 1978.

51 **Smith, T.** Violence and children. (Comment on the Select Committee on Violence in the Family's report.) Journal of Medical Ethics, 3 (3), Sep 1977, 146-147.

52 **Somerset Area Review Committee for Non-Accidental Injury to Children** Report of the review panel (on the case of) Wayne Brewer. Taunton: the Committee, 1977. (Chairman D.J.R. Clark.)

53 **Stainton, M.C.** Non-accidental trauma in children. Canadian Nurse, 71 (10), Oct 1975, 26-29.

54 **Stevenson, O.** Social services and child abuse: some dilemmas and opportunities. Royal Society of Health Journal, 97 (5), Oct 1977, 205-209.

55 **Thomas, T.** Blinded by the light when the red button is pushed. (Dangers of invoking formal procedures unnecessarily in cases of suspected child abuse.) Health and Social Service Journal, 90, 18 Jul 1980, 950-951.

d NON-ACCIDENTAL INJURY: NURSES' ROLE

1 **AORN Journal** Five articles on child abuse, with special refernece to the nurse's role in recognition, reporting and prevention. AORN Journal, 27 (4), Mar 1978, 631-656.

2 **Black, P.M.** The child at risk—interprofessional co-operation. (Baillière's prize for nursing studies—3rd prize.) Nursing Mirror, 144, 14 Apr 1977, 61-64; 21 Apr 1977, 56-61.

3 **Bysshe, J.** A battered baby. (A case study.) Nursing Times, 72, 24 Jun 1976, 986-987.

4 **Cooper, W.** Why battered children are our business. (Advice for community nurses on detecting physical abuse.) Journal of Community Nursing, 2 (1), Jul 1978, 4-5.

5 **England, F.E.C.** Detection of non-accidental injury. (With case study of care of child in accident and emergency department.) Nursing Times, 75, 25 Oct 1979, 1858-1861.

6 **Fitzpatrick, M.** Recognition and prevention of child abuse or non-accidental injury. Queen's Nursing Journal, 19 (7), Oct 1976, 203-205.

6 **Friedman, A.L. and others** Nursing responsibility in child abuse. Nursing Forum, 15 (1), 1976, 95-112.

7 **Gilbert, M.T.** Behavioural approach to the treatment of child abuse. (Behaviour modification administered by a clinical psychologist and a nurse to establish a link between a child abusing parent and her daughter.) Nursing Times, 72, 29 Jan 1976, 140-143.

8 **Gilbert, M.T.** Child abuse. (Symposium paper on the nurse therapist.) Nursing Mirror, 144, 12 May 1977, 50-51.

9 **Gower, M.D.** Non-accidental injury and the health visitor. Nursing Times, 72 (40), 7 Oct 1976, 1563-1564.

10 Greary, E. Health visitors and the courts. (Legal advice in child abuse cases. Letter.) Health Visitor, 50 (8), Aug 1977, 268, 269.

11 Hagar, L. The nursing process a tool to individualized care. (Case study with four-year-old child abuse victim.) Canadian Nurse, 73 (10), Oct 1977, 38-41.

12 Hardy, M. and others Prevention of baby battering. (Project in Coventry by GP and HVs in a health centre.) Practitioner, 222, Feb 1979, 243-245, 247.

13 Hurwitz, A. Child abuse: a program for intervention. (Course for student nurses involving fieldwork with potential abusive families.) Nursing Outlook, 25 (9), Sep 1977, 575-577.

14 Hutchings, J. and Hughes, N. Community nursing and psychology. 6: Child abuse. Journal of Community Nursing, 2 (7), Jan 1979, 14-15.

15 Hyman, C.A. Non-accidental injury. (Report of research study involving the completion of questionnaires by health visitors.) Health Visitor, 51 (5), May 1978, 168-172.

16 Josten, L. Out-of-hospital care for a pervasive family problem—child abuse. (Role of community nurse.) American Maternal-Child Nursing Journal, 3 (2), Mar/Apr 1978, 111-116.

17 Journal of Practical Nursing The abused child: the abused adult. (Two articles, including nurses' index of suspicions of child abuse.) Journal of Practical Nursing, 28 (9), Sep 1978, 24-29, 37.

18 Krige, P.D. Child abuse. (Review of suggested causes and outline of role of nurse.) South African Nursing Journal, 44 (5), May 1977, 7, 29.

19 Leaman, K. The sexually abused child. (Families' need for counselling and the nurse's role.) Nursing, 77, 7 (5), May 1977, 68, 70-72.

20 McKeel, N.L. Child abuse can be prevented. (Nurse's role.) American Journal of Nursing, 78 (9), Sep 1978, 1478-1482.

21 Martin, A. The nurse and the law: err on the side of caution. (With reference to child abuse.) Journal of Community Nursing, 3 (3), Sep 1979, 10.

22 Nursing (U.S.) Recognizing and helping the abused child. Nursing (U.S.), 9 (2), Feb 1979, 64-67.

23 Nursing Times Care teams must exchange facts on 'at risk' children. Nursing Times, 72, 12 Feb 1976, 202.

24 Nursing Times HV made 'no error' in child killing case. (Implications of the health visitor in the child killing case of Oliver Jackson.) Nursing Times, 72, 5 Aug 1976, 1181.

25 Patchett, S. Legal proceedings and health visitors. (Problems these cause for access to children at risk. Letter.) Health Visitor, 50 (6), Jun 1977, 189.

26 Robinson, J. Interdisciplinary in-service education and training in child abuse. (Research study of health visitor and social worker training and communication.) Health Visitor, 52 (4), Apr 1979, 126-127, 129.

27 Scharer, K.M. Rescue fantasies: pro-

fessional impediments in working with abused families. (Nurses' need to save child and danger of their negative responses towards the parents.) American Journal of Nursing, 78 (9), Sep 1978, 1483-1484.

28 Slack, P. Planning training for coping with non-accidental injury. Nursing Times, 72, 7 Oct 1976, 1561-1563.

29 Snyder, C. and Spietz, A. Characteristics of abuse: a report of five families. (Project to demonstrate the effectiveness of family assessment by nurse.) Nurse Practitioner, 2 (8), Nov/Dec 1977, 23-27.

30 Tagg, P.I. Nursing intervention for the abused child and his family. Pediatric Nursing, 2 (5), Sep/Oct 1976, 36-39.

31 Thomas, J.N. Yes, you can help a sexually abused child. RN Magazine, 43 (8), Aug 1980, 23-29.

32 Weller, C.M.R. Assessing the non-accidental injury. (Role of nurse in E.D. and common symptoms to be looked for.) Journal of Emergency Nursing, 3 (2), Mar/Apr 1977, 17-26.

e NON-ACCIDENTAL INJURY: PARENTS AND PREVENTION

1 Appleton, P. and others Group treatment for families having severe handling difficulties with a preschool child: its role in the prevention of child abuse. (Scheme at Bethel Hospital, Norwich.) British Journal of Occupational Therapy, 41 (6), Jun 1978, 200-206.

2 Ashley, A. Voluntary self-help for parents under stress in Britain. (To prevent child abuse.) Midwife, Health Visitor and Community Nurse, 16 (6), Jun 1980, 244, 246.

3 Bedford, A. Behaviour modification in child protective social work. (Techniques used by an NSPCC special unit working with abusing families.) Social Work Today, 10, 3 Oct 1978, 27-28.

4 Beswick, K. and others Child abuse and general practice. (Preventive scheme at Didcot Health Centre, Broadway, Didcot, Oxon.) British Medical Journal, 2, 2 Oct 1976, 800-802.

5 Bushweller, E. The nurse who came to play. (Community nurse used play therapy to help break the cycle of the abused teenage mother who became a child abuser herself.) RN Magazine, 40 (12), Dec 1977, 48-49.

6 Carr, J.L. Communicating with the child-abusing family. Topics in Clinical Nursing, 1 (3), Oct 1979, 41-48.

7 Cater, J.I. and Easton, P.M. Separation and other stress in child abuse. (Factors which predispose towards battering.) Lancet, 1, 3 May 1980, 972-973.

8 Cunningham, R. Child abuse and family—centred care. Toronto: University of Toronto, Faculty of Nursing, 1979. (Literature review monograph; 1.)

9 Doyle, C. and Oates, M. Child abuse: when to tread a careful path between parent and child. (Types of parents who abuse children and how to establish relationship with them.) Social Work Today, 12, 30 Sep 1980, 12-15.

10 Health Visitor Accident surveillance system. (Description of scheme in Surrey AHA to detect and prevent child abuse.) Health Visitor, 52 (12), Dec 1979, 511.

11 Hill, A. Prevention is better: nipping child abuse in the bud. (Project in Bradford to follow up families after the birth of a baby to study factors in child abuse.) Social Work Today, 11, 22 Jul 1980, 6-7.

12 Jackson, B. Self help for parents. (Parents Helpline groups for parents with violent feelings towards their children.) New Society, 43, 12 Jan 1978, 65-69.

13 Johnston, D.W. and Guest, J.C. Team work with the army in child care. (Problems army families experience with reference to the prevention of child abuse.) Midwife, Health Visitor and Community Nurse, 16 (1), Jan 1980, 17-18, 20.

14 Kitchen, M. Breaking the vicious circle of battering. (Family centre in Harrow for families where children have been physically injured.) Social Work Today, 11, 15 Jan 1980, 8-9.

15 Lynch, M. and Roberts, J. Predicting child abuse. (Report of research by Human Development Research Unit, Park Hospital for Children, Oxford.) Nursing Mirror, 145, 22 Sep 1977, 18-19.

16 Lynch, M.A. and Roberts, J. Predicting child abuse: signs of bonding failure in the maternity hospital. (Survey at the Park Hospital for Children, Oxford.) British Medical Journal, 1, 5 Mar 1977, 624-626.

17 Meadow, R. Munchausen syndrome by proxy. The hinterland of child abuse. (Parents who by falsifying symptoms cause their children needless hospital investigations.) Lancet, 2, 13 Aug 1977, 343-345.

18 Melville, J. A parents' lifeline. (Child abuse and services for parents at risk.) New Society, 45, 14 Sep 1978, 567-568.

19 Mercer, R.T. Nursing care for parents at risk. Thorofare: Slack, 1977.

20 Nix, H. Why parents anonymous? (Group approach to deal with child abuse.) Journal of Psychiatric Nursing, 18 (10), Oct 1980, 23-28.

21 Ortman, E. Attachment behaviors in abused children. (Research study of differences in mother/child relationships between abused and non-abused children.) Pediatric Nursing, 5 (4), Jul/Aug 1979, 25-29.

22 Roberts, J. and others Prevention of child abuse: group therapy for mothers and children. (Project set up by Didcot practice and research team from Park Hospital for Children, Oxford.) Practitioner, 219, Jul 1977, 111-115.

23 Social Work Today Child abuse registers. Social Work Today, 9, 21 Mar 1978, 14-17.

24 Social Work Today Consumer's viewpoint by a battering parent. Social Work Today, 7 (3), 29 Apr 1976, 78.

f NURSERIES, PLAYGROUPS, CHILD MINDERS

1 Andrews, G.M. Occupational therapy in an opportunity playgroup (to integrate normal and handicapped children.) British Journal of Occupational Therapy, 40 (4), Apr 1977, 83-84.

2 Bone, M. Pre-school children and the need for day-care: a survey carried out on behalf of the Department of Health and Social Security. HMSO, 1977.

3 Brain, J. and Martin, M.D. Child care and health for nursery nurses. Amersham: Hulton Educational Publications, 1980.

4 Brunell, R.D. and others Who looks after the children. (Survey by HV students to discover incidence of child-minding.) Health Visitor, 52 (11), Nov 1979, 458-461.

5 Bryant, B. and others Children and minders. Grant McIntyre, 1980. (Oxford preschool research project; 3.)

6 Campbell, C. Bowling from the nursery end. (Criticism by second-year student nurse of poorly planned secondment to day nursery.) Nursing Mirror, 150, 24 Jan 1980, 14.

7 Cunningham, P.J. editor Nursery nursing. 3rd ed. Faber, 1977.

8 Garland, C. and White, S. Children and day nurseries: management and practice in nine London day nurseries. Grant McIntyre, 1980. (Oxford preschool research project; 4.)

9 Hannon, P. Society at work. Minders of our future? (Present state of child minding.) New Society, 44, 11 May 1978, 304-305.

10 Herrman, S. An introduction to nursery nursing. Heinemann Educational, 1979.

11 Hughes, B. Reassessing the role of pre-school play groups. (In care of the deprived child.) Social Work Today, 9, 9 May 1978, 23-25.

12 Inner London Pre-School Playgroups Association Playgroups: a shared adventure. The Association, 1976.

13 Jackson, B. Towards a policy for the under-fives. (Views on child minding.) Nursing Times, 72 (5), 5 Feb 1976, 168.

14 Jackson, B. and Jackson, S. Childminder: a study in action research. Routledge and Kegan Paul, 1979.

15 Johnson, R. Childminding and day care. The needs of the child. Royal Society of Health Journal, 96 (3), Jun 1976, 114-117.

16 Mack, J. A day nursery for the whole family. (Rydevale day nursery set up by Wandsworth community relations council.) New Society, 47, 22 Feb 1979, 422-423.

17 Mack, J. A new class of minders. (Work of local authority child minders, advisers and home school liaison teachers in deprived areas of Birmingham.) New Society, 38, 9 Dec 1976, 517.

18 Moss, O.M. and Van Emden, J. Get the grown ups out of the nursery—they want to help. (Role of nursery nurse.) Journal of Community Nursing, 3 (1), Jul 1979, 16, 20.

19 Moss, P. and Plewis, IL. Who wants nurseries? (Study by the Thomas Coram Research Unit investigating the potential use of nurseries in Bloomsbury and North Paddington.) New Society, 36, 22 Apr 1976, 188-189.

20 Royal Society of Health Journal Child-minding and day care. (Three articles.) Royal Society of Health Journal, 96 (3), Jun 1976, 114-128.

21 Stapleton, P. Culture clashes and the childminder: problems relating to African families and the provision of day care. Social Work Today, 7 (9), 22 Jul 1976, 271-272.

22 Stroud, J. Some thoughts on child minding. (Its role and value.) Midwife, Health Visitor and Community Nursing, 13 (8), Aug 1977, 249-251.

23 Sylva, K. and others Childwatching at playgroup and nursery school. Grant McIntyre, 1980. (Oxford preschool research project; 2.)

24 Thayer, P. Childminding and day care. Where is he best cared for: child-minder, day nursery or daycare centre? Royal Society of Health Journal, 96 (3), Jun 1976, 118-121.

25 Woodhead, M. Intervening in disadvantage: a challenge for nursery education. A review of British research into pre-school education for disadvantaged children. NFER, 1976.

g HOSPITAL DAY NURSERIES

1 Eardley, A. and Simpson, S. Hospital day nurseries: a survey. Health and Social Service Journal, 90, 25 Jan 1980, Centre eight papers, A35-A39.

2 Hollins, S. and others Hospital day nurseries. (For children of staff. Letter.) British Medical Journal, 1, 15 Apr 1978, 991.

ELDERLY AND DISABLED

52 ELDERLY AND RETIRED

a GENERAL

1 Agate, J. Geriatrics for nurses and social workers. 2nd ed. Heinemann Medical, 1979.

2 Age Concern Profiles of the elderly. Vol.1. Mitcham: Age Concern, 1977. (Age Concern research publications.)

3 American Journal of Nursing Staying well while growing old. (Seven articles including pre-retirement counselling, drugs, sex and skin changes.) American Journal of Nursing, 78 (8), Aug 1978, 1334-1354.

4 Anderson, F. An Institute of Gerontology. (Campaign conference for Age Action Year.) Nursing Mirror, 143, 15 Jul 1976, 40-41.

5 Anderson, F. Preventive geriatric medicine. Midwife, Health Visitor and Community Nurse, 12 (6), Jun 1976, 187-189.

6 Anderson, F. and Cowan, N.R. Survival of healthy older people. (Survey of people attending the Rutherglen Consultative Health Centre for Older People.) British Journal of Preventive and Social Medicine, 30 (4), Dec 1976, 231-232.

7 Anderson, W.F. Practical management of the elderly. 3rd ed. Oxford: Blackwell, 1976.

8 Arekalian, M. Extending health care to the elderly. (Including discussion of definition of 'levels of wellness'.) Nursing Forum, 18 (3), 1979, 253-262.

9 Barrowclough, F. and Pinel, C. All nurses must share in the care of the old. (Review of physiological and social aspects of ageing.) Nursing Mirror, 148, 4 Jan 1979, 13-16.

10 Bozian, M.W. and Clark, H.M. Counteracting sensory changes in the aging. American Journal of Nursing, 80 (3), Mar 1980, 473-476.

11 Brocklehurst, J.C. editor Geriatric care in advanced societies. Lancaster: MTP, 1975.

12 Brocklehurst, J.C. editor Textbook of geriatric medicine and gerontology. 2nd ed. Churchill Livingstone, 1978.

13 Bromley, D.B. Speculations in social and environmental gerontology. Nursing Times, 73, 21 Apr 1977, Occ. papers, 53-56.

14 Caird, F.I. Diagnosis in old people. Physiotherapy, 62 (6), Jun 1976, 178-179.

15 Carver, V. and Liddiard, P. editors An ageing population: a reader and sourcebook.

Hodder and Stoughton in association with Open University Press, 1978.

16 Chalmers, G.L. Caring for the elderly sick. Tunbridge Wells: Pitman Medical, 1980.

17 Coleman, P.G. Health expectations are the key to well-being in old age. (Report of two research studies in the Netherlands.) Modern Geriatrics, 9 (3), Mar 1979, 57-58.

18 Community Outlook An ageing population. (Feature on various aspects of ageing.) Nursing Times, 74, 10 Aug 1978, Community Outlook, 221, 223-225, 227, 229-230.

19 Coni, N. and others Lecture notes on geriatrics. Blackwell, 1977.

20 Cross, V.H. Geriatric medicine—death and rebirth. (The role and status of the geriatrician.) British Medical Journal, 2, 24 Sep 1977, 816-817.

21 Dunn, A. Giants of geriatrics. (Interview with Professor Bernard Isaacs.) Nursing Times, 72, 11 Mar 1976, 362-363.

22 Exton-Smith, A.N. and Evans, J.G. editors Care of the elderly: meeting the challenge of dependency. Proceedings of a conference, Washington DC, 17-19 May 1976. Academic Press, 1977.

23 Exton-Smith, A.N. and Overstall, P.W. Geriatrics. Lancaster: MTP Press, 1979. (Guidelines in medicine; 1.)

24 Fuller, S.S. and Larson, S.B. Life events, emotional support, and health of older people. (Mainly over 65 years old.) Research in Nursing and Health, 3 (2), Jun 1980, 81-89.

25 Garland, M.H. The challenge of geriatric medicine. (Symposium on care of the elderly.) Nursing Mirror, 145, 3 Nov 1977, 15-16.

26 Gore, I. The generation jigsaw. Allen and Unwin, 1976.

27 Gore, I. Physical activity in old age. Nursing Mirror, 142, 19 Feb 1976, 48-49.

28 Hall, M.R.P. and others Medical care of the elderly. Aylesbury: HM & M, 1978. (For nurses and others.)

29 Hawker, M. Keep-fit exercises for geriatric patients. Nursing Mirror, 142, 19 Feb 1976, 50-51.

30 Help the Aged Cry, and you cry alone: a disturbing new report. Help the Aged, 1977.

31 Hetherington, R.J. Fallacies in geriatrics. Today the aged are the outcasts of society. Such

hostility is in part the antithesis of the cult of youth, in part misunderstood economics. Nursing Times, 75, 26 Apr 1979, 718-719.

32 Hobman, D. Is geriatrics the answer to the problems of old age? 3. Attitudes (of society to the elderly.) Journal of Medical Ethics, 2 (4), Dec 1976, 196-199.

33 Hobman, D. editor The social challenge of ageing. Croom Helm, 1978.

34 Hodkinson, H.M. Common symptoms of disease in the elderly. Oxford: Blackwell, 1976. 2nd ed. 1980.

35 Irvine, R.E. and others The older patient: a textbook of geriatrics. 3rd ed. Hodder and Stoughton, 1978. (Modern nursing series.)

36 Isaacs, B. editor Recent advances in geriatric medicine. 1. Churchill Livingstone, 1978.

37 Millard, P.H. Is geriatrics the answer to the problem of old age? 1. Thoughts of a geriatrician. Journal of Medical Ethics, 2 (4), Dec 1976, 193-195.

38 Morden, P. A self-help guide to the aging process. (Chart prepared for use as a learning tool or as audio-visual aid.) Canadian Nurse, 76 (7), Jul/Aug 1980, 19-25.

39 National Corporation for the Care of Old People Old age: a register of social research 1976-1977. The Corporation, 1977.

40 Physiotherapy Issue on geriatric medicine. Physiotherapy, 62 (5), May 1976, 146-159.

41 Pinel, C. Geriatrics as a specialty. (The development of social reform, geriatric medicine, gerontology and geriatric nursing.) Nursing Times, 72, 14 Oct 1976, 1601-1603.

42 Puner, M. To the good long life: what we know about growing old. Macmillan, 1978. (Open University set book.)

43 Rai, G.S. and Pearce, V. Databook on geriatrics. Lancaster: MTP, 1980.

44 Royal College of Physicians of London Report of the Working Party on Medical Care of the Elderly. The College, 1977. (Chairman Sir Cyril Clarke). Reprinted with editorial comment in Lancet, 1, 21 May 1977, 1091-1095.

45 Royal Society of Health Journal Practical care of geriatric patients. (Five articles.) Royal Society of Health Journal, 95 (1), Feb 1975, 21-37.

46 Simpson, R.G. Geriatric perspectives. (Changing pattern of management in modern geriatric care.) Nursing Mirror, 143, 30 Sep 1976, 54-56.

47 Whitehead, J.A. It's due to your age dear. (Inadequacies in the diagnosis of elderly patients' problems.) Nursing Times, 72, 9 Sep 1976, 1412-1413.

b MIDDLE AGE AND RETIREMENT

1 Ashton, K. The graceful art of retiring. (Work of David Simmonds who leads a project to set up groups for retired NHS staff.) Nursing Times, 74, 21/28 Dec 1978, 2089.

2 Benson, J.T. Retirement. An end or a beginning? Royal Society of Health Journal, 97 (2), Apr 1977, 74-76.

3 Best, P. Promoting good health in retirement—a team effort. (Education, screening and rehabilitation.) Modern Geriatrics, 8 (12), Dec 1978, 19-20, 23.

4 Bungay, G.T. and others Study of symptoms in middle life with special reference to the menopause. (Survey of men and women.) British Medical Journal, 281, 19 Jul 1980, 181-183.

5 Collin, A. 'Mid-life crisis' and its implications in counselling. British Journal of Guidance and Counselling, 7 (2), Jul 1979, 144-152.

6 Dodsworth, A.J. Preventive medicine in geriatrics—2. Preparing for retirement. (Using a scheme at Joseph Lucas Ltd. as an example of pre-retirement course.) Nursing Times, 72, 17 Jun 1976, 943-949.

7 Earland, M. 'The best is yet to be.' (Small survey as part of JBCNS course project on attitudes towards and policies on preparation for retirement.) Nursing Mirror, 149, 13 Dec 1979, 28-31.

8 Estes, D. Pre-retirement series for hospital personnel. (In Omaha, Nebraska.) Journal of Gerontological Nursing, 4 (1), Jan/Feb 1978, 15-19.

9 Gaston, S.K. Death and midlife crisis. Journal of Psychiatric Nursing, 18 (1), Jan 1980, 31-35.

10 Hemming, J. Perspective for retirement. Royal Society of Health Journal, 97 (2), Apr 1977, 76-78.

11 Jones, S. Fostering mutual help for the elderly. (The case for providing training opportunities for retired people.) Health and Social Service Journal, 89, 11 May 1979, 574-576.

12 McKinnon, R. Occupational health—the final function. (Pre-retirement courses for employees.) Occupational Safety and Health, 8 (6), Jun 1978, 12-13.

13 OCTOBER teach-ins for the autumn years. (Pre-retirement courses at Addenbrookes Hospital, Cambridge, for hospital staff including nurses.) Health and Social Service Journal, 89, 14 Sep 1979, 1161.

14 Smith, D. Don't kick the work habit when the axe falls. (Experimental fellowship organisation for retired NHS staff in Gloucestershire.) Health and Social Service Journal, 88, 15 Dec 1978, 1418-1419.

15 Smith, S.A. The eligibility of older people

for community services: mental health aspects: roles and attitudes toward retirement and pre-retirement counseling. Occupational Health Nursing, 26 (10), Oct 1978, 11-14.

c SERVICES

1 Abrams, M. The elderly: an overview of current British social research. National Corporation for the Care of Old People/Age Concern, 1978.

2 Baker, D.E. The elderly: a challenge to nursing—16. Future care for the elderly. Nursing Times, 74, 9 Feb 1978, 237-238.

3 British Medical Association. Board of Science and Education Report of the working party on services for the elderly. BMA, 1976. (Chairman Sir Ferguson Anderson.)

4 Burrows, J. The elderly: a challenge to nursing—2. The elderly in our society. (Life expectancy and demands on health services.) Nursing Times, 73, 27 Oct 1977, 1670-1674.

5 Central Office of Information. Reference Division Care of the elderly in Britain. 2nd ed. HMSO, 1977. (Reference pamphlet no.121.)

6 Chisholm, M. Caring services for the elderly. Nursing Mirror, 142, 27 May 1976, 62-64.

7 Clift, D. Following the split, unity. (Geriatric liaison team from health and social services to promote common approach to planning geriatric services.) Health and Social Service Journal, 89, 14 Sep 1979, 1174.

8 Clode, D. Oh, what a frustrating war at the front line. (Report of Age Concern conference.) Health and Social Service Journal, 87, 11 Nov 1977, 1558-1559.

9 Cowper-Smith, F. A recipe for planned care for the elderly. (Report on recent conference.) Nursing Times, 75, 13 Dec 1979, 2146-2147.

10 Cruise, V.J. Better geriatric care—making it happen. (Report of attempts in Exeter Health Care District to implement better standards of care, as part of DHSS project.) Nursing Times, 74, 21 Sep 1978, 1563-1564.

11 Davidson, N. Self-service grannycare. (Heinz Wolff of M.R.C.'s project to promote wider availability of and changed attitudes towards aids.) Health and Social Service Journal, 90, 25 Apr 1980, 553-554.

12 Davidson, N. The words and the reality of that happy old age. (Assessment of the growth in size and needs of the elderly population.) Health and Social Service Journal, 88, 15 Dec 1978, 1410-1411.

13 Department of Health and Social Security and Welsh Office A happier old age: a discussion document on elderly people in our society. HMSO, 1978.

14 Department of Health and Social Security. Development Group—Social Work Service A life style for the elderly: report of a seminar... 18-20 July, 1974. HMSO, 1976.

15 Dodd, K. and others Misplacement of the elderly in hospitals and residential homes: a survey and follow-up. (One-day census in Leicestershire and six-month follow-up survey.) Health Trends, 3 (12), Aug 1980, 74-76.

16 GRANDPA or grand person—do we really care? (Ways of maintaining quality of life and independence of elderly people, by seven student nurses from Gloucestershire Royal School of Nursing.) Nursing Times, 74, 5 Oct 1978, 1626-1627.

17 Heath, J. compiler Care of the elderly: a guide for personnel involved in teaching in hospital and community. Sheffield: NHS Learning Resources Unit, 1979.

18 Hobman, D. The elderly and their world. (Suggests sixteen measures to relieve problems facing elderly.) Social Work Today, 10, 9 Jan 1979, 20.

19 Hobman, D. Practical care of geriatric patients. (a) An old person's view of the health services. Royal Society of Health Journal, 95 (1), Feb 1975, 21-25.

20 Hunt, A. Some aspects of the health of elderly people in England. (With reference to author's survey based on informants' own descriptions.) Health Trends, 1 (11), Feb 1979, 21-23.

21 Isaacs, B. and Neville, Y. The measurement of need in old people. Scottish Home and Health Department, 1976. (Scottish health service studies, no.34.)

22 Kaye, V. Picking their old chestnuts and taking their choice. (DHSS seminar on the needs of the elderly.) Health and Social Service Journal, 87, 5 Aug 1977, 1124-1125.

23 Leonard, J.C. Can geriatrics survive? (Proposals for integrating the care of the elderly into general medicine thus doing away with separate geriatric units.) British Medical Journal, 1, 29 May 1976, 1335-1336.

24 McGilloway, F.A. Care of the elderly: a national and international issue. Journal of Advanced Nursing, 4 (5), Sep 1979, 545-554.

25 Muir Gray, J.A. 'Section 47': an ethical dilemma for doctors. (Compulsory removal from home of physically incapable people under Section 47 of National Assistance Act 1948.) Health Trends, 3 (12), Aug 1980, 72-74.

26 Norton, D. Care of the elderly. (Policies and implications for nursing care.) World Health, Dec 1978, 18, 20-21.

27 Orriss, H.D. Dual care of the elderly. (Separation of the planning and management of hospital medical care and local authority residential care.) Nursing Times, 72, 27 May 1976, 820-821.

28 Packwood, T. Rehabilitating these departments back to the front line. (Problems in the provision of care for the elderly.) Health and Social Service Journal, 87, 25 Mar 1977, 526-527.

29 Robinson, W. Improving geriatric care. (Rcn and British Geriatric Society conference.) Nursing Mirror, 143, 9 Dec 1976, 37.

30 Traill, L. and McEwan, C. How participation figures in their lives. (Pilot project in part of Forth Valley Health Board area to publicise facilities for the elderly and involve them in promotion and maintenance of their own health.) Health and Social Service Journal, 89, 1 Mar 1979, 209-212.

31 Williams, L. Care of the elderly—back to

basics. Journal of Community Nursing, 2 (10), Apr 1979, 10-11.

32 Williamson, J. Problems in care of the elderly. Health Bulletin, 34 (6), Nov 1976, 312-316.

d SERVICES: OVERSEAS COUNTRIES

1 Benson, E.R. Care for the elderly in Yugoslavia. International Nursing Review, 23 (2), Mar/Apr 1976, 55-56.

2 Chye, T.C. Home nursing care for the aged and chronic sick. (The Home Nursing Federation of Singapore.) Nursing Journal of Singapore, 18 (2), Nov 1978, 66.

3 Devine, B.A. China's 'House of Respect'. (Care of elderly in China.) Journal of Gerontological Nursing, 6 (6), Jun 1980, 338-340.

4 Evason, E. and Edwards, G. Social policy and the elderly in the GDR. Social Work Today, 8, 25 Jan 1977, 13-15.

5 Flynn, A. Yesterday's workers. (Winston Churchill Memorial Trust scholarship tour studying care of the elderly in Scandinavia.) Health Visitor, 49 (2), Feb 1976, 45-46.

6 Franck, P. A survey of health needs of older adults in Northwest Johnson County, Iowa. Nursing Research, 28 (6), Nov/Dec 1979, 360-364.

7 Godber, C. Danes' single door approach. (Danish system of residential care for the elderly.) Health and Social Service Journal, 89, 1 Feb 1979, 100-103.

8 Hamilton, L. 'HAP'—One response to the 'Medical Nemesis'. (Health Activation Programs to encourage the elderly to look after their health and reduce their dependence on professionals.) Journal of Gerontological Nursing, 3 (2), Mar/Apr 1977, 52-53.

9 McClelland, M. Japan's modern approach to an age-old problem. (Report of study tour looking at geriatric care.) Nursing Mirror, 147, 17 Aug 1978, 13-15.

10 Melin, R.C. and Hymans, D.J. Developing a health care model for long-term care facilities. (Nursing homes for elderly people.) Journal of Nursing Administration, 7 (8), Oct 1977, 12-14.

11 Moss, F.E. and Halamandaris, V.J. Too old, too sick, too bad: nursing homes in America. Germantown, Md.: Aspen Systems, 1977.

e HOSPITAL CARE

1 Adams, J. A change of scene—1. Ridge Hill—a home, not a ward. The effect on a group of elderly female patients who were moved to temporary bungalow accommodation while their hospital wards were being upgraded. Nursing Times, 75, 27 Sep 1979, 1659-1661.

2 Agate, J. Long stay hospital care of older patients. Nursing Mirror, 145, 8 Dec 1977, 15-17.

3 Alvermann, M.M. Toward reducing stress in the institutionalized elderly—therapeutic tape recordings. Journal of Gerontological Nursing, 5 (6), Nov/Dec 1979, 21-26.

4 Anderson, A.M. and others Three system built units for geriatric patients—a preliminary report. Health Bulletin, 37 (2), Mar 1979, 67-70.

5 Bagnall, W.E. and others Geriatric medicine in Hull: a comprehensive service. (Partially age-related 'single-ward' scheme for treatment and rehabilitation led to reduction in admissions to general medical wards.) British Medical Journal, 2, 9 Jul 1977, 102-104.

6 Barrowclough, F. Design for geriatric care. (Ways in which the geriatric ward design used by the West Midlands Regional Health Authority fails to meet present needs.) Nursing Times, 72, 26 Aug 1976, 1330-1331.

7 Barrowclough, F. The elderly in institutions. (General discussion.) Nursing Mirror, 145, 15 Dec 1977, 27-28.

8 Binks, F.A. Changing the subject. (Effect of past system of compulsion and custody on care of the elderly.) Lancet, 2, 1 Jul 1978, 32-34.

9 Cairns, J. Treating long-term patients as individuals. (Scheme at Belhaven Hospital, Dunbar to encourage elderly people to participate in community life.) Nursing Times, 75, 21 Jun 1979, 1058-1059.

10 Castledine, G. The great age-old problem. (Problems of institutionalisation of elderly chronic sick.) Nursing Mirror, 150, 31 Jan 1980, 14.

11 Chang, B.L. Generalized expectancy, situational perception, and morale among institutionalized aged. Nursing Research, 27 (5), Sep/Oct 1978, 316-324.

12 Chang, B.L. Locus of control, trust, situational control and morale of the elderly. (With reference to the quality of life of the institutionalised elderly.) International Journal of Nursing Studies, 16 (2), 1979, 169-181.

13 Davies, J.E. A change of scene—2. Effects of the new home on patients and nurses. (Move for group of geriatric patients to temporary accommodation at Ridge Hill Mental Handicap Unit.) Nursing Times, 75, 4 Oct 1979, 1725-1726.

14 Dent, R.V. Geriatric care in hospital. (Four factors important to the quality of life and their implications for staff.) Nursing Times, 73, 29 Sep 1977, 1507-1509.

15 Department of Health and Social Security A programme for improving geriatric care in hospital: report of a working group. DHSS, 1978. (Chairman M. Heath) (Enclosed with HN(79)35.)

16 Department of Health and Social Security Summary report of a working group on a programme for improving geriatric care in hospital. (Function of DHSS/NHS group was to help implement report of joint working party of Rcn and British Geriatrics Society, 1975.) Journal of Advanced Nursing, 4 (5), Sep 1979, 581-587.

17 Dobson, A. Showers for the elderly. (Successfully introduced in a new hospital.) Nursing Times, 75, 17 May 1979, 841-842.

18 Gregory, J. and McDonnel, T. A sense of achievement. (Adult education classes in geriatric and psychiatric hospitals.) Nursing Mirror, 151, 14 Aug 1980, 26-27.

19 Higham, S. and McVittie, K. Advice on geriatric care. (Improvements in geriatric care in

the Newcastle group of hospitals resulting from advice from a Hospital Advisory Service team.) Nursing Times, 72, 29 Jan 1976, 152-155.

20 HILLCREST Hospital. Nursing Times, 73, 14 Apr 1977, Archive, 13-16.

21 Holland, G.P. The elderly—a challenge to nursing—12. Clothing and the elderly. (Its importance in long term hospital care.) Nursing Times, 74, 12 Jan 1978, 69-70.

22 Howells, S. New hospitals from old stock. (How existing hospital can be adapted with reference to the change of use of the Nelson Hospital to provide beds for geriatric patients.) Health and Social Service Journal, 89, 23 Nov 1979, 1512-1513.

23 Hyde, A. Away from the workhouse. (Care of the elderly in two community hospitals.) Health and Social Service Journal, 89, 4 May 1979, 508-511.

24 Kemp, J. The elderly: a challenge to nursing—15. Planning hospital care. Nursing Times, 74, 2 Feb 1978, 198-199.

25 Kennedy, R.D. and Acland, S.M.S. Attitudes of the elderly and their relatives to geriatric admission. (Survey at Stobhill General Hospital, Glasgow.) Health Bulletin, 34 (4), Nov 1976, 320-324.

26 Lysak, A. and others The pub as a therapeutic force. (Within a long-stay hospital for elderly patients.) Health Care in Canada, 20 (12), Dec 1978, 38-39.

27 MacKinnon, M. Take one empty ward: an experiment in redeployment of resources. (Scheme to use temporarily an empty ward for short-term admissions of the ill elderly.) Nursing Times, 74, 16 Mar 1978, 437.

28 Millard, P.H. To rehabilitate or to vegetate? A scathing look at some of the equipment in use in geriatric units. Nursing Mirror, 146, 16 Mar 1978, 14-16.

29 Moore, D. Geriatrics—country style. (History and current use of Newholme Hospital in Bakewell, Derbyshire.) Nursing Times, 74, 6 Jul 1978, 1139-1141.

30 Orr, J.G. Care of the elderly patient in hospital. (Using Maslow's pyramid of needs as a guide: personal development, status, comfort, companionship and basic needs.) Nursing Times, 73, 7 Jul 1977, 1028-1032.

31 Pullen, B. Keeping the long-stay patients in touch with 'the good old days'. (Ways of avoiding institutionalisation in long-stay geriatric patients.) Health and Social Service Journal, 88, 30 Jun 1978, 738-739.

32 Rudd, T.N. Providing a humane environment (for geriatric patients in hospital). Health and Social Service Journal, 86, 20 Mar 1976, 548.

33 Rudd, T.N. Workload in geriatric departments. (Relationship between bed complement and staffing.) Health and Social Service Journal, 86, 10 Apr 1976, 674.

34 Towell, D. and Dartington, T. Encouraging innovations in hospital care. (Principles for planning improved hospital care illustrated by two reports, King Edward's Hospital Fund 'Living in hospital' and the British Geriatric Society and Rcn, 'Improving geriatric care in hospital'.) Journal of Advanced Nursing, 1 (5), Sep 1976, 391-398.

35 Waters, J.E. The social ecology of long-term care facilities for the aged: a case example. (Research study on people interacting with their social and physical environments.) Journal of Gerontological Nursing, 6 (3), Mar 1980, 155-160.

36 West, J. Modern geriatric unit — Tolworth Hospital. Nursing Mirror, 142, 4 Mar 1976, 67-69.

f ACCIDENTS AND ABUSE

1 Andrews, K. Old age. Falls in the elderly. (Causes.) British Journal of Occupational Therapy, 41 (7), Jul 1978, 231.

2 Baker, A. 'Granny battering' — 3. (Lack of awareness in health professionals and relatives of elderly people's feelings and needs.) Midwife, Health Visitor and Community Nurse, 14 (5), May 1978, 147-148.

3 Barrowclough, F. Ward accidents: danger! Why old people fall. (Includes prevention.) Nursing Mirror, 148, 14 Jun 1979, 28-29.

4 Boardman, K.P. Fractures in an elderly population in a psychiatric hospital. Nursing Mirror, 144, 3 Mar 1977, 52-57.

5 Daly, J. Getting the elderly back on their feet after an accident. Nursing Mirror, 148, 15 Mar 1979, 28-30.

6 Felstein, I. Nurses and accident prevention. (With reference to the young and elderly.) Midwife, Health Visitor and Community Nurse, 15 (9), Sep 1979, 342, 344-345.

7 Illing, M. Comment...on how we can identify those at risk. (Granny-bashing.) Nursing Mirror, 145, 22 Dec 1977, 34.

8 Isaacs, B. Don't get up — you'll fall! (Reasons why hospitalised geriatric patients fall.) Nursing Mirror, 149, 18 Oct 1979, 40-41.

9 Isaacs, B. Don't let her walk — she'll fall! (Methods of restoring independent walking to unstable old people.) Nursing Mirror, 149, 25 Oct 1979, 26-27.

10 Isaacs, B. and Hayward, C. Guidelines for reducing the risk of disability. (From falls. Based on research.) Geriatric Medicine, 10 (2), Feb 1980, 19-20, 23.

11 Johnson, D.G. Abuse and neglect — not for children only! (With proposed model for abuse and neglect of the elderly.) Journal of Gerontological Nursing, 5 (4), Jul/Aug 1979, 11-13.

12 Livesley, B. If the blood does not circulate. (Falls and fractures in the elderly.) Journal of Community Nursing, 1 (3), Sep 1977, 5, 8.

13 Morfitt, J.M. Accidents to old people in residential homes. Public Health, 93 (3), May 1979, 177-184.

14 Morfitt, J.M. Residential homes for the elderly — which are the safest? (Survey of incidence of accidents in Wolverhampton.) Public Health, 94 (4), Jul 1980, 223-228.

15 Open University Abuse of old people. (Excerpt from course on conflict in the family.)

Nursing Times, 76, 11 Sep 1980, Community Outlook, 262.

16 Price, J.H. Unintentional injury among the aged. (Includes methods of prevention of falls, burns and car accidents.) Journal of Gerontological Nursing, 4 (3), May/Jun 1978, 36-41.

17 Scott, C.J. Accidents in hospital with special reference to old people. Health Bulletin, 34 (6), Nov 1976, 330-335.

18 Seabrook, J. Young against old. (Cruelty towards elderly people.) New Society, 47, 15 Feb 1979, 345-346 .

19 Smith, C. Refresher course. Accidents and the elderly. Nursing Times, 42, 2 Dec 1976, 1872-1874.

20 Walshe-Brennan, K. Granny bashing. Nursing Mirror, 145, 29 Dec 1977, 32-34.

g DRUG ADMINISTRATION

1 Arie, T. Overdrugged old people. (Review of problems.) Geriatric Medicine, 10 (8), Aug 1980, 24-25.

2 Baxendale, C. and others A self-medication retraining programme. (For elderly patients at Southern General Hospital, Glasgow for use while in hospital and after discharge.) British Medical Journal, 2, 4 Nov 1978, 1278-1279.

3 Bishop, T. Drugs and the elderly: a breeding-ground for mishaps. (Problems of drug administration and role of nurses, with report of small survey of elderly people.) Nursing Mirror, 147, 23 Nov 1978, 49-50.

4 Brock, A.M. Self-administration of drugs in the elderly. Nursing Forum, 18 (4), 1979, 340-351.

5 Crome, P. and others Drug compliance in elderly hospital in-patients: trial of the Dosett box. (Self-medication scheme at Guy's Hospital.) Practitioner, 224, Aug 1980, 782-785.

6 Cullen, A.M.S. Medication programme in homes for the elderly. (Letter describing scheme in Derbyshire to appoint staff pharmacist (social services).) Nursing Times, 76, 11 Dec 1980, 2191.

7 Das, B.C. and others Labelling medicines: a new system evaluated. (To improve compliance in elderly people.) Geriatric Medicine, 10 (9), Sep 1980, 82-83, 85.

8 Dittmar, S.S. and Dulski, T. Early evening administration of sleep medication to the hospitalized aged. A consideration in rehabilitation. (Research study.) Nursing Research, 26 (4), Jul/Aug 1977, 299-303.

9 Edwards, I.R. Weaning elderly patients off barbiturates. (With outline of risks.) Geriatric Medicine, 10 (6), Jun 1980, 65-66, 68, 70.

10 Garland, M.H. Drugs and the elderly: prescribing for the elderly should take into account their changed metabolism and their degree of mental alertness. Nursing Times, 75, 1 Mar 1979, NT Extra, 3-6.

11 Isaacs, B. Don't trust him — he can't cope! (Value of self-medication for elderly patients.) Nursing Mirror, 149, 11 Oct 1979, 24-25.

12 Judge, T.G. and Caird, F.I. Drug treatment of the elderly patient. Pitman, 1978.

13 Lamy, P.P. Drugs and the elderly: what the nurse should know. Journal of Practical Nursing, 30 (8), Aug 1980, 15-19.

14 Law, R. and Chalmers, C. Medicines and elderly people: a general practice survey. (Survey of 150 patients in Inner London examining the taking of prescribed and purchased medicines and drug hoarding.) British Medical Journal, 1976, 1, 6 Mar 1976, 565-568.

15 Macdonald, E.T. and others Improving drug compliance after hospital discharge. (Assessment of the effect on medication errors of counselling elderly people.) British Medical Journal, 2, 3 Sep 1977, 618-621.

16 McLennan, W. Dangerous drugs. (Problems for the elderly.) Nursing Times, 72 (28), 15 Jul 1976, Care of the elderly supplement, xii.

17 Moon, D. Drug treatment in the elderly: the pharmacist's role in dispensing to the elderly. Nursing Times, 74, 8 Jun 1978, 972-973.

18 Plant, J. Educating the elderly in safe medication use. (Seniors' Health Program, Chicago, based on a hospital and health care centre, organised health education in the community.) Hospitals, 51 (8), 15 Apr 1977, 97-102.

19 Playfer, J.R. Drug treatment in the elderly. Reactions to drugs. Nursing Times, 74, 8 Jun 1978, 971.

20 Ramsay, A.G. and Ballinger, B.R. Drug distribution and identifying psychogeriatric patients. (Research study to investigate problems faced by nursing staff.) Nursing Mirror, 145, 7 Jul 1977, 21.

21 Ramsay, A. and others Individual drug supply in a psychogeriatric ward. An evaluation of the system. Nursing Times, 73, 14 Apr 1977, 537-539.

22 RN Magazine Teaching the elderly to avoid accidental drug abuse. (Descriptions by two nurses of successful methods.) RN Magazine, 40 (11), Nov 1977, 39-42.

23 Roberts, R. Self-medication trial for the elderly. (Scheme in Royal Devon and Exeter Hospital (Heavitree) for patients.) Nursing Times, 74, 8 Jun 1978, 976-977.

24 Rodman, M.J. Drug therapy today. Adjusting medications for the needs of the elderly. RN Magazine, 38 (5), May 1975, 65-66, 68, 70, 72, 74, 76, 78, 80, 82, 84, 86, 89.

25 Shaw, S.M. and Opit, L.J. Need for supervision in the elderly receiving long term prescribed medication. (Survey of 127 patients in a group practice with four district nurses and two health visitors attached and an additional seconded research nurse to help with the project.) British Medical Journal, 1, 28 Feb 1976, 505-507.

26 Wandless, I. and Davis, J.W. Can drug compliance in the elderly be improved? (Comparison of three instruction schemes.) British Medical Journal, 1, 5 Feb 1977, 359-361.

h SEX AND THE ELDERLY

1 Brower, H.T. and Tanner, L.A. A study of older adults attending a program on human sexuality: a pilot study. Nursing Research, 28 (1), Jan/Feb 1979, 36-39.

2 Eastman, M. A new look at old love. (Sexuality in the elderly.) Health and Social Service Journal, 88, 13 Oct 1978, 1170-1172.

3 Falk, G. and Falk, U.A. Sexuality and the aged. (With special reference to nursing homes.) Nursing Outlook, 28 (1), Jan 1980, 51-55.

4 Felstein, I. When the music goes off-key... (Sexual problems in middle age with some reference to diabetics and the disabled.) Nursing Mirror, 148, 22 Feb 1979, 16-18.

5 Fox, N. and others Sexuality among the aging. Journal of Practical Nursing, 28 (6), Jun 1978, 16-18.

6 Friedeman, J.S. Development of a sexual knowledge inventory for elderly persons. (To test sexual knowledge in elderly persons.) Nursing Research, 28 (6), Nov/Dec 1979, 372-374.

7 Friedeman, J.S. Factors influencing sexual expression in aging persons: a review of the literature. Journal of Psychiatric Nursing and Mental Health Services, 16 (7), Jul 1978, 34-47.

8 Friedeman, J.S. Sexuality in older persons: implicaions for nursing practice. Nursing Forum, 18 (1), 1979, 92-101.

9 Stanford, D. All about sex...after middle age. (Sexual activity in the elderly.) American Journal of Nursing, 77 (4), Apr 1977, 608-611.

10 Whitton, J. The forgotten need. (Sexual activity among elderly people.) Health and Social Service Journal, 87, 25 Nov 1977, 1624-1625.

53 NURSING THE ELDERLY

a GENERAL

1 Baltes, M.M. and Zerbe, M.B. Re-establishing self-feeding in a nursing home resident. Nursing Research, 25 (1), Jan-Feb 1976, 24-26.

2 Barrowclough, F. and Pinel, C. Geriatric care for nurses. Heinemann Medical, 1979.

3 Boylan, A. and Marbach, B. Dehydration: subtle, sinister...preventable. (In geriatric patients.) RN Magazine, 42 (8), Aug 1979, 36-41.

4 Brimmer, P.F. Past present and future in gerontological nursing research. Journal of Gerontological Nursing, 5 (6), Nov/Dec 1979, 27-34.

5 Brislen, W. A study to identify the expectations of selected elderly patients and their relatives for their nursing care in hospital. MSc thesis, University of Manchester, Department of Nursing, 1978.

6 Burnside, I.M. editor Nursing and the aged. New York: McGraw-Hill, 1976.

7 Carnevali, D.L. and Patrick, M. editors Nursing management for the elderly. Philadelphia: Lippincott, 1979.

8 Castledine, G. A home away from home. (Nursing care of elderly couple in hospital with assessment of nursing problems.) Nursing Mirror, 149, 20/27 Dec 1979, 30-31.

9 Chisholm, M.K. The nurse's responsibilities when caring for the elderly. Nursing Times, 73, 29 Sep 1977, 1509-1510.

10 Conahan, J.M. Helping your elderly patients: a guide for nursing assistants. New York: Tiresias Press, 1976.

11 Cupit, S. Nursing care study. A solitary, sad old lady. (Day-to-day nursing care and treatment of a patient in a long-stay ward.) Nursing Mirror, 149, 25 Oct 1979, 44-46.

12 CURRENT practice in gerontological nursing. 1, 1979. St. Louis: Mosby, 1979. (Mosby's current practice and perspectives in nursing series.)

13 Dodsworth, T. The qualities of nursing (needed for nursing geriatric patients). Nursing Mirror, 142, 6 May 1976, 71.

14 Eliopoulos, C. Gerontological nursing. New York: Harper and Row, 1979.

15 Epstein, C. Learning to care for the aged. Reston, Virginia: Reston Publishing Co., 1977. (For nurses.)

16 Flanagan, D. Nursing care study. Mrs. Brown, not 'old' at 92. Nursing Mirror, 148, 24 May 1979, 42-43.

17 Grant, P.M. Nursing care study. Hospitalisation—and the elderly patient. Nursing Times, 72, 11 Mar 1976, 379-382.

18 Harris, G. Nursing care study. A goal reached. (Care of elderly lady in rehabilitation ward of general hospital including use of habit retraining chart for incontinence.) Nursing Times, 74, 14 Sep 1978, 1524-1526.

19 Hooker, S. Caring for elderly people: understanding and practical help. Routledge and Kegal Paul, 1976.

20 Isaacs, B. Don't tell her. She'll worry! (What nurses and doctors say to elderly patients facing death.) Nursing Mirror, 149, 4 Oct 1979, 27-29.

21 Journal of Gerontological Nursing Issue on group work with the elderly. Journal of Gerontological Nursing, 2 (6), Nov/Dec 1976, 14-40.

22 Lamprill, J. Nursing care study. Geriatric nursing: Alice—not in Wonderland. (102-year-old lady in long-stay ward of geriatric hospital.) Nursing Mirror, 147, 28 Dec 1978, 29-30.

23 Lore, A. Supporting the hospitalized elderly person. American Journal of Nursing, 79 (3), Mar 1979, 496-499.

24 Macdonald, M.I. Practical concerns for nursing the elderly in an institutional setting. Canadian Nurse, 73 (4), Apr 1977, 25-30.

25 McKenzie, J. Nursing care study. Multiple pathology in old age. (Partially blind lady with general malnutrition and dehydration. By student nurse.) Nursing Times, 76, 24 Jan 1980, 149-151.

26 McLeod, F. Geriatric care. Aylesbury: HM & M, 1976. (Nursing modules series.)

27 Mezey, M. and others The health history of the aged person. (Methods for adapting usual interviewing techniques.) Journal of Gerontological Nursing, 3 (3), May/Jun 1977, 47-51.

28 Murray, R.B. and others The nursing process in later maturity. Englewood Cliffs, N.J.: Prentice-Hall, 1980.

29 Norton, D. The elderly: a challenge to nursing. 1. Geriatric nursing—what it is, and what it is not. Nursing Times, 73, 20 Oct 1977, 1622-1623.

30 Norwich, H.S. A study of nursing care in geriatric hospitals. (In NE Thames region into factors affecting care and to produce dependency measures.) Nursing Times, 76, 14 Feb 1980, 292-295.

31 Nursing Clinics of North America Symposium on gerontologic nursing. Nursing Clinics of North America, 14 (4), Dec 1979, 577-664.

32 Nursing Clinics of North America Symposium on gerontological nursing. Nursing Clinics of North America, 11 (1), Mar 1976, 115-206.

33 Nursing Mirror A symposium on care of the elderly. (Six articles.) Nursing Mirror, 145, 3 Nov 1977, 15-20, 23-26, 29-32, 35.

34 Nursing Times The caring team for the elderly—the nursing contribution. (Summary of functions of the various types of nurse in the caring team.) Nursing Times, 73, 22 Sep 1977, Occ. papers, 128.

35 Nursing Times The elderly: a challenge to nursing. Macmillan Journals, 1978.

36 Reinhardt, A.M. editor Current practice in gerontological nursing. 1. St. Louis: Mosby, 1979. (Mosby's current practice and perspectives in nursing series.)

37 Roberts, R. and Wright, W.B. Ban the bib—it's worth the effort. (Scheme in Exeter to replace bibs by large cloth napkins.) Modern Geriatrics, 9 (3), Mar 1979, 2.

38 Roberts, T. Should geriatric nursing be a specialty? Nursing Times, 73, 6 Oct 1977, 1566-1568.

39 Rogers, J.C. Advocacy: the key to assessing the older client. Journal of Gerontological Nursing, 6 (1), Jan 1980, 33-36.

40 Royal College of Nursing. Society of Geriatric Nursing Healthy future for geriatric nursing. (Report of first AGM and conference.) Nursing Mirror, 144, 28 Apr 1977, 36-37.

41 Rudd, T.N. Should the case conference replace the ward round? (For non-medical staff including hospital and community nurses.) Modern Geriatrics, 9 (2), Feb 1979, 84, 87.

42 Scottish Health Education Unit Caring with confidence: a guidance manual for those caring for the elderly. Edinburgh: the Unit, 1979.

43 Smith, C.E. and others Differences in importance ratings of self-care geriatric patients and the nurses who care for them. (Research study to identify what nursing care activities are seen as important by patients and nurses.) International Journal of Nursing Studies, 17 (3), 1980, 145-153.

44 Stevens, P. Nursing care study. Lily—a long-stay patient. Nursing Times, 72, 19 Feb 1976, 254-256.

45 Stickland, M.E. The elderly: a challenge to

nursing—6. Problems of locomotion. Nursing Times, 73, 24 Nov 1977, 1841-1842.

46 Storrs, A.M.F. Geriatric nursing. Baillière Tindall, 1976. (Nurses' aids series.) 2nd ed. 1980.

47 Sullivan, J.A. Effects of differing nursing approaches on residents in housing units for the elderly. (Summary of research project.) Nursing Research Report, 12 (3), Dec 1977, 5, 11.

48 Wainwright, H. Feeding problems in elderly disabled patients. (In continuing care wards of geriatric units.) Nursing Times, 74, 30 Mar 1978, 542-543.

49 Wells, T.J. Problems in geriatric nursing care: a study of nurses' problems in care of old people in hospitals. Edinburgh: Churchill Livingstone, 1980.

50 World Health Organization. Regional Office for Europe Nursing aspects on the care of the elderly: report on a working group, West Berlin, 29 Nov-3 Dec 1976. Copenhagen: WHO, 1977. Summary in Nursing Times, 74, 13 Apr 1978, 626-630; Journal of Advanced Nursing, 3 (4), Jul 1978, 407-415.

b ATTITUDES

1 Baker, D.E. Attitudes of nurses to the care of the elderly. PhD thesis, University of Manchester, Faculty of Medicine, 1978.

2 Brock, A.M. and Madison, A.S. The challenge in gerontological nursing. (Nurses' lack of interest in the care of the aged and the increase in the elderly population.) Nursing Forum, 16 (1), 1977, 95-105.

3 Chamberland, G. and others Improving students' attitudes toward aging. (Curriculum developments at Troy State University, Alabama.) Journal of Gerontological Nursing, 4 (1), Jan/Feb 1978, 44-45.

4 Devine, B.A. Old age stereotyping: a comparison of nursing staff attitudes toward the elderly. (Research study.) Journal of Gerontological Nursing, 6 (1), Jan 1980, 25-32.

5 Dye, C.A. Attitude change among health professionals: implications for gerontological nursing. Journal of Gerontological Nursing, 5 (5), Sep/Oct 1979, 31-35.

6 Fraser, M. Thinking for action. (Nurses' attitudes to elderly patients at Walnuttree Hospital, Sudbury.) Nursing Times, 72, 19 Feb 1976, 246-247.

7 Futrell, M. and Jones, W. Attitudes of physicians, nurses, and social workers toward the elderly the health maintenance services for the aged: implications for health manpower policy. (Research study.) Journal of Gerontological Nursing, 3 (3), May/Jun 1977, 42-46.

8 Hart, L.K. and others Changing attitudes toward the aged and interest in caring for the aged. (Study of students attitudes at the University of Iowa College of Nursing.) Journal of Gerontological Nursing, 2 (4), Jul/Aug 1976, 10-16.

9 Hatton, J. Nurses' attitude toward the aged: relationship to nursing care. (Research study.) Journal of Gerontological Nursing, 3 (3), May/Jun 1977, 21-26.

10 Hawkins, K. Prisoners of their disabilities.

(A student's view of geriatric nursing and the need for change.) Nursing Mirror, 149, 23 Aug 1979, 10.

11 Heller, B.R. and Walsh, F.J. Changing nursing students' attitudes toward the aged. (Developing a 45-hour teaching unit 'Basic concepts in nursing the aged'). Journal of Nursing Education, 15 (1), Jan 1976, 9-17.

12 Hooper, J.E. An exploratory study of student and pupil nurses' attitudes towards, and expectations of, nursing geriatric patients in hospital. MSc thesis, Surrey University, 1979.

13 Isaacs, B. Don't expect...at her age! (Attitudes towards the elderly.) Nursing Mirror, 149, 20 Sep 1979, 22-23.

14 Isaacs, B. May I leave the room, nurse? (An attempt by author to imagine what it would be like to be a geriatric patient or his relative. See also editorial on p.1.) Nursing Mirror, 147, 23 Nov 1978, 24-25.

15 Lillie, D. Attitudes in geriatrics. Nursing Times, 72 (28), 15 Jul 1976, Care of the elderly supplement, iii, v, vii.

16 Robb, S.S. Attitudes and intentions of baccalaureate nursing students towards the elderly. Nursing Research, 28 (1), Jan/Feb 1979, 43-50.

17 Seigel, H. Baccalaureate education and gerontology. (Ways of developing positive attitudes towards the elderly.) Journal of Nursing Education, 18 (7), Sep 1979, 4-6.

18 Sellman, D. The nurse's dilemma. What should the nurse's attitude be towards an elderly patient who want to be ill? (Case study.) Nursing Times, 42, 2 Dec 1976, 1894-1895.

19 Wilhite, M.J. and Johnson, D.M. Changes in nursing students' stereotypic attitudes toward old people (after an eight week educational program). Nursing Research, 25 (6), Nov-Dec 1976, 430-432.

20 World of Irish Nursing What do you see nurse? (Poem written by old woman and a nurse's reply.) World of Irish Nursing, 9 (7/8), Jul/Aug 1980, 7.

c EDUCATION AND TRAINING

1 Bahr, R.T. and Gress, L.D. Course description. The nursing process: ethnicity and aging. Journal of Gerontological Nursing, 6 (4), Apr 1980, 210-213.

2 Bishop, V. Studying an age-old problem. (Description of JBCNS course in geriatric nursing in Hastings Health District.) Nursing Mirror, 150, 3 Apr 1980, 45-46.

3 Braverman, A.M. and others The teaching of geriatrics to health visitor students. Health Visitor, 49 (5), May 1976, 148.

4 Brock, A.M. Improving nursing care of the elderly: an educational task. (Courses at the University of Maryland School of Nursing.) Journal of Gerontological Nursing, 3 (1), Jan-Feb 1977, 26-28.

5 Brower, H.T. A study of content needs in graduate gerontological nursing curriculum. Journal of Gerontological Nursing, 5 (5), Sep/Oct 1979, 21-28.

6 Elder, M.T.K. and others Five on a course. (Account of authors' experiences on JBCNS course in geriatric nursing.) Nursing Times, 75, 30 Aug 1979, 1504-1505.

7 Etten, M.J. Gerontological nursing education at the associate degree and diploma levels. (Course at St Petersburg Junior College with review of research.) Journal of Gerontological Nursing, 5 (4), Jul/Aug 1979, 32-39.

8 Everson, S.J. and Mealey, A.R. Baccalaureate nursing students as leaders in geriatric groups. (Method of giving students experience in group work which resulted in improved client behaviour.) Journal of Nursing Education, 17 (7), Sep 1978, 17-26.

9 Garrett, G.E.R. Educational aspects of a geriatric secondment: a scheme for student nurses in the Bristol Health District. Nursing Times, 75, 30 Aug 1979, 1501-1502.

10 Gress, L.D. Governance and gerontological nursing in schools of nursing. (With review of literature on development of curriculum.) Journal of Gerontological Nursing, 5 (6), Nov/Dec 1979, 44-48.

11 Gunter, L.M. and Estes, C.A. Education for gerontic nursing. New York: Springer, 1979. (Springer series on the teaching of nursing; v.5.)

12 Gunter, L.M. and Ryan, J.E. Self-assessment of current knowledge in geriatric nursing: 1,311 multiple choice questions and referenced answers. Flushing: Medical Examination Publishing Co., 1976.

13 Hannon, J. Effect of a course on aging in a graduate nursing curriculum: a small descriptive study. Journal of Gerontological Nursing, 6 (10), Oct 1980, 604, 611-615.

14 Hildick-Smith, M. and Hodson, J. Your tomorrow. (In-service training programme on the care of the elderly for staff in Nunnery Fields Hospital and Haine Hospital in Kent.) Nursing Times, 74, 29 Jun 1978, 1076-1077.

15 Hutt, A. Shared learning for shared care. (Account of a pilot multidisciplinary course in geriatric care for medical, nursing and physiotherapy students at the Middlesex Hospital, London.) Journal of Advanced Nursing, 5 (4), Jul 1980, 389-396.

16 Joint Board of Clinical Nursing Studies 1. Geriatric nursing. Nursing Mirror, 143 (5), 29 Jul 1976, Nursing care supplement, 2, i-iv.

17 NEW slant on geriatric care at The Middlesex. (Joint teaching of medical and nursing students in geriatric care.) Nursing Mirror, 143, 21 Oct 1976, 36-38.

18 Radford, K.M. and Fenwick, G. Non-clinical projects for trainee nurses. (Scheme in Redhills Hospital, Exeter, to encourage learners to look critically at aspects of long-stay geriatric care.) Nursing Times, 74, 21 Sep 1978, 1564-1565.

19 Williams, E. First impressions. (Methods used at the West Suffolk Hospital to introduce learners to the care of the elderly.) Nursing Mirror, 148, 26 Apr 1979, 32-34.

d MANAGEMENT AND STAFFING

1 Abdellah, F.G. and others PACE: an

approach to improving the care of the elderly. (Patient Appraisal, Care Planning and Evaluation.) American Journal of Nursing, 79 (6), Jun 1979, 1108-1110.

2 Brower, T.F. and others The geriatric nurse practitioner: an expanded role for the care of the older adult. (Project at the University of Miami School of Nursing.) Journal of Gerontological Nursing, 2 (4), Jul/Aug 1976, 17-20.

3 Corbus, H.F. and others The problem oriented medical record in long-term facilities: a teaching method. (Evaluation of quality of care via patient care audit.) Journal of Gerontological Nursing, 3 (4), Jul/Aug 1977, 24-31.

4 Davies, A.D.M. and Crisp, A.G. Setting performance goals in geriatric nursing. (Use of behavioural techniques, with reference to teaching workshop.) Journal of Advanced Nursing, 5 (4), Jul 1980, 381-388.

5 Gabbett, M.C. and others Adaptation—key to problem-oriented documentation in geriatrics. Journal of Gerontological Nursing, 6 (2), Feb 1980, 91-93.

6 Gunter, L.M. and others Issues and ethics in gerontic nursing. Journal of Gerontological Nursing, 5 (6), Nov/Dec 1979, 15-20.

7 Gunter, L.M. and Miller, J.C. Toward a nursing gerontology. (Scientific study of the nursing care of the elderly.) Nursing Research, 26 (3), May/Jun 1977, 208-221.

8 Hirschfeld, M.J. Research in nursing gerontology. (Scientific study of nursing care of the elderly.) Journal of Advanced Nursing, 4 (6), Nov 1979, 621-626.

9 Jannelli, L.M. Utilizing Roy's adaptation model from a gerontological perspective. Journal of Gerontological Nursing, 6 (3), Mar 1980, 140-142, 147-150.

10 Orstein, S. Establishing a therapeutic climate for geriatric care. (Evolving patterns of new ideas and changing standards of care.) Journal of Gerontological Nursing, 2 (4), Jul/Aug 1976, 30-36.

11 Pepper, G.A. and others Geriatric nurse practitioner in nursing homes. (Two year project in Salt Lake City to replace physicians with nurses.) American Journal of Nursing, 76 (1), Jan 1976, 62-64.

12 Pinel, C. and Seriki, C. Nursing establishments in geriatric hospitals. (Recommendations for staffing based on a study of the existing establishment at North Manchester General Hospital.) Nursing Times, 72, 3 Jun 1976, 850-853.

13 Price, F. Initiation and development of individualized patient care plans. Journal of Gerontological Nursing, 2 (4), Jul/Aug 1976, 24-26.

14 Rhys Hearn, C. Staffing geriatric wards. Trials of a 'package'. (Formula based on prescriptions of care and work measurement.) Nursing Times, 75, 26 Apr 1979, Occ. papers, 45-48; 3 May 1979, Occ. papers, 52.

15 Sweeney, S.B. Manpower utilisation and quality control. (With discussion of patient dependency index for geriatric nursing home patients.) Lamp, 37 (5), May 1980, 5-10.

16 Yurick, A.G. and others The aged person

and the nursing process. New York: Appleton-Century-Crofts, 1980.

e NURSE PATIENT RELATIONSHIP

1 Boore, J. The elderly: a challenge to nursing—4. Old people and sensory deprivation. Nursing Times, 73, 10 Nov 1977, 1754-1755.

2 Brislen, W. A study to identify the expectations of selected elderly patients and their relatives for their nursing care in hospital. MSc thesis, Manchester University Department of Nursing, 1978.

3 Burnside, I.M. Recognizing and reducing emotional problems in the aged. Nursing, 7 (3), Mar 1977, 56-60.

4 Chaisson, G.M. Life-cycle: a social-stimulation game to improve attitudes and responses to the elderly. (Among health professionals.) Journal of Gerontological Nursing, 6 (10), Oct 1980, 587-592.

5 Coleman, P.G. Capitalising on what we know of the ageing personality. Geriatric Medicine, 9 (7), Jul 1979, 60-61.

6 Corder, J. The good old days take on a new life for old stagers. (Fair Old Times Reminiscence Theatre Company, a troupe of actors who visit residential homes for the elderly for reminiscence therapy.) Health and Social Service Journal, 89, 13 Jul 1979, 874-875.

7 Davidson, N. Life on our side of the fence. (Problems faced by the elderly illustrated by interviews with five Glaswegians.) Health and Social Service Journal, 88, 22/29 Dec 1978, 1442-1445.

8 Davison, W. Stress in the elderly. Physiotherapy, 64 (4), Apr 1978, 113-115.

9 Dietsche, L.M. Facilitating the life review through group reminiscence. (Discussion group at a geriatric day care centre.) Journal of Gerontological Nursing, 5 (4), Jul/Aug 1979, 43.

10 Edsall, J.O. and Miller, L.A. Relationship between loss of auditory and visual acuity and social disengagement in an aged population. Nursing Research, 27 (5), Sep/Oct 1978, 296-298.

11 Fielding, P. An exploratory investigation of self concept in the institutionalised elderly, and a comparison with nurses' conceptions and attitudes. (Study in four settings, a day hospital, an assessment ward, a rehabilitation ward and a long term care ward.) International Journal of Nursing Studies, 16 (4), 1979, 345-354.

12 Fitzpatrick, J.J. and Donovan, M.J. Temporal experience and motor behavior among the aging. (Study to compare institutionalised and non-institutionalised people.) Research in Nursing and Health, 1 (2), Jul 1978, 60-68.

13 Gresham, M.L. The infantilization of the elderly: a developing concept. (Recognition of infant-like behaviour in the elderly.) Nursing Forum, 15, 1976, 195-210.

14 Henthorn, B.S. Disengagement and reinforcement in the elderly. (Survey of two elderly groups to explore relationship between degree of disengagement and self-reported reinforcement.) Research in Nursing and Health, 2 (1), Mar 1979, 1-18.

15 Jacobs, B.P. When age brings a crisis, the nurse can restore hope. (Causes of loneliness in old people and the nurse's role in combating it.) Nursing Mirror, 147, 12 Oct 1978, 25-27.

16 Jones, E. Refresher course. Immobilisation syndrome in the elderly. Nursing Times, 72, 1 Jul 1976, 1009-1011.

17 Keywood, O. 'Sans everything'—not yet. (Plea for greater sensitivity in approaches to care for the elderly.) Nursing Times, 74, 18 May 1978, 820-821.

18 Kiesel, M. and Bininger, C. An application of psycho-social role theory to the aging. (Role possibilities of the elderly in nurse-patient interactions.) Nursing Forum, 18 (1), 1979, 80-91.

19 Kratz, C.R. Sensory deprivation—3. In the elderly. Nursing Times, 75, 22 Feb 1979, 330-332.

20 McNulty, B. The elderly: a challenge to nursing—9. Longevity and loss. (Emotional needs of elderly and coping with various types of loss.) Nursing Times, 73, 15 Dec 1977, 1967-1968.

21 Munns, B. Problems and satisfactions of the elderly person's perceptions of their main life concerns with comparisons in certain areas between these perceptions and those of nurse interviewers. MSc thesis, Surrey University, 1980.

22 Thurmott, P. The elderly: a challenge to nursing—7. Isolation and loneliness. Nursing Times, 73, 1 Dec 1977, 1884-1886.

23 Wahl, P.R. Therapeutic relationships with the elderly. Journal of Gerontological Nursing, 6 (5), May 1980, 260-266.

24 Wilkin, D. and Jolley, D.J. Mental and physical impairment in the elderly in hospital and residential care. 1. Old people in two long-stay geriatric wards, one long-stay psychogeriatric ward and 14 local authority residential homes were assessed during 1977 using the Crichton Royal Behavioural Rating Scale. Nursing Times, 74, 19 Oct 1978, Occ. papers, 117-120; 26 Oct 1978, Occ. papers, 124.

25 Wilkin, D. and others Changes in behavioural characteristics of elderly populations of local authority homes and long-stay hospital wards, 1967-7. (Assessment using Crichton Royal Behavioural Rating scale showing the need for a reappraisal of present patterns of care.) British Medical Journal, 2, 4 Nov 1978, 1274-1276.

54 COMMUNITY CARE

a GENERAL

1 Alexander, J.R. and Eldon, A. Characteristics of elderly people admitted to hospital, Part III Homes, and sheltered housing. (Dependency characteristics and medical problems.) Journal of Epidemiology and Community Health, 33 (1), Mar 1979, 91-95.

2 Allen, V. A plant for Sam. (District nursing care study of elderly man who had neglected himself and had ulcerated legs.) Nursing Times, 76, 18/25 Dec 1980, 2225-2229.

3 Anderson, F. Helping old people to continue living at home. The doctor and the old person in the community. Royal Society of Health Journal, 98 (1), Feb 1978, 3-5.

4 Armitage, M. The cost of caring for the elderly. (Domiciliary social services.) Social Work Today, 10, 5 Jun 1979, 15-16.

5 Agate, J. Taking care of old people at home. Unwin Paperbacks, 1979.

6 Auckland, A. Community nursing care study. Mr. Hogg—chairman. (An elderly man dependent on the voluntary home help and the local community hospital.) Nursing Times, 73, 12 May 1977, 703-704.

7 Baker, A.A. Slow euthanasia—or 'she will be better off in hospital'. (Frail and neglected elderly people living in their own homes do not always benefit from being moved into hospital.) British Medical Journal, 2, 4 Sep 1976, 571-572.

8 Bosanquet, N. Inside the social services: community care for the elderly. Nursing Times, 73, 26 May 1977, 791-792.

9 Bradshaw, J. and others Found dead: a study of old people found dead. Mitcham: Age Concern, 1978. (Occasional paper, no.5.)

10 British Association of Social Workers Social work with the elderly. Guidelines from BASW. Social Work Today, 8, 12 Apr 1977, 7-15.

11 Burgess, K. Community nursing care study. My Mrs. Masters. Nursing Times, 73, 6 Jan 1977, 34.

12 Challis, D. and others Bringing better community care to fragile elderly people. (Community Care Project in Kent.) Social Work Today, 11, 5 Feb 1980, 14-16.

13 Chapman, P. Unmet needs and the delivery of care: a study of the utilisation of social services by old people. Social Administration Research Trust, 1979. (Occasional papers on social administration; 61.)

14 Christie, L. The case for a Central Advisory Service for the Elderly. (In each town, to coordinate provision of information on financial, health and welfare matters.) Nursing Mirror, 147, 13 Jul 1978, 22-23.

15 Chow, R.K. Quality of care: a present and future challenge for all nurses. (Patient Care Management System for elderly people in the community.) Journal of Gerontological Nursing, 6 (5), May 1980, 255-259.

16 Clark, A.N.G. Diogenes syndrome: how to assess severe, self-imposed neglect. Geriatric Medicine, 10 (2), Feb 1980, 65-67.

17 Collins, A. Social services and care of the elderly. (By student nurse on community care option.) Nursing Mirror, 145, 27 Oct 1977, 37.

18 Craigmile, W.M.M. and others Domiciliary care of the elderly. (Survey in Aberdeen of dependency characteristics and other features.) Nursing Times, 74, 2 Feb 1978, Occ. papers, 13-15.

19 Cruise, J. Better geriatric care: making it happen. (Report of DHSS-sponsored project in Exeter.) Health Trends, 4 (10), Nov 1978, 92-95.

20 Davidson, N. Ageing ghettos feeling the pressure. (Provision for the elderly in Norfolk including voluntary organisations.) Health and Social Service Journal, 89, 8 Feb 1979, 130-133.

21 Department of Health and Social Security. Social Work Service Development Group Growing old in Brighton: a development group exercise in Brighton in 1977-79. HMSO, 1980.

22 Faulkner, H. Breaking down the prison of a pensioner's loneliness. (Activities of Help the Aged, by its director.) Health and Social Service Journal, 87, 18 Nov 1977, 1594-1595.

23 Gray, N. Community nursing. Nursing a geriatric patient at home. Nursing Mirror, 145, 27 Oct 1977, 40.

24 Gunshon, B. Nursing care study. United in caring. (Care of two elderly people by the Bury district nursing service.) Nursing Times, 73, 24 Mar 1977, Health Centre, xx, xxii, xxiv.

25 Hall, J.E. But the gas fire never arrived: a case study of Sam. (Role of HV with elderly man, by student nurse on community option.) Health Visitor, 51 (12), Dec 1978, 471-472.

26 Jarvis, J. Care of the elderly in the community. (King's Fund study day reported by Wendy Robinson.) Nursing Mirror, 144, 26 May 1977, 6-9.

27 Lewis, S. Building a care service on rock foundations. (Home care service for the elderly in Bromley AHA.) Health and Social Service Journal, 89, 13 Apr 1979, 416-417.

28 Luker, K.A. Health visiting and the elderly. (Observation of home visits suggests that health visitors' visits lacked a clear aim and structure.) Midwife, Health Visitor and Community Nurse, 15 (11), Nov 1979, 457-459.

29 Luker, K.A. Health visiting and the elderly: an experimental study to evaluate the effects of focused health visitor intervention on elderly women living alone at home. PhD thesis, University of Edinburgh, 1980.

30 Lyons, H. Updating Greek legends. (How Kensington and Chelsea and Westminster AHA (Teaching) used the Delphi technique to make strategy for development of services for the elderly.) Health and Social Service Journal, 89, 18 May 1979, 600-603.

31 Marks-Maran, H.C. The wheelchair arrived... (Community nursing care study of elderly man with pulmonary fibrosis, osteoporosis of the spine and peripheral vascular disease.) Nursing Times, 74, 13 Jul 1978, 203-204, 207.

32 Marshall, M. Community nursing care study. With the old folks at home. (Caring for an elderly Scottish lady at home.) Nursing Times, 73, 2 Jun 1977, 819-821.

33 Marshall, S. A processed approach to Annie. (District nursing care study with care plan for 80-year-old patient with range of problems.) Nursing Mirror, 151, 11 Sep 1980, Supplement, ix-xi.

34 Millard, P.H. Geriatric care in the community. Midwife, Health Visitor and Community Nurse, 12 (4), Apr 1976, 109, 111, 113.

35 Morris, J. Problems in old people. (Living at home.) Midwife, Health Visitor and Community Nurse, 14 (4), Apr 1978, 106-107.

36 Muir Gray, J.A. and Gayler, I. Mixed bathing. (Survey of the time spent by district nurses and nursing auxiliaries in Oxfordshire bathing elderly patients.) Queen's Nursing Journal, 19 (9), Sep 1976, 169-170.

37 Muir Gray, J.A. Nursing the elderly in the community: who should do what? (Overlapping roles of health visitor and district nurse.) Nursing Mirror, 146, 18 May 1978, 42-44.

38 Oliver, V.A. Community nursing care study. Her final choice. (Elderly patient who discharged herself from hospital and died at home.) Nursing Times, 73, 16 Jun 1977, 900-901.

39 Opit, L.J. and Shaw, S.M. Care of the elderly sick at home, whose responsibility is it? (Need for a unified administration combining medical and social services.) Lancet, 2, 20 Nov 1976, 1127-1129.

40 Opit, L.J. Domiciliary care for the elderly sick: economy or neglect? (Costs of the home nursing service in the Central Birmingham Health District.) British Medical Journal, 1, 1 Jan 1977, 30-33.

41 Plank, D. Caring for the elderly: report of a study of various means of caring for dependent elderly people in eight London boroughs. Greater London Council, 1977. (Research memorandum.)

42 Roberts, I. The elderly: a challenge to nursing—14. Planning care at home. Nursing Times, 74, 26 Jan 1978, 154-156.

43 Roberts, V. and De Berker, A. Home care: a joint task for the family practice and social workers. (Multidisciplinary project in Waltham Forest involving health and social services staff.) Health and Social Service Journal, 88, 4 Aug 1978, 875-876.

44 Robertson, C. and others Domiciliary health and welfare services for the elderly in Glasgow: use and need. Community Health, 7 (3), Jan 1976, 128-133.

45 Royal Society of Health Journal Helping old people to continue living at home. (Five articles on nursing and medical care, social services, occupational therapy and the role of the day hospital.) Royal Society of Health Journal, 98 (1), Feb 1978, 3-18.

46 Sullivan, J.A. and Armignacco, F. Effectiveness of a comprehensive health program for the well-elderly by community health nurses. (Evaluation of three nursing approaches.) Nursing Research, 28 (2), Mar/Apr 1979, 70-75.

47 Toll, P. Community nursing care study. Mrs. Jones. (Case study undertaken while on district nurse training.) Nursing Times, 72 (34), 26 Aug 1976, 1306-1307.

48 Truscott, D. For freedom and dignity in old age. (Self help groups of pensioners and role of voluntary worker.) Health and Social Service Journal, 87, 27 May 1977, 860-861.

49 White, C.A. Community nursing care study. Aided independence. (Study of elderly lady by student nurse.) Nursing Times, 72, 11 Nov 1976, 1758-1760.

50 Williams, I. The care of the elderly in the community. Croom Helm, 1979.

51 Yeadon, J. Community nursing care study. Fergus. (Elderly man.) (Second prize in a

Nursing Times essay competition.) Nursing Times, 72, 30 Sep 1976, 1513-1514.

b DAY HOSPITALS AND SHORT STAY

1 Bowl, R. Day danger of reflecting that old block mentality. Review of some current research in day care for the elderly. Health and Social Service Journal, 87, 7 Oct 1977, 1410-1411.

2 Brocklehurst, J.C. and Tucker, J.S. Progress in geriatric day care. King Edward's Hospital Fund for London, 1980.

3 Comben, S. and McNicoll, M. Geriatric day hospital: remedial or social centre? British Journal of Occupational Therapy, 42 (9), Sep 1979, 211-212.

4 Cornforth, G. and Chew, K. A joint approach: cross-financing at work. (Scheme in Driffield which allows elderly patients to become day residents in two homes while still under hospital care.) Health and Social Service Journal, 86, 10 Jul 1976, 1256.

5 Dall, J.L.C. Helping old people to continue living at home. The contribution of the day hospital. (With elderly patients.) Royal Society of Health Journal, 98 (1), Feb 1978, 10-11.

6 Furbank, M.E. Combined day hospital/day centre. (At Liskeard, Cornwall, for the rehabilitation and assessment of elderly patients and to relieve relatives.) Nursing Times, 73, 22/29 Dec 1977, Occ. papers, 161-162.

7 Gooch, L.A. and Luxton, D.E.A. A new geriatric day hospital. (Attached to Tower Hospital, Ely.) Nursing Mirror, 145, 21 Jul 1977, 36-38.

8 Griffiths, R.A. and Cosin, L.Z. The floating bed. (Admission of geriatric patients for 2 nights out of every fortnight in the Oxford region.) Lancet, 1, 27 Mar 1976, 684-685.

9 Hewinson, E.E. The GP hospital: one example of an ideal arrangement. (In Tamworth, offering short-term holiday care for the elderly.) Modern Geriatrics, 8 (12), Dec 1978, 10-11.

10 Hornby, M. and Brown, M. The night comes alive with laughter. (Evening group for elderly people organised at Castleford Geriatric Day Hospital to provide care and relieve relatives.) Health and Social Service Journal, 89, 5 Oct 1979, 1286-1287.

11 Irvine, R.E. Geriatric day hospitals: present trends. (With statistics on attendances and costs.) Health Trends, 3 (12), Aug 1980, 68-71.

12 Kaim-Caudle, P. The chat shop on wheels. (Assessment of the experimental provision of a mobile day centre for the elderly in Sunderland.) Health and Social Service Journal, 88, 6 Jan 1978, 11.

13 Keetch, J. The long weekend. (Problems of home care of geriatric patients during weekends and holidays illustrated by two case studies.) Queen's Nursing Journal, 19 (2), May 1976, 38-39.

14 McNicoll, M. and Comben, S.C. Geriatric day hospital—remedial or social centre? Physiotherapy, 65 (7), Jul 1979, 210-211.

15 Marston, P.D. Day hospitals: a physiotherapist's view. (Burton House Day Hospital, University Hospital of South Manchester.) Physiotherapy, 62 (5), May 1976, 151-152.

16 Martin, A. and Millard, P.H. Day hospitals for the elderly: therapeutic or social? St. George's Hospital Geriatric Teaching and Research Unit, 1978.

17 Moore, J. and Mellotte, C. Day services can be a realistic alternative to residential care. (For handicapped adults and the elderly, with reference to a survey in Kirklees.) Health and Social Service Journal, 88, 17 Nov 1978, 1314-1315; 24 Nov 1978, 1346-1347.

18 National Corporation for the Care of Old People Day care for the elderly: the role of residential homes. NCCOP, 1976. (Home advice broadsheets, no.2.)

19 National Corporation for the Care of Old People Provision of transport to outpatient departments and day hospitals: problems and possibilities: report of the two conferences... The Corporation, 1978.

20 Robinson, W. Experiment in geriatric care. (Geriatric day unit at South Western Hospital, Stockwell.) Nursing Mirror, 144, 20 Jan 1977, 39-41.

21 Schattschneider, H. Community resources for the elderly: 2 programs. (Day Therapy Centre, Hamilton, Ontario, and the Day Hospital in Edmonton, Alberta.) Canadian Nurse, 73 (4), Apr 1977, 47-51.

22 Tyndall, R.M. Day hospital dilemma: when patients refuse. Lack of attendance at day hospitals may mean the referrals were not appropriate. Modern Geriatrics, 8 (2), Feb 1978, 34-35, 37.

c FAMILY

1 Archbold, P.G. Impact of parent caring on middle-aged offspring. (Six families with elderly parent one or more years post-stroke.) Journal of Gerontological Nursing, 6 (2), Feb 1980, 78-85.

2 Bergmann, K. How to keep the family supportive. (Of elderly relatives.) Geriatric Medicine, 9 (8), Aug 1979, 53-54, 57.

3 Boyd, R.V. and Woodman, J.A. The Jekyll-and-Hyde syndrome: an example of disturbed relations affecting the elderly. (Difference in capability of the disabled when supervised by trained staff and when at home with relatives.) Lancet, 2, 23 Sep 1978, 671-672.

4 Deeping, E. Caring for elderly parents. Constable, 1979.

5 Felstein, I. Continuing care and holiday relief (for relatives of the elderly chronically sick). Midwife, Health Visitor and Community Nurse, 13 (3), Mar 1977, 75-76.

6 Franks, H. Your parent—your problem: the relative burden of old age. (Stress in families looking after elderly relatives.) Mind Out, 17, Jul/Aug 1976, 11-13.

7 Isaacs, B. Don't expect relatives to help. (In care of the elderly.) Nursing Mirror, 149, 27 Sep 1979, 25-26.

8 Isaacs, B. Geriatric patients: do their families care? (Admission of old people to a geriatric unit in Glasgow when home care was not possible.) British Medical Journal, 4, 30 Oct, 282-286.

9 Keddie, K.M.G. Action with the elderly: a handbook for relatives and friends. Oxford: Pergamon, 1978. (Problems and progress in development series.)

10 Kratz, C. The elderly: a challenge to nursing—3. Old people and their families. (Review of studies of support given by families of old people.) Nursing Times, 73, 3 Nov 1977, 1719-1720.

11 McKenzie, H. GP guidance can relieve the daughter's burden. (Survey by National Council for the Single Woman and her Dependants.) Geriatric Medicine, 9 (12), Dec 1979, 4.

12 McKenzie, H. Help for the single woman with elderly dependants. (By administrative director of the National Council for the Single Woman and her Dependants.) Nursing Times, 74, 16 Feb 1978, 292-293.

13 McMurray, M. Mr. Poot and family. (Care study of elderly man living with relatives outlining roles of primary health care team.) Nursing Times, 76, 14 Aug 1980, Community Outlook, 224-226, 238.

14 Sandford, J.R.A. Tolerance of debility in elderly dependants by supporters at home: its significance for hospital practice. (Survey at University College and Whittington Hospitals analysing the problems which, if alleviated, would restore a tolerable situation at home.) British Medical Journal, 3, 23 Aug, 471-473.

d SCREENING, SURVEYS AND 'AT RISK'

1 Abrams, M. Beyond three-score and ten: a first report on a survey of the elderly. Mitcham: Age Concern, 1978. (Age Concern Research Publication.)

2 Barber, J.H. and Wallis, J.B. An information system on the needs of the elderly. (Geriatric assessment programme, Woodside Health Centre developed so health visitors could assess needs objectively.) Health Bulletin, 34 (6), Nov 1976, 324-330.

3 Barber, J.H. and Wallis, J.B. Looking after the old 2. The benefits to an elderly population of continuing geriatric assessment. Journal of the Royal College of General Practitioners, 28, Jul 1978, 425-429.

4 Barber, J.H. and Wallis, J.B. Screening in general practice. Assessment of the elderly in general practice. (Assessment programme by health visitors at Woodside Health Centre, Glasgow.) Journal of the Royal College of General Practitioners, 26, Feb 1976, 106-114.

5 Barber, J.H. and others A postal screening questionnaire in preventive geriatric care. (Survey in Woodside Health Centre which had response rate of 81%.) Journal of the Royal College of General Practitioners, 30, Jan 1980, 49-51.

6 Best, P. The elderly: a challenge to nursing—13. Health promotion for the elderly. (Health education and screening.) Nursing Times, 74, 19 Jan 1978, 111-114.

7 Buckley, E.G. Personal points of view—the

role of the general practitioner in the geriatric assessment unit. Health Bulletin, 35 (6), Nov 1977, 323-326.

8 **Caird, F.I. and Judge, T.G.** Assessment of the elderly patient. 2nd ed. Tunbridge Wells: Pitman Medical, 1979.

9 **Chang, B.L.** Perceived situational control of daily activities: a new tool. (For assessing the elderly.) Research in Nursing Health, 1 (4), Dec 1978, 181-188.

10 **Charlewood, J.E.** Screening: first 'tame' the beast. (How four GPs in Newcastle-upon-Tyne set up screening service.) Geriatric Medicine, 9 (10), Oct 1979, 25-27.

11 **Colt, A.M. and others** Home health care is good economics. (Report of project to determine the demand for and costs of domiciliary services for the elderly.) Nursing Outlook, 25 (10), Oct 1977, 632-636.

12 **Cook, J.** A search for minor but remedial complaints. (Prize-winning entry in screening competition outlining procedures and involving GP or practice nurse.) Geriatric Medicine, 10 (4), Apr 1980, 70.

13 **Davidson, P. and others** Asking questions in the house. (Survey by Solihull health care planning team into needs of elderly for hearing aids and chiropody.) Health and Social Service Journal, 89, 17 Aug 1979, 1045-1046.

14 **Dodsworth, A.L.** Preventive medicine in geriatrics — 1. Screening the elderly. Nursing Times, 72, 10 Jun 1976, 909-910.

15 **Douglas-Jones, A.** Screening for a health future. (Prize-winning entry in competition.) Geriatric Medicine, 10 (5), May 1980, 67-68.

16 **Dunt, D.R. and others** A technique for precisely measuring activities of daily living. (In the elderly in three situations — without physical aids and personal assistance and with both aids and assistance.) Community Medicine, 2 (2), May 1980, 120-121.

17 **Epps, B.M.** Counting the cost of old age. (Stockport's dependency scale and services.) Health and Social Service Journal, 90, 22 Aug 1980, 1096-1099.

18 **Felstein, I.** Screening in later life. (Description of some screening schemes for the elderly with three readers' letters on p.306, 309.) Nursing Times, 75, 11 Oct 1979, Community Outlook, 305-306.

19 **Figgins, P.** Screen now — benefit later. (Setting up of screening clinics for the over-fifties involving HVs.) Nursing Mirror, 149, 30 Aug 1979, 24-25.

20 **Fordyce, I.D. and Russell, E.M.** A sample survey: older people at home. (Aberdeen.) Community Medicine, 2 (4), Nov 1980, 291-297.

21 **Frazer, F.W.** Assessment of elderly patients. (Tool for use by doctor and physiotherapist, including distress and disability classifications.) Physiotherapy, 65 (7), Jul 1979, 212-213.

22 **Freedman, G.R. and others** Looking after the old. 1. Screening the aged in general practice. Journal of the Royal College of General Practitioners, 28, Jul 1978, 421-425.

23 **Goble, R.E.A. and others** Functional assessment of the elderly: occupational therapy in general practice. British Journal of Occupational Therapy, 42 (9), Sep 1979, 207-210.

24 **Hall, M.R.P.** The assessment of disability in the geriatric patient. Rheumatology and Rehabilitation, 15 (2), May 1976, 59-64.

25 **Hay, E.H.** A geriatric survey in general practice. (Screening survey of 300 patients by doctors and nurses at Shirebrook Health Centre, Mansfield.) Practitioner, 216, Apr 1976, 443-447.

26 **Henderson, P.A.** Problems of a survey of the elderly in a general practice. (Based on visits by health visitors.) Practitioner, 222, Jan 1979, 19-21.

27 **Hoadley, D.M.** Survey of nursing and social needs of the elderly in a group practice. (Crawley, Sussex.) Nursing Times, 72, 4 Nov 1976, 1731-1732.

28 **Hunt, A.** The elderly at home: a survey... HMSO, 1978.

29 **Isaacs, B. and Neville, Y.** The needs of old people. The 'interval' as a method of measurement. (Survey of the elderly in the west of Scotland to measure needs for residential and domiciliary services.) British Journal of Preventive and Social Medicine, 30 (2), Jun 1976, 79-85.

30 **Luker, K.A.** Measuring life satisfaction in an elderly female population. (Use of Life Satisfaction Index in pilot study for research on health visitor intervention.) Journal of Advanced Nursing, 4 (5), Sep 1979, 503-511.

31 **McNab, A. and Philip, A.E.** Screening an elderly population for psychological well-being. (Survey by community nurses using a Personal Disturbance Scale (SAD).) Health Bulletin, 38 (4), Jul 1980, 160-162.

32 **Pike, L.A.** Screening the elderly in general practice. Journal of the Royal College of General Practitioners, 26, Sep 1976, 698-703.

33 **Rauckhorst, L.M. and others** Community and home assessment. Journal of Gerontological Nursing, 6 (6), Jun 1980, 319-327.

34 **Rowe, J. and Vernon, R.** Registering need. (Simple scheme for compiling an Elderly at Risk register.) Nursing Times, 74, 10 Aug 1978, Community Outlook, 238.

35 **Shaw, S.** The role of the nurse in assessing the health of elderly people in McLachlan, G. editor. Probes for health. Oxford University Press, 1975. Chapter 6, 109-123.

36 **Stokes, S.A. and others** Health assessment — considerations for the older individual. Journal of Gerontological Nursing, 6 (6), Jun 1980, 328-337.

e HYPOTHERMIA

1 **Age Concern Westminster. Heating Liaison Officer** How to keep warm. The Author, 1979.

2 **Bangs, C.** Do's and dont's of immediate treatment. (Of hypothermic patient.) RN Magazine, 42 (11), Nov 1979, 42-44.

3 **Collins, K.J. and others** Accidental hypothermia and impaired temperature homoeostatis in the elderly. British Medical Journal, 1, 5 Feb 1977, 353-356.

4 **Green, D.** Keeping your client warm. (Methods of cash help and material aid available.) Nursing Mirror, 148, 4 Jan 1979, 30-32.

5 **Green, M.** Home heating. (Effect of hypothermia on elderly and means of prevention.) Royal Society of Health Journal, 97 (4), Aug 1977, 177-183, 186-187.

6 **Gupta, K.** Managing the patient with accidental hypothermia. Geriatric Medicine, 9 (12), Dec 1979, 51-52.

7 **Hayter, J.** Hypothermia hyperthermia in older persons. Journal of Gerontological Nursing, 6 (2), Feb 1980, 65-68.

8 **Health Education Council. Medical and Research Division** Hypothermia in the elderly. The Health Education Council's 'Cold Kills the Old' campaign. Health Education Journal, 36 (2), 1977, 49-54.

9 **Help the Aged** Death in winter: a special report on inadequate heating conditions amongst the old. Help the Aged, 1978.

10 **Keywood, O.** Too cold or too hot? (Hypo- and hyperthermia in elderly people.) Nursing Mirror, 147, 5 Oct 1978, 55.

11 **Ledingham, I.M. and others** Central rewarming system for treatment of hypothermia. Lancet, 1, 31 May 1980, 1168-1169.

12 **Lye, M.** Heatwaves bring high mortality to elderly. (Hyperthermia.) Health and Social Service Journal, 88, 26 May 1978, 612.

13 **Millard, P.H.** Hypothermia in the elderly. (Symposium on care of the elderly.) Nursing Mirror, 145, 3 Nov 1977, 23-25.

14 **Rautray, R.C. and Jones, B.** Fighting hypothermia. (Causes and management of the elderly with hypothermia.) Nursing Mirror, 147, 31 Aug 1978, 22.

15 **Shearer, A.** Elderly. (Campaign in Birmingham to prevent hypothermia.) New Society, 35, 1 Jan 1976, 17.

16 **West, J.** The chill wind of approaching old age. (Hypothermia in the elderly with reference to role of district nurse and her use of metallised thermal blankets.) Journal of Community Nursing, 3 (7), Jan 1980, 4-5.

17 **Wicks, M.** Old and cold: hypothermia and social policy. Heinemann, 1978. (Studies in social policy and welfare.)

18 **Wicks, M. and Donnison, D.** Out in the cold? A debate on hypothermia. (With reference to supplementary benefits.) New Society, 44, 15 Jun 1978, 597-599.

f NUTRITION AND DIET

1 **Allard, J. and others** Malnutrition and neglect. (In the elderly at home.) Nursing Mirror, 146, 5 Jan 1978, 18-20.

2 **Booth, T.** Nutrition survey strikes a warning note for elderly. The dietary effects of the meals on wheels service. Health and Social Service Journal, 87, 15 Jul 1977, 1050-1051.

3 **Davies, L. and Holdsworth, M.D.** A tech-

nique for assessing nutritional 'at risk' factors in residential homes for the elderly. Journal of Human Nutrition, 33 (3), Jun 1979, 165-169.

4 Debry, G. Nutrition of the elderly. (Survey in France.) Journal of Human Nutrition, 31 (3), Jun 1977, 195.

5 Department of Health and Social Security. Committee on Medical Aspects of Food Policy Nutrition and health in old age: the cross-sectional analysis of the findings of a survey made in 1972/3 of elderly people who had been studied in 1967/8. HMSO, 1979. (Report on health and social subject; 16.)

6 Dickerson, J.W.T. Nutrition, aging and the elderly. Royal Society of Health Journal, 98 (2), Apr 1978, 81-83, 95.

7 Garland, M.H. Problems in the elderly. 6. Malnutrition in the elderly. Hospital Update, 5 (4), Apr 1979, 337-338, 340.

8 Judge, T.G. Nutrition of the elderly. Physiotherapy, 62 (6), Jun 1976, 178-179.

9 Kemm, J.R. Meals-on-wheels and Luncheon Clubs. (Demand for and value of these services.) Health Trends, 4 (11), Nov 1979, 90-92.

10 Leslie, J. Nutrition and diet. 6. The elderly. Nursing Mirror, 145, 25 Aug 1977, 31-33.

11 MacLennan, B. Malnutrition: cause or effect. (In the elderly.) Health and Social Science Journal, 87, 16 Sep 1977, 1328.

12 Nursing Three articles on nutrition in the elderly with one on the work of the geriatric visitor. Nursing, 12, Apr 1980, 517-520.

13 Pollman, J.W. and others Is fiber the answer to constipation problems in the elderly? A review of literature. International Journal of Nursing Studies, 15 (3), 1978, 107-114.

14 Stanley, G. and Lutz, W. Meals services for the elderly in Scotland. Edinburgh: Scottish Home and Health Department, 1976. (Scottish health service studies, no.35.)

g REHABILITATION

1 Ager, G. Aides for the elderly during inclement times. (Aides based in hospital social work department who visit elderly patients after discharge.) Health and Social Service Journal, 89, 29 Jun 1979, 806-807.

2 Blair, P. When the elderly go home. (Continuing Care Project in Birmingham looking at ways of helping discharged patients.) Health and Social Service Journal, 89, 4 May 1979, 517.

3 Bhowmick, D.K. and Arnold, J.P. Half-way house in geriatric practice. (Home for elderly patients fit to leave hospital but not yet ready to return home.) British Medical Journal, 2, 31 Jul 1976, 293-294.

4 Christie, A. Holiday exchange success. (Involving geriatric patients at Cameron Hospital, Fife and Roadmeetings Hospital, Carluke.) Nursing Times, 74, 31 Aug 1978, 1453-1454.

5 Davidson, N. You can't buy dignity on the cheap. (Ways of meeting health needs of elderly population with reference to Birmingham-based

Continuing Care Project.) Health and Social Service Journal, 89, 22 Feb 1979, 160-161.

6 Felce, D. and Jenkins, J. Engagement in activities by old people in residential care. (Descriptive and experimental studies in a geriatric hospital and two residential homes.) Health and Social Service Journal, 89, 2 Nov 1979, Centre eight papers, E23-E28.

7 Goldstone, H. Helping old people to continue living at home. Stop, Look, Listen. (Occupational therapy and rehabilitation.) Royal Society of Health Journal, 98 (1), Feb 1978, 15-18.

8 Griffiths, A. and Bhowmick, B.K. Sick role status and the elderly discharged from hospital. (Suggest that elderly people stagnate or regress socially on discharge.) Practitioner, 221, Dec 1978, 926-928.

9 Jones, C.T. and Dent, A.M. Occupational therapy in residential homes for the elderly. (Scheme in Mid Derybshire Division of Derbyshire Social Services Dept.) British Journal of Occupational Therapy, 43 (1), Jan 1980, 16.

10 Keywood, O. Preparing the elderly to return home. (Rehabilitation of hospital patients.) Nursing Mirror, 147, 7 Sep 1978, 42-44; 14 Sep 1978, 38-40.

11 National Corporation for the Care of Old People Organising aftercare: an examination of ways in which aftercare arrangements for elderly hospital patients could be improved... NCCOP, 1979. (Continuing care project.)

12 Partridge, C. and Wright, B. Helping patients to help themselves. 4. The elderly patient. (Advice on rehabilitation for community nurses.) Nursing Mirror, 146, 29 Jun 1978, 38-39.

13 Rees, J. Rehabilitation of an elderly patient back into the community. Nursing Times, 74, 16 Mar 1978, 448-452.

14 REHABILITATION service in an acute medical geriatric unit. (Amersham, Bucks.) British Journal of Occupational Therapy, 40 (8), Aug 1977, 183-186.

15 Slack, G. A 'hospital' for the elderly patient in the comfort of his own home. (Work of the Continuing Care Project and findings of recent studies.) Health and Social Service Journal, 88, 14 Jul 1978, 791-792.

16 Smith, J. A special kind of package deal... (Hotel at St. Leonards owned by Hackney Borough Council providing holidays for their elderly citizens.) Health and Social Service Journal, 88, 21 Jul 1978, 826-828.

17 Struthers, T. Old—but they keep a purpose in life. (Rehabilitation programme in a residential home.) British Journal of Occupational Therapy, 39 (2), Feb 1976, 44-45.

18 Thursfield, P.J. The hospital that doesn't say 'goodbye'! (Scheme to provide continuity of care for elderly patients discharged from hospital and awaiting admission.) Nursing Mirror, 148, 8 Feb 1979, 50-52.

19 Williams, L.V. Occupational therapy for the elderly. (Nurse's role and care plan based on the nursing process.) Nursing Times, 75, 25 Jan 1979, 167-169.

h RESIDENTIAL CARE AND HOUSING

1 Baines, G. Where cutting costs can mean a deadly risk of life. (Fire hazards in old people's homes.) Health and Social Service Journal, 87, 13 May 1977, 808-809.

2 Bosanquet, N. Inside the social services. Residential care for the elderly. Nursing Times, 73, 28 Apr 1977, 615-616.

3 Brearley, C.P. Residential work with the elderly. Routledge and Kegan Paul, 1977.

4 Brenner, D. Equipment research. (Scheme in Southwark to equip handicapped elderly people with a radio contact alarm system.) Health and Social Service Journal, 89, 24 Aug 1979, 1068-1069.

5 Butler, A. and Oldman, C. The ringing of false alarm bells. (Alarm systems for the elderly.) Health and Social Service Journal, 89, 31 Aug 1979, 1112-1113.

6 Chippendale, A. A warden's day. (In a sheltered housing scheme for the elderly, showing the health problems of residents.) New Society, 45, 7 Sep 1978, 508-509.

7 Clarke, A.K. E.M.M.A.: a comprehensive alarm system for the elderly infirm and disabled who live alone. British Journal of Occupational Therapy, 42 (9), Sep 1979, 214.

8 Clarke, M. and others The elderly in residential care: patterns of disability. (One-day census of elderly people in institutional care provided by NHS, social service department, and voluntary and private agencies.) Health Trends, 1 (11), Feb 1979, 17-20.

9 Coakley, D. and Woodford-Williams, E. Effects of burglary and vandalism on the health of old people. Lancet, 2, 17 Nov 1979, 1066-1067.

10 Davidson, N. What outlook for sheltered housing? Health and Social Service Journal, 89, 25 Jan 1979, 77.

11 Department of Health and Social Security A classification of staff in homes for the elderly. HMSO, 1977. (Statistical and research report series, no.18.)

12 Department of Health and Social Security and Welsh Office Residential homes for the elderly: arrangements for health care. A memorandum of guidance. DHSS, 1977.

13 Dickson, N. An alternative to the service 'too young to benefit from lessons in its own history'. (History of Springbok House, an experimental rest home for the infirm elderly opened in 1952 and its relevance to today's needs.) Health and Social Service Journal, 88, 3 Nov 1978, 1254-1255.

14 Dodd, K. and others A census of elderly people in care. (Census in Leicestershire aimed to measure how residents were able to cope with daily living and staff's attitudes.) Social Work Today, 10, 31 Jul 1979, 10-13.

15 Fry, L. Aftermath. Implications of the recent fire at Wensley Lodge old people's home. Health and Social Service Journal, 87, 14 Jan 1977, 48-49.

16 Gibberd, K. Unnatural homes. (Residential homes for the elderly.) New Society, 38, 2 Dec 1976, 462-463.

17 Gore, L. Richmond Hill climb up a better type of service. (Using management by objectives to improve care in an old people's home.) Health and Social Service Journal 86, 4 Mar 1977, 388-389.

18 Grier, M.R. Choosing living arrangements for the elderly. (Descriptive studies of decision making process.) International Journal of Nursing Studies, 14 (2), 1977, 69-76.

19 Grier, M.R. Living arrangements for the elderly. (Survey of how nurses and elderly people make decisions about choosing living arrangements for the elderly.) Journal of Gerontological Nursing, 3 (4), Jul/Aug 1977, 19-22.

20 Hain, M.J. and Chen, S.P.C. Health needs of the elderly (in two high rise apartments, Erie, Pennsylvania). Nursing Research, 25 (6), Nov-Dec 1976, 433-438.

21 Hardie, M. The elderly: a challenge to nursing—10. Housing and the elderly. Nursing Times, 73, 22/29 Dec 1977, 1996-1998.

22 Harris, D. A question of life and death in the home. (Attitudes to death of residents and staff in homes for the elderly.) Social Work Today, 11, 8 Jul 1980, 25.

23 Harris, H. Workhouse? Hotel?—it's still just the bleedin' same! (Homes for the elderly, which in spite of hotel-like surroundings erode residents' privacy and power.) Social Work Today, 9, 1 Nov 1977, 13-15.

24 Harrisson, S. and Ayton, M. Dependency of elderly people in homes on staffing ratios. (Survey including need for professional nursing care.) Health and Social Service Journal, 89, 3 Aug 1979, Centre eight papers, E15-E20.

25 Hartie, M. Elderly couple require small council house. . . (Case study showing problems in rehousing, by a health visitor.) Nursing Mirror, 147, 14 Dec 1978, 58-60.

26 Lewis, R.J. Flying warden answers 80-year-old's Mayday call. (Scheme in Stockport involving domiciliary care teams and assistants to back up wardens in sheltered housing.) Modern Geriatrics, 9 (3), Mar 1979, 27-30, 33.

27 Lewis, R.J. Is this home the place for the very frail elderly? Stockport social services and the AHA are running an experimental home with more nursing and double the usual number of care assistants. Geriatric Medicine, 9 (4), Apr 1979, 17-18.

28 Lindars, M.E. Residential homes for the elderly. (Role of the professional nurse.) Nursing Mirror, 146, 19 Jan 1978, 41.

29 Lipman, A. and Slater, R. Building high to avoid confusing the elderly confused. (Some problems of spatial disorientation in building accommodation for the elderly based on recent research.) Health and Social Service Journal, 86, 11 Sep 1976, 1634-1635.

30 Lodge, B. and Parker, F. The resident's role in residential homes for the elderly. (With 24-hour programme of activity and leisure including orientation in time and space.) Nursing Times, 76, 21 Aug 1980, 1495-1500.

31 McKay, R. Private lives. . . (Increased use of private residential accommodation by local authorities and inadequacy of statutory controls.) Health and Social Service Journal, 89, 25 Jan 1979, 74-76.

32 Miller, P. and Russell, D.A. Elements promoting satisfaction as identified by residents in the nursing home. (Research study using Life Satisfaction Index.) Journal of Gerontological Nursing, 6 (3), Mar 1980, 121-129.

33 Orriss, H.D. Fire precautions in old people's homes. Nursing Times, 72, 18 Nov 1976, 1812-1814.

34 Peace, S. Life in old people's homes. (Report of survey of elderly people's opinions in attempt to measure 'quality of life'.) Mind Out, 33, Mar/Apr 1979, 21.

35 Petrie, J. Building up a challenge to traditional care of the elderly: the design of a newly built home for the elderly. Health and Social Service Journal, 87, 8 Apr 1977, 628-629.

36 Roe, P. and Guillem, V. The need for medical supervision in homes. (Survey of residential homes for the elderly in Somerset revealed the extent of unmet medical need.) Health and Social Service Journal, 88, 10 Feb 1977, 168-169.

37 Rogers, P.J. The elderly: a challenge to nursing—11. Furniture and the elderly. (Choice and arrangement for optimum mobility.) Nursing Times, 74, 5 Jan 1978, 32-34.

38 Rose, V. Catering for old age: Whiteley Village community. Nursing Mirror, 142, 15 Apr 1976, 70-72.

39 Turner, J. The last refuges, where all too many old people go to die. (Private old people's homes.) New Society, 47, 25 Jan 1979, 183-186.

40 University of Keele. Department of Adult Education The quality of life of the elderly in residential homes and hospitals: report of a seminar. . .25-27 Mar 1977. Stoke-on-Trent: Beth Johnson Foundation/University of Keele, 1977.

41 Ward, P. Quality of life in residential care. Personal Social Service Council, 1980.

42 West, J. Nursing homes and the care of the elderly. Nursing Mirror, 142, 11 Mar 1976, 56.

43 Whitton, J. How to quench the last flames of independence in old age: the erosion of personal autonomy in residential homes for the elderly. Health and Social Service Journal, 87, 3 Jun 1977, 894-895.

55 PSYCHOGERIATRICS

a GENERAL

1 Beck, C. Mental health and the aged: a values analysis. Advanced in Nursing Science, 1 (3), Apr 1979, 79-87.

2 British Medical Journal Dementia—the quiet epidemic. (Diagnosis and treatment, including role of community nurse.) British Medical Journal, 1, 7 Jan 1978, 1-2.

3 British Medical Journal Management of elderly demented patients. British Medical Journal, 1, 21 May 1977, 1301.

4 Cowper-Smith, F. The ageing brain: the problem before us. (Report of conference on psychogeriatric care.) Nursing Times, 75, 12 Jul 1979, 1166.

5 Davidson, R. The elderly disturbed patient. (Assessment and treatment.) Nursing Mirror, 146, 6 Apr 1978, 23-24.

6 Davidson, R. The problem of senile dementia. Nursing Times, 74, 1 Jun 1978, 932-933.

7 Fine, W. Cerebral symptomatology in old age. Nursing Mirror, 146, 11 May 1978, 33-36.

8 Gilleard, C.J. and others Behavioural disabilities in psychogeriatric patients and residents of old people's homes. (With reference to assessment using CAPE behaviour rating scale.) Journal of Epidemiology and Community Health, 34 (2), Jun 1980, 106-110.

9 Godber, C. The confused elderly. Nursing Times, 72 (28), 15 Jul 1976, Care of the elderly supplement, vii, viii, x.

10 Godber, C. Demented—or just a scapegoat? (Evaluation of mental state of elderly patients with list of diagnostic pointers.) Nursing Mirror, 149, 19 Jul 1979, 29-30.

11 Hare, M. Clinical check list for diagnosis of dementia. (Study in a psychogeriatric unit.) British Medical Journal, 2, 22 Jul 1978, 266-267.

12 Hirschfeld, M.J. The cognitively impaired older adult. American Journal of Nursing, 76 (12), Dec 1976, 1981-1984.

13 Jolley, D. Dementia in old age: an outline of current issues. Health Trends, 12 (1), Feb 1980, 1-4.

14 Jones, G. Elderly confused people: a study of a multidisciplinary unit in action. Social Work Service, 23, Jun 1980, 27-33.

15 Jones, I.H. Senile dementia. Nursing Times, 75, 18 Jan 1979, 104-106.

16 Miller, A.E. Geriatrics in psychiatry. Nursing Mirror, 142, 3 Jun 1976, 52-54.

17 MIND Mental health of elderly people: Mind's response to the DHSS discussion paper 'A happier old age'. Mind, 1979.

18 Norberg, A. and others Ethical problems in feeding patients with advanced dementia. (Study in Sweden of patients difficult to spoon feed with reference to psychological model of 'double-binding'.) British Medical Journal, 281, 27 Sep 1980, 847-848.

19 Pasker, P. and others The elderly mentally ill—whose responsibility? (A census in North-East Essex to evaluate needs.) British Medical Journal, 2, 17 Jul 1976, 164-166.

20 Presly, A.S. and others An evaluation of the reduction in patient number in psychogeriatric wards. (Assessment of regrouping of patients from two wards to three new wards.) Health Bulletin, 38 (1), Jan 1980, 32-36.

21 Shaw, J. A literature review of treatment options for mentally disabled old people. Journal of Gerontological Nursing, 5 (5), Sep/Oct 1979, 36-42.

22 Smith, T.C.G. Chronic brain syndrome. (In the elderly. Discussion of Crichton Geriatric Behavioural Rating Scale.) Journal of Community Nursing, 1 (3), Sep 1977, 28.

23 Thomson, I. Integration of psychiatric assessment for the elderly. (With that of younger patients in the Isle of Wight.) Lancet, 2, 30 Jul 1977, 239-240.

24 Wattis, J.P. Mental problems in the elderly. (Brief mention of HV's role.) Midwife, Health Visitor and Community Nurse, 16 (5), May 1980, 214, 216.

25 Whitehead, T. Confusing causes of confusion. (Acute confusional states in the elderly.) Nursing Mirror, 147, 21 Sep 1978, 29-30.

26 Whitehead, T. Confusing the causes of confusion. (Acute confusion due to underlying medical condition or to emotional states, eg severe anxiety and mixed manic depressive state.) Nursing Mirror, 151, 17 Jul 1980, 38-39.

27 Whitehead, T. In the service of old age: the welfare of psychogeriatric patients. 2nd ed. Aylesbury: HM & M, 1978.

28 Whitehead, T. Psychiatric disorders in old age: a handbook for the clinical team. 2nd ed. Aylesbury: HM & M, 1979. (For nurses and others.)

29 Worth, D. Not in their perfect mind. (Mental deterioration in the elderly.) Nursing Mirror, 147, 2 Nov 1978, 50-52.

b NURSING

1 Black, S. and Simon, R. The specialist nurse, support care and the elderly mentally infirm. (Service in Bucks based on Tindal General Hospital involving community psychiatric nursing, admission unit and long stay provision.) Nursing Times, 76, 14 Feb 1980, Community Outlook, 45-46.

2 Blair, S.E.E. Supportive psychotherapy groups with the elderly. (In a psychogeriatric admission unit.) British Journal of Occupational Therapy, 42 (6), Jun 1979, 137-138.

3 Brown, E. Psychogeriatrics: on the right track. (Psychogeriatric assessment ward at Bangour Village Hospital, West Lothian.) Nursing Mirror, 149, 6 Sep 1979, 50-51.

4 Chivers, T. Introduction of care plans in a psychogeriatric ward. (At the London Hospital.) Nursing Times, 74, 30 Nov 1978, Supplement, 21-24.

5 Christie, L.S. Some thoughts after 30 years nursing: planning based on realistic information is the only way we can build an adequate service to provide care for the elderly mentally ill in psychiatric hospitals. Nursing Times, 75, 16 Aug 1979, 1398-1399.

6 Conroy, C. and Clarke, P.J. Reality orientation: a basic rehabilitation technique for patients suffering from memory loss and confusion. (For confused elderly patients.) British Journal of Occupational Therapy, 40 (10), Oct 1977, 250-251.

7 Degun, C. Reality orientation: a multidisciplinary therapeutic approach. (A controlled study with 18 geriatric patients at Warley Hospital, Brentwood, of a therapeutic orientation method initiated in the United States.) Nursing Times, 72 (33), 19 Aug 1976, Occ. papers, 117-120.

8 Evans, P.J. Thinking of Maslow. (Discussion of patients' psychological needs with reference to Maslow's hierarchy of needs applied to psychogeriatric nursing. By a student nurse.) Nursing Times, 76, 24 Jan 1980, 163-165.

9 Fairbairn, H.A. Reality orientation with geriatrics: a three month project at the Geriatric Unit, Newtown Hospital, Worcester. British Journal of Occupational Therapy, 43 (6), Jun 1980, 204-205.

10 Goble, I.W.J. Nursing care study. Chronic brain syndrome: a challenge to nursing skills. (In 69 year old man.) Nursing Mirror, 147, 7 Dec 1978, 47-49.

11 Gray, P. and Stevenson, J.S. Changes in verbal interaction among members of resocialization groups. (Group therapy in nursing home with confused elderly people.) Journal of Gerontological Nursing, 6 (2), Feb 1980, 86-90.

12 Haber, L.C. and others The effect of short term group psychotherapy on the elderly. Canadian Journal of Psychiatric Nursing, 18 (1), Jan-Feb 1977, 8-11.

13 Hahn, K. Using 24-hour reality orientation. Journal of Gerontological Nursing, 6 (3), Mar 1980, 130-135.

14 Heaney, M.W. and Brooks, M. Never too old to climb. (A nurse administered program designed to help elderly psychiatric patients achieve more independence.) Journal of Psychiatric Nursing and Mental Health Services, 13 (6), Nov/Dec 1975, 37-41.

15 Hector, L. Nursing care study. A time for caring. (For elderly lady in psychogeriatric hospital.) Nursing Times, 74, 4 May 1978, 750-752.

16 Hefferin, E.A. and Hunter, R.E. Reality orientation. How we turned the idea into a program. (Implementing better patient care through research on nursing care plans.) Nursing, 77 7 (5), May 1977, 10-12.

17 Hettiaratchy, P. Group psychotherapy is unorthodox, but it works. (In psychogeriatric unit with non-demented day patients.) Geriatric Medicine, 9 (5), May 1979, 61-62.

18 Hillman, D. Stimulation of the long-stay and psychogeriatric patient. Nursing Times, 72, 21 Oct 1976, 1648-1649.

19 Hogstel, M.O. Use of reality orientation with aging confused patients. Nursing Research, 28 (3), May/Jun 1979, 161-165.

20 Holden, U.P. A flexible technique for rehabilitating the confused. (Reality orientation.) Geriatric Medicine, 9 (7), Jul 1979, 49-50.

21 Holden, U.P. Return to reality. (Reality orientation for withdrawn, confused and depressed old people.) Nursing Mirror, 149, 22 Nov 1979, 26-29.

22 Hunt, P. The elderly: a challenge to nursing—8. Confusion in the elderly. Nursing Times, 73, 8 Dec 1977, 1928-1929.

23 Isaacs, B. Don't bother—she won't notice! (Causes of dementia and nursing care.) Nursing Mirror, 149, 1 Nov 1979, 24-25.

24 Jackson, B.S. The role of the psychiatric nurse specialist in caring for the institutionalized aged. Journal of Psychiatric Nursing, 17 (11), Nov 1979, 21-23.

25 Lee, R.E. Reality orientation. Restoring the senile to life. Journal of Psychiatric Nursing, 26 (1), Jan 1976, 28-29, 35, 37; (2), Feb 1976, 30-31.

26 McDonnell, P. Nursing care study. Senile dementia: a restless, lonely old lady. Nursing Mirror, 149, 6 Sep 1979, 46-49.

27 McMordie, W.R. and Blom, S. Life review therapy: psychotherapy for the elderly. (Emphasising 'positive' reminiscing.) Perspectives in Psychiatric Care, 17 (4), Jul/Aug 1979, 162-166.

28 Matthews, R. and Kemp, M. Rooms of the past strike a chord in the mentally infirm. (Decoration of day rooms in styles from Victorian/Edwardian era to 1950s to test patients' response to surroundings, at Powick Mental Hospital.) Geriatric Medicine, 9 (6), Jun 1979, 37-38, 41.

29 Miller, A.E. Evaluation of the care provided for patients with dementia in six hospital wards. MSc thesis, University of Manchester, Department of Nursing, 1978.

30 Nursing Times Embarrassment of male nurses. (Problems in female psychogeriatric wards at Warlingham Park Hospital.) Nursing Times, 76, 27 Mar 1980, 533.

31 Potter, A. Nursing care study. In a world of her own. (Advanced senile dementia.) Nursing Mirror, 150, 3 Apr 1980, 48-49.

32 Powter, S. Senile dementia. Nursing care study. (Symposium on care of the elderly.) Nursing Mirror, 145, 3 Nov 1977, 31-32, 35.

33 Rampersad, M. Annie is demented. (Hospital care.) Nursing Times, 75, 18 Jan 1979, 106-107.

34 Scott, D. and Crowhurst, J. Reawakening senses in the elderly. (Sensory retraining in a psychiatric setting using activities such as singing, tasting and marching.) Canadian Nurse, 71 (10), Oct 1975, 21-22.

35 Stevens, P. Problems with Emily. (Community psychiatric nursing care of the elderly lady.) Nursing Times, 74, 27 Apr 1978, 721-723.

36 Todd, J. Water depletion in mentally disturbed elderly patients. (Details of three patients.) Nursing Mirror, 142, 29 Apr 1976, 60-61.

37 Trick, K.L.K. and Daisley, R.A. A handbook of psychogeriatric care. Tunbridge Wells: Pitman Medical, 1980.

38 Twist, R.L. Psychogeriatric patients need encouragement and acceptance. Canadian Journal of Psychiatric Nursing, 18 (2), Mar-Apr 1976, 8-10.

39 Voelkel, D. A study of reality orientation and resocialization groups with confused elderly. (Research study.) Journal of Gerontological Nursing, 4 (3), May/Jun 1978, 13-18.

40 Walker, M. and Nepom, R. Reality orientation: establishing a climate of trust in geriatric care. Canadian Nurse, 76 (7), Jul/Aug 1980, 26-27.

41 Wilkinson, I.M. and Graham-White, J. Dependency rating scales: for use in psychogeriatric nursing. (Development of scale by researchers at Royal Edinburgh Hospital.) Health Bulletin, 38 (1), Jan 1980, 36-41.

c SERVICES

1 Anderson, C.J. Issues in the treatment of psychiatric-geriatric patients: a brief review of the literature. (American practice in dealing with elderly mentally ill.) Journal of Gerontological Nursing, 3 (3), May/Jun 1977, 32-41.

2 Chivers, T. and Westwater, J. Hospital care of confused elderly people. Nursing, 9, Jan 1980, 393-396.

3 Cowper-Smith, F. 'I think you're wonderful'. (Report of visit to and work on psychogeriatric unit at Netherne Hospital, Surrey.) Nursing Times, 75, 16 Aug 1979, 1393-1397.

4 Hanley, T. Practical care of geriatric patients. (d) The organization of psychogeriatric care. Royal Society of Health Journal, 95 (1), Feb 1975, 31-35.

5 Haurheeram, I. Integrated geriatric wards. (Mixed sex psychogeriatric ward at Fairfield Hospital, Herts.) Nursing Times, 75, 8 Mar 1979, 406.

6 Jolley, D. Hospital inpatient provision for patients with dementia. British Medical Journal, 1, 21 May 1977, 1335-1336.

7 Milne, J.S. and Robinson, R.A. New referrals during one year to a psychiatric service for the elderly. (Royal Victoria Hospital, Edinburgh.) Health Bulletin, 35 (2), Mar 1977, 84-88.

8 Murray, P. Failing to count the days. (The present state of psychogeriatric services.) Health and Social Service Journal, 89, 15 Feb 1979, 157-159.

9 Savage, B.J. and Wright, A.L. Shared care of the elderly. (Joint project between Fulbourn Hospital and Cambridgeshire Social Services Department in psychiatric care.) Nursing Times, 73, 31 Mar 1977, 465-468.

10 Shulman, K. and Arie, T. Fall in admission rate of old people in psychiatric units. British Medical Journal, 1, 21 Jan 1978, 156-158.

11 Whitehead, T. A general hospital service for the elderly mentally ill. (Includes description of unit in Brighton.) Hospital and Health Services Review, 73 (9), Sep 1977, 306-308.

12 Whitehead, T. Running a special unit for the elderly mentally ill. (In Brighton health district.) Modern Geriatrics, 9 (2), Feb 1979, 59-60.

d COMMUNITY AND DAY HOSPITALS

1 Ainsworth, D. The community nurse in a developing psychogeriatric service. (Based on Withington Hospital, Manchester.) Nursing Times, 74, 25 May 1978, 873-874.

2 Ball, T. A share in the caring. (How ambulance staff were trained and involved with psychogeriatric day hospital patients in Bingley, West Yorkshire.) Health and Social Service Journal, 90, 13 Jun 1980, 776-778.

3 Brown, C. Community psychiatric nursing. A psychogeriatric day unit. (Stepping Stones House, Bromley.) Nursing Times, 72, 4 Nov 1976, 1711-1713.

4 Brunt, P. and Simmons, R. Caring for the elderly mentally ill in old people's homes. (Pilot scheme in a residential home in Buckinghamshire.) Health and Social Service Journal, 86, 10 Dec 1976, 2196-2197.

5 Burkitt, P.A. Community nursing care study. 'My Wilfred.' (Male nurse's care of elderly man with senile dementia. First prize in a Nursing Times essay competition.) Nursing Times, 72, 30 Sep 1976, 1511-1513.

6 Crawford, M. Occupational therapy with the elderly mentally ill and infirm. (In local authority home.) British Journal of Occupational Therapy, 43 (1), Jan 1980, 17-19.

7 Davies, V. Psychogeriatrics. Finding the best home for the confused elderly. (Six-bed psychogeriatric unit in Denbigh.) Nursing Mirror, 147, 26 Oct 1978, 51-53.

8 Fottrell, E. and others 'Asset stripping' the declining mental hospital. A psychogeriatric day hospital was developed from a long-stay back ward of a large mental hospital. (Tooting Bec.) British Medical Journal, 280, 12 Jan 1980, 89-90.

9 Fuller, J. and others Dementia: supportive groups for relatives. (Scheme at the German Hospital in East London.) British Medical Journal, 1, 23 Jun 1979, 1684-1685.

10 Godber, C. Dementia in the elderly: don't overwhelm the family. (Management of the confused elderly patient at home including support for relatives.) Nursing Mirror, 149, 26 Jul 1979, 30-32.

11 Godber, C. Managing psychogeriatric problems: don't wait until the relatives are desperate. (Short-stay relief scheme in Southampton.) Modern Geriatrics, 9 (3), Mar 1979, 47-48.

12 Heaslewood, J. Home helps problems swept under the carpet. (Call for increased numbers and specialised training with reference to the care of the mentally confused elderly.) Health and Social Service Journal, 89, 5 Jan 1979, 15.

13 Hemsi, L. Psychogeriatric care in the community. (With reference to setting up new department in an Inner London Borough.) Health Trends, 12 (2), May 1980, 25-29.

14 Hunt, P. A community psychiatric nurse describes her job. (With special reference to care of elderly people.) Geriatric Medicine, 9 (4), Apr 1979, 41-43.

15 Hunt, P. Dementia in the elderly: the caring family needs support. (Role of community psychiatric nurse with psychogeriatric patients and relatives.) Nursing Mirror, 149, 2 Aug 1979, 24-25.

16 Journal of the Royal College of General Practitioners Brain failure. (Care of elderly with senile dementia in the community.) Journal of the Royal College of General Practitioners, 27, Aug 1977, 451-453.

17 Lodge, B. and Parker, F. Environmental modification in day care. (Using Forest Day Hospital for patients with senile dementia at Carlton Hayes Hospital, as an example.) Social Work Today, 8, 22 Mar 1977, 14-15.

18 McNicholas, W. A home for the confused elderly. (Ullswater House, London.) Nursing Times, 73, 19 May 1977, 747-750.

19 Manning, M. I don't want to be a burden. (The community psychogeriatric service in Southampton featured in a BBC TV documentary.) Nursing Mirror, 146, 26 Jan 1978, 6-8.

20 Masters, P. Senile dementia — community support. (Role of community psychiatric nurse.) Nursing Times, 76, 12 Jun 1980, 1065.

21 Savage, B.J. and Wright, A.L. Shared care of the elderly. (Co-operation between a psychogeriatric ward at Fulbourn Hospital, Cambridge, and Cambridgeshire Social Service Department.) Health and Social Service Journal, 86, 8 May 1976, 840-841.

22 Sidell, M. Confused elderly people and community care. (Community psychogeriatric nursing service in Cambridgeshire.) Nursing, 9, Jan 1980, 399-402.

23 Sykes, P. Residential care of the elderly mentally handicapped. Royal Society of Health Journal, 98 (1), Feb 1978, 30-31.

24 Tippings, R. and White, D.M.D. New community nursing service for the elderly mentally ill. (In Hereford Health District.) Nursing Times, 74, 19 Oct 1978, 1719-1720.

25 Tough, H. and others Surgery-attached psychogeriatric nurses: an evaluation of psychiatric nurses in the primary care team. (Survey of five nurses' work with 50 patients.) Journal of the Royal College of General Practitioners, 30, Feb 1980, 85-89.

26 Winbow, A. Home visits by hospital team can help psychogeriatric patients. (To assess patients.) Modern Geriatrics, 8 (2), Feb 1978, 19-20, 23.

27 World Health Organization. Regional Office for Europe Psychogeriatric care in the community. Copenhagen: WHO, 1979. (Public health in Europe; 10.)

56 DISABLED

a GENERAL

1 Agerholm, M. Classification of intrinsic handicaps. (Disadvantage arising from individual's own characteristics as opposed to environment or circumstances.) Nursing Times, 75, 4 Oct 1979, Occ. papers, 108.

2 Agerholm, M. Handicap: the way to better understanding. (Definitions and classifications of handicaps with checklist of difficulties for use in assessment.) Nursing Mirror, 149, 19 Jul 1979, 37-39.

3 Agerholm, M. Handicaps and the handicapped: a nomenclature and classification of intrinsic handicaps. Royal Society of Health Journal, 95 (1), Feb 1975, 3-8.

4 Bamford, T. Integrating the disabled. Alf Morris: champion under attack. Social Work Today, 8, 19 Apr 1977, 6-7.

5 Banham, B.J. Practical assistance for the handicapped. (Work of Disabled Living Foundation.) Midwife, Health Visitor and Community Nurse, 15 (6), Jun 1979, 240-241.

6 Bebbington, A.C. Scaling indices of disablement. (In assessing the personal independence of subjects in research surveys.) British Journal of Preventive and Social Medicine, 31 (2), Jun 1977, 122-126.

7 Blaxter, M. The meaning of disability: a sociological study of impairment. Heinemann, 1976.

8 Bosanquet, N. Inside the social services... The blind, the deaf and the physically handicapped. Nursing Times, 73, 30 Jun 1977, 1006-1007.

9 Buchanan, J.M. and Chamberlain, M.A. Survey of the mobility of the disabled in an urban environment. Royal Association for Disability and Rehabilitation, 1978.

10 Burningham, S. The right to take risks. (Current progress towards freedom of access for the disabled.) Health and Social Service Journal, 88, 4 Aug 1978, 882-884.

11 Campling, J. Better lives for disabled women. Virago, 1979.

12 Chartered Society of Physiotherapy Handling the handicapped: a guide to the lifting and movement of disabled people. 2nd ed. Cambridge: Woodhead-Faulkner, 1980.

13 Creese, A.L. and Fielden, R. Hospital or home care for the severely disabled: a cost comparison. British Journal of Preventive and Social Medicine, 31 (2), Jun 1977, 116-121.

14 Davis, M. The institutional tradition. (The faults of hospital treatment for the physically handicapped.) Nursing Mirror, 143, 23 Sep 1976, 65-67.

15 DECLARATION of Rights of Deaf-Blind Persons. (Adopted by the Helen Keller World Conference on Services to Deaf-Blind Youths and Adults in 1977.) International Nursing Review, 25 (4), Jul/Aug 1978, 121.

16 DIRECTORY for the disabled: a handbook of information and opportunities for the disabled and handicapped. Woodhead-Faulkner/Multiple Sclerosis Society, 1977.

17 Disabled Living Foundation Coping with disablement. Heinemann Medical, 1979.

18 Gungadin, G. Patient care study. Life in a wheelchair. Queen's Nursing Journal, 18 (11), Feb 1976, 298, 302.

19 Gunn, A.D.G. Aspects of student health. Problems of disabled students. British Medical Journal, 1976, 2, 18 Dec 1976, 1498-1499.

20 Health and Social Service Journal Education and the disabled. (Six articles dealing with physical and mental handicap, deafness and blindness.) Health and Social Service Journal, 87, 4 Nov 1977, 1524-1532, 1535-1538.

21 Kiernan, C. The hands say it all. (Use of sign language and symbol systems by the handicapped.) Nursing Mirror, 151, 25 Sep 1980, 16-20.

22 KING's Fund directory of organisations for patients and disabled people. King Edward's Hospital Fund for London, 1979.

23 Kowalsky, E.L. The nurse's role in health maintenance of the physically disabled client. AORN Journal, 4 (1), Jan/Feb 1979, 12-15.

24 Kushlick, A. Some ways of setting, monitoring and attaining objectives for services for disabled people. (Research being undertaken by the Wessex Regional Health Authority.) British Journal of Mental Subnormality, 21 (2), Dec 1975, 84-102.

25 McCarthy, B.P. The management of menstrual flow in disabled women. (Preliminary findings from Disabled Living Foundation project.) Nursing Times, 76, 6 Mar 1980, 409-411.

26 Marais, E. and Marais, M. Lives worth living: the right of all the handicapped. Souvenir Press, 1976. (Human horizons series.)

27 Marshall, M. Engineering help for disabled people. (Work of REMAP, Rehabilitation Engineering Movement Advisory Panels.) Nursing Times, 76, 11 Dec 1980, Community Outlook, 371.

28 Mattingly, S. The Disabled Persons Register. Health Trends, 10 (1), Feb 1978, 19-20.

29 Morris, A. 'I'm arguing for a photo finish, not for a level start.' (Interview with the Minister for the Disabled.) Health and Social Service Journal, 87, 22 Jul 1977, 1072-1075.

30 Nursing Mirror A symposium on caring for the severely handicapped. From a Study Day held at the Royal Hospital and Home for Incurables, Putney. Nursing Mirror, 145, 8 Dec 1977, 13-25.

31 Nursing Times Disability without handicap. A special supplement on practical help for disabled people. Nursing Times, 74, 17 Aug 1978, Supplement, 3-4, 6, 8, 11, 14, 16-17, 19-20.

32 Office of Health Economics Physical impairment: social handicap. OHE, 1977. (Studies of current health problems, no.60.)

33 Orriss, H. Putting the elderly into a balanced perspective. (A plea for other deprived groups such as the disabled, mentally ill and handicapped who do not receive the same publicity as the elderly.) Health and Social Service Journal, 86, 4 Feb 1977, 202-203.

34 Osborne, P. Learning from experience. (Report of study tour to Denmark, Holland and Sweden to study the care of the disabled, accompanied by a tetraplegic friend.) Nursing Mirror, 146, 23 Feb 1978, 26-29.

35 Perry, E.L. The ethics of caring. (For handicapped people.) Nursing Mirror, 145, 8 Dec 1977, 20-22.

36 Rostron, J. and Rostron, P.M. Services for the disabled. Part 2. Implications of research study and assessment of areas of need uncovered. Nursing Mirror, 146, 16 Feb 1978, 49-50.

37 Smith, R.T. and Midanik, L. The effects of social resources on recovery and perceived sense of control among the disabled. (Primary group affiliations and formal group relationships.) Sociology of Health and Illness, 2 (1), Mar 1980, 48-63.

38 Topliss, E. Provision for the disabled. 2nd ed. Oxford: Basil Blackwell; Martin Robertson, 1979.

39 Veal, B. DIG—an organisation of the disabled. (Disablement Income Group.) Nursing Mirror, 143 (14), 30 Sep 1976, 66-67.

40 Warren, M.D. Identifying handicapped people in general practice. (The use of the age sex register as a basis for locating the handicapped.) Journal of the Royal College of General Practitioners, 26, Nov 1976, 828-836.

41 Working Party on Integration of the Disabled Report. National Fund for Research into Crippling Diseases, 1976. (Chairman: The Earl of Snowdon.)

b AIDS, EQUIPMENT AND CLOTHING

1 Bowell, R. The disabled who help themselves. (Activities of the Possum Users' Association and details of the Cordent-Possum project to develop equipment for people with very limited movement.) Nursing Mirror, 145, 29 Dec 1977, 14-17.

2 Burningham, S. Always reinventing the wheel. (Pilot scheme in Redbridge of appointment of designer to design and make aids for the disabled.) Health and Social Service Journal, 89, 17 Aug 1979, 1043.

3 Carpenter, E.M. An inflatable bath aid. (Airlift MK 7, for handicapped children and adults.) British Journal of Occupational Therapy, 41 (12), Dec 1978, 409.

4 Chamberlain, M.A. Aids centres: what they do. (Survey of 13 centres.) Health Trends, 12 (2), May 1980, 39-40.

5 Chamberlain, M.A. and others Evaluation of aids and equipment for bath and toilet. (Survey in Leeds and recommendations for improved continuity of care for discharged patients.) Rheumatology and Rehabilitation, 17 (3), Aug 1978, 187-194.

6 Community Outlook Getting the right piece in the right place. (Article and fact sheet on equipment for the disabled.) Nursing Times, 75, 8 Feb 1979, Community Outlook, 33, 35-37, 39-40, 42.

7 Cowper-Smith, F. Active leisure for the handicapped. (Through games, toys, and other equipment. Report of a seminar held by the organisation 'Active.') Nursing Times, 73, 26 May 1977, 774-776.

8 Cowper-Smith, F. A life of your own. (Report of Naidex, exhibition of aids for the disabled.) Nursing Times, 74, 5 Oct 1978, 1628-1631.

9 Cowper-Smith, F. Moving towards independence. (Report of visit to Naidex 77, exhibition of aids for the disabled.) Nursing Times, 73, 1 Dec 1977, 1863-1866.

10 Cumbie, A. Express delivery. (New department run by Red Cross centralising the supply of all home aids for Leicestershire AHA's medical and social services.) Health and Social Service Journal, 88, 26 May 1978, 606.

11 **Diamond, J.** Aiding detached in a semi. (Rehabilitation house in Lancaster for assessment and training in activities of daily living.) Health and Social Service Journal, 88, 3 Feb 1978, 132-133.

12 **Disabled Living Foundation** The importance of clothing in the care of long-term patients. Report of a workshop held on hospital clothing by the Disabled Living Foundation at the King's Fund Centre, London. British Journal of Occupational Therapy, 40 (4), Apr 1977, 88-89.

13 **Feeney, R.** Aids for living (for the disabled). Nursing Times, 42, 2 Dec 1976, 1884-1885.

14 **Fowler, I.** Sharing fifty-fifty all the way for Hastings. (Pilot scheme organised jointly by health and social services in Hastings for the supply and distribution of nursing aids.) Health and Social Service Journal, 89, 19 Oct 1979, 1352-1353.

15 **Gardiner, R.** Provision of aids and equipment for the elderly and disabled in the community. (Description of distribution service of Fife Health Board.) Health Bulletin, 36 (6), Nov 1978, 310-312.

16 **Haworth, R.J. and Nichols, P.J.R.** Hoists in the home: their recommendation and use. Rheumatology and Rehabilitation, 19 (1), Feb 1980, 42-57.

17 **Hinks, M.D.** Clothing and the long-term patient. (Disabled Living Foundation workshop.) Nursing Mirror, 144, 10 Mar 1977, 39-41.

18 **Jay, P.** Clean living: some of the most practical bathing aids available. Nursing Mirror, 146, 6 Apr 1978, 40.

19 **Jay, P.** Medical concerns. (Suitable clothing for the handicapped.) Nursing Mirror, 146, 20 Apr 1978, 36.

20 **Jefcoate, R.** Roger: I know you can do it. (Interview with Roger Jefcoate, consultant assessor on technical aids for the disabled.) Nursing Times, 73, 10 Feb 1977, 212-213.

21 **Jefcoate, R.** Using technology to add life to years. (Electronic aids for the handicapped.) Journal of Community Nursing, 3 (2), Aug 1979, 11, 32.

22 **Morris, M.A.** Aid for the disabled. (Vac-Pac system of envelope filled with polystyrene beads to help muscular dystrophy patients maintain comfortable position.) British Medical Journal, 1, 7 Jan 1978, 25-26.

23 **Office of Population Censuses and Surveys. Social Survey Division** Wheelchairs and their users: a survey. HMSO, 1977.

24 **Orriss, H.** A lone crusader breaking the cruel bonds of handicap. (The work of Roger Jefcoate, independent consultant and assessor of electronic aids.) Health and Social Service Journal, 87, 14 Jan 1977, 52-53.

25 **Page, M. and Feeney, R.J.** Measurement and assessment techniques for WC and bath aids for the disabled: a survey carried out by the Institute for Consumer Ergonomics in Loughborough. Nursing Times, 76, 7 Aug 1980, 1404-1408.

26 **Pepmiller, E.G.** Selecting a wheelchair. Helping your patient make the best choice. (With section on nursing considerations for wheelchair-bound patients.) Journal of Practical Nursing, 29 (2), Feb 1979, 12-13, 30.

27 **Pepmiller, E.** Take a seat . . . assessing your patient's wheelchair comfort. Journal of Practical Nursing, 30 (2), Feb 1980, 17-18.

28 **POSSUM.** (Electronic aid systems for the physically handicapped.) Nursing Times, 76, 28 Aug 1980, Supplement, 7-8.

29 **Robertson, J.C. and Haines, J.R.** A community/hospital home aids loan scheme (based on a Rehabilitation Demonstration Centre). (In Salisbury.) Health Trends, 10 (1), Feb 1978, 15-16.

30 **Robinson, W.** Aids for the disabled. Nursing Mirror, 146, 16 Feb 1978, Supplement, i, iii, v, vii, ix, xi, xiii, xv.

31 **Robinson, W.** Possum means 'I can.' (Work of the Possum Controls Ltd factory producing electronic aids for the disabled.) Nursing Mirror, 144, 3 Feb 1977, 45-47.

32 **Rose, V.** Apprentices design handicap aids. (British Aircraft Corporation.) Nursing Mirror, 143, 11 Nov 1976, 59-61.

33 **Ruston, R. and others** Dressing for disabled people: a manual for nurses and others. Disabled Living Foundation, 1977.

34 **Savage, J.H.** Reading aids for handicapped patients. Book-rest, page holder, and page-turner. Nursing Mirror, 144, 5 May 1977, 60-62.

35 **Savage, J.H.** A simple aid to page turning. (To help disabled people to read books and magazines.) Nursing Mirror, 144, 28 Apr 1977, 46-47.

36 **Savage, J.H.** Wheelchair loading aid. (For loading wheelchairs into cars. Details of construction.) Nursing Mirror, 144, 16 Jun 1977, 34-35.

37 **Selby, M.** Phones for the disabled. (Research project run by DHSS and GPO.) Nursing Mirror, 145, 20 Oct 1977, 45-46.

38 **Sinnott, G.** Stairlifts: a report on the findings of a survey made in cooperation with the Department of Health and Social Security on the use of stairlifts in the home. (In Liverpool.) British Journal of Occupational Therapy, 41 (10), Oct 1978, 334-335.

39 **Tarling, C.** Hoists and their use. Heinemann Medical for Disabled Living Foundation, 1980.

40 **Thornely, G. and others** Evaluation of aids and equipment for the bath and toilet. A report on the findings of a survey funded by the DHSS. British Journal of Occupational Therapy, 40 (10), Oct 1977, 243-246.

41 **Thornton, M.** Clothing for the handicapped. Midwife, Health Visitor and Community Nurse, 16 (2), Feb 1980, 67, 70.

42 **Tudor, M.A.** Wheelchairs. (Rules and guidelines for use and various types available.) Nursing Mirror, 145, 8 Dec 1977, 22-25.

43 **Ward, P.R.** Recovery and reuse of aids for disabled people: the costs and value. Health Trends, 12 (1), Feb 1980, 14-15.

44 **Wilson, D.** Helping the handicapped: 7. Household help. (Aids). 8. Eating and drinking aids. Journal of Community Nursing, 3 (7), Jan 1980, 28-30; (9), Mar 1980, 17-18.

c COMMUNITY AND HOME CARE

1 **Baker, M.R. and others** Planning for the physically handicapped of working age: whose needs? (In a survey severity of handicap as assessed by GPs and independent observer was greater than that perceived by the handicapped themselves.) Health Trends, 3 (12), Aug 1980, 55-56.

2 **Battye, L.** A residential care situation. (A comparison of two Cheshire Homes by a resident.) Social Work Service, 9, Apr 1976, 14-18.

3 **Collins, M. and Collins, D.** Kith and kids: self-help for families of the handicapped. Souvenir Press, 1976. (Human horizons series.)

4 **CONSUMER's viewpoint.** Unanswered questions on my mother's death. (Experiences of social and health services for a disabled patient.) Social Work Today, 8 (4), 26 Oct 1976, 9-10.

5 **Davis, A.J.** Disability, home care and the care-taking role in family life. (Research study with families who decided to keep a disabled adult at home.) Journal of Advanced Nursing, 5 (5), Sep 1980, 475-484.

6 **Department of Health and Social Security** Physically disabled people living at home: a study of numbers and needs. HMSO, 1978. (Report on health and social subjects; 13.)

7 **Foott, S.** Handicapped at home. Design Council/Disabled Living Foundation, 1977.

8 **Frost, W.** Community nursing and the physically handicapped. Nursing Mirror, 144, 3 Mar 1977, 66-68.

9 **Gordon, D.** Social starvation that is beginning of the end. (Report of Greater London Association for the Disabled symposium on the disabled in the community.) Health and Social Service Journal, 87, 25 Nov 1977, 1612-1613.

10 **Greater London Association for the Disabled** The disabled person in the community: who cares? Symposium papers, 25 May 1977 . . . The Association, 1977.

11 **Johnson, A.** The Star and Garter Home for Disabled Sailors, Soldiers and Airmen. Nursing Times, 73, 24 Nov 1977, Archive, 37-40.

12 **Murray, A.D.** How one local authority helps its disabled. (Day centres in Croydon.) Social Work Today, 8 (9), 30 Nov 1976, 13-15.

13 **Newby, J.A.** No room for the disabled? The work of the registered housing associations and their relevance to the disabled. Nursing Times, 73, 8 Dec 1977, Community Outlook, 125, 127-128, 130.

14 **Osborne, P.** Crossroads care attendant scheme: two-year pilot scheme designed to help relatives caring for a disabled person at home. Nursing Mirror, 143 (6), 5 Aug 1976, 60-61.

15 **Rostron, J.** Assessing the needs of the handicapped. The rehousing of and adaptation of accommodation for severely physically disabled adults. Nursing Mirror, 146, 9 Mar 1978, 44-46.

16 **Rostron, J.** Assessing the physically

disabled: social factors in rehousng. Public Health, 92 (5), Sep 1978, 246-250.

17 Rostron, J. Going home: a brief commentary on certain services available to traumatically disabled patients on discharge from hospital. British Journal of Occupational Therapy, 40 (11), Nov 1977, 281-282.

18 Rostron, J. Integrating the disabled. A house without assistance. (The environmental problems facing the disabled.) Social Work Today, 8, 19 Apr 1977, 8-11.

19 Rostron, J. and Rostron, P.M. Assessment techniques for rehousing or adaptations for severely physically disabled adults. International Journal of Nursing Studies, 15 (4), 1978, 203-209.

20 Rostron, J. and Rostron, P.M. Services for the disabled. Part 1. Some of the services available for traumatically disabled patients on discharge from hospital. (Research study.) Nursing Mirror, 146, 9 Feb 1978, 43-44.

21 Royal Assocation for Disability and Rehabilitation Crossroads care attendant scheme trust. RADAR, 1977.

22 Weightman, G. Home winner. (Growth of crossroads care attendance schemes which provide help for relatives with severely disabled people at home.) New Society, 43, 2 Mar 1978, 490-491.

d PSYCHOLOGICAL AND SEXUAL ASPECTS

1 Baxter, R.T. and Linn, A. Sex counselling and the SCI patient. (Importance of emphasising psychological rather than physical aspects.) Nursing, 8 (9), Sep 1978, 46, 48-52.

2 Billington, R. Sexual self image and physical disability. (Work of the counsellor among couples where one or both are disabled.) Midwife, Health Visitor and Community Nurse, 13 (2), Feb 1977, 46-49.

3 Blanchard, M.G. Sex education for spinal cord injury patients and their nurses. Supervisor Nurse, 7 (2), Feb 1976, 20-22, 24-26, 28.

4 Campling, J. Sexuality and the disabled woman. Nursing Times, 76, 28 Aug 1980, Supplement, 14.

5 Craft, M. Sexual problems of the disabled. Psychological aspects. Royal Society of Health Journal, 96 (3), Jun 1976, 110-113.

6 Eardley, A. and Thornton, M. Postsurgical problems. (Symposium paper on sexual problems of the disabled.) Nursing Mirror, 142, 5 Feb 1976, 58-59.

7 Eisenberg, M.G. Psychological aspects of physical disability: a guide for the health care educator. New York: National League for Nursing, 1977.

8 Elyan, P.H. Sexual problems of the disabled. Counselling the handicapped. Royal Society of Health Journal, 96 (3), Jun 1976, 103-105.

9 Fozzard, E.L. The psychosexual needs of the neurologically disabled. Journal of Neurosurgical Nursing, 10 (3), Sep 1978, 92-94.

10 Greengross, W. Entitled to love: the sexual

and emotional needs of the handicapped. Malaby Press/National Fund for Research into Crippling Diseases, 1976.

11 Hamilton, A. The sexual problems of the disabled. Nursing, 5, Aug 1979, 220-225.

12 Hodges, L.C. Human sexuality and the spinal cord injured: role of the clinical nurse specialist. Journal of Neurosurgical Nursing, 10 (3), Sep 1978, 125-129.

13 Holden, T. Patiently speaking. (Paralysed patient's account of dealing with emotional stresses of illness.) Nursing Times, 76, 12 Jun 1980, 1035-1036.

14 Morgan, M.R. Patients with cerebral palsy. (Symposium paper on the sexual problems of the disabled.) Nursing Mirror, 142 (5), 5 Feb 1976, 56-57.

15 Nursing Mirror Sex counsellors for the disabled. Notes on conferences and training courses organised by the Committee on Sexual Problems for the Disabled (SPOD.) Nursing Mirror, 142, 5 Feb 1976, 42.

16 Nursing Mirror A symposium on sexual problems of the disabled. Nursing Mirror, 142, 5 Feb 1976, 47-59.

17 Ogionwo, W. The self-concept of disadvantage: factors which facilitate or hinder change. (How acquired social and psychological factors affect the performance of handicapped people.) International Journal of Health Education, 22 (4), 1979, 216-226.

18 Richards, B. The social and psychological aspects of sexuality. (Symposium paper on the sexual problems of the disabled.) Nursing Mirror, 142, 5 Feb 1976, 50-52.

19 Royal Society of Health Journal Disability and sexual problems. (Four articles on counselling and other aspects.) Royal Society of Health Journal, 98 (1), Feb 1978, 36-48.

20 Royal Society of Health Journal The sexual problems of the disabled. (Five articles.) Royal Society of Health Journal, 96 (3), Jun 1976, 100-113.

21 Silver, J.R. and Owens, E. Sexual problems of the disabled. Psychological reactions. Royal Society of Health Journal, 96 (3), Jun 1976, 108-110.

22 Smith, J. and Bullough, B. Sexuality and the severely disabled person. American Journal of Nursing, 75 (12), Dec 1975, 2194-2197.

23 Stewart, B. Breaking the social taboo on sexual rights of the disabled. Health and Social Service Journal, 86, 29 Oct 1976, Rehabilitation supplement, 6-7.

24 Stewart, W.F.R. Disability and problems of sex—the work of SPOD. (Comments on Sexual Problems of the Disabled.) Midwife, Health Visitor and Community Nurse, 12 (10), Oct 1976, 313, 315-316.

25 Stewart, W.F.R. Sexual rehabilitation—a gap in provision for the disabled. (Symposium paper.) Nursing Mirror, 142 (5), 5 Feb 1976, 48-49.

26 Stewart, W.F.R. The sexual problems of the disabled. Sex and the physically handicapped. Royal Society of Health Journal, 96 (3), Jun 1976, 100-103.

27 Stewart, W.F.R. The sexual side of handicap: a guide for the caring professions. Cambridge: Woodhead-Faulkner, 1979.

28 Task Force on Concerns of Physically Disabled Women Towards intimacy: family planning and sexuality concerns of physically disabled women. 2nd ed. New York: Human Sciences Press, 1978.

29 Task Force on Concerns of Physically Disabled Women Within reach: providing family planning services to physically disabled women. 2nd ed. New York: Human Sciences Press, 1978.

30 Torkildsen, M. Handicapped patients and their special needs. (Sexual problems.) Midwife, Health Visitor and Community Nurse, 14 (6), Jun 1978, 183-184.

31 Walsh, J.J. The spinal cord disabled. (Symposium paper on the sexual problems of the disabled.) Nursing Mirror, 142, 5 Feb 1976, 53.

32 Wilke, H. Psychological aspects of physical disability: a personal approach. Rehabilitation, 98, Jul-Sep 1976, 5-12.

e REHABILITATION AND EMPLOYMENT

1 Blackford, N. Mind over body. (Sport for the disabled.) Nursing Mirror, 151, 17 Jul 1980, 28-29.

2 Bodington, M. Holidays for the severely disabled (from the Royal Hospital and Home for Incurables, Putney). Nursing Mirror, 144, 27 Jan 1977, 68-69.

3 Brosnan, B. Servite House—a home for individuals. (In Ealing, for handicapped men and women.) Nursing Mirror, 145, 25 Aug 1977, 42-44.

4 Brosnan, B. Yoga benefits the disabled. Nursing Mirror, 148, 11 Jan 1979, 16-19.

5 Community Outlook Job sheet. (Assistance for disabled people seeking employment with profiles of six disabled people's experience on p.43.) Nursing Times, 76, 14 Feb 1980, Community Outlook, 40-41.

6 Community Outlook Work—the current state of play. (Employment of disabled people.) Nursing Times, 76, 14 Feb 1980, Community Outlook, 37-38.

7 Cooper, N.E. Vocational reintegration of handicapped workers with assistance devices. International Labour Review, 115 (3), May/Jun 1977, 343-352.

8 Dickinson, M. Integrating the disabled. Rehabilitating the traumatically disabled adult. Social Work Today, 8, 19 Apr 1977, 12-13.

9 Durrant, K.J. Activities for the severely handicapped. (The Elizabeth Centre for training and rehabilitation attached to Little High Wood Hospital, Essex.) Nursing Times, 72, 10 Jun 1976, 911-912.

10 Evans, C. Down the avenues of choice. (Research into the rehabilitation of the handicapped at the Royal Hospital and Home for Incurables, Putney.) Nursing Mirror, 150, 24 Jan 1980, 28.

11 Fairbrother, C. Riding high. (Riding for

the Disabled Association.) Nursing, 5, Aug 1979, 229-230.

12 **Gallop, S.** Integrating the disabled. Two crosses to bear. (Problems of employment for the disabled.) Social Work Today, 8, 19 Apr 1977, 14.

13 **Gunn, A.D.G.** University education for the physically disabled. Journal of the Royal College of General Practitioners, 27, Mar 1977, 161-166.

14 **Hall, E.M.** Rudiments of care 3. Helping the patient with work, or productive occupation. (History and current schemes of rehabilitation of the disabled.) Nursing Times, 75, 21 Jun 1979, 1061-1062.

15 **Hudson, R.** Time to rethink policy for forgotten jobless. Causes for the reduction in registered disabled and the implications of this for employment opportunities. Health and Social Service Journal, 87, 16 Dec 1977, 1702-1704.

16 **Mohr, D.H.** Education and disabled people. Social Service Quarterly, 49 (4), Apr-Jun 1976, 141-143.

17 **Morris, K.** Across to Rome. (Report of bus trip with Across Trust's handicapped passengers in Jumbulance.) Nursing Mirror, 148, 22 Feb 1979, 24-26.

18 **Nursing Times** Wakerley Lodge. (Unit for the young disabled with seven articles on aspects of the work including rehabilitation.) Nursing Times, 73, 12 May 1977, 673, 688-692, 696, 697-699.

19 **Physiotherapy** Recreation for disabled people. (Six articles in each issue.) Physiotherapy, 64 (10), Oct 1978, 289-301; (11), Nov 1978, 324-329.

20 **Robinson, W.** A holiday centre for spastics. (Lanlivery, Cornwall.) Nursing Mirror, 142 (16), 15 Apr 1976, 65-67.

21 **Schlesinger, H.** Breaking barriers to the employment of the disabled. British Journal of Occupational Therapy, 41 (11), Nov 1978, 372-374.

22 **Simpson, R.** Don't quota me. (Quota scheme for employment of disabled people.) New Society, 43, 23 Mar 1978, 668-669.

23 **Turner, A. and Norman, J.** Chair dancing. (For people in wheelchairs.) British Journal of Occupational Therapy, 40 (11), Nov 1977, 270-271.

24 **Warren, M.D.** Disability and rehabilitation: research programme of the health services research unit, University of Kent. (Symposium on rehabilitation in the community.) Rheumatology and Rehabilitation, 16 (4), Nov 1977, 248-249.

25 **WHO Chronicle** Disability prevention and rehabilitation. WHO Chronicle, 30 (8), Aug 1976, 324-328.

MEDICINE AND THERAPEUTICS

57 MEDICINE AND SCIENCE

a ANATOMY AND PHYSIOLOGY

1 Buisseret, P. The cavities of the body. Nursing Mirror, 144, Nursing Care Supplement series 4.
1. The head and neck. 19 May 1977, i-iv.
2. The thoracic cavity. 26 May 1977, i-iv.
3. The mediastinal cavity. 2 Jun 1977, i-iv.
4. The gastrointenstinal tract. 9 Jun 1977, i-iv.
5. The hepatobiliary system. 16 Jun 1977, i-iv.
6. The pelvic cavity. 23 Jun 1977, i-iv.

2 Burgess, A. The nurse's guide to fluid and electrolyte balance. 2nd ed. New York: McGraw-Hill, 1979.

3 Burke, S.R. The composition and function of body fluids. 2nd ed. St. Louis: Mosby, 1976.

4 Cohen, S. Programmed instruction. Metabolic acid-base disorders. American Journal of Nursing, 78.
2. Physiological abnormalities and nursing actions. (1), Jan 1978, P.I., 1-20.
3. Clinical and laboratory findings. (3), Mar 1978, P.I., 1-16.

5 Glenister, T.W.A. and Ross, J.R.W. Anatomy and physiology for nurses. 3rd ed. Heinemann Medical, 1980.

6 Green, J.H. Basic clinical physiology. 3rd ed. Oxford University Press, 1978. (For nurses and others.)

7 Green, J.H. An introduction to human physiology. 4th S.I. ed. Oxford University Press, 1976.

8 Guyton, A.C. Physiology of the human body. 5th ed. Philadelphia: Saunders, 1979.

9 Hull, J. and Isaacs, B. Healing of wounds: a programmed text. Sheffield: NHS Learning Resources Unit, 1978.

10 Iveson-Iveson, J. Anatomy and physiology. Nursing Mirror, 148.
The accessory organs of digestion. 19 Apr 1979, 24-25.
The digestive tract. 5 Apr 1979, 38-39; 12 Apr 1979, 31-32.
The ear. 15 Feb 1979, 26-23.
The eye. 22 Feb 1979, 31-33.
The nervous system. 25 Jan 1979, 20-23; 1 Feb 1979, 26-28; 8 Feb 1979, 31-33.
The respiratory system. 8 Mar 1979, 29-31.
The skeleton. 17 May 1979, 30-32; 24 May 1979, 34-35.
The urinary system. 15 Mar 1979, 31-32.

11 Joseph, J. Essential anatomy. 2nd ed. Lancaster: MTP, 1979. (For nurses and others.)

12 Lever, J.D. Introducing anatomy. Heinemann Medical, 1980.

13 McNaught, A.B. Companion to 'illustrated physiology'. 3rd ed. Churchill Livingstone, 1976.

14 Mayers, C.P. Pathology. 2nd ed. Hodder and Stoughton, 1977. (Modern nursing series.)

15 MONITORING fluid and electrolytes precisely. Horsham: Intermed Communications Inc., 1978. (Nursing skillbook series.)

16 Nursing Issue on fluids in balance. Nursing, 13, May 1980, 541-584.

17 Nursing Clinics of North America Symposium on fluid, electrolyte and acid-base balance. (8 articles.) Nursing Clinics of North America, 15 (3), Sep 1980, 535-646.

18 Nursing Mirror The six senses. (A series of five supplements reprinted from Nursing Mirror, Jan and Feb 1978.) NM, 1978.

19 Nursing Times Systems of life. No.30. Respiration—3. Control of respiration. Nursing Times, 73, 2 Jun 1977, (4)p.

20 Nursing Times Systems of life. Nos.31-32. Nervous system—1 and 2. Nursing Times, 73, 7 Jul 1977, (4); 4 Aug 1977, (4).

21 Nursing Times Systems of life: part 3. Macmillan Journals, 1977.

22 Piper, M.E. Fluid and electrolyte balance. Nursing Mirror, 143 (18), 28 Oct 1976, 55-57.

23 Porth, C.M. Physiological coping: a model for teaching pathophysiology. Nursing Outlook, 25 (12), Dec 1977, 781-784.

24 Reed, G.M. and Sheppard, V.F. Regulation of fluid and electrolyte balance: a programed instruction in clinical physiology. 2nd ed. Philadelphia: Saunders, 1977.

25 Riddle, J.T.E. Elementary textbook of anatomy and physiology applied to nursing. 5th ed. Churchill Livingstone, 1977.

26 Roberts, A. Body fluids. 9. Seminal fluid and hydrocele. (Includes methods of contraception and investigations of infertility.) Nursing Times, 74, 16 Feb 1978, Body Fluids, 33-36.

27 Roberts, A. Body fluids. 11. Amniotic fluid. Nursing Times, 74, 20 Apr 1978, Body Fluids, 41-44.

28 Roberts, A. Body fluids. 18. Body water and its control. (Includes assessment of a patient's fluid balance.) Nursing Times, 74, 23 Nov 1978, Body Fluids, 69-72.

29 Roper, N. Man's anatomy, physiology, health and environment. 5th ed. Churchill Livingstone, 1976.

30 Selkurt, E.E. editor Physiology. 4th ed. Boston: Little, Brown and Co., 1976.

31 Smith, K. Fluids and electrolytes: a conceptual approach. New York: Churchill Livingstone, 1980.

32 Stroot, V.R. and others Fluids and electrolytes: a practical approach. 2nd ed. Philadelphia: Davis, 1977. (For nurses.)

33 Twombly, M. The shift into third space. (Shift of fluid from vascular to interstitial space.) Nursing, 8 (6), Jun 1978, 38-41.

34 Worthington, L. What those blood gases can tell you. RN Magazine, 42 (10), Oct 1979, 23-27.

b DIAGNOSTIC TECHNIQUES

1 Blood, A. Pigeon post. Pioneering work in the Plymouth Health District aimed at providing a flying specimens service. Nursing Mirror, 145, 11 Aug 1977, 8.

2 Brian, V.A. The new fangled contrivance: the story of the stethoscope. Nursing Mirror, 142, 20 May 1976, 62-64.

3 Canadian Nurse Your guide to clinical laboratory procedures. Canadian Nurse, 75 (8), Sep 1979, 25-40.

4 Carlson, M. Demystifying diagnostic procedures. Hospital admission. 3. Urinalysis. 4. EKGs. Journal of Practical Nursing, 29 (7), Jul 1979, 31-33, 40; (8), Aug 1979, 26-29.

5 Cruickshank, J. The computer: a third person in medical diagnosis. Journal of Community Nursing, 3 (11), May 1980, 20, 22; (12), Jun 1980, 18-20.

6 Evans, D.M.D. Special tests and their meanings. 10th ed. Faber, 1976.

7 Eymontt, M.J. Preparing your patient for nuclear medicine: the safe diagnostic tool. Nursing, 7 (12), Dec 1977, 46-49.

8 French, R.M. Guide to diagnostic procedures. 4th ed. New York: McGraw-Hill, 1975. 5th ed. 1980.

9 Highet, A.S. and Champion, R.H. Procedures in practice. Skin biopsy. British Medical Journal, 280, 24 May 1980, 1259-1260; 31 May, 1980, 1312-1313.

10 Marchiondo, K. The very fine art of

collecting culture specimens. Nursing (U.S.), 9 (4), Apr 1979, 34-43.

11 Pearson, M.C. Needle biopsies (of the lung). Nursing Mirror, 142, 20 May 1976, 50-52.

12 Sachdev, Y. and others Programmed investigation unit. (Ward used to investigate patients needing minimum nursing care at Royal Victoria Infirmary, Newcastle upon Tyne.) British Medical Journal, 2, 10 Jul 1976, 91-93.

13 Simpson, J.D. New techniques in nuclear medicine. (Diagnostic procedures based on monitoring radioactivity.) Nursing Times, 73, 3 Nov 1977, 1716-1718.

14 Strand, M.M. and Elmer, L.A. Clinical laboratory tests: a manual for nurses. St. Louis: Mosby, 1976. 2nd ed. 1980.

15 Williams, A.R. Medical photography—a personal view. Nursing Mirror, 144, 6 Jan 1977, 37-42.

c GENETICS AND GENETIC COUNSELLING

1 Arnold, A. and Moseley, R. Ethical issues arising from human genetics. (Function of genetic counsellors and types of screening programmes to ensure the birth of normal children.) Journal of Medical Ethics, 2 (1), Mar 1976, 12-17.

2 Aulberg, B.J.M. Genetic diseases in general practice. (Role of G.P.) Journal of the Royal College of General Practitioners, 27, Oct 1977, 592-595.

3 Canadian Nurse Dilemma. (Faced by families confronted with selective abortion after antenatal genetic tests.) Canadian Nurse, 72 (8), Aug 1976, 51-56.

4 Carter, C.O. Recent advances in genetic counselling. Nursing Times, 75, 18 Oct 1979, 1795-1798.

5 Clayton, R.P. Gene manipulation: the risks and proposals for their control. Occupational Health, 29 (6), Jun 1977, 254-257.

6 Cohen, F.L. Genetic knowledge possessed by American nurses and nursing students. (Research study.) Journal of Advanced Nursing, 4 (5), Sep 1979, 493-501.

7 Cowie, V. Chromosomes. Nursing Mirror, 143, 7 Oct 1976, 50-52.

8 Cowie, V. Genetics. The shape of things to come. (Includes prenatal diagnosis and genetic counselling.) Nursing Mirror, 149, 22 Nov 1979, 16-18; 29 Nov 1979, 28-30; 6 Dec 1979, 22-24; 13 Dec 1979, 20-22.

9 Dunlop, J.M. Genetic engineering. Nursing Times, 72, 5 Feb 1976, 169-171.

10 Emery, A.E.H. Elements of medical genetics. 5th ed. Churchill Livingstone, 1979.

11 Emery, A.E.H. and others Prospective study of genetic counselling. British Medical Journal, 1, 12 May 1979, 1253-1256.

12 Fielding, D.W. Genetic counselling in 1977. Queen's Nursing Journal, 19 (14), May 1977, 401-404.

13 Fitzsimmons, B. The one-in-four risk of a rare disease. (Genetic counselling of young Muslim couple who both carried abnormal gene of Roberts' syndrome.) Nursing Mirror, 150, 31 Jan 1980, 40-42.

14 Gray, A. DNA—the amazing helix. Midwife, Health Visitor and Community Nurse, 16 (7), Jul 1980, 295, 298.

15 Greenaway, P. Test-tube organisms. (Genetic manipulation.) Nursing Mirror, 151, 11 Dec 1980, 36-38.

16 Jones, I.H. Genetics and inherited diseases. Nursing Times, 74, 9 Mar 1978, 392-395.

17 Lythgoe, E. and Weetman, M. The HV in the department of medical genetics. (Genetic counselling by HVs attached to Department of Medical Genetics in Manchester.) Nursing Times, 76, 10 Jan 1980, Community Outlook, 15-16, 19.

18 Maclean, D.E. Recent advances in human genetics—implications for nursing education curriculum. Journal of Advanced Nursing, 1 (4), Jul 1976, 303-310.

19 Malter, S. Genetic counselling: a responsibility of health care professionals. Nursing Forum, 16 (1), 1977, 27-35.

20 Matthews, D.R. Genetics: your fate in your genes. Nursing Mirror, 147, 12 Oct 1978, 30-34.

21 Nevin, N.C. Screening for children: the importance of screening for genetic diseases. (Includes neural tube defects.) Royal Society of Health Journal, 99 (1), Feb 1979, 37-40.

22 Ross, T. The blueprint for a more certain future. (Role of nurse who runs genetic counselling clinic at Nottingham's City Hospital.) Nursing Mirror, 150, 31 Jan 1980, 38-39.

23 Skinner, R. Genetic counselling. Midwife, Health Visitor and Community Nurse, 15 (4), Apr 1979, 132, 134, 136, 138, 140.

24 S.A. Nursing Journal Special issue on genetic diseases. S.A. Nursing Journal, 44 (11), Nov 1977, 6-46.

25 Wenlock, J. Clinical genetics. Health Trends, 12 (4), Nov 1980, 83-84.

26 WHO Chronicle Genetic engineering: benefits and dangers. WHO Chronicle, 32 (12), Dec 1978, 465-468.

27 Williamson, R. Genetic engineering. Nursing Mirror, 145, 1 Sep 1977, 23-24.

d MATHEMATICS AND METRICATION

1 Arton, M. Teachers' page. 13. A brief look at SI Units. Midwives Chronicle, 88, Nov 1975, 370-371.

2 Craig, J. and Page, G.C. SI for you and me. (History of measurement and explanation of SI units with diagrams.) Canadian Nurse, 75 (2), Feb 1979, 16-21.

3 Jefferies, P.M. Mathematics in nursing. 5th ed. Baillière Tindall, 1978. (Nurses' aids series.)

4 Knapp, R.G. Basic statistics for nurses. New York: Wiley, 1978.

5 Kviz, F.J. and Knafl, K.A. Statistics for nurses: an introductory text. Boston: Little, Brown and Co., 1980.

6 Lipsey, S.I. Mathematics for nursing science: a programmed text. 2nd ed. New York: Wiley, 1977.

7 Martinson, I.M. and Kepner, G.R. Mathematics for health professionals. New York: Springer, 1977.

8 Metrication Board How to write metric: a style guide for teaching and using SI units. HMSO, 1977.

9 Miller, V. SI—the easy way. (Two-hour teaching programme.) Nursing Times, 76, 10 Jan 1980, Community Outlook, 11-13.

10 Phillips, D.S. Basic statistics for health science students. San Francisco: Freeman, 1978.

11 Routh, J.I. Mathematical preparation for the health scineces. 2nd ed. Philadelphia: Saunders, 1976.

12 Sackheim, G.I. and Robins, L. Programmed mathematics for nurses. 4th ed. New York: Macmillan, 1979. (Programmed text.)

13 Saxton, D.F. and others Programmed instruction in arithmetic, dosages and solutions. 4th ed. St. Louis: Mosby, 1977.

14 SI UNITS are simply metric units. Queen's Nursing Journal, 18 (10), Jan 1976, 280-281.

15 Swinscow, T.D.V. Statistics at square one. 4th ed. British Medical Association, 1978. (Reprinted from the British Medical Journal.)

16 Taylor, C.E. Mathematics for nursing. Boston: Little, Brown and Co., 1978.

17 Watchorn, G.W. Medical calculations for nurses. 2nd ed. Faber, 1976.

18 World Health Organization The SI for the health professions. Geneva: WHO, 1977.

19 WHO Secretariat SI Units: how to make the change. (Advice to institutions on planning for metrication.) WHO Chronicle, 32 (3), Mar 1978, 92-98.

e MEDICINE

1 Burton, J.L. Aids to medicine for nurses. Edinburgh: Churchill Livingstone, 1976.

2 Cooke, R.G. A summary of medicine for nurse and medical auxiliaries. 7th ed. Faber, 1977.

3 Croft, D. Nuclear medicine in district general hospitals. British Medical Journal, 2, 24 Nov 1979, 1336-1338.

4 Fairley, B. Medical spin-offs from space: many useful by-products of the US space programme. Nursing Mirror, 143 (27), 30 Dec 1976, 33-36.

5 Gibson, J. Common symptoms described for nurses. Oxford: Blackwell, 1976. 2nd ed. 1978.

6 **Gibson, J.** Modern medicine for nurses. 4th ed. Blackwell, 1979.

7 **Golding, A.M.B. and Tosey, D.** The cost of high technology medicine. Lancet, 2, 12 Jul 1980, 195-197.

8 **Gurr, M.R.** Understanding medical terminology. (With examples and answers.) Nursing Times, 74, 8 Jun 1978, 978-979.

9 **Harrison, R.J.** Textbook of medicine with relevant physiology and anatomy. Hodder and Stoughton, 1977. 2nd ed. 1980. (Modern nursing series.)

10 **Hector, W. and Malpas, J.S.** Textbook of medicine for nurses. 3rd ed. Heinemann, 1977.

11 **Hopkins, H.H.** The development of the modern endoscope. NATNews, 17 (8), Aug 1980, 18-22.

12 **Houston, J.C. and White, H.H.** Principles of medicine and medical nursing. 4th ed. Hodder and Stoughton, 1975. 5th ed. 1979. (Modern nursing series.)

13 **Houston, J.C. and others** A short textbook of medicine. 5th ed. Hodder and Stoughton, 1979.

14 **Iveson-Iveson, J.** Disease: its cause and effect. 1. Introduction of medical model and nursing process. 2. Inherited and congenital disorders; 12. Idiopathic disease. Nursing Mirror, 149, 13 Sep 1979, 24-25; 20 Sep 1979, 26-28; 20 Nov 1979, 24.

15 **Kennedy, I.** The 1980 Reith lectures. The Listener, Nov-Dec, 1980.

16 **McKeown, T.** The role of medicine: dream, mirage or nemesis? Nuffield Provincial Hospitals Trust, 1976. (The Rock Carling Fellowship, 1976.) Revised ed. 1979.

17 **Morris, J.F. and Small, J.C.** Revision notes for senior nurses: medicine. Heinemann, 1976-1978. 2 vols.

18 **Nursing Times** Vivisection. (Three articles by A. Whittaker, B. McMillan, and J. Eagles.) Nursing Times, 75, 8 Mar 1979, 395-399.

19 **Robinson, W.** Clinical research at Northwick Park—what's new. Nursing Mirror, 144, 5 May 1977, 57-59.

20 **Robinson, W.** Towards tomorrow: the latest developments at the National Institute for Medical Research, Mill Hill. Nursing Mirror, 146, 9 Mar 1978, 8-10.

21 **Sears, W.G. and Winwood, R.S.** Medicine for nurses. 13th ed. Edward Arnold, 1979.

22 **Swales, J.D.** Thoughts on the Reith lectures. Lancet, 2, 20/27 Dec 1980, 1348-1350.

23 **Toohey, M.** Medicine for nurses; edited by Arnold Bloom. 12th ed. Churchill Livingstone, 1978.

24 **WHO Chronicle** Biomedical research: a revised code of ethics. WHO Chronicle, 30 (9), Sep 1976, 360-362.

f MEDICINE, ALTERNATIVE

1 **Agarwal, A.** New respectability for 'witch doctors'. (WHO's programme of primary health care which includes traditional healer.) New Scientist, 79, 10 Aug 1978, 413-415.

2 **Armstrong, M.E.** Use of altered states of awareness in nursing practice. (Using meditation and biofeedback as examples.) AORN Journal, 25 (1), Jan 1977, 49-53.

3 **Basmajian, J.V.** Biofeedback: the clinical tool behind the catchword. AORN Journal, 2 (5), Sep/Oct 1977, 10, 14, 22.

4 **Blackie, M.G.** The patient, not the cure: the challenge of homeopathy. Macdonald and Jane's, 1976.

5 **British Medical Journal** Hypnosis in the NHS. (Its current status.) British Medical Journal, 2, 7 Oct 1978, 978.

6 **Casey, B.** Homeopathy. Nursing Mirror, 142, 1 Apr 1976, 74-75.

7 **Collins, J. and others** Acupuncture and pain. American Association of Nurse Anethetists Journal, 44, Feb 1976, 62-64.

8 **Davies, G.** The hands of the healer: has faith a place? Journal of Medical Ethics, 6 (4), Dec 1980, 185-189.

9 **Dove, C.I.** Alternative medicine. Osteopathy. Nursing Times, 72, 29 Jan 1976, 129-131.

10 **Duffin, D.** Acupuncture past and present. Physiotherapy, 64 (7), Jul 1978, 203-207.

11 **Felstein, I.** Water provides a cure. (Development of spas and their use today for conditions including rheumatism, psoriasis and dyspepsia.) Nursing Mirror, 149, 13 Dec 1979, 24-25.

12 **Fozzard, E.L.** Clinical applications of biofeedback training. (Research study of its short- and long-term effectiveness.) AORN Journal, 4 (5), Sep/Oct 1979, 4-6.

13 **Harvey, D.** Biofeedback—a signal technique. (Its implications for psychiatry.) Mind Out, 22, May/Jun 1977, 13-14.

14 **Harvey, P.G.** Biofeedback: trick or treatment? Nursing Mirror, 146, 27 Apr 1978, 15-17.

15 **Healing Research Trust** A nature cure? (Extracts from evidence to the Royal Commission on the NHS.) Nursing Times, 73, 19 May 1977, 726-727.

16 **Inglis, B.** Self diagnosis: self medication. Methods ancient and modern. Royal Society of Health Journal, 97 (4), Aug 1977, 156-158.

17 **Lovejoy, N.C.** Biofeedback: a growing role in holistic health. Advances in Nursing Science, 2 (4), Jul 1980, 83-93.

18 **Mann, F.** Acupuncture. Nursing Mirror, 143, 28 Oct 1976, 61-63.

19 **Mendiratta, S.** The point about acupuncture... (Its use in modern medicine.) Nursing Mirror, 149, 9 Aug 1979, 30-31.

20 **Phillips, K.C.** Biofeedback: what is it? Nursing, 10, Feb 1980, 431.

21 **Putt, A.M.** A biofeedback service by nurses. (For stress-related disorders.) American Journal of Nursing, 79 (1), Jan 1979, 88-89.

22 **Rose-Neil, S.** Alternative medicine. Acupuncture. Nursing Times, 72, 6 May 1976, 687-689.

23 **Ross, T.** Alien medicine from Asia. ('Hakims' and 'Vaids', Asian folk healers in Britain.) Nursing Mirror, 150, 28 Feb 1980, 21-23.

24 **Ross, T.** The serene way to fitness. (Yoga.) Nursing Mirror, 151, 3 Jul 1980, 24-26.

25 **Ryan, B.J.** Biofeedback training: the voluntary control of mind over body and mind. Nursing Forum, 14, 1975, 48-55.

26 **Searle, C.** The power of the folk healer. (Role of the traditional healer in treatment of cancer in isolated rural communities of Africa.) Nursing Mirror, 151, 4 Dec 1980, 30-34.

27 **Stein, R.F. and Kim, K.C.** Psychological and sociological aspects of patients receiving acupuncture treatments. (Research study.) International Journal of Nursing Studies, 15 (4), 1978, 171-192.

28 **Strutt, M.** Behind the mirror. (Spiritual healing.) Nursing Times, 72, 12 Aug 1976, 1226-1227.

29 **Tamez, E.G. and others** Relaxation training as a nursing intervention versus pro re nata medication. Nursing Research, 27 (3), May/Jun 1978, 160-165.

30 **Thomas, D. and Abbas, K.A.** Comparison of transcendental meditation and progressive relaxation in reducing anxiety. British Medical Journal, 2, 23/30 Dec 1978, 1749.

31 **Thomson, W.A.R.** Spas that heal. Black, 1978.

32 **Twentyman, L.R.** Homeopathy. Nursing Mirror, 144, 31 Mar 1977, 45-47; 7 Apr 1977, 65-67; 14 Apr 1977, 55-57.

33 **Wilcox, J.** Alternative medicine. Radionics. (Use of extra sensory perception and machines to determine energy changes in the human body.) Nursing Times, 72, 15 Apr 1976, 568-570.

34 **World Health** Issue on traditional medicine (including WHO's programme). World Health, Nov 1977, 3-30.

35 **World Health Organisation** The promotion and development of traditional medicine. Geneva: WHO, 1978. (Technical report series, no.622.)

g MICROBIOLOGY AND PARASITOLOGY

1 **Akinsanya, J.A.** Microbiology, health and hygiene. Macmillan, 1980. (Macmillan tropical nursing and health science series.)

2 **Beishir, L.** Microbiology in practice: individualized instruction for the allied health sciences. 2nd ed. San Francisco: Canfield, 1977.

3 **Burton, G.R.** Microbiology for the health sciences. Philadelphia: Lippincott, 1979.

4 **Campbell, L.** Microbiology: a bit of both. (Organisms which share characteristics of both plants and animals.) Nursing Mirror, 151, 21 Aug 1980, 38.

5 **Cowper-Smith, F.** Research for survival.

(Microbiological Research Establishment, Porton Down.) Nursing Times, 42, 2 Dec 1976, 1876-1878.

6 Cronholm, L.S. and Metz, M.C. Microbiology made relevant. (Creating the hospital environment in a classroom setting by designing laboratory exercises at the University of Louisville.) Nursing Outlook, 24 (4), Apr 1976, 247-250.

7 Fawzy, M.E. Hydatid disease. (Hydatid cysts caused by tapeworms.) Nursing Mirror, 144, 5 May 1977, 48-49.

8 Fryer, J. Bacterial resistance to antibiotics. Nursing Mirror, 142, 26 Feb 1976, 50-52.

9 Gibson, J.M. Modern microbiology and pathology for nurses. Oxford: Blackwell Scientific, 1979.

10 Hare, R. and Cooke, E.M. Bacteriology and immunity for nurses. 4th ed. Churchill Livingstone, 1977. 5th ed. 1979.

11 Iveson-Iveson, J. 7. Parasites and man. Nursing Mirror, 143 (15), 7 Oct 1976, Nursing care supplement series 3, i-iv.

12 Maunder, J.W. Parasites and man. Human lice — biology and control. Royal Society of Health Journal, 97 (1), Feb 1977, 29-32.

13 Parker, M.J. Microbiology for nurses. 5th ed. Baillière Tindall, 1978. (Nurses' aids series.)

14 Simmons, N.A. editor An introduction to microbiology for nurses. 3rd ed. Heinemann Medical, 1980. Earlier editions entitled 'Bacteriology for nurses' by G. Taylor.

15 Tomkins, A.M. Giardiasis. (Diarrhoea and malabsorption caused by parasite.) Nursing Times, 73, 9 Jun 1977, 876-877.

16 Watson, K.L. Medical microbiology. Nursing Mirror, 146.
1. History and basic organisms. 19 Jan 1978, 14-16.
2. Culture media and the recognition and properties of viruses. 26 Jan 1978, 24-26.
3. The destruction of micro-organisms. 2 Feb 1978, 32-33.
4. Antimicrobial therapy and antibiotic use and misuse. 9 Feb 1978, 30-32.
5. Parasitic organisms that invade man. 16 Feb 1978, 27-28.
6. Infections in communities. 23 Feb 1978, 30-32.
7. Resistance and immunity to infection. 2 Mar 1978, 30-31.
8. The basis of acquired immunity. 9 Mar 1978, 30-33.
9. Some applications of microbiology to nursing. 16 Mar 1978, 32-33.

17 Watson, K.L. Parasitology. 5. A fluke of nature. Nursing Mirror, 151, 4 Dec 1980, 28-29.

18 Winner, H.I. Microbiology in patient care. 2nd ed. Hodder and Stoughton, 1978. (Modern nursing series.)

h RADIOLOGY AND RADIO-THERAPY

1 Allen, M. A job in focus. (Phyllis Briggs, radiographer at Bromley Hospital.) Nursing Mirror, 148, 26 Apr 1979, 26-27.

2 Anderson, W. Technology in nursing. Radiotherapy. 12. Radiation protection methods. Nursing Times, 76, 17 Jan 1980, Scan, 45-48.

3 Armstrong, P. X-ray in focus. (Aspects involved in interpreting X-rays.) Nursing Times, 72, 15 Jan 1976, Post-basic, 1-4.

4 Baker, J. Technology in nursing. Radiotherapy. 10. Implants and applicators. Nursing Times, 75, 29 Nov 1979, Scan, 37-40.

5 Barnett, J.W. Patients' emotional responses to barium X-rays. (Study to test the effect of giving patients information on their reactions before and during the procedure.) Journal of Advanced Nursing, 3 (1), Jan 1978, 37-46.

6 Burrows, E.H. Myelography. Nursing Mirror, 144, 17 Mar 1977, 64-66.

7 Carlson, M. Demystifying diagnostic procedures. Part II: Hospital admission — chest X-rays. (With section on nursing considerations.) Journal of Practical Nursing, 29 (6), Jun 1979, 15-17, 40.

8 Carmichael, J.H.E. and Berry, R.J. Diagnostic X-rays in late pregnancy and in the neonate. (A survey of current practice in teaching and non-teaching hospitals throughout the U.K.) Lancet, 1, 14 Feb 1976, 351-352.

9 Cattell, A. Technology in nursing. Radiotherapy. Nursing Times, 75.
6. Moulds and makers. 26 Jul 1979, Scan, 21-24.
7. Simulators. 30 Aug 1979, Scan, 25-28.
8. Dosimetry. 4 Oct 1979, Scan, 29-32.
9. Telepathy. 1 Nov 1979, Scan, 33-30.

10 Chajek, T. and others New diagnostic method for Wilson's disease. (Diagnostic X-ray spectometry (DXS).) Nursing Mirror, 145, 27 Oct 1977, 22-23.

11 Chesney, D.N. and Chesney, M.O. Care of the patient in diagnostic radiography. 5th ed. Blackwell, 1978.

12 Cosgrove, D.O. Technology in nursing. Radiotherapy. Nursing Times, 75.
4. Ultrasound in tumour localisation. 24 May 1979, Scan, 13-16.
5. Radioisotopes in tumour localisation. 28 Jan 1979, Scan, 17-20.

13 Deeley, T.J. A guide to the radiotherapy and oncology department. Bristol: Wright, 1979. (For nurses and others.)

14 Goldman, M. A guide to the X-ray department. Bristol: Wright, 1978.

15 Greenwood, D.P. Radiography. Nursing Times, 72.
1. Investigations associated with the urinary tract. 8 Jul 1976, 1040-1042.
2. Retrograde pyelography, cystography and urethrography. 15 Jul 1976, 1096-1097.
3. Angiography and other radiographic investigations. 22 Jul 1976, 1126-1128.

16 Harmer, C. Technology in nursing. Radiotherapy. 11. Unsealed radioactive isotopes in treatment. Nursing Times, 75, 20/27 Dec 1979, Scan, 41-44.

17 Haynes, P. Radiography in the operating theatre. NATNews, 12 (5), Jul 1975, 12-14.

18 Hugh, A.E. Radiography in the home. (Use of portable X-ray units.) Journal of the Royal College of General Practitioners, 26, Dec 1976, 917-920.

19 Husband, J.E. Computed tomography: a new technique in radiology. (With illustrations.) Midwife, Health Visitor and Community Nurse, 15 (12), Dec 1979, 486-489.

20 Kendall, B. Computed tomography: a giant step forward in neurology. (Method of radiography with reference to brain and cerebrospinal fluid.) Nursing Mirror, 148, 22 Feb 1979, 35-38.

21 Kiff, M.L. The CAT. (Computerised axial tomography.) Journal of Practical Nursing, 27 (6), Jun 1977, 18-19, 35.

22 Kreel, L. Computerised transverse axial tomography.) Journal of Practical Nursing, 27 1976, Key clinical, 17-20.

23 Kreel, L. and Meire, H.B. The diagnostic process: a comparison of scanning techniques. (Including ultrasound and computerised tomography.) British Medical Journal, 2, 24 Sep 1977, 809-811.

24 Leahy, I.M. and others The nurse and radiotherapy: a manual for daily care. St. Louis: Mosby, 1979.

25 Long, N. How to see your patient safely through an angiogram. RN Magazine, 41 (10), Oct 1978, 60-62.

26 Madeja, C. Computerized tomography: an introduction. Journal of Neurosurgical Nursing, 9 (2), Jun 1977, 87-89.

27 Mears, D. Technology in nursing. Radiotherapy. 3. Computerised axial tomography. Nursing Times, 75, 26 Apr 1979, Scan, 9-12.

28 Nursing Times X-rays in focus. Macmillan Journals, 1977. 17 leaflets. Articles in Nursing Times, 72, 1976, 12 Feb, 11 Mar, 15 Apr, 13 May, 10 Jun, 8 Jul, 12 Aug, 9 Sep, 14 Oct, 11 Nov. Post Basic, 5-44.

29 Nursing Times X-rays in focus. Radiology of the stomach and duodenum. Nursing Times, 73, 21 Apr 1977, Post Basic, 13-16.

30 Nursing Times Scan technology in nursing. Macmillan Journals, 1979. (Series of articles by T.J. Coady and A. Bennet reprinted from Nursing Times.)

31 Reeves, K.R. This CAT is a revolutionary scanner. (Computerized axial tomography.) RN Magazine, 39 (8), Aug 1976, 41-43.

32 Stone, B.H. Computerized transaxial brain scan. (Including patient preparation and case study.) American Journal of Nursing, 77 (10), Oct 1977, 1601-1604.

33 Tealey, A.R. Getting children to keep still during radiotherapy. Maternal-Child Nursing Journal, 2 (3), May/Jun 1977, 178-181.

34 Thomson, L. Side-effects of radiotheraopy. Nursing Times, 76, 15 May 1980, 877-881.

35 Tiffany, R. Technology in nursing. Radiotherapy. 1. Introduction. Nursing Times, 75, 22 Feb 1979, Scan, 1-4.

36 Tinker, J.H. Understanding chest X-rays. American Journal of Nursing, 76 (1), Jan 1976, 54-58.

37 **Unwin, S.** Technology in nursing. Radiotherapy. 2. Radiobiology. (Study of the effect of ionising radiation on cells and tissues.) Nursing Times, 75, 15 Mar 1979, Scan, 5-8.

38 **Weir, J. and Abrahams, P.** X-ray anatomy 1. (20° occipitofrontal view of skull, anteroposterior view of internal carotid arteriogram—arterial phase with subtraction, veins on the neck.) Nursing Times, 76, 31 Jan 1980, (7).

39 **Weir, J. and Abrahams, P.** X-ray anatomy. 2. (Left ventricular angiocardiogram, aortic arch arteriogram and aortic and iliac arteriogram.) Nursing Times, 76, 27 Mar 1980, (7).

40 **Weir, J. and Abrahams, P.** X-ray anatomy. 3. (Anteroposterior view of pelvis, anteroposterior amniogram in third trimester and posteroanterior view of thorax.) Nursing Times, 76, 29 May 1980, (7).

41 **Weir, J. and Abrahams, P.** X-ray anatomy. 4. (Right anterior oblique barium study of stomach and duodenum, splenoportagram and lymphangiogram (first day).) Nursing Times, 76, 31 Jul 1980, (7).

42 **Weir, J. and Abrahams, P.** X-ray anatomy. 5. (Intravenous pyelogram, retrograde pyelogram and renal arteriogram.) Nursing Times, 76, 25 Sep 1980, (7).

i SCIENCE

1 **Flitter, H.H.** An introduction to physics in nursing. 7th ed. St. Louis: Mosby, 1976.

2 **Gibson, J.** Human biology: elementary anatomy and physiology for students and nurses. 3rd ed. Faber, 1978.

3 **Jensen, J.T.** Physics for the health professions. 2nd ed. Philadelphia: Lippincott, 1976.

4 **Keily, D.** Programmed basic chemistry for allied health students. St. Louis: Mosby, 1978.

5 **Kilgour, O.F.G.** An introduction to the biological aspects of nursing science. Heinemann, 1978.

6 **Kilgour, O.F.G.** An introduction to the physical aspects of nursing science. 3rd ed. Heinemann, 1978.

7 **Lankford, T.R.** Integrated science for health students. 2nd ed. Reston, Va.: Reston Pub., 1979.

8 **Nave, C.R. and Nave, B.C.** Physics for the health sciences. Philadelphia: Saunders, 1975. 2nd ed. 1980.

9 **Robinson, W.** Molecular research—progress and the future. (Molecular Biology Research Unit, Cambridge.) Nursing Mirror, 143, 5 Aug 1976, 39-41.

10 **Routh, J.I.** Introduction to biochemistry. 2nd ed. Philadelphia: Saunders, 1978. (For nurses and others.)

11 **Sackheim, G.I. and Schultz, R.M.** Chemistry for the health sciences. 3rd ed. Collier Macmillan, 1977.

12 **Shugar, G. and others** Health sciences chemistry. Philadelphia: Davis, 1978.

13 **Strouth, C.** A survey of amino acid and protein chemistry. Journal of Nursing Care, 12 (10), Oct 1979, 25-27, 29.

14 **Wilson, K.J.W.** A study of the biological sciences in relation to nursing. (Rcn Research Society summary of PhD thesis, Edinburgh University, published by Churchill Livingstone, 1975.) Nursing Times, 73, 9 Jun 1977, Occ. papers, 84.

15 **Wittman, K.S.** Basic sciences for health careers. New York: McGraw-Hill, 1976. (Nursing and allied health series.)

j TROPICAL MEDICINE

1 **Adams, A.R.D. and Maegraith, B.G.** Tropical medicine for nurses. 5th ed. edited by Brian Maegraith and H.M. Giles. Oxford: Blackwell Scientific, 1980.

2 **Bhanderi, P.** Communicable diseases. 6. Marburg virus disease. Midwife, Health Visitor and Community Nurse, 14 (2), Feb 1978, 49.

3 **Blandart, P.** Communicable diseases. 3. Lassa fever. Midwife, Health Visitor and Community Nurse, 13 (1), Jan 1977, 12-13.

4 **Crichton, M.A.** Nursing care study. A patient with yaws. Nursing Times, 75, 17 May 1979, 830-832.

5 **Department of Health and Social Security and Welsh Office** Memorandum on lassa fever. HMSO, 1976.

6 **Nzeribe, N.** Basic tropical nursing. Baillière Tindall, 1978.

7 **Raeburn, P.** Lassa fever. Nursing Times, 72 (34), 26 Aug 1976, ICNA Supplement, 37-38.

8 **Shankey, P.** Nursing of patients with Marburg fever. Nursing Mirror, 144, 26 May 1977, 16-18.

9 **Simpson, D.I.H.** Marburg fever. Nursing Mirror, 144, 26 May 1977, 13-15.

10 **Southgate, B.A.** Bancroftian filariasis. Nursing Times, 72, 22 Jan 1976, 107-108.

11 **Vella, E.E.** Marburg disease. Nursing Times, 73, 27 Jan 1977, 120-122.

12 **Wright, S.G.** Rare virus infections from the tropics. (Lassa fever and Marburg virus disease.) Nursing Times, 74, 12 Jan 1978, 74-76.

13 **Wright, W.J.** Lassa fever. Nursing Times, 72, 15 Apr 1976, 578-579.

58 PHARMACOLOGY

a GENERAL AND TEXTBOOKS

1 **Adamson, L.** Control of medicines in the UK. (Medicines Commission and Medicines Division of the DHSS.) Nursing Times, 74, 8 Jun 1978, 973-975.

2 **Albanese, J.A.** Nurses' drug reference. New York: McGraw-Hill, 1979.

3 **Allwood, M.C. and Fell, J.T. editors** Textbook of hospital pharmacy. Oxford: Blackwell Scientific, 1980.

4 **American Journal of Nursing** Nurses work in clinical research team: test drugs, develop drug delivery systems. (Expanded role of nurses.) American Journal of Nursing, 77 (12), Dec 1977, 1983, 1990.

5 **Anderson, E.M. and Vervoren, T.M.** Workbook of solutions and dosage of drugs including arithmetic. 10th ed. St. Louis: Mosby, 1976.

6 **Asperheim, M.K. and Eisenhauer, L.A.** The pharmacologic basis of patient care. 3rd ed. Philadelphia: Saunders, 1977.

7 **Bergersen, B.S.** Pharmacology in nursing. 13th ed. St. Louis: Mosby, 1976.

8 **Binns, T.B.** Clinical pharmacology. The Committee on Review of Medicines. British Medical Journal, 281, 13 Dec 1980, 1614-1615.

9 **British Medical Journal** Expanding role for pharmacists. British Medical Journal, 2, 30 Sep 1978, 911-912.

10 **Brooks, R.V.** Anabolic steroids: their use and abuse. Nursing Mirror, 143, 9 Dec 1976, 54-55.

11 **Brooks, S.M. editor** Nurses' drug reference. Boston: Little, Brown and Co., 1978.

12 **Brown, A.** Debendox in the dock. Nursing Mirror, 150, 21 Feb 1980, 8-9.

13 **Community Outlook** Fact sheet: anaphylaxis. Nursing Times, 75, 8 Mar 1979, Community Outlook, 64-65.

14 **Cooper, P.** Progress in therapeutics. Drowsiness from drugs. Midwife, Health Visitor and Community Nurse, 12 (6), Jun 1976, 196.

15 **Davies, D.M.** Anaphylaxis and the community nurse. (Report of survey on drugs used for treating anaphylactic shock and instruction given. Reprinted from Adverse Drug Reaction Bulletin.) Journal of Community Nursing, 1 (3), Sep 1977, 15-16; Nursing Mirror, 145, 8 Sep 1976, 41-42.

16 **Davies, D.M. and others** Comprehensive clinical drug information service: first year's experience. (Northern Regional Health Authority.) British Medical Journal, 1, 8 Jan 1977, 89-90.

17 **Dison, N.,** Simplified drugs and solutions for nurses, including arithmetic. 6th ed. St. Louis: Mosby, 1976. 7th ed. 1980.

18 **Falconer, M.W. and others** The drug, the nurse, the patient. 6th ed. Philadelphia: Saunders, 1978.

19 **Falconer, M.W.** Patient studies in pharmacology: a guidebook. Philadelphia: Saunders, 1976.

20 **Gibberd, F.B. and Tonkin, R.D.** Nurses handbook of current drugs. 3rd ed. Heinemann, 1978.

21 **Gibson, J.** The nurse's materia medica. 4th ed. Blackwell, 1976. 5th ed. 1980.

22 **Govoni, L. and Hayes, J.E.** Drugs and nursing implications. 3rd ed. New York: Appleton-Century-Crofts, 1978.

23 **Hindmarch, I.** Calling time on hypnotic drugs. (The effect of hypnotic medication on

performance.) Nursing Mirror, 150, 13 Mar 1980, 37-38.

24 Drugs and pharmacology for nurses. 7th ed. Churchill Livingstone, 1979. (Churchill Livingstone nursing texts.)

25 Johns, M.P. Drug therapy and nursing care. Collier Macmillan, 1979.

26 Jones, B.R. Pharmacology for student and pupil nurses and students in associated professions. 2nd ed. Heinemann, 1978.

27 Journal of Community Nursing Drugs in district nursing. Chemotherapeutic agents. Journal of Community Nursing, 1 (4), Oct 1977, 20; (5), Nov 1977, 14.

28 Keane, C.B. and Fletcher, S.M. Drugs and solutions: a programmed introduction. 4th ed. Philadelphia: Saunders, 1980.

29 Lancet Drug use in the third world. Lancet, 2, Dec 1980, 1231-1232.

30 Laurence, D.R. and Black, J.W. The medicine you take: benefits and risks of modern drugs. Croom Helm, 1978.

31 Leach, F.N. The regional drug information service: a factor in health care? (Functions, and analysis of inquiries received by the North-Western Regional Drug Information Service.) British Medical Journal, 1, 25 Mar 1978, 766-768.

32 Lesser, F. How we keep unsafe drugs off the market. (Interview with Sir Eric Scowen, first chairman of Committee on Safety of Medicines.) New Scientist, 88, 4 Dec 1980, 634-636.

33 Rose, K. The stress of chemotherapy. (Physiological effects and nursing implications.) Canadian Nurse, 74 (5), May 1978, 18-21.

34 Scott, J. Trial jargon made easy. (Terminology used in clinical trials of drugs.) Nursing Mirror, 147, 28 Sep 1978, 7.

35 Sears, W.G. and Winwood, R.S. Materia medica for nurses: a textbook of drugs and therapeutics. 8th ed. Arnold, 1976. 9th ed. 1980.

36 Smith, S.E. How drugs act series 2. 4th ed. Macmillan Journals, 1976.

37 Smith, S.E. How drugs act — 30. The safety of drugs. Nursing Times, 72, 22 Jan 1976, 114-115.

38 Smith, T. Fifty years of penicillin. (History of its discovery in the 1930s.) Journal of Community Nursing, 1 (12), Jun 1978, 28-29.

39 Squire, J.E. and Welch, J.M. Basic pharmacology for nurses. 6th ed. St. Louis: Mosby, 1977.

40 Swonger, A.K. Nursing pharmacology: a systems approach to drug therapy and nursing practice. Boston: Little, Brown and Co., 1978.

41 Trounce, J.R. Pharmacology for nurses. 7th ed. Churchill Livingstone, 1977.

42 Turner, P. and Volans, G.N. The drugs handbook. Macmillan, 1978. (For nurses and others.)

43 Wiener, M.B. and others Clinical pharmacology and therapeutics in nursing. New York: McGraw-Hill, 1979.

b ADVERSE REACTIONS AND INTERACTIONS

1 Black, C.D. and others Drug interactions in the GI tract. American Journal of Nursing, 77 (9), Sep 1977, 1426-1428.

2 Bourne, D. Incompatibilities of additives to intravenous infusion fluids. Australian Nurses Journal, 6 (6 and 7), Dec 1976-Jan 1977, 23, 35.

3 Brown, M.M. and others Drug—drug interactions among residents in homes for the elderly. (A subclass of adverse drug responses.) Nursing Research, 26 (1), Jan-Feb 1977, 47-52.

4 Coomes, E.N. Iatrogenic disease: doctor-induced illness. Nursing Mirror, 147, 21 Sep 1978, 13-15.

5 D'Arcy, P.F. Iatogenic disease: a hazard of multiple drug therapy. Royal Society of Health Journal, 96 (6), Dec 1976, 277-283.

6 Dickerson, J.W.T. Some adverse effects of drugs on nutrition. Royal Society of Health Journal, 98 (6), Dec 1978, 261-265.

7 Greenan, E. Drug therapy in child care. (Study at the Royal Hospital for Sick Children, Glasgow, monitoring adverse drug reactions which highlighted the role of drugs taken before admission.) Nursing Times, 72, 8 Apr 1976, 538-539.

8 Iveson-Iveson, J. Disease: its cause and effect. 10. Iatrogenic disease. Nursing Mirror, 149, 15 Nov 1979, 22-23.

9 Joyce, C.R.B. 'Side' effects: a misnomer. (Additional effects of drugs.) Journal of Medical Ethics, 2 (3), Sep 1976, 112-117.

10 Karch, A.M. Mixing drugs may be hazardous to your patient's health. (With table of common drug interactions.) Journal of Practical Nursing, 29 (6), Jun 1979, 18-20.

11 Karch, F.E. and Lasagna, L. Evaluating adverse drug reactions. Adverse Drug Reaction Bulletin, 59, Aug 1976, 204-207.

12 Lawson, D.H. Risks of drug treatment. (Methods of detecting adverse effects of drugs.) Nursing Mirror, 146, 26 Jan 1978, 41-42.

13 LeSage, J., Beck, C. and Johnson, M. Nursing diagnosis of drug incompatibility: a conceptual process. Advances in Nursing Science, 1 (2), Jan 1979, 63-77.

14 Lesser, F. Patient scrutiny for drug side effects. (Patients monitor their own reactions to a new drug.) New Scientist, 77, 5 Jan 1978, 16-17.

15 Parker, W.A. Medication histories. (Prevention of adverse drug reactions by comprehensive assessment of medication histories as part of patients' records.) American Journal of Nursing, 76 (12), Dec 1976, 1969-1971.

16 Pearson, R.M. and Nestor, P. Drug interactions. Nursing Mirror, 145, 10 Nov 1977, Supplement, i-ii, iv-vi.

17 Smith, S.E. How drugs act — 28. Drug inter-actions. Nursing Times, 72, 1/8 Jan 1976, 33-34.

18 Steane, M.A. Drug interactions: problems of multiple drug therapy. Queen's Nursing Journal, 19 (12), Mar 1977, 326-327.

19 Whiting, B. and Goldberg, A. The drug disc: a drug interaction warning system United Kingdom trial and subsequent development. Health Bulletin, 34 (3), May 1976, 167-171.

c DRUG ADMINISTRATION

1 Apple, J.L. The classification of medication errors. (Scheme at Forsyth Memorial Hospital, North Carolina.) Supervisor Nurse, 7 (12), Dec 1976, 23, 25, 28-29.

2 Applewhite, K. and others Dispensing for individual inpatients. (A report of the Ross system of individual dispensing services on geriatric, surgical and medical wards in Salford AHA.) Nursing Mirror, 144 (77), 28 Apr 1977, 62.

3 Bajaj, P.S. and McDermott, D. Investigating unit dose feasibility. (Study at Ottawa General Hospital.) Hospital Administration in Canada, 17 (5), May 1975, 40-44.

4 Barley, S.L. Why not a nurses' formulary? (Advocates nurses' being allowed to prescribe certain drugs and equipment.) Journal of the Royal College of General Practitioners, 30, Feb 1980, 101.

5 Batty, C.R. The dilemma of the unit-dose pharmacy system. Hospital Administration in Canada, 17 (11 and 12), Nov/Dec 1975, 49-50.

6 Bellerby, M. A new system for administering cytotoxic drugs. (New apparatus which is safer for staff and patients.) Nursing Times, 76, 3 Jul 1980, 1168-1169.

7 Brown, G.C. Medication errors: a case study. (To analyse and solve problem.) Hospitals, 53 (20), 16 Oct 1979, 61-62, 65.

8 Bryar, R. Beginning research. Self medication in a student population. (A study of the literature and a sample of students from one university.) Nursing Times, 73, 13 Jan 1977, 52-55.

9 Carr, J.J. and others How to solve dosage problems in one easy lesson. (Dialogue between instructor and nurses.) American Journal of Nursing, 76 (12), Dec 1976, 1934-1939.

10 Castledine, G. Patients and their drugs. (Problems of drug administration for nurses.) Nursing Mirror, 147, 16 Nov 1978, 14.

11 Chalmers, H. Return to basics. 6. 'First, do no harm.' (Administration of drugs.) Nursing Mirror, 145, 11 Aug 1977, Nursing care supplement series 5, i-ii, iv.

12 Chamberlain, S.L. Low-dose heparin therapy. (With instructions on way to give abdominal injections.) American Journal of Nursing, 80 (6), Jun 1980, 1115-1117.

13 Crooks, J. Drug administration — 2. The contribution of the computer. (Nursing Mirror Forum 1976.) Nursing Mirror, 142, 1 Apr 1976, 55-57.

14 Department of Health and Social Security Security. (Circular HC(77)16 on Controlled Drugs with details of accompany memorandum.) Nursing Mirror, 145, 10 Nov 1977, supplement xi.

15 **Hallett, R.** Unit dose system can improve service. (Report of research study.) Dimensions in Health Service, 54 (4), Apr 1977, 11.

16 **Hartley, B.** Now you're on cortisone. A teaching package. (Includes survey of patients' knowledge and teaching package for patients on cortisone.) Canadian Nurse, 74 (2), Feb 1978, 16-27.

17 **Henney, C.** Drug administration. 1. (Research study into computer based system. Nursing Mirror Forum 1976.) Nursing Mirror, 142, 1 Apr 1976, 52-54.

18 **Inoue, F.** How clinical pharmacy practice benefits hospital and patient. (Active participation of pharmacists in drug therapy involving consultation with other members of the health care team.) Hospital Administration in Canada, 18 (11), Nov 1976, 32-33.

19 **Jolly, S.C.** Government to invoke new British Standard for child resistant containers for medicines. BSI News, Dec 1975, 6-7.

20 **Lowther, R.** How to forecast staff needs. (The cost of providing pharmaceutical services in wards.) Health and Social Service Journal, 89, 13 Apr 1979, 406-407.

21 **Lundin, D.V.** You *can* inject heparin subcutaneously. (Procedure to reduce risk of haematomas.) RN Magazine, 41 (12), Dec 1978, 51-54.

22 **National Joint Committee of the Medical and Pharmaceutical Professions on the Dispensing of NHS Prescriptions in Rural Areas** Report. Department of Health and Social Security, 1977. (Chairman: C.M. Clothier.)

23 **Newton, M. and Newton, D.W.** Guidelines for handling drug errors. Nursing, 7 (9), Sep 1977, 62-68.

24 **Palmer, D.A.** Unit dose. (Advantages and drawbacks.) American Journal of Nursing, 80 (11), Nov 1980, 2062-2063.

25 **Parker, W.A.** Drugs brought in by patients: the need for control. Hospital Administration in Canada, 19 (11), Nov 1977, 32-33.

26 **Rosenman, H. and others** Improving general drug distribution through nursing-pharmacy co-operation. (System developed at Kingsbrook Jewish Medical Center, New York.) Hospital Topics, 55 (5), Sep/Oct 1977, 30-33.

27 **Royal College of Nursing** Drug administration—a nursing responsibility. Rcn, 1980.

28 **Royal Society of Medicine. Medico-Pharmaceutical Forum** Dangerous mistakes in drug administration: report of a working party. The Forum, 1979. Summary of this report on problems encountered by anaesthetists in identifying dispensed medicines in NATNews, 17 (2), Feb 1980, 8, 10.

29 **Self, T.H. and others** Systematic patient medication record review: a manual for nurses. St. Louis: Mosby, 1980.

30 **Smith, A. and others** Clinical pharmacology clinics in general practice. (Description of pilot scheme and analysis of its effects on prescribing.) British Medical Journal, 2, 16 Jul 1977, 169-170.

31 **Stewart, D.Y. and others** Unit-dose medication: a nursing perspective. (System at University Hospital, London, Ontario.) American Journal of Nursing, 76 (8), Aug 1976, 1308-1310.

32 **Thomas, S.** Practical nursing. Medicines: care and administration. Nursing Mirror, 148, 12 Apr 1979, 28-30.

33 **Thomson, W.** Closed circuit television prescribing: time saving prescription dispensing system in use at St. Thomas' Hospital, London. Nursing Mirror, 142, 17 Jun 1976, 64-65.

34 **Trudeau, T.W.** Establishing a computer based total unit dose drug distribution system. Hospital Topics, 54 (3), May/Jun 1976, 40-44.

35 **Vendura, N.** Pharmacology program produces results. (Inservice education programme based on adult education principles.) Journal of Nursing Administration, 9 (9), Sep 1979, 34-39.

36 **Walters, S. and others** Joint nursing-pharmacy program helps reduce medication errors. (Through total patient care, audits, reminder cards and computer system, using unit-dose system.) Hospitals, 53 (6), 16 Mar 1979, 141, 143-144.

37 **White, S.J.** Unit dose innovations. American Journal of Hospital Pharmacy, 32, Aug 1975, 814-817. (Reprint file.)

38 **Wilson, B.S.** Medication error policy. (Definition of medication errors, reporting procedures and disciplinary steps.) Supervisor Nurse, 9 (5), May 1978, 53-54, 56.

d INTRAVENOUS THERAPY

1 **Albert, T.** The research that got away. (Failure of experiment, owing to doctors' attitudes to keep patients on IV infusions during daylight hours only, using team of nurses to put them up and take them down.) World Medicine, 15 (20), 12 Jul 1980, 25-26.

2 **American Journal of Nursing** Intravenous therapy: a special feature. (Five articles including how to insert an IV, IV drug incompatibilities and guide to combining IV medications.) American Journal of Nursing, 79 (7), Jul 1979, 1267-1296.

3 **Amonsen, S. and Gren, J.E.** Relationship between length of time and contamination in open intravenous solutions. Nursing Research, 27 (6), Nov/Dec 1978, 372-374.

4 **Bessette, M.C.** A hazard of intravenous therapy—corded particles. Canadian Nurse, 73 (6), Jun 1977, 34-35.

5 **Bodnar, A. and D'Agostino, J.** IV therapy. 2. Preventing problems and ensuring safety. Journal of Practical Nursing, 27 (9), Sep 1977, 24-27.

6 **Boore, J.** Types of intravenous fluids used. Nursing, 13, May 1980, 584.

7 **Bowell, E. and Armstrong, J.** Pictures in nursing. Management of intravenous therapy. Nursing, 13, May 1980, 579-583.

8 **Coco, C.D.** Intravenous therapy: a handbook for practice. St. Louis: Mosby, 1980.

9 **Dinel, B.** Hazards surround IV admixtures. Hospital Administration in Canada, 20 (9), Sep 1978, 21, 23.

10 **Gahart, B.L.** Intravenous medications: a handbook for nurses and other allied health personnel. 2nd ed. St. Louis: Mosby, 1977.

11 **Grossman, S.B.** I.V. nurses accept a challenge. (Canadian Intravenous Nurses Association.) Hospital Administration in Canada, 18 (10), Oct 1976, 61-62.

12 **Hanson, R.L.** Heparin-lock or keep-open I.V.? (Study to compare two intravenous routes.) American Journal of Nursing, 76 (7), Jul 1976, 1102-1103.

13 **Hart, G.D.** The I.V. nurse. Hospital Administration in Canada, 18 (10), Oct 1976, 62, 64.

14 **Huxley, V.D.** Heparin lock: how, what, why. (Intermittent infusion reservoir used in intravenous therapy.) RN Magazine, 42 (10), Oct 1979, 36-41.

15 **James, M.F.** Guidelines for nurses. The administration of intravenous drugs through an established intravenous pathway. (Example of extended role of nurse. For letter on this article, see Nursing Mirror, 12 Jan 1978, 12.) Nursing Mirror, 145, 10 Nov 1977, Supplement, viii, x.

16 **Jenner, E.A.** Intravenous infusion—a cause for concern? (Survey of control of infection procedures adopted by 191 hospitals with regard to intravenous fluid administration.) Nursing Times, 73, 3 Feb 1977, 156-158.

17 **Lafferty, M.K.** 'Don't tell me that drip has run out again'—or Whatever happened to that revolutionary intravenous regulator? (Device to improve intravenous therapy control.) Australian Nurses Journal, 5 (3), Sep 1975, 30-31.

18 **Lawson, M. and others** Long-term I.V. therapy: a new approach. (Peripherally inserted central venous catheters.) American Journal of Nursing, 79 (6), Jun 1979, 1100-1103.

19 **Luken, L.** IV therapy: a practical approach to nursing care. Journal of Practical Nursing, 29 (8), Aug 1979, 20-22, 35.

20 **Marks, M.** Straight to the veins: extending the role of the nurse in intravenous therapy. (Includes total parenteral nutrition.) Nursing Mirror, 149, 16 Aug 1979, Supplement, i, iii-vi, viii, xi.

21 **Michael, S.L.** Home I.V. therapy. American Journal of Nursing, 78 (7), Jul 1978, 1223-1226.

22 **Montgomery, C.** I.V. nursing teams try to solve problems. (Report of Canadian Intravenous Nurses Association seminar.) Dimensions in Health Service, 54 (4), Apr 1977, 43-44.

23 **Nursing Times** IV infusion techniques 'not clever but lucky.' (Conference on microbiological hazards of infusion therapy.) Nursing Times, 72, 1 Apr 1976, 478.

24 **Parfitt, D. McC. and Thompson, D.V.** Pediatric home hyperalimentation: educating the family. Maternal-Child Nursing Journal, 5 (3), May/Jun 1980, 196-202.

25 **Poole, H.H.** Drugs in infusion fluids.

Adverse Drug Reaction Bulletin, 62, Feb 1977, 216-219.

26 Royal College of Midwives Report of the Working Party on the addition of drugs to intravenous fluids—RCM comments. Midwives Chronicle, 89, Jan 1976, 8.

27 Rushton, E.A. Intravenous: past and present. (Work of IV team at University Hospital, London, Ontario.) Hospital Administration in Canada, 19 (10), Oct 1977, 69, 71.

28 Sager, D.P. and Bomar, S.K. Intravenous medications: a guide to preparation, administration and nursing management. Philadelphia: Lippincott, 1980.

29 Thomas, S. Practical nursing. Intravenous infusion. Nursing Mirror, 148, 5 Apr 1979, 34-37.

30 Thomson, L. Home I.V. saves money and frees beds. Health Care in Canada, 21 (6), Jun 1979, S6.

31 Ungvarski, P.J. Parenteral therapy. What to do before and during I.V. therapy to decrease the possibilities of contamination. American Journal of Nursing, 76 (12), Dec 1976, 1974-1977.

32 Wark, E. Chemotherapy and the nurse. 2. The interaction of drugs and intravenous fluids. (Treatment for cancer patients at Royal Marsden Hospital.) Nursing Mirror, 142 (13), 25 Mar 1976, 46-49.

33 Wells, J.M. Chemotherapy and the nurse. 1. A policy for intravenous drugs. (Treatment for cancer patients at Royal Marsden Hospital.) Nursing Mirror, 142, 25 Mar 1976, 45-47.

34 White, S.J. IV fluids and electrolytes: how to head off the risks. (Nursing implications of twelve products.) RN Magazine, 42 (11), Nov 1979, 60-63.

35 Yu Keng Teo, M. Calibrating the infusion bottle. Nursing Times, 73, 6 Jan 1977, 32-33.

e PATIENT TEACHING AND COMPLIANCE

1 American Society of Hospital Pharmacists Medication teaching manual: a guide for patient counselling. Washington: The Society, 1978.

2 Aslam, M. and others Compliance in medication by Asian immigrants. Doctors may overestimate the level of medical knowledge and literacy of Asian patients. (Two pilot studies at Dudley Road Hospital, Birmingham.) Nursing Times, 75, 31 May 1979, 931-932.

3 Barofsky, I. editor Medication compliance: a behavioural management approach. Thorofare: Slack, 1977. (Includes the role of the nurse.)

4 Blackwell, B. Counselling and compliance. (Counselling patients to improve compliance in taking medications.) Patient Counselling and Health Education, 1 (2), Fall 1978, 45-49.

5 Bodnar, E.M. Employees on continued medication: identification and discussion of problems with employees, continuing on medication, as noted on the occupational health scene. Occupational Health Nursing, 26 (7), Jul 1978, 11-15.

6 Caplan, R.D. and others Adhering to medical regimens: pilot experiments in patient education and social support. Ann Arbor: University of Michigan, Institute for Social Research, 1976.

7 Cohen, S.J. editor New directions in patient compliance. Lexington, Mass.: Lexington Books, 1979.

8 Covington, T.R. and Porter, M.E. Improper prescription instructions: a factor in patient compliance. (Research study.) Patient Counselling and Health Education, 1 (3), Winter/Spring 1979, 97-100.

9 D'Altroy, L.H. and others Patient drug self-administration improves regimen compliance. Hospitals, 52 (21), 1 Nov 1978, 131-132, 134-136.

10 Del Bueno, B.J. Continuing education. Spinach and other good things. (Study to test effectiveness of continuing education programs in modifying nurses' medication information-giving behaviour.) Journal of Nursing Administration, 7 (4), Apr 1977, 32-34.

11 Gaines, H.P. Why patients learn...why patients fail...: factors that influence patient compliance. (Changes in attitudes and behaviour as well as adherence to drug regime.) Journal of Practical Nursing, 29 (9), Sep 1979, 22-24, 39.

12 Graham, J.M. and Suppree, D.A. Improving drug compliance in general practice. (Reasons for the problem and survey of various measures.) Journal of the Royal College of General Practitioners, 29, Jul 1979, 399, 402-404.

13 Gulko, C.S. and Butherus, C. Toward better patient teaching. (Reprinted from Nurses' Drug Alert Mar 1977.) Journal of Practical Nursing, 27 (7), Jul 1978, 18-24.

14 Gulko, C.S. and Butherus, C. Toward better patient teaching. Part 3. (With reference to drugs, including insulin and oral contraceptives.) Journal of Practical Nursing, 28 (9), Sep 1978, 33-34, 40.

15 Hannary, D.G. Self-medication: a developing concept in future hospital planning service. (Study in London, Ontario, with long term patients in a rehabilitation ward to increase self reliance and decrease instructional dependence.) Hospital Administration in Canada, 19 (1), 1977, 33, 36-37.

16 Hermann, F. and others Package inserts for prescribed medicines: what minimum information do patients need? (Guide to help patients take and store drugs and recognise problems.) British Medical Journal, 2, 21 Oct 1978, 1132.

17 Hood, J.C. and Murphy, J.E. Patient non-compliance can lead to hospital readmissions. Study shows that discharge counselling and a starter supply of medications can reduce patient noncompliance. Hospitals, 52, 1 Jan 1978, 79-82, 84.

18 Hussar, D.A. Your role in patient compliance. (Predicting likely noncompliers and suggestions for encouraging compliance with treatment.) Nursing (U.S.), 9 (11), Nov 1979, 48-53.

19 Iveson-Iveson, J. Is your medicine really necessary? (Report on a symposium entitled 'Medicines, information and the patient'.) Nursing Mirror, 147, 3 Aug 1978, 9.

20 Kaufman, R.L. and others Medication discharge counselling program developed by pharmacists. Hospitals, 52, 1 Jan 1978, 89-92.

21 Kyi, K.K. and others Minimum information for sensible use of self-prescribed medicines: an international consensus. Report by an Ad-Hoc Working Group. Lancet, 2, 12 Nov 1977, 1017-1019.

22 Ley, P. Memory for medical information. (With reference to doctor/patient communication and patient compliance.) British Journal of Social and Clinical Psychology, 18 (2), Jun 1979, 245-255.

23 Parkin, D.M. and others Deviation from prescribed drug treatment after discharge from hospital. British Medical Journal, 2, 18 Sep 1976, 686-688.

24 Parkin, D.M. Survey of the success of communications between hospital staff and patients. (Over one third did not know how to manage their own drug therapy at home.) Public Health, 90 (5), Jul 1976, 203-209.

25 Romankiewicz, J.A. To improve patient adherence to drug regimens: an interdisciplinary approach. (Using patient medication instruction cards.) American Journal of Nursing, 78 (7), Jul 1978, 1216-1219.

26 Royal Society of Medicine. Medico-Pharmaceutical Forum Drug information for patients: keep it simple. (Meeting discussing need for well-designed leaflets.) British Medical Journal, 280, 14 Jun 1980, 1393.

27 Sclafani, M. Medication classes for the emotionally ill. (To inform patients about the medication they are taking and the necessity for continuing it as prescribed.) Journal of Psychiatric Nursing and Mental Health Services, 15 (4), Apr 1977, 13-16.

28 Sechrist, K.R. The effect of repetitive teaching on patient's knowledge about drugs to be taken at home. (Study carried out by nursing students at the University of Ibadan.) International Journal of Nursing Studies, 16 (1), 1979, 51-58.

29 Sharpe, D. The general practice pharmacist's viewpoint. (On self medication.) Royal Society of Health Journal, 97 (4), Aug 1977, 165-166, 187.

30 Smith, A. Medicine and the media. (List of patients' booklets issued by drug companies.) British Medical Journal, 281, 6 Sep 1980, 674-675.

31 Smith, A. and others Compliance with drug treatment. British Medical Journal, 1, 19 May 1979, 1335-1336.

32 Smith, D.L. Providing pharmacy service to ambulatory patients. (Patient education program at Sunnybrook Medical Centre, Toronto.) Hospital Administration in Canada, 17 (11 and 12), Nov/Dec 1975, 35-39, 41.

33 Smith, S.E. How drugs act—29. Patients do not always take their drugs. Nursing Times, 72, 15 Jan 1976, 72-73.

34 Toledo, J.R. and others Management of non-compliance to medical regimen: a suggested methodological approach. International Journal of Health Education, 22 (4), 1979, 232-241.

35 Weber, C.E. and Sather, M.R. Discharge

medication counselling. How to enhance patient compliance with prescribed medication regimens. Hospital Topics, 54 (6), Nov/Dec 1976, 39-42.

f DRUG MISUSE

1 Central Office of Information. Reference Division The prevention and treatment of drug misuse in Britain. HMSO, 1979.

2 Committee on the Review of Medicines Recommendations on barbiturate preparations. British Medical Journal, 2, 22 Sep 1979, 719-720.

3 Connell, P.H. What is barbiturate dependence and who is at risk? Journal of Medical Ethics, 2 (2), Jun 1976, 58-62.

4 Cust, G. Respect for medicines. (Problems associated with the use of drugs.) Midwife, Health Visitor and Community Nurse, 15 (3), Mar 1979, 97-98, 100.

5 D'Orban, P.T. Barbiturate abuse. Journal of Medical Ethics, 2 (2), Jun 1976, 63-67.

6 Jones, M. Uses and abuses of psychotropic drugs: a successful drug reduction project. (At St. George's Hospital, Morpeth, Northumberland.) Nursing Times, 75, 1 Mar 1979, NT Extra, 7-8, 10.

7 Sandroff, R. The potent placebo. (With reference to New Mexico survey showing placebo abuse by nurses and physicians.) RN Magazine, 43 (4), Apr 1980, 35-37, 88, 90, 92, 94, 96.

8 Webb, R.A.J. Drug abuse in hospitals. Australian Nurses Journal, 5 (8), Feb 1976, 27-28, 36.

g POISONING AND SELF-POISONING

1 Blake, D.R. and Bramble, M.G. Self-poisoning: psychiatric assessment by junior staff. (Research study.) British Medical Journal, 1, 30 Jun 1979, 1763.

2 Blake, D.R. and Mitchell, J.R.A. Self-poisoning: management of patients in Nottingham, 1976. (Survey which revealed lack of psychiatric evaluation and after care.) British Medical Journal, 1, 22 Apr 1978, 1032-1035.

3 Blake, D.R. and others Is there excessive use of gastric lavage in the treatment of self-poisoning? Lancet, 2, 23/30 Dec 1978, 1362-1364.

4 British Medical Journal Policies on self-poisoning. (Review of schemes at Addenbrooke's Hospital and elsewhere, including projects involving initial assessments by nurses.) British Medical Journal, 2, 3 Nov 1979, 1091-1092.

5 Catalan, J. The assessment of patients following a deliberate self-poisoning: a comparison of the assessment by doctors and nurses. MSc thesis, Oxford University, 1979.

6 Catalan, J. and others The role of the nurse in the management of deliberate self-poisoning in the general hospital. (Description of nurse's work and training and reference to results of evaluative studies in this area.) International Journal of Nursing Studies, 17 (4), 1980, 275-282.

7 Chase, R. and North, P. Nursing care

study. Blindness averted. (Intensive care nursing of child with accidental quinine poisoning.) Nursing Mirror, 146, 30 Mar 1978, 17-18.

8 CIBA Clinical Symposia Issue on the treatment of poisoning. CIBA Clinical Symposia, 30 (2), 1978, 4-47.

9 Department of Prices and Consumer Protection Child poisoning from household products: a report based on a detailed investigation into suspected child poisoning in the home. The Department, 1976.

10 Edmonds, O.P. Case history. Scrombotoxic poisoning. (Food poisoning from infected mackerel with role of OH staff outlined.) Occupational Health, 32 (5), May 1980, 247-249.

11 Erb, H.L. Emergency treatment of drug overdose. Canadian Nurse, 75 (5), May 1979, 30-35.

12 Gardner, R. and others Consultation-liaison scheme for self-poisoned patients in a general hospital. (Assessment of need for psychiatric treatment and after-care by medical teams including nurses at Addenbrooke's Hospital, Cambridge.) British Medical Journal, 2, 18 Nov 1978, 1392-1394.

13 Gardner, R. and others Psychological and social evaluation in cases of deliberate self-poisoning admitted to a general hospital. (By medical teams and nursing staff.) British Medical Journal, 2, 17 Dec 1977, 1567-1570.

14 Gazzard, B.G. and others Why do people use paracetamol for suicide? (Survey by questionnaire of 107 patients admitted after an overdose.) British Medical Journal, 1, 24 Jan 1976, 212-213.

15 Goulding, R. and others Household products and poisoning. (Two complementary studies.) British Medical Journal, 1, 4 Feb 1978, 286-287.

16 Graham, J.D.P. and Hitchins, H.A.N. The National Poisons Information Service and hospital admissions for children—the experience in Wales of the Cardiff Centre. British Medical Journal, 2, 19 Nov 1977, 1339-1340.

17 Graham, J.D.P. and others Self poisoning—a decennial survey from Cardiff. Public Health, 93 (4), Jul 1979, 223-229.

18 Hawton, K. and Blackstock, E. Attempted suicide. Deliberate self-poisoning: implications for psychotropic drug prescribing in general practice. (Survey of 130 patients and 122 GPs and suggested alternative methods of management.) Journal of the Royal College of General Practitioners, 27, Sep 1977, 560-563.

19 Ives, G. Nurse could you care more? (Nurses' unsympathetic attitudes towards overdose patients.) Nursing Times, 75, 30 Aug 1979, 1475.

20 Jensen, S. The initial management of acute poisoning. Journal of Emergency Nursing, 3 (4), Jul/Aug 1977, 13-16.

21 Jones, D.R. A follow-up of self-poisoned patients. (At either outpatient clinic or home to identify problems and help needed.) Journal of the Royal College of General Practitioners, 27, Dec 1977, 717-719.

22 Jones, D.I.R. Self-poisoning with drugs:

the past 20 years in Sheffield. British Medical Journal, 1, 1 Jan 1977, 28-29.

23 Jozwiak, J.S. Acetaminophen overdose: a new and treacherous care problem. (Paracetamol. Includes care plan for the overdose patient in hepatic coma.) RN Magazine, 41 (12), Dec 1978, 56, 58-62.

24 Kerfoot, M. Self-poisoning by children and adolescents. (Research study.) Social Work Today, 10, 24 Jul 1979, 9-11.

25 Kingston, B. and Hawton, K. Under paracetamol tragedy. (How to prevent increasing number of overdoses with brief case history.) Nursing Times, 73, 24 Feb 1977, 272.

26 Lawson, A.A.H. and McCallum, C.J. Trends in acute poisoning in a District Medical Unit. Health Bulletin, 37 (4), May 1979, 121-127.

27 McLean, W. Child poisoning in England and Wales: some statistics on admissions to hospital, 1964-76. Health Trends, 12 (1), Feb 1980, 9-12.

28 Macey, A.M. Preventing hepatotoxicity in acetaminophen overdose. (Paracetamol.) American Journal of Nursing, 79 (2), Feb 1979, 301-303.

29 Matthew, H. and Lawson, A.A.H. Treatment of common acute poisonings. 4th ed. Edinburgh: Churchill Livingstone, 1979.

30 Mennear, J.H. The poisoning emergency. (Including table of poisons and suggested general treatment for poisoning management.) American Journal of Nursing, 77 (5), May 1977, 842-844.

31 Meredith, T. and Vale, A. Poisons. Nursing Mirror, 147.
1. Acute poisoning. 12 Oct 1978, Supplement, i-iv.
2. Haemoperfusion—a new technique. 19 Oct 1978, Supplement, i-iv.
3. Are household products really hazardous? 26 Oct 1978, Supplement, i-iv.

32 Musson, V.J. Nursing care study. Haemoperfusion in the treatment of severe barbiturate poisoning. Nursing Times, 72, 16 Dec 1976, 1956-1958.

33 Nursing Poisoning. (Classification, prevention and treatment.) Nursing, 15, Jul 1980, 668-671.

34 O'Brien, S.E.M. and Stoll, K.A. Attitudes of medical and nursing staff towards self-poisoning patients in a London hospital. International Journal of Nursing Studies, 14 (1), 1977, 29-35.

35 O'Connor, B. Accidental poisoning in children—a review. (An analysis of the problem at Queen Elizabeth Hospital for Children, Hackney.) Nursing Times, 72 (43), 28 Oct 1976, ABPN Supplement, 7-8.

36 Panrucker, R. Nursing care study. Botulism: a team effort to save the poison salmon victims. (In Birmingham.) Nursing Mirror, 147, 14 Dec 1978, 32-35.

37 Proudfoot, A.T. and Park, J. Changing patterns of drugs used in self-poisoning. (Analysis of admissions to the Regional Poisoning Treatment Centre at Edinburgh Royal Infirmary.) British Medical Journal, 1, 14 Jan 1978, 90-93.

38 Robertson, J. The epidemiology of self-poisoning. Public Health, 91, (2), Mar 1977, 75-82.

39 Rogers, D. and others Non-accidental poisoning: an extended syndrome of child abuse. (Six cases at the Hospital for Sick Children, Great Ormond Street.) British Medical Journal, 1, 3 Apr 1976, 793-796.

40 Seche, J. Nursing decisions: emergency care of an aspirin overdose patient. RN Magazine, 41 (10), Oct 1978, 83-87, 93.

41 Sencicle, L. Jean's taken an overdose. (Community psychiatric nursing care study of woman following overdose.) Nursing Mirror, 147, 7 Dec 1978, 58-60.

42 Sibert, J.R. and others Child-resistant packaging and accidental child poisoning. (Effectiveness assessed.) Lancet, 2, 6 Aug 1977, 289-290.

43 Stevens, B.C. Preventing fatal overdose. (Review of research into self-poisoning and suicide prevention.) Nursing Mirror, 145, 15 Dec 1977, 47-48.

44 Stoddart, J.C. Treatment of poisoning in the ITU. (Self-poisoning.) Nursing Times, 74, 9 Nov 1978, 1846-1848.

45 Vale, J.A. Medical treatment of acute poisoning. Nursing Times, 72, 16 Dec 1976, 1954-1955.

46 Vale, J.A. Paracetamol poisoning. Nursing Times, 73, 28 Jul 1977, 1163-1164.

47 Vale, J.A. Paraquat poisoning. Nursing Times, 73, 3 Feb 1977, 154-155.

48 Vale, A. and Meredith, T. Poisons. Nursing Mirror, 147.
4. Paraquat: is there any treatment? 9 Nov 1978, Supplement, i-iv.
5. How safe is paracetamol? 16 Nov 1978, Supplement, i-iv.
6. How poisonous are 'poisonous plants?' 23 Nov 1978, Supplement, i-iv.

49 Watson, J. Over to you. (Drugs taken and factors involved in overdose.) Nursing Times, 72, 1/8 Jan 1976, 35-36.

h OXYGEN THERAPY

1 British Medical Journal Domiciliary oxygen. (Review of oxygen therapy and need for domiciliary service.) British Medical Journal, 2, 9 Jul 1977, 77-78.

2 Freedman, B.J. Oxygen therapy in hospital practice: the indications for oxygen therapy and its safe application. Nursing Times, 74, 14 Dec 1978, 2072-2076.

3 Greenberg, D.A. and others Hyperbaric oxygen: exciting new clinical results. (High pressure oxygen therapy for range of conditions.) RN Magazine, 42 (9), Sep 1979, 53-57.

4 Jones, M.M. and others How patients use domiciliary oxygen. (Survey in Southampton.) British Medical Journal, 1, 27 May 1978, 1397-1400.

5 Moran, P. Methods for giving oxygen to infants and children. Nursing Mirror, 145, 7 Jul 1977, 10-12.

6 Thomas, S. The administration of oxygen. (Detailed guidance for nurses.) Nursing Mirror, 148, 22 Mar 1979, 30-32.

59 PAIN

a GENERAL

1 British Medical Journal The gate control theory of pain. British Medical Journal, 2, 26 Aug 1978, 586-587.

2 Condon, P. Pain relief—the nurse's role. Nursing Times, 76, 12 Jun 1980, 1052-1054.

3 Copp, L.A. Interview—Laurel Archer Copp (discussing her research into pain). Nursing Times, 73, 7 Apr 1977, 496-497.

4 Davitz, L.L. Black and white nurses' inferences of suffering. (Research study.) Nursing Times, 74, 27 Apr 1978, 708-710.

5 Davitz, L.L. and others Cross-cultural inferences of physical pain and psychological distress. (A study of reactions to patient suffering in nurses from six different cultures.) Nursing Times, 73, 14 Apr 1977, 521-523; 21 Apr 1977, 556-558.

6 Davitz, L.J. and others Suffering as viewed in six different cultures. (A study of nurses' perception of patient's pain in Korea, Japan, Taiwan, Thailand, Puerto Rico, and the U.S.A.) American Journal of Nursing, 76 (8), Aug 1976, 1296-1297.

7 Doherty, G. The patient in pain: handling the guilt feelings. Canadian Nurse, 75 (2), Feb 1979, 31.

8 Dudley Hart, F. Pain as an old friend. (Chronic pain and pain as a career which fills social need for patient.) British Medical Journal, 1, 26 May 1979, 1405-1407.

9 Duncan, C. The nurse and the patient in pain. ONA Journal, 6 (6), Jun 1979, 242-244.

10 Fagerhaugh, S.Y. and Strauss, A. Politics of pain management: staff-patient interaction. Menlo Park, California: Addison-Wesley, 1977.

11 Graffam, S. Nurse response to patients in pain: an analysis and an imperative for action. Nursing Leadership, 2 (3), Sep 1979, 23-25.

12 Green, D.E. Pain and the hospitalised patient. New Zealand Nursing Journal, 71 (8), Aug 1978, 3-6; (9), Sep 1978, 7-10.

13 Hedlin, A. and Dostrovsky, J. Understanding the physiology of pain. Canadian Nurse, 75 (2), Feb 79, 28-30.

14 Hunt, J.M. and others Patients with protracted pain: a survey conducted at The London Hospital. (Patients' views and doctors' and nurses' efforts and attitudes.) Journal of Medical Ethics, 3 (2), Jun 1977, 61-73.

15 Hutchinson, J.T. The psychological aspects. (Symposium paper on pain.) Nursing Mirror, 144, 10 Mar 1977, 50-52.

16 Jacox, A.K. Assessing pain. American Journal of Nursing, 79 (5), May 1979, 895-900.

17 Jacox, A.K. editor Pain: a source book for nurses and other health professionals. Boston: Little, Brown and Co., 1977.

18 Kim, S. Pain: theory, research and nursing practice. Advances in Nursing Science, 2 (2), Jan 1980, 43-59.

19 Lewis, G. The place of pain in human experience. Journal of Medical Ethics, 4 (3), Sep 1978, 122-125.

20 McCauley, K. and Polomano, R.C. Acute pain: a nursing perspective with cardiac surgical patients. Topics in Clinical Nursing, 2 (1), Apr 1980, 45-56.

21 McGough, A. The nurse's role. (Symposium paper on pain.) Nursing Mirror, 144, 10 Mar 1977, 62-64.

22 McMahon, M.A. and Miller, P. Pain response: the influence of psycho-social-cultural factors. Nursing Forum, 17 (1), 1978, 58-71.

23 Mehta, M. The principles of pain. (Symposium paper.) Nursing Mirror, 144, 10 Mar 1977, 48-50.

24 Merskey, H. The patient with chronic pain. Practitioner, 220, Feb 1978, 237-242.

25 Nursing Coping with pain. Nursing, 1, Apr 1979, 1-52; 2, May 1979, 55-108.

26 Nursing Clinics of North America Symposium on impressions of pain: a nursing diagnosis. Nursing Clinics of North America, 12 (4), Dec 1977, 609-696.

27 Nursing Mirror A symposium on pain. Nursing Mirror, 144, 10 Mar 1977, 47-64.

28 Nursing Times Pain: some aspects. Articles reprinted from Nursing Times. Macmillan Journals, 1977.

29 Pace, J.B. Helping patients overcome the disabling effects of chronic pain. Nursing, 77 7 (7), Jul 1977, 38-43.

30 Reading, A.E. and others Measuring the subjective aspects of pain. (Methods used in the Dept of Obstetrics and Gynaecology at King's College Hospital with patients with dysmenorrhoea and post-IUD insertion.) Nursing Mirror, 147, 28 Sep 1978, 13-15.

31 Roland, R.J. Nursing care for patients with pain. (Using the nursing process.) AORN Journal, 27 (6), May 1978, 1180, 1182, 1184, 1186, 1188, 1190, 1192, 1194.

32 Rosen, M. Assessing pain. (Symposium paper.) Nursing Mirror, 144, 10 Mar 1977, 52-54.

33 Storlie, F. Pointers for assessing pain. Nursing, 8 (5), May 1978, 37-39.

34 Trethowan, W.H. Pain. (Theories of pain transmission and psychological processes involved.) Nursing Mirror, 145, 11 Aug 1977, 37-38.

35 Winslow, L.S. Pain: a personalized approach. (Using the nursing process to determine patients' needs.) Journal of Practical Nursing, 27 (2), Feb 1977, 16-17, 34, 41.

b PAIN RELIEF

1 American Journal of Nursing The management of pain. (Two articles, a reference guide to analgesics and using analgesics effectively.)

American Journal of Nursing, 79 (1), Jan 1979, 74-78.

2 Barnard, J.D.W. and Lloyd, J.W. Cryo-analgesia. (Pain relief through extreme low temperature.) Nursing Times, 73, 16 Jun 1977, 897-899.

3 Brewer, C. Pain at the Mayo. (New approaches to relief of pain at the Mayo Clinic in Rochester, Minnesota.) World Medicine, 15 (2), 20 Oct 1979, 34-35.

4 British Medical Journal Postoperative pain. (Review of analgesics.) British Medical Journal, 2, 19 Aug 1978, 517-518.

5 Budd, K. The concept of chronic pain relief. (Role of pain relief clinics.) Health Trends, 3 (11), Aug 1979, 69-71.

6 Church, J.J. Continuous narcotic infusions for relief of postoperative pain. British Medical Journal, 1, 14 Apr 1979, 977-979.

7 Copperman, H. Use of morphine: lifting the mantle of mystery. Nursing Mirror, 149, 5 Jul 1979, 40-41.

8 Coyle, N. Analgesics at the bedside. (Self-medication programme for hospitalised patients with chronic pain.) American Journal of Nursing, 79 (9), Sep 1979, 1554-1557.

9 Davis, A.J. Teaching your patients to use electricity to ward off pain. (Transcutaneous nerve stimulation.) RN Magazine, 41 (2), Feb 1978, 43-45.

10 Dunbar, N. Percutaneous stimulation in the treatment of acute and chronic pain. Journal of Neurosurgical Nursing, 8 (2), Dec 1976, 105-112.

11 Everall, M. Cold therapy. (Application of cold packs and ice for pain relief in joints and muscles.) Nursing Times, 72, 29 Jan 1976, 144-145.

12 Fordyce, W.E. Behavioral methods for chronic pain and illness. St. Louis: Mosby, 1976.

13 Frazer, F.W. Persistent post-sympathetic pain treated by connective tissue massage. Physiotherapy, 64 (7), Jul 1978, 211-213.

14 Fry, E.N.S. Postoperative analgesia. (System developed in the North Tees General Hospital involving self-demand techniques without expensive equipment.) Nursing Times, 73, 5 May 1977, 655-656.

15 Goloskov, J.W. and LeRoy, P.L. The evolving role of the nurse and the neurosurgical physician's assistant in the treatment of intractable pain states. Journal of Neurosurgical Nursing, 7 (2), Dec 1975, 107-115.

16 Goodall, J. Analgesics—the choice. Queen's Nursing Journal, 19 (4), Jul 1976, 109-110.

17 Gramse, C.A. For control of severe pain: dorsal column stimulation. (Battery device to block pain impulses to the spinal cord.) American Journal of Nursing, 78 (6), Jun 1978, 1022-1025.

18 Hannington-Kiff, J.G. Counterpains. (The relief of chronic pain by counter-irritants.) Nursing Times, 73, 3 Mar 1977, 312-313.

19 James, C.D.T. Pain clinics. (For chronic pain.) Nursing Mirror, 143, 9 Dec 1976, 56-57.

20 Johnson, I. Transcutaneous electrical stimulation. (Use of electricity to relieve pain.) Journal of Neurosurgical Nursing, 7 (2), Dec 1975, 87-90.

21 Lamb, S. Neuroaugmentation for the chronic pain patient. (Implantation of electrodes into the brain.) Journal of Neurosurgical Nursing, 11 (4), Dec 1979, 215-220.

22 Lancet Intravenous salicylates for postoperative pain? Lancet, 2, 20/27 Dec 1980, 1346-1347.

23 Lancet Patient-controlled analgesia. (Review of literature on electronically controlled devices for intravenous drug administration used especially for post-operative pain.) Lancet, 1, 9 Feb 1980, 289-290.

24 Linchitz, R. Nursing care of the patient with brain stimulation for pain control. (Chronic electrical stimulation of the brain by surgically implanted electrodes.) AORN Journal, 25 (4), Mar 1977, 651-661.

25 Lipton, S. The control of chronic pain. Edward Arnold, 1979. (Current topics in anaesthesia; 2.)

26 Lipton, S. Recent advances in pain relief. (Symposium paper.) Nursing Mirror, 144, 10 Mar 1977, 57-59.

27 Lloyd, J.W. Conservative methods of pain control. (Work of the Oxford Regional Pain Relief Unit, Abingdon.) Nursing Mirror, 144, 10 Mar 1977, 54-56.

28 Lloyd, J.W. Use of anaesthesia: the anaesthetist and the pain clinic. British Medical Journal, 281, 9 Aug 1980, 432-434.

29 McCaffery, M. How to relieve your patients' pain fast and effectively...with oral analgesics. Nursing (U.S.), 10 (11), Nov 1980, 58-63.

30 McCaffery, M. Pain relief for the child. Problem areas and selected nonpharmacological methods. Pediatric Nursing, 3 (4), Jul/Aug 1977, 11-16.

31 McCaffery, M. and Hart, L.L. Undertreatment of acute pain and narcotics. American Journal of Nursing, 76 (10), Oct 1976, 1586-1591.

32 Mehta, M. Treating intractable pain: changing attitudes and alternatives. Nursing Times, 72, 12 Aug 1976, 1236-1237.

33 Miles, J. Pain relief: electrical stimulation. Nursing Mirror, 150, 14 Feb 1980, 46-47.

34 Mushin, W.W. and others The Pain centre. Practitioner, 218, Mar 1977, 439-442.

35 Ostrowski, M.J. Pain control in advanced malignant disease using transcutaneous nerve stimulation. British Journal of Clinical Practitioners, 33 (6), Jun 1979, 157-162.

36 Ostrowski, M.J. and Dodd, V.A. Transcutaneous nerve stimulation for relief of pain in advanced malignant disease. Nursing Times, 73, 11 Aug 1977, 1233-1238.

37 Rosenburgh, S.P. Pain—theories and treatment by cutaneous afferent stimulation.

Journal of Neurosurgical Nursing, 8 (2), Dec 1976, 80-84.

38 Rutter, P.C. and others Morphine: controlled trial of different methods of administration for postoperative pain relief. British Medical Journal, 280, 5 Jan 1980, 12-13.

39 Staples, D. Behavioural treatment for chronic pain. (Neck pain.) Physiotherapy, 65 (4), Apr 1979, 110-113.

40 Stewart, D. and others Acupuncture analgesia: an experimental investigation. (Study to establish whether acupuncture has any analgesic properties beyond those of suggestion.) British Medical Journal, 1, 8 Jan 1977, 67-70.

41 Stewart, E. To lessen pain: relaxation and rhythmic breathing. American Journal of Nursing, 76 (6), Jun 1976, 958-959.

42 Swerdlow, M. The value of clinics for the relief of chronic pain. Journal of Medical Ethics, 4 (3), Sep 1978, 117-118.

43 Topics in Clinical Nursing Pain management. (Book reviews, 89-95.) Topics in Clinical Nursing, 2 (1), Apr 1980, xi, 88.

44 Yanchinski, S. Finger-tip pain relief. (Electrical nerve stimulation to relieve back pain.) New Scientist, 79, 10 Aug 1978, 395-397.

c TERMINAL AND CANCER PAIN

1 AORN Journal Analgesics may be only treatment for cancer pain. (Report of studies of analgesic drug efficiency at Sloan Kettering Institute for Cancer Research, New York City.) AORN Journal, 26 (4), Oct 1977, 802-804.

2 British Medical Journal Pain and the dissatisfied dead. (Control of terminal pain with reference to hospice care.) British Medical Journal, 1, 25 Feb 1978, 457-460.

3 Hannington-Kiff, J.G. Pain control and terminal care. South West Thames Regional Cancer Services, 1976.

4 Hoy, A.M. Terminal pain. Nursing Mirror, 144, 10 Mar 1977, 60-62.

5 Journal of Community Nursing Drugs in district nursing: drugs for the dying. Journal of Community Nursing, 3 (2), Aug 1979, 12.

6 Lamerton, R. Care of the dying. 6. The pains of death. Nursing Times, 69, 11 Jan 1973, 56-57.

7 Lancet Peace at last? (Pain control in terminal cancer.) Lancet, 1, 1 Apr 1978, 698-700.

8 Leung, J.C.K. Terminal pain. Nursing Times, 76, 12 Jun 1980, 1050-1051; 19 Jun 1980, 1101-1102; 26 Jun 1980, 1145-1147.

9 Lloyd, J. and others The pain of cancer. (Analysis of admissions to Pain Relief Unit, Abingdon.) Practitioner, 220, Mar 1978, 453-456.

10 Rankin, M. The progressive pain of cancer. Topics in Clinical Nursing, 2 (1), Apr 1980, 57-73.

11 Saunders, C. Care of the dying—4. Control of pain in terminal cancer. Nursing Times, 72, 22 Jul 1976, 1133-1135.

12 Saunders, C. Listening a key to control of terminal patients' pain. (Seminar report.) Nursing Times, 72, 27 May 1976, 796.

13 Twycross, R.G. The assessment of pain in advanced cancer. Journal of Medical Ethics, 4 (3), Sep 1978, 112-116.

14 Twycross, R.G. The target is a pain-free patient. (Relief of pain in advanced cancer.) Nursing Mirror, 147, 14 Dec 1978, 38-39.

15 Valentine, A.S. Pain relief for cancer patients. (Double blind randomized study to test efficiency of elixir including methadone.) American Journal of Nursing, 78 (12), Dec 1978, 2054-2056.

16 Vere, D.W. The hospital as a place of pain. (Reasons why terminal pain is not relieved adequately in hospital, as opposed to hospice, care.) Journal of Medical Ethics, 6 (3), Sep 1980, 117-119.

17 Young, J.L. The pain of a terminally ill patient in the home. Nursing Clinics of North America, 12 (4), Dec 1977, 653-662.

60 PRESSURE SORES

1 Agate, J. Pressure sores. Mechanical and medical factors. Nursing Mirror, 144, 17 Mar 1977, Supplement, i, iii, vii.

2 Agris, J. and Spira, M. Pressure ulcers: prevention and treatment. CIBA Clinical Symposia, 31 (5), 1979, 1-32.

3 Barbenel, J.C. and others Incidence of pressure sores in the Greater Glasgow Health Board area. (Survey of hospital inpatients and patients visited by district nurse.) Lancet, 2, 10 Sep 1977, 548-550.

4 Bardsley, J.I. Investigations into movement related to the aetiology of pressure sores. PhD thesis, University of Strathclyde, 1977.

5 Barton, A.A. and Barton, M. Drug based prevention of pressure sores. (A double blind clinical trial was carried out in 85 patients undergoing surgery to the upper shaft of the femur and to the hip joint and the administration of A.C.T.H. proved effective.) Lancet, 1976, 2, 28 Aug 1976, 443-444.

6 Barton, A.A. Prevention of pressure sores. (Pathogenesis and drug based prevention.) Nursing Times, 73, 13 Oct 1977, 1593-1595.

7 Barton, A.A. Stop! Drugs at work on pressure sores. (Research showing that pre-operative administration of Acthar Gel reduced incidence of pressure sores postoperatively.) Nursing Mirror, 149, 16 Aug 1979, 40.

8 Baum, M.E. Flexible decubitus treatment: adapting peristomal skin care products and treatment to decubitus ulcers. Nursing Care, 9 (7), Jul 1976, 24-27.

9 Baxter, B. Strathclyde bioengineering seminar. Biomechanics of tissue viability and clinical application. (Problems and prevention of pressure sores.) NATNews, 13 (6), Aug 1976, 18-20.

10 Bayliss, D. Nursing care study. Decubitus ulcer: a secondary problem is cured. Nursing Mirror, 148, 17 May 1979, 45-48.

11 Berglas, C. and Sullivan, O. Decubitus ulcers: a nursing care study. (Research study to test the effectiveness of collagenase, an enzymatic debriding agent.) Journal of Nursing Care, 13 (4), Apr 1980, 16-17, 30.

12 Bliss, M. and Murray, E. The use of Ripple beds. (To prevent and treat pressure sores.) Nursing Times, 75, 15 Feb 1979, 280-283.

13 Bowker, P. and Davidson, L.M. Development of a cushion to prevent ischial pressure sores. (Made of thixotropic gel.) British Medical Journal, 2, 20 Oct 1979, 958-961.

14 British Medical Journal Treating pressure sores. (Review of methods.) British Medical Journal, 1, 13 May 1978, 1232.

15 Cameron, G. Pressure sores: what to do when prevention fails. (With coloured illustrations of treatment of stages 1-4 pressure sores and development of pressure sore record.) Nursing (U.S.), 9 (1), Jan 1979, 42-47.

16 Chrisp, M. New treatment of pressure sores. (Trials of new occlusive dressing, Op-site at Prudhoe Hospital.) Nursing Times, 73, 4 Aug 1977, 1202-1205.

17 Clark, M.O. and others Pressure sores. Findings of a survey carried out in Glasgow to determine the incidence of pressure sores in the patient community of Greater Glasgow Health Board. Nursing Times, 74, 2 Mar 1978, 363-366.

18 Constantian, M.B. editor Pressure ulcers: principles and techniques of management. Boston: Little, Brown and Co., 1980.

19 Coombs, R.M. Supporting patients on air: an answer to pressure sores. (Low Air Loss Bed System.) Nursing Mirror, 142 (4), 29 Jan 1976, 45-46.

20 Cowper-Smith, F. The greatest challenge. (Report of conference on pressure sores at Northwick Park Hospital.) Nursing Times, 75, 2 Aug 1979, 1294-1295.

21 Dalkin, M. Nursing care study: sometimes, you just can't win! (Care of varicose ulcers by district nurse.) Journal of Community Nursing, 2 (6), Dec 1978, 21-22.

22 Denne, W.A. An objective assessment of the sheepskins used for decubitus sore prophylaxis. (Concluded that natural sheepskins were better than simulations.) Rheumatology and Rehabilitation, 18 (1), Feb 1979, 23-29.

23 Department of Biomedical Engineering Institute of Orthopaedics Nursing instructions for the Low Air Bed System LALBS Mk 4. (For treatment of pressure sores.) Nursing Mirror, 142 (4), 29 Jan 1976, 47-48.

24 Di Mascio, S. Debrisan for decubitus ulcers. (Report of small trial.) American Journal of Nursing, 79 (4), Apr 1979, 684-685.

25 Dolphin, S. and Walker, M. Healing accelerated by Ionozone therapy. (Trial of apparatus producing steam consisting of ionised water, ozone and oxygen to treat ulcers and pressure sores.) Physiotherapy, 65 (3), Mar 1979, 81-82.

26 Dyson, R. Bed sores—the injuries hospital staff inflict on patients. (Report of research project in the Bath group of hospitals.) Nursing Mirror, 146, 15 Jun 1978, 30-32.

27 Eales, H.J. and McPherson, G.A.D. Varicose ulcers—treatment on an outpatient basis. (At South Middlesex Hospital, Isleworth.) Nursing Times, 74, 21/28 Dec 1978, 2104-2106.

28 Easterby, M. A treatment for pressure sores and statis ulcers. Nursing Times, 73, 14 Apr 1977, 519-520.

29 Ferguson-Pell, M.W. Critical assessment of the effects of pressure with special reference to the development of pressure sores. PhD thesis, University of Strathclyde, 1977.

30 Finn, E. Outpatient treatment of leg ulcers using pigskin. Nursing Times, 74, 26 Jan 1978, 136-139.

31 Fisher, M.V. Pressure sores. Treatment using ultrasound. Nursing Times, 72 (8), 26 Feb 1976, 302.

32 Fugill, G.C. Pressure sores. (Prevention and treatment.) Physiotherapy, 66 (2), Feb 1980, 46-47.

33 Gerber, R.M. and Rowe Van Ort, S. Topical application of insulin in decubitus ulcers. (Experimental study which did not show clinical effectiveness of insulin therapy.) Nursing Research, 28 (1), Jan/Feb 1979, 16-19.

34 Gibbs, J.R. Net suspension beds for managing threatened and established pressure sores. Lancet, 1977, 1, 22 Jan 1977, 174-175.

35 Goldstone, L.A. and Roberts, B.V. A preliminary discriminant function analysis of elderly orthopaedic patients who will or will not contract a pressure sore. (Assessment of patients using Norton scale.) International Journal of Nursing Studies, 17 (1), 1980, 17-23.

36 Grahame, R. The water bed on active service. (The Beaufort-Winchester Flotation Bed, used in the conservative and surgical management of pressure sores.) Nursing Mirror, 139 (5), 2 Aug 1974, 62-63.

37 Green, M.F. Pressure sores. The team approach. Nursing Times, 72, 26 Feb 1976, 292-294.

38 Gruis, M. and Innes, B. Assessment: essential to prevent pressure sores. American Journal of Nursing, 76 (11), Nov 1976, 1762-1764.

39 Hammond, M.A. Breaking down the dry barrier. (Use of Op-Site for pressure sores and wounds.) Nursing Mirror, 149, 1 Nov 1979, 38-40.

40 Hansard Pressure sores—cost in nursing time and money. Hansard (House of Commons), 13 Nov 1979, WA, 585-6.

41 Hibbert, D.L. A sore point at home. (Survey of management of pressure sores in the community based on questionnaire completed by district nurses.) Nursing Mirror, 151, 7 Aug 1980, 40-41.

42 Jellis, A.J. Pressure sores. Way of prevention. Nursing Times, 72 (8), 26 Feb 1976, 291-292.

43 Jones, E. Prevention of pressure sores: the clinical score chart. (To identify patients at risk and using Norton scale.) Nursing Times, 76, 27 Mar 1980, 565-566.

44 Kavchak-Keyes, M.A. Four proven steps

for preventing decubitus ulcers. Nursing, 7 (9), Sep 1977, 58-61.

45 **Kavchak-Keyes, M.A.** Treating decubitus ulcers using four proven steps. Nursing, 7 (10), Oct 1977, 44-45.

46 **Kerr, J.C. and others** Pressure sores: nurses' knowledge, attitudes and clinical judgement—a preliminary investigation. Edmonton: University of Alberta, Faculty of Nursing, 1980.

47 **Lancet** Leaving no ripple. (Unpopularity of ripple beds in spite of their effectiveness in preventing pressure sores.) Lancet, 2, 29 Jul 1978, 247-248.

48 **Lancet** Sore points. (Review of prevention of and treatment for pressure sores.) Lancet, 1977, 1, 14 May 1977, 1042-1043.

49 **Love, C.** Nursing care study. A problem sore. (Pressure sore causing osteomyelitic lesion and sinus in paralysed lady. By clinical teacher.) Nursing Times, 76, 27 Mar 1980, 560-564.

50 **Lowthian, P.** Practical nursing. Turning clock system to prevent pressure sores. (24-hour clock system for manual turning of patients.) Nursing Mirror, 148, 24 May 1979, 30-31.

51 **Lowthian, P.** Pressure sore prevalence: a survey of sores in orthopaedic patients. (A one-day survey at the Royal National Orthopaedic Hospital, Stanmore.) Nursing Times, 75, 1 Mar 1979, 358-360.

52 **Lowthian, P.** Pressure sores. (Letter explaining tissue damage caused by pressure.) Nursing Times, 73, 4 Nov 1977, 1712-1713.

53 **Lowthian, P.T.** Pressure sores. Practical prophylaxis. (Preventive methods particularly suitable for elderly patients.) Nursing Times, 72 (8), 26 Feb 1976, 295-298.

54 **Lowthian, P.T.** A review of pressure sore prophylaxis. Nursing Mirror, 144, 17 Mar 1977, Supplement, vii, ix, xi, xiii, xv.

55 **Lowthian, P.** Sheepskins and underpads for pressure sores. (Letter.) Nursing Times, 73, 21 Jul 1977, 1125.

56 **Lowthian, P.T. and others** Underpads for preventing pressure sores. (Pilot study of three nursing underpads at Northwick Park, Central Middlesex and Watford General Hospitals.) Nursing Mirror, 144, 10 Mar 1977, 66-69.

57 **McClemont, E.J.W. and others** Pressure sores: a new method of treatment. (Debrisan.) British Journal of Clinical Practice, 33 (1), Jan 1979, 21-26.

58 **Mackinnon, A.** Management of pressure areas—a nurse's plea. (Advocates use of Op-Site dressing.) Lamp, 35 (7), Jul 1978, 16-18.

59 **Midwife, Health Visitor and Community Nurse** New Pulsair for pressure sores. (Description and photo of new medium-cell ripple mattress.) Midwife, Health Visitor and Community Nurse, 16 (3), Mar 1980, 121.

60 **Mikulic, M.A.** Treatment of pressure ulcers. (Review of methods of prevention and treatment, with extensive bibliography.) American Journal of Nursing, 80 (6), Jun 1980, 1125-1128.

61 **Mykyta, L.J.** The treatment of pressure

sores. Australian Nurses Journal, 7 (1), Jul 1977, 35-36.

62 **Nightingale, K.** Pressure sores. (General review of causes and treatment.) Health and Social Service Journal, 88, 10 Mar 1978, 286.

63 **Northwick Park Hospital. Nursing Practice Research Unit** and **Department of Health and Social Security** The prevention of pressure sores: proceedings of a conference... DHSS, 1979.

64 **Nursing Mirror** Pressure sores. Nursing Mirror, 144, 17 Mar 1977, Supplement, i-xv.

65 **Nursing Times** Pressure sores. A national problem. Nursing Times, 72 (8), 26 Feb 1976, 290.

66 **Parr, E.** Nursing care study. A patient with pressure sores: management of this elderly lady included consideration of her social situation. Nursing Times, 75, 1 Mar 1979, 369-372.

67 **Pinel, C.** Refresher course. Pressure sores. Nursing Times, 72 (5), 5 Feb 1976, 172-174.

68 PREPARATIONS for pressure sores. Drug and Therapeutics Bulletin, 15, 2 Sep 1977, 69-71.

69 **Rampino, E.** Did we do that to him? (Prevention and treatment of pressure sores.) Journal of Practical Nursing, 26 (6), Jun 1976, 18-21.

70 **Ramsay, B.M.** Pressure sores in para- and tetraplegic patients: porcine dermis stimulated healthy granulation and controlled infection. (Trial of Corethium 2 Lyophilised porcine skin (Dermis).) Nursing Times, 75, 1 Mar 1979, 361-364.

71 **Relph, E.J.** Pressure sores. Treatment using micropore. Nursing Times, 72, 26 Feb 1976, 301.

72 **Rhodes, B. and others** The treatment of pressure sores in geriatric patients: a trial of sterculia powder. (Karaya gum powder.) Nursing Times, 75, 1 Mar 1979, 365-368.

73 **Robinson, W.** Beware of the hospital bed? (Interview with Professor John Scales who has been studying the problems of wound dressing and pressure sores.) Nursing Mirror, 144, 3 Mar 1977, 39-41.

74 **Ryan, D.M.** Pressure sores. Treatment using Stomahesive. Nursing Times, 72, 26 Feb 1976, 299-300.

75 SEATING the disabled. (With reference to the prevention of pressure sores.) British Medical Journal, 280, 5 Apr 1980, 963-964.

76 **Snowden, D.** Decubitus ulcer. (History and pathology and report of survey of preventive and curative methods used at Chapel Allerton Hospital, Leeds.) Nursing Mirror, 148, 1 Feb 1979, 22-25; 8 Feb 1979, 26-30.

77 **Stapleton, M.** An evaluation of the Pneumatress: a study of the effectiveness of a posture-changing mattress in preventing the incidence of pressure sores. Nursing Times, 75, 1 Feb 1979, 198-201.

78 **Taylor, V.** Intact heel decubitus: an innovative treatment with a special cleansing sponge. AORN Journal, 4 (6), Nov/Dec 1979, 9-10.

79 **Ternouth, A.** Nursing care study. Healing a deep sacral sore (in a patient with multiple sclerosis). Nursing Times, 73, 27 Jan 1977, 135-136.

80 **Van Ort, S.R. and Gerber, R.M.** Topical application of insulin in the treatment of decubitus ulcers: a pilot study. Nursing Research, 25 (1), Jan-Feb 1976, 9-12.

81 **Wall, B.** The pathology of pressure sores, and factors which influence their healing. Chiropodist, 33 (12), Dec 1978, 442-445.

82 **Wright, W.B. and Radford, K.** Pressure sores: sensible precautions which aid prevention. Geriatric Medicine, 10 (2), Feb 1980, 9.

61 NUTRITION AND DIET

a GENERAL

1 **Bender, A.E.** Nutrition policies and population policies. Journal of Human Nutrition, 34 (6), Dec 1980, 417-428.

2 **Bogan, K.A.** Nutrition and mental health: what is the relationship? Occupational Health Nursing, 24 (2), Feb 1976, 17-20.

3 **British Nutrition Foundation and others** Nutrition education: report of a working party. HMSO, 1977. (Chairman: T.B. Williamson and J.B. Sharp.)

4 **Burkitt, D.P.** Two blind spots in medical knowledge. What is the role played by non-nutritious roughage in our diet? Nursing Times, 72, 1/8 Jan 1976, 24-27.

5 **Community Outlook** Fat sheet. (Advice on reducing saturated fat, increasing polyunsaturates and cutting down cholesterol.) Nursing Times, 76, 13 Mar 1980, Community Outlook, 72-73.

6 **Department of Health and Social Security** Prevention and health: eating for health. A discussion booklet. HMSO, 1978.

7 **Elliot, E. and others** A survey of dietitians' work in hospitals in the United Kingdom. Journal of Human Nutrition, 32 (3), Jun 1978, 187-193.

8 **Fawns, H.T.** Vitamin A1. Discovery and isolation of the vitamin. Vitamin A2. Consequences of deficiency. Nursing Times, 74, 16 Feb 1978, 286-289; 23 Feb 1978, 331-332.

9 **Fawns, H.T.** Vitamin E. Its discovery and uses. Nursing Times, 75, 19 Apr 1979, 664-666.

10 **Fawns, H.T.** Vitamin K and blood clotting. (Therapeutic agent for haemorrhagic diseases.) Nursing Times, 74, 26 Oct 1978, 1764-1766.

11 **Fielden, H.** When roughage is the fibre of health. Nursing Mirror, 151, 7 Aug 1980, 32-34.

12 **Hayter, J.** Trace elements: implications for nursing. (Their value in diet and adverse effects of certain elements.) Journal of Advanced Nursing, 5 (1), Jan 1980, 91-101.

13 **Krebs, H.** Citric acid cycle: a chemical reaction for life. (Chemical changes affecting food as it is oxidised.) Nursing Mirror, 149, 16 Aug 1979, 30-32.

14 Leeds, A.H. Dietary fibre—a review of current and potential therapeutic uses. Queen's Nursing Journal, 19 (14), May 1977, 386-389.

15 Leslie, J. Common sense guide to good and healthy eating. (With 'nutrition at a glance' chart.) Nursing Mirror, 147, 16 Nov 1978, 27-30.

16 Leslie, J. Nutrition and diet. 5. Prevention is better than cure. (Nutrient value of foods.) Nursing Mirror, 145, 11 Aug 1977, 25-27.

17 Mackie, A. How fed up can you get? (Commercial influences on food we eat, by Director General of Health Education Council.) Nursing Mirror, 150, 17 Apr 1980, 17-18.

18 Mann, J.I. A prudent diet for the nation. (Nutritional factors in the aetiology of disease.) Journal of Human Nutrition, 33 (1), Feb 1979, 57-63.

19 May, M. Eat, drink and be healthy. Nursing Mirror, 151, 31 Jul 1980, 28-29.

20 Moore, T. Vitamin intake. Journal of Community Nursing, 4 (2), Aug 1980, 12-14.

21 Newland, P.M. Therapeutic dietetics since the inception of the National Health Service: a review. Journal of Human Nutrition, 34 (1), Feb 1980, 17-22.

22 Passmore, R. and others Prescription for a better British diet. British Medical Journal, 1, 24 Feb 1979, 527-531.

23 Potterton, D. Good diet, bad diet. (Work of McCarrison Society and details of McCarrison's views on nutrition.) Nursing Times, 74, 7 Dec 1978, 2035.

24 Ross, T. A changeable feast. (Changing and contradictory theories of nutrition over the years.) Nursing Mirror, 150, 17 Apr 1980, 22-24.

25 Schwarz, V. Malnutrition in our society. Fats or oils? Iron and vitamin deficiencies. Health Visitor, 49 (10), Oct 1976, 325-326.

26 Scott, J. Nutrition and weight control in Canada and USA. (Study tour of Winston Churchill fellow of 1975.) Nursing Times, 73, 19 May 1977, 756-757.

27 Shaper, A.G. and Marr, J.W. Dietary recommendations for the community towards the postponement of coronary heart disease. (A review of recommendations over the last ten years.) British Medical Journal, 1, 2 Apr 1977, 867-871.

28 Swaffield, L. Fats and fiction. (Controversy over effects of dietary fats.) Nursing Times, 76, 13 Mar 1980, Community Outlook, 69-70, 75-76, 79.

29 Thomas, J. The place of education in a national nutrition policy. Royal Society of Health Journal, 99 (5), Oct 1979, 189-195.

30 Thompson, D.R. Fats and heart disease: a point for controversy. Nursing Times, 76, 31 Jul 1980, 1360-1361.

31 Turner, R.W.D. Fats and heart disease: points for controversy. (Review of recent research and outline of 'prudent diet'.) Nursing Times, 76, 11 Dec 1980, 2189-2190.

32 Ward, R. Foods of the future. Nursing Mirror, 143, 30 Dec 1976, 37-39.

33 Wilkinson, R.G. Dear David Ennals... (Health differences between upper and lower classes with particular reference to diet.) New Society, 38, 16 Dec 1976, 567-568.

34 Winckler, I. Nutrition today. Nursing Times, 72.
The importance of good nutrition. 2 Dec 1976, 1890-1891.
Moderation in all things. 9 Dec 1976, 1917-1918.
This slimming business. 16 Dec 1976, 1968-1969.

b COMMUNITY SERVICES

1 Dobson, A.M. and Mann, P.G. Introducing dietetics into general practice. (Scheme in Bolton.) Journal of Human Nutrition, 32 (6), Dec 1978, 467-471.

2 Elliott, E. and others Thin spread of dietitians. (Report of investigation into the deployment of dietitians in the NHS and the extent to which auxiliary staff might be used.) Health and Social Service Journal, 88, 6 Jan 1978, 14.

3 Felstein, I. A dietitian in the team? (Report of experimental project involving dietary advice clinic in a Bolton group practice.) Nursing Times, 76, 10 Jul 1980, Community Outlook, 211-212.

4 Griffin, J.F. The role of the dietitian in industry. (Personal comment on the role, responsibilities, opportunities and problems of the dietitian working in the food and pharmaceutical industry.) Journal of Human Nutrition, 34 (6), Dec 1980, 450-451.

5 Pawan, A.E. Dietetics in the community. Journal of Community Nursing, 1 (10), Apr 1978, 27-28.

6 Queen's Nursing Journal Bedford Sick Diet Guild. A description from the December 1904 issue of Queen's Nursing Magazine of the forerunner of meals on wheels. Queen's Nursing Journal, 19 (15), Jun 1977, 422.

c NURSING

1 Beck, M.E. Nutrition and dietetics for nurses. 5th ed. Churchill Livingstone, 1977.

2 Buckley, J.E. and others Feeding patients with dysphagia. Nursing Forum, 15 (1), 1976, 69-85.

3 Donovan, L. Is the doctor starving your patient? and are you contributing to the problem? Here's how to recognize the signs of 'physician-induced' malnutrition. RN Magazine, 41 (7), Jul 1978, 36-40.

4 Havard, A. and Mincher, R.F. Special diets in hospital: a problem or not? Nursing Times, 72, 25 Mar 1976, 470-471.

5 Hessor, I.B. Detecting deficient energy and protein intake in hospital patients: a simple record method. (Study in Denmark in which patient, relatives and nurses recorded food intake.) British Medical Journal, 1, 24 Jun 1978, 1667-1668.

6 Hirschhorn, M. Who sees what a patient eats? Nursing Mirror, 149, 12 Jul 1979, Supplement, ii-iii, v.

7 Johnston, M. Behavioural treatment of an eating problem. (Oral feeding of an adolescent girl who had been tube fed for four months following a road accident.) Nursing Times, 72, 15 Jul 1976, 1098-1099.

8 Jones, A.M. Overcoming the feeding problem of the mentally and the physically handicapped. (Children and adults.) Journal of Human Nutrition, 32 (5), Oct 1978, 359-367.

9 Jones, D. Careful diet. (Importance of patients' diet in nursing care.) Nursing Mirror, 151, 24 Jul 1980, 30-32.

10 Keithley, J.K. Proper nutritional assessment can prevent hospital malnutrition. Nursing (U.S.), 9 (2), Feb 1979, 68-72.

11 McBride Schreier, A, and Lavenia, J. The nurse's role in nutritional management of radiotherapy patients. Nursing Clinics of North America, 12 (1), Mar 1977, 173-182.

12 MacDougall, V. Nutritional assessment of the ICU patient. Canadian Nurse, 75 (5), May 1979, 39-43.

13 MacMillan, P. Give us this day. (Malnutrition in hospital patients.) Nursing Times, 75, 5 Jul 1979, 1126-1227.

14 Milner, A. Spread the word! (Advice on teaching patients about nutrition.) Nursing Mirror, 151, 10 Jul 1980, 24-26.

15 Mock, J. The role of the health visitor in nutrition education. MSc thesis, University of Manchester, Department of Community Medicine, 1976.

16 Nursing Issue on nutrition and health, with introduction on p.463-464 summarising nurse's role and responsibilities. Nursing, 11, Mar 1980, 463-504.

17 Nursing Issue on nutrition and illness. (With articles on the nurse nutritionist and alternative methods of feeding.) Nursing, 12, Apr 1980, 505-540.

18 O'Connor, H.M. and others Preventive nutrition in the nursing curriculum? (Role of nurse in nutrition advice.) Journal of Practical Nursing, 28 (8), Aug 1977, 31-33.

19 Porter, S.W. Intensive care 3. Feeding critically ill patients. Nursing Times, 74, 2 Mar 1978, 355-359.

20 Rose, J.C. Nutritional problems in radiotherapy patients. American Journal of Nursing, 78 (7), Jul 1978, 1194-1196.

21 Salmond, S.W. How to assess the nutritional status of acutely ill patients. American Journal of Nursing, 80 (5), May 1980, 922-924.

22 Schneggenburger, C. and Nolan, B.S. Diet teaching at Dustin House. (Long term psychiatric patients.) Journal of Psychiatric Nursing and Mental Health Services, 15 (5), May 1977, 18-22.

23 Shackleton, A.D. and Poleman, C.L. Practical nurse nutrition education. 4th ed. Philadelphia: Saunders, 1979.

24 Soukop, M. and Calman, K.C. Nutritional support in patients with malignant disease. Journal of Human Nutrition, 33 (3), Jun 1979, 179-188.

25 Willans, J.H. Appetite in the terminally ill

patient. (Provision of meals in a hospice.) Nursing Times, 76, 15 May 1980, 875-876.

26 **Williams, S.R.** Nutrition and diet therapy: a learning guide for students. 3rd ed. St. Louis: Mosby, 1977.

d PARENTERAL NUTRITION

1 **Amos, A.** Parenteral nutrition 2. The nurse's role. Nursing Times, 72, 29 Jul 1976, 1153-1155.

2 **Bateman, E.C.** Clinical nutrition in current practice. Tube feeding. Journal of Human Nutrition, 31 (2), Apr 1977, 85-93.

3 **Bodnar, A. and Agostino, J.D.** IV therapy. 1. Infection control. Journal of Practical Nursing, 27 (8), Aug 1977, 18-21.

4 **Borgen, L.** Total parenteral nutrition in adults. American Journal of Nursing, 78 (2), Feb 1978, 224-228.

6 **British Medical Journal** Deficiencies in parenteral nutrition. British Medical Journal, 2, 30 Sep 1978, 913-914.

7 **Bush, J.** Cervical esophagostomy to provide nutrition. (Including nursing care.) American Journal of Nursing, 79 (1), Jan 1979, 107-109.

8 **Callaghan, K.A.** Psychological care of the child on long term IV nutrition. Australasian Nurses Journal, 4 (10), Apr 1976, 45-47.

9 **Candy, D.C.A.** Parenteral nutrition in paediatric practice: a review. Journal of Human Nutrition, 34 (4), Aug 1980, 287-296.

10 **Clark, H.** A review of total parenteral nutrition. American Association of Nurse Anesthetists Journal, 47 (3), Jun 1979, 313-322.

11 **Colley, R. and Wilson, J.** Meeting patients' nutritional needs with hyperalimentation. Nursing (U.S.), 9.
How to begin hyperalimentation therapy. 9 (5), May 1979, 76-87.
Managing the patient on hyperalimentation. (6), Jun 1979, 57-61.

12 **Colley, R. and others** Meeting patients' nutritional needs with hyperalimentation. Providing hyperalimentation for infants and children. Nursing (U.S.), 9 (7), Jul 1979, 50-52.

13 **Desomery, C.H. and Hansen, B.W.** Regulation of appetite during total parenteral nutrition. Nursing Research, 27 (1), Jan/Feb 1978, 19-24.

14 **Duffy, T.J. and Fischer, H.B.J.** Parenteral nutrition in adults. (The need, principles and patient management.) Nursing Times, 76, 29 May 1980, 968-971.

15 **Ellis, B.W. and others** A rational approach to parenteral nutrition. British Medical Journal, 1, 5 Jun 1976, 1388-1391.

16 **Englert, D.M. and Dudrick, S.J.** Principles of intravenous hyperalimentation. AORN Journal, 25 (7), Jun 1977, 1253-1267.

17 **Goy, J.A.E.** Parenteral nutrition 1. Theoretical aspects. Nursing Times, 72, 29 Jul 1976, 1150-1152.

18 **Grant, J.P.** Handbook of total parenteral nutrition. Philadelphia: Saunders, 1980.

19 **Griggs, B.A. and Hoppe, M.C.** Nasogastric tube feeding. American Journal of Nursing, 79 (3), Mar 1979, 481-485.

20 **Hales, D.R.** Parenteral nutrition: first decade, trends. Hospitals, 53 (23), 1 Dec 1979, 100-102.

21 **Hanson, R.L.** New approach to measuring adult nasogastric tubes for insertion. (To aid location of end of tube in fundus of stomach.) American Journal of Nursing, 80 (7), Jul 1980, 1334-1335.

22 **Heatley, R.** Intravenous feeding. Nursing Mirror, 144, 6 Jan 1977, 46-48.

23 **Iveson-Iveson, J.** Intravenous therapy: a two day symposium 'Microbiological hazards of infusion therapy' held recently by Travenol Laboratories Ltd. Nursing Mirror, 142, 3 Jun 1976, 65-66.

24 **Ivey, M.F.** The status of parenteral nutrition. Nursing Clinics of North America, 14 (2), Jun 1979, 285-304.

25 **Johnston, I.D.A. editor** Advances in parenteral nutrition: proceedings of an international symposium held in Bermuda, 16-19 May, 1977. Lancaster: MTP, 1978.

26 **Johnston, I.D.A.** Parenteral nutrition in the cancer patient. Journal of Human Nutrition, 33 (3), Jun 1979, 189-196.

27 **Keighley, B.D. and MacGregor, A.R.** Total parenteral nutrition at home: the implications for a rural practice. Journal of the Royal College of General Practitioners, 30, Jun 1980, 354-357.

28 **Kubo, W. and others** Fluid and electrolyte problems of tube-fed patients. American Journal of Nursing, 76 (6), Jun 1976, 912-916.

29 **Ladefoged, K. and Jarnum, S.** Long-term parenteral nutrition. (At home.) British Medical Journal, 2, 22 Jul 1978, 262-266.

30 **Manzi, C.C. and Masoorli, S.** Troubles with I.V.s? Try these tips and techniques... Nursing, 8 (10), Oct 1978, 78-82, 84.

31 **Milewski, P.J. and others** Parenteral nutrition at home in management of intestinal failure. (Study of five patients.) British Medical Journal, 280, 7 Jun 1980, 1356-1357.

32 **Miller, V.** Intravenous alimentation in paediatric practice. Nursing Times, 73, 1 Dec 1977, 1874-1877.

33 **Nielsen, T.** A study of the nursing problems that are experienced by patients receiving intravenous feeding. MSc thesis, University of Manchester, Department of Nursing, 1978.

34 **Powell-Tuck, J. and others** Team approach to long-term intravenous feeding in patients with gastrointestinal disorders. (At St. Mark's Hospital, consisting of clinician, specialist nurse and pharmacist.) Lancet, 2, 14 Oct 1978, 825-828.

35 **Prescott, R.W.G. and Stoddart, J.C.** Unrecognised dehydration during parenteral nutrition. British Medical Journal, 1, 22 Mar 1980, 847.

36 **Priestnal, K.W. and Rutter, L.** Parenteral nutrition via a subclavian line. Nursing Times, 76, 10 Jan 1980, 78-81.

37 **Rubenstein, R.B. and Woods, D.** Hyperalimentation: your role in an innovative procedure. Journal of Practical Nursing, 27 (5), May 1977, 26-29.

38 **Silk, D.B.A.** Enteral nutrition. Hospital Update, 6 (8), Aug 1980, 761-763, 765-766, 768, 772-774, 776.

39 **Skoutakis, V.A.** Team approach to total parenteral nutrition. American Journal of Hospital Pharmacy, 32, Jul 1975, 693-697. (Reprint file.)

40 **Thomas, P.M. and Cosh, D.G.** Parenteral nutrition with special reference to the paediatric age group. Australasian Nurses Journal, 4 (10), Apr 1976, 28-32, 34-36.

41 **Todd, V.E.** The team approach to total parenteral nutrition. (Report of symposium, with special reference to infection control procedures.) Nursing Times, 74, 31 Aug 1978, Contact, 4.

42 **Varcoe, I.M.** Nursing care of children undergoing parenteral nutrition. Australasian Nurses Journal, 4 (10), Apr 1976, 39-41.

43 **Vernall, S.W.** Parenteral nutrition. (History, uses and nurse's role.) New Zealand Nursing Journal, 72 (11), Nov 1979, 10-13.

e MALNUTRITION AND DEVELOPING COUNTRIES

1 **Behar, M.** Nutrition and the future of mankind. WHO Chronicle, 30 (4), Apr 1976, 140-143.

2 **Gopalan, E.** The fight against malnutrition in the world. (Based on conclusions and recommendations of the Thirtieth World Health Assembly discussions.) WHO Chronicle, 31 (7), Jul 1977, 276-278.

3 **Iveson-Iveson, J.** The spectre at our dining table. (Malnutrition in developing countries.) Nursing Mirror, 151, 18 Sep 1980, 21-23.

4 **Laugesen, M.** Child's bangle for the diagnosis of undernutrition. Nursing Journal of India, 66 (8), Aug 1975, 176-177.

5 **Morley, D. and Harman, P.** The Third World: what the child eats and how this has changed our approach to malnutrition. Nursing Times, 75, 1 Nov 1979, 1881-1883.

6 **Peel, S.** Famine relief. Discusses a new Oxfam booklet on selective feeding procedures. Nursing Mirror, 144, 14 Apr 1977, 39-40.

7 **Roberts, A.M.** Obesity in malnourished children. (In an orphanage in Colombia, South America.) Nursing Times, 74, 2 Feb 1978, 194-197.

8 **World Health** Issue on malnutrition and ways of combating it. World Health, Aug/Sep 1979, 2-35.

9 **World Health** Issue on nutrition in developing countries. World Health, May 1977, 3-29.

10 World Health Organisation The management of nutritional emergencies in large populations. Geneva: WHO, 1978.

f SPECIAL DIETS AND DEFICIENCY DISEASES

1 Bennett, S. Vitamin 'D' deficiency, rickets and osteomalacia. Health Visitor, 50 (6), Jun 1977, 180-182.

2 British Medical Journal Exotic diets and the infant. (Cult diets and those governed by religious beliefs.) British Medical Journal, 1, 1 Apr 1978, 804-805.

3 Community Outlook Asian diet fact sheet + Food talk. An English/Asian vocabulary compiled by the Commission for Racial Equality to help professionals to discuss food values with their Asian clients. Nursing Times, 73, 10 Nov 1977, Community Outlook, 108-110.

4 Cranston, D. and Williams, G.L. Moat versus rickets. (Study at Moat Girls' School, Leicester, to investigate the part which could be played by the school medical service in alleviating the incidence of rickets.) New Society, 38, 9 Dec 1976, 511-512.

5 Dawar, A. Food for thought in work with immigrants. (Diet of ethnic minority groups with reference to HV's role.) Nursing Mirror, 149, 18 Oct 1979, 27-30.

6 Department of Health and Social Security Topics of our time. 1: vitamin D deficiency and osteomalacia. HMSO, 1976.

7 Fawns, H.T. B-group vitamins and pellagra. Nursing Times, 72, 1 Apr 1976, 496-498.

8 Fawns, H.T. Vitamin D and rickets. Nursing Times, 74, 5 Oct 1978, 1648-1651.

9 Felstein, I. Community care in deficiency diseases. Midwife, Health Visitor and Community Nurse, 12 (12), Dec 1976, 395-396.

10 Ford, J.A. High risk for Asian immigrants in Britain. (Rickets and osteomalacia.) Nursing Mirror, 149, 1 Nov 1979, 36-37.

11 Garrett, G.E.R. The coeliac child. (Investigation and treatment, with outline of gluten-free diet.) Nursing Times, 73, 3 Nov 1977, 1708-1710.

12 Health and Social Service Journal When it's all a matter of eating habits. Diets for the sick minorities. Health and Social Service Journal, 89, 13 Apr 1979, 404-405.

13 Henry, C.L. Patients' view of a gluten-free diet. (Survey of 62 patients.) Journal of Human Nutrition, 34 (1), Feb 1980, 50-51.

14 Hunt, S. Traditional Asian food customs. (Food and diet for Asians. British Diabetic Association Study day.) Journal of Human Nutrition, 31 (4), Aug 1977, 245-258.

15 Hunt, S.P. and others Vitamin D status in different subgroups of British Asians. (A study of 32 Ugandan families in Greater London.) British Medical Journal, 2, 4 Dec 1976, 1351-1354.

16 Leighton, K. Coeliac disease and the Coeliac Society. Health Visitor, 53 (2), Feb 1980, 50, 54.

17 McCreery, M. Diet: first line defence against coeliac disease. RN Magazine, 39 (2), Feb 1976, 50-52, 56, 58.

18 McKay, R. What kind of welcome? (Rickets among Asians.) Health and Social Service Journal, 88, 1 Dec 1978, 1364-1366.

19 Moncrieff, M. Rickets. Nursing Times, 73, 10 Feb 1977, 199-201.

20 Pearson, D. and others Dietary survey of immigrant schoolgirls in Leicester. (With special reference to vitamin D intake.) Journal of Human Nutrition, 31 (5), Oct 1977, 362-384.

21 Polanska, N. and Wills, M.R. Factors contributing to osteomalacia in the elderly and in the Asian communities in the United Kingdom. Journal of Human Nutrition, 30 (6), Dec 1976, 371-376.

22 Potterton, D. Growing up a vegetarian. (Value of a vegetarian diet.) Nursing Times, 74, 30 Mar 1978, Supplement, viii, x-xi.

23 Ross, T. Animal, vegetable, mineral. (Value of vegetarian diet on nutritional and ecological grounds.) Nursing Mirror, 151, 10 Jul 1980, 22-24.

24 Sanders, T.A.B. How adequate are vegan diets for children? Health Visitor, 53 (8), Aug 1980, 319, 322.

25 Singleton, N. and Tucker, S.M. Vitamin D status of Asian infants. (Survey in Southall.) British Medical Journal, 1, 11 Mar 1978, 607-610.

26 Van Den Berghs and Jurgens Limited Asians in Britain: a study of their dietary patterns in relation to their cultural and religious backgrounds. Burgess Hill: The Company, 1976.

62 REHABILITATION

a GENERAL

1 Alaszewski, A. and Meltzer, H. The relationship between qualified and unqualified workers in health care: the case of the remedial therapy professions. Sociology of Health and Illness, 1 (3), Dec 1979, 284-305.

2 Blair, P. Rehabilitation the real way. (Scheme at Tyrone and Fermanagh Hospital to involve employers in rehabilitation of patients.) Health and Social Service Journal, 89, 1 Jun 1979, 672.

3 Brewerton, D.A. and Nichols, P.I.H. Return to work. (Problems due to gap between medical and employment services.) British Medical Journal, 2, 15 Oct 1977, 1006-1007.

4 British Medical Journal Accident and emergency services. Rehabilitation. By a special correspondent. British Medical Journal, 2, 17 Nov 1979, 1267-1269.

5 Campling, J. Society at work. Getting back to work. (Employment rehabilitation centres.) New Society, 36, 1 Apr 1976, 17-18.

6 Campling, J. Thirty years of words but little or no action. (Rehabilitation services.) Health and Social Service Journal, 90, 4 Apr 1980, 457-458.

7 Clarke, A.K. Let's be realistic about rehabilitation. (Suggestions for improvement in services.) Journal of Community Nursing, 1 (4), Oct 1977, 24-25.

8 Council for Professions Supplementary to Medicine. Working Party on higher and further education PSM education and training: the next decade. The Council, 1979. (Chairman: M.J. Davies.)

9 Darnbrough, A. Miracles for the many. (Report on recent World Congress of Rehabilitation International.) Nursing Mirror, 151, 14 Aug 1980, 28-29.

10 Donald, B. Professions auxiliary, supplementary or complementary to medicine. (Development of the eight paramedical professions.) Health Trends, 10 (1), Feb 1978, 5-9.

11 Glanville, H.J. New lamps for old. (Developments in education and research for the remedial professions at Southampton University.) Physiotherapy, 63 (1), Jan 1977, 9-12.

12 Glanville, H.J. What is rehabilitation? An inaugural lecture (at the University of Southampton). Rehabilitation, 100, Jan-Mar 1977, 13-25.

13 Hume, C.A. Long term patients—1. Remember how the world has changed. (Problems on discharge from hospital encountered by the rehabilitation team at the Royal Edinburgh Hospital.) British Journal of Occupational Therapy, 39 (8), Aug 1976, 195-196.

14 Johnson, H. and others A comparative study of the jobs of occupational therapists, physiotherapists and remedial gymnasts. Polytechnic of Central London, 1976.

15 Joint Working Party of the Remedial and Nursing Professions Report. The Working Party, 1977. (Chairmen: E.L. McMillan, R.B. Mayoh.)

16 King's Fund Centre and Polytechnic of Central London Training for the remedial professions: report of a working party. KEHF, 1976. (King's Fund Project Paper, no.13.) (Chairman: A.F. Gray.)

17 Lane, K. Interface. Resettlement officer. (Work of a job resettlement service at Northwick Park Hospital.) Nursing Times, 72, 24 Jun 1976, 969-970.

18 Ludkin, S. Employment rehabilitation. 2. Report of a study carried out at the Queen Elizabeth Hospital, Gateshead in 1977. (To assess effect of publicising the availability of rehabilitation and resettlement services including function of DRO.) Health Trends, 1 (11), Feb 1979, 23-26.

19 Mattingly, S. editor Rehabilitation today. Update Publications, 1977.

20 Meade, T.W. Problems for the research worker in rehabilitation studies. Rheumatology and Rehabilitation, 16 (4), Nov 1977, 254-256.

21 Medlock, E.J. Employment rehabilitation. 10. The hospital resettlement officer. Health Trends, 8 (2), May 1976, 22.

22 Moyes, J.E. Rehabilitation—an experiment in communication between hospital and primary care teams from the Department of Rehabilitation, South Tees Health District, Middlesbrough, Cleveland. (Display, lecture and discussion period organised by rehabilitation department in GP's premises.) British Journal of Occupational Therapy, 43 (9), Sep 1980, 301.

23 Simpson, J. Rehabilitation and primary care. (Scheme of daily clinics for admission to rehabilitation programme to which GP's referred patients.) Health Bulletin, 35 (4), Jul 1977, 166-171.

24 Singer, N. Education and training in the remedial professions. Physiotherapy, 62 (2), Feb 1976, 62-65.

25 Smith, D. A surfeit of opinion and a dearth of fact. (Comment on recent working party report on the training of the professions supplementary to medicine.) Health and Social Service Journal, 90, 25 Jan 1980, 125-126.

26 Stocking, B. 'The next decade.' A critique of the CPSM report. (Council for the Professions Supplementary to Medicine report on education and training.) Health Services Manpower Review, 6 (2), May 1980, 11-14.

27 Weightman, G. The road back to town. (Successful rehabilitation in the community for patients at Herrison Hospital, Dorset.) New Society, 39, 3 Mar 1977, 440-441.

28 Winship, H. Rehabilitation. (Role of Employment Rehabilitation Centres.) Nursing Mirror, 145, 27 Oct 1977, 20-21.

29 Woodcock, D. Bridging the back-to-work gap in Newcastle-upon-Tyne and in Wakefield. (Work of hospital resettlement officer in Wakefield.) Nursing Times, 74, 17 Aug 1978, 1361.

30 Young, H. D.O.C.T.A.: a project. (Department of Combined Therapeutic Activities at Botleys Park Hospital.) British Journal of Occupational Therapy, 42 (1), Jan 1979, 19-20.

b NURSING

1 Arndt, K. and others Interdisciplinary rehabilitation modules. (Multidisciplinary team care in rehabilitation unit.) Supervisor Nurse, 9 (2), Feb 1978, 18-19.

2 Australian Nurses Journal 1. Unit management committee. 2. Nursing—the positive approach. (Two articles on the team concept in a rehabilitation unit.) Australian Nurses Journal, 7 (7), Feb 1978, 38-40.

3 Boroch, R.M. Elements of rehabilitation in nursing: an introduction. St. Louis: Mosby, 1976.

4 Boucher, R.J. and Dittmar, S. Rehabilitation nursing and related readings: bibliography. Part 1. AORN Journal, 4 (4), Jul/Aug 1979, 22.

5 Burgher, D. and Hanson, R.L. Patient classification for nurse staffing in rehabilitation. AORN Journal, 5 (3), May/Jun 1980, 16-20.

6 Capell, P.T. and Case, D.B. Ambulatory care manual for nurse practitioners. Philadelphia: Lippincott, 1976.

7 Chamberlain, M.A. The value of health visitors in rehabilitation in the community. Rheumatology and Rehabilitation, 16 (4), Nov 1977, 250-253.

8 Daubert, E.A. Patient classification system

and outcome criteria. (Assessment of rehabilitation potential by community nurses.) Nursing Outlook, 27 (7), Jul 1979, 450.

9 Deutsch, B.L. Ambulatory care nursing procedure and employee health service manual. Flushing: Medical Examination Publishing Co., 1977.

10 Edmonds-Hill, P.A. Only a team can win the struggle for rehabilitation. (Report of study visit to look at the role of nurses in rehabilitation hospitals.) Australian Nurses Journal, 6 (11), May 1977, 31-33, 37.

11 Engstrand, J.L. Primary nursing. (Scheme in a rehabilitation centre to implement primary nursing.) AORN Journal, 2 (5), Sep/Oct 1977, 3-4, 7-8.

12 Erickson, R. and others Employing reality orientation in a short term setting. (For patients with CVAs, post head injury syndromes and various neurological conditions.) AORN Journal, 3 (6), Nov/Dec 1978, 18-21.

13 Fenwick, A.M. An interdisciplinary tool for assessing patients' readiness for discharge in the rehabilitation setting. Journal of Advanced Nursing, 4 (1), Jan 1979, 9-21.

14 Firth, D. and others The assessment of the value of health visitors in the rehabilitation team (to bridge the gap between hospital and community at Ida Hospital, Leeds.) Rheumatology and Rehabilitation, 15 (3), Aug 1976, 188-190.

15 Firth, D. and others Health visitors in a rehabilitation unit. (Attachment to unit in Leeds.) Nursing Times, 74, 9 Feb 1978, 249-250.

16 McCay, J. Patient rehabilitation—the nurse's role. Nursing, 5, Aug 1979, 217-219.

17 Murray, P. editor Current perspectives in rehabilitation nursing. 1. St. Louis: Mosby, 1979. (Mosby's current practice and perspectives in nursing series.)

18 Nursing Clinics of North America Symposium on care of the ambulatory patient. Nursing Clinics of North America, 12 (4), Dec 1977, 539-608.

19 O'Neal, E.A. A framework for ambulatory care evaluation. Journal of Nursing Administration, 8 (7), Jul 1978, 15-20.

20 Partridge, C. and Wright, B. Helping patients to help themselves. (Rehabilitation for district nurses.) Nursing Mirror, 146.
2. Patients with bronchitis and rheumatoid arthritis. 15 Jun 1978, 40.
3. Patients with Parkinsonism and multiple sclerosis. 22 Jun 1978, 38.

21 Payne, M.E. The nurse as patient advocate in the rehab setting. AORN Journal, 4 (5), Sep/Oct 1979, 9-11.

22 Riffle, K.L. editor Rehabilitative nursing case studies: a compilation of 30 case histories. New York: Medical Examination Pub.Co., 1979.

23 Schorr, T.M. Where nurses have autonomy and patients have authority. (Editorial on the Loeb Center for Nursing and Rehabilitation.) American Journal of Nursing, 76 (2), Feb 1976, 219.

24 Siegele, D.S. A study of baccalaureate students in a rehabilitation setting. (Research

study of students' impressions and grasp of rehabilitation concepts.) AORN Journal, 3 (1), Jan/Feb 1978, 15-17, 19.

25 Simmon, M.J. The rehabilitation liaison nurse. (To coordinate hospital and home care.) ONA Journal, 4 (1), Jan 1977, 7-8.

26 Starck, P.L. A model for emphasizing rehabilitation in the nursing process. (Use of nursing process with patients with long-term illnesses.) AORN Journal, 3 (2), Mar/Apr 1978, 10-15.

27 Stryker, R.P. Rehabilitative aspects of acute and chronic nursing care. 2nd ed. Philadelphia: Saunders, 1977.

c OCCUPATIONAL THERAPY

1 Adamson, G. Horticulture as therapy. Social Service Quarterly, 52 (3), Spring 1979, 95-97.

2 Aina, B. The occupational therapist in the community. British Journal of Occupational Therapy, 43 (9), Sep 1980, 295-297.

3 Aitken, C. Rehabilitation. Facts and fantasies about occupational therapy. British Journal of Occupational Therapy, 39 (7), Jul 1976, 172-174.

4 Andrews, K. Research and the therapist. British Journal of Occupational Therapy, 42 (2), Feb 1979, 44-45.

5 Atkinson, L. Unique to occupational therapy. (Lecture reviewing history of profession and current role.) British Journal of Occupational Therapy, 43 (7), Jul 1980, 221-224.

6 Benjamin, J. The Northwick Park A.D.L. index. (Method of measuring 'quality of life'— necessary activities during daily living.) British Journal of Occupational Therapy, 39 (12), Dec 1976, 301-306.

7 Cornell, A. and others Useful assessment form. (Of ADL.) British Journal of Occupational Therapy, 40 (8), Aug 1977, 190-191.

8 Dick, D. The profession of occupational therapy. Health Services Manpower Review, 5 (4), Nov 1979, 17-20.

9 Evans, C. Development of A.D.L. indices. (Activities of daily living.) British Journal of Occupational Therapy, 39 (12), Dec 1976, 307-308.

10 Green, M. Development or oblivion? (Occupational therapy as a profession.) British Journal of Occupational Therapy, 40 (12), Dec 1977, 300-301.

11 Greenhalgh, L.M. Rehabilitation and occupational therapy. Nursing, 5, Aug 1979, 243-247.

12 Grove, E. Occupational therapy in the United Kingdom. (Paper presented at 1st European Congress at Edinburgh.) British Journal of Occupational Therapy, 40 (7), Jul 1977, 157-159.

13 Jones, M.S. An approach to occupational therapy; revised by Peggy Jay. 3rd ed. Butterworth, 1977.

14 Macdonald, E.M. editor Occupational therapy in rehabilitation: a handbook for occupational therapists, students and others interested in this aspect of reablement. 4th ed. Baillière Tindall, 1976.

15 **Malcolm, M.L.** Occupational therapy techniques. British Journal of Occupational Therapy, 40 (10), Oct 1977, 236-238.

16 **Nichols, P.J.R.** Are ADL indices of any value? (Activities of daily living.) British Journal of Occupational Therapy, 39 (6), Jun 1976, 160-163.

17 **Orriss, H.D.** Rehabilitation and the occupational therapist. (With reference to the 1976 report of the Hospital Advisory Service.) Journal of Occupational Therapy, 41 (2), Feb 1978, 73-74.

18 **Ravetz, C.** Occupational therapy: an organisational perspective: (Sociological analysis.) British Journal of Occupational Therapy, 41 (11), Nov 1978, 369-370.

19 **Savage, J.H.** Household assessment cabinet. (For use in evaluation of patients' ability to cope with activities of daily living.) Nursing Mirror, 144, 23 Jun 1977, 31-32.

20 **Shopland, A.J. and others** Refer to occupational therapy. 2nd ed. Churchill Livingstone, 1979.

21 **Sym, D.M.** A review of occupational therapy — changing attitudes in a developing profession. British Journal of Occupational Therapy, 43 (5), May 1980, 149-151.

22 WORLD Federation of Occupational Therapists Seventh International Congress March 12-17, 1978, Jerusalem, Israel. Theme — Models for occupational therapy in a changing world. British Journal of Occupational Therapy, 40 (7), Jul 1977, 165-166.

23 **Zinovieff, A.** Occupational therapy in the treatment of physical disability: a modern approach. (Techniques of functional assessment and remedial activities.) Rehabilitation, 99, Oct-Dec, 1976, 10-15.

d PHYSIOTHERAPY

1 **Bryant, B.** The roots of a profession. (History, present and future of physiotherapy.) Health and Social Service Journal, 90, 6 Jun 1980, 746-748.

2 **Bryant, R.J.S.** The physiotherapy profession. Health Services Manpower Review, 5 (2), May 1979, 13-15.

3 **Craven, J.** Getting them back on their feet. (Work of senior physiotherapist.) Nursing Mirror, 148, 7 Jun 1979, 26-27.

4 **Downie, P.A.** Interface. The physiotherapist. (Co-operation between nurses and physiotherapists.) Nursing Times, 72, 27 May 1976, 809-811.

5 **Farrow, G.** A unique school. (The North London School of Physiotherapy for the Visually Handicapped.) Nursing Times, 74, 15 Jun 1978, 991-993.

6 **Frazer, F.W.** Community physio: a new colleague for the district nurse. (Project in South Birmingham Health District to evaluate the benefit to the elderly of a domiciliary physiotherapy service.) Nursing Mirror, 147, 19 Oct 1978, 58-60.

7 **Glossop, E.S. and Smith, D.S.** A new service for the disabled in Harrow. (Domiciliary physiotherapy service based at Northwick Park Hospital.) Rheumatology and Rehabilitation, 16 (4), Nov 1977, 253.

8 **Grant, D.** The physiotherapist as patient counsellor. Physiotherapy, 65 (7), Jul 1979, 218-220.

9 **Haycock, E.** The physiotherapist and the paraplegic patient. Queen's Nursing Journal, 19 (5), Aug 1976, 128-129.

10 **Hayne, C.R.** Physiotherapy for occupational health nurses. Nursing Mirror, 147. 1. Introduction. 10 Aug 1978, Supplement, i-iv. 2/3. Therapeutic heat and cold. 17 Aug 1978, Supplement, i-iv; 24 Aug 1978, Supplement, i-iv. 4. Massage. 7 Sep 1978, Supplement, i-iv. 5. The use of exercise. 14 Sep 1978, Supplement, i-iv. 6. Employee fitness. 28 Sep 1978, Supplement, i-iv.

11 **Hayne, C.R.** Safe...sure? (Applications of the Health and Safety at Work Act to physiotherapy.) Physiotherapy, 64 (1), Jan 1978, 10-13.

12 **Hazell, J.** Physiotherapy with alcoholics and drug-dependent patients. Nursing Mirror, 142, 15 Jan 1976, 62-63.

13 **Holgate, B.** Report on a pilot scheme for a domiciliary physiotherapy service. (In Manchester for elderly people.) Chest, Heart and Stroke Journal, 2 (4), Winter 1977/1978, 38-42.

14 **Jarvis, R.E.** Physiotherapy for children and young adults with arthritis. Physiotherapy, 64 (5), May 1978, 143-145.

15 **Lee, J.M. editor** Aids to physiotherapy. Churchill Livingstone, 1978.

16 **Mercer, J.** Physiotherapy as a profession. (Based on author's PhD thesis.) Physiotherapy, 66 (6), Jun 1980, 180-184.

17 **Partridge, C.J. and Warren, M.D.** Physiotherapy in the community: a descriptive study of fourteen schemes. Canterbury: Health Services Research Unit, 1977.

18 **Pennefather, M.E. and Tanner, E.R.** Physiotherapy in a group practice. (Scheme in South London.) Practitioner, 221, Dec 1978, 824-826.

19 **Physiotherapy** Congress lectures. Four articles on physiotherapy in the community in Canterbury, West Berkshire, South Lothian and Cheltenham. Physiotherapy, 63 (11), Nov 1977, 352-359.

20 **Physiotherapy** Physiotherapy in the community (including paediatric physiotherapy.) Three articles. Physiotherapy, 66 (1), Jan 1980, 2-14.

21 **Pratt, J.W.** A psychological view of the physiotherapist's role. Physiotherapy, 64 (8), Aug 1978, 241-242.

22 **Ricketts, E.O.S. and Delpak, K.** The role of the physiotherapist in an addiction unit. Physiotherapy, 66 (12), Dec 1980, 409-410.

23 **Sloan, A.W.** The physiological basis of physiotherapy and other professions related to medicine. Baillière Tindall, 1979.

24 **Struthers, T.** The role of the male occupational therapist. British Journal of Occupational Therapy, 43 (6), Jun 1980, 189-190.

25 **Sutcliffe, B.J.** Physiotherapy in the community. Midwife, Health Visitor and Community Nurse, 16 (4), Apr 1980, 166, 168, 170.

26 **Ward, W.M.** Physiotherapists — career patterns and attitudes. (Survey.) Health Trends, 1 (11), Feb 1979, 14-17.

27 **Ward, A.W.M. and others** Physiotherapists' careers: survey of former students at St. Thomas' Hospital, London and Sheffield. Physiotherapy, 63 (10), Oct 1977, 314-315.

28 **Ward, A.W.M. and others** Physiotherapists who trained at Sheffield and St. Thomas' 1952-1970. (Survey of attitudes towards the profession and current activity.) Health and Social Service Journal, 87, 18 Nov 1977, F.17-F.24.

29 **Warren, M.D.** The right treatment in the right place: the need for comprehensive and integrated community care. (With reference to developing a district-wide physiotherapy service.) Physiotherapy, 63 (11), Nov 1977, 350-351.

30 **Waterson, M.** Hot and cold therapy. Nursing, 8 (10), Oct 1978, 46-49.

e SPEECH THERAPY

1 **Bull, T.R. and Cook, J.L.** Speech therapy and ENT surgery. Blackwell, 1976.

2 **Calnan, M. and Richardson, K.** Speech problems among children in a national survey: associations with hearing, handedness and therapy. Community Health, 8 (2), Oct 1976, 101-105.

3 **Evesham, M.** Stuttering. (Recent developments in treatment.) Midwife, Health Visitor and Community Nurse, 16 (1), Jan 1980, 23-24.

4 **Fox, M.J.** Patients with receptive aphasia: they really don't understand. American Journal of Nursing, 76 (10), Oct 1976, 1596-1598.

5 **Kirby, J.** A slipping tongue. (Treatment programme at the City Literary Institute and the work of the Association of Stammerers.) New Society, 40, 30 Jun 1977, 658.

6 **Gough, D.** Aphasia and the nurse. Nursing Mirror, 147, 3 Aug 1978, 28-29; 10 Aug 1978, 29-30.

7 **Hollingworth, C.** Domiciliary speech therapy. Chest, Heart and Stroke Journal, 1 (1), Spring 1976, 22-24.

f ART, MUSIC AND DRAMA THERAPY

1 **Affleck, I.S.** Poetry as medium in a unit for the treatment of alcoholism. (At the Royal Edinburgh Hospital.) British Journal of Occupational Therapy, 40 (11), Nov 1977, 277.

2 **Allen, P.** A musical box of therapy. (Music therapy.) Nursing Mirror, 149, 13 Sep 1979, 31-32.

3 **Alvin, J.** Music therapy for the autistic child. Oxford University Press, 1978.

4 Alvin, J. Principles of music therapy. Physiotherapy, 64 (3), Mar 1978, 77-79.

5 Atack, S.M. Art activities for the handicapped. Souvenir Press, 1980. (Human horizons series.)

6 Bull, C. Bringing a little colour to brighten our lives. (Peter Senior's hospital arts project has already had a beneficial impact in staff and patient areas of St. Mary's Hospital, Manchester and is now expanding its efforts to the Manchester Royal Infirmary.) Health and Social Service Journal, 89, 6 Apr 1979, 370-371.

7 Burwell, D. Psychodrama and the depressed elderly. Canadian Nurse, 73 (4), Apr 1977, 54-55.

8 Byrne, P. Art in therapy. (Review.) Royal Society of Health Journal, 97 (6), Dec 1977, 288-290.

9 Campbell, C.M. Puppetry as an aid in treatment and training. British Journal of Occupational Therapy, 42 (12), Dec 1979, 329-330.

10 Darby, C. Vital links: the art of self-expression. (Work of senior art therapist at St. Lawrence's Hospital, Caterham for the mentally handicapped.) Nursing Mirror, 149, 21 Jun 1979, 20-21.

11 Dollin, L. Art as a treatment medium in the psychiatric hospital. British Journal of Occupational Therapy, 39 (9), Sep 1976, 225-230.

12 Drummond, P. Painting a picture of care. (Manchester Hospitals Art Project which promote a more visually stimulating environment for patients and staff and exploits the therapeutic quality of art.) Health and Social Service Journal, 80, 19/26 Dec 1980, 1618-1619.

13 Dyson, R.A. Psychodrama: developments and applications. Psychiatric Nursing, 16 (1), Jan-Feb 1975, 8-9, 13-14.

14 Eskow, L. Drama and movement in therapy. Physiotherapy, 64 (3), Mar 1978, 70-73.

15 Gerace, L. and Rosenberg, L. The use of art prints in group therapy with aftercare patients. Perspectives in Psychiatric Care, 17 (2), Mar/Apr 1979, 83-86.

16 Goldsmith's College As we see it: approaches to art as therapy. The College, 1977.

17 Gordon, D. Psychotherapy: psychodrama—an emotional outlet. (Programme at Stobhill Hospital, Glasgow.) Nursing Mirror, 148, 15 Mar 1979, 36-38.

18 Granger, B. Sound health with music. (Letter describing value of music, with mention of author's 'Sound Health' advisory service. (Nursing Times, 76, 21 Aug 1980, 1474.)

19 Hardgrove, C. Children respond to therapeutic art. Hospitals, 54 (8), 16 Apr 1980, 67-69.

20 Healey, A.R. Sculpting as a group technique for increasing awareness. (Form of art therapy.) Perspectives in Psychiatric Care, 15 (3), 1977, 118-121.

21 Heath, T. The talking pictures. (Art therapy with adolescents.) Nursing Mirror, 150, 13 Mar 1980, 30-32.

22 Herth, K. The therapeutic use of music. (In general hospitals with stroke and post-operative patients.) Supervisor Nurse, 9 (9), Oct 1978, 22-23.

23 Hinds, P.S. Music: a milieu factor with implications for the nurse-therapist. (Research study of group play therapy with children.) Journal of Psychiatric Nurse, 18 (6), Jun 1980, 28-33.

24 Hyman, R. Choosing art for your hospital: some basic do's and don't's. Hospitals, 53 (6), 16 Mar 1979, 95-98.

25 Jeavons, T. Art therapy: multiple handicap and art structure. (With mentally and physically handicapped children.) Physiotherapy, 64 (3), Mar 1978, 74-76.

26 Jones, H.V.R. Psychodrama with adolescents. Nursing Times, 74, 14 Dec 1978, 2052-2054.

27 Karp, M. Psychodrama. Social Work Today, 7 (7), 24 Jun 1976, 201.

28 Kartman, L.L. The use of music as a program tool with regressed geriatric patients. Journal of Gerontological Nursing, 3 (4), Jul/Aug 1977, 38-42.

29 King, B. Getting in shape. (Work of Shape, a group offering music, art, dance and poetry therapy to groups and institutions.) Nursing Times, 76, 3 Apr 1980, 607-609.

30 Lindsay, S. Music in hospitals. (Work of the Council for Music in Hospitals.) Social Service Quarterly, 49 (3), Jan/Mar 1976, 101-102.

31 Macmillan, M. Madness—or just a case of sadness? (Psychodrama with psychiatric patients.) Nursing Times, 76, 24 Jul 1980, 1310-1313.

32 Marcovitch, H. Acting out. (Holwell Centre for Psychodrama in North Devon.) World Medicine, 14 (25), 22 Sep 1979, 53-54, 56.

33 Mason, C. Musical activities with elderly patients. Physiotherapy, 64 (3), Mar 1978, 80-82.

34 Masters, G. Learning to communicate. (Technique of drama therapy with psychiatric patients.) Nursing Times, 74, 2 Mar 1978, 350-352.

35 Minas, S.C. Dance as a therapy. British Journal of Occupational Therapy, 41 (3), Mar 1978, 101-103.

36 Misner, S.J. Using art therapy techniques in staff and patient education. (To encourage expression of feelings regarding matters such as death.) Nursing Outlook, 27 (8), Aug 1979, 536-539.

37 Mitchell, R. Establishing a therapy group. (Drama therapy with psychiatric patients at Hardmanflat Hospital, East Lothian.) Nursing Times, 74, 2 Mar 1978, 352-354.

38 Monroe, C.J. and Herron, S. Projective art used as an integral part of an intensive group therapy experience. (At psychiatric day hospital, Belfast.) British Journal of Occupational Therapy, 43 (1), Jan 1980, 21-24.

39 Nursing Times Making art work. (Conference on the role of art, dance and music therapy in hospital.) Nursing Times, 73, 28 Jul 1977, 1142-1143.

40 Nursing Times Muzak while you work? (Two letters on use of music in wards.) Nursing Times, 76, 24 Jul 1980, 1305.

41 Philpott, A.R. compiler Puppets and therapy. Educational Puppetry Association, 1976.

42 Priestley, M. Another creative therapy. (Music.) British Journal of Occupational Therapy, 40 (9), Sep 1977, 213-214.

43 Priestley, M. Music, Freud and the port of entry. (The use of music in self-expression.) Nursing Times, 72, 9 Dec 1976, 1940-1941.

44 Priestley, M. Music therapy. New Psychiatry, 3 (5), 4 Mar 1976, 12-13.

45 Ricketts, L. Music and handicapped children. Journal of the Royal College of General Practitioners, 26, Aug 1976, 585-587.

46 Shaw, H. 'Anti-stress' art. (Conference on the role of the artist in the hospital environment.) Nursing Times, 72, 24 Jun 1976, 960-961.

47 Thomas, K. Art for the elderly. (Scheme at the Western Hospital in South Hammersmith Health District.) British Journal of Occupational Therapy, 41 (5), May 1978, 169.

48 Turner, I. and Gale, M. Drama and movement therapy in a continuing care ward. (Scheme at Herne Hospital, Kent.) Nursing Times, 75, 22 Mar 1979, 478-480.

SURGERY, ACCIDENTS AND EMERGENCIES

63 SURGERY

a GENERAL

1 Aries, J.M. Haemostasis in surgery. (History and current methods.) NATNews, 15 (9), Sep 1978, 22-23, 25, 28, 30, 32.

2 Barlett, D. Operating theatre lighting. NATNews, 15 (11), Nov 1978, 24, 26, 28, 30.

3 Brand, J.C. and Tolins, S.H. The nursing student's guide to surgery. Boston: Little, Brown and Co., 1979.

4 Butler, C. Surgery—before and after penicillin. British Medical Journal, 2, 25 Aug 1979, 482-483.

5 Clemons, B. Lister's day in America. (Development of antiseptic surgery.) AORN Journal, 24 (1), Jul 1976, 43-51.

6 Dixon, E. Design for 2001. (Likely changes of approach to surgery in the 21st century.) Nursing Mirror, 148, 15 Mar 1979, Supplement xii, xv.

7 Dixon, E.P. An introduction to the operating theatre. Edinburgh: Churchill Livingstone, 1976.

8 Ellis, H. and Wastell, C. General surgery for nurses. Blackwell, 1976. 2nd ed. 1980.

9 Grubb, R.D. and others Operating room guidelines: an illustrated manual. St. Louis: Mosby, 1979.

10 Henderson, M.A. Essential surgery for nurses. Edinburgh: Churchill Livingstone, 1980.

11 Higson, R. Types of hernia. Nursing Mirror, 146, 23 Feb 1978, 14-18.

12 Lamont, S. New Zealand. (Report on visit to theatres in New Zealand to study thermal comfort and compare basic standards.) NATNews, 14 (9), Dec 1977, 14-15.

13 MacClelland, D.C. Music in the operating room. AORN Journal, 29 (2), Feb 1979, 252-260.

14 McDermott, A. Changed for the better? (Change in operating theatres during the last twenty years.) Nursing Times, 72, 16 Dec 1976, 1981.

15 McDowall, R.A.W. Specialised care. 10. Microvascular surgery. Nursing Mirror, 145, 24 Nov 1977, Nursing care supplement series 6, i-iv.

16 McFarland, J. editor Basic clinical surgery for nurses and medical students. 2nd ed. Butterworth, 1980.

17 Macfarlane, D.A. and Thomas, L.P. editors Textbook of surgery. 4th ed. Churchill Livingstone, 1977.

18 Metheny, N.A. and Snively, W.D. Perioperative fluids and electrolytes. American Journal of Nursing, 78 (5), May 1978, 840-845.

19 Moroney, J. Surgery for nurses. 13th ed. Churchill Livingstone, 1975. 14th ed. 1978.

20 Nash, D.F. The principles and practice of surgery for nurses and allied professions. 6th ed. Arnold, 1976.

21 Nursing Times Safe practice in the operating theatre. (Five articles.) Nursing Times, 74, 2 Nov 1978, Theatre nursing 5-6, 11-12, 15, 17-18, 20.

22 Oliver, J.D. Staff needs considered in OR design. AORN Journal, 23 (2), Feb 1976, 212-217.

23 Pachniuk, L.H. Theatre nursing care study. Bilateral hernia repair. Nursing Times, 72, 4 Nov 1976, 1720-1721.

24 Phillips, J. Big is best? A study into the optimum size of multi-suite operating departments. NATNews, 17 (5), May 1980, 7-8, 10-11, 13-14.

25 Plant, J.A. and Devlin, H.B. Planned early discharge of surgical patients. (System at North Tees General Hospital.) Nursing Times, 74, 2 Mar 1978, Occ. papers, 25-28.

26 Taylor, S. Principles of surgery and surgical nursing. 3rd ed. Hodder and Stoughton, 1977. (Modern nursing series.)

27 Tinckler, L.F. The surgery of groin hernia. Nursing Times, 74, 14 Sep 1978, 1519-1523.

b TRANSPLANTS AND REPLANTATION

1 Bailey, C.C. Bone marrow transplants in the 1980s. World Medicine, 15 (5), 3 May 1980, 54-56.

2 Calne, R. and others Pancreatic transplantation: the start of something new. (Procedure and nursing care studies of two patients at Addenbrooke's Hospital, Cambridge.) Nursing Mirror, 151, 25 Sep 1980, 36-41.

3 Chambers, J. Bone marrow transplantation: a nursing challenge. Nursing Mirror, 144, 17 Mar 1977, 39-41.

4 Death, A. Nursing care study. Reimplantation of fingers. (At Odstock Hospital Plastic Surgery Unit.) Nursing Mirror, 146, 20 Apr 1978, 15-17.

5 Department of Health and Social Security The removal of cadaveric organs for transplantation: a code of practice. HMSO, 1979. (Chairman: Lord Smith of Marlow.)

6 Edwards, J. Bone marrow transplantation: transatlantic comparisons. (Comparison of methods used at the Royal Marsden Hospital and a Seattle cancer centre.) Nursing Mirror, 148, 7 Jun 1979, 31-32.

7 Fairhead, S. The background. (Principles behind bone marrow transplantation.) Nursing Times, 73, 17 Feb 1977, 225-227.

8 Geyer, B. A nursing challenge: replantation of a severed arm. (In two-year old child.) Canadian Nurse, 72 (4), Apr 1976, 19-22.

9 Lander, H. Bone marrow transplantation. Australian Nurses Journal, 8 (7), Feb 1979, 44-48.

10 McDowell, R.A.W. Replantation surgery. Nursing Mirror, 142, 1 Jan 1976, 55-57.

11 Watson, J.G. Aspects of bone marrow grafting in childhood. Nursing Times, 73, 17 Feb 1977, 235-236.

c DAY AND SHORT STAY SURGERY

1 Cliff, K.S. A computer model for a five-day surgical ward. (Based on grouping of operative procedures by length of stay.) Public Health, 93 (1), Jan 1979, 4-10.

2 Cliff, K.S. The use of Hospital Activity Analysis data in assessing operative procedures suitable for five-day care. Health and Social Service Journal, 89, 27 Apr 1979, Centre eight papers A29-A32.

3 Dilnot, G.E. The benefits of day unit surgery. (History of concept, description of unit at Warneford Hospital and survey of other hospitals' practice.) NATNews, 16 (12), Dec 1979, 12, 16-17, 19-20, 25.

4 Garraway, W.M. and others Consumer acceptability of day care after operations for hernia or varicose veins. Journal of Epidemiology and Community Health, 32 (3), Sep 1978, 219-221.

5 Garraway, W.M. and others General practitioners' response to day care surgery. (Survey in Edinburgh.) Practitioner, 221, Jul 1978, 22-23, 25.

6 O'Donovan, T.R. Ambulatory surgery.

Royal Society of Health Journal, 96 (3), Jun 1976, 129-133, 146.

7 Ogg, T.W. Assessment of preoperative cases. (Patients undergoing day surgery in Aberdeen complete a questionnaire.) British Medical Journal, 1, 10 Jan 1976, 82-83.

8 Prescott, R.J. and others Economic aspects of day care after operations for hernia or varicose veins. (Costs of staff including district nurses.) Journal of Epidemiology and Community Health, 32 (3), Sep 1978, 222-225.

9 Ruckley, C.V. and others The community nurse and day surgery. (Survey of nurses taking part in scheme in Edinburgh.) Nursing Times, 76, 7 Feb 1980, 255-256.

10 Scobie, W.G. and Garraway, W.M. Day case surgery for children. (Pilot study in North Lothian district.) Nursing Times, 75, 8 Feb 1979, 252-254.

11 Shaw, L.M. Designing an outpatient surgery program. AORN Journal, 31 (5), Apr 1980, 900, 902, 906, 908, 910, 912, 914, 916.

d ANAESTHESIA

1 Austin, P. The pharmacology of some common anaesthetic drugs. NATNews, 14 (8), Nov 1977, 27-28.

2 Austin, T.R. General anaesthetic techniques. NATNews, 14 (7), Sep 1977, 29-30.

3 Baskett, P.J.F. Use of anaesthesia. The anaesthetist in the accident and emergency service. British Medical Journal, 281, 26 Jul 1980, 287-289.

4 Bellerby, S. Induction of anaesthesia in emergency procedures. NATNews, 16 (8), Aug 1979, 12-13, 16-17, 20.

5 Campbell, D. and Spence, A. Norris and Campbell's anaesthesia, resuscitation and intensive care. 5th ed. Edinburgh: Churchill Livingstone, 1978.

6 Horton, J.M. Use of anaesthesia. Care of the unconscious. British Medical Journal, 281, 5 Jul 1980, 38-40.

7 O'Daniel, L. Anesthetic management of the alcoholic patient. American Association of Nurse Anesthetists Journal, 48 (5), Oct 1980, 445-451.

8 Office of Health Economics Anaesthesia. OHE, 1976. (Studies in current health problems, no.55.)

9 Richards, R.S. Anesthesia for the patient with cardiac disease. American Association of Nurse Anesthetists Journal, 44 (2), Apr 1976, 147-161.

10 Spence, A.A. Uses of anaesthesia. Postoperative care. British Medical Journal, 281, 2 Aug 1980, 367-368.

11 Telfer, A.B.M. Use of anaesthesia. Intensive care. British Medical Journal, 280, 28 Jun 1980, 1593-1595.

12 White, M.J. and Wolf-Wilets, V.C. Memory loss following halothane anesthesia. (Research study with surgical patients.) AORN Journal, 26 (6), Dec 1977, 1053-1064.

13 Yates, E. Pioneer in anaesthesia. (Crawford Long, who was first to use anaesthetic during surgery in 1842.) Nursing Mirror, 147, 24 Aug 1978, 20.

e ANAESTHESIA: NURSE'S ROLE

1 AANA Journal A survey of nurse anaesthetists — 1975. (To establish an accurate profile of AANA members.) American Association of Nurse Anesthetists Journal, 43 (6), Dec 1975, 586-605.

2 AANA Journal A survey of nurse anaesthetists 1976 — a condensed report, by J.H. Goff. American Association of Nurse Anesthetists Journal, 45 (2), Apr 1977, 143-169.

3 AANA Journal A survey of nurse anaesthetists — 1977. A condensed review. American Association of Nurse Anesthetists Journal, 47 (6), Dec 1979, 663-673; 48 (2), Apr 1980, 124-132.

4 Asken, M.J. and Wilders, J.L. Medical psychology curriculum objectives for a school of anesthesia. (To prepare nurse anaesthetists to understand patients' reactions to illness and surgery.) American Association of Nurse Anesthetists Journal, 47 (4), Aug 1979, 425-430.

5 Baida, M.R. Nursing care in use of local anesthesia. AORN Journal, 28 (5), Nov 1978, 855-858.

6 Biebuyck, J.F. Role of the nurse in modern anaesthesia. Address given at symposium 'Science with Humanity' organised by the Nursing Staff, Groote Schuur Hospital, February 1976. S.A. Nursing Journal, 44 (2), Feb 1977, 27-29.

7 Brown, B. and Rowland, S. The role of the nurse in the anaesthetic room. (Research study.) NATNews, 17 (9), Sep 1980, 37-43.

8 Carrington, A.C. The role of the nurse in the anaesthetic room. NATNews, 15 (8), Aug 1978, 12.

9 Davenport, H.T. and Crampton-Smith, A. The nurse in a British department of anaesthetics. NATNews, 12 (5), Jul 1975, 4.

10 Easton, J. Study day for anaesthetic nurses. (Report.) NATNews, 15 (11), Nov 1978, 8-9.

11 Garde, J.F. Identity and involvement. (Role of CRNA (Certified Registered Nurse Anesthetist) as nurse practitioner.) American Association of Nurse Anesthetists Journal, 45 (4), Aug 1977, 375-385.

12 Ginsberg, H. The nurse anaesthetist. S.A. Nursing Journal, 43 (2), Feb 1976, 16-17.

13 Heggarty, J.M. The British anaesthetic nurse — her role, value and future. Nursing Mirror, 145, 6 Oct 1977, 25-27.

14 Holloway, A.M. Is a sister in charge of anaesthetics necessary in the operating theatre? S.A. Nursing Journal, 44 (6), Jun 1977, 10-11.

15 Liddicott, D.G. and Williams, M.J. Anaesthetic nurse, or operating department assistant? (Letter on respective roles and training.) Nursing Mirror, 145, 1 Dec 1977, 11.

16 Lucas, B.G.B. Are nurses of value in anaesthesia? NATNews, 15 (10), Oct 1978, 43, 45.

17 Millington, C. Clinical nurse consultant in anaesthetics. (Symposium paper.) Nursing Mirror, 142, 13 May 1976, 49-50.

18 Millington, C. The clinical nurse consultant specialty anaesthetic nursing. Johnson & Johnson Scholar Award Project 1976. (Study to investigate the need for a consultant in anaesthetics.) NATNews, 13 (9), Dec 1976, 18-22.

19 Nightingale, K.M. Waiting for the anaesthetic. (Role of nurse in anaesthetic room.) Nursing Times, 75, 18 Oct 1979, Theatre nursing, 8, 10.

20 Roddy, P.C. and Hambleton, R. Need, supply and distribution of anesthesiologists and nurse anesthetists in the U.S., 1972 and 1980. Medical Care, 15 (9), Sep 1977, 750-766.

21 Serafin, D. The nurse anesthetist, a changing role: past, present and future. American Association of Nurse Anesthetists Journal, 47 (5), Oct 1979, 533.

22 Smith, B.J. Anesthesia — a nursing process. American Association of Nurse Anesthetists Journal, 44 (4), Aug 1976, 397-400.

23 Smith, B.J. Safeguarding your patient after anesthesia. Nursing, 8 (10), Oct 1978, 53-56.

24 Smith, B.J. Should you become a nurse anesthetist? (Role outlined.) Nursing, 7 (11), Nov 1977, 22-23.

25 Wachstein, J. Anaesthesia and recovery room techniques. 2nd ed. Baillière Tindall, 1976. (Nurses aids series.)

f EQUIPMENT

1 AORN Journal Standards for sponge, needle, and instrument procedures. AORN Journal, 23 (6), May 1976, 971-973.

2 Baxter, B. Disposable drapes. NATNews, 11 (7), Sep 1975, 32.

3 Beck, W.C. and Nora, P.F. ASTM standard for surgical gloves. (American Society for Testing and Materials.) AORN Journal, 25 (5), Apr 1977, 869-872.

4 Crawford, M.L. Surgical instruments in America. AORN Journal, 24 (1), Jul 1976, 150, 152-154, 156.

5 Desmond, S. Some observations on the supply of surgical gauze and associated hospital products. NATNews, 12 (1), Jan 1975, 5-7.

6 Duffin, N. Recycling oxygen masks in the recovery room. Nursing Times, 74, 11 May 1978, 801-802.

7 Fletcher, V.S. A history of the operation gown and mask — from frock coat to disposables. NATNews, 14 (4), May 1977, 19-22, 24.

8 Iveson-Iveson, J. Lasers: a major advance in surgery. Nursing Mirror, 143, 21 Oct 1976, 66-67.

9 Hammond, M.A. Refuse disposal — 1978. (Development of Barnet Box for disposal of 'sharps' and discussion of other types of waste disposal.) Nursing Times, 74, 7 Dec 1978, Contact 8-9.

10 Hearn, L. Sophisticated nuts and bolts— or beds of nails? (Review of equipment used in theatre.) Nursing Mirror, 149, 11 Oct 1979, Supplement xix, xxii, xxiv, xxvi-xxviii.

11 Redstone, J.M. A sharp reminder. (Need for system of safe disposal of sharp instruments to prevent injury to theatre staff.) NATNews, 17 (6), Jun 1980, 8, 10.

12 Standring, J.A. Disposable gloves: a study of the uses, relative advantages and cost of disposable gloves. (In wards and departments.) Nursing Times, 76, 21 Aug 1980, ICNA, 15, 17-18.

13 Teasdale, J. Disposables: their use in operating theatres. (Research study by Johnson and Johnson 1977 Scholar Award Winner.) NATNews, 15 (5), May 1978, 17, 20.

g HAZARDS TO STAFF

1 Adler, G.R. Electrical safety in the operating room. American Association of Nurse Anesthetists Journal, 44 (6), Dec 1976, 619-629.

2 AORN Journal Samplings in ORs shows high level of trace gases. (Findings of the American Society of Anesthesiologists.) AORN Journal, 22 (6), Dec 1975, 1010.

3 Armstrong, R.F. and others Anaesthetic waste gas scavenging systems. (A comparison of five devices reducing concentrations of halothane in the atmosphere.) British Medical Journal, 1977, 1, 9 Apr 1977, 941-943.

4 Cooke, L. Historical development and overview of electrical safety in the operating room. Australasian Nurses Journal, 7 (5), Dec 1977, 17-19.

5 Davenport, H.T. and others Measurement and reduction of occupational exposure to inhaled anaesthetics. British Medical Journal, 2, 20 Nov 1976, 1219-1221.

6 Department of Health and Social Security Pollution of operating departments etc by anaesthetic gases. The Department, 1976. (HC(76)38). See Nursing Times, 72, 12 Aug 1976, 1220.

7 Donn, M.C. Chairman's letter. (To members of NATN re Health Notice HC(76)38 'Pollution of operating theatres etc. by Anaesthetic Gases.' NATNews, 14 (5), Jul 1977, 12.

8 Gamberale, F. The effect of anesthetic gases on the psychomotor and perceptual functions of anesthetic nurses. Work-Environment—Health, 11 (2), 1974, 108-113. (Reprint file.)

9 Gange, M.A. Protection for theatre staff against halothane pollution. (Mask worn by recovery room nurse.) Nursing Times, 74, 28 Sep 1978, 1600.

10 Halliday, M.M. and others Survey of operating room pollution within an N.H.S. district. Lancet, 1, 9 Jun 1979, 1230-1232.

11 Jones, M. Identifying electrical hazards and implementing safety measures: the theatre nurse's role. Australasian Nurses Journal, 7 (5), Dec 1977, 22-24.

12 Light, S. Staff face danger in the operating theatre. (Pollution by anaesthetic gases.) Nursing Mirror, 148, 11 Jan 1979, 20-22.

13 McCutcheon, R. Eliminating gas pollution in the O.R. Dimensions in Health Services, 57 (3), Mar 1980, 11-12.

14 Mainland, J.F. and Dudley, H.A.F. editors Safety in the operating theatre. Arnold, 1976.

15 Milliken, R.A. and Rendell-Baker, L. Anesthetic pollution: the smog we live in. (Summarises sources of pollution and evidence of disease caused by them.) Hospital Topics, 55 (2), Mar/Apr 1977, 28, 32, 33.

16 Pharoah, P.O.D. and others Outcome of pregnancy among women in anaesthetic practice. (Survey of 5700 women doctors registered since 1950.) Lancet, 1, 1 Jan 1977, 34-36.

17 Plant, J. Despite equivocal data, activity to curb waste gases mounts. (Health hazards of waste anaesthetic gases.) Hospitals, 52, 1 Jan 1978, 93-95, 98-99.

18 Sabo, B. Hazards of macroshock, microshock in the OR. AORN Journal, 24 (5), Nov 1976, 892-898.

19 Seufert, H.J. A review of occupational health hazards associated with anesthetic waste gases. AORN Journal, 24 (4), Oct 1976, 744-746, 748-749, 752.

20 THEATRE staff in danger of cancer and abortion from waste gases. Nursing Mirror, 142, 11 Mar 1976, 35; Nursing Times, 72, 11 Mar 1976, 360.

21 Tomlin, P.J. Health problems of anaesthetists and their families in the West Midlands. British Medical Journal, 1, 24 Mar 1979, 779-784.

22 Vaughan, R.S. Theatre pollution and its possible effects on personnel. (Atmospheric contamination with anaesthetic agents and policies to control it.) NATNews, 15 (6), Jun 1978, 16-18.

23 Wilson, D. 'Clean up' operations in the theatre (to prevent occupational hazards to operating theatre personnel.) NATNews, 13 (4), May 1976, 17-18.

24 Wright, S.A. Operating room pollution— or is it contamination? (Review of research.) American Association of Nurse Anesthetists Journal, 47 (3), Jun 1979, 313-322.

h HAZARDS TO PATIENTS

1 Abbey, T. Accidents to patients in the operating theatre. Nursing Times, 74, 2 Nov 1978, Theatre nursing, 5-6, 8.

2 Dixon, E. The legal aspects of surgery. (Research study to discover views of doctors, theatre nurses and patients.) NATNews, 15 (11), Nov 1978, 12-14, 16, 18-20.

3 Dobbie, A.K. Accidental lesions in the operating theatre. NATNews, 11 (9), Dec 1974, 10, 12, 13.

4 Donn, M. Theatre nursing. (Interview with Mary Donn, member of committee of inquiry into Shewan anaesthetic accident. Procedure to check nitrous oxide and oxygen machines.)

Nursing Times, 73, 6 Oct 1977, Theatre Nursing, 1, 3.

5 King's Health District (Teaching) Report of a committee appointed to enquire into a situation within the main operating theatre suite at Dulwich Hospital. The District, 1978. (Case of Elizabeth Shewan.) Abridged report in Health and Social Service Journal, 87, 22 Jul 1977, 1070-1071, Comment, 1064-1065; NATNews, 14 (6), Aug 1977, 5-7; Editorial in Lancet, 2, 23 Jul 1977, 175-176.

6 Medical Defence Union and Royal College of Nursing Joint memorandum on safeguards against failure to remove swabs and instruments from patients. Revised ed. MDU and Rcn, 1978.

7 Medical Defence Union and Royal College of Nursing Joint memorandum on safeguards against wrong operations. Revised ed. MDU and Rcn, 1978.

8 Nightingale, K.M. Out of sight: out of mind. An enquiry into the incidence of pressure injuries in the operating department. NATNews, 15 (8), Aug 1978, 22-26; (9), Sep 1978, 15-18.

9 Shewan, J. It must never happen again. (Letter from father of woman who suffered brain damage in an accident in operating theatre on ways of preventing such accidents.) Nursing Mirror, 145, 4 Aug 1977, 11.

10 Truesdell, S. and Wood, T. Communication: key to efficient patient care. (Programme to reduce incidence of postoperative chest infection through improving nurses' skills and teaching patients.) Nursing, 7 (8), Aug 1977, 52-53.

11 Zelechowski, G.P. Hidden killer: malignant hyperthermia. (During anaesthesia.) Nursing, 7 (9), Sep 1977, 35.

64 SURGICAL NURSING

a GENERAL AND TEXTBOOKS

1 Chang, L.F. How to succeed with wet-to-dry dressings. (Used for surgical, traumatic and chronic open wounds which must heal by secondary intention.) RN Magazine, 42 (1), Jan 1979, 63-66.

2 Conradie, M.E. 'Excellence in nursing.' A study in the art and science principles in nursing in general and applied in the care of the surgical patient in particular. (Includes pre-operative teaching and use of nursing process.) S.A. Nursing Journal, 44 (7), Jul 1977, 7-10.

3 Desharnais, A. Review of surgical nursing. New York: McGraw-Hill, 1979. (Multiple choice questions.)

4 Fish, E.J. Surgical nursing. 10th ed. Baillière Tindall, 1979. (Nurses' aids series.)

5 Frazier, C.A. The allergic surgical patient. AORN Journal, 26 (4), Oct 1977, 790, 792, 794, 796, 798.

6 Fream, W.C. Notes on surgical nursing. 2nd ed. Churchill Livingstone, 1978.

7 Hall, S.E. Caring for wounds: the nurse's responsibility towards her patients with wounds, to assist good healing. Nursing Mirror, 146, 9 Mar 1978, Supplement, ix, xi, xiii.

8 Harding, K. and Richardson, G. Silastic foam elastomer for treating open granulating wounds. Nursing Times, 75, 27 Sep 1979, 1679-1682.

9 Haywood, G. Porcine skin: a way to help the healing... Nursing Mirror, 148, 22 Mar 1979, 37-38.

10 Hodkinson, L. The bandage and bandaging. From cotton strip to plastic aerosol. (History of bandaging and developments since World War II.) Nursing Mirror, 148, 26 Apr 1979, Supplement, i-ii, iv, vi-vii, x, xii, xiv-xv.

11 Holford, C.P. Bandages—friends or enemies? (Functions and advice on application.) Nursing Times, 73, 14 Jul 1977, 1092-1093.

12 Hopkins, S.J. Biological wound dressing. Nursing Mirror, 142, 3 Jun 1976, 56-59.

13 Iveson-Iveson, J. The development of surgical dressings. Nursing Mirror, 142, 24 Jun 1976, 63.

14 Leddy, S. Nursing decisions: experiences in clinical problem solving. A parent requiring a cholecystectomy. RN Magazine, 39 (2), Feb 1976, 43-49.

15 Lukacs, R. and Dormer, M. A dressing room for tariff system. (Poor standard of dressing provision in the community.) Health and Social Service Journal, 89, 25 May 1979, 638.

16 MacFie, J. and others Foam elastomer dressing: a liquid alternative to gauze. (Used in treatment of open granulating wounds.) Nursing Mirror, 149, 2 Aug 1979, 30-32.

17 Meshelany, C.M. Post-op wound dressings: your guide to impeccable technique. (Including how to dress a closed surgical wound.) RN Magazine, 42 (5), May 1979, 22-33.

18 Morgan, M.E. Surgical nurse clinical specialist. AORN Journal, 23 (4), Mar 1976, 638, 640, 642, 644.

19 Murchie, M. and McGillivray, A. Nursing care of the draining wound. Nursing Times, 72, 16 Dec 1976, 1959-1960.

20 NATNews Surgical dressings in hospital environment. NATNews, 12 (5), Jul 1975, 11.

21 Nursing Clinics of North America Symposium on wound healing. Nursing Clinics of North America, 14 (4), Dec 1979, 665-778.

22 O'Malley, P. Managing the difficult draining wound. (Description of one method.) Nursing (U.S.), 9 (12), Dec 1979, 40-41.

23 Roaf, R. and Hodkinson, L. Basic surgical care. 2nd ed. Pitman, 1978. (For nurses and others.)

24 Sanderson, B.A. An advance in wound care. (Advantages of Op-Site wound dressing—a self-adhesive plastic film.) Queen's Nursing Journal, 19 (9), Dec 1976, 253-254.

25 Soul, J. A trial of Debrisan in the cleansing of infected surgical wounds. (Showed marked reduction in oedema, erythema and rest pain.) British Journal of Clinical Practice, 32 (6), Jun 1978, 172-173.

26 Steele, B.G. Self-assessment of current knowledge in general surgical nursing: 1,228 multiple choice questions and referenced answers. Garden City: Medical Examination Publishing Co., 1978.

27 Thomas, S. and others A critical evaluation of some extensible bandages in current use. (Comparison showed that cotton crepe or cotton stretch bandages perform better and are less expensive than crepe bandages.) Nursing Times, 76, 26 Jun 1980, 1123-1126.

28 Tinckler, L.F. A vacuum suction bottle holder. An answer to the problem of hanging bottles for wound drainage. Nursing Times, 75, 4 Jan 1979, 25.

29 Turner, T.D. A look at wound dressings. Contemporary surgical dressings are regularly evaluated in Wales. Health and Social Service Journal, 89, 4 May 1979, 529-531.

30 Tweedle, D. Tissue repair: how the metabolism reacts to injury. (How nutritional support plays important part in healing process.) Nursing Mirror, 147, 23 Nov 1978, 34-36.

31 Westaby, S. and Everett, W.G. The wound irrigation device: a new technique for managing troublesome wounds. (Using Stomahesive.) Nursing Times, 75, 1 Mar 1979, 351-353.

32 Whiteside, J.E. Surgical nursing. 2nd ed. Sydney: Angus and Robertson, 1975.

33 Wilson, D. Debrisan, the drug with a difference. (New wound cleansing agent for infected wounds, pressure sores, burns and venous ulcers.) Journal of Community Nursing, 1 (8), Feb 1978, 16-17.

34 Winter, G.D. Wound healing. (The process of tissue regeneration.) Nursing Mirror, 146, 9 Mar 1978, Supplement, i, iii-iv, vii-viii.

b PREOPERATIVE AND POST-OPERATIVE CARE

1 Andrews, S.J. Post operative nursing in the theatre unit. (Survey of procedures in ten hospitals.) NATNews, 14 (3), Apr 1977, 10-11, 14, 16, 18, 22.

2 AORN Journal Remember...to your patient you don't really look like you think you look. (Patients' feelings on the way to surgery. Mainly illustrations.) AORN Journal, 23 (7), Jun 1976, 1198-1201.

3 AORN Journal Standards of nursing practice: recovery room. (Three articles.) AORN Journal, 31 (5), Apr 1980, 795-813.

4 Aw, A.C. The recovery room. (Its planning and equipment, and care of patients.) NATNews, 14 (5), May 1977, 15-17, 24.

5 Chalmers, H. Return to basics. 4. Preoperative and post-operative care. Nursing Mirror, 145, 28 Jul 1977, Nursing care supplement series 5, i-iv.

6 Crick, E. Patients wait for surgery in 'twilight zone'. (Pre-operative waiting room provides quiet, restful atmosphere where nurses can talk to patients.) AORN Journal, 22 (6), Dec 1975, 980, 982.

7 Croushore, T.M. Postoperative assessment: the key to avoiding the most common nursing mistakes. Nursing (U.S.), 9 (4), Apr 1979, 47-51.

8 Cullen, D.J. Recovery room complications. AORN Journal, 26 (4), Oct 1977, 746, 750-751, 754-755, 758-759, 762-763.

9 Donn, M.C. The nurse's role in immediate postoperative care. (Letter giving present position regarding training.) British Medical Journal, 1, 11 Jun 1977, 1537.

10 Drain, C.B. and Shipley, S.B. The recovery room. Philadelphia: W.B. Saunders, 1979.

11 Fawcett, P. The patient comes to theatre. (Role of escort nurse with reference to scheme in use at York District Hospital.) Nursing Times, 75, 18 Oct 1979, Theatre nursing, 7-8.

12 Felton, G. and others Preoperative nursing intervention with the patient for surgery: outcomes of three alternative approaches. (Research study.) International Journal of Nursing Studies, 13 (2), 1976, 83-96.

13 Finn, K.L. How's your post-op ambulation technique? (Helping and teaching patients to cough and move around.) RN Magazine, 42 (9), Sep 1979, 69-72.

14 Flaherty, G.G. and Fitzpatrick, J.J. Relaxation technique to increase comfort level of postoperative patients: a preliminary study. (To reduce muscular tension during first attempt at getting out of bed.) Nursing Research, 27 (6), Nov/Dec 1978, 352-355.

15 Fraser, I. Early postoperative bathing: challenging traditional methods. Nursing Times, 72, 25 Nov 1976, 1844.

16 Groah, L. Do patients value preoperative assessments? (Research study.) AORN Journal, 29 (7), Jun 1979, 1250-1256.

17 Hercules, P.R. Nursing in the postoperative care unit: a review. 1: Respiratory complications. 2: Other complications. AORN Journal, 28 (6), Dec 1978, 1042-1052.

18 Hersey, F. and O'Neill, P. Reducing postoperative hospital stays. Dimensions in Health Service, 57 (3), Mar 1980, 22-23.

19 Hill, G.L. Surgical malnutrition. (Survey of surgical patients in Leeds General Infirmary.) Nursing Mirror, 145, 17 Nov 1977, 17-19.

20 Hill, G.L. and others Malnutrition in surgical patients: an unrecognised problem. Lancet, 1, 26 Mar 1977, 689-692.

21 Hoo, A.S. A study into the concept of mobilization of patients post-operatively. MSc thesis, University of Manchester, Department of Nursing, 1979.

22 Hospital Administration in Canada Preoperative assessment unit takes fear out of patient care. (Halifax Infirmary Hospital.) Hospital Administration in Canada, 19 (3), Mar 1977, S14-S15.

23 Howe, P. The respiratory effects of surgery. (Pre- and post-operative nursing care.) Nursing, 7, Nov 1979, 324-327.

24 Kapsar, P.P. The preoperative visit—O.R. nurses and patients interact. Surgical nurses' integral role in caring for patients before, during and after surgery. Hospitals, 50 (8), 16 Apr 1976, 87-88.

25 Keighley, M.R.B. and others Evaluation

of single-dose hypnotic treatment before elective operation. (A prospective randomised double-blind controlled trial to evaluate a single dose of triazolam, flurazepam, and placebo on the evening before an operation.) British Medical Journal, 281, 27 Sep 1980, 829-831.

26 McConnell, E.A. Nursing audit for recovery room. AORN Journal, 26 (3), Sep 1977, 525-528, 530.

27 McConnell, E.A. Primary nursing in the recovery room. AORN Journal, 30 (5), Nov 1979, 1007-1008, 1010.

28 McConnell, E.A. Toward complication-free recoveries for your surgical patients. RN Magazine, 43 (6), Jun 1980, 31-33, 82-84, 86, 90; (7), Jul 1980, 35-38, 70, 73, 76.

29 Marcott, M. There's more to post-op extubation than just pulling out a tube. (Guidelines for removing endotracheal tubes, an extension to nurse's role in parts of U.S.A.) RN Magazine, 40 (9), Sep 1977, 43-47.

30 Murphy, M. and Roglitz, C. Preoperative teaching, integration of nursing and social work services. (At St. Joseph Mercy Hospital, Ann Arbor, Michigan, with reference to neurosurgical patients.) Journal of Neurosurgical Nursing, 9 (1), Mar 1977, 5-11.

31 Ozuna, J.M. A study of surgical patients' temperatures: effects of preoperative procedures on patients' body temperatures. AORN Journal, 28 (2), Aug 1978, 240-245.

32 Sharp, E. Check lists for theatre patients. (Devised at Newcastle General Hospital to ensure adequate preparation of patients for theatre.) Nursing Times, 74, 9 Mar 1978, 422-423.

33 Stephens, D.S.B. and Boaler, J. The nurse's role in immediate postoperative care. (A survey of the knowledge and attitudes of 163 nurses discusses the need for recovery nurses and more training for this work.) British Medical Journal, 1, 7 May 1977, 1199-1202. Reprinted in Nursing Mirror, 145, 29 Sep 1977, 20-23.

34 Welsh, J. America 1976. (Report of study tour looking at pre and post operative visits by theatre nurses.) NATNews, 14 (7), Sep 1977, 14-15, 17.

35 Welsh, J. and Richardson, A. How well do you know your patient, nurse? (Advantages and disadvantages of pre- and post-operative visits by theatre nurses.) NATNews, 13 (5), Jul 1976, 12-15.

36 Zorab, J.S.M. It's the normal routine. (Criticism of aspects of preoperative preparation including shaving and fasting.) World Medicine, 13 (19), 28 Jun 1978, 26-28.

c PREOPERATIVE TEACHING AND PATIENT ANXIETY

1 Arnold, R. Pre-op visit calms fears. (By theatre nurse.) Hospital Administration in Canada, 20 (4), Apr 1978, 28-30.

2 Axford, R. and Cutchen, L. Using nursing research to improve preoperative care. (Implementation and evaluation of teaching programme.) Journal of Nursing Administration, 7 (10), Dec 1977, 16-20.

3 Barron, J. Modern surgery—a personal view. (Patients' fears about various aspects of surgery.) NATNews, 16 (3), Mar 1979, 13-16.

4 Boore, J.R.P. Nursing surgical patients in acute pain. (Includes preoperative preparation and patient instruction sheet for better recovery after surgery.) Nursing, 1, Apr 1979, 37-43.

5 Boore, J. Information—a prescription for recovery? (Description of author's research.) Nursing Mirror, 151, 11 Dec 1980, 32-35.

6 Boore, J. Pre-operative care of patients. (A review of research and theoretical work carried out with particular reference to psychological preparation.) Nursing Times, 73, 24 Mar 1977, 409-411.

7 Boore, J. Pre-operative information and post-operative recovery. (Author's research.) NATNews, 17 (1), Jan 1980, 16-17, 19.

8 Boore, J.R.P. Prescription for recovery: the effect of pre-operative preparation of surgical patients on post-operative stress, recovery and infection. Royal College of Nursing, 1978. (Research series.) Summary in Nursing Times, 76, 17 Apr 1980, Occ. papers, 44. Based on 'An investigation into the effects of some aspects of pre-operative preparation of patients on post-operative stress and recovery'. PhD thesis, University of Manchester, 1976.

9 Crabtree, M. Application of cost-benefit analysis to clinical nursing practice: a comparison of individual and group preoperative teaching. Journal of Nursing Administration, 8 (12), Dec 1978, 11-16.

10 Donn, M. Communication—the key to preparation for surgery. Nursing Mirror, 143, 21 Oct 1976, 46-47.

11 Dunkelman, H. Patients' knowledge of their condition and treatment: how it might be improved. (Report of research study by author, a nurse, and suggested checklist to record information given and booklet explaining pre- and post-operative care.) British Medical Journal, 2, 4 Aug 1979, 311-314.

12 Dziurbejko, M.M. and Larkin, J.C. Including the family in preoperative teaching. (Report of experimental study.) American Journal of Nursing, 78 (11), Nov 1978, 1892-1894.

13 Fortin, F. and Kerouac, S. A randomized controlled trial of preoperative patient education. (Sacre-Coeur of Cartierville Hospital, Montreal.) International Journal of Nursing Studies, 13 (1), 1976, 11-24.

14 Fortin, F. and Kerouac, S. Validation of questionnaires on physical function. (Assessment of a preoperative educational program by studying physical functions after surgery and at home.) Nursing Research, 26 (2), Mar-Apr 1977, 128-135.

15 Goodwin, J.O. Programmed instruction for self-care following pulmonary surgery. (The effectiveness of a booklet developed at the University of Michigan is tested on groups of patients.) International Journal of Nursing Studies, 16 (1), 1979, 29-40.

16 Gruendemann, B.J. Preoperative group sessions part of nursing process. AORN Journal, 26 (2), Aug 1977, 257-262.

17 Haag, M.G.P. and Adamski, J.A. Uncovering preoperative anxiety. (Q-sort, a method for patients to pick out statements most reflecting their concerns about surgery.) American Association of Nurse Anesthetists Journal, 46 (6), Dec 1978, 615-621.

18 Hartson, D. and Hartson, K. The five-minute interview. (Preoperative interview by nurse.) AORN Journal, 31 (4), Mar 1980, 606-608.

19 Hewitt, D. Is that pre-op patient terrified? (Assessment guide to measure anxiety levels.) RN Magazine, 42 (9), Sep 1979, 44-47.

20 Hoopes, N.M. and McConnell, M. An approach to preoperative visits. (At Johns Hopkins Hospital, Baltimore.) AORN Journal, 26 (6), Dec 1977, 1048-1052.

21 Howells, J.G. editor Modern perspectives in the psychiatric aspects of surgery. Macmillan, 1978. (Modern perspectives in psychiatry; 7.)

22 Hughes, J. Overcoming fear: the pre-operative visit. (Value of ward visit by theatre nurses with brief reference to scheme at Royal Shrewsbury Hospital.) Nursing Times, 75, 18 Oct 1979, Theatre nursing, 4, 6.

23 Johnson, J.E. and others Altering patients' responses to surgery: an extension and replication. (Study to determine reliability of the effects of preoperative preparation on post-operative recovery observed in previous study.) Research in Nursing Health, 1 (3), Oct 1978, 111-121.

24 Johnson, J.E. and others Sensory information, instruction in a coping strategy, and recovery from surgery. (Study of 81 cholecystectomy patients.) Research in Nursing Health, 1 (1), Arp 1978, 4-17.

25 Kinney, M.R. Effects of preoperative teaching upon patients with different modes of response to threatening stimuli. International Journal of Nursing Studies, 14 (1), 1977, 49-59.

26 Kleinbeck, S.V.M. SOAPing the pre-operative interview. (Advice on interviewing and recording interview.) AORN Journal, 28 (6), Dec 1978, 1031-1035.

27 Klos, D. and others A comparison of two methods of delivering presurgical instructions. (Pamphlet and/or nurse visit.) Patient Counselling and Health Education, 2 (1), First Quarter 1980, 6-13.

28 LeBourdais, E. Pre-operative teaching makes happier patients. Dimensions in Health Service, 54 (1), 1977, 13.

29 Leigh, J.M. and others Effect of pre-operative anaesthetic visit on anxiety. (Research study showing its importance and suggesting anaesthetic nurse should visit patient if anaesthetist is too busy.) British Medical Journal, 2, 15 Oct 1977, 987-989.

30 Marcinek, M.B. Stress in the surgical patient. (Physiological effects.) American Journal of Nursing, 77 (11), Nov 1977, 1809-1911.

31 Phippen, M.L. Nursing assessment of preoperative anxiety. AORN Journal, 31 (6), May 1980, 1019-1026.

32 Ridgeway, M. Preop interviews assure quality care. AORN Journal, 24 (6), Dec 1976, 1083-1084.

33 Schrader, E.S. Counseling helps gyn patients handle surgery. (Preoperative teaching by theatre nurse.) AORN Journal, 30 (2), Aug 1979, 233-241.

34 Schrader, E.S. Group teaching can supplement patient interviews. (Preoperative visits.) AORN Journal, 26 (2), Aug 1977, 223-224, 226.

35 Schrankel, D.P. Pre-operative teaching. (Advice on implementing programme.) Supervisor Nurse, 9 (5), May 1978, 82, 85-86, 89-90.

36 Silva, M.C. Preoperative teaching for spouses. (Research study and teaching programme.) AORN Journal, 27 (6), May 1978, 1081-1086.

37 Silva, M.C. Spouses need nurses too. (Interviews with spouses of surgical patients revealed stresses experienced.) Canadian Nurse, 73 (12), Dec 1977, 38-41.

38 Skillings, I.L. Emotional support for surgery patients. (Preoperative group teaching programme.) AORN Journal, 26 (2), Aug 1977, 263-265.

39 Voshall, B. The effects of preoperative teaching on postoperative pain. Topics in Clinical Nursing, 2 (1), Apr 1980, 39-43.

40 Wassner, A. Patient care for safety. (Pre-operative teaching.) International Nursing Review, 23 (5), Sep-Oct 1976, 144-147.

41 Waters, W. and Macintyre, I.M.C. Attitudes and criticisms of surgical in-patients. (Study at Leith Hospital, Edinburgh.) Practitioner, 218, Feb 1977, 269-272.

42 Wiley, L. Nursing grand rounds. Dealing with depression after radical surgery. (Case study.) Nursing (U.S.), 9 (2), Feb 1979, 47-51.

65 THEATRE NURSING

a GENERAL

1 Adeloye, A. The nurse and the operating theatre: past, present and future. Nigerian Nurse, 8 (2), Apr/Jun 1976, 18-21.

2 Arnold, R. Nurses need to focus attention on expertise in operating room. Hospital Administration in Canada, 19 (3), Mar 1977, S18-S20.

3 Association of Operating Room Nurses Operating room nursing: peri-operative role. (Report of an AORN working party.) AORN Journal, 27 (6), May 1978, 1156, 1161-1162, 1164-1165, 1168, 1170, 1175.

4 Brigden, R.J. Operating theatre technique: a textbook for nurses... 4th ed. Edinburgh: Churchill Livingstone, 1980.

5 Campbell, M.H. Theatre routine. 2nd ed. Heinemann Medical, 1979. (Modern practical nursing series; 2.)

6 Davies, A.C. Total patient care in theatre— an idea. (Report of project and visit to U.S.A.) NATNews, 17 (1), Jan 1980, 10, 12-13.

7 Davis, J.E. Why a mandate for the circulator. (The function of the operating room nurse as circulator for surgical procedures.) AORN Journal, 23 (7), Jun 1976, 1185-1193.

8 Dudley, H.A.F. Micro-ergonomics: an analysis of hand movements in the passage of instruments from theatre nurse to surgeon. Nursing Mirror, 144, 27 Jan 1977, 48-49.

9 Dudley, H.A. Operative ergonomics. (Illustrating the poor positions taken up by surgeon and nurse and the inadequate work space.) Nursing Mirror, 143, 28 Oct 1976, 53-54.

10 Dudley, H.A.F. What I expect from my scrub nurse. (By a surgeon.) NATNews, 15 (6), Jun 1978, 10-11.

11 Griffith, D.L. Refresher course. Nursing care in the operating theatre. Nursing Times, 74, 2 Feb 1978, 186-187.

12 Gruendemann, B.J. and others The surgical patient: behavioural concepts for the operating room nurse. 2nd ed. St. Louis: Mosby, 1977.

13 Hill, S. Working in the operating department in Italy and Greece. NATNews, 11 (4), May 1974, 15-16.

14 Hunt, A. The individual approach. (Use of nursing process in operating department.) Nursing Mirror, 149, 11 Oct 1979, Supplement, x, xii.

15 Iihama, S. and Kubota, U. Operating room nursing in Japanese hospitals. AORN Journal, 28 (5), Nov 1978, 848-854.

16 Jordan, C.H. Awareness for action. (The role of the operating room nurse now and in the future.) AORN Journal, 25 (7), Jun 1977, 1317-1336 (9 p.)

17 Kneedler, J.A. Perioperative role in three dimensions. (Pre and postoperative care by theatre nurses in addition to care during surgery.) AORN Journal, 30 (5), Nov 1979, 859-874.

18 Larke, G.A. Perioperative charting: OR nursing on display. AORN Journal, 31 (2), Feb 1980, 194-198.

19 Latz, P.A. and others A framework for primary OR nursing. AORN Journal, 29 (5), Apr 1979, 959-960, 964, 968, 972.

20 Lemaitre, G. and Finnegan, J.A. The patient in surgery: a guide for nurses. 4th ed. Philadelphia: Saunders, 1980.

21 Lindeman, C. and others AORN-WICHE report. Relationship between OR nursing activities and patient outcomes. (Includes preoperative, intraoperative and postoperative phases of care.) AORN Journal, 27 (2), Feb 1978, 203-218.

22 Miles, B.F. An American experience. (Study tour of theatre nursing in America.) New Zealand Nursing Journal, 69 (12), Dec 1976, 11-13.

23 Nolan, M.G. AORN survey of members listed as CNS. (To determine if nurses were functioning as clinical nurse specialists in theatre.) AORN Journal, 26 (6), Dec 1977, 1034-1041.

24 Nolan, M.G. A master nurse clinician for intraoperative care. Nursing Clinics of North America, 10 (4), Dec 1975, 645-653.

25 Nolan, M.G. Potentials in OR nursing. AORN Journal, 23 (4), Mar 1976, 583-590.

26 Nursing Clinics of North America Symposium on perspectives in operating room nursing. Nursing Clinics of North America, 10 (4), Dec 1975, 613-686.

27 Phippen, M.L. Intraoperative nursing assessment. (Application of first stage of nursing process.) AORN Journal, 28 (1), Jul 1978, 160, 162, 164, 166.

28 Porter-O'Grady, T. and Carter, J.A. Bringing the nursing process into the OR. AORN Journal, 30 (5), Nov 1979, 898-899, 902-903, 906-907, 910, 913-914.

29 Quayle, S. Care and safety of the patient in the operating department. (Prize-winning essay.) NATNews, 17 (3), Mar 1980, 14-16.

30 Schrader, E.S. The case for the clinical nurse specialist in the OR. (Editorial.) AORN Journal, 23 (4), Mar 1976, 547-548.

31 Schrader, E.S. The clinical nurse specialist in the OR. (Work of one clinical specialist in Daniel Freeman Hospital, Inglewood, California, including teaching and research activities.) AORN Journal, 23 (4), Mar 1976, 571-582.

32 Schrader, E.S. Japan. Nurses struggle to show that OR nursing is nursing. (Report of visit to theatres in Tokyo hospitals.) AORN Journal, 26 (3), Sep 1977, 501-510.

33 Shaw, H. The nursing process, the operating theatre, and the patient. (Pre-operative assessment, theatre care and post-operative evaluation.) NATNews, 13 (8), Nov 1976, 20, 22.

34 Warren, M.C. The receiving nurse in the operating theatre. (Reception of patient and checking of identity. Includes preoperative check list for use by ward nurse.) NATNews, 15 (11), Nov 1978, 10-11.

35 Warren, M.C. A study of the utilisation of the nursing process in operating theatre nursing in the United States and Canada. (Based on visits and questionnaires.) NATNews, 17 (12), Dec 1980, 16-18, 20.

36 Wells, P. 'Confine and contain' approach to OR cleanup. (Procedures for cleaning between operations.) AORN Journal, 25 (1), Jan 1977, 60-65.

b PROFESSIONAL ASPECTS

1 AORN Nursing Research Committee Bibliography of OR nursing research. (Masters and PhD theses.) AORN Journal, 27 (5), Apr 1978, 960-963.

2 Association of Operating Room Nurses Standards of administrative nursing practice: operating room. AORN Journal, 23 (7), Jun 1976, 1202-1208.

3 Association of Operating Room Nurses and American Nurses Association Standards of nursing practice: operating room. Kansas City: ANA, 1975. Reprinted in: AORN Journal, 24 (4), Oct 1976, 798, 800, 802, 804, 806, 808.

4 Brigden, R.J. and Scott, S.B.R. Research and theatre nursing. (The Theatre Nursing, Education and Research Fellowship Fund.) NATNews, 17 (3), Mar 1980, 12.

5 Cowper-Smith, F. It's different—but is it better? (Report of visit to Association of

Operating Room Nurses conference in U.S.A.) Nursing Times, 76, 5 Jun 1980, 990-992.

6 **Cowper-Smith, F.** Theatre nurses face life and death issues. (Report of NATN conference.) Nursing Times, 73, 27 Oct 1977, 1658-1659.

7 **Donn, M.** Don't write our requiem. (Role of theatre nurses and ODAs in the future with reference to current views of various organisations.) Nursing Mirror, 149, 11 Oct 1979, Supplement, ii-iii, v.

8 **Donn, M.C.** Theatre nurses meet changing social needs. (Paper describing theatre nursing in Britain presented at 1978 AORN congress.) AORN Journal, 28 (3), Sep 1978, 411-415.

9 **Driscoll, J.** OR nurses as researchers. AORN Journal, 23 (2), Feb 1976, 206-208.

10 **Dunn, A.** Gateway to power. (Report on annual congress of the Association of Operating Room Nurses.) Nursing Times, 75, 29 Mar 1979, 523-525.

11 **Dunn, M.** Keynote speech. (Annual congress speech describing theatre developments—in particular the emergence of the Operating Department Assistant.) NATNews, 13 (9), Dec 1976, 13-14.

12 **Lamb, K.A.** Factors motivating nurses to work in the OR. AORN Journal, 25 (7), Jun 1977, 1338-1354 (8 p.)

13 **Lofthouse, B.** The origins of NATN. NATNews, 14 (7), Sep 1977, 11-12.

14 **McCarville, M.** Maintaining standards in the OR. Dimensions in Health Service, 54 (3), Mar 1977, 30-37.

15 **National Association of Theatre Nurses** Annual congress. NATNews.
Twelfth. 13 (8), Nov 1976.
Thirteenth. 14 (8), Nov 1977, 12-13, 15-16, 18, 20-21.

16 **National Association of Theatre Nurses** 12th Annual Congress. Professional status under threat from ODAS, claim theatre nurses, by M. Dunn. Nursing Mirror, 143, 4 Nov 1976, 35-37.

17 **National Association of Theatre Nurses** Code of practice. (Guidelines on standards of theatre practice.) NATNews, 12 (4), May/Jun 1975, 10, 12-13.

18 **National Association of Theatre Nurses** Staffing and Training Sub-committee Codes of practice: guidelines to the total patient care and safe practice in operating theatres. Harrogate: NATN, 1977.

19 **Nursing Mirror** Theatre horizons, theatre people. A special supplement on the occasion of the National Association of Theatre Nurses 13th Annual Congress, Harrogate, October 12-14, 1977. (Interviews with a nurse, surgeon, anaesthetist and operating department assistant, by T. Ross.) Nursing Mirror, 145, 6 Oct 1977, iii, v, vii, x. Also 27 Oct 1977, 4-5.

20 **Nursing Times** Theatre nursing. A special supplement to mark next week's conference of NATN. Nursing Times, 73, 6 Oct 1977, Theatre Nursing, 1, 3, 5-6, 8, 9-10, 12, 14.

21 **Poole, D.L.** Do we still care?: a debate held at Congress in 1978. (Changes in role of theatre nurse.) NATNews, 16 (3), Mar 1979, 8-9, 11-12.

22 **Squires, N-M** Sliding standards are deep concern. (Report of conference of Canadian theatre nurses.) Hospital Administration in Canada, 20 (7), Jul/Aug 1978, 26-29.

c EDUCATION AND TRAINING

1 **Berchem, R.** Three approaches to specialty courses in OR nursing. Self study course in Wisconsin for all nurses. AORN Journal, 24 (5), Nov 1976, 907, 909, 911.

2 **Cowell, R.** Behavioural objectives for post basic students in the operating department. NATNews, 12 (5), Jul 1975, 15, 19.

3 **Crawford, M.E.** Three approaches to specialty courses in OR nursing, Critical need for ORN's motivates Seattle program. (Eight week course introducing the operating room.) AORN Journal, 24 (5), Nov 1976, 905, 906.

4 **Deets, C.A.** Evaluating CE programs. (In-service education, with reference to theatre nursing.) AORN Journal, 26 (1), Jul 1977, 152, 154, 156, 158, 160, 162, 164, 166, 168.

5 **Dixon, E.** A formal future for the student. (Education of future theatre nurse.) Nursing Mirror, 149, 11 Oct 1979, Supplement, vi, ix-x.

6 **Donn, M.C.** Training of theatre staff. (Includes a list of Joint Board of Clinical Nursing Studies, courses for SRN's and SEN's.) NATNews, 13 (2), Feb 1976, 11-13.

7 **Drake, J.** Report on operating theatre staff training and conditions in Holland. (Study visit with a grant from the Theatre Nursing Education and Research Fellowship Fund.) NATNews, 12 (7), Sep 1975, 24, 26.

8 **Groah, L.** Staff development—reality oriented. (Guidelines for orientation programmes in the operating theatre.) AORN Journal, 24 (6), Dec 1976, 1063-1068.

9 **Knowles, P.** Three approaches to specialty courses OR nursing. Twin Cities nurses learn OR skills in classroom, lab. (Course for qualified nurses with OR experience in Minneapolis.) AORN Journal, 24 (5), Nov 1976, 900-901, 903, 905.

10 **Konda, N.L.** Staff development for OR nurses. (Nursing process as framework for developing in-service training for recovery room nurses.) AORN Journal, 26 (4), Oct 1977, 664-667.

11 **Metzger, R.S.** The beginning of OR nursing education. AORN Journal, 24 (1), Jul 1976, 73, 76, 80-81, 84-85, 88, 90.

12 **Miller, A.** Post basic courses. Methods of assessment. (Operating Department technique courses.) NATNews, 13 (6), Aug 1796, 11-12, 14-16.

13 **Nursing Mirror** Joint Board of Clinical Nursing Studies. 7. Operating department nursing. Nursing Mirror, 143 (11), 9 Sep 1976, Nursing care supplement series 2, i-iv.

14 **Peers, J.G.** Operating room staff development. (Reprinted from AORN Journal.) NATNews, 14 (4), May 1977, 10-12.

15 **Pounds, E.** Assessing learning needs of OR nurses. (Study sponsored by the AORN Research Committee.) AORN Journal, 24 (3), Sep 1976, 433-436.

16 **Puetz, B.E.** Continuing education and OR and RR nurses. (Results of 1978 survey in Indiana.) AORN Journal, 31 (4), Mar 1980, 652, 654, 656, 658, 660, 662.

17 **Redstone, J.M.** The problems involved in the instruction of different grades of learners within the operating department. NATNews, 16 (4), Apr 1979, 8-12.

18 **Warren, M.C.** Post-registration courses for operating theatre nursing in the countries of the European Economic Community. (Research study of courses in Belgium, Denmark, Ireland and Italy.) NATNews, 15 (6), Jun 1978, 20-23.

d MANAGEMENT AND STAFFING

1 **AORN Journal** Is physician/nurse relationship deteriorating? (Editorial.) AORN Journal, 23 (1), Jan 1976, 11-12.

2 **AORN Journal** OR nursing notes form, guidelines. (Guidelines to assist nurses in recording patient information, in the University Hospitals of Cleveland.) AORN Journal, 26 (3), Sep 1977, 513, 516, 518, 520.

3 **AORN Journal** Should OR nurses act as first assistant? (To surgeon, assisting with suturing etc. Views for and against and discussion of role of nurse.) AORN Journal, 26 (5), Nov 1977, 890-891, 894-895, 898-899, 903-904, 908-909, 912.

4 **AORN Journal** Physicians respond to question of first assistant. (Comments by three surgeons on possible new role for theatre nurses.) AORN Journal, 27 (2), Feb 1978, 242-244, 247-250.

5 **Armstrong, D.M.** Nursing administrator's expectations of OR leader. AORN Journal, 25 (5), Apr 1977, 859-864.

6 **Bennett, B.M.** Deviant behavior in the OR. (The particular problems of interaction between nurses and doctors in the theatre.) AORN Journal, 25 (5), Apr 1976, 786-790, 792, 794.

7 **Best, R.** POMR for operating and recovery rooms. Supervisor Nurse, 7 (8), Aug 1976, 19-22.

8 **Chvala, C.** OR supervisor's role in planning the surgical suite. AORN Journal, 23 (1), Jun 1976, 1238-1239, 1242-1243, 1246-1247, 1252, 1254.

9 **Coffey, M.** 'Unhappiness' in Royal Northern theatres. (Report of a Committee of Inquiry.) Nursing Times, 72, 5 Aug 1976, 1180.

10 **Craig, B.J.** Team leader concept implemented in the OR. AORN Journal, 28 (4), Oct 1978, 726, 728, 730, 732.

11 **Davis, J.E.** Revising the OR record. (Experience of author.) AORN Journal, 26 (5), Nov 1977, 877-883.

12 **Dixon, E.** Programme for today. (The basic plan of today's theatre, equipment and the training of staff.) Nursing Mirror, 148, 15 Mar 1979, Supplement, ix-x, xii.

13 **Elliot, M.D.** Assertion opens options for OR nurses. AORN Journal, 28 (2), Aug 1978, 219-226.

14 Freeman, D.M. Operating theatre suites staff workload comparisons. NATNews, 14 (7), Sep 1977, 19-20, 22.

15 Heggs, P.M. The state enrolled nurse in theatre—past, present and future. NATNews, 13 (7), Sep 1976, 15-16, 18.

16 Hickey, P. High-speed life in operating theatres. (Some of the problems besetting nurse managers in theatre.) Health and Social Service Journal, 88, 3 Nov 1978, 1250-1251.

17 House, J.L.M. Group theatres—area or division? (Organisation of group theatres in Plymouth Health District.) Nursing Times, 72, 15 Apr 1976, 594-595.

18 Hulme, M. Theatre staffing—what now? (Describes staffing arrangements 25 years ago.) NATNews, 16 (8), Aug 1979, 19-20.

19 Jacob, J.L. and others Documenting patient care in the OR. (Importance of accurate and detailed records in general, with example of theatre nurse's record.) AORN Journal, 26 (4), Oct 1977, 659-663.

20 Joyce, P.M. Utilization of personnel in the operating suite. (Includes technicians.) Australian Nurses Journal, 7 (9), Apr 1978, 40-43.

21 Kneedler, J.A. Corrective action completes audit cycle. (Implementation of audit information.) AORN Journal, 26 (3), Sep 1977, 485-494.

22 Lewin, W. Five years on. 1. (Views on the implementation of the Lewin report.) Nursing Times, 72, 21 Oct 1976, Theatre nursing supplement, 3.

23 Litterst, T. A proposal; OR consulting team. (To provide consultancy services in theatre management and nursing practice.) AORN Journal, 26 (5), Nov 1977, 870-876.

24 Luttman, P.A. OR/RR nursing record improves care. AORN Journal, 22 (6), Dec 1975, 909-912.

25 Maguire, J.M. Planning an operating theatre suite. S.A. Nursing Journal, 43 (4), Apr 1976, 27-29, 11.

26 Michau, E. Functions of the operating room personnel. (Organisation and management and roles of various grades of nurse.) NATNews, 17 (9), Sep 1980, 24-25, 27.

27 National Association of Theatre Nurses The Lewin report. (On theatre staffing including the role of the ODA. Report of final session of NATN conference 1978.) NATNews, 15 (12), Dec 1978, 16, 20, 23, 25, 27.

28 National Association of Theatre Nurses Operating theatre area management. (Working Party on Staffing Norms and Grading.) NATNews, 15 (2), Feb 1978, 8-9.

29 NATNews Pointing system for theatre staffing. (Editorial.) NATNews, 13 (2), Feb 1976, 3.

30 NATNews The PRN scheme and the theatre. Impressions on the use of a pool of reserve nurses within operating theatres in the Bromley Area Health Authority. NATNews, 12 (4), May/Jun 1975, 17, 19-20.

31 Nolan, M.G. Study of role of OR nurse, technician raises questions. (Study of Seattle in 1975.) AORN Journal, 24 (4), Oct 1976, 645-646.

32 Organ, C.H. OR nurse, surgeon: common areas of concern. AORN Journal, 22 (6), Dec 1975, 898-902.

33 Quayle, S.N. Efficient costing and budgeting in the operating theatre. (By winner of Johnson & Johnson Fellow Award 1977.) NATNews, 15 (2), Feb 1978, 11-14.

34 Overman, M. The endless advantages of the octagonal OR. Dimensions in Health Service, 53 (2), Feb 1976, 39-40, 42.

35 Rait, A. After Lewin. (Functions of the operating department manager.) Nursing Times, 72, 12 Feb 1976, 208.

36 Rait, A. Operating department budgeting. (Study of systems in the United States and their application for the U.K.) Nursing Times, 72 (42), 21 Oct 1976, Theatre nursing supplement, 20, 22.

37 Reed, E.A. OR nursing audit becomes a reality. AORN Journal, 26 (3), Sep 1977, 479-484.

38 Richman, J. and Balcombe, M. Organisation theory revisited: is it an essential skill for OH nurses? Occupational Health, 32 (5), May 1980, 252-256.

39 Riley, J.A. The integration of nursing, para-medical and auxiliary/ancillary staff into a single grading structure. Technic, 22, Mar 1980, 7.

40 Rosenkoetter, M.M. and Price, D.L. OR of the future: implications for design. AORN Journal, 24 (2), Aug 1976, 241-245, 248.

41 Smith, M.L. Bringing the OR closer to nursing. (Attempt to integrate theatre nurses with other nursing specialties and promote communication with the director of nursing.) AORN Journal, 31 (4), Mar 1980, 664, 666-667.

42 Trouten, A.F. The operating room door is open. (Theatre nurses' increased communication with other hospital staff due to rapid technological advances necessitating greater specialization.) Hospital Administration in Canada, 19 (3), Mar 1977, S8-S9, S11.

43 Wall, T. Report on the Workshop for Nurses in functional control of operating departments. (Rcn workshop for operating department managers.) NATNews, 13 (9), Dec 1976, 23, 25, 27.

e OPERATING DEPARTMENT ASSISTANTS

1 Brett, H. Five years on—2. (Action taken on operating department assistants after the Lewin report recommendations.) Nursing Times, 72 (42), 21 Oct 1976, Theatre nursing supplement, 5.

2 Cowie, A.G.A. The future of the ODA. NATNews, 15 (4), Apr 1978, 12.

3 Davies, A.J. A training scheme for senior operating department assistants. (In South West Thames RHA.) NATNews, 17 (2), Feb 1980, 17-18, 20.

4 Department of Health and Social Security Training of operating department assistants. STM (75) 39. Extracts in NATNews, 12 (7), Sep 1975, 12.

5 National Association of Theatre Nurses Lewin and all that. (Report of NATN London Branch study day.) NATNews, 15 (8), Aug 1978, 20-21.

6 National Association of Theatre Nurses Some thoughts on the national training of operating department personnel: a provocative document from some members of the Surrey Branch. NATNews, 12 (7), Sep 1975, 17-18.

7 NATNews Report of the workshop for visiting assessors. (Training of ODAs.) NATNews, 15 (3), Mar 1978, 10-14.

8 Nursing Times The ODA is here to stay. (Seven articles on the history and current role of the operating department assistant.) Nursing Times, 74, 19 Oct 1978, 1710-1718.

9 Royal College of Nursing 'Are ODAs really necessary?' Nurses discuss problems of administration in theatres. (Rcn workshop.) Nursing Times, 72, 5 Aug 1976, 1182.

10 Suddes, G. Look again at ODAs. (Their role, by secretary of the British Association of ODAs.) Nursing Mirror, 147, 13 Jul 1978, 7.

11 Williams, M. Theatre of protest among the ODAs. (Frustrations ODAs face and four-point plan for improved training.) Nursing Mirror, 148, 15 Mar 1979, 20-22.

66 INFECTION AND STERILISATION

a GENERAL AND INFECTION CONTROL

1 Abrams, J. and others Infection surveillance prepares for move to new facility. (Team evaluates potential infection hazards.) Hospitals, 51, 16 Sep 1977, 177-178, 180.

2 American Hospital Association Infection control in the hospital. 4th ed. Chicago: the Association, 1979.

3 AORN Journal Standards for infection control in recovery room nursing. AORN Journal, 29 (7), Jun 1979, 1305, 1308, 1312.

4 Ashton, K. Our dirty hospitals. (Report of address at study day on infection control.) Nursing Times, 75, 21 Jun 1979, 1035.

5 Aspinall, M.J. Scoring against nosocomial infections. (Analysis of causes of infection and programme to prevent infection.) American Journal of Nursing, 78 (10), Oct 1978, 1704-1707.

6 Ayliffe, G.A.J. Screening of hospital staff for staphylococcus aureus. (Answer to question on value of taking nasal swabs from theatre staff.) Nursing Times, 74, 6 Apr 1978, Contact 6.

7 Ayliffe, G.A.J. and others Decline of the hospital staphylococcus? Incidence of multi-resistant staph. aureus in three Birmingham hospitals. Lancet, 1, 10 Mar 1979, 538-541.

8 Babcock, J.B. Some practical problems and trouble shooting. (Effective surveillance, analysis and evaluation of data for an infection control program.) Hospitals, 50 (6), 16 Mar 1976, 133-134, 138.

9 Bakels, M. and Anspach, W.E. Is clean air necessary? NATNews, 11 (7), Sep 1974, 25, 27, 30.

10 Bennett, J.V. and Brachman, P.S. editors Hospital infections. Boston: Little, Brown and Co., 1979.

11 Bolton, J. Special environments for health care. (Including control of infections.) Health and Social Service Journal, 90, 12 Sep 1980, M2-M8.

12 Brandt, S.L. and Benner, P. Infection control in hospitals: what are the challenges? American Journal of Nursing, 80 (3), Mar 1980, 432-434.

13 Carbary, L.J. Hospital acquired infections. (Methods of preventing infections.) Nursing Care, 8 (12), Dec 1975, 28-32.

14 Central Sterilising Club The microbial hazards of the hospital environment. (Papers given at the 1976 annual meeting.) Health and Social Service Journal, 86, 26 Jun 1976, Supplement, 3-15.

15 Chavigny, K.H. Microbial infections in hospitals: a review of the literature and some suggestions for nursing research. International Journal of Nursing Studies, 14 (1), 1977, 37-47.

16 Chewick, S. Infection control. Infection control demands administrative support. Dimensions in Health Service, 52 (12), Dec 1975, 40-41.

17 Connell, A.D. Controlling operating room related infection in cancer patients. Nursing Clinics of North America, 7 (4), Dec 1975, 667-678.

18 Cowper-Smith, F. A safer place for patients. (Report of two conferences on infection control.) Nursing Times, 75, 11 Oct 1979, 1742-1744.

19 Cox, R.N. The human micro environment and its role in the operating theatre. NATNews, 11 (5), Jul 1974, 13-16.

20 Cragg, C.E. Cross infection: a new approach to an old problem. (Education programme for nurses to reduce rate of cross infection on a paediatric ward.) Canadian Nurse, 75 (2), Feb 1979, 40-45.

21 Department of Health and Social Security Working Party to Formulate a Code of Practice for the Prevention of Infection in Clinical Laboratories Report. DHSS, 1978. (Chairman: Sir James Howie.)

22 Dubay, E.C. and Grubb, R.D. Infection: prevention and control. 2nd ed. St. Louis: Mosby, 1978.

23 Ehrenkranz, N.J. and others Consortium upgrades 12 hospitals' infection control programs. (South Florida Hospital Consortium using infection control nurse and physician epidemiologists.) Hospitals, 53 (1), 1 Jan 1979, 82-84.

24 Environmental Health Officers Association The unhealthy state of hospital hygiene. (Draft report by the Environmental Health Officers Association.) Health and Social Service Journal, 87, 25 Mar 1977, 520-521.

25 Gibala, D. Infection control. Training supportive personnel on the environmental aspects of infection control. Hospital Topics, 54 (5), Sep/Oct 1976, 1-2, 46-48.

26 Gibson, G.L. The bedpan and cross infection. (Infection hazards and disposal systems.) Nursing Times, 72, 5 Aug 1976, 1198-1200.

27 Gibson, N. Hospital infection. (Historical development of infection control with current methods and future plans.) Australian Nurses Journal, 6 (2), Aug 1976, 27-30.

28 Goad, D.M. and Thomas, W.R.G. Physiotherapy pool safety test. (Investigation into existing infection control procedures.) Nursing Times, 72, 14 Oct 1976, 1615.

29 Gray, M.J. The challenge of infection control. Hospital Topics, 58 (2), Mar/Apr 1980, 21-22.

30 Grimes, M.J. An infection control program, the first step toward quality assurance. Hospital Topics, 55 (4), Jul/Aug 1977, 6-8.

31 Howie, J.W. and Collins, C.H. The Howie Code for preventing infection in clinical laboratories: comments on some general criticisms and specific complaints. British Medical Journal, 280, 19 Apr 1980, 1071-1074.

32 James, C.D.T. Our Listerian heritage. Nursing Mirror, 145, 6 Oct 1977, 28-30.

33 Lacey, R.W. Cross infection. Changes in staphylococcal infections and new anti-staphylococcal antibiotics. Nursing Times, 72, 4 Mar 1976, 327-329.

34 Lancet Viral cross infections in children's wards. Lancet, 1, 26 Jun 1976, 1391-1393.

35 Lewis, J.F. Infections associated with the administration of anesthesia. American Association of Nurse Anesthetists Journal, 44 (2), Apr 1976, 166-173.

36 McInnes, B. Controlling the spread of infection: a programmed presentation. 2nd ed. St. Louis: Mosby, 1977.

37 MacKay, J.P. The microbial hazards of the hospital environment: the message to nurses. Health and Social Service Journal, 86, 26 Jun 1976, Supplement, 13.

38 Maurer, I.M. Hospital hygiene. 2nd ed. Arnold, 1978. (For nurses and others.)

39 Nightingale, K.M. Carbolic to carelessness? (Problems involved in encouraging staff to observe infection control measures.) Nursing Times, 74, 6 Apr 1978, Contact, 7-8.

40 Parker, M.T. editor Hospital—acquired infections: guidelines to laboratory methods. Copenhagen: WHO, Regional Office for Europe, 1978. (WHO regional publications European series; 4.)

41 Parker, M.T. The hospital environment as a source of septic infection. (Review of research with 51 references.) Royal Society of Health Journal, 98 (5), Oct 1978, 203-209.

42 Polakavetz, S.H. and others Nosocomial infection: the hidden cost in health care. (Ways to reduce incidence of infection.) Hospitals, 52 (10), 16 Aug 1978, 101-102, 104, 106.

43 Rice, W.W. and Darr, K. Infection control: beyond surveillance and record keeping. (Study of current practices of infection control committees in small to medium community hospitals.) Hospital Progress, 57 (11), Nov 1976, 82-85, 104.

44 Spiers, A.S.D. Antibacterial sink helps combat nosocomial infection. Hospitals, 52, 16 Jan 1978, 87-89.

45 Stronge, J.L. and Meers, P.D. Hospitals... should do the sick no harm. (Series on infection.) Nursing Times, 76, 24 Jan 1980; 21 Feb 1980; 20 Mar 1980; 17 Apr 1980; 15 May 1980; 19 Jun 1980; 21 Aug 1980.

46 Stronge, J.L. From trolls to tulips. (Study tour of infection control procedures in Scandinavia and Holland.) Nursing Times, 73, 24 Feb 1976, ICNA Supplement, 47-48.

47 Taylor, M.R.H. and others Simple and effective measures for control of enteric cross-infection in a children's hospital. Lancet, 1, 21 Apr 1979, 865-867.

48 Thomas, M. Stamping out the source. (Role of microbiologist in operating theatre.) Health and Social Service Journal, 87, 21 Oct 1977, 1471-1472.

49 Tring, F.C. Cross infection. The danger of scaly skin, (as a major source of dissemination of infection). Nursing Times, 72, 4 Mar 1976, 330-331.

50 Wahba, A.H.W. Hospital infections: a continuing danger to patients and staff. (Current WHO research activities.) WHO Chronicle, 31 (2), Feb 1977, 63-66.

51 Watkin, B. Hospital-acquired infection. Nursing Mirror, 142, 5 Feb 1976, 39.

52 Whitehead, P.D. Control of hospital infection. Nursing Mirror, 143, 9 Dec 1976, 62-64.

53 Williams, J.D. editor Modern topics in infection. Heinemann, 1978.

b INFECTION CONTROL SISTER

1 Barrett-Connor, E. and others, editors Epidemiology for the infection control nurse. St. Louis: Mosby, 1978.

2 Beaufoy, A. and Ratsoy, M.B. Man versus microbe: a case for the infection control nurse. Canadian Nurse, 76 (11), Dec 1980, 30-32.

3 Chavigny, K.H. Hospital epidemiology: a challenge to nursing education. (Education of nurses for infection control posts.) Nursing Education, 4 (1), Jan/Feb 1979, 28-34.

4 Chelgren, G. and LaForce, F.M. Limited periodic surveillance proves practical and effective. (Monitoring of hospital-acquired infections by nurses at Veterans Administration Hospital, Denver.) Hospitals, 52 (6), 16 Mar 1978, 151-152, 154.

5 Emery, H.C. Safety—a concern for the infection control nurse. Hospital Topics, 56 (3), May/Jun 1978, 41-43.

6 Evans, C.S. Communication in infection control. (Charts outlining infection control procedures generally and those specific to each department.) Supervisor Nurse, 8 (9), Sep 1977, 48-49.

7 **Griggs, B.M.** A systems approach to the development and evaluation of a minicourse for nurses: (in nosocomial infections associated with respiratory equipment.) Nursing Research, 26 (1), Jan-Feb 1977, 34-41.

8 **Hindley, K.P.** 100 years' war: the work of the infection control nurse in hospitals. Nursing Mirror, 142, 8 Apr 1976, 67-68.

9 **Infection Control Nurses Association** Contact. Nursing Times, ICNA Supplement.
4. 72, 15 Apr 1976, Supplement, 25-32.
5. 72, 26 Aug 1976, Supplement, 33-40.
6. 73, 24 Feb 1977, Supplement, 41-48.
7. 73, 25 Aug 1977, Supplement, 49-56.
8. 74, 6 Apr 1978, Contact, 1-8.
9. 74, 31 Aug 1978, Contact, 1-8.
10. 74, 7 Dec 1978, Contact, 1-10.
11. 75, 15 Feb 1979, Contact, 1-8.
12. 75, 6 Sep 1979, Contact, 3, 5-6, 8, 10, 13, 15-16, 18-19.

10 **Infection Control Nurses Association** Contact No.12, Sep 1979. (Report of tenth annual symposium at Durham University.) Nursing Times, 75, 6 Sep 1979, Contact, 3, 5-6, 8, 10, 13, 15-16, 18-19.

11 **Journal of Infection Control Nursing** No. 13. February 1980. Nursing Times, 76, 28 Feb 1980, JICN, 1-8.

12 **Katz, E.** The isolation of the infection control officer. Dimensions in Health Service, 56 (12), Dec 1979, 18-20, 22.

13 **Loxton, E.** The infection control sister — aims and objectives. Australian Nurses Journal, 6 (6 and 7), Dec 1976-Jan 1977, 24-25.

14 **Mabbett, A.N.** Infection control: the need for environmental control officers in hospitals. Hospital Topics, 54 (3), May/Jun 1976, 1-3.

15 **Nadolny, M.D.** Infection control in hospitals: what does the infection control nurse do? American Journal of Nursing, 80 (3), Mar 1980, 430-431.

16 **Nursing Times** Infection control training 'does not exist.' Conference urged to implement proposed JBCNS course. Nursing Times, 72, 9 Sep 1976, 1373.

17 **Osborn, P.H.** Developing and maintaining an infection control program. Supervisor Nurse, 8 (12), Dec 1977, 16-18.

18 **Parker, M.** Clinical nurse consultant in infection control. (Symposium paper.) Nursing Mirror, 142, 13 May 1976, 51-53.

19 **Picton, S.J.** JBCNS course no.910 on principles of infection control. (Description of course run at the Royal Free Hospital.) Health Care World Wide, 47, 1, 4.

20 **Stamm, W.E.** Elements of an active, effective infection control program. (Work of an infection control nurse, epidemiologist, and infection control committee.) Hospitals, 50 (23), 1 Dec 1976, 60, 62, 64.

21 **Taylor, L.J.** 910 — the first sixteen. (Report of first JBCNS course on the principles of infection control.) Nursing Times, 74, 31 Aug 1978, Contact, 8.

22 **Trussell, P.M. and Crow, S.** Medical

asepsis, research and continuing education. (Report of research study on effectiveness of continuing education programme.) Journal of Continuing Education in Nursing, 8 (2), Mar-Apr 1977, 17-21.

23 **Turner, J.G.** The nurse epidemiologist: selection and preparation. (Education of infection control nurse.) Supervisor Nurse, 9 (4), Apr 1978, 33-36, 38, 41.

24 **White, P.** Infection control. Epidemiology and infection control. (Four basic epidemiology tools to be used by the infection control officer.) Dimensions in Health Service, 52 (12), Dec 1975, 34, 37, 39.

c CENTRAL STERILE SUPPLY

1 **Alexander, M.** Managing a sterile supply service. Nursing Times, 72 (42), 21 Oct 1976, Theatre nursing supplement, 16, 18, 20.

2 **Association of Sterile Supply Administrators** The management of theatre sterile supply units is the responsibility of the Sterile Supply Manager. NATNews, 13 (3), Apr 1976, 13-16.

3 **Central Sterilising Club** Clean-up. (Report of meeting.) Health and Social Service Journal, 87, 21 Oct 1977, 1467-1474.

4 **Cox, M.** Taking stock of costing. Costing systems for CSSD packs. Health and Social Service Journal, 87, 27 May 1977, 858-859.

5 **Department of Health and Social Security** Steering Committee on the Standardisation of Supplies from Central Sterile Supply Departments Report. DHSS, 1976. (Summarised in HC(78)43.)

6 **Ditchburn, R.** Is a registered nurse justified in today's central supply department? Hospital Administration in Canada, 18 (1), Jan 1976, 20-21.

7 **George, J.C.S.** Some guidance and basic information relating to the washing process of equipment in the CSSD. NATNews, 13 (3), Apr 1976, 19, 21.

8 **Jupp, M.R.** Sterile supplies. Feasibility of CSSD supply to health centres. (Research study of pilot schemes in two health centres in Croydon.) Nursing Times, 75, 6 Dec 1979, 2124-2127.

9 **Keesee, M.A.** Central sterile work core adds space, reduces contamination. (Design of a central sterile corridor to solve problems of overcrowding and rapid growth.) Hospitals, 50 (6), 16 Mar 1976, 119-120, 124, 126-127.

10 **McDougall, S.M.** Standards and standardisation. (Implications of Cunliffe report on CSSDs.) Health and Social Service Journal, 89, 4 May 1979, 543.

11 **Ryan, P.** In-hospital packaging rationale. (Factors considered by the AORN Technical Standards Committee when developing standards for sterile equipment packaging and use.) AORN Journal, 23 (6), May 1976, 980-988.

12 **Tallett, E.H.** Containing sterile fluids: methods and materials available for packaging sterile fluids. Health and Social Service Journal, 87, 21 Oct 1977, 1469.

13 **Webster, H.J.** Quality assurance in the central service department. (Policies for a central

sterile supply department.) Hospital Administration in Canada, 18 (1), Jan 1976, 16-18.

d DISINFECTION AND STERILISATION

1 **Adler, V.G.** Letting off steam in a highly successful technique: the history of low temperature steam and formaldehyde disinfection techniques at Bristol hospitals. Health and Social Service Journal, 87, 21 Oct 1977, 1470-1471.

2 **AORN Journal** Are lab coats acceptable to cover scrub attire? (Policy on operating room wearing apparel.) AORN Journal, 23 (2), Feb 1976, 177-179.

3 **AORN Journal** Guidelines for cleaning and disinfection of flexible fiberoptic endoscopes (FFE) used in GI endoscopy. AORN Journal, 28 (5), Nov 1978, 907, 910.

4 **Brunt, M.** Intensive care — 10. Bacteriological control in intensive therapy. Nursing Times, 74, 20 Apr 1978 , 670-672.

5 **Clarke, B.H.** Thirteen steps to a clean OR. A single decontamination procedure — practical, swift and safe — plus an alert circulating nurse is the most effective combination of all OR cases. Modern Healthcare, 4 (2), Aug 1975, 82-83.

6 **Collins, B.J. and others** A survey of the use and abuse of bedpan macerators. Nursing Times, 76, 28 Feb 1980, JICN 4-6.

7 **Department of Health and Social Security** Sterilizers. HMSO, 1980. (Health technical memorandum; 10.)

8 **Dixon, E.** Aseptic techniques — safeguards for the patient. (In theatre.) Nursing Mirror, 147, 2 Nov 1978, Supplement, ix.

9 **Everall, P.H.** The quality control of sterilization. NATNews, 13 (1), Jan 1976, 7-8, 10-11, 13.

10 **Geelhoed, G.W.** Isolate the infection, not the patient. (Management of sepsis following surgery.) AORN Journal, 28 (1), Jul 1978, 54-61.

11 **Grant, E.M.** The bedpan round. (Letter on danger of infection in present system and need for new equipment.) British Medical Journal, 1, 14 May 1977, 1283.

12 **Haglof, K.** Cleaning, disinfection and handling of fibre optic equipment. Nursing Times, 72 (15), 15 Apr 1976, ICNA Supplement, 30-32.

13 **Hanwell, A.E.** Disinfection of fibreoptic endoscopes. Health and Social Service Journal, 89, 4 May 1979, 544.

14 **Hawkins, C.M.** A survey of systems in use for disposal/disinfection of bedpans and associated equipment. Nursing Times, 75, 6 Sep 1979, Contact 13, 8, 16.

15 **Hawkins, C. and others** Use and abuse of phenolic disinfectants: a preliminary investigation into the possibility of overexposure of babies to phenols. (By infection control nurses in Bristol.) Nursing Times, 74, 6 Apr 1978, Contact, 4-5.

16 **Huth, M.E.** Principles of asepsis. AORN Journal, 24 (4), Oct 1976, 790, 792-793, 796.

17 Kowaksli, J. and Peck, P. Standards needed for sterilization monitoring. (Sterilization control program at St. Mary's Hospital, Milwaukee.) Hospital Progress, 57 (4), Apr 1976, 52-54.

18 MacClelland, D.C. Sterilization by ionizing radiation. AORN Journal, 26 (4), Oct 1977, 675-680, 683-684.

19 McGuiness, W.J. Alternative method of drying. (Arklone drying process for surgical instruments.) Health and Social Service Journal, 87, 21 Oct 1977, 1472-1473.

20 McLauchlan, J. Aseptic micro-environments for joint replacement surgery. Nursing Mirror, 142, 15 Jan 1976, 47-49.

21 Meers, P.D. Hospitals...should do the sick no harm. 5. Combating infection by disinfection. Nursing Times, 76, 15 May 1980, (4).

22 Mitchell, N.J. Disposable clothing in operating theatres and its effectiveness in reducing aerial microbial contamination. NATNews, 15 (10), Oct 1978, 22, 24.

23 Mitchell, N.J. Is theatre clothing any use? (Experiments with design and fabric.) Nursing Mirror, 147, 2 Nov 1978, Supplement, iv, vii.

24 Mitchell, N.J. and others Reduction of skin bacteria in theatre air with comfortable, non-woven disposable clothing for operating-theatre staff. British Medical Journal, 1, 18 Mar 1978, 696-698.

25 Mullick, A. Control of airborne infection using a mobile horizontal laminar air-flow system. NATNews, 15 (7), Jul 1978, 10-12.

26 NATNews A fresh look at antiseptics in hospital. NATNews, 13 (7), Sep 1976, 30-31.

27 Nelson, J.P. Effectiveness, costs of clean rooms, helmet aspirators. (Used in orthopaedic operations.) AORN Journal, 27 (4), Mar 1978, 718, 720, 722, 724, 726, 728, 730, 732, 734.

28 Noy, M. and others Disinfection of plastic aprons. Nursing Times, 72 (34), 26 Aug 1976, ICNA Supplement, 39-40.

29 Public Health Laboratory Service Communicable Disease Surveillance Centre A salmonella outbreak. (Spread by bedpan washers.) British Medical Journal, 2, 10 Sep 1977, 713.

30 Richardson, A.M. The importance of being well-dressed in the theatre. (In order to prevent cross-infection.) NATNews, 15 (4), Apr 1978, 14-15, 17.

31 Schrader, E.S. What price asepsis? (The problem of wound infection in the surgery patient, the burn patient, and the immuno-suppressed patient.) AORN Journal, 25 (1), Jan 1977, 136, 138, 140, 142.

32 Seaman, R.E. The challenge of barrier testing. (Testing effectiveness of materials in blocking pathogens with reference to gowns, caps, drapes, etc.) AORN Journal, 31 (2), Feb 1980, 213-214, 216, 218, 220.

33 Shepherd, B.J. Closed-glove technique. (Letter commenting on its use as part of aseptic procedure.) NATNews, 14 (5), Jul 1977, 16, 18.

34 Shepherd, B.J. To continue—closed glove technique. NATNews, 14 (9), Dec 1977, 8.

35 Shepherd, B.J. The importance of being well-dressed in the theatre. (To prevent cross-infection.) NATNews, 15 (7), Jul 1978, 6, 8.

36 Silvester, J.C. The use of isolators in surgery. (To control sterility of the operating field, with reference to hip surgery.) Nursing Times, 74, 24 Aug 1978, 1411-1413.

37 Skingle, D. Ethylene oxide gas sterilisation meets a growing need. NATNews, 17 (1), Jan 1980, 8-9.

38 Smith, B.J. Closed gowning and gloving technique. (With ten photographs.) NATNews, 14 (6), Aug 1977, 12, 14.

39 Stronge, J.L. Hospitals...should do the sick no harm. 4. Combating infection. 1. Introduction, and sterilisation. Nursing Times, 76, 17 Apr 1980, (4).

40 Tabb, J.M. Non-touch technique for putting on sterile gloves. (With diagrams.) NATNews, 14 (9), Dec 1977, 10-11.

41 Tomalin, C. Hospital cleaning and patient infections. (King's Fund conference.) Health and Social Service Journal, 86, 24 Jan 1976, 163.

42 White, D.A. Are telephones an infection hazard? British Medical Journal, 1, 8 Mar 1980, 696-697.

43 Williams, S.C.H. and Mansell, R. Fluid-ised sand beds—a cross infection risk? A study of bacterial dissemination among patients nursed on sand beds. Nursing Times, 75, 22 Mar 1979, 489-490.

44 Woodside, W. Sterile fluids—recent developments. NATNews, 16 (5), May 1979, 10, 12.

e DISINFECTION OF THE SKIN

1 Amortegui, A.J. and Buffenmyer, C. Comparison of the antiseptic effect of two iodophor preparations on hand washing in a well-baby nursery. (Betadine and Prepodyne.) Journal of Gynecological and Neonatal Nursing, 7 (6), Nov/Dec 1978, 35-38.

2 AORN Journal Question and answer on value of pre-operative shaving with references. AORN Journal, 30 (2), Aug 1979, 266, 268.

3 AORN Journal Standards for preoperative skin preparation of patients. AORN Journal, 23 (6), May 1976, 974-975.

4 AORN Journal Standards for surgical hand scrubs. AORN Journal, 23 (6), May 1976, 976-977.

5 Breitung, J. Are you fudging on hand-washing routines? (Pathogens transmitted and recommended washing procedure.) RN Magazine, 40 (6), Jun 1977, 71.

6 Casewell, M. and Phillips, I. Hands as routes of transmission for Klebsiella species. (Cross infection in intensive care unit.) British Medical Journal, 2, 19 Nov 1977, 1315-1317.

7 Flournoy, D.J. and others Nosocomial infection linked to handwashing. (Report of study.) Hospitals, 53 (15), 1 Aug 1979, 105-107.

8 Krutz, J.B. and Boxall, J. Cross infection. A

partial substitute for hand washing. (A study comparing normal hand washing with the application of a disinfectant—alcoholic chlorhexidine.) Nursing Times, 72 (9), 4 Mar 1976, 332-333.

9 Moore, M. and Abbott, N.K. Can hand-washing practices be changed? (Short account of research study.) American Journal of Nursing, 80 (1), Jan 1980, 80.

10 Powis, S.J.A. and others Preoperative skin preparation: clinical evaluation of depilatory cream. (Comparison with routine shaving.) British Medical Journal, 1976, 2, 13 Nov 1976, 1166-1168.

11 Taylor, L.J. An evaluation of handwashing techniques. Nursing Times, 74, 12 Jan 1978, 54-55; 19 Jan 1978, 108-110.

12 Wilson, V. Routine shaving and wound infection. (History, research and AORN recommendations.) AORN Journal, 28 (4), Oct 1978, 762, 764, 766, 768, 770.

f ISOLATION UNITS AND BARRIER NURSING

1 Ayliffe, G.A.J. and others A unit for source and protective isolation in a general hospital. (Study of cross-infection, techniques of isolation nursing and assessment of value of isolation unit.) British Medical Journal, 2, 25 Aug 1979, 461-465.

2 Bagshawe, K.D. and others Isolating patients in hospital to control infection. British Medical Journal, 2.
1. Sources and routes of infection. 26 Aug 1978, 609-612.
2. Who should be isolated, and where? 2 Sep 1978, 684-686.
3. Design and construction of isolation accommodation. 9 Sep 1978, 744-748.
4. Nursing procedures. 16 Sep 1978, 808-811.
5. An isolation system. 23 Sep 1978, 879-881.

3 Brewis, E.L. and others Practical aspects of nursing children under the laminar flow 1. (Unit at the Royal Hospital for Sick Children, Yorkhill, Glasgow, where leukaemia patients are nursed in pathogen-free environment.) Nursing Times, 73, 21 Jul 1977, 1120-1124.

4 Brewis, E.L. and others Nursing children under the laminar flow 2. A boy with leukaemia. (Case study of child in hospital and at home.) Nursing Times, 73, 28 Jul 1977, 1154-1156.

5 Chambers, J. Leslie's story. (Experience of Leslie Dewhurst in an isolator unit following bone marrow transplant.) Nursing Times, 73, 17 Feb 1977, 221-225.

6 Demetriou, A. and others A secure isolation unit in Manchester. (To deal with patients suspected of having dangerous imported infections, eg Lassa fever.) Nursing Times, 75, 15 Feb 1979, 274-276.

7 Fradd, E.H. Containment of salmonellosis in a baby ward. Barrier nursing using an isolator tent. Nursing Times, 75, 12 Apr 1979, 630-632.

8 Quirk, P. Very clean food for the very special patient. (For use with children in isolator tents at Westminster Children's Hospital who undergo bone marrow transplantation.) Health and Social Service Journal, 88, Jan 1978, 106-108.

9 Riemensnider, D.K. and Richards, R.F. Providing supportive information to the patient in isolation. 'Educational prescription' form aids in explaining isolation procedures, precautions to patient and his family. Hospitals, 51 (11), 1 Jun 1977, 103-104, 106.

10 Stronge, J.L. Hospitals...should do the sick no harm. 12. Controlling infection by isolation 2. Nursing Times, 76, 18/25 Dec 1980, (4).

11 Tyrrell, D.A.J. and others An isolation unit in a district general hospital. (Northwick Park.) British Medical Journal, 2, 6 Aug 1977, 373-374.

12 Walters, E.M. Barrier nursing...superstition or science? Nursing Times, 72 (34), 26 Aug 1976, ICNA Supplement, 35.

67 ACCIDENTS AND EMERGENCIES

a SERVICES

1 Ashton, K. Immediate care in the country. (Report on conference organised by South Powys Rcn centre, involving ambulance personnel and medical staff as well as nurses.) Nursing Times, 74, 10 Aug 1978, 1313.

2 Atherley, G.R.C. Accidents and failing to cope disease. Occupational Health, 29 (3), Mar 1977, 115-117.

3 Brett, T. Flying squad to the rescue. (Operated by Derbyshire Royal Infirmary.) Health and Social Service Journal, 90, 29 Aug 1980, 1131-1133.

4 British Medical Journal Accident and emergency services. British Medical Journal, 2. Introduction. 6 Oct 1979, 837-839.
The network of services. 13 Oct 1979, 917-919.
Disasters, flying squads and immediate care. 20 Oct 1979, 973-975.
How should accident and emergency departments be run? 27 Oct 1979, 1051-1053.
The staffing of departments. 3 Nov 1979, 1119-1121.
Design of departments. 10 Nov 1979, 1204-1207.
The needs of the community. 24 Nov 1979, 1348-1350.

5 Brown, P.T. and Murray, A. The modern ambulance service. Nursing Times, 72, 29 Apr 1976, 649-650.

6 Burges, S.H. Interface. The police surgeon. Nursing Times, 72, 25 Nov 1976, 1845-1848.

7 Cowley, A. Ambulanceman. Nursing Mirror, 143, 9 Dec 1976, 47-48.

8 Cowper-Smith, F. Mobile accident unit at East Birmingham Hospital. Nursing Times, 42, 2 Dec 1976, 1868-1869.

9 Davy, R.G. Mobile accident team. (Hillingdon Hospital.) Nursing Mirror, 144, 27 Jan 1977, 39-40.

10 Devlin, R. How an air ambulance brings a new heart. (Work of Scottish Air Ambulance Service.) Nursing Mirror, 150, 19 Jun 1980, 18-21.

11 Dow, A.R. Better wise before the event.

(Problems in integrating new accident and emergency unit into Sunderland District General Hospital.) Health and Social Service Journal, 89, 14 Dec 1979, 1608-1609.

12 Easton, K. editor Rescue emergency care. Heinemann, 1977.

13 Fletcher, S.B. A different approach to accident and emergency services—the French experience. Hospital and Health Services Review, 74 (5), May 1978, 152-156.

14 Gage, B. Steering the fleet towards a smoother running service. (Efficient management of the NHS ambulance service.) Health and Social Service Journal, 87, 15 Apr 1977, 662-663.

15 Gardiner, J. Advanced ambulance training. (Training scheme in Gloucestershire and care of patient by ambulancemen in mobile resuscitation unit.) Nursing Times, 75, 12 Jul 1979, 1168-1171.

16 Harris, N. Rough start but wheels of progress show promise. (West Midlands ambulance control system.) Health and Social Service Journal, 86, 28 Aug 1976, 1548-1549.

17 Health and Social Service Journal Six articles on the ambulance service. Health and Social Service Journal, 89, 25 Jan 1979, 58-72.

18 Hospital and Health Services Review The work and organisation of the ambulance service. Hospital and Health Services Review, 73 (4), Apr 1977, 141-143.

19 Hoy, M. Not 'just another casualty'. (Role of multidisciplinary team in A and E department including deciding priorities of care.) Nursing, 15, Jul 1980, 633-634, 637.

20 Hyde, A. Giving help at high speed. (Work of accident and emergency department at Luton and Dunstable Hospital with statistics on costs.) Health and Social Service Journal, 90, 4 Jan 1980, 26-27.

21 Ingham, M. Anatomy of an emergency service. (Accident flying squad in Lincolnshire.) Health and Social Service Journal, 88, 3 Nov 1978, 1245-1246.

22 Joint Consultative Committee Accident and emergency services: report on staffing. Has some comment on facilities and postregistration training of nursing staff.) British Medical Journal, 2, 18 Nov 1978, 1447-1448.

23 Kaye, V. Six hundred square miles that add up to a heavy workload. (The London Ambulance Service.) Health and Social Service Journal, 87, 7 Oct 1977, 1402-1403.

24 Lilley, W. Interface. The ambulanceman. Nursing Times, 72, 29 Apr 1976, 647-649.

25 May, D. Ty Bronna—the vital link. (New H.Q. for South Glamorgan ambulance service operating the first integrated radio control centre for local NHS transport.) Nursing Mirror, 143, 9 Sep 1976, 62-64.

26 Morris, J.B. and Hird, M.D. A survey of new attenders at the accident and emergency department of the small specialist hospital—Angus District. (Involved nurses in data collection and studies need for assessment by doctor or nurse.) Health Bulletin, 37 (4), May 1979, 108-116.

27 Mouzas, G.L. A handbook for the

accident and emergency department. Heinemann Medical, 1979.

28 Nursing Saving lives. Part 1. Nursing, 14, Jun 1980, 585-628.

29 Nursing Times London Ambulance Service. (History from 1882 and service today.) Nursing Times, 73, 22 Sep 1977, Archive, 29-32.

30 Oakes, A.R. Trauma: twentieth century epidemic. (History, present and future.) Heart Lung, 8 (5), Sep/Oct 1979, 918-922.

31 O'Flanagan, P. The work of an accident and emergency department. (Survey of patients seen in a six month period in one hospital.) Journal of the Royal College of General Practitioners, 26, Jan 1976, 54-60.

32 Pollard, M. Steering clear of hazards in the drive for safety first. (Health and Safety policy for ambulancemen.) Health and Social Service Journal, 87, 26 Aug 1977, 1214-1215.

33 Rains, A.J.H. and others Emergency and acute care. Hodder and Stoughton, 1976.

34 Rawlins, T. Problems of extreme weather in Sweden. (How accident and emergency services cope.) Nursing Times, 76, 31 Jul 1980, 1367-1368.

35 Salvage, J. Under fire from all sides. (Problems facing the ambulance service.) Nursing Mirror, 151, 31 Jul 1980, 8.

36 Scott, S. The mobile accident unit. (At East Birmingham Hospital. Symposium paper.) Nursing Mirror, 145, 6 Oct 1977, 14-15.

37 Shirvore, R.S. Patient management on the road. (The difference in the working environment between the hospital and incident situation.) Nursing Mirror, 143, 9 Dec 1976, 45-46.

38 Snook, R. and Pacifico, R. Ambulance ride: fixed or floating stretcher? British Medical Journal, 2, 14 Aug 1976, 405-407.

39 Weeks, L. The ambulance service. Nursing, 14, Jun 1980, 592-594.

40 Wilson, D.H. and Hall, M.H. Casualty officer's handbook. 4th ed. Butterworths, 1979.

b NURSING

1 Albin, S.L. and others Evaluation of emergency room triage performed by nurses. (Bronx Municipal Hospital Center, New York.) Hospital Tropics, 55 (1), Jan/Feb 1977, 45-50.

2 Bailey, J.A. Development of a regional trauma center: nursing approach. (At University Hospital, San Diego, California.) Nursing Clinics of North America, 13 (2), Jun 1978, 255-265.

3 Barber, J.M. and Budassi, S.A. Mosby's manual of emergency care: practices and procedures. St. Louis: Mosby, 1979.

4 Barry, J. editor Emergency nursing. New York: McGraw-Hill, 1978.

5 Bradley, D. Accident and emergency nursing. Baillière Tindall, 1980. (Nurses' aid series: special interest texts.)

6 Bucknall, T.E. ASSIST. (Order of priorities for nursing care of patients with severe multiple injuries.) Nursing Times, 75, 1 Nov 1979, 1902-1903.

7 Caldwell, P. Continuing education for emergency nurses (California-Style.) Journal of Emergency Nursing, 3 (4), Jul/Aug 1977, 27-32.

8 Calkin, J.D. and Gulbrandsen, M.W. Nursing practice decisions in emergencies: a course and how it was designed. Journal of Nursing Education, 17 (9), Nov 1978, 30-37.

9 Dyck, K. and others Sample standard nursing care plans for patients in emergency departments: a working document. Vancouver: Registered Nurses' Association of British Columbia, 1977.

10 Everett, P. A case for justice. (Forensic medicine and advice to accident and emergency nurses on dealing with murdered patients.) Nursing Mirror, 149, 15 Nov 1979, 30-31.

11 GIVING emergency care competently. Horsham: Intermed Communications Inc., 1978. (Nursing skillbook series.)

12 Harrison, M. Role of the nurse in resuscitation and intensive care. (Symposium on road traffic accidents.) Nursing Mirror, 145, 6 Oct 1977, 16-17.

13 Howell, R.G. Accident and emergency services: how does your department compare? (Operational research study of time spent by patients in A & E department.) Hospital and Health Services Review, 74 (4), Apr 1978, 116-118.

14 Huckstep, R.L. A simple guide to trauma. 2nd ed. Churchill Livingstone, 1978.

15 Iveson-Iveson, J. Disease: its cause and effect. 8. Induced disease. (Treatment and nursing care of trauma.) Nursing Mirror, 149, 1 Nov 1979, 20-21.

16 Karn, H.M. The nurse and the provision of primary care in accident departments. (Includes advice on management of department and treatment including triage.) New Zealand Nursing Journal, 71 (9), Sep 1978, 20-23.

17 Lanros, N.E. Assessment and intervention in emergency nursing. Bowie, Maryland: Brady, 1978.

18 Lewin, D.C. The nursing management of major accidents. The author, 1976. (Leverhulme Nursing Fellowship, 1976.)

19 McMorrow, G. An emergency room audit for a small hospital. Supervisor Nurse, 9 (8), Aug 1978, 33-35.

20 Mann, J.K. and Oakes, A.R. Critical care nursing of the multi-injured patient. Philadelphia: Saunders, 1980.

21 Marsh, T.O. A nurses' guide to sleuthing (or, how to collect evidence, hospital style). (Importance of careful observation of patients with injuries where violence is the suspected cause.) RN Magazine, 41 (8), Aug 1978, 48-50.

22 Mathewson, H.S. Organizing your acute care teams. RN Magazine, 39 (11), Nov 1976, OR 6-7.

23 Milde, F.K. and others Continuing education needs of registered nurses in Iowa Hospital emergency departments. (Research

study.) Journal of Continuing Education in Nursing, 11 (1), Jan/Feb 1980, 29-35.

24 Molyneux-Luick, M. The ABCs of multiple trauma. Nursing, 7 (10), Oct 1977, 30, 32-36.

25 Norman, J. and Moles, T.M. editors Management of the injured patient. Macmillan Journals, 1978.

26 Nursing Clinics of North America Symposium on trauma. Nursing Clinics of North America, 13 (2), Jun 1978, 175-265.

27 Paxton, J. Pictures in nursing. Emergency resuscitation. Nursing, 15, Jul 1980, 649-651.

28 Pink, N. Triage in the accident and emergency department. (Putting patients into three categories of priority.) Australian Nurses Journal, 6 (9), Mar 1977, 35-36.

29 Roberts, K.M. and others Changing perceptions of organizational communication: can short term intervention help? (A training program in an emergency room of a large metropolitan hospital.) Nursing Research, 25 (3), May/Jun 1976, 197-200.

30 Simchuk, C.J. Development of criteria for emergency department nursing audit. Journal of Emergency Nursing, 3 (5), Sep/Oct 1977, 47-49.

31 Stanley, L. 'Expanded-role' nursing hits the hospitals. (Nurse practitioner in accident and emergency department.) RN Magazine, 41 (10), Oct 1978, 57-59.

32 Stevenson, J.S. and others A plan for nurse staffing in hospital emergency services. New York: National League for Nursing, 1978.

33 Waeckerle, J.F. and others The emergency nurse as a primary health care provider: a retrospective study. (Expanded role of nurse in triage in emergency department.) Journal of Emergency Nursing, 3 (4), Jul/Aug 1977, 21-25.

34 Warner, C.G. editor Emergency care: assessment and intervention. 2nd ed. St. Louis: Mosby, 1978.

35 Williams, M. Birmingham Accident nurses. AGM. (Occupational Health Nurses Association, Birmingham Accident Hospital conference.) Occupational Health, 28 (5), May 1976, 253-254.

36 Wood, K.M. Nurse-patient communication in an accident department. MSc thesis, University of Manchester, Department of Nursing, 1979.

c PATIENT AND FAMILY

1 Ahamed, M. Follow-up of children age 0-5 years seen in accident and emergency unit. (Report of two surveys by HVs.) Health Visitor, 51 (3), Mar 1978, 84-86.

2 Andrianos, A.F. and Swain, C.R. Interfacing the role of a psychiatric clinical nurse specialist with a hospital emergency room setting. Journal of Psychiatric Nursing, 17 (4), Apr 1979, 24-27.

3 Brown, E.A. Psychiatric problems in A & E departments. Nursing Times, 74, 17 Aug 1978, 1369-1371.

4 Burgess, A.W. and Johansen, P.M. Assault:

patterns of emergency visits. (Survey at Boston City Hospital of the number and patterns of victimization over a monthly period.) Journal of Psychiatric Nursing and Mental Health Services, 14 (11), Nov 1976, 32-36.

5 Canright, P. and Campbell, M.J. Nursing care of the child and his family in the emergency department. Pediatric Nursing, 3 (4), Jul/Aug 1977, 43-45.

6 Cowper-Smith, F. Violence in casualty departments. (Evidence from The Middlesex, East Birmingham, Liverpool and Maudsley Hospitals.) Nursing Times, 73, 7 Apr 1977, 482-485.

7 Darby, C. Nurses, surgeons clash on A & E violence report. (Report of meeting of Rcn Accident and Emergency Forum and Casualty Surgeons Association.) Nursing Mirror, 146, 11 May 1978, 2. Also reported in Nursing Times, 74, 11 May 1978, 774.

8 Eggland, E.T. The anxious family in the emergency room. (Nurse's role in care.) Nursing Care, 8 (11), Nov 1975, 28-29, 31-32.

9 Hankoff, L.D. and others Crisis intervention in the emergency room. (Counselling by nurses of emergency room patients.) Nursing Digest, 2 (8), Oct 1974, 11-13.

10 Jackson, R.H. and Wilkinson, A.W. Why don't we prevent childhood accidents? (Analysis of main causes and suggestions for prevention.) British Medical Journal, 1, 22 May 1976, 1258-1262.

11 Jeffery, R. Normal rubbish: deviant patients in casualty departments. (Attitudes of staff to certain types of patients such as drunks, tramps and people who have taken overdoses.) Sociology of Health and Illness, 1 (1), Jun 1979, 90-107.

12 McFarlane, J.M. Pediatric care in the emergency room. A contemporary re-evaluation. Pediatric Nursing, 2 (2), Mar/Apr 1976, 22-25.

13 McKnight, W. Understanding the patient in emergency. (Psychosocial care.) Canadian Nurse, 72 (7), Jul 1976, 20-23.

14 Miller, M. Patient teaching in the emergency department. Journal of Emergency Nursing, 4 (1), Jan/Feb 1978, 21-23.

15 Nicklin, W. McK. The role of the family in the emergency department. (With reference to nurse's role in teaching relatives.) Canadian Nurse, 75 (4), Apr 1979, 40-43.

16 Nyberg, J. Perception of patient problems in the emergency department. (Research study of nurses and patients to discover how the two groups rated the severity of problems.) Journal of Emergency Nursing, 4 (1), Jan/Feb 1978, 15-19.

17 Pisarcik, G. and others Psychiatric nurses in the emergency room. (Part of emergency department staff at Boston City Hospital who interview patients with emotional or psychiatric problems.) American Journal of Nursing, 79 (7), Jul 1979, 1264-1266.

18 Royal College of Nursing. Joint Working Party on Violence in the Accident and Emergency Department Discussion paper. Rcn, 1978.

19 Royal Society of Health Strict measures proposed to reduce A & E violence. (Report of Royal Society of Health conference on violence in the general hospital.) Nursing Times, 74, 2 Mar 1978, 342.

20 Royal Society of Health Journal Violence in the general hospital. (Two articles with reference to accident and emergency departments.) Royal Society of Health Journal, 98 (4), Aug 1978, 187-190, 198.

21 Sharer, P.S. Helping survivors cope with the shock of sudden death. (With reference to the emergency department.) Nursing (U.S.), 9 (1), Jan 1979, 20-21.

22 Sherber, J. and Russell, H.J. Emotional aspects of trauma and treatment, too. (Work of a counsellor trained in crisis intervention.) Modern Healthcare, 5 (6), Jun 1976, 37-39.

23 Speich, P.L. Taking a psychosocial stress 'pulse'. (Advice to emergency nurses on assessment of patients' stress levels.) Journal of Emergency Nursing, 5 (4), Jul/Aug 1979, 43-47.

24 Valman, H.B. Accident and emergency paediatrics. 2nd ed. Oxford: Blackwell, 1979.

25 Whitehead, T. A & E departments need psychiatric nurse back-up. (Talk on 'The violent patient in hospital.') Nursing Times, 73, 15 Dec 1977, 1938.

26 Whitehead, T. A psychiatric presence in the accident and emergency department. World Medicine, 13 (16), 17 May 1978, 93, 95.

27 Whitehead, T. Psychiatry as an emergency service: the growing need for psychiatrically trained staff in every accident and emergency department. Nursing Mirror, 147, 10 Aug 1978, 17.

28 Wilson, D.H. Every emergency department should have one—an interview room. British Medical Journal, 1, 10 Jan 1976, 87-88.

29 Winterbottom, S. Violence in the accident and emergency department. Nursing Mirror, 146, 15 Jun 1978, 21-23.

d FIRST AID

1 Andrew, R. First aid in pictures. Wolfe, 1976.

2 Barrett, J. Bandaging techniques and treatment for other minor injuries. (Use in accident and emergency departments.) Nursing Times, 76, 26 Jun 1980, 1127-1132.

3 Emerson, E. If only... (Details of Heimlich Maneuver with choking patients.) Journal of Practical Nursing, 27 (8), Aug 1977, 14-15.

4 Gardner, A.W. and Roylance, P.J. New advanced first aid. 2nd ed. Bristol: Wright, 1977.

5 Glendon, I. and McKenna, S. Attitudes to first aid. (Report of research project—FACT (UK).) Occupational Health, 30 (12), Dec 1978, 605-607.

6 Haghenbeck, K. Quick! What's your first move when a patient chokes? RN Magazine, 42 (12), Dec 1979, 55-59, 61-62.

7 Homewood, J. The role of the first aider in small industries. (Report of survey.) Occupational Health, 30 (12), Dec 1978, 581-584.

8 Jacka, S.M. and Griffiths, D.G. Treatment room nursing: a handbook for nursing sisters working in general practice, schools and industry. Blackwell, 1976.

9 Lucas, B. editor First aid in the home. St. John Ambulance Association and Brigade, 1978.

10 McKenna, S.P. and others First aid training—does it really make you safer? (Findings of three research studies in factories.) Occupational Safety and Health, 8 (5), Sep 1978, 28-30.

11 Marsden, N. Diagnosis before first aid: a manual for emergency care workers. Churchill Livingstone, 1978.

12 Nicholson, H.M. Dress rehearsal for calamity. (Work of the Casualties Union—teaching first aid and simulating emergency situations.) Journal of the Society of Occupational Medicine, 27 (1), Jan 1977, 31-33.

13 Occupational Health Occupational first aid. Occupational Health, 31.
3. Choking. (Includes Heimlich manoeuvre.) (1), Jan 1979, Suppl. (4).
4. Dressings. (2), Feb 1979, Suppl. (4).
5. Control of bleeding. (3), Mar 1979, Suppl. (4).
6. Unconsciousness. (5), May 1979, Suppl. (4).

14 Occupational Health Occupational first aid. Occupational Health, 32.
12. New legislation. (1), Jan 1980, Suppl. (4).
13. New legislation—reactions. 1. (Rcn comments.) (6), Jun 1980, Suppl. (4).

15 Proctor, H. and London, P.S. Principles of first aid for the injured. 3rd ed. Butterworth, 1977.

16 Richards, N.C.G. Treatment of choking. A new first aid method. Nursing Times, 73, 9 Jun 1977, 856-857.

17 Ruben, H. and Macnaughton, F.I. The treatment of food-choking. (Comparison of Heimlich's manoeuvre with other first-aid measures.) Practitioner, 221, Nov 1978, 725-729.

18 Skeet, M. First aid in the street and home. Nursing, 14, Jun 1980, 615-620.

19 Skeet, M. Principles and practice of first aid. Nursing Mirror, 146, Supplement, i-iv.
1. Coronary occlusion and other emergencies. 23 Feb 1978.
2. Preventing the need for first aid. 2 Mar 1978.
4. Transport of casualties. 23 Mar 1978.
5. Fractures. 30 Mar 1978.
6. The control of bleeding. 20 Apr 1978.
7. Poisoning and other emergencies. 27 Apr 1978.

20 Swanson, I. First aid rooms. (Comprehensive advice.) Occupational Health, 29 (7), Jul 1977, 292-301.

21 University of Aston Department of Safety and Hygiene First aid training and its effect on safety. (In industry.) Occupational Health, 29 (10), Oct 1977, 426-431.

e HEAD INJURIES

1 Adams, J.H. Patients who talk and die after a non-missile head injury. Nursing Mirror, 142, 22 Apr 1976, 55-56.

2 Anwar, M. Head injury: nurses found Flora's way home. (Rehabilitation of elderly car crash victim in geriatric unit.) Nursing Mirror, 149, 23 Aug 1979, 34-35.

3 Bailey, J. Head trauma: when careful assessment's a matter of life and death. RN Magazine, 42 (5), May 1979, 44-54.

4 Caswell, A. Nursing care study. Skull fracture: emergency in the Falklands! (Care of 22-month-old child.) Nursing Mirror, 149, 30 Aug 1979, 30-32.

5 Coplestone, J.A. Nursing care study. Head injury. (By student nurse.) Nursing Times, 76, 3 Apr 1980, 591-595.

6 Cross, A. Nursing care of patients with head injuries. (Symposium paper.) Nursing Mirror, 145, 13 Oct 1977, 21-24.

7 Field, J.H. Epidemiology of head injuries in England and Wales with particular application to rehabilitation. Department of Health and Social Security, 1976.

8 Gordon, D. Depressed fractures and missile wounds of the skull. Nursing Mirror, 142, 26 Feb 1976, 45-46.

9 Humphrey, M. and Oddy, M. The social costs of head injuries. (Research study with patients and relatives by two psychologists.) New Society, 45, 31 Aug 1978, 452-453.

10 Jones, C. Monitoring recovery after head injury: translating research into practice. (Use of Glasgow Coma Scale, Galveston Orientation and Amnesia Test and Glasgow Outcome Scale.) Journal of Neurosurgical Nursing, 11 (4), Dec 1979, 192-198.

11 Kendall, T. and Taurah, H. Head injury complicated by urinary tract infection and possible renal failure. (Care of Rampton Hospital patient at Rampton and two other hospitals.) Nursing Times, 76, 19 Jun 1980, 1099-1100.

12 Kunkel, J. and Wiley, J.K. Acute head injury: what to do when...and why. Nursing (U.S.), 9 (3), Mar 1979, 23-33.

13 Lewin, W. Changing attitudes to the management of severe head injuries. British Medical Journal, 2, 20 Nov 1976, 1234-1239.

14 Lincoln, N.B. Behaviour modification in physiotherapy. (Techniques used at Rivermead Rehabilitation Centre, Oxford, with head-injured patients.) Physiotherapy, 64 (9), Sep 1978, 265-267.

15 Murdoch, A.E. A patient with a depressed fracture of the skull. Advances in surgery and supportive treatment saved a victim of the troubles in Northern Ireland from a vegetative existence. Nursing Times, 76, 29 May 1980, 972-975.

16 Proctor, H. Management of head injuries. (Symposium paper.) Nursing Mirror, 145, 13 Oct 1977, 19-21.

17 Roach, J. Head injuries and the theatre nurse. NATNews, 14 (1), Jan 1977, 10, 12-13, 17.

18 Rose, J. and others Avoidable factors contributing to death after head injury. (Review of 116 patients.) British Medical Journal, 2, 3 Sep 1977, 615-618.

f HOME ACCIDENTS

1 Adair, D. and others A project on home accidents. (Survey by student HVs.) Health Visitor, 53 (5), May 1980, 158-160.

2 Department of Prices and Consumer Protection A commentary on electrical fatalities in the home 1974-75. The Department, 1976.

3 Guy, C.J. Home accidents—could they be reduced? (Survey of 2,563 accidents treated at Bedford General Hospital 1972-1974.) Health and Social Service Journal, 86, 10 Jan 1976, 62.

4 Mackessack Deitch, K. Domestic accidents: their cause and prevention. Journal of the Royal College of General Practitioners, 28, Jan 1978, 38-40, 42-43, 45.

5 Occupational Health Home, hazardous home. (Proposals for a national survey of home accidents by the Department of Prices and Consumer Protection.) Occupational Health, 28 (4), Apr 1976, 179-181.

g INJURIES: MISCELLANEOUS

1 Archer, R. Nursing care study. Snakebite. Nursing Times, 73, 10 Feb 1977, 206-209.

2 Baughman, D. The frozen patient: handle with care. (Hypothermia, with extensive bibliography.) RN Magazine, 42 (11), Nov 1979, 38-42.

3 Budassi, S.A. Chest trauma. Nursing Clinics of North America, 13 (3), Sep 1978, 533-541.

4 Chhabra, S.L. Injuries to the elbow. Nursing Times, 74, 27 Jul 1978, 1252-1254.

5 Dickins, B.F. David: a case for ventilation. (Care in A and E department and ITU of man with chest injuries.) Nursing, 7, Nov 1979, 310-314.

6 Fernsebner, B. A protocol for malignant hyperthermia. AORN Journal, 31 (5), Apr 1980, 814-818.

7 Fryer, J.A. Crush injury to the arm. Nursing Times, 72 (42), 21 Oct 1976, Theatre nursing supplement, 11-14.

8 Graff, C. Warning: don't jump to conclusions when a patient's in shock. RN Magazine, 42 (8), Aug 1979, 23-28.

9 Hartley, M.B. Hypothermia. AORN Journal, 24 (4), Oct 1976, 764, 766-767, 769.

10 Hedberg, D.T. Shock. American Association of Nurse Anesthetists Journal, 44 (5), Oct 1976, 508-512.

11 Holt, D. Anaphylactic shock. A shock that's easy to see. Nursing Mirror, 148, 31 May 1979, 32-34.

12 Hulme, J. How to remove fish-hooks. Nursing Mirror, 145, 29 Dec 1977, 23.

13 Jackson, H. Nursing care of patients with chest injuries. (With section on central venous pressure.) Nursing, 7, Nov 1979, 303-309.

14 Katsaros, C. and Bobb, J. Shock—the critical hour. (Time when resuscitation efforts are likely to succeed.) Journal of Emergency Nursing, 4 (5), Sep/Oct 1978, 45-50.

15 Maclean, D. and Emslie-Smith, D. Accidental hypothermia. Blackwell, 1977.

16 McMaster, P. Major hepatic injury: liver injuries shouldn't be such a killer. Better management to cut deaths. Nursing Mirror, 147, 12 Oct 1978, 37-39.

17 Nairn, D. Hypovolaemic shock. Bleeding: a shock to the system. Nursing Mirror, 148, 22 Mar 1979, 40-42.

18 Nursing Mirror Nursing Mirror Forum 77, Birmingham. Road traffic accidents. Nursing Mirror, 145, 6, 13, 20 and 27 Oct 1977. Includes: Harrison, M. Nursing care of chest injuries. 20 Oct 1977, 22-24.
Horner, M. Nursing care of abdominal and pelvic injuries. 20 Oct 1977, 28-29.
London, P.S. The management of multiple injuries. 27 Oct 1977, 17-19.
Thomas, C. Effects of shock on the human body. 3 Oct 1977, 17-19, and Management of chest injuries. 20 Oct 1977, 19-21.
Tubbs, N. Management of abdominal and pelvic injuries. 20 Oct 1977, 25-27.

19 Owens, E.R. Road traffic accident—case report. (By ambulanceman.) Nursing Mirror, 145, 25 Aug 1977, 16-18.

20 Pattison, B. Nursing care study. Emergency call. (Plank from a fence driven through the chest wall in a car accident.) Nursing Times, 42, 2 Dec 1976, 1870-1871.

21 Reason, J. Absent minds. (Research into accidents caused by mental lapses.) New Society, 38, 4 Nov 1976, 244-245.

22 Reid, H.A. Snakebite in Britain. Nursing Mirror, 143, 16 Sep 1976, 48-52.

23 Richardson, S. Nursing care study. Lacerations to left groin. (Care in theatre and postoperatively of 11-year-old girl.) Nursing Times, 75, 8 Feb 1979, 234-236.

24 Sabey, B. and Wall, J.G. Seat belts and survival. New Society, 35, 26 Feb 1976, 433-434.

25 Southwood, W.F.W. Closed abdominal injuries. (Diagnosis, treatment and management.) Nursing Times, 73, 12 May 1977, 700-702.

26 Stambaugh, D. and Wallace, C. What every nurse needs to know about massive chest damage. RN Magazine, 40 (7), Jul 1977, 40-43.

27 Thair, S. Nursing care study. Adder snake bite: poison in the grass. Nursing Mirror, 150, 20 Mar 1980, 34.

28 Thompson, M.A. Shock syndrome: mechanisms and manifestations, nursing assessment intervention and evaluation. Menlo Park, Cal: Addison-Wesley, 1978. (Personal resources in nursing module series.)

29 Watson, M. Hand injuries. Nursing Times, 74.
1. Primary care. 16 Feb 1978, 276-278.
2. Amputations. 23 Feb 1978, 321-322.
3. Principles of the management of complicated injuries. 2 Mar 1978, 360-362.

30 Webb, K.A. Nursing care study.

Accidental burial. (Intensive care of unconscious man following accidental burial while digging in disused tip.) Nursing Times, 74, 2 Nov 1978, 1794-1798.

31 Wright, W.J. Adder bites. Nursing Times, 74, 4 May 1978, 747-749.

32 Wynn Parry, C.B. and others Rehabilitation of the injured hand. Nursing Times, 74, 7 Sep 1978, 1483-1489.

33 Young, J.F. How the brain recognises and responds to shock. Journal of Neurosurgical Nursing, 8 (1), Jul 1976, 37-44.

34 Young, S. Preventing the adult respiratory distress syndrome. ('Shock lung.' Preventative treatment of shock in the A & E department.) Journal of Emergency Nursing, 5 (1), Jan/Feb 1979, 17-22.

h RAPE

1 Allgaier, A. Hospitals respond to rising rape rate. Proper evidence collection and sympathetic care can help law enforcement officials as well as victims. Hospitals, 53 (15), 1 Aug 1979, 65-68.

2 Blair, M.L. The problem of rape (and the role of the nurse in counselling victims). Midwife, Health Visitor and Community Nurse, 12 (9), Sep 1976, 284-286.

3 Burgess, A.W. and Holmstrom, L.L. Recovery from rape and prior life stress. (Longitudinal study.) Research in Nursing Health, 1 (4), Dec 1978, 165-174.

4 Clark, T.P. Primary health care. Counseling victims of rape. (Yale New Haven Hospital.) American Journal of Nursing, 76 (12), Dec 1976, 1964-1966.

5 COMMUNICATION breakdown: I was a rape victim. (Personal account by social worker and plea for more sensitive approach by health professionals.) Nursing Mirror, 147, 9 Nov 1978, 21.

6 Gottesman, S.T. Police attitudes toward rape before and after a training program. (Exploratory research study on police training programmes.) Journal of Psychiatric Nursing and Mental Health Services, 15 (12), Dec 1977, 14-18.

7 Hall, J. Rape and some of its effects. (Rape Crisis Centre in London.) Midwife, Health Visitor and Community Nurse, 13 (4), Apr 1977, 96, 99-100.

8 Huerd, D. How a rape advocacy service works. (Rape relief project, Yakima, Washington.) Hospital Progress, 58 (12), Dec 1977, 70, 77.

9 Huntington, K. Forensic gynaecology. (The nurse's role in initial help for the sexually assaulted patient.) Nursing Mirror, 143, 30 Sep 1976, 57-58.

10 Ipema, D.K. Rape: the process of recovery. (Analysis of tape-recorded interviews with victims.) Nursing Research, 28 (5), Sep/Oct 1979, 272-275.

11 Journal of Practical Nursing Rape. (Three articles, including nursing implications and treatment programme at Beth Israel Hospital,

Boston.) Journal of Practical Nursing, 28 (11), Nov 1978, 13-19.

12 Katz, S. and Mazur, M.A. Understanding the rape victim: a synthesis of research findings. New York: Wiley Interscience, 1979. (Wiley series on personality processes.)

13 LeBourdais, E. Rape victims: the unpopular patients. Dimensions in Health Service, 53 (3), Mar 1976, 12-14.

14 Lefort, S. Care of the rape victim in emergency. Canadian Nurse, 73 (2), Feb 1977, 42-45.

15 Moynihan, B. and Coughlin, P. Sexual assault: a comprehensive response to a complex problem. Journal of Emergency Nursing, 4 (6), Nov/Dec 1978, 22-26.

16 Phillips, M. and Bearney, C. Understanding patients charged with rape. Dimensions in Health Service, 55 (12), Dec 1978, 22-24.

17 Plant, J. and Wood, E.C. E.D. involvement in audit activities, rape treatment. Hospitals, 51 (7), 1 Apr 1977, 107-109, 110, 112.

18 Toner, B. The facts of rape. Arrow, 1977.

19 Van Dyke, C. Why a Catholic hospital provides rape relief. (Care for rape victims at St. Elizabeth Hospital, Yakima, Washington.) Hospital Progress, 58 (12), Dec 1977, 64-69.

20 Welch, M.S. Rape and the trauma of inadequate care. Nursing Digest, 5 (1), Spring 1977, 50-52.

21 West, D.J. Rape as revenge. New Society, 45, 28 Sep 1978, 684-686.

22 Wright, R. The English rapist. (Survey of cases in six countries 1972-76.) New Society, 53, 17 Jul 1980, 124-125.

i RED CROSS AND ST. JOHN

1 THE INTERNATIONAL Red Cross. (History and current role.) Nursing Times, 74, 15 Jun 1978, Occ. papers, 61-63.

2 RED CROSS nursing: born on the battlefield. (History and current role.) World Health, Dec 1978, 29.

j ROAD ACCIDENTS

1 Bennett, J. Nursing care study. A road traffic accident victim. Intensive nursing care of a child with head injuries. Nursing Times, 75, 19 Apr 1979, 656-659.

2 British Medical Journal Road accidents— priorities and possibilities. (By a special correspondent. See also editorial on p.287-288.) British Medical Journal, 1, 3 Feb 1979, 328-331.

3 British Medical Journal Motorcycle and bicycle accidents. British Medical Journal, 1, 6 Jan 1979, 39-41.

4 Bull, J.P. How accidents happen. (Symposium on road traffic accidents.) Nursing Mirror, 145, 6 Oct 1977, 13-14.

5 Christian, M.S. Non-fatal injuries sustained by seatbelt wearers: a comparative study. British Medical Journal, 2, 27 Nov 1976, 1310-1311.

6 Cliff, K.S. Accounting for accidents. (Cost to NHS of treating people involved in road traffic accidents.) Health and Social Service Journal, 90, 7 Mar 1980, 323-325.

7 Dryden, K.G. Motor car accidents. (District nurses and the law series.) Queen's Nursing Journal, 18 (10), Jan 1976, 284-285.

8 Fox, J. Nursing care study. Splenectomy and nephrectomy: ten days' trauma—and he still wants another motorbike! (Care of road traffic accident victim in casualty, ward and ITU.) Nursing Mirror, 148, 18 Jan 1979, 25-30.

9 Franklin, D. Crash! stay calm and think ahead. (Advice on action at the scene of a road traffic accident including first aid.) Nursing Mirror, 149, 6 Sep 1979, 34, 36-37.

10 Hopkins, P. Causes and prevention of road accidents. Nursing Times, 74, 28 Sep 1978, 1594-1596.

11 Lucas, B. Nursing care study. Pregnant car crash victim. Nursing Times, 72, 25 Mar 1976, 451-453.

12 McFarland, M.B. Fat embolism syndrome. (Case study of trauma following a car accident leading to respiratory distress.) American Journal of Nursing, 76 (12), Dec 1976, 1942-1944.

13 Malley, W. and Michel, J. Road traffic accidents. Nursing Mirror, 142 (25), 17 Jun 1976, Nursing care supplement, 5, i-iv.

14 Schneider, C. Nursing care study. Rupture of profunda femoris artery. It's all go for one busy hour. (Care of motorcycling accident patient in emergency department.) Nursing Mirror, 150, 17 Jan 1980, 42-43.

15 Skeet, M. Principles and practice of first aid. 3—Road accidents. Nursing Mirror, 146, 16 Mar 1978, Supplement, i-iv.

16 Van Emden, J. The after-effects of road accidents. (Psychological effects and legal aspects.) Journal of Community Nursing, 1 (9), Mar 1978, 29-30.

17 Walker, R. Nursing care study. A patient with traumatic rupture of the right main bronchus. (Intensive care after motor cycle accident. By staff nurse.) Nursing Times, 76, 17 Jan 1980, 102-104.

k SPORT AND HOLIDAYS

1 Adams, I.D. Skateboard injuries. (And the possibility of epiphyseal injuries.) Nursing Times, 75, 26 Apr 1979, 707-708.

2 Bennett, R.M. Drowning and near drowning: etiology and pathophysiology. American Journal of Nursing, 76 (6), Jun 1976, 919-921.

3 Burnett, R. Mountain rescue. Health and Social Service Journal, 86, 17 Apr 1976, 716-717.

4 Caudle, J.T. Emergency nursing of near drowning victims. American Journal of Nursing, 76 (6), Jun 1976, 922-923.

5 Clarke, C.R.A. The care of the mountaineer. Practitioner, 217, Aug 1976, 235-239.

6 Cowper-Smith, F. Mountain rescue in North Wales. (The Llanberis team and co-ordinated operations with R.A.F.) Nursing Times, 73, 8 Dec 1977, 1904-1906.

7 Fingland, F. Shark attack victim. (In South Africa.) Nursing Times, 74, 25 May 1978, 868-869.

8 Gunn, A.D.G. Sport? It's a pain. (Sports injuries.) Journal of Community Nursing, 2 (8), Feb 1979, 25-26.

9 Illingworth, C. and others Skateboard injuries: preliminary report. British Medical Journal, 2, 24/31 Dec 1977, 1636.

10 Isler, C. Don't act thunderstruck: save victims of lightning. RN Magazine, 39 (8), Aug 1976, 37-39.

11 Kemm, I. Skateboard injuries. (Survey of casualty department attendances at Sheffield Royal Infirmary.) British Medical Journal, 1, 8 Apr 1978, 894.

12 Lee, R.M. Lightning injuries. AORN Journal, 23 (7), Jun 1976, 1316-1318, 1320, 1322, 1324.

13 Maitra, A.K. Skateboard injuries. British Journal of Clinical Practitioners, 33 (10), Oct 1979, 281-282, 288.

14 Molyneux-Luick, M. Water-sports injuries: the old and the new. Nursing, 8 (8), Aug 1978, 50-55.

15 Physiotherapy Issue on sports medicine. Physiotherapy, 62 (8), Aug 1976, 245-265.

16 Rivers, R.P.A. and others Falls from equipment as a cause of playground injury. Community Health, 9 (3), Feb 1978, 178-179.

17 Tobin, N. Fireworks—the need for reform. Nursing Mirror, 143 (18), 28 Oct 1976, 46-47.

18 Woolstone, A.S. Injuries of professional football. Nursing Times, 73, 19 May 1977, 728-729.

19 Wright, D. Prevention of injuries in sport. Physiotherapy, 65 (4), Apr 1979, 114-119.

20 Wynn-Davies, B. Lethal leisure. (Accidents connected with sports.) Nursing Mirror, 145, 18 Aug 1977, 13-14.

21 Yuill, G.M. Icarus's syndrome: new hazards in flight. (Dangers of hang gliding.) British Medical Journal, 1977, 1, 26 Mar 1977, 823-825.

68 BURNS AND PLASTIC SURGERY

a GENERAL AND NURSING

1 Artz, C.P. and others, editors Burns: a team approach. Philadelphia: W.B. Saunders, 1979. (Includes a section on nursing care.)

2 Australasian Nurses Journal Issue on burns. (Seven articles including care of adolescents and children and pre-hospital care.) Australasian Nurses Journal, 7 (3), Oct 1977, 3-4, 6-15.

3 Buckle, V. Use of polythene gloves in

treating burns of the hand. Nursing Times, 73, 3 Feb 1977, 170.

4 **Busby, H.C.** Nursing management of the acute burn patient and nursing management of optimal burn recovery. Journal of Continuing Education in Nursing, 10 (4), Jul/Aug 1979, 16-30.

5 **Charlesworth, D.** 'The silent epidemic.' (Burns Unit, Texas Institute of Rehabilitation.) S.A. Nursing Journal, 43 (7), Jul 1976, 17, 16.

6 **Christopher, K.L.** The use of a model for hemodynamic balance to describe burn shock. Nursing Clinics of North America, 15 (3), Sep 1980, 617-627.

7 **Dhurmadut, B.** Fluid replacement with special reference to burned patients. Nursing Times, 73, 10 Mar 1977, 337-338.

8 **Doswell, W.M.** Nursing decisions. Experiences in clinical problem solving. Series 2, number 7. Karen A. A patient with burns. RN Magazine, 40 (5), May 1977, 59-64, 66-67, 68.

9 **Ewers, D.** Smoke inhalation: assessment and management. (Respiratory tract injury in burn victims.) Journal of Emergency Nursing, 5 (1), Jan/Feb 1979, 5-9.

10 **Hayter, J.** Emergency nursing care of the burned patient. Nursing Clinics of North America, 13 (2), Jun 1978, 223-234.

11 **Hyde, A.** Open for business as usual. (Burns unit at Mount Vernon Hospital, Northwood.) Health and Social Service Journal, 90, 22 Feb 1980, 246-247.

12 **Jacoby, F.C.** Individualized burn wound dressings. (Selection of right type of dressing for the type of wound.) Nursing 77, 7 (6), Jun 1977, 62-63.

13 **Jacoby, F.G.** Nursing care of the patient with burns. 2nd ed. St. Louis: Mosby, 1976.

14 **Jones, C.A.** Burns. The home stretch... rehabilitation. Nursing, 7 (12), Dec 1977, 54, 56-57.

15 **Jones, C.A. and others** Burns. What to do during the first crucial hours. Nursing Care, 7 (3), Mar 1977, 23-31.

16 **Kinzie, V.** What to do for the severely burned. RN Magazine, 43 (4), Apr 1980, 47-51, 104, 106, 108, 110.

17 **Lawrence, J.C.** Minor burns. (A report of a trial in which tulle gras medicated with chlorexidine was compared with a non-medicated tulle gras.) Nursing Mirror, 144, 28 Apr 1977, 58-60.

18 **Lawrence, J.** Pig skin beats burns. (Found to have advantages over traditional dressings in clinical trials.) Nursing Mirror, 151, 3 Jul 1980, 28-29.

19 **Marvin, J.A.** Burn nursing as a speciality. (History from 1938 and future directions.) Heart Lung, 8 (5), Sep/Oct 1979, 913-917.

20 **Millership, R.** Nursing care of the burned patient. UNA Nursing Journal, 74 (2), Mar-Apr 1976, 16-19.

21 **Minar, V.** Fluid resuscitation of the burn patient. Journal of Emergency Nursing, 4 (5), Sep/Oct 1978, 39-43.

22 **Physiotherapy** Five articles on burns. Physiotherapy, 63 (5), May 1977, 146-158.

23 **Rogenes, P.R. and Moylan, J.A.** Restoring fluid balance in the patient with severe burns. American Journal of Nursing, 76 (12), Dec 1976, 1952-1957.

24 **Small, A.** Early surgery for electrical mouth burns. AORN Journal, 23 (1), Jan 1976, 126, 128, 130, 132, 134, 138, 140.

25 **Swift, W.** Emotional care and support. An overseas tour around burns units and centres (in America and England). Australian Nurses Journal, 6 (5), Nov 1976, 31-33.

26 **Wagner, M.M.** Emergency care of the burned patient. American Journal of Nursing, 77 (11), Nov 1977, 1788-1791.

27 **Wright, D.** The burn wound: topical therapy for infection control. Australian Nurses Journal, 8 (5), Jan 1979, 25-26.

b CHILDREN

1 **Aston, S.** Burns in children. CIBA Clinical Symposia, 28 (4), 1976, 2-38.

2 **Burgdorf, M.M.** Coping behaviors of a school age child hospitalized with burns. Maternal-Child Nursing Journal, 7 (1), Spring 1978, 11-19.

3 **Campbell, L.** Special behavioral problems of the burned child. American Journal of Nursing, 76 (2), Feb 1976, 220-224.

4 **Chapman, C.E.** Nursing care study. Burns. (Three year old girl with 75% burns.) Nursing Mirror, 146, 9 Feb 1978, 18-20.

5 **Emig, E. and Lloyd, J.R.** How to get burned children home sooner. (Through nurses' teaching parents the right way to care for their children.) RN Magazine, 40 (7), Jul 1977, 37-39.

6 **Isler, C.** A mouth burn need not disfigure a child. RN Magazine, 39 (12), Dec 1976, 31-34.

7 **Kessler, R.L.** Nursing care study. Care of a scalded child. Nursing Times, 75, 12 Apr 1979, 619-624.

8 **Lamont, J.** Nursing care study. Scalds: a frame-up for Stuart... (Care of fifteen-month-old boy on burns frame and care of skin graft.) Nursing Mirror, 149, 2 Aug 1979, 34-36.

9 **Learmonth, A.** Factors in child burn and scald accidents in Bradford 1969-73. (Survey which found correlation with New Commonwealth immigrants and overcrowding.) Journal of Epidemiology and Community Health, 33 (4), Dec 1979, 270-273.

10 **Maternal-Child Nursing Journal** The severely burned child. (Three articles.) Maternal-Child Nursing Journal, 2 (4), Jul/Aug 1977, 220-227.

11 **Savedra, M.** Coping with pain: strategies of severely burned children. Maternal-Child Nursing Journal, 5 (3), Fall 1976, 197-203.

12 **Talabere, L. and Graves, P.** A tool for assessing families of burned children. American Journal of Nursing, 76 (2), Feb 1976, 225-227.

c PATIENT AND FAMILY

1 **American Journal of Nursing** Psychiatric nurse works with burn patients. (Counselling patients and their families.) American Journal of Nursing, 80 (1), Jan 1980, 124, 126.

2 **Bernstein, N.R.** Emotional care of the facially burned and disfigured. Boston: Little, Brown and Co., 1976.

3 **Mieszala, P. and Hartmann, R.** Burn prevention group teaching for victims. (Cook County Hospital, Chicago.) Supervisor Nurse, 7 (6), Jun 1976, 66-69.

4 **Peeling, B.** One day at a time on a burn unit. (Psychological needs of burn patients illustrated by case studies.) Canadian Nurse, 74 (10), Nov 1978, 38-41.

5 **Swift, W.** Impressive results were obtained when they devised a staff teaching programme in the burn unit. (Survey regarding programme of experience for student nurses.) Australian Nurses Journal, 8 (2), Aug 1978, 45, 59.

6 **Singletary, Y.** More than skin deep. (Emotional needs and psychological problems resulting from severe burns.) Journal of Psychiatric Nursing and Mental Health Services, 15 (2), Feb 1977, 7-13. Reproduced in Occupational Health Nursing, 25 (7), Jul 1977, 15-20.

d INDUSTRIAL BURNS

1 **Cumming, D.** Nursing care study. Phenol burns: carbolic acid strikes fast. (Care of diabetic patient who suffered phenol burns at work.) Nursing Mirror, 149, 27 Sep 1979, 40-42.

e PLASTIC SURGERY

1 **Bucy, N. and others** Lead your maimed patient back to independence. (Nursing care following plastic surgery to crushed hands.) RN Magazine, 40 (6), 15 Jun 1977, 29-32.

2 **Chouinard, F. and others** Vigilant nursing care after reconstructive microsurgery. (Care study of patient with reconstruction of large concave scar on leg.) Nursing (U.S.), 9 (6), Jun 1979, 18-25.

3 **Dunwoody, H.** Theatre nursing care study. Microvascular free groin flap. A technique which shortens dramatically a patient's stay in hospital. Nursing Times, 75, 26 Apr 1979, 702-706.

4 **Finn, K.L.** Rebuilding skin. Part 1. A successful graft may be up to you. (How skin grafts work and role of the nurse.) RN Magazine, 40 (10), Oct 1977, 41-45.

5 **Finn, K.L.** Rebuilding skin. Part 2. Meeting the challenges of flap care. (Used in cases where grafts would not take.) RN Magazine, 40 (11), Nov 1977, 47-52.

6 **Jones, C.A. and Feller, I.** Burns. Avoiding and coping with complications before and after grafting. Nursing, 7 (11), Nov 1977, 72-81.

7 **Kamer, F.M. and others** Specialty office surgery. (Plastic surgery performed in an outpatient clinic.) AORN Journal, 23 (7), Jun 1976, 1256, 1258, 1260, 1262, 1264, 1266.

8 **King, T. and others** The defeated patient, her worries come first. (Care of patient following

plastic surgery to chest wall.) Nursing 77, 7 (4), Apr 1977, 29-31, 33.

9 McCredie, V. and Bailey, B.N. Microvascular surgery in plastic surgery. (Techniques and nursing care.) Nursing Times, 74, 21/28 Dec 1978, 2095-2100.

10 Morgan, E.B. An improved vacuum splint for a cross-leg flap. Nursing Times, 74, 14 Dec 1978, 2077-2078.

11 Pughe, H.M. Nursing care study. Split skin grafting: why it's safer to graft on the ward. Nursing Mirror, 147, 28 Dec 1978, 27-28.

12 Reid, W.H. Free grafts—skin and other tissues. Nursing Times, 73, 20 Oct 1977, 1627-1630.

13 Roberts, M. The skin bank. Nursing Mirror, 143, 2 Sep 1976, 52-57.

14 Stuart, M.S. Skin flaps and grafts after head and neck surgery. (For cancer.) American Journal of Nursing, 78 (8), Aug 1978, 1368-1374.

15 Trust, D.S. Skin deep: an introduction to skin camouflage and disfigurement therapy. Edinburgh: Paul Harris, 1977.

16 Wooldridge, M. and Surveyer, J.A. Skin grafting for full-thickness burn injury. American Journal of Nursing, 80 (11), Nov 1980, 2000-2004.

17 Yiacoumettis, A.M. and Neuman, M. Better results from delayed primary skin grafting. Nursing Mirror, 147, 24 Aug 1978, 28-30.

69 DISASTER AND WAR

a DISASTER MANAGEMENT

1 Adams, P. Major incident procedures. (With reference to Redhill General Hospital.) Nursing, 14, Jun 1980, 623-625.

2 Bander, K.W. Hospital structures guidelines for coping with snowstorms. Hospitals, 52 (21), 1 Nov 1978, 123-124, 126, 128, 130.

3 Bickerton, J. Volunteer in Guatemala. (Nurse's experiences following 1976 earthquake.) Nursing Times, 74, 7 Sep 1978, 1500-1502.

4 Bond, I. Violent event. (Emergency care at the Notting Hill Carnival.) Nursing Times, 72, 23 Sep 1976, 1464-1465.

5 Ciuca, R. and others When disaster happens. How do you meet emotional needs? (Work of a mental health team after a school bus disaster in California.) American Journal of Nursing, 77 (3), Mar 1977, 454-456.

6 Crooks, L. and others Disaster planning: a team effort. (With worksheets and charts for recording supplies/instruments and patients' valuables.) AORN Journal, 28 (3), Sep 1978, 395-410.

7 Davies, R. Accidents and disasters—the victim speaks. (Work being carried out within the NCSS on the social consequences of disasters.) Social Service Quarterly, 49 (4), Apr-Jun 1976, 127-130.

8 Davies, R. Social care in disaster management. (Role of social services.) Social Service Quarterly, 51 (2), Oct/Dec 1977, 57-60.

9 Davis, R.W. Three mile island: a nursing dilemma. (Evacuation of pregnant women and pre-school children following nuclear accident and plans for mass evacuation.) Supervisor Nurse, 10 (12), Dec 1979, 12-15.

10 Dawber, N.M. Disaster planning for hospitals. S.A. Nursing Journal, 44 (8), Aug 1977, 24-26.

11 Department of Health and Social Security Health service arrangements for dealing with major accidents. DHSS, 1977. (HC(77)1.)

12 Edwards, J.G. Psychiatric aspects of civilian disasters. British Medical Journal, 1, 17 Apr 1976, 944-947.

13 Friedman, E. Updating disaster plans: a tale of three hospitals. Hospitals, 52 (9), 1 May 1978, 95-96, 98, 100-102.

14 Gibson, W.H. Disaster planning. Journal of the Society of Occupational Medicine, 26 (4), Oct 1976, 136-138.

15 Hargreaves, A.G. Coping with disaster. American Journal of Nursing, 80 (4), Apr 1980, 683.

16 Henderson, M. Disaster planning—Britain lags behind. (International conference—Action for Disaster.) Health and Social Service Journal, 86, 1 May 1976, 789.

17 Isler, C. Could you cope with a nuclear accident? (Guide to immediate action.) RN Magazine, 42 (6), Jun 1979, 66, 71, 73-74, 77.

18 Jackson, J. Notting Hill carnival 1977—a hospital version. (Administrative plans for reception of casualties.) Hospital and Health Services Review, 74 (1), Jan 1978, 13-16.

19 Jones, J.R. It can happen to you! (Disaster planning is essential). (Fire and explosions at petrol service station with 34 casualties.) Journal of Emergency Nursing, 4 (1), Jan/Feb 1978, 24-27.

20 Jones, K.S. Mass disaster organisation and advances in emergency care. Australasian Nurses Journal, 5 (8), Mar 1977, 11-13, 34.

21 League of Red Cross Societies Guidelines for nurses in disaster preparedness and relief. (Extracts.) Nursing Journal of India, 49 (6), Jun 1978, 141-142.

22 Leamons, E.P. Mass casualty alert program. (Role of OH nurse in planning disaster procedure.) Occupational Health Nursing, 25 (5), May 1977, 13-16.

23 McClelland, M. Hiroshima—the effects of the atom bomb. (Report of visit in June to Radiation Effects Research Foundation and Red Cross Hospital.) Nursing Mirror, 145, 1 Sep 1977, 19-22.

24 Miles, I.M. The role of the nurse in floods and earthquakes. S.A. Nursing Journal, 43 (6), Jun 1976, 27-29.

25 Montgomery, C. Post mortem on a disaster. (Mock disaster at Toronto International Airport to test procedures.) Dimensions in Health Service, 53 (12), Dec 1976, 31-33.

26 Palmer, E.L. Student reactions to disaster. (Effects of tornadoes in Wichita Falls, Texas.) American Journal of Nursing, 80 (4), Apr 1980, 680-682.

27 Porat, A. Planning for emergencies. (Disaster planning.) Occupational Health, 32 (9), Sep 1980, 463-466.

28 Rawlins, T. A study of major accident planning (in Sweden). The Author, 1980. (3M Travel award for accident and emergency nursing.)

29 Royal College of Nursing Coping with catastrophe. (Account of disaster procedure at Sheffield's adult general hospitals, described at Rcn Centre meeting.) Nursing Mirror, 145, 1 Dec 1977, 4.

30 Savage, P.E.A. Disasters—hospital planning: a manual for doctors, nurses and administrators. Oxford: Pergamon, 1979.

31 Seaver, D.J. Coping with internal disaster is a hospital priority. Hospitals, 51 (14), 16 Jul 1977, 167-168, 170, 172.

32 Sharma, L. Nursing preparedness in disaster relief. (Part 2 covers integration into nursing curriculum.) Nursing Journal of India, 66 (10), Oct 1975, 223-224; (11), Nov 1975, 249-250.

33 Skeet, M. Manual for disaster relief work. Churchill Livingstone, 1977. (For nurses and others.)

34 Skeet, M. When disaster strikes. (Plans for coping with disasters.) Journal of Community Nursing, 1 (9), Mar 1978, 12-13.

35 S.A. Nursing Journal Issue on disaster nursing. S.A. Nursing Journal, 43 (6), Jun 1976, 6-31.

36 Starling, C. Dissecting a disaster. (Watford General Hospital's disaster plan is revised following a major train crash in 1975.) Health and Social Service Journal, 88, 7 Jul 1978, 760-761.

37 Strickler, A. The case for disaster site medical teams. Dimensions in Health Service, 53 (2), Feb 1976, 30-32.

38 Vinsel, D.B. Hospitals must plan for nuclear accidents. Hospitals, 54 (16), 16 Aug 1980, 113-114, 116, 118, 121.

39 Wert, B.J. Stress due to nuclear accident: a survey of an employee population. (Survey of employees in the Harrisburg area following the accident at Three Mile Island power station.) Occupational Health Nursing, 17 (9), Sep 1979, 16-24.

40 Wiener, P. Setting up an external disaster procedure and the role of the nursing service supervisor. Hospital Topics, 54 (3), Jul/Aug 1976, 22, 24-25.

41 Wightman, C. Simulated disaster highlights problems. Dimensions in Health Service, 57 (4), Apr 1980, 14-15.

42 Woodbridge, R. Nursing in a famine. (Oxfam nurses in Ethiopia.) Nursing Times, 72, 5 Feb 1976, 166-167.

43 WHO Chronicle Emergency care in natural disasters: view of an international seminar. (Held in Manila in 1978.) WHO Chronicle, 34 (3), Mar 1980, 96-100.

44 Yatzie, N. Help! (Simulated disaster game to teach nurse learners how to organise emergency care, including triage.) Canadian Nurse, 76 (6), Jun 1980, 33-36.

b WAR AND CONFLICT

1 Cook, A. Settling down in a new country. (Health care of 74 Vietnamese refugees in a Save the Children Fund project in Warwick.) Nursing Mirror, 149, 23 Aug 1979, 17-18.

2 Cowan, N. After the bullets. (Resettlement plan for Eritrean refugees in Sudan.) Nursing Mirror, 151, 18/25 Dec 1980, 30-31.

3 Devlin, A. Nursing care study. Innocent victim—shot before birth. (Victim of unrest in Northern Ireland.) Nursing Mirror, 143, 18 Nov 1976, 45-47.

4 Devlin, D. Nursing care study. Victim of circumstance. (Depression arising from civil conflict in Belfast.) Nursing Times, 72, 12 Feb 1976, 215-216.

5 Dunn, A. Save the children. (Work of Save the Children Fund in relief work overseas.) Nursing Times, 76, 28 Aug 1980, 1514.

6 Fink, K.P. Victims of political-racial persecution. Awareness of these unfortunate people's background can help the medical team to cope with their otherwise inexplicable behaviour. Nursing Times, 75, 22 Mar 1979, 496-499.

7 Godfrey, L. What will you do in the war, doctor? (Proposals for health services during nuclear war.) World Medicine, 15 (14), 19 Apr 1980, 86-87, 89, 91.

8 Hirschfeld, M.J. Care of the aging holocaust survivor. A nurse in Israel describes how care must be modified to meet the special needs of the survivors of Nazi persecution. American Journal of Nursing, 77 (7), Jul 1977, 1187-1189.

9 Illman, J. The hazards of surviving. (Long term effects on prisoners of war and concentration camp survivors.) World Medicine, 13 (15), 3 May 1978, 57-58, 61.

10 Kalter, S. Operating theatre management in wartime in the fighting area. (Israel.) S.A. Nursing Journal, 42 (11), Nov 1975, 15-17.

11 Lewin, D.C. Picking up after the terrorist. (Nurse's role in the treatment of the victims of violence.) Nursing Mirror, 148, 12 Apr 1979, 36-37.

12 McAlister, E. Nursing care of bomb and bullet victims. Nursing Mirror, 146, 15 Jun 1978, 19-21.

13 Melville, J. The scars of the survivors. (Psychological problems in survivors of Vietnam, Hiroshima or concentration camp.) New Society, 50, 18 Oct 1979, 124-126.

14 Nuttall, P. Light years away from the NHS. (Report of course to prepare health professionals for work in refugee camps.) Nursing Times, 76, 10 Jul 1980, 1206.

15 Ochberg, F.M. The victim of terrorism. Practitioner, 220, Feb 1978, 293-302.

16 Pearson, R. Health visiting with a difference. (Work in reception centre for Vietnamese refugees.) Health Visitor, 53 (7), Jul 1980, 257-258.

17 Philpot, T. A harbour of love. (Visit to two camps in Hong Kong for the Vietnamese Boat People.) Nursing Mirror, 151, 18/25 Dec 1980, 24-26.

18 Podgorny, G. and Stanley, L. Dealing with the special dangers of gunshot wounds. (Care in the casualty departments.) RN Magazine, Oct 1977, 62-71.

19 Roberts, I.G. Health problems associated with nuclear war. Midwife, Health Visitor and Community Nurse, 16 (3), Mar 1980, 113-114, 116.

20 Royal Victoria Hospital, Belfast A 'war zone' hospital in the front line of achievement. Health and Social Service Journal, 86, 24/31 Dec 1976, 2284-2285.

21 Rutherford, W. The nature of injuries caused by bombs and bullets. Nursing Mirror, 146, 15 Jun 1978, 16-18.

22 Simpson, M. The story of a seventies soldier. ('Shell-shock' and stress among today's soldiers.) New Society, 47, 8 Mar 1979, 546-548.

23 Teare, R.D. Ballbearing-bomb injuries. British Medical Journal, 1, 7 Feb 1976, 310-311.

24 Thomas, L. Dust of life: children of the Saigon streets. (A nurse's experiences in Vietnam.) Hamish Hamilton, 1977.

25 White, K.M. Evaluating the trauma of gunshot wounds. American Journal of Nursing, 77 (10), Oct 1977, 1589-1593.

c FORCES NURSING

1 American Journal of Nursing Military nurses are different today, Corps Chiefs agree. American Journal of Nursing, 80 (3), Mar 1980, 382, 384.

2 Cowper-Smith, F. RAF flies home the sick. N.M.'s reporter travels with a RAF Aeromed Team bringing patients home from Germany. Nursing Mirror, 142, 24 Jun 1976, 55-58.

3 Cowper-Smith, F. RAF nurses training for in-flight care. Nursing Mirror, 142, 11 Mar 1976, 47-48.

4 Hall, C. Selection in QARANC. (A two-way selection process involving a 24 hour visit to the QARANC training centre for job briefing, selection, tests and interviewing.) Nursing Mirror, 142 (6), 12 Feb 1976, 66-67.

5 Ingham, M.J. Down to earth structure for high flying professionals. (RAF hospital organisation seen at Nocton Hall, near Lincoln.) Health and Social Service Journal, 86, 28 Jan 1977, 150-151.

6 Young, P. Army nurses in Belfast. (Description of visit to the Military Wing of Musgrave Park Hospital.) Nursing Mirror, 145, 15 Sep 1977, 6-9.

7 Young, P. Nursing with the Forces. 1. The RAF. (Princess Mary's Royal Air Force Nursing Service.) Nursing Focus, 1 (9), Jun 1980, 390-392.

8 Young, P. Nursing with the Forces. 2. The QAs. (Queen Alexandra's Royal Army Nursing Corps.) Nursing Focus, 1 (11), Jul 1980, 434-436.

9 Young, P. Nursing with the forces. 3. The QARNNS. Nursing Focus, 1 (12), Aug 1980, 471-473.

OCCUPATIONAL HEALTH

70 OCCUPATIONAL HEALTH

a GENERAL

1 Amis, R.H. Health and safety at work: the employer's view. (By Chairman of CBI Health, Safety and Welfare Committee.) Journal of the Society of Occupational Medicine, 30 (3), Jul 1980, 98-102.

2 Arlidge, J.T. Dr. J.T. Arlidge (1822-99). (Contribution to occupational health.) Occupational Health, 29 (7), Jul 1977, 316-318.

3 Ashford, N.A. Crisis in the workplace: occupational disease and injury. A report to the Ford Foundation. MIT Press, 1976.

4 Bernhardt, J.H. Anticipated benefits from an effective occupational health program. Occupational Health Nursing, 24 (9), Sep 1976, 9-14.

5 Black, D. The spirit of occupational medicine. (Survey of pioneers with brief comment on present and future trends.) British Medical Journal, 2, 22/29 Dec 1979, 1622-1626.

6 British Medical Journal EEC occupational health charter. British Medical Journal, 280, 16 Feb 1980, 499.

7 Campbell, Y. Report on the XVIII International Congress on Occupational Health held from 14-19 September 1975 in Brighton, England. S.A. Nursing Journal, 43 (3), Mar 1976, 16-17.

8 Dawson, H. A meeting of minds: Avon's OH society. (New multidisciplinary society which started in December 1975.) Occupational Health, 32 (9), Sep 1980, 468-472.

9 Department of Employment Gazette Research developments in workplace health and safety. Department of Employment Gazette, 86 (12), Dec 1978, 1395-1396.

10 Duncan, K. Occupational health: a science? Occupational Health, 31 (8), Aug 1979, 397-401.

11 El Batawi, M. Work-related diseases. World Health, Jun 1978, 10-13.

12 Gardner, A.W. editor Current approaches to occupational medicine. Bristol: Wright, 1979.

13 Hamilton, M. OH research at Northwick Park. (Four projects recently investigated: high pressure in diving: effect of night work on nurses: cross infection hazards of clothing: protective clothing for helicopter crews.) Occupational Health, 29 (3), mar 1977, 108-112.

14 Hunter, D. The diseases of occupations. 6th ed. Hodder and Stoughton, 1978.

15 Hunter, W.J. The work of the Commission of the European Communities on health and safety. Journal of the Society of Occupational Medicine, 28 (3), Jul 1978, 101-108.

16 International Congress on Occupational Health 19th: 1978: Dubrovnik. Proceedings of the xix international congress on occupational health 25-30 Sept., 1978, Dubrovnik edited by R. Plestina. Zagreb: Institute for Medical Research and Occupational Health, 1980. 4 vols. (Archives of industrial hygiene and toxicology.)

17 International Labour Conference Proposed action by H.M. Government...on two conventions and two recommendations adopted at the 63rd session (1977) of the International Labour Conference. HMSO, 1978. (Cmnd.7420)

18 Krekel, S. The union's role in occupational health. Occupational Health Nursing, 24 (10), Oct 1976, 13-14.

19 McCleeland, E. and Van Hoozer, H. Occupational factors affecting health. Occupational Health Nursing, 24 (12), Dec 1976, 19-22.

20 Orriss, H.D. Days lost through illness. Sickness Benefits payments recorded in Social Security Statistics 1974. Occupational Health, 28 (6), Jun 1976, 290-294.

21 Preece, A. Surrey: one of industry's universities. (Research into health and safety and plans for a new Institute.) Occupational Health, 30 (7), Jul 1978, 314-317.

22 Ross, D. Bernardino Ramazzini (1633-1714). (The 'father of occupational medicine'.) Occupational Health, 31 (3), Mar 1979, 136-141.

23 Schilling, R.S.F. The future of occupational medicine. Journal of the Society of Occupational Medicine, 26 (4), Oct 1976, 120-126.

24 Simson, R.E. International trends in occupational health. (Address to Second Australian Convention: Occupational health nursing.) Australasian Nurses Journal, 6 (9), Apr 1977, 18-19, 22-23.

25 Smith, J.M. The psychology of changing attitudes. (With reference to health education and occupational health.) Occupational Health, 30 (10), Oct 1978, 468-473.

26 Teeling-Smith, G. Sickness and discontent. Occupational Health, 24 (5), May 1972, 153-154.

27 Trades Union Congress TUC handbook on safety and health at work. TUC, 1978.

28 Tyrer, F.H. Occupational medicine today: talking to the unions. Journal of the Society of Occupational Medicine, 30 (3), Jul 1980, 103-108.

29 Waldron, H.A. Lecture notes on occupational medicine. Blackwell, 1976. 2nd ed. 1979.

30 Waldron, H.A. and Harrington, J.M. editors Occupational hygiene: an introductory text. Oxford: Blackwell Scientific, 1980.

31 World Health Organization. Regional Office for Europe Health aspects of wellbeing in working places: report on a WHO working group 18-20 Sept, 1979 in Prague. Copenhagen: WHO, 1980.

32 WHO Chronicle Occupational health problems and their control. WHO Chronicle, 30 (8), Aug 1976, 318-324.

33 Zenz, C. Developments in occupational medicine. Chicago: Yearbook Medical Publishers, 1980.

b LEGISLATION

1 Bell, J.D. The Health and Safety at Work Act (1974) and its application to infection control. Nursing Times, 73, 25 Aug 1977, ICNA 50-52.

2 Boucher, B.J. Guidance on preparing local rules to help implement the Health and Safety at Work etc Act. (Guidance notes devised by Tower Hamlets District Safety Committee.) British Medical Journal, 1, 3 Mar 1979, 599-601.

3 Breckin, M. Does too much law cause apathy? (Review of safety legislation from 19th century.) Occupational Health, 32 (1), Jan 1980, 33-35.

4 Broadhurst, A. The health and safety at work act in practice. Heyden, 1978.

5 Cartwright, P.A. Occupational health and safety. (Aspects of Health and Safety at Work Act 1974 which affect community health workers.) Community Health, 9 (1), Aug 1977, 2-10.

6 Chartered Society of Physiotherapy The Health and Safety at Work Act 1974: policy statements and codes of safe practices. (Lists hazards and safety precautions.) Physiotherapy, 65 (1), Jan 1979, 17-28.

7 Farndale, W.A.J. and Russell, S. Law on

accidents to health service staff and volunteers. Beckenham: Ravenswood, 1977.

8 Finch, J. Law and the nurse. Who is responsible for health and safety? Nursing Mirror, 151, 25 Sep 1980, 26-27.

9 Health and Safety Executive The factories act 1961: a short guide. HMSO, 1977.

10 Health and Safety Executive A guide to the 1963 OSRP (Offices, Shops and Railway Premises) Act. HMSO, 1979. (HS(R)4).

11 Jackson, J. Health and safety—the law. New Commercial Pub. Co., 1979.

12 Nixon, C. Take a closer look at Eliz. 2 c37. (Health and Safety at Work Act 1974.) British Journal of Occupational Therapy, 39 (10), Oct 1976, 252-256.

13 Powell-Smith, V. A protection handbook: questions and answers on the health and safety at work act. 3rd ed. Osborne, 1977.

14 Williams, B. Putting health and safety into practice. (Interpretation of the Health and Safety at Work Act 1974 by Kensington, Chelsea and Westminster Area Health Authority.) Health and Social Service Journal, 86, 24 Jul 1976, 1346-1347.

c SERVICES

1 Atherley, G.R.C. and others An approach to the financial evaluation of occupational health services. Journal of the Society of Occupational Medicine, 26 (1), Jan 1976, 21-30.

2 Boydstun, S.M. Design of an occupational health unit. Occupational Health Nursing, 27 (1), Jan 1979, 7-11.

3 Coppin, M. Profile of an industrial health service. (Service at Slough for small firms.) Occupational Safety and Health, 9 (12), Dec 1979, 40-41.

4 Cox, R.A.F. The role of the company medical officer. Health Education Journal, 38 (2), 1979, 53-55.

5 Duncan, K.P. Health care of people at work in Britain. Occupational health services. Journal of the Society of Occupational Medicine, 26 (1), Jan 1976, 31-34.

6 Elliott, P.M. Harlow industrial health service. (Group health service.) Journal of the Society of Occupational Medicine, 28 (1), Jan 1978, 16-19.

7 Gough-Thomas, H. The evolution of joint occupational health services. (Conference paper.) Community Health, 7 (3), Jan 1976, 171-177.

8 Hamblett, E.P. Occupational health services for local authorities. (Conference paper.) Community Health, 7 (3), Jan 1976, 169-171.

9 Health and Safety Commission Prevention and health. Occupational health services: the way ahead. HMSO, 1977.

10 Health and Safety Executive. H.M. Factory Inspectorate. Industry and services: annual report 1975. HMSO, 1977.

11 Heathershaw, R. The way ahead—

perhaps! (Critical look at the EMAS discussion document on OH services.) Occupational Safety and Health, 8 (3), Mar 1978, 38-39.

12 McVicar, J. Peripatetic medicine. (OH services for small organisation provided by group services such as the West Midlands Industrial Health Service.) Industrial Society, 62, Jan/Feb 1980, 24.

13 Murray, R. The ethics of the industrial physician. Occupational Health, 31 (7), Jul 1979, 342-344.

14 Occupational Health OH cover for exhibitions. (Occupational health service at the National Exhibition Centre, Birmingham.) Occupational Health, 28 (8), Aug 1976, 382-386.

15 Occupational Health Scotland's OH dream comes true. (Opening of Wolfson Institute of Occupational Health at Ninewells Hospital, Dundee.) Occupational Health, 30 (1), Jan 1978, 4-5.

16 Royal College of Nursing. Society of Occupational Health Towards a national OH service. (Rcn views on guidelines issued by the Employment Medical Advisory Service.) Occupational Health, 28 (7), Jul 1976, 340-341.

17 SOCIETY of Occupational Medicine. View on Future Relationships between Occupational Medicine and the National Health Service. Journal of the Society of Occupational Medicine, 29 (2), Apr 1979, 43-44.

18 Stewart, D.M. The role of an information officer in an occupational health service. (1975 Congress paper.) Occupational Health Nursing, 24 (1), Jan 1976, 13-14.

19 Turpin, J. and Richards, M. Sharing a service. (Small factories share GKN's medical services in mid-Wales.) Occupational Health, 28 (10), Oct 1976, 473-474.

20 Tyrer, F.H. Group occupational health services. (History and description of current services.) Journal of the Society of Occupational Medicine, 30 (3), Jul 1980, 118-122.

21 University of Aston in Birmingham. Department of Safety and Hygiene Evaluating an OH service. Occupational Health, 28 (11), Nov 1976, 529-530.

22 University of Aston in Birmingham. Department of Safety and Hygiene Trends of employment of doctors in industry. Occupational Health, 29 (2), Feb 1977, 67-69.

23 White, D.A. The East of Scotland Occupational Health Service. (A group occupational health service serving a wide range of organisations.) Journal of the Society of Occupational Medicine, 27 (2), Apr 1977, 67-71.

d EMPLOYMENT MEDICAL ADVISORY SERVICE

1 Bibbings, R.E. Health and safety at work: the trade union view. (With reference to future role of EMAS.) Journal of the Society of Occupational Medicine, 30 (3), Jul 1980, 90-97.

2 Duncan, K. Health at work—the contribution of EMAS. (Employment Medical Advisory Service.) Department of Employment Gazette, 87 (4), Apr 1979, 350-354.

3 Duncan, K. Recent developments in the Employment Medical Advisory Service. Health Trends, 12 (1), Feb 1980, 16-18.

4 Duncan, K. and Radwanski, D. Plugged in. (Discussion about the day to day running of the Employment Medical Advisory Service.) Occupational Health, 28 (3), Mar 1976, 134-137.

5 Employment Medical Advisory Service Report 1975-1976. HMSO, 1977.

6 Orriss, H. Dealing with the hazards. (Structure of the Employment Medical Advisory Service and the range of its work in the field of occupational health.) Health and Social Service Journal, 88, 10 Feb 1978, 166.

7 Orriss, H. Employment Medical Advisory Service: first two years. Health and Social Service Journal, 86, 3 Apr 1976, 639.

e SERVICES OVERSEAS

1 De Glanville, H. and others, editors Occupational health: a manual for health workers in developing countries. Nairobi: African Medical and Research Foundation, 1979. (Rural health series; 11.)

2 Hamilton, M. OH cover for all workers—the Finnish approach. Occupational Health, 29 (8), Aug 1977, 332-335.

3 International Labour Office Migrant workers: occupational safety and health. Geneva: ILO, 1977. (Occupational safety and health series; no.34.)

4 Plant, J. Small firms look to hospitals for occupational health services. (System at Salem Hospital, Milwaukee.) Hospitals, 52 (6), 16 Mar 1978, 135-137.

f ENVIRONMENT, ERGONOMICS, SHIFTWORK

1 Bolton, C.H. Functional clothing design. (Industrial clothing designed by the Royal Aircraft Establishment, Farnborough, to give greater freedom of movement.) Occupational Health, 28 (2), Feb 1976, 79-85.

2 Colover, J. VDUs—a suitable case for treatment? (Problems and optimum conditions for use.) Occupational Health, 31 (7), Jul 1979, 366-372.

3 THE COMPRESSED work week. (Effects of 10 hour, 4 day week on health of workers.) Occupational Health Nursing, 25 (7), Jul 1977, 36-37.

4 De Trense, M. Design for working. (The reduction of job dissatisfaction and absenteeism by improving the working environment.) Occupational Health, 28 (12), Dec 1976, 559-562.

5 Gilbert, P. Visual display units—are they safe? (With operator's view on p.363.) Occupational Health, 30 (8), Aug 1978, 357-363.

6 Hamilton, M. An inspectorate's dilemma. (Annual report of the Alkali and Clean Air Inspectorate.) Occupational Health, 29 (7), Jul 1977, 284-286.

7 Hammond, J. Human engineering cuts stress and accidents. (Ergonomics and advice on lifting.) Occupational Safety and Health, 9 (5), May 1979, 14-16.

8 Hartley, C. Applying TLVs. (Threshold limit values, measure of airborne concentration of substances.) Occupational Health, 32 (6), Jun 1980, 301-303.

9 Hawkins, L.H. Circadian rhythms and shiftworking. Occupational Health, 32 (1), Jan 1980, 14-18; (2), Feb 1980, 86-90.

10 Hayne, C.R. Ergonomics—made to measure. Occupational Health, 32 (11), Nov 1980, 556-567.

11 Hayne, C.R. Ergonomics—the team approach. Occupational Health, 32 (5), May 1980, 228-232.

12 Hayne, C.R. Pass on the lifting message. (Organisation of a seminar on safe manual handling techniques.) Occupational Health, 31 (7), Jul 1979, 351-355.

13 Jacques, P. Dust and fibres in the environment. (a) Trade Unions and the working environment. (b) Particular matter in the atmosphere. (c) Health risks from inhaled dusts and fibres. Royal Society of Health Journal, 97 (3), Jun 1977, 95-105.

14 Lavery, I. Safe use of lasers. Occupational Health, 30 (5), May 1978, 220-222.

15 Lee, W.R. Some ethical problems of hazardous substances in the working environment. British Journal of Industrial Medicine, 34 (4), Nov 1977, 274-280.

16 Lobstein, R. Monitoring discomfort. (Use of heart rate measuring and palmar sweating for monitoring discomfort with the environment.) Occupational Health, 28 (7), Jul 1976, 349-353.

17 Lyons, S. Industry must understand more about lighting. Occupational Health, 24 (5), May 1972, 157-63.

18 Manenica, I. Fatigue. (Causes of fatigue in light repetitive work.) Occupational Health, 28 (5), May 1976, 228-233.

19 Mitchell, L.J. Making work more human: the case for group technology. Occupational Health, 32 (5), May 1980, 235-239.

20 Office of Population Censuses and Surveys. Social Survey Division Women and shiftwork: the protective legislation survey carried out for the Equal Opportunities Commission. HMSO, 1979.

21 Ross, D.S. Case history. Two cases of trigger finger. (1. A caulker/burner, and 2. A vegetable peeler, with general discussion.) Occupational Health, 30 (1), Jan 1978, 34-38.

22 STOP the conveyor—I want to get off. (Research sponsored by the International Institute of Labour Studies into the quality of working life and dehumanisation of work.) Occupational Health, 29 (4), Apr 1977, 143-149.

23 Tyler, G. Clockwise: a guide to working flexible hours. Occupational Health, 32 (8), Aug 1980, 413-415.

24 University of Aston in Birmingham. Department of Safety and Hygiene Effect of heat and its control. Occupational Health, 28 (8), Aug 1976, 390-393.

25 University of Aston in Birmingham. Department of Safety and Hygiene Human kinetics and good movement. (With reference to occu-

pational safety.) Occupational Health, 30 (1), Jan 1978, 22-25.

26 University of Aston in Birmingham. Department of Safety and Hygiene Lighting the workplace. (Implications for safety and health.) Occupational Health, 29 (11), Nov 1977, 474-477.

27 Voke, J. VDUs—a health hazard? (Including checklist prepared by the Industrial Society's Occupational Health Advisory Committee.) Industrial Society, 62, Sep 1980, 31-33.

28 Ward Gardner, A. and Dagnall, B.D. The effect of twelve-hour shift working on absence attributed to sickness. British Journal of Industrial Medicine, 34 (2), May 1977, 148-150.

g INDUSTRIAL INJURIES AND ACCIDENTS

1 Bartrip, P. Injured at work: the battle for compensation. (Historical survey in the light of the Pearson report.) New Society, 43, 16 Mar 1978, 595-597.

2 Bell, R. How much risk to the pound? (Problems of implementing Health and Safety at Work Act illustrated by one industrial tribunal's judgements.) Occupational Health, 32 (3), Mar 1980, 132-134.

3 Breckin, M.J. Joint consultation at Bournville—50 years ago. (Formation of an Accidents Committee.) Occupational Health, 29 (5), May 1977, 209-211.

4 Brown, G.N. Disaster planning for industry. Occupational Health, 29 (9), Sep 1977, 385-392.

5 Hale, A.R. Accident investigation: collecting the facts? (Reason why it is useful for organisations.) Occupational Health, 29 (9), Sep 1977, 400-403.

6 Kingsford, D.J. Case history. Ultra-violet radiation: an environmental hazard. (In three laboratory workers.) Occupational Health, 30 (2), Feb 1978, 74-80.

7 McMillan, G.H.G. Looking at problems—a new approach to injury records. Occupational Health, 32 (6), Jun 1980, 286-298.

8 Nedved, M. Burning issues. (Fires in industry.) Occupational Health, 32 (2), Feb 1980, 96-98.

9 Nedved, M. Explosions—prevention and control. Occupational Health, 32 (7), Jul 1980, 358-362.

10 Nedved, M. Reducing the risk of fire. Occupational Health, 32 (5), May 1980, 243-246.

11 Proctor, T.B. and Cutts, N.J. A novel method of collecting information. (A questionnaire machine for collecting accident details developed at the Safety in Mines Research Establishment.) Occupational Health, 28 (6), Jun 1976, 302-307.

12 Whincup, M. Compensation for negligence. Occupational Health, 32 (4), Apr 1980, 177-183.

13 Woodward, E. Nursing care study: nursing a case of severe industrial injury at

home. (Care of a severe sacral wound.) Journal of Community Nursing, 2 (2), Aug 1978, 4-5.

h MENTAL HEALTH AND STRESS

1 Anderson, W.A. Recognising stress. The man who couldn't say no! Occupational Health, 31 (9), Sep 1979, 396-402.

2 Ardis, M. Stress at work: a comparison of attitudes between the psychiatric and non-psychiatric short stay patients. (A survey by questionnaire to hospitals in Hull.) Journal of the Society of Occupational Medicine, 26 (1), Jan 1976, 13-20.

3 Baughn, S.L. The role of the nurse in dealing with stress in the industrial setting. Occupational Health Nursing, 24 (4), Apr 1976, 15-16.

4 Brook, A. Coping with the stress of change at work. Health Trends, 4 (10), Nov 1978, 80-84.

5 Cooper, C.L. and Payne, R. editors Stress at work. Chichester: Wiley, 1978. (Studies in occupational stress series.)

6 Cox, T. and others Job stress: the effects of repetitive work. Department of Employment Gazette, 87 (12), Dec 1979, 1234-1237.

7 de Trensé, M. How can work stress be tackled? Occupational Health, 29 (5), May 1977, 198-199.

8 Dixon, W.M. Occupational mental health in the United Kingdom. Journal of the Society of Occupational Medicine, 27 (4), Oct 1977, 143-147.

9 Erskine, J.F. and Brook, A. A method of developing the psychiatric resources of an occupational health team. (A psychiatrist spends half a day weekly with the team at the South Eastern Region, Central Electricity Generating Board.) Journal of the Society of Occupational Medicine, 26 (4), Oct 1976, 132-135.

10 Fletcher, B. Occupational psychology—an unexploited resource. Occupational Health, 31 (8), Aug 1979, 415-421.

11 Fletcher, B. Stress, illness and social class. (Concludes that blue-collar stress is a serious problem and executive stress a myth.) Occupational Health, 31 (9), Sep 1979, 405-411.

12 Fletcher, B. and others Exploding the myth of executive stress. Personnel Management, 11 (5), May 1979, 30-34.

13 Frankenhaeuser, M. Coping with stress at work. (Psychobiological approach.) Nursing Mirror, 148, 4 Jan 1979, 11-12.

14 Hall, D. Why work and job satisfaction are vital to mental health. (Report of MIND annual conference.) Health and Social Service Journal, 87, 21 Oct 1977, 1456-1457.

15 Halse, H. Stress at work. (Report of survey in Australia and ways to reduce stress.) Industrial Society, 60, Nov/Dec 1978, 17-18, 24.

16 Hunt, C. The cause and effect of stress on young people at work. (1975 Congress paper.) Occupational Health Nursing, 24 (1), Jan 1976, 17-18.

17 Kinsler, D.D. Relaxation: key to stress

reduction. Occupational Health Nursing, 25 (7), Jul 1977, 7-8.

18 Lader, M.M. Anxiety: measuring the effects. (Includes sources of stress at work.) Journal of the Society of Occupational Medicine, 27 (3), Jul 1977, 107-113.

19 Martin, I.C.A. Clinical parable. Rolls-Royce syndrome. (Executive stress causing complete physical and mental exhaustion.) Nursing Times, 73, 27 Oct 1977, 1688-1689.

20 Melhuish, A.H. Causes and prevention of executive stress. (Findings of a trial project.) Occupational Health, 29 (5), May 1977, 193-197.

21 Rowntree, G.R. The troubled employee in industry. (1975 Congress paper.) Occupational Health Nursing, 24 (1), Jan 1976, 26-27.

22 Sheahan, J. Mental distress at work. (Includes stress in general.) Nursing Mirror, 148, 25 Jan 1979, 16-19.

23 Smith, J.M. The occupational psychologist and health and safety: the psychologist's part in the prevention of accidents and stress diseases. Occupational Health, 27 (4), Apr 1977, 150-155.

24 Trachtenberg, D. Early behavioral manifestations of emotional disorders. (Role of occupational health nurse.) Occupational Health Nursing, 25 (9), Sep 1977, 16-19.

i NOISE AND OCCUPATIONAL DEAFNESS

1 Atherley, G.R.A. and Noble, W.G. Occupational hearing loss: the Industrial Injuries scheme. Occupational Health, 28 (4), Apr 1976, 182-188.

2 Barnard, J. Employing the deaf and hard of hearing. Occupational Health, 29 (3), Mar 1977, 91-95.

3 Bradley, L.P.N. Understanding hearing loss. (Role of nurse with special reference to industry.) Journal of Practical Nursing, 30 (5), May 1980, 27-29.

4 Brenny, A.A. A hearing conservation program: general considerations for the occupational health nurse. Occupational Health Nursing, 27 (12), Dec 1979, 16-20.

5 Dye, B.J. Hearing conservation education program. (Scheme at Brooks Air Force Base, Texas.) Occupational Health Nursing, 27 (1), Jan 1979, 12-14.

6 Faiers, M.C. Noise deafness and the employer's liability. Journal of the Society of Occupational Medicine, 28 (1), Jan 1978, 20-24.

7 Esler, A. Attitude change in an industrial hearing conservation program: comparative effects of directives, educational presentations and individual explanations as persuasive communications. (Research study by OH nurse.) Occupational Health Nursing, 26 (12), Dec 1978, 15-20.

8 Health and Safety Executive Audiometry in industry: discussion document. HMSO, 1978.

9 Hibbs, G.M. Audiometry on wheels. (Mobile audiometric unit established by Cadbury Schweppes to cover remote factories.) Occupational Health, 30 (5), May 1978, 213-217.

10 International Labour Office Protection of workers against noise and vibration in the working environment. Geneva: ILO, 1977. (ILO codes of practice.)

11 Kenyon, D. Unlocking silence. (Difficulties of the deaf at work.) Industrial Society, 59, Jul/Aug 1977, 14, 16.

12 McGinty, L. Noise: a standard error. While a government working party on noise at work is shaken by disagreements, workers are still inadequately protected against noise by current standards. New Scientist, 43, 24 Feb 1977, 452-454.

13 May, J. The noise problem in industry: what it is and how it can be controlled. Occupational Safety and Health, 9 (2), Feb 1979, 16-19.

14 Martin, A. Tuning in to hearing hazards. (Occupational deafness and education in its prevention.) Personnel Management, 11 (11), Nov 1979, 42-46.

15 Merriman, R. DeciBels made simple. Occupational Health, 31 (3), Mar 1979, 116-120.

16 Moller, A. How good are work noise standards? New Scientist, 73, 27 Jan 1977, 192-194.

17 Orriss, H.D. New noise legislation? (Report of the Industrial Health Advisory Subcommittee on Noise.) Occupational Health, 28 (1), Jan 1976, 24-26.

18 Society of Occupational Medicine Written evidence by the Society of Occupational Medicine to the Industrial Diseases Subcommittee on Occupational Deafness. Journal of the Society of Occupational Medicine, 27 (4), Oct 1977, 151-152.

19 Somerville, E.T. Noise induced hearing loss and industrial audiometry. (Hearing Conservation Programme adopted by the Metal Box Company Ltd.) Journal of the Royal College of General Practitioners, 26, Oct 1976, 770-780.

20 Sutton, P. The protection handbook of industrial noise control. 2nd ed. Osborne, 1977.

21 Tempest, W. The assessment of hearing handicap. (In occupational health.) Journal of the Society of Occupational Medicine, 27 (4), Oct 1977, 134-137.

22 University of Aston in Birmingham. Department of Safety and Hygiene The proposed noise legislation. Occupational Health, 28 (3), Mar 1976, 156-158.

j SAFETY AND ACCIDENT PREVENTION

1 Atherley, G. Proven or political? (Personal view of the HSC consultative document on safety representatives.) Occupational Health, 28 (1), Jan 1976, 18-20.

2 Benedictus, R. Safety representatives. Sweet and Maxwell, 1980. (Law at work series.)

3 Booth, R. Safety. (University of Aston in Birmingham Department of Occupational Health and Safety.) Occupational Health, 32 (11), Nov, 583-584.

4 Booth, R. Safety: too important a matter to be left to the engineers? (Inaugural lecture of

Professor of Safety and Hygiene at Aston University.) Occupational Health, 31 (4), Apr 1979, 174-179; 31 (5), May 1979, 228-234.

5 Bush, D. These hazards are not academic. (Accident prevention at Birmingham University.) Occupational Safety and Health, 7 (6), Jun 1977, 14-16.

6 Cameron, J. All set for the coming of the safety man. (How Cleveland area set up an effective safety system.) Health and Social Service Journal, 88, 15 Sep 1978, 1042-1043.

7 Else, D. Fitting British Standard man. (With reference to protective equipment.) Occupational Health, 30 (10), Oct 1978, 498-501.

8 Emery, M. Changing attitudes to safety... 1. (Strategy for behaviour change with reference to prevention of occupational accidents.) Occupational Safety and Health, 8 (5), Sep 1978, 31-33.

9 Glendon, A.I. Accident prevention and safety—whose responsibility? (With questionnaire for readers on p.37.) Occupational Health, 31 (1), Jan 1979, 31-36.

10 Glendon, A.I. The role and training of safety representatives. Occupational Safety and Health, 7 (11), Nov 1977, 35-36; (12), Dec 1977, 37-39.

11 Glendon, A.I. Whose responsibility? 2. (Results of survey of 30 readers on responsibility for safety and accident prevention.) Occupational Health, 32 (8), Aug 1980, 409-412.

12 Green, J. Designing hazard data sheets. (Information system for employees.) Occupational Health, 30 (12), Dec 1978, 596-604.

13 Hamilton, M. How others see us—the OH nurse's view of the safety officer. (Based on views of OH nurses in various settings.) Occupational Health, 31 (6), Jun 1979, 290-294.

14 Hamilton, M. No mere 'scrap of paper'. (Need for written safety policy under HASWA.) Occupational Safety and Health, 9 (6), Jun 1979, 10-13, 15.

15 Handley, W. editor Industrial safety handbook. 2nd ed. McGraw-Hill, 1977.

16 Health and Safety Commission Health and safety at work: safety representatives and safety committees. HMSO, 1976.

17 Health and Safety Commission Advisory Committee on Major Hazards. First report. HMSO, 1976. Second report, 1979.

18 Health and Safety Executive. Accident Prevention Advisory Unit Success and failure in accident prevention. HMSO, 1976.

19 Hesmondhalgh, S. Safety training from top to bottom. (Role of the personnel manager in safety training.) Personnel Management, 8 (12), Dec 1976, 32-35.

20 Janner, G. Enter the union safety representative. How safety representatives will interrelate with existing health and safety professionals in the workplace. Occupational Health, 30 (3), Mar 1978, 110-113.

21 McKenna, S. When are safety posters effective? (In occupational health.) Occupational Health, 30 (11), Nov 1978, 552-555.

22 Occupational Health Comments on the document. (Comments by the individuals on the Health and Safety Commission proposals on safety representatives and safety committees.) Occupational Health, 28 (5), May 1976, 234-240.

23 Occupational Health Employees join the team. (Comments upon the HSC consultative document on safety representatives and safety committees.) Occupational Health, 28 (1), Jan 1976, 11-13.

24 Occupational Health Enforcement officers may be used as 'pawns'. (With reference to safety representatives, trade unions and the Health and Safety at Work Act.) Occupational Health, 30 (11), Nov 1978, 516-517.

25 Occupational Health Guide to the document: (on safety representatives and safety committees issued by HSC). Occupational Health, 28 (1), Jan 1976, 14-17.

26 Orriss, H. Protection from ourselves. (Comments on first report of Health and Safety Executive.) Health and Social Service Journal, 87, 18 Nov 1977, 1591.

27 Perusse, M. Counting the near misses. (The Hazard and Accident Card as a method of encouraging workers to report dangerous incidents and hazards.) Occupational Health, 30 (3), Mar 1978, 123-126.

28 Raafat, H. Basic concepts of hazards. Occupational Health, 30 (9), Sep 1978, 439-441.

29 Riley, J.D. Safety committees/safety reps: who does what? (Explanation of relevant sections of the Health and Safety at Work Act.) Occupational Health, 30 (2), Feb 1978, 67-71.

30 Rose, P. Safety at work. (The present success of the Health and Safety Executive.) New Society, 37, 22 Jul 1976, 182.

31 Rose, P. Surveying the new safety structure. (The effectiveness of legislation resulting from the Robens Report.) Personnel Management, 8 (11), Nov 1976, 34-37.

32 Royal College of Nursing Health and safety at work etc Act 1974: safety representatives' handbook. Rcn, 1980.

33 Royal College of Nursing. Society of Occupational Health Nursing The Rcn and the document. (Comments on the Health and Safety Commission's consultative document on safety representatives and committees.) Occupational Health, 28 (4), Apr 1976, 202-204.

34 Royal College of Physicians Assessment of health risks at work. Report of a recent symposium at the Royal College of Physicians. (With sections on understanding the hazards, value of screening and scheme to reduce heart attacks.) Occupational Health, 30 (1), Jan 1978, 40-43.

35 Royal Society for the Prevention of Accidents Safety 77: occupational conference papers. RoSPA, 1977.

36 Smith, A. Caught out in the Act. (Progress of safety reps and committees.) Health and Social Service Journal, 90, 12 Sep 1980, 1192-1193.

37 University of Aston in Birmingham. Department of Safety and Hygiene Inside information. (Problems in providing information about health hazards to employees.) Occupational Health, 28 (5), May 1976, 256-258.

38 University of Aston in Birmingham. Department of Safety and Hygiene The new representatives. (Comments on 'The Safety Representatives and Safety Committee Regulations, 1976.') Occupational Health, 28 (10), Oct 1976, 488-490.

39 University of Aston in Birmingham. Department of Safety and Hygiene Questions which need to be asked about personal protection schemes. (e.g. respirators and hearing protectors.) Occupational Health, 29 (8), Aug 1977, 344-347.

40 University of Aston in Birmingham. Department of Safety and Hygiene Safety. Where research is needed. Occupational Health, 28 (4), Apr 1976, 205-207.

41 University of Aston in Birmingham. Department of Safety and Hygiene Safety. Who is really responsible? Occupational Health, 28 (2), Feb 1976, 100-102.

42 University of Aston in Birmingham. Department of Safety and Hygiene The safety of fixed machinery guards. Occupational Health, 27 (4), Apr 1977, 168-171.

43 University of Aston in Birmingham. Department of Safety and Hygiene Safety representatives: who should train and who should pay? Occupational Health, 29 (7), Jul 1977, 304-307.

44 University of Aston in Birmingham. Department of Safety and Hygiene Who is the safety officer? Occupational Health, 28 (12), Dec 1976, 580-582.

45 Wilkinson, W.R. Our brother's keeper. Some thoughts on safety representatives and recent safety legislation. Occupational Health and Safety, 7 (8), Aug 1977, 30-31.

46 Wilkinson, W.R. Safety memo. (Hints on running training sessions.) Industrial Society, 59, Nov/Dec 1977, 15.

71 OCCUPATIONAL HEALTH NURSING

a UNITED KINGDOM

1 Casteledine, G. Occupied with the staff's welfare. (Eight elements within role of OH nurse.) Nursing Mirror, 151, 10 Jul 1980, 12.

2 Grayham, D. Organisation theory—an essential skill for OH nurses? Occupational Health, 31 (12), Dec 1979, 562-565.

3 Hamilton, M. How others see us—the safety officer's view of the OH nurse. Occupational Health, 31 (2), Feb 1979, 68-72.

4 Harrison, B.M. Into Europe—6. United Kingdom. (Occupational health services and OH nursing.) Occupational Health, 30 (9), Sep 1978, 424-436.

5 Hill, C. Taking treatment to the shop floor: a day in the life of an industrial health service nurse. (At the West Midlands Industrial Health Service in West Bromwich.) Occupational Safety and Health, 8 (1), Jan 1978, 18-19.

6 Jarman, B.M. The extending role of the British occupational health nurse. Doctor? Safetyworker? Nurse? Journal of Advanced Nursing, 3 (2), Mar 1978, 189-198.

7 Justham, D. How OH nurses affect referrals to casualty. (Research study.) Occupational Health, 31 (10), Oct 1979, 472-478.

8 May, G. Nursing 2500 men on a vast North Wales power site. (Dinorwic pumped storage station.) Nursing Standard, 72, May 1978, 7.

9 Melville, J. Nurses at large. (The work of occupational health nurses.) New Society, 40, 21 Apr 1977, 115.

10 Occupational Health Checklist. A check list has recently been devised for use by occupational health staff from the Central Middlesex Industrial Health Service when visiting premises of member firms for the first time. Occupational Health, 28 (12), Dec 1976, 563-567.

11 Radwanski, D. Nursing and occupational health. In Gardner, A. Ward, editor Current approaches to occupational medicine. Bristol: Wright, 1979. Ch.13, 218-229.

12 Royal College of Nursing Society of Occupational Health Nursing Annual National Conference. Nursing Mirror, 145, 15 Dec 1977, 3-4.

13 Royal College of Nursing. Society of Occupational Health Nursing Professionals at work. (OH annual conference.) Occupational Health, 28 (1), Jan 1976, 37-42.

14 Royal College of Nursing. Society of Occupational Health Nursing Rcn Society. (Objectives and future activities of the Rcn Society of Occupational Health Nursing including an interview with Paul Lloyd.) Occupational Health, 28 (4), Apr 1976, 192-201.

15 Slaney, B. editor Occupational health nursing. Croom Helm, 1980.

16 Slaney, B. Saving lives at work. (Role of the OH nurse.) Nursing, 14, Jun 1980, 606-608.

b UNITED STATES

1 American Association of Industrial Nurses Issue giving papers from the 23rd AAIN Annual President's meeting with the theme 'AAIN action line for '76.' Occupational Health Nursing, 23 (12), Dec 1975, 9-36.

2 American Association of Industrial Nurses The nurse in industry: a history of the American Association of Industrial Nurses, Inc. New York: AAIN, 1976.

3 American Association of Industrial Nurses Philosophy of AAIN. Adopted by the AAIN Board of Directors, 24 April 1976. Occupational Health Nursing, 24 (6), Jun 1976, 37.

4 American Association of Industrial Nurses Principles of management-nurse relationship in industry and commerce. Occupational Health Nursing, 24 (7), Jul 1976, 26-27.

5 American Association of Occupational Health Nurses Principles of the nurse-physician relationships in an occupational health service. Occupational Health Nursing, 25 (1), Jan 1977, 17-18.

6 American Association of Occupational

Health Nurses Objectives of an occupational health nursing service. Occupational Health Nursing, 25 (1), Jan 1977, 24.

7 American Journal of Nursing Occupational health nurse promotes health in workplace. (Work of Anne Murphy.) American Journal of Nursing, 80 (3), Mar 1980, 502, 506.

8 Bender, J. and Fagerlund, P. A profile of industrial nursing practices in North Dakota. (Survey conducted by interviews with 14 occupational health nurses.) Occupational Health Nursing, 24 (5), May 1976, 20-22.

9 Benfield, L.M. The evolution of a health department. (Setting-up of department in an international corporation by an OH nurse.) Occupational Health Nursing, 27 (10), Oct 1979, 15-18.

10 Bill, S.A. A glimpse into AAIN's past. Occupational Health Nursing, 23 (12), Dec 1975, 20-22.

11 Brown, M.L. The implications of research for occupational health nursing practice. (1975 Congress paper.) Occupational Health Nursing, 24 (1), Jan 1976, 10-12.

12 Carew, H.M. Occupational health nursing: a view from within. Occupational Health Nursing, 24 (9), Sep 1976, 19-21.

13 Fish, M.S. Rights and responsibilities of occupational health nurses: the role and need for insurance. Occupational Health Nursing, 25 (11), Nov 1977, 11-12.

14 Leamons, E.P. Recruit another nurse: opportunities offered in the occupational health field. (Lists varied roles of OH nurses and describes pilot programme of student nurse visits to factory.) Occupational Health Nursing, 26 (11), Nov 1978, 11-13.

15 Lee, J.A. The nurse in industry: a guide for the newly employed occupational health nurse. Cincinnati, Ohio: United States Department of Health, Education and Welfare, 1978.

16 Lopez, E.A. Who am I? How am I seen? What can I do about it? (Views of OH nurse's role by ANA and management.) Occupational Health Nursing, 27 (8), Aug 1979, 9-13.

17 Phaneuf, M.C. Occupational health nursing: a perspective for 1980. (Catherine R. Dempsey Memorial Lecture.) Occupational Health Nursing, 28 (7), Jul 1980, 9-13.

18 Rose, S.I. A comparison study of occupational health nursing in a hospital setting as opposed to an industrial setting. (Research study in Florida.) Occupational Health Nursing, 24 (3), Mar 1976, 9-18.

19 Saller, D.M. Occupational health nursing of the future. Occupational Health Nursing, 24 (11), Nov 1976, 24-26.

20 Saller, D.M. United we stand. (Functions of American Association of Occupational Health Nurses.) Occupational Health Nursing, 25 (11), Nov 1977, 20-23.

21 Tinkham, C.W. Occupational health nursing in the 1980s. (Catherine R. Dempsey Memorial Lecture.) Occupational Health Nursing, 25 (6), Jun 1977, 7-13.

22 Weaver, B.R. Where do we go from here? The future of nursing: (with particular reference to occupational health nursing). Occupational Health Nursing, 24 (7), Jul 1976, 7-13.

23 Wirthlin, J.S. The industrial nurse's role as seen by a lawyer. Occupational Health Nursing, 24 (11), Nov 1976, 20-23.

c OTHER COUNTRIES

1 Bond, H. Into Europe. 2. Italy. (Occupational health services and nursing.) Occupational Health, 30 (5), May 1978, 226-235.

2 Buck, V. Into Europe—5. West Germany. Occupational Health, 30 (8), Aug 1978, 384-391.

3 Bundle, N. Legal aspects of occupational health nursing. (In New South Wales.) Lamp, 34 (1), Jan 1977, 7, 9, 11, 13; Australian Nurses Journal, 6 (9), Mar 1977, 37-39.

4 Bundle, N. Occupational health nurses... their role in Australia's industry. Lamp, 35 (6), Jun 1978, 10-12.

5 Craw, H. and Humphries, A. Occupational health nursing in New South Wales. (1975 Congress paper.) Occupational Health Nursing, 24 (1), Jan 1976, 19-20.

6 Cullen, M. Into Europe—3. Eire. (Occupational health and OH nursing.) Occupational Health, 30 (6), Jun 1978, 274-278.

7 Curran, I. Obituary: Sister Ida Curran. (The last serving of the six pioneer industrial nurses in New Zealand.) New Zealand Nursing Journal, 70 (8), Aug 1978, 18-19.

8 Duque, E.E. and Yabes, J.J. Occupational health nursing in the Philippines. (Research study.) Philippine Journal of Nursing, 49 (1), Jan/Mar 1979, 16-20.

9 Greenstreet, I.N. Occupational health nursing. Not just dispensing Bandaids and Disprin. (Account of a day's work.) New Zealand Nursing Journal, 70 (7), Jul 1977, 14-15.

10 Hayman, M.J. The occupational health nurse in the work environment. Canadian Nurse, 72 (7), Jul 1976, 36-41.

11 Homewood, J. Into Europe. 1. Denmark. (Occupational health services and nursing.) Occupational Health, 30 (4), Apr 1978, 167-176.

12 Jinadu, M.K. Occupational health and the nurse in developing and industrializing countries. Royal Society of Health Journal, 99 (5), Oct 1979, 219-221.

13 Matthew, S. and Williams, M.M. Into Europe. 4. Belgium. (Occupational health and OH nursing.) Occupational Health, 30 (7), Jul 1978, 322-327.

14 Mellish, J.M. The birth, growth and development and future dimensions of occupational health nursing. (With some reference to South Africa.) Curationis, 3 (2), Sep 1980, 48-53.

15 Newberry, A. and Fernie, A. 2nd Australian Convention on Occupational Health Nursing. New Zealand Nursing Journal, 70 (7), Jul 1977, 12-13.

16 Nursing News To keep SA working. (History of OH nursing in South Africa.) Nursing News, 3 (2), May 1980, 6-7.

17 Occupational Health OH nursing in the Middle East. (Advice from male nurse who has worked in Jordan and Saudi Arabia.) Occupational Health, 32 (2), Feb 1980, 60.

18 O'Sullivan, J. Legal areas affecting the occupational health nurse. Australasian Nurses Journal, 6 (9), Apr 1977, 16-18.

19 Oxer, M.E.M. Establishment of a part-time nursing service for small enterprises in Australia. (1975 Congress paper.) Occupational Health Nursing, 24 (1), Jan 1976, 15-16.

20 Parker, B. Occupational health nursing in South Australia—before and after the occupational health legislation. Australian Nurses Journal, 8 (2), Aug 1978, 33-36.

21 Williams, M.M. OH nursing in Europe. (Background to forthcoming series on the state of OH nursing in some of the EEC countries.) Occupational Health, 30 (3), Mar 1978, 130-131.

d EDUCATION AND TRAINING

1 American Association of Occupational Health Nurses AAOHN plan for continuing education in nursing. (American Association of Occupational Health Nurses' standards and assessment factors for continuing education programmes.) Occupational Health Nursing, 25 (5), May 1977, 9-12.

2 Brown, E.M. Summary of descriptive study of the occupational health nursing content in baccalaureate curricula of selected schools of nursing. Occupational Health Nursing, 24 (10), Oct 1976, 9-12.

3 Dorward, A.L. and Johnson, I.W.B. Where there's a will—there's a new OH nursing course. (Development of course at Foresterhill College, Aberdeen.) Occupational Health, 30 (7), Jul 1978, 300-305.

4 Hamilton, M. On course at Keele. (Week's study course for occupational health nurses held by the Rcn.) Occupational Health, 28 (5), May 1976, 244-247.

5 Holgate, P.D. and others Evaluation of day release as a scheme of study. (Survey of ten years of the Royal College of Nursing occupational health nursing course.) Occupational Health Nursing, 24 (2), Feb 1976, 14-16.

6 Homewood, J.V. The role of the occupational health nurse in education within the occupational health team. (1975 Congress paper.) Occupational Health Nursing, 24 (1), Jan 1976, 28-29.

7 Klutas, E.M. Reflections on certification. (History of examination system for OH nurses in USA with outlines of scope of examinations.) Occupational Health Nursing, 25 (10), Oct 1977, 26-34.

8 McCarthy, N.A. and Detherage, K.S. Learning primary preventive nursing intervention in the occupational health setting. (Student experience in occupational health at Boston College of Nursing.) Occupational Health Nursing, 24 (7), Jul 1976, 16-19.

9 Nursing Times Occupational hazards. (Editorial on occupational health nurses' case for mandatory training or statutory committee.) Nursing Times, 74 (3), 19 Jan 1977, 83.

10 Occupational Health Learning from each

other. (Report of the Rcn study course for OH nurses at Newcastle upon Tyne.) Occupational Health, 29 (6), Jun 1977, 243-247; (7), Jul 1977, 287-291.

11 **Puetz, B.E.** Continuing education participation of occupational health nurses in Indiana. (Research study.) Occupational Health Nursing, 27 (10), Oct 1979, 24-28.

12 **Radwanski, D.** An experiment in occupational health nursing teaching. (Course at Dundee University which was combined with the medical Diploma of Industrial Hygiene—1975 Congress paper.) Occupational Health Nursing, 24 (1), Jan 1976, 21-22.

13 **Sullivan, H.G.** A student nurse in industry. (Six-week clinical project.) Occupational Health Nursing, 25 (9), Sep 1977, 11-12.

e MANAGEMENT AND ROLE

1 **Baughn, S.L.** A nursing theory and model for occupational health nursing. Occupational Health Nursing, 25 (1), Jan 1977, 7-12.

2 **Bridges, H.M.** A survey report on the expanding role of the industrial nurse. Occupational Health Nursing, 24 (10), Oct 1976, 22-26.

3 **Brooks, J.A. and Holle, M.L.** Physical assessment for nurses employed in industrial medicine departments. (Report of course.) Occupational Health Nursing, 28 (6), Jun 1980, 7-8.

4 **Burkeen, O.E.** The nurse and industrial hygiene. Occupational Health Nursing, 24 (4), Apr 1976, 7-10.

5 **Cahall, J.B.** The use of the nursing process in the industrial setting. Occupational Health Nursing, 24 (11), Nov 1976, 9-13.

6 **Davis, R.L.** The occupational health audit. (Collection and analysis of information needed to develop an effective occupational health service.) Occupational Health Nursing, 24 (2), Feb 1976, 10-12.

7 **Gonzalez, P.** Bioethics and the occupational health nurse. (Catherine R. Dempsey Memorial Lecture.) Occupational Health Nursing, 17 (9), Sep 1979, 11-15.

8 **Goodwin, J.S. and Horner, S.O.** Applying management principles to the occupational health unit. Occupational Health Nursing, 24 (6), Jun 1976, 13-15.

9 **Graham, T.** The nursing process and OH. Occupational Health, 31 (12), Dec 1979, 556-560.

10 **Hagey, A. Capt.** Charting simplified. (Of periodic health examinations for US Army employees.) Occupational Health Nursing, 26 (4), Apr 1978, 16-19.

11 **Hagey, A.** An occupational health 'table of contents'. (Chart to list employee's work experience and exposure to occupational hazards.) Occupational Health Nursing, 26 (11), Nov 1978, 19-21.

12 **Hannigan, L.** Is there a need for expansion of the nurse's role in occupational health? Occupational Health Nursing, 24 (3), Mar 1976, 19-21.

13 **Holgate, P.** Health screening at work. (Role of occupational health nurse.) Occupational Health, 29 (9), Sep 1977, 373-377.

14 **Hutchinson, M.E.** Efficient occupational health service management. Occupational Health Nursing, 24 (2), Feb 1976, 7-9.

15 **Jacobi, E.M.** Professional accountability. (Lecture at annual conference.) Occupational Health Nursing, 26 (6), Jun 1978, 7-11.

16 **Keith, T.A.** Role of the industrial health professional in the screening and monitoring of systemic hypertension.) Occupational Health Nursing 25 (8), Aug 1977, 16-18.

17 **Klutas, E.M.** Confidentiality of medical information. (In occupational health nursing.) Occupational Health Nursing, 25 (4), Apr 1977, 14-17.

18 **Krikorian, M.** The occupational health nurse's emerging role in administering the plant employee protection program. (Safety programmes.) Occupational Health Nursing, 26 (8), Aug 1978, 20-21.

19 **McClure, M.L.** The occupational health nurse as a primary care provider. (With discussion of concept of nurse practitioner.) Occupational Health Nursing, 25 (11), Nov 1977, 16-19.

20 **Manuel, J.** Rehabilitation: the nurse's role. (Occupational health nurses' work at the Central Electricity Generating Board, Midlands Region.) Occupational Health, 28 (9), Sep 1976, 418-419.

21 **Murray, M.E.** C.A.R.P.—a new way to learn. (Ways of making annual safety review more interesting and successful.) Canadian Nurse, 76 (6), Jun 1980, 42-44.

22 **Occupational Health Nursing** Standards, interpretations, and audit criteria for performance of occupational health programs; nursing. (Extract from manual showing audit procedures in detail.) Occupational Health Nursing, 25 (4), 1977, 20-36.

23 **Rohan, J.T.** Updating medical files. (Form asking employees to complete brief details of health history.) Occupational Health Nursing, 26 (5), May 1978, 23-25.

24 **Schwartz, L.** The patient history: an outline for data collection. Occupational Health Nursing, 26 (10), Oct 1978, 17-20.

25 **Silberstein, C.A.** Implementing and evaluating the nursing process in the occupational health unit. Occupational Health Nursing, 24 (11), Nov 1976, 14-19.

26 **Simons, R.S.** The occupational health nurse: safety's overlooked resource. (Survey of safety-related activities.) Occupational Health Nursing, 28 (5), May 1980, 7-12.

27 **Sterner, P.L.** Quality assurance in occupational health nursing. Occupational Health Nursing, 25 (4), Apr 1977, 7-11.

28 **Trail, I.D.** Primary care: an expanded role for the occupational health nurse. Occupational Health Nursing, 24 (6), Jun 1976, 7-10.

f COUNSELLING AND PSYCHIATRIC ASPECTS

1 **American Association of Occupational Health Nurses** A guide to interviewing and counseling for the occupational health nurse. New York: AAIN, 1977.

2 **Bostwick, J.A.** Death—what should you do? (Responsibilities of OH nurse.) Occupational Health, 30 (9), Sep 1978, 418-421.

3 **Christie, E.** All in a day's work. (Case histories illustrating the job of occupational health nurses counselling workers in Northern Ireland.) Nursing Times, 72, 12 Feb 1976, 212-214.

4 **Community Outlook** The OH nurse as educator. (West Midlands Industrial Health Service.) Nursing Times, 74 (6), 9 Feb 1978, Community Outlook, 31, 33-35.

5 **Etherton, T.** How much time is spent counselling? (MIND research study with OH nurses.) Occupational Health, 31 (2), Feb 1979, 79-82.

6 **Hagen, E.L.** The counselling of female employees. Occupational Health Nursing, 25 (5), May 1977, 19-21.

7 **Hannigan, L.** The psychiatric aspects of occupational health nursing. Occupational Health Nursing, 27 (1), Jan 1979, 15-16.

8 **Heckler, L.M.** Employee education programs—one aspect of a nurse's expanded role in an occupational health program. (With reference to a smoking cessation programme.) Occupational Health Nursing, 28 (8), Aug 1980, 25-29.

9 **Hines, J.** Counselling: the case for the specialist. Occupational Health, 32 (11), Nov 1980, 577-581.

10 **Kuchinski, B.B. and Colligan, M.J.** Psychogenic illness in industry and the role of the occupational health nurse. Occupational Health Nursing, 27 (7), Jul 1979, 7-17.

11 **Rappaport, M.** Psychological nursing in industry. Occupational Health Nursing, 26 (5), May 1978, 26-29.

12 **Salotti, R.A.** The occupational health nurse as a mental health counsellor. Occupational Health Nursing, 24 (12), Dec 1976, 23-26.

13 **Schwartz, R.M.** Sexual freedom—how does the occupational health nurse handle it? Occupational Health Nursing, 24 (4), Apr 1976, 11-14.

14 **Settino, J.** Reflections from a new nurse in industry. (A new preventive role for Oh nurse—assisting employees with general health problems.) Occupational Health Nursing, 25 (4), Apr 1977, 18-19.

15 **Stewart, B.** Guide to counselling. (Based on Wessex RHA handbook.) Occupational Health.
1. 30 (11), Nov 1978, 542-547.
2. 30 (12), Dec 1978, 586-593.
3. Interaction. 31 (1), Jan 1979, 44-49.
4. Communication. 31 (2), Feb 1979, 96-100.
5. 31 (3), Mar 1979, 128-131.
6. Conclusion. 31 (4), Apr 1979, 202-206.

16 **Tubbs, A.L.** The occupational health nurse as counselor—learning to listen. Occupational Health Nursing, 28 (6), Jun 1980, 13-14.

17 Turvey, M.K. and Marshall, A.M. The influence of the occupational health nurse as an educator. (1975 Congress paper.) Occupational Health Nursing, 24 (1), Jan 1976, 23-25.

18 Williams, M.M. A study of counselling by occupational health nurses in hospital and other occupational health services. MPhil thesis, University of London, 1979.

19 Williams, M.M. What is meant by 'counselling'. (Research study into what OH nurses understand by counselling and how much they do.) Occupational Health, 32 (1), Jan 1980, 38-43.

72 OCCUPATIONAL HEALTH IN THE HEALTH SERVICE

a GENERAL AND UNITED KINGDOM

1 Blackadder, E.S. Health and safety at work for the healthcare industry. (Review of Government and Health and Safety Executive policy.) Royal Society of Health Journal, 99 (4), Aug 1979, 137-139.

2 British Medical Journal From the OH Committee. Occupational health service for NHS. (Report of recent meeting including discussion of delegation to nurses.) British Medical Journal, 1, 11 Mar 1978, 664-665.

3 British Medical Journal Health and safety at work. (Comment on HSE's pilot study 'Working conditions in the medical service'.) British Medical Journal, 2, 9 Sep 1978, 715-716.

4 Cameron, D. Doctors and nurses deserve health care too. (Review of Scottish Home and Health Department study of hospital occupational health services in Scotland.) Health and Social Service Journal, 86, 21 Jan 1977, 94-95.

5 Clark, L. OH care for NHS staff. Nursing Times 74.
1. Occupational health in the NHS: an introduction. 20 Jul 1978, 1196-1197.
2. Health supervision. 27 Jul 1978, 1255-1256.
3. Health and safety at work. 3 Aug 1978, 1285-1286.
4. Counselling, absenteeism and research. 10 Aug 1978, 1337-1338.
5. Towards an effective service. (Operational policy). 17 Aug 1978, 1372.

6 Clode, D. At risk—the health of hospital workers. (Report on pilot study by HSE.) Health and Social Service Journal, 88, 16 Jun 1978, 684.

7 Clode, D. Danger: major obstacles ahead. (Report on the HSE pilot study on health and safety in hospitals.) Health and Social Service Journal, 88, 4 Aug 1978, 872-874.

8 Clode, D. Explosive mix of power and suspicion. (Implementation of the Health and Safety at Work Act in the NHS. See also p.894.) Health and Social Service Journal, 88, 11 Aug 1978, 902-905.

9 Dennis, H.L. Safety representatives... warts and all. (Health service managers' responsibilities.) Nursing Times, 76, 21 Aug 1980, 1503-1505.

10 Department of Health and Social Security The functions of occupational health services for the employees of health authorities. (Appendix to draft guidelines for OH services in the NHS.) Occupational Health, 29 (10), Oct 1977, 434-437.

11 Gregory, J. OH in the health service. Occupational Health, 32 (4), Apr 1980, 196-201.

12 Hammond, G. The establishment and development of an occupational health service in hospitals and community service. (With historical review from 1964.) World of Irish Nursing, 9 (5/6), May/Jun 1980, 2, 4.

13 Harvey, J. Covering all the ground to reduce working risks. (Health and safety programme at Camden and Islington AHA (T).) Health and Social Service Journal, 87, 18 Mar 1977, 476-477.

14 Health and Safety Executive Pilot study: working conditions in the medical service. (Using North West Thames region.) Health and Safety Executive, 1978.

15 Healy, G. Health and safety regulations: a catalyst for conflict? (Operation of Health and Safety at Work Act in the NHS and how introduction of safety representatives may bring conflict.) Health and Social Service Journal, 88, 18 Aug 1978, Centre eight papers, F29-F32.

16 Johnson, G.A.E. Safety at work pilot scheme. (Letter describing pilot scheme for the Health and Safety at Work Act in Hither Green Hospital.) Health and Social Service Journal, 88, 20 Oct 1978, 1198.

17 Jones, V.E. Is your service really necessary? (The birth and early development of an OH service at Charing Cross Hospital.) Occupational Health, 29 (11), Nov 1977, 462-467.

18 Jones, V.E. Is your service really necessary? Caring for a multidisciplinary society: the OH nurse's role. 2. The occupational health service at the Charing Cross Hospital. Occupational Health, 29 (12), Dec 1977, 518-523.

19 Jones, V.E. Is your service really necessary? 3. Risks to hospital staff at Charing Cross Hospital and the role of the occupational health nurse in dealing with them. Occupational Health, 30 (1), Jan 1978, 26-33.

20 Jones, V.E. Is your service really necessary? 4 and 5. Operational policy. (Principles, aims and functions of the OH unit at Charing Cross Hospital.) Occupational Health, 30 (2), Feb 1978, 84-90; 30 (3), Mar 1978, 134-137.

21 Jones, V.E. Is your service really necessary? 6. Proving the need. (OH unit at Charing Cross Hospital.) Occupational Health, 30 (4), Apr 1978, 184-188.

22 Jones, V.E. Teaching hospital porters to lift patients safely. (Project at Charing Cross Hospital.) Occupational Health, 31 (1), Jan 1979, 23-30.

23 Kearney, J.M. Sickness absence patterns in hospital staff. (Survey by the Highland Health Board.) Occupational Health, 27 (4), Apr 1977, 162-165.

24 Lancet Commentary from Westminster. Health and safety in medical establishments. (Five-year programme of hospital inspection to be undertaken by HSE.) Lancet, 2, 9 Sep 1978, 586.

25 Lancet Commentary from Westminster. The safety of hospital workers. (Comment on pilot study by HSE in North West Thames region.) Lancet, 1, 10 Jun 1978, 1270-1271.

26 Nursing Mirror Inspectors slam 'below standard' conditions. (Report on HSE pilot study on hospitals in the North West Thames Region.) Nursing Mirror, 146, 22 Jun 1978, 4.

27 Nursing Times NHS pilot schemes will point the way to enforcing the Health and Safety Act. Nursing Times, 72, 25 Nov 1976, 1824.

28 Nursing Times Occupational health service for NHS workers—on a shoestring. (Draft circular for consultation.) Nursing Times, 74, 15 Sep 1977, 1417.

29 Nursing Times OH—what a lovely war. (Editorial on current impasse in providing OH service for NHS staff.) Nursing Times, 74, 20 Jul 1978, 1183.

30 Nursing Times Nursing Times explains. Safety representatives in the NHS. Nursing Times, 74, 5 Oct 1978, 1623.

31 Occupational Health At last the DHSS guidelines on OH services. (For NHS staff. Summary of draft circular issued in August.) Occupational Health, 29 (9), Sep 1977, 364-365.

32 Occupational Health Physician heal thyself. (Editorial on OH services in the NHS.) Occupational Health, 29 (7), Jul 1977, 275.

33 Pavitt, L. The pending file. (Occupational health services for NHS staff.) Nursing Times, 76, 14 Aug 1980, 1423.

34 Pearson, J.C.G. and others Survey of present health care provisions for staff of health boards. Scottish Home and Health Department, 1976. (Scottish health service studies, no.36.)

35 Royal College of Nursing Long overdue, but still welcome. (Comments by the Rcn Society of OH Nursing on the DHSS draft circular on NHS OH services.) Occupational Health, 29 (11), Nov 1977, 460-461.

36 Royal Institute of Public Health and Hygiene Occupational health and the National Health Service. Papers presented at annual conference. Community Health, 8 (4), May 1977, 221-225.

37 Smythe, T. The NHS and the psychiatrically ill worker. Occupational Health, 32 (8), Aug 1980, 394-401.

38 Swarbrick, P. Developing a good OH service in the NHS. Occupational Health, 31 (5), May 1979, 240-245.

b OVERSEAS COUNTRIES

1 Glover, N.J. The occupational health service for employees of Gisborne Hospital Board. New Zealand Nursing Journal, 70 (3), Mar 1977, 6-7.

2 McEwen, J. An employee fitness program. (At Ottawa Civic Hospital.) Canadian Nurse, 76 (4), Apr 1980, 36-38.

3 Morgan, J.A. and Wozniak, P.R. Reducing direct and indirect losses. The hospital safety program. (At Little Company of Mary Hospital, Evergreen Park, Illinois.) Hospital Progress, 58 (11), Nov 1977, 88-89, 106.

4 Osborn, P. Employee health service in a hospital. (Range of work.) Supervisor Nurse, 10 (10), Oct 1979, 40-42.

c HAZARDS

1 Armand Smith, N.G. Tuberculin testing of a general hospital staff. (Survey at Northern General Hospital, Edinburgh.) Health Bulletin, 37 (4), Jul 1979, 174-179.

2 British Medical Journal Tuberculin testing in hospital staff. British Medical Journal, 2, 3 Sep 1977, 592.

3 Brown, P.M. and Souter, R.V. Health and safety in hospital laboratories. (Report of inspection of hospital laboratories in the Hull area.) Journal of the Society of Occupational Medicine, 27 (4), Oct 1977, 148-150.

4 Clark, L. Laboratory hazards (in hospitals). Occupational Health, 28 (2), Feb 1976, 86-95.

5 Dempster, G. Infection control. Protection from carriers of hepatitis B. (Safety precautions for staff dealing with hepatitis cases.) Dimensions in Health Service, 52 (12), Dec 1975, 27-29.

6 Donn, M.C. Report on symposium on environmental hazards (for hospital staff). NATNews, 13 (6), Aug 1976, 21-23.

7 Flury, P.A. Environmental health and safety in the hospital laboratory. Springfield: Thomas, 1978.

8 Harrington, J.M. and Shannon, H.S. Incidence of tuberculosis, hepatitis, brucellosis and shigellosis in British medical laboratory workers. British Medical Journal, 1, 27 Mar 1976, 759-762.

9 Hendrick, D.J. and Lane, D.J. Occupational formalin asthma. (Found in nursing staff at the haemodialysis unit, Churchill Hospital, Oxford.) British Journal of Industrial Medicine, 34 (1), Feb 1977, 11-18.

10 Hicks, C. Occupational hazards. (Work-in at Etwall Hospital, Derbyshire.) Nursing Times, 76, 3 Apr 1980, 579-580.

11 Holgate, P. Safety in the NHS. Nursing, 14, Jun 1980, 602-605.

12 Milliken, R.A. and others Hospital environmental pollution and employee health hazards. Hospital Topics, 55 (2), Mar/Apr 1977, 22, 24, 26, 27.

13 Murray, W.G.D. Health hazards in hospital. (Conference paper.) Community Health, 7 (3), Jan 1976, 166-169.

14 Nevenheim, A. Tests measure ethylene oxide risk to hospital's central supply staff. Hospitals, 53 (6), 16 Mar 1979, 147-148, 150.

15 Peters, D. Job perils in the nursing service. (Report of questionnaire survey into hazards faced by hospital nurses and their attitudes to health and safety.) Occupational Safety and Health, 9 (2), Feb 1979, 23-24, 42.

16 Royal College of Nursing Acquired infection in the NHS and its prevention: a suggested code of practice for occupational health and NHS staff. Rcn, 1978.

17 Salvage, J. Danger! nurses at work. (Occupational hazards to hospital staff.) Nursing Mirror, 148, 22 Mar 1979, 12.

18 Samuels, T.M. Personnel exposures to ethylene oxide in a central service assembly and sterilisation area. Hospital Topics, 56 (3), May/Jun 1978, 27-33.

19 Skinner, M. Safety fights against all the odds. (Safety in pathology laboratories with reference to the Howie recommendations.) Health and Social Service Journal, 89, 1 Feb 1979, 88-89.

d RADIATION

1 Dunster, H.J. Radiation protection standards. Community Health, 8 (3), Jan 1977, 124-131.

2 Lavery, I. A model code of practice. (Regulations on exposure to ionising radiations.) Occupational Health, 32 (4), Apr 1980, 187-191.

3 Lloyd, D. Radiation exposure and chromosome damage. Occupational Health, 31 (11), Nov 1979, 504-509.

4 McKinlay, A. and Harlen, F. Ultra violet radiation in the workplace. Occupational Health, 31 (10), Oct 1979, 454-461.

5 Minder, W. and Osborn, S.B. Manual on radiation protection in hospitals and general practice. Vol.5: personnel monitoring services. Geneva: WHO, 1980.

6 Mould, R.F. Danger! Guard against radiation. (Protective procedures in hospital.) Nursing Mirror, 147, 31 Aug 1978, 15-18; 7 Sep 1978, 23-25.

7 Mould, R.F. Radiation protection for nurses. IPC Business Press, 1978. Based on articles in Nursing Mirror, 31 Aug 1978, 15-18; 7 Sep 1978, 23-25.

8 Occupational Health Radiation research. A review of the latest projects being carried out by the National Radiological Protection Board. Occupational Health, 29 (5), May 1977, 200-205.

9 Scott, E. Radiation protection for nurses. Nursing Times, 75, 15 Mar 1979, 441-445.

10 Spoor, N. Health care of people at work. Safety in the handling of radionuclides. Journal of the Society of Occupational Medicine, 26 (2), Apr 1976, 43-49.

11 Weeks, J.L. Radiation exposure in the laboratory (including a case study report). Journal of the Society of Occupational Medicine, 26 (1), Jan 1976, 9-12.

73 OCCUPATIONAL HEALTH IN SPECIAL AREAS

a AGRICULTURE

1 British Medical Journal Country health. (Occupational hazards of agriculture.) British Medical Journal, 2, 24/31 Dec 1977, 1621-1622.

2 Elliott, C.K. The farmer, his health and that of his family. Rehabilitation, 100, Jan-Mar 1977, 31-35.

3 Helmsman, A. Safe and sound. (Noise level safety for tractors.) Occupational Health, 28 (11), Nov 1976, 514-517.

4 International Labour Office Guide to health and hygiene in agricultural work. Geneva: ILO, 1979.

5 Martin, M. Why forestry needs OH nurses. (Study of the need for occupational health services for Forestry Commission employees.) Occupational Health, 28 (9), Sep 1976, 424-438; (10), Oct 1976, 477-486.

6 Miller, C.H.W. Diseases of sprout pickers. (A Bedfordshire GP writes about his experience of the food industry.) Occupational Health, 28 (6), Jun 1976, 300-301.

7 Occupational Safety and Health Agricultural safety supplement. Occupational Safety and Health, 9 (7), Jul 1979, 37-40; (10), Oct 1979, 43-46.

8 Ross, D.S. The straw plaiters. (Conditions of work and occupational health aspects of a cottage industry.) Occupational Health, 29 (8), Aug 1977, 350-352.

9 Smith, D.M. Health care of people at work. Agricultural workers. (Hazards and suggested health precautions.) Journal of the Society of Occupational Medicine, 27 (3), Jul 1977, 87-92.

b ASBESTOS

1 British Medical Journal Exposure to asbestos dust. British Medical Journal, 1, 5 Jun 1976, 1361.

2 Dalton, J.P. Asbestos: killer dust. British Society for Social Responsibility in Science, 1978.

3 Elmes, P.C. Asbestos—health hazards in perspective. Current information on the health risk of asbestos. Royal Society of Health Journal, 96 (6), Dec 1976, 248-252.

4 Health and Safety Executive Asbestos: (summary of reports by the Health and Safety Commission and the Advisory Committee on Asbestos.) HSE, 1979.

5 Kelly, R.T. Asbestos—health hazards in perspective. Constructional uses. Royal Society of Health Journal, 96 (6), Dec 1976, 246-248.

6 Kelly, R.T. GLC code on asbestos. Occupational Health, 28 (10), Oct 1976, 475-476.

7 Lancet Asbestos. (Review of studies of asbestos-associated disorders.) Lancet, 2, 10 Dec 1977, 1211-1213.

8 Mann, B. Asbestosis—the killer disease. Nursing Mirror, 143, 15 Jul 1976, 54-56.

9 Nursing Times 'An acceptable level of risk.' (Ombudsman's report on cases of asbestosis at Acre Mill, Hebden Bridge, Yorkshire.) Nursing Times, 72, 6 May 1976, 684. See also Lancet, 1, 1 May 1976, 944-945.

10 Ross, D.S. An early case of asbestosis. (Its detection in a fitter and problems of telling him about his condition.) Occupational Health, 30 (6), Jun 1978, 258-260.

11 Shield, A.C. Deadly asbestos. Australian Nurses Journal, 5 (3), Sep 1975, 33-34.

12 Tait, N. Asbestos killer. (Report of two campaigns to highlight the hazards of asbestos.) Nursing Times, 72, 6 May 1976, 682-683.

13 Taylor, N.R.W. Hazards to health from the use of asbestos. Health Trends, 9 (3), Aug 1977, 54-55.

14 Wagg, R.M. Asbestos—health hazards in perspective. Safety measures when handling asbestos. Royal Society of Health Journal, 96 (6), Dec 1976, 252-255.

15 Wright, W.J. Asbestosis—the symptoms and course of the disease. Nursing Times, 72, 6 May 1976, 685-686.

c CHEMICAL

1 Booth, C.M. High pressure paint gun injuries. British Medical Journal, 19 Nov 1977. Reprinted in Occupational Health, 30 (11), Nov 1978, 558-563.

2 Bourne, M.S. and others Asthma due to industrial use of chloramine. (Used as sterilising agent in breweries.) British Medical Journal, 2, 7 Jul 1979, 10-12.

3 Burge, P.S. Occupational asthma in the electronics industry. (Includes general discussion of occupational asthma.) Occupational Health, 30 (9), Sep 1978, 411-417.

4 Cohen, R. Industrial toxicology: a practical approach. Occupational Health Nursing, 28 (6), Jun 1980, 9-12.

5 Crow, K. Chloracne: the chemical disease. New Scientist, 78, 13 Apr 1978, 78-80.

6 Ffrench, G. Guide to gases which threaten your life. (The detection and avoidance of dangerous gases and treatment and management of chemical poisoning, physical injuries and infection.) Nursing Mirror, 148, 15 Feb 1979, 32-37.

7 Donovan, L. Polyvinyl chloride. (Nursing care of victims of toxic fumes.) RN Magazine, 41 (2), Feb 1978, 58-63.

8 Fox, A.J. and Collier, P.F. Mortality experience of workers exposed to vinyl chloride monomer in the manufacture of polyvinyl chloride in Great Britain. British Journal of Industrial Medicine, 34 (1), Feb 1977, 1-10.

9 Gardiner, J.S. Health care of people at work. The toxicological screening of industrial chemicals. Journal of the Society of Occupational Medicine, 27 (1), Jan 1977, 13-19.

10 Gill, J. and Martin, K. Safety management: reconciling rules with reality. (Survey of safety policy in a large chemical plant.) Personnel Management, 8 (6), Jun 1976, 36-39.

11 Hall, J.A. Vinyl chloride: a hazard of the seventies. Occupational Health, 31 (5), May 1979, 251-257.

12 Iveson-Iveson, J. The price of progress. (Visit to BASF, a large chemical company in West Germany renowned for its occupational health service.) Nursing Mirror, 151, 4 Dec 1980, 24-26.

13 Kornbacher, G. The nurse's role in toxicology. Occupational Health Nursing, 24 (8), Aug 1976, 24-26.

14 Law, G. Nursing care study. Arsine poisoning. Nursing Mirror, 143, 11 Nov 1976, 46-47.

15 Le Quesne, P. Dangerous substances at work. (Toxicology.) Nursing Mirror, 151, 7 Aug 1980, 28-30.

16 Mendis, R. Common accidents in a brewery. (Based on analysis of accident records.) Nursing Mirror, 146, 6 Apr 1978, 35.

17 Montgomery, R.R. and Reinhardt, C.F. A capsule dose of toxicology. (A brief guide to toxic substances.) Occupational Health Nursing, 24 (5), May 1976, 7-16.

18 Nedved, M. The electrochemical industry: a survey of the hazards. Occupational Health, 31 (2), Feb 1979, 88-90.

19 Proctor, N.H. and Hughes, J.P. editors Chemical hazards of the workplace. Philadelphia: Lippincott, 1978.

20 Raniere, T.M. Chemical hazard identification—our need to work together. (Need for nurse, doctor and environmental safety experts to work together.) Occupational Health Nursing, 26 (9), Sep 1978, 19-21.

21 Rubenstein, R. and Bellin, J.S. Chemical hazards in the workplace. Occupational Health Nursing, 24 (10), Oct 1976, 16-21.

22 University of Aston in Birmingham. Department of Safety and Hygiene Difficulties in monitoring toxic substances in air. Occupational Health, 28 (7), Jul 1976, 362-364.

23 University of Aston in Birmingham. Department of Safety and Hygiene The lessons of Flixborough. Occupational Health, 28 (1), Jan 1976, 45-47.

24 University of Aston in Birmingham. Department of Safety and Hygiene Testing chemicals for cancer risk. Occupational Health, 28 (8), Sep 1976, 442-445.

25 Vale, P.T. and Kipling, M.D. Miscellaneous symptoms occurring in workers engaged in the manufacture of PVC. Journal of the Society of Occupational Medicine, 26 (3), Jul 1976, 95-97.

26 Wright, W. Clouds of misery. (Dangers of dioxin, used as chemical warfare agent and in industrial processes.) Nursing Mirror, 151, 21 Aug 1980, 24-25.

d CONSTRUCTION

1 Abeytunga, P.K. Constructive criticism. (Hazards on construction sites and ways to improve situation.) Occupational Health, 31 (6), Jun 1979, 302-305.

2 Hamilton, M. Construction defaults on health care for employees. (Report of recent construction industry safety conference.) Occupational Health, 31 (11), Nov 1979, 532-534.

3 Health and Safety Executive. HM Factory Inspectorate One hundred fatal accidents in construction. HMSO, 1978.

4 Lancet Whole body vibration. (Review of research.) Lancet, 1, 14 May 1977, 1040-1041.

5 Ross, D.S. Low haemoglobin/high altitude.

Unusual symptoms which affected a construction supervisor working at altitude. Occupational Health, 28 (10), Oct 1976, 493-496.

6 Royal Society of Health Journal Accidents in the building industry. (Four articles on implementing the Health and Safety at Work Act.) Royal Society of Health Journal, 97 (6), Dec 1977, 245-252.

7 White, T.G. and Wicks, R.P. Heart failure in industry? (Using electrical impedance plethysmography to detect possible heart failure in crane drivers.) Occupational Health, 28 (2), Feb 1976, 70-77.

e METALS AND MINING

1 Antrobus, M. Lead poisoning. (A case study of industrial poisoning.) Nursing Times, 72 (47), 25 Nov 1976, 1832-1834.

2 Archibald, R.M. Medicine for the mines. 1. (Medical services.) 2. (Nursing service.) Health and Social Service Journal, 86, 3 Apr 1976, 628-629; 15 May 1976, 886-887.

3 Coombs, D. Precision foundry hazards. Occupational Health, 32 (3), Mar 1980, 123-127.

4 Critchley, J. Cadmium—working with a poison. (Includes screening programme at Johnson Matthey Metals Ltd.) Occupational Health, 32 (7), Jul 1980, 341-346.

5 Health and Safety Executive Airborne dust in quarries: health precautions. HMSO, 1976. (Health and safety executive guidance note.)

6 Kowalski, A. Production pressures put lives of Polish miners at risk. Occupational Health, 32 (3), Mar 1980, 145-147.

7 McIvor, J. Flying to work. (Occupational health nurses working in uranium mine in Northern Canada.) Canadian Nurse, 73 (12), Dec 1977, 34-36.

8 Mooney, F.S. Coal dust: source of pneumoconiosis and lung cancer. Nursing Mirror, 142, 12 Feb 1976, 46-47.

9 Moore, M.R. Occupational health. 6. The silent epidemic. (Lead poisoning.) Nursing Mirror, 151, 4 Sep 1980, 26-28.

10 Morris, E. Lead poisoning: an historic view. Occupational Health, 32 (9), Sep 1980, 449-459.

11 Payne, L.R. The hazards of cobalt. Journal of the Society of Occupational Medicine, 27 (1), Jan 1977, 20-25.

12 Ross, D.S. and Hewitt, P.J. Welding fumes and welders' health. Occupational Health, 28 (11), Nov 1976, 520-527.

13 Sloan, D. The health hazards of welding. Occupational Safety and Health, 8 (6), Jun 1978, 28-29; (7), Jul 1978, 44-45.

14 Walder, D. Can uranium trigger 'bends'? Occupational Health, 28 (12), Dec 1976, 557-558.

f OIL

1 Berrie, P. Occupational health. 1. Diving

into deep water. (Causes and effects of decompression sickness with care study of victim.) Nursing Mirror, 151, 31 Jul 1980, 18-22.

2 **British Medical Journal** Medicine in the 'Seventies. The North Sea. British Medical Journal, 1, 20 Mar 1976, 705-706.

3 **British Society for Social Responsibility in Science** Oil: a worker's guide to the health hazards and how to fight them. The Society, 1976.

4 **Crosbie, W.A. and Clarke, M.B.** Physical characteristics and ventilatory function of 404 commercial divers working in the North Sea. British Journal of Industrial Medicine, 34 (1), Feb 1977, 19-25.

5 **Douglas, R.** Safety in a hostile marine environment: how construction workers cope with North Sea hazards. Occupational Safety and Health, 8 (5), May 1978, 66-67.

6 **Evans, M.J.** Helicopter supply and evacuation. (Problems of North Sea medical emergencies for helicopters.) Journal of the Society of Occupational Medicine, 26 (3), Jul 1976, 89-91.

7 **Gardiner, R.W.K.** Work on Uncle John. (Author's work as a nurse on a North Sea oil rig including his role as caisson master in charge of life support equipment for divers.) Nursing Times, 74, 18 May 1978, 827-829.

8 **Golden, F.S.C.** Hypothermia: a problem for North Sea industries. Journal of the Society of Occupational Medicine, 26 (3), Jul 1976, 85-88.

9 **Hamilton, M.** Compressed air code. (Medical code of practice for work in compressed air formulated by the Medical Research Council decompression sickness panel.) Occupational Health, 28 (4), Apr 1976, 208-209.

10 **Hamilton, M.** Lifeline for North Sea Divers. (Proposal for transferring injured divers via a pressurised transfer chamber to a hyperbaric hospital.) New Scientist, 72, 2 Dec 1976, 516-518.

11 **Iveson-Iveson, J.** Nursing in the North Sea. (Occupational health nursing in the oil industry.) Nursing Mirror, 146, 16 Mar 1978, 28-29.

12 **James, P.B.** Medical training for the diving industry. (In the North Sea.) Nursing Times, 74, 18 May 1978, 824-826.

13 **Nimmo, A. and Innes, G.** A survey of in-patients from the oil related industries in North-East Scotland. (Admitted to the Grampian, Orkney and Shetland Health Board Areas 1976/1977.) Health Bulletin, 37 (1), Jan 1979, 20-23.

14 **Occupational Health** Facing up to North Sea hazards. (Institute of Petroleum Safety.) Occupational Health, 28 (11), Nov 1976, 535-538.

15 **Proctor, D.M.** Medicine and the North Sea: hospital support in off-shore emergencies. Journal of the Society of Occupational Medicine, 26 (2), Apr 1976, 53-56.

16 **Robinson, W.** Decompression sickness. (Developments supported by the Medical Research Council.) Nursing Mirror, 143, 16 Dec 1976, 39-40.

17 **Ross, B.C.** Noise on offshore platforms. Occupational Health, 30 (11), Nov 1978, 524-527.

18 **Royal College of Nursing** Comments on Health and Safety Executive recommendations for the training of offshore sick bay attendants (rig medics.) Rcn, 1978.

19 **Shepherd, F.G.G.** Medicine and the North Sea: emergencies for the general practitioner. Journal of the Society of Occupational Medicine, 26 (2), Apr 1976, 50-52.

20 **Swiss, M.** Why these divers died. (Lessons to be learnt from details of North Sea diving accidents issued by the Department of Energy.) Occupational Health, 28 (7), Jul 1976, 343-347.

g STUDENT HEALTH

1 **Bourke, J.B. and others** The use and value of a University Health Centre with attached beds in the management of general surgical patients. (Nottingham.) Health Trends, 2 (10), May 1978, 42-44.

2 **Brian, V.A.** Undergrads' nurse: self-confidence rewarded. (Based on author's experience when in charge of the vaccination and injection clinic in a large university health service.) Nursing Mirror, 147, 20 Jul 1978, 38.

3 **British Medical Journal** Health services in higher education. British Medical Journal, 281, 12 Jul 1980, 96-97.

4 **Bush, D.** Aspects of student health. Health and safety in a university. British Medical Journal, 2, 4 Dec 1976, 1369-1371.

5 **Committee of Vice-Chancellors and Principals of the Universities of the United Kingdom** Safety in universities: notes of guidance. Part 2: 1 Lasers. Association of Commonwealth Universities, 1978.

6 **Dickinson, K.G.** Aspects of student health. Student health services. British Medical Journal, 2, 13 Nov 1976, 1177-1178.

7 **Edmonds, O.P.** University nurses in Canada. (Study tour examining the role of the college health nurse.) Occupational Health, 28 (3), Mar 1976, 152-155.

8 **Finlay, S.E.** Aspects of student health. Physical diseases in university students. (Result of a study of university entrants at Nottingham University.) British Medical Journal, 2, 27 Nov 1976, 1312-1314.

9 **Goldsmith, M.** A senior nursing sister's work (in student health) *in* Wilkinson, A. editor Student health practice. Pitman, 1979. Ch.8, 58-68.

10 **Hamilton, M.** University health and safety service—a blueprint for others. (Work of Manchester University's occupational health service.) Occupational Health, 29 (3), Mar 1977, 96-97.

11 **Mackenzie, L.** College health. (Occupational health service in Cambridgeshire College of Arts and Technology with aspects of current work.) Occupational Health, 29 (1), Jan 1977, 13-21; (2), Feb 1977, 54-61.

12 **MacMaster, E.** Sources of stress in university nursing students. (Research study.) Nursing Papers, 11 (4), Winter 1979, 87-96.

13 **Pashley, B.W.** Counselling in an educational community: a case study. (Research study carried out 1972 to 1975 at Hull University to ascertain students' perceptions of counselling services provided.) Community Health, 8 (3), Jan 1977, 143-154.

14 **Pashley, B.** Student health services: how educational? Health Education Journal, 36 (3), 1977, 70-76.

15 **Rees, W.D.C.** Counselling in colleges of education. (Survey of student welfare services, including use of college nurse as confidant.) British Journal of Guidance and Counselling, 5 (1), Jan 1977, 65-72.

16 **Thorne, B.** Aspects of student health. Counselling and the student. British Medical Journal, 2, 20 Nov 1976, 1245-1246.

17 **Veasey, H.E.M.** Aspects of student health. Specific psychological problems. British Medical Journal, 1, 1 Jan 1977, 26-28.

18 **Wilkinson, A. editor** Student health practice. Pitman, 1979.

h TRANSPORT, TRAVEL AND SPORT

1 **Airline Users Committee** Care in the air: advice for handicapped passengers. The Committee, 1977.

2 **Ashworth, N.W.** Implications to industrial organizations. (Of travel abroad by employees.) Royal Society of Health Journal, 97 (5), Oct 1977, 221-224.

3 **Castledine, G.** Why sport? Five articles on sports medicine including one on the value of exercise. Nursing, 4, Jul 1979, 155-168, 170, 173.

4 **Clark, D.** St. John Ambulance spreads its wings. (Aeromedical service escorting patients across the world.) Nursing Times, 74, 24 Aug 1978, 1398-1399.

5 **Cowan, J.M.C.** In-flight treatment. (Study of medical training of aircraft cabin crew for in-flight emergencies.) Occupational Health, 28 (12), Dec 1976, 570-576.

6 **Duff, J.** Medicine on Everest. (Experiences of a member of the successful South-West face expedition in 1975.) Nursing Mirror, 142, 24 Jun 1976, 46-48. Reprinted in Nursing Mirror, 143, 2 Sep 1976, 68-70.

7 **Gunn, A.D.G.** Holidays—the shot in the arm we all need. (With table showing international travel immunisations.) Journal of Community Nursing, 2 (10), Apr 1979, 4-5.

8 **Haward, L.R.C.** Pilot beware! (Occupational stress in pilots.) Nursing Mirror, 146, 22 Jun 1978, 13-15.

9 **Lover, J.** Homeward bound. (Volunteer nurse's work with St. John Ambulance Aeromedical Service.) Nursing Mirror, 150, 19 Jun 1980, 21-22.

10 **Morris, P.** The trouble with trucks. (Survey of the occupational hazards of heavy goods vehicle drivers.) Occupational Health, 28 (6), Jun 1976, 285-289.

11 **Neustatter, P.** Travel medicine. Midwife, Health Visitor and Community Nurse, 16 (8), Aug 1980, 324-327.

12 **Owen, J.R.** The care of athletes on tours abroad. Practitioner, 217, Aug 1976, 240-245.

13 **Ross, T.** Sky-high care at Heathrow. (Medical screening and care of employees and passengers.) Nursing Mirror, 151, 4 Sep 1980, 18-20.

14 **Royal College of Physicians of London** The cardiovascular fitness of airline pilots: report of a working party. British Medical Association, 1978. (Reprinted from British Heart Journal, 40 (4), Mar 335-350.) (Chairman: J.F. Goodwin.)

15 **Smith, J. and Gardner, S.** Health at London Airport. (Letter describing a visit to the Health Control Section at Heathrow.) Health Visitor, 49 (3), Mar 1976, 91.

16 **Sperryn, P.N.** Aspects of student health. Sports medicine and the student. British Medical Journal, 1, 19 Feb 1977, 502-503.

17 **Sperryn, P.N.** Medical aspects of major games. (Problems of Olympic teams in Montreal.) Nursing Times, 72, 22 Jul 1976, 1114-1116.

18 **Sperryn, P.N.** Overuse injuries in sport. Nursing Mirror, 143, 1 Jul 1976, 51-52.

19 **Steele, V.** St. James' Hospital NHS Sports Medicine Clinic. Physiotherapy, 62 (8), Aug 1976, 246-250.

20 **Turner, A.C.** The health of the traveller and the spread of disease. (Advice on immunisation, comfort during journey and possible infections.) Royal Society of Health Journal, 97 (5), Oct 1977, 210-213.

21 **Williams, J.G.P.** Sports medicine. Nursing Mirror, 143, 1 Jul 1976, 48-50.

i OTHER AREAS

1 **Brooker, B.** Saving lives at Pilkington. (Role of the OH nurse in glass-manufacturing industry.) Nursing, 14, Jun 1980, 610-612.

2 **Clayton, R.** Improving the lot of the homeworker. (Risks to health and prospects for protection through legislation.) Occupational Health, 30 (7), Jul 1978, 331-333.

3 **Green, A.** Working in a cold environment. (Problems and precautions needed in sub-zero conditions (T. Wall and Sons (Ice Cream) Ltd).) Occupational Health, 30 (8), Aug 1978, 366-371.

4 **Harding, L.** Hotel nurse. (Work at the London Tara Hotel, Kensington.) Nursing Mirror, 144, 13 Jan 1977, 65-66.

5 **Howell, C.M.** The glass industry: a glimpse into industrial nursing. Nursing Times, 76, 28 Feb 1980, 383-384.

6 **Lever Industrial Advisory Bureau** The Lever industrial guide to health, safety and welfare for the hotel and catering industry. Lever Industrial Limited, 1976.

7 **Posner, E.** Stopping the potter's rot. (Development of silicosis prevention since the 1920s.) Occupational Health, 28 (5), May 1976, 247-250.

8 **Roth, A.** MPs under strain. New Society, 36, 29 Apr 1976, 228-230.

9 **Smith, C.A.** Fire, mist and vapours. (Health and safety aspects of printing industry.) Occupational Health, 32 (7), Jul 1980, 364-368; (8), Aug 1980, 417-420.

10 **Taylor, P.J.** Occupational and regional associations of death, disablement and sickness absence among post office staff 1972-75. British Journal of Industrial Medicine, 33 (4), Nov 1976, 230-235.

11 **Taylor, P.J.** The Post Office Occupational Health Service. Journal of the Society of Occupational Medicine, 26 (2), Apr 1976, 65-68.

PSYCHIATRY

74 PSYCHIATRIC SERVICES

a PSYCHIATRIC SERVICES AND MENTAL HEALTH

1 Altschul, A.T. Psychiatry under review. 1. The care of the mentally disordered: three approaches. (Medical, social and psychological models.) Nursing Times, 76, 13 Mar 1980, 452-454.

2 Altschul, A. Psychiatry under review. 3. The role of professionals. Nursing Times, 76, 27 Mar 1980, 555-556.

3 Altschul, A. Psychiatry under review. 8. The team approach to psychiatric care. Nursing Times, 76, 1 May 1980, 797-798.

4 Baker, A.A. editor Comprehensive psychiatric care. Blackwell, 1976.

5 Barter, J. Beneath all the bustle have attitudes really changed? (MIND's current initiatives in the mental health field.) Health and Social Service Journal, 88, 6 Oct 1978, 1140-1141.

6 British Medical Journal Clinical responsibility: 2. Where does the patient stand. Working paper by A.W. Clare. When did you last see your psychiatrist? (Multidisciplinary team in psychiatry, with discussion including nurse staffing levels and role of unions.) British Medical Journal, 2, 24/31 Dec 1977, 1637-1642.

7 Brough, D.J. and Watson, J.P. Psychiatric facilities in an 'over-resourced' NHS region. (Survey in South-East Thames RHA revealed deficiencies in provision.) British Medical Journal, 2, 1 Oct 1977, 905-906.

8 Davidson, J. The cracks in the facade of a crumbling white paper. (Lack of progress in breaking down large mental hospitals into smaller units.) Health and Social Service Journal, 87, 16 Sep 1977, 1326-1327.

9 DeCato, C.M. and Wicks, R.J. Psychological testing referrals: a guide for psychiatrists, psychiatric nurses, physicians in general practice and allied health personnel. Journal of Psychiatric Nursing and Mental Health Nursing, 14 (6), Jun 1976, 24-30.

10 Department of Health and Social Security Better services for the mentally ill. (Cmnd. 6233). HMSO, 1975.

11 Department of Health and Social Security. Standing Mental Health Advisory Committee The role of psychologists in the health services: report of the sub-committee. HMSO, 1977. (Chairman: W.H. Trethowan.)

12 Grimes, J.A. The probability of admission to a mental illness hospital or unit. (Mental health statistics.) Health Trends, 10 (1), Feb 1978, 13-14.

13 Hill, D. Progress but in slow tempo. (Advance since 1930 in the care of the mentally ill.) Health and Social Service Journal, 90, 11 Jul 1980, 904-906.

14 Jones, J. Last again in the priority race. (On the effect of financial cutbacks on facilities for the mentally ill.) Health and Social Service Journal, 77, 29 Apr 1977, 744.

15 Jowell, T. 'Joint planning hasn't gone to the roots of the way mental health services are constructed'. (Interview with MIND's assistant director.) Health and Social Service Journal, 88, 6 Jan 1978, 8-10.

16 Knight, L. Thirty years on . . . (Mental health services since 1948.) Mind Out, 30, Jul/Aug 1978, 20-22.

17 Lloyd, W.A. Better services for the mentally ill and handicapped: paving the way. (Changes in mental health services in the United Kingdom.) Australian Nurses Journal, 6 (5), Nov 1976, 34-38; Lamp, 34 (4), Apr 1977, 5, 7, 9.

18 Lusher, A.E. Mental health emergencies. (Survey in Surrey of communication between social workers and GPs, psychiatrists and mental hospitals.) Health and Social Service Journal, 86, 29 May 1976, 982.

19 Mattingly, R. Better service for the mentally ill? (Comments upon the White Paper.) Health and Social Service Journal, 85, 20/27 Dec 1975, 2795.

20 Meacher, M. editor New methods of mental health care. Oxford: Pergamon, 1979.

21 MIND A small step forward: comments on 'The way forward'. Mind, 1978.

22 Nichols, K. Introducing the mind. (Need for health education on mental health.) New Society, 45, 21 Sep 1978, 624-625.

23 Rollin, H.R. Treatment in psychiatry: from nihilism to cautious optimism. (Changes in treatment over the last fifty years.) Practitioner, 224, Jun 1980, 645, 647, 649.

24 Ross, T. Looking on the bright side. (Psychiatric services in Scotland with reference to community psychiatric nursing service.) Nursing Mirror, 148, 29 Mar 1979, 28-29.

25 Sainty, A. Mental Health Week—let's care more, not less. (MIND's manifesto of priorities in mental health services.) Nursing Mirror, 145, 20 Oct 1977, 15-17.

26 Shering, A. Psychiatric research in the MRC Brain Metabolism Unit. (Edinburgh.) Nursing Times, 72, 23 Sep 1976, 1466-1467.

27 Smythe, T. Politicians have not been helped by the confusion of mental health professionals. (Last of series of interviews with MIND staff, with its director.) Health and Social Service Journal, 884, 13 Jan 1978, 38-40.

28 Tancredi, L.R. and Slaby, A.E. Ethical policy in mental health care: the goals of psychiatric intervention. Heinemann, 1977.

29 Tizzard, K. A local management information system for the mental health services. (Computer based system for mental hospitals in Cornwall.) Hospital and Health Services Review, 72 (1), Jan 1976, 7-11.

30 Towell, D. Developing services based on large institutions: some organisational requirements. (With reference to comprehensive services for two or more health districts.) Health Services Manpower Review, 4 (2), May 1978, 3-6.

31 Towell, D. Large institutions—problems and solutions. (With reference to the mentally ill.) Hospital and Health Services Review, 74 (10), Oct 1978, 359-365.

32 Walshe-Brennan, K. Needs that fall through the net of psychiatric services: a survey of the need for psychiatric facilities in the Oxford region revealed many gaps in provision. Health and Social Services Journal, 87, 25 Mar 1977, 522-523.

33 Woodmansey, A.C. First things first: a blueprint for mental health. (Advocates psychotherapy and outlines roles of midwife, HV and social worker.) Public Health, 93 (3), May 1979, 131-139.

34 World Health Issue on mental health. World Health, Dec 1977, 2-34.

35 Young, K. Discharge and be damned. Heads you win—tails I lose. (Trends in the treatment of mental illness.) Royal Society of Health Journal, 98 (3), Jun 1978, 112-115.

b LEGISLATION

1 Bosanquet, N. Stimulus for disagreement. (A review of the Mental Health Act 1959.) Nursing Times, 72 (35), 2 Sep 1976, 1340-1341.

2 Campaign for the Mentally Handicapped Mental handicap and mental health legislation: a response to the DHSS consultative document 'A review of the mental health act 1959.' CMH, 1977.

3 **Caulfield, C.** Suitable case for consent. (Legal position regarding treatment and detention of psychiatric patients.) Health and Social Service Journal, 88, 28 Apr 1978, 486.

4 **Clare, A.W.** In defence of compulsory psychiatric intervention. (Reply to Szasz's views.) Lancet, 1, 3 Jun 1978, 1197-1198.

5 **Day, P.** Admission of confusion. (Comments on the consultative document on the Mental Health Act 1959.) Health and Social Service Journal, 89, 21 Aug 1976, 1504.

6 **Department of Health and Social Security** A review of the Mental Health Act 1959. (Consultative document.) HMSO, 1976.

7 **Department of Health and Social Security and others** Review of the mental health act 1959. HMSO, 1978. (Cmnd 7320)

8 **Edwards, A.H.** Shaw's guide to mental health services. Shaw, 1976.

9 **Gostin, L.O.** 'I could write a book on sections of law that cause the problems.' (Interview with legal and welfare rights officer of MIND by D. Ball.) Health and Social Service Journal, 87, 16 Dec 1977, 1698-1700.

10 **Gostin, L.O.** A human condition: the law relating to mentally abnormal offenders. Observations, analysis and proposals for reform. Vol.2. Mind, 1977. (A MIND special report.)

11 **Gostin, L.O.** The mental health act 1959: is it fair? MIND, 1978.

12 **Harding, T.W. and Curran, W.J.** Promoting mental health through the law. (Some of the main findings of a WHO international survey of mental health legislation.) WHO Chronicle, 32 (3), Mar 1978, 109-113.

13 **Health and Social Service Journal** Five articles on the new White Paper on the reform of the Mental Health Act. Health and Social Service Journal, 88, 22 Sep 1978, 1072-1075.

14 **Hoggett, B.M.** Mental health. Sweet and Maxwell, 1976. (Social work and law series.)

15 **Hospital and Health Services Review** Mental disorder: freedom or restraint? (Problems arising from the law of mental disorder.) Hospital and Health Services Review, 72 (12), Dec 1976, 443-446.

16 **Hospital and Health Services Review** Notes for students. Review of the Mental Health Act 1959. Hospital and Health Services Review, 75 (6), Jun 1979, 223-224; (7), Jul 1979, 258-260.

17 **Hospital and Health Service Review** Trends and developments in the law relating to the treatment of mental disorder. Hospital and Health Services Review, 72 (1), Jan 1976, 34-36.

18 **Lancet** Law and mental disorder. (Comment on White Paper.) Lancet, 1, 7 Apr 1979, 759-761.

19 **Martin, A.** Feeble review: bland outlook. (Comments on the consultative document on the Mental Health Act 1959.) Health and Social Service Journal, 89, 21 Aug 1976, 1505.

20 **Martin, A.J.** A human condition. (Comments on 'A human condition' vol 2, the law relating to the mentally abnormal offender, by L. Gostin.) Nursing Times, 73, 21 Apr 1977, 550-551.

21 **Martin, A.** Nurses and the law—5. The Mental Health Act. Nursing Times, 74, 10 Aug 1978, 1343-1344.

22 **Martin, A.J.** Reviewing the Act. Consultative document on the Mental Health Act. Nursing Times, 72, 19 Aug 1976, 1262-1263.

23 **Martin, A.** This is not an act of convenience. (Legal aspects for staff of administration of compulsory treatment to psychiatric patients.) Health and Social Service Journal, 87, 30 Sep 1977, 1372.

24 **MIND** Observations...on the DHSS consultative document 'A review of the mental health act 1959'. Mind, 1976.

25 **National Schizophrenia Fellowship** Comments on the 'DHSS review of the mental health act 1959'. Surbiton: The Fellowship, 1976.

26 **National Society for Mentally Handicapped Children** Review of the mental health act 1959: report of the working party. NSMHC, 1977. (Chairman: Rolf Hermelin.)

27 **Nursing Times** Mental Health Act: Ennals hears views on detention. (Conference report.) Nursing Times, 72, 4 Nov 1976, 1701.

28 **Price, C.** Mental health and Parliament. The central issues for parliamentary debate contained in the new White paper on the Mental Health Act. (By an M.P.) Nursing Times, 74, 5 Oct 1978, 1625.

29 **Rollin, H.R.** Confidentiality in psychiatric practice. Nursing Times, 74, 13 Jul 1978, 1161, 1163.

30 **Royal Society of Health Journal** Review of the Mental Health Act, 1959. (Views of a doctor and a social worker.) Royal Society of Health Journal, 99 (5), Oct 1979, 213.

31 **Social Work Today** Compulsory admission of the mentally ill. (Three articles.) Social Work Today, 9, 4 Jul 1978, 19-25.

32 **Spencer, D.A.** The revision of the Mental Health Act, 1959. Should the mentally handicapped be excluded? Royal Society of Health Journal, 98 (2), Apr 1978, 84-87, 92.

33 **Sumner, E.** Bordering on bedlam. (Part 1 History of mental health legislation.) Nursing Mirror, 151, 4 Dec 1980, 16-18.

34 **Sumner, E.** Psychiatry. 2. Loosening the legal straitjacket. (Comment on consultative document's and White Paper's proposed changes in 1959 Mental Health Act.) Nursing Mirror, 151, 11 Dec 1980, 28-30.

35 **Turner, J.** Under the lunatic law. (Work of the Court of Protection, which deals with the property and personal affairs of the long-term mentally ill.) New Society, 43, 19 Jan 1978, 127-128.

36 **Walshe-Brennan, K.S.** Legal problems in psychiatry. Nursing Mirror, 142, 6 May 1976, 73-74.

c COMMUNITY SERVICES

1 **Agulnik, P. and others** The Isis Centre: a counselling service within the National Health Service. (Oxford.) British Medical Journal, 2, 7 Aug 1976, 355-357.

2 **Ashton, J.R.** Community care in psychiatry — is it a myth? Community Health, 9 (4), May 1978, 211-215.

3 **Berke, J.** I haven't had to go mad here. (Arbours Crisis Centre in North London.) Mind Out, 36, Sep./Oct 1979, 19-20.

4 **Berry, C. and Gordo, B.** Community care for the mentally ill. (Queen's Road Day Centre, Coventry.) Nursing Times, 72, 27 May 1976, 804-805.

5 **Brook, A.** An aspect of community mental health: consultative work with general practice teams. (Psychiatrist with psychotherapeutic skills.) Health Trends, 10 (2), May 1978, 37-39.

6 **Brook, A. and Temperley, J.** The contribution of a psychotherapist to general practice. (A study in four group practices conducted by the Tavistock Clinic.) Journal of the Royal College of General Practitioners, 26, Feb 1976, 86-94.

7 **Cohen, D.** Psychiatry at home. (Experiment in community psychiatry at Napsbury Hospital, Herts.) New Society, 43, 2 Mar 1978, 486-487.

8 **Cole, A.** Alternatives to mental hospitals. (Report of international conference held in Ghent, Belgium.) Nursing Times, 76, 17 Apr 1980, 673-674. (See also Health and Social Service Journal, 90, 25 Apr 1980, 538-540.)

9 **Corser, C.M. and Ryce, S.W.** Community mental health care: a model based on the primary care system. (Craigshill Health Centre, Livingston New Town.) British Medical Journal, 2, 8 Oct 1977, 936-938.

10 **Donnelly, G.** Mental health care in the community. Nursing Mirror, 145, 8 Dec 1977, 43.

11 **Gillard, R.E.** The Worcester Development Project. Newtown Hospital. Nursing Times, 73, 14 Jul 1977, 1074-1075.

12 **Goldberg, D. and Huxley, P.** Mental illness in the community: the pathway to psychiatric care. Tavistock, 1980.

13 **Harris, J. and Mills, G.** Family psychiatry: communicating with the network. Practitioner, 221, Dec 1978, 829-831, 835.

14 **Hassall, C. and Stilwell, J.A.** Family doctor support for patients on a psychiatric case register. (Part of Worcester Development Project.) Journal of the Royal College of General Practitioners, 27, Oct 1977, 605-608.

15 **Kilroy-Silk, R.** Now is the hour for action. (Lack of progress in providing day care facilities for the mentally ill.) Health and Social Service Journal, 89, 24 Aug 1979, 1075.

16 **Lancet** Community psychiatry depolarised. (Review of its current status.) Lancet, 1, 20 May 1978, 1079-1080.

17 **Lancet** Is there a life after hospital? (Psychiatric patients in the community.) Lancet, 2, 27 Sep 1980, 682-683.

18 **Leopoldt, H.** Counting the cost of change. (Statistics from Littlemore Hospital illustrate changes following increased community mental health care.) Health and Social Service Journal, 87, 22 Jul 1977, 1081.

19 Lloyd, T. The Worcester Development Project. Planning and co-ordination. Nursing Times, 73, 14 Jul 1977, 1064-1066.

20 Lloyd, W.A. Practical aspects of care. (Worcester Development Project, England and the growth of the community psychiatric nurse.) Lamp, 33 (12), Dec 1976, 15-22.

21 Melville, J. Helping people to survive a crisis. (Arbours crisis centre in North London providing therapy to people with emotional crises.) New Society, 46, 12 Oct 1978, 78-79.

22 Melville, J. Nobody labels us here. (Brecknock Road Community Centre, a mental health project in London.) Mind Out, 40, May/Jun 1980, 14-16.

23 New Society Out of hospital. (Community care for the mentally ill.) New Society, 35, 25 Mar 1976, 673.

24 Nursing Times The Worcester Development Project. Sponsored by the DHSS, it seeks to provide a fully comprehensive local service for the mentally ill in the Worcester and Kidderminster Health Districts. (Six articles.) Nursing Times, 73, 14 Jul 1977, 1064-1079.

25 Oldfield, S. Counselling experiment. (Isis Centre, Oxford National Health Service Counselling Centre.) New Society, 38, 14 Oct 1976, 81.

26 Pullen, I. Description of an extramural service for psychiatric emergencies. (Experimental service in Edinburgh aiming to deal with patients in their homes.) Health Bulletin, 38 (4), Jul 1980, 163-166.

27 Ross, T. In time of trouble. (Psychiatric emergency clinic at St. Clement's Hospital in East London.) Nursing Mirror, 151, 4 Dec 1980, 22-23.

28 Scott, R.D. A family oriented psychiatric service to the London Borough of Barnet. Health Trends, 3 (12), Aug 1980, 65-68.

29 Social Work Today Feature of five articles on the Worcester Development Project providing community care for the mentally ill. Social Work Today, 11, 12 Feb 1980, 10-15.

30 Sykes, P. Integrated psychiatric care. (Development in community care and general hospital psychiatry.) Medical Record, 17 (2), May 1976, 124-132.

31 Todd, N.A. Psychiatric consultation in a health centre. A comparison of out-patients seen in health centre, general hospital and mental hospital settings. Health Bulletin, 36 (3), May 1978, 115-119.

32 Walshe-Brennan, K.S. Community care—fact or fiction? (For psychiatric patients.) Nursing Mirror, 143, 22 Jul 1976, 67-68.

33 Walshe-Brennan, K.S. Conflicts in community psychiatry. Community Health, 9 (1), Aug 1977, 35-40.

34 Whitfield, M.J. and Winter, R.D. Psychiatry and general practice: results of a survey of Avon general practitioners. (Their views on psychiatry and the psychiatric services available.) Journal of the Royal College of General Practitioners, 30, Nov 1980, 682-686.

d OVERSEAS COUNTRIES

1 Baasher, T.A. and others, editors Mental health services in developing countries: papers presented at a WHO seminar... Addis Ababa, 27 Nov-4 Dec 1973. Geneva: World Health Organization, 1975. (WHO offset publication, no.22.)

2 Baasher, T.A. Mental health services in Eastern Mediterranean countries. WHO Chronicle, 30 (6), Jun 1976, 234-239.

3 Bloch, S. and Reddaway, P. Russia's political hospitals: the abuse of psychiatry in the Soviet Union. Gollancz, 1977.

4 Canadian Council on Hospital Accreditation Guide to accreditation of Canadian mental health services. Toronto: the Council, 1975.

5 Clayton, P. Psychiatric care in Pakistan: the good (what little there is), the bad, and the horrifying. (Report of study tour.) Nursing Mirror, 146, 1 Jun 1978, 22-24.

6 Climent, C.E. and others Mental health in primary health care. (Interim results of WHO study in seven developing countries.) WHO Chronicle, 34 (6), Jun 1980, 231-236.

7 Coleman, J.V. and Patrick, D.L. Integrating mental health services into primary medical care. Medical Care, 14 (8), Aug 1976, 654-661.

8 David, H.F. Mental health services in the developing countries. WHO Expert Committee on Mental Health. Journal of Psychiatric Nursing and Mental Health Services, 14 (1), Jan 1976, 24-29.

9 Draper, J. Mental health is a top priority in the USA. (New American Mental Health Systems Bill.) Mind Out, 38, Jan/Feb 1980, 12-16.

10 Dressler, D.M. and others Hospital, nursing homes become partners in psychiatric care. (Psychiatric outreach programme in Connecticut offered by a general hospital to local nursing homes.) Hospitals, 52 (5), Mar 1978, 93-94, 96.

11 Dudley, A. Psychiatry—the American approach. Describes the organisation of psychiatric facilities in Kansas, and compares them with their British counterparts. Nursing Mirror, 143, 11 Nov 1976, 64-66.

12 Forrest, L.M. Paraprofessionals can be taught to deliver professional-level care. (Scheme to teach mental health technicians to give improved patient care.) Nursing, 8 (9), Sep 1978, 22-23.

13 Gallagher, R.M. Development of a mental health programme in the Central Coast of New South Wales, Australia. (With reference to the role of the nurse in the community.) Journal of Advanced Nursing, 5 (4), Jul 1980, 397-407.

14 Grant, E.E. A model for an extended comprehensive emergency screening service in an urban mental health care and treatment facility. Journal of Psychiatric Nursing and Mental Health Services, 16 (5), May 1978, 23-27.

15 Jablensky, A. Racism, apartheid and mental health. (Mental health care in South Africa.) World Health, Dec 1977, 16-21.

16 Low-Beer, G.A. A message to all British

nurses and to their professional organisations and trade unions, from Leonid Plyushch. (Illegal use of psychiatry in the USSR.) Nursing Mirror, 142, 15 Apr 1976, 47-48.

17 McEvoy, P.J. and McEvoy, H.F. Management of psychiatric problems in a Kenyan mission hospital. (With an emphasis on nursing and other staff training.) British Medical Journal, 1, 12 Jun 1976, 1454-1456.

18 Martin, D. Family care for the mentally disordered in Belgium. (Fostering of mentally, physically, socially or emotionally handicapped adults.) Health and Social Service Journal, 89, 7 Dec 1979, Centre eight papers, C33-C40.

19 May, A.R. Mental health services in Europe: a review of data collected in response to a WHO questionnaire. Geneva: World Health Organisation, 1976. (WHO offset publication, no.23.)

20 Mellor, P. ICN Tokyo. Psychiatric care in Japan. (Report on visit to hospital and rehabilitation centre.) Nursing Times, 73, 28 Jul 1977, 1170-1172.

21 Nursing Times Psychiatry abuse. (Russia.) Nursing Times, 72, 25 Nov 1976, 1828.

22 Townsend, J.A. Psychiatric inpatient unit and outpatient clinic liaison service. Journal of Psychiatric Nursing and Mental Health Services, 14 (3), Mar 1976, 7-9.

23 Van Lier, M. The care of the psychiatric patient today. (New Zealand.) New Zealand Nursing Journal, 69 (11), Nov 1976, 22-26.

75 PSYCHIATRIC NURSING

a TEXTBOOKS

1 Aguilera, D.C. Review of psychiatric nursing. St. Louis: Mosby, 1977.

2 Altschul, A. Psychiatric nursing. 5th ed. Baillière Tindall, 1977. (Nurses' aids series.)

3 Bagg, C. Handbook of psychiatry for social workers and health visitors. Constable, 1977.

4 Burgess, A.W. and Lazare, A. Psychiatric nursing in the hospital and the community. 2nd ed. Englewood Cliffs, N.J.: Prentice-Hall, 1976.

5 Burr, J. and Budge, U.V. Nursing the psychiatric patient. 3rd ed. Baillière Tindall, 1976.

6 Doona, M.E. Travelbee's intervention in psychiatric nursing. 2nd ed. Philadelphia: F.A. Davis, 1979.

7 Dreyer, S. Guide to nursing management of psychiatric patients. 2nd ed. St. Louis: Mosby, 1979.

8 Dunlap, L.C. Mental health concepts applied to nursing. New York: Wiley, 1978.

9 Gibson, J. Mental nursing examinations questions and answers. 4th ed. Faber, 1978.

10 Gibson, J. Psychiatry for nurses. 4th ed. Oxford: Blackwell Scientific, 1979.

11 Haber, J. and others Comprehensive

psychiatric nursing. New York: McGraw-Hill, 1978.

12 **Irving, S.** Basic psychiatric nursing. 2nd ed. Philadelphia: Saunders, 1978.

13 **Joel, L.A. and Collins, D.I.** Psychiatric nursing: theory and application. New York: McGraw-Hill, 1978.

14 **Kneisl, C.R. and Wilson, H.S. editors** Current perspectives in psychiatric nursing: issues and trends. St. Louis: Mosby, 1976-1978. 2 vols. (Current practice and perspectives in nursing series.)

15 **Koshy, K.T.** Revision notes on psychiatry. Hodder and Stoughton, 1977. (Modern nursing series.)

16 **Kreigh, H.Z. and Perko, J.E.** Psychiatric and mental health nursing: a commitment to care and concern. Reston, Va.: Reston Publishing, 1979.

17 **Kyes, J.J. and Hofling, C.K.** Basic psychiatric concepts in nursing. 4th ed. Philadelphia: Lippincott, 1980.

18 **Lancaster, J.** Adult psychiatric nursing. New York: Medical Examination Pub.Co.; Kimpton, 1980. (Current clinical nursing series.)

19 **Manfreda, M.L. and Krampitz, S.D.** Psychiatric nursing. 10th ed. Philadelphia: Davis, 1977.

20 **Marram, G.D.** The group approach in nursing practice. 2nd ed. St. Louis: Mosby, 1978.

21 **Mereness, D.A. and Taylor, C.M.** Essentials of psychiatric nursing. 10th ed. St. Louis: Mosby, 1978.

22 **Minski, L.** Handbook of psychiatry for students and nurses. 7th ed. by R.G. Priest and G. Woolfson. Heinemann, 1978.

23 **Morgan, H.G. and Morgan, M.H.** Aids to psychiatry. Edinburgh: Churchill Livingstone, 1979. ('Aides to' series.)

24 **Pothier, P.C. editor** Psychiatric nursing: a basic text. Boston: Little, Brown & Co., 1980.

25 **Robinson, L.** Psychiatric nursing as a human experience. 2nd ed. Philadelphia: Saunders, 1977.

26 **Rodgers, J.A. and McGovern, W.N.** Psychiatric/mental health nursing review. New York: Arco, 1976. (Arco nursing review series.)

27 **Sim, M. and Gordon, E.B.** Basic psychiatry. 3rd ed. Edinburgh: Churchill Livingstone, 1976.

28 **Snell, H.** Mental disorder: an introductory textbook for nurses. Allen and Unwin, 1977.

29 **Stoltzfus, D.J.** Self-assessment of current knowledge in mental health nursing. New York: Medical Examination Publishing, 1979. (Multiple choice questions.)

30 **Stuart, G.W. and Sundeen, S.J.** Principles and practice of psychiatric nursing. St. Louis: Mosby, 1979.

31 **Topalis, M. and Aguilera, D.C.** Psychiatric nursing. 7th ed. St. Louis: Mosby, 1978.

32 **Trick, K.L.K. and Obcarskas, S.** Understanding mental illness and its nursing. 2nd ed. Pitman, 1976.

33 **Watkins, P.N. and Goodchild, J.L.** The care of distressed and disturbed people: a workbook for students of nursing. Heinemann Medical, 1980.

b GENERAL

1 **Altschul, A.T.** Use of the nursing process in psychiatric care. Nursing Times, 73, 8 Sep 1977, 1412-1413.

2 **Altschul, A.T.** A systems approach to the nursing process. (With reference to psychiatric patients.) Journal of Advanced Nursing, 3 (4), Jul 1978, 333-340.

3 **Auld, M.** The Scottish situation. (Trends in psychiatric nursing.) Nursing Mirror, 150, 26 Jun 1980, Supplement, ii-iv.

4 **Beadle, E.** What is the future for psychiatric services? (Problems facing psychiatric nursing with need for change in management and training.) Mind Out, 43, Nov 1980, 21-22.

5 **Broome, A.** Observation in a psychiatric hospital. (Study in a male chronic ward, St. George's Hospital, Morpeth.) Nursing Times, 73, 2 Jun 1977, 837-838.

6 **Clarke, R.** Assessment in psychiatric hospitals. (Methods of assessing patients' needs and reference to geriatric, long-stay and acute admission patients.) Nursing Times, 75, 5 Apr 1979, 590-592.

7 **Darcy, P.T.** Psychiatric nursing today. 3. Care conflicts. 4. Training and career development. Nursing Mirror, 147, 20 Jul 1978, 26-27.

8 **Downing, A.R. and Brockington, I.F.** Nurse-rating of psychotic behaviour. (Evaluation of six schedules.) Journal of Advanced Nursing, 3 (6), Nov 1978, 551-561.

9 **Ellis, S.** Building an identity. (Rcn Welsh Board conference on psychiatric nursing.) Nursing Times, 75, 17 May 1979, 820.

10 **Fautrel, F.** Nursing: not just a first aid job. (Changes in hospital structures and attitudes necessary to improve nursing care of psychiatric patients.) Mind Out, 23, Jul/Aug 1977, 8-9, 17.

11 **Goldstone, L.A.** Long stay female population in a psychiatric hospital. (Includes an assessment of nursing care required.) Nursing Mirror, 144, 17 Mar 1977, 67-68; 24 Mar 1977, 71-72.

12 **Jones, M.P.** The nursing process in psychiatry. (With description of its implementation at Winterton Hospital, Stockton-on-Tees.) Nursing Times, 76, 17 Jul 1980, 1273-1275.

13 **Mitchell, B. and Hughes, J.** Psychiatric nursing—what future? (With survey of 415 learners and 288 ward sisters/charge nurses.) Nursing Focus, 1 (6), Feb 1980, 234-237; (7), Mar 1980, 276-277.

14 **Napsbury Hospital** Standard guidelines for nursing staff. St. Albans: the Hospital, 1978.

15 **Nursing Mirror** Where now for psychiatric nursing? (Four articles.) Nursing Mirror, 150, 26 Jun 1980, Supplement, i-vii, x-xii, xiv-xvi.

16 **Nursing Times** Psychiatric nursing for the eighties. (Reports of international congress organised by Nursing Times.) Nursing Times, 76, 11 Sep 1980, 1594-1595; 18 Sep 1980, 1638-1641.

17 **Reid, H.** A nurse's objectives for newly arrived patients. (With reference to psychiatric hospitals. By a student nurse.) Nursing Times, 76, 24 Jan 1980, 165-166.

18 **Ryan, L.J. and others** From personal responsibility to professional accountability in psychiatric nursing. Journal of Psychiatric Nursing and Mental Health Services, 15 (6), Jun 1977, 19-24.

19 **Schrock, R.A.** Psychiatry under review. 6. Planning nursing care for the mentally ill. Nursing Times, 76, 17 Apr 1980, 704-706.

20 **Smith, L.** Psychiatry under review. 7. A nursing history and data sheet. Nursing Times, 76, 24 Apr 1980, 749-754.

21 **Sugden, J.** Nursing activity and some variables in the psychiatric treatment process. MPhil thesis, University of Edinburgh, 1980.

22 **Syson-Nibbs, L.** Progress through a planned approach. (Research study on the use of the nursing process on a psychiatric ward.) Nursing Mirror, 150, 14 Feb 1980, 42-44.

23 **Thompson, A.** The nursing process. 1. Its value for special hospital patients. (Security hospitals, eg Rampton.) Nursing Mirror, 148, 1 Mar 1979, 20-21.

24 **Warcaba, B.** Charting change in nursing. (Sample survey at St. Crispin and Princess Marina Hospitals, Northampton, investigating changes in psychiatric nursing.) New Psychiatry, 3, 29 Apr 1976, 12-13.

25 **Wilkinson, T.** The problems and the values of objective nursing observations in psychiatric nursing care. (Description of drug trial which illustrates problems involved in objective nursing recordings to assess response to a specific treatment.) Journal of Advanced Nursing, 4 (2), Mar 1979, 151-159.

c OVERSEAS COUNTRIES

1 **Berezowsky, J.B.** Nursing the acutely psychotic patient. Canadian Nurse, 73 (2), Feb 1977, 23-25.

2 **Brown, R.** The future of psychiatric nursing—a New South Wales view. Australian Nurses Journal, 8 (8), Mar 1979, 39-40.

3 **Bonk, J.R.** Don't pass the buck! The full moon is not responsible for an increase in the occurrence of untoward events in a hospital setting! (Research study.) Journal of Psychiatric Nursing, 17 (5), May 1979, 33-36.

4 **Canadian Journal of Psychiatric Nursing** Special issue on the psychiatric nurse in Canada. (Including history 5-8.) Canadian Journal of Psychiatric Nursing, 20 (4), Jul/Aug 1979, 5-18.

5 **Conroy, J.B.** The future of mental health nursing—case of sink or swim. Lamp, 33 (11), Nov 1976, 5, 7, 9.

6 **Cormack, D.** Psychiatric nursing in the USA. (Report of an eight week study tour.) Journal of Advanced Nursing, 1 (5), Sep 1976, 399-409.

7 Doona, M.E. and others Professional affirmation in nursing care. (Development of professional skills by two psychiatric nurses.) Journal of Psychiatric Nursing and Mental Health Services, 15 (8), Aug 1977, 16-23.

8 Edmonds, J. The future model of mental health nursing in N.S.W. Lamp, 34 (3), Mar 1977, 27-28.

9 Fried, A.L. and Fried, F.E. Hospital and community psychiatric nursing. Journal of Psychiatric Nursing and Mental Health Services, 14 (12), Dec 1976, 31-36.

10 Gardner, K.G. Levels of psychiatric nursing practice in an ambulatory setting. (Descriptive model.) Journal of Psychiatric Nursing and Mental Health Services, 15 (9), Sep 1977, 26-29.

11 Green, N.C. A psychiatric assessment tool for staff and students. Journal of Psychiatric Nursing, 17 (4), Apr 1979, 28-31.

12 Janzen, S. Taxonomy for development of perceptual skills. (Framework for teaching perception in mental health context and nursing interaction model.) Journal of Nursing Education, 19 (1), Jan 1980, 33-40.

13 Jones, B.E. and Miles, J.E. The nurse and the hospitalized mentally ill physician. (Observation study at the Health Sciences Centre Hospital, University of British Columbia.) American Journal of Nursing, 76 (8), Aug 1976, 1314-1317.

14 Krall, M.L. Guidelines for writing mental health treatment plans. American Journal of Nursing, 76 (2), Feb 1976, 236-237.

15 Moran, J.C. An alternative to constant observation: the behavioral check list. (For monitoring patients in acute psychiatric unit.) Perspectives in Psychiatric Care, 17 (3), 1979, 114-117.

16 Nursing Clinics of North America Symposium on directions in psychiatric nursing. Nursing Clinics of North America, 13 (4), Dec 1978, 641-716.

17 Osted, A. What way the future? (For the psychiatric nursing profession in Canada.) Psychiatric Nursing, 16 (1), Jan-Feb 1975, 6-7.

18 Psychiatric Nurses Association of Canada Standards of practice for registered psychiatric nurses. Canadian Journal of Psychiatric Nursing, 19 (1), Jan/Feb 1978, 13; (2), Mar/Apr 1978, 5.

19 Solomon, J.A. My experience of nursing and more specifically in psychiatric nursing in Baltimore, U.S.A. S.A. Nursing Journal, 43 (8), Aug 1976, 25-26.

20 Torkington, J.R. Psychiatric nursing approaches and outcomes. Australian Nurses Journal, 9 (5), Nov 1979, 31-32, 37.

21 Tregunna, Mrs. Evaluating health care services. (Registered Nurses Association of British Columbia's quality assurance programme.) Canadian Journal of Psychiatric Nursing, 19 (3), May/Jun 1978, 8-12.

22 World Health Organization. Regional Office for Europe Role of nursing in psychiatric and mental health care: report on a working group, Saarbrücken, 10-13 March, 1975. Copenhagen: WHO, 1976.

23 Wylie, D. Goals for the future provision of effective nursing care. Canadian Journal of Psychiatric Nursing, 17 (1), Jan-Feb 1976, 7-8.

d ATTITUDES

1 Astor, A. and Frois, M. A change for the better. (Change in attitudes and regime in a long-term psychiatric ward at Fulbourn Hospital.) Nursing Times, 76, 28 Aug 1980, 1534-1535.

2 Barnes, R. To know them is to love them... (Survey of psychiatric nurse students' perceptions of psychiatric social workers' activities.) Health and Social Service Journal, 89, 19 Oct 1979, 1351.

3 Brady, M.M. Nurses' attitudes towards a patient who has a psychiatric history. (Study of 128 nurses in a New York hospital.) Journal of Advanced Nursing, 1 (1), Jan 1976, 11-23.

4 Creech, S.K. Changes in attitudes about mental illness among nursing students following a psychiatric affiliation. (Twelve week placement in mental hospital.) Journal of Psychiatric Nursing and Mental Health Services, 15 (6), Jun 1977, 9-14.

5 Crum, M.R. and Rowlands, E.E. Open-mindedness, rigidity, and the tendency to change inferences among psychiatric nursing staff: a pilot study. Nursing Research, 27 (1), Jan/Feb 1978, 42-47.

6 Fautrel, F. Why don't nurses complain? Part 1. (Survey of nurses' attitudes in hospitals for the mentally handicapped and mentally ill.) Mind Out, 22, May/Jun 1977, 5-7.

7 Ferguson, A. Psychiatric nursing: the myth today. (Low morale caused by disparity between teaching and practice.) Nursing Times, 74, 7 Sep 1978, 1474-1475.

8 Flaskerud, J.H. A tool for comparing the perceptions of problematic behavior by psychiatric professionals and minority groups. (Structured personal interview.) Nursing Research, 29 (1), Jan/Feb 1980, 4-9.

9 Gutierrez, J.L.A. and Ruiz, J.S. Comparative study of the psychiatric nurses' atittudes towards mental patients. (Survey of nurses and university students in Madrid to analyse the effect of professional training on tolerance of mental disorders.) International Journal of Social Psychiatry, 24 (1), Spr 1978, 47-52.

10 Harding, A.V. and Keats, D.M. Nurses' attitudes to psychiatric treatment. (Research study using Attitudes to Treatment Questionnaire.) Australasian Nurses Journal, 9 (3), Jan/Feb 1980, 28-30.

11 Kahn, A.M. Relationship between nurses' opinions about mental illness and experience. (Experimental psychiatric nurses and medical-surgical nurses compared along the five dimensions of the Opinions about Mental Illness Scale.) Nursing Research, 25 (2), Mar-Apr 1976, 136-140.

12 Morrison, J.K. and others The attitudes of nursing students and others about mental illness. (Student nurses compared with psychiatric nurses and students in psychiatry, psychology and education.) Journal of Psychiatric Nursing and Mental Health Services, 14 (4), Apr 1976, 17-19.

13 Olade, R.A. Attitudes towards mental illness: a comparison of post-basic nursing students with science students. (Nigerian university students.) Journal of Advanced Nursing, 4 (1), Jan 1979, 39-46.

14 Pallis, D.J. Psychiatric treatment: the question of attitudes. (Review of studies of attitudes of patients and staff including nurses.) International Journal of Social Psychiatry, 24 (4), Winter 1978, 281-286.

15 Reich, S. and Geller, A. The self-image of nurses employed in a psychiatric hospital. (Survey in New York City.) Perspectives in Psychiatric Care, 15 (3), 1977, 126-128.

16 Smith, E. Attitudes of student psychiatric nurses towards mental illness. (Research study.) Nursing Times, 73, 28 Jul 1977, 1174-1175.

17 Vousden, M. Far from the madding crowd? (Resistance to change among psychiatric nurses.) Nursing Mirror, 150, 10 Jan 1980, 12.

18 Watt, J. and Martin, C.J. It takes more than a move to rid mental illness of stigma. (Survey of staff and patient opinions of the psychiatric unit at Gartnavel General Hospital, Glasgow.) Health and Social Service Journal, 86, 29 Oct 1976, 1936-1937.

19 Whitehead, T. Difficult patients. (The problem of public and professional attitudes towards psychiatric patients.) Health and Social Service Journal, 86, 31 Jul 1976, 1397.

20 Whitehead, T. Stop the roundabout before we are caught in chains again. (The danger of a regressive attitude towards mental illness among health professionals.) Health and Social Service Journal, 86, 18 Feb 1977, 298-299.

21 Wold, C.N. Relationship of staff development activity to opinions about mental illness. (Study of psychiatric aides at Topeka State Hospital before and after a continuing education programme.) Nursing Research, 25 (2), Mar-Apr 1976, 98-104.

22 Wolf, M.F. The effect of education on nurses' views of a therapeutic milieu. (Views of optimum psychiatric environments.) Journal of Psychiatric Nursing and Mental Health Services, 16 (8), Aug 1978, 29-33.

e ROLE

1 Bayer, M. Psych patients are people, too! (Six skills of psychiatric nursing—patience, persistence, potential, peer relationship, practice and prevention.) Nursing Care, 9 (4), Apr 1976, 22-24.

2 Cangas, J. de Care vs. custodialism. (Objectives of psychiatric nursing.) Canadian Nurse, 73 (6), Jun 1977, 36-37.

3 Del Campo, E.J.H. Psychiatric nursing therapy: philosophy and methods. Journal of Psychiatric Nursing and Mental Health Services, 16 (8), Aug 1978, 34-37.

4 Dumas, R.G. Expanding the theoretical framework for effective nursing. (With reference to psychiatric nursing and need to develop clearer conceptions of authority, power and leadership.) Nursing Clinics of North America, 13 (4), Dec 1978, 707-716.

5 Fleming, J. Greenbank revolution. To make full use of the changing role of the psychiatric nurse would revolutionise the psychiatric side of medicine. Nursing Times, 73, 3 Feb 1977, 152-153.

6 Gardner, K.G. Supportive nursing: a critical review of the literature. Journal of Psychiatric Nursing, 17 (10), Oct 1979, 10-16.

7 Hayes, E.W. Antipsychiatric nursing: a personal overview. (Challenges several aspects of psychiatric nurse's duties.) Canadian Journal of Psychiatric Nursing, 20 (4), Jul/Aug 1979, 16-18.

8 Hessler, I. Psychiatry under review. 2. Roles, status and relationships in psychiatric nursing. Nursing Times, 76, 20 Mar 1980, 508-509.

9 Hocking, I.L. and others Willingness of psychiatric nurses to assume the extended role. (Survey to identify these characteristics.) Nursing Research, 25 (1), Jan-Feb 1976, 44-48.

10 Iveson-Iveson, J. The role of the psychiatric nurse. (Report of symposium organised by Community Psychiatric Nurses Association.) Nursing Mirror, 146, 23 Feb 1978, 37.

11 Littlefield, N. The psychiatric nurse as a change agent. Nursing Clinics of North America, 14 (2), Jun 1979, 373-382.

12 McIvor, D.L. Psychiatric nurses provide leadership. (A psychologist's view of psychiatric nurses.) Canadian Journal of Psychiatric Nursing, 16 (6), Nov/Dec 1975, 7.

13 Mansfield, E. A conceptual framework for psychiatric-mental health nursing. Journal Psychiatric Nursing, 18 (6), Jun 1980, 34-41.

14 Peplau, H. Psychiatric nursing: role of nurses and psychiatric nurses. (Those with basic and post-basic training.) International Nursing Review, 25 (2), Mar/Apr 1978, 41-47.

15 Plutchik, R. and others Role of the psychiatric nurse. (Study at Jacobi Hospital, New York, of which functions psychiatric nurses and non-nursing personnel considered most important.) Journal of Psychiatric Nursing and Mental Health Services, 14 (9), Sep 1976, 38-43.

16 Powers, M.E. Universal utility of psycho-analytic theory for nursing practice models. Journal of Psychiatric Nursing, 18 (4), Apr 1980, 28-30.

17 Sullivan, M.E. Processes of change in an expanded role in nursing in a mental health setting. Journal of Psychiatric Nursing and Mental Health Services, 15 (2), Feb 1977, 18-24.

18 Ulsafer, J. A relationship of existential philosophy to psychiatric nursing. Perspectives in Psychiatric Care, 14 (1), Jan-Mar 1976, 23-28.

f CLINICAL NURSE SPECIALIST

1 Ballard, K.A. New York State Nurses Association certification: its history and progress. (Psychiatric clinical nurse specialists.) Perspectives in Psychiatric Care, 14 (3), Jul-Sep 1976, 112-114.

2 Gelperin, E.A. Psychotherapeutic intervention by nurse clinical specialist. (Study of the effect of nursing intervention in a group of institutionalised chronically ill patients.) Journal of Psychiatric Nursing and Mental Health Services, 14 (3), Mar 1976, 16-18.

3 Goldstein, S. The psychiatric clinical specialist in the general hospital. Journal of Nursing Administration, 9 (3), Mar 1979, 34-37.

4 Kolson, G. Mental health nursing consultation: a study of expectations. Journal of Psychiatric Nursing and Mental Health Services, 14 (8), Aug 1976, 24, 31-32.

5 Kuntz, S. and others The psychiatric clinical specialist: the progression of a specialty. (Outline of trends based on review of journal articles, which are not listed.) Perspectives in Psychiatric Care, 18 (2), Mar/Apr 1980, 90-92.

6 Lamberton, M.M. Primary health care. Adult nurse clinician on a psychiatric unit. American Journal of Nursing, 76 (12), Dec 1976, 1961-1963.

7 Lathrop, V.G. A nurse-directed psychiatric intensive treatment unit. (With outline of role of psychiatric nurse clinical specialist.) Nursing Clinics of North America, 13 (4), Dec 1978, 673-683.

8 Palermo, E. Mental health consultation in a home care agency. (Role of psychiatric nurse specialist.) Journal of Psychiatric Nursing, 16 (9), Sep 1978, 21-23.

9 Pettengill, M.M. Development of a system for State Certification. (The Society for Certified Clinical Specialists in Psychiatric Nursing of the New Jersey State Nurses Association.) Perspectives in Psychiatric Care, 14 (3), Jul-Sep 1976, 107-111.

10 White, E.A. The clinical specialist on the mental health team. Journal of Psychiatric Nursing and Mental Health Services, 14 (11), Nov 1976, 7-12.

g EDUCATION AND TRAINING

1 Allen, J. and others Doing something about it—and quickly too. (Research study at Fulbourn psychiatric hospital by student nurses into the attitudes of learners to teaching sessions.) Nursing Times, 75, 14 Jun 1979, 1003-1005.

2 Association of Psychiatric Nurse Tutors (Scotland) Statement of current policy. Nursing Mirror, 143, 21 Oct 1976, 41; Nursing Times, 72, 7 Oct 1976, 1542.

3 Barber, P. An educational approach towards the development of interpersonal relationship skills in psychiatric nursing. The author, 1976.

4 Darcy, P.T. Psychiatric nursing today. 5. Better than Briggs. (Basic curriculum integration using modules based on care factors.) Nursing Mirror, 147, 27 Jul 1978, 26-27.

5 Denny, E.O. and Denny, J.A. A comparison of mental health nursing education in the United Kingdom and the psychiatric component of a baccalaureate program in the United States. Journal of Nursing Education, 18 (1), Jan 1979, 42-49.

6 Dietrich, G. Teaching psychiatric nursing in the classroom. (Description of practice at the Bethlem Royal and The Maudsley Hospital School of Nursing.) Journal of Advanced Nursing, 3 (6), Nov 1978, 525-534.

7 French, H.P. and Jones, G.E. Behavioural objectives for practical experience in psychiatric nurse education. (Production of booklet for

learners.) Nursing Times, 76, 14 Feb 1980, 298-301.

8 French, H.P. and Jones, G.E. A student learning package. (In psychiatric nursing module at Durham AHA Combined Schools of Nursing.) Nursing Focus, 1 (3), Nov 1979, 120.

9 Gannon, R.A. Teaching group therapy to learner psychiatric nurses: a basic guide. Nursing Times, 75, 6 Dec 1979, 2128-2129.

10 General Nursing Council Educational policy: mental and mental subnormality nurse training. GNC, 1978. (Circular 78/6 + enclosures A-D.)

11 Heywood Jones, I. and Masters, G. Group project. (Project by psychiatric nursing students to examine group dynamics.) Nursing Times, 75, 25 Jan 1979, 163-166.

12 Hooper, A. Student psychiatric nurses: a repertory grid study. MSc thesis, University of Manchester, Department of Nursing, Oct 1978.

13 Jones, I.H. Orientation of student psychiatric nurses. (Organisation of introductory six week block.) Nursing Mirror, 145, 14 Jul 1977, 30-32.

14 Mitchell, W. Assessment in psychiatric nursing. (Student assessment at St. Luke's Woodside Hospital, London.) Nursing Times, 72, 4 Mar 1976, 350-352.

15 Mitchell, W. Assessment in psychiatric nursing. Communication and organisation. (St. Luke's-Woodside Hospital, London.) Nursing Times, 72, 6 May 1976, 709-710.

16 Newall, E. Psychiatric nursing—how much do you know? (Multiple-choice questions and answers.) Nursing Mirror, 147, 31 Aug 1978, 28-29, 34.

17 Simpson, R. Psychiatry under review. 12. Psychiatric nursing—what now? (History of psychiatric nurse training and current dissatisfactions.) Nursing Times, 76, 5 Jun 1980, 1020-1021.

18 Smyth, T. Instant replay. (Use of video recording, with special reference to psychiatric nurse training.) Nursing Times, 76, 4 Sep 1980, 1585-1588.

h EDUCATION AND TRAINING: OVERSEAS COUNTRIES

1 Adelowo, E.O. Psychiatric nursing education in Nigeria. Nigerian Nurse, 10 (1), Jan/Mar 1978, 46-49.

2 Carser, D. and Doona, M.E. Alienation: a nursing concept. (Teaching programme.) Journal of Psychiatric Nursing, 16 (9), Sep 1978, 33-40.

3 Coser, R.L. Training in ambiguity: learning through doing in a mental hospital. New York: Free Press, 1979.

4 Cowell, D. The practice of nursing. Psychiatric care. (Future training of psychiatric nursing as seen by the 'Goals in nursing education' report.) Australian Nurses' Journal, 5 (3), Sep 1975, 9-12.

5 Davidhizar, R. A nursing student experience in a psychiatric activity program. (Participation in group therapy and occupational therapy in acute care psychiatric unit.) Journal of Nursing Education, 18 (7), Sep 1979, 56-59.

6 Davidhizar, R.E. Use of simulation games in teaching psychiatric nursing. Journal of Nursing Education, 16 (5), May 1977, 9-12.

7 Hartig, E. Developing a psychiatric nursing curriculum incorporating the standards of practice for the registered psychiatric nurse... (Based on the nursing process.) Canadian Journal of Psychiatric Nursing, 19 (1), Jan/Feb 1978, 6-7.

8 Holden, J. The role of the clinical instructor. (Supervising general nurse students during psychiatric placement.) Australian Nurses Journal, 7 (11), Jun 1978, 48-50.

9 Jansson, D.P. Student consultation: a liaison psychiatric experience for nursing students. (In psychiatric module using other students as consultants.) Perspectives in Psychiatric Care, 17 (2), Mar/Apr 1979, 77-82.

10 Kerr, N.J. Discussion of common errors in communication made by students in psychiatric nursing. Perspectives in Psychiatric Care, 16 (4), Jul/Aug 1978, 184-187.

11 Kornfield-Jacobs, G. and Karshmer, J.F. A collaborative model for university nursing education and agency staff development. (To integrate the education of senior nursing students and staff at a psychiatric hospital.) Journal of Psychiatric Nursing and Mental Health Services, 15 (11), Nov 1977, 15-22.

12 Lahey, E.M. and Lahey, J.B. The use of imagery in teaching psychiatric nursing. Journal of Practical Nursing, 26 (5), May 1976, 28-29.

13 Lasor, B. Time out! The use of simulation in teaching psychiatric nursing. Canadian Nurse, 75 (9), Oct 1979, 36-38.

14 Miller, T.W. and Orsolits, M.B. A model for training nursing staff as primary counselors for psychiatric service. Journal of Psychiatric Nursing and Mental Health Services, 16 (6), Jan 1978, 28-33.

15 Sayre, J. Common errors in communication made by students in psychiatric nursing. (With examples of exchanges where the goal of therapeutic interaction is not achieved.) Perspectives in Psychiatric Care, 16 (4), Jul/Aug 1978, 175-183.

16 Seeno, M.E. The effectiveness of teaching psychiatric nursing within a surgical unit. Journal of Psychiatric Nursing and Mental Health Services, 15 (3), Mar 1977, 15-18.

17 Tilden, V.P. and Gustafson, L. Termination in the student-patient relationship: use of a teaching tool. (Psychotherapeutic relationship in psychiatric nursing.) Journal of Nursing Education, 18 (8), Oct 1979, 9-13.

18 Williams, M.L. Effects of clinical setting on anxiety and achievement in psychiatric nursing education. (Research study.) Journal of Nursing Education, 18 (2), Feb 1979, 4-14.

i MANAGEMENT AND STAFFING

1 Apostoles, F.E. and others Developing a psychiatric nursing audit. Journal of Psychiatric Nursing and Mental Health Services, 15 (5), May 1977, 9-15.

2 Broome, A.K. and Weaver, S.M. Nursing in mental hospitals: who cares for the patients? (Observational study by two psychologists of nurses and other staff's activities on a ward, with discussion of method for allocating staff and resources.) Nursing Mirror, 146, 8 Jun 1978, 16-18.

3 Cormack, D. Psychiatric nursing observed: a descriptive study of the work of the charge nurse in acute admission wards of psychiatric hospitals. Royal College of Nursing, 1976. (Research series.)

4 Benfer, B.A. Clinical supervision as a support system for the care-giver. Perspectives in Psychiatric Care, 17 (1), Jan/Feb 1979, 13-17.

5 DeGiovanni, I.S. and others Beyond outcomes: evaluating staff functioning on an inpatient psychiatric ward. (Report of evaluation project.) Journal of Psychiatric Nursing and Mental Health Services, 16 (4), Apr 1978, 28-31.

6 Fielding, S. Night duty in a comprehensive psychiatric unit. Nursing Mirror, 144, 17 Feb 1977, 69-70.

7 Goodwin, G. Ward policies in psychiatric hospitals. (King's Fund conference on the experience of Fulbourn Hospital, Cambridge, and Harrison Hospital, Dorchester.) Nursing Times, 72, 7 Oct 1976, 1573.

8 Hambleton, B. Staffing inflation. (Factors affecting staffing needs in psychiatric hospitals.) Nursing Mirror, 144, 5 May 1977, 68-70.

9 Hazzard, M.E. and O'Farrell, E. Personality testing for better staffing in mental health facilities. (Research study to identify personality characteristics of auxiliaries working in a private psychiatric hospital in USA.) Journal of Psychiatric Nursing, 16 (9), Sep 1978, 41-57.

10 Laing, M.M. and others The planning and implementation of a psychiatric self-care unit. Journal of Psychiatric Nursing and Mental Health Services, 15 (7), Jul 1977, 30-34, 37.

11 McWhirt, F.D. Staffing in a psychiatric unit: a study to determine adequate staffing patterns. Supervisor Nurse, 8 (12), Dec 1977, 27-31.

12 Morgan, R. Must the ward mental nurse remain confined to the ward? (Clinical organisation at St. Wulstan's Hospital, Malvern, where ward nurses provide workshop supervision.) Nursing Mirror, 144, 5 May 1977, 63-64.

13 Puskar, K.R. A psychiatric clinic as a system having six organizational variables. (Analysis of organisation and suggestions for restructuring in order to avoid worker alienation and job dissatisfaction.) Journal of Psychiatric Nursing and Mental Health Services, 15 (8), Aug 1977, 9-15.

14 Sharpe, D. The appointment of charge nurses in psychiatric hospitals. (Survey of the prevalence of appointing charge nurses to designated posts or grades within the psychiatric division.) Nursing Mirror, 144, 31 Mar 1977, 57-58.

15 Sharpe, D. Male and female nurse ratios in a psychiatric hospital. (Report of research study.) Nursing Times, 74, 5 Oct 1978, 1656.

16 Stybel, J.L. Organic organizational research in a psychiatric inpatient setting. Journal of Psychiatric Nursing and Mental Health Services, 14 (5), May 1976, 18-22.

17 Walsh, P.A. 'Mental illness', 'mental handicap' and the nursing service establishment—an alternative approach. (A comparison between the medical and behavioural approach to establishment.) Journal of Advanced Nursing, 1 (4), Jul 1976, 283-292.

j NURSE PATIENT RELATIONSHIP

1 Altschul, A.T. Psychiatry under review. 5. Hints on maintaining patient-nurse interaction. Nursing Times, 76, 10 Apr 1980, 650-652.

2 Blacker, H.R. Talking to patients. (Skills of dealing with psychiatric patients.) Nursing Times, 72, 5 Aug 1976, 1212-1214.

3 Boettcher, E.G. Nurse-client collaboration: dynamic equilibrium in the nursing care system. (Involving patient in setting goals.) Journal of Psychiatric Nursing, 16 (12), Dec 1978, 7-15.

4 Coltrane, F. and Pugh, C.D. Danger signals in staff/patient relationships in the therapeutic milieu. (Indicating social rather than professional relationship.) Journal of Psychiatric Nursing and Mental Health Services, 16 (6), Jan 1978, 34-36.

5 Crawford, D.A. Social skills training for psychiatric patients. Nursing Times, 74, 10 Aug 1978, 1322-1323.

6 THE CURATIVE relationship—a nursing care study. (An outline of the clinical application of nurse-patient relationship therapy.) Nursing Mirror, 143, 16 Dec 1976, 53-55.

7 Fulton, J. Nurse-patient relationship therapy. (Therapeutic use with psychiatric patients.) Nursing Mirror, 143, 16 Dec 1976, 51-52.

8 Hall, B.A. The effect of interpersonal attraction on the therapeutic relationship: a review and suggestions for further study. Journal of Psychiatric Nursing and Mental Health Services, 15 (9), Sep 1977, 18-23.

9 Johnson, M.N. Self-disclosure: a variable in the nurse-client relationship. (Research study.) Journal of Psychiatric Nursing, 18 (1), Jan 1980, 17-20.

10 Karshmer, J.F. and others Casual attributions: bias in the nurse-patient relationship. (Research study of ways of explaining behaviour.) Journal of Psychiatric Nursing, 18 (5), May 1980, 25-30.

11 Licker, L. and others It's the staff that keeps the patient talking. (Study showing the importance of staff presence when encouraging chronic psychiatric patients to speak in a group setting.) Journal of Psychiatric Nursing and Mental Health Services, 14 (5), May 1976, 11-14.

12 Macklin, D. Psychosocial nursing. Trouble stirring in the kitchen. (System, developed at The Cassel Hospital, which employs psychological understanding of the nurse/patient relationship.) Nursing Mirror, 148, 24 May 1979, 38-39.

13 Randolph, B.M. and Bernau, K. Dealing with resistance in the nursing care conference. (Interpersonal relationships in clinical conference discussions.) American Journal of Nursing, 77 (12), Dec 1977, 1955-1958.

14 Simmons, J.A. The nurse-client relationship in mental health nursing. 2nd ed. Philadelphia: Saunders, 1976. (Workbook guides to understanding management.)

15 Stegne, L.R. A positive approach to negative behaviour. (Programme of education and management at St. Thomas Psychiatric Hospital, Ontario, to help staff cope with aggressive, angry or hostile patients.) Canadian Nurse, 74 (6), Jun 1978, 44-48.

k PSYCHIATRIC CARE IN PHYSICAL ILLNESS

1 De Cambra, B. Re-making the bedside manner. (Work of the general nurse in psychiatric team.) Australian Nurses Journal, 6 (3), Sep 1976, 22-23.

2 Freeman, C.K. Transactional analysis: a model for psychiatric consultation in the general hospital. Nursing Forum, 18 (1), 1979, 43-51.

3 Garant, C.A. The psychiatric liaison nurse—an interpretation of the role. (Acting as consultant in non-psychiatric units on psychological aspects of patient care.) Supervisor Nurse, 8 (4), Apr 1977, 75-78.

4 Hedlund, N.L. Mental health nursing consultation in the general hospital. (Through individual consultation and group discussions nurses increased skills in handling psychosocial aspects of patient care.) Patient Counselling and Health Education, 1 (2), Fall 1978, 85-88.

5 Hospitals Support team helps patients cope with stress. (Psychiatric support of the physically ill patient in Chicago.) Hospitals, 53 (12), 16 Jun 1979, 93-94.

6 Howard, J.S. Liaison nursing. (Nurse clinician as psychiatric consultant to staff regarding psychosocial aspects of patient care.) Journal of Psychiatric Nursing and Mental Health Services, 16 (4), Apr 1978, 35-37.

7 Langman-Dorwart, N. A model for mental health consultation to the general hospital. (Meetings of psychiatric nurse consultant and general nurses to discuss problems of emotional needs of their patients.) Journal of Psychiatric Nursing, 17 (3), Mar 1979, 29-33.

8 Lucas, M.J. and Folstein, M.F. Nursing assessment of mental disorders on a general medical unit. (Research study using Mini-Mental Status Examination.) Journal of Psychiatric Nursing, 18 (5), May 1980, 31-33.

9 Meredith, L. and Weatherhead, R. Psychiatric consultation liaison nursing: 18 months later. (Report of scheme to help reduce anxiety of nurses through discussion of problems related to care of particular patients.) Lamp, 37 (6), Jun 1980, 19-20.

10 Nelson, J.K.N. and Davis, D.S. Educating the psychiatric liaison nurse. (Consultants to non-psychiatric nurses and patient populations.) Journal of Nursing Education, 18 (8), Oct 1979, 14-20.

11 Nelson, J.K.N. and Schilke, D.A. The evolution of psychiatric liaison nursing. (A survey of the development of psychiatric nurse consultants for physically ill patients.) Perspectives in Psychiatric Care, 14 (2), Apr-Jun 1976, 61-65.

12 Wolff, P.I. Psychiatric nursing consultation: a study of the referral process. (In a general hospital.) Journal of Psychiatric Nursing and Mental Health Services, 16 (5), May 1978, 42-47.

76 PSYCHIATRIC NURSE THERAPIST

a GENERAL

1 Aylett, M.J. The nurse as psychotherapist. General Practice Team, 55, Mar 1976, 2.

2 Barker, P. Behaviour therapy in psychiatric and mental handicap nursing. (Survey of students six months after taking Scottish Committee for Clinical Nursing Studies course.) Journal of Advanced Nursing, 5 (1), Jan 1980, 55-69.

3 Barker, P. and others The future of nurse therapists. (Letter.) Nursing Mirror, 144, 16 Jun 1977, 11-12.

4 Broome, A.K. and others Long-term behaviour problems in psychiatric hospitals. (Problems in implementing behaviour therapy programmes.) Nursing Times, 75, 22 Mar 1979, 493-495.

5 Broome, A. and Collis, B. A patient for behaviour modification. (Case study of a disturbed and violent woman who had been hospitalised for 18 years.) Nursing Times, 72, 15 Apr 1976, 580-581.

6 Brown, M. The hospital setting. (Symposium paper on the nurse therapist.) Nursing Mirror, 144, 12 May 1977, 51-52.

7 Butler, R.J. and Rosenthall, G. Behaviour and rehabilitation: behavioural treatment for long-stay patients. Bristol: Wright, 1978. (For nurses.)

8 Butler, R.J. and Rosenthall, G. Behaviour and rehabilitation: development of an in-service training course. (Course in behaviour modification for qualified and student nurses at Stanley Royal Hospital, Yorkshire.) Nursing Times, 72, 5 Feb 1976, 191-193.

9 Cox, M. Coding the therapeutic process. Emblems of encounter: a manual for counsellors and therapists. Oxford: Pergamon, 1978.

10 Crisp, A.H. Interpersonal psychotherapies in medicine. (Origins and descriptions of different types.) Lancet, 2, 24/31 Dec 1977, 1342-1345.

11 Darcy, P.T. Psychiatric nursing today. 1. Protecting the patients. 2. Behaviour therapy and the nurse. Nursing Mirror, 147, 13 Jul 1978, 31-32.

12 Davies, K. A day treatment centre. (Symposium paper on the nurse therapist.) Nursing Mirror, 144, 12 May 1977, 54-55.

13 Enelow, A.J. Elements of psychotherapy. Oxford University Press, 1977.

14 Fraser, D. and others Against the odds: the results of a token economy programme with long term psychiatric patients. International Journal of Nursing Studies, 13 (1), 1976, 55-63.

15 Gomersall, J. Back into time. (Regression therapy.) Nursing Mirror, 150, 17 Jan 1980, 38-40.

16 Hallam, R.S. and others Behavioural nurse therapists? 1. Why train nurses. (Pioneer work at The Maudsley Hospital.) Nursing Times, 72, 6 May 1976, Occ. papers, 67-68.

17 JOINT Board of Clinical Nursing Studies. 10. Behaviour modification. Nursing Mirror, 143, 30 Sep 1976, Nursing care supplement series 2, i-iv.

18 Joint Working Party on Statutory Registration of Psychotherapists Report. Tavistock Centre, 1978. (Chairman: Paul Sieghart.)

19 McPherson, F.M. and others A course in behaviour modification. (Six-month course for qualified psychiatric and mental subnormality nurses organised by Tayside Area Clinical Psychology Department.) Nursing Times, 74, 20 Jul 1978, 1207-1209.

20 Markham, G. Changing scenes. (How nurses have become more involved in behaviour therapy.) Nursing Mirror, 150, 26 Jun 1980, Supplement, xiv-xvi.

21 Marks, I.M. Overview of a new clinical specialty. (Symposium paper on the nurse therapist.) Nursing Mirror, 144, 12 May 1977, 46-47.

22 Marks, I.M. and others Behavioural nurse therapists? 2. The implications. (Results of using nurses to treat adult neurotic problems at the Maudsley Hospital.) Nursing Times, 72, 13 May 1976, Occ. papers, 69-71.

23 Marks, I.M. and others Nursing in behavioural psychotherapy: an advanced clinical role for nurses. Royal College of Nursing, 1977. (Research series.)

24 Murphy, M. Community links. (Symposium paper on the nurse therapist.) Nursing Mirror, 144, 12 May 1977, 55-56.

25 Nursing Mirror A symposium on the developing role of the nurse therapist. (Papers read at the Second Annual National Conference on Nurse Therapy.) Nursing Mirror, 144, 12 May 1977, 45-56.

26 Oozeer, I. and others A role for a nurse therapist in a psychiatric outpatient clinic. (Research study at Guy's Hospital.) Journal of Advanced Nursing, 3 (1), Jan 1978, 47 54.

27 Orwin, A. Psychiatric nurses as behavioural therapists. (Work of the Hollymoor Clinic psychiatric unit over a ten year period.) Nursing Times, 72, 25 Mar 1976, 461-464.

28 Ramsay, M. Outpatient treatment. (Symposium paper on the nurse therapist.) Nursing Mirror, 144, 12 May 1977, 53-54.

29 Robertson, J.M. Ideas for materials and social skills assessment. (Social skills therapy for long-term psychiatric patients at Whitchurch Hospital, Cardiff.) British Journal of Occupational Therapy, 41 (11), Nov 1978, 365-367.

30 Rosen, B. Contract therapy. (Psychotherapy for patients with neurotic and personality disorders.) Nursing Times, 73, 19 Jan 1978, 119-121.

31 Stoll, K. Breaking the habit: a look at

behaviour modification. Mind Out, 22, May/Jun 1977, 8-10.

32 Storr, A. The art of psychotherapy. Secker and Warburg; Heinemann Medical, 1979.

33 Toman, A.M. Autogenic training. (Psychophysiological form of therapy for psychiatric disorders.) Nursing Times, 76, 21 Aug 1980, 1488-1492.

34 Watkins, D. Franz Anton Mesmer—founder of psychotherapy. Nursing Mirror, 142, 27 May 1976, 66-67.

35 Watts, M. Total care in Cambridge Ward. (Behavioural psychotherapy unit at the Middlesex Hospital.) Nursing Focus, 1 (8), Apr 1980, 312-313.

b OVERSEAS COUNTRIES

1 Bailey, D.S. and Dreyer, S.O. Therapeutic approaches to the care of the mentally ill. Philadelphia: Davis, 1977. (For nurses and others.)

2 Berni, R. and Fordyce, W.E. Behavior modification and the nursing process. 2nd ed. St. Louis: Mosby, 1977.

3 Branson, H.K. The nurse's role in behavior modification. Nursing Care, 8 (12), Dec 1975, 21-23.

4 Burdis, C. Biofeedback—does it work? (Its use in psychiatry, with reference to study at Behaviour Modification Treatment Unit at University Hospital, London, Ontario.) Canadian Nurse, 76 (2), Feb 1980, 44-46.

5 Carruth, B.D. Modifying behavior through social learning. (Graduate course in psychiatric nursing at the University of Texas School of Nursing to teach behavior therapy.) American Journal of Nursing, 76 (11), Nov 1976, 1804-1806.

6 Davidson, K.R. and others A descriptive study of the attitudes of psychiatrists toward the new role of the nurse therapist. Journal of Psychiatric Nursing, 16 (11), Nov 1978, 24-28.

7 Dienemann, J. The application of psychotherapeutic conceptual models in nursing practice. Journal of Psychiatric Nursing and Mental Health Services, 14 (5), May 1976, 28-30.

8 Goodwin, C.E. and Taaffe, C.H. Sex-typing and consumer preference for a male or female psychotherapist. (Research study.) Journal of Psychiatric Nursing, 18 (5), May 1980, 21-24.

9 Hauser, M.J. Nurses and behavior modification: resistance, ignorance or both. (Questions why nurses have not learned and used this technique.) Journal of Psychiatric Nursing and Mental Health Services, 16 (8), Aug 1978, 17-19.

10 Hill, S. and Hoch, M. 12-hour psychotherapy. (Twelve sessions of psychotherapy by nurses.) Canadian Nurse, 72 (5), May 1976, 30-31, 34.

11 Klingbeil, G.A. and Alvandi, O.M. Concepts of transactional analysis and anxiety with persons in crisis. (A study to compare different approaches to group therapy.) Journal of Psychiatric Nursing and Mental Health Services, 13 (6), Nov/Dec 1975, 5-10.

12 Knapp, T.J. and Peterson, L.W. Behavior analysis for nursing somatic disorders. Review of the literature. (Behavior therapy in physical disorders.) Nursing Research, 26 (4), Jul/Aug 1977, 281-287.

13 LeBow, M.D. Approaches to modifying patient behavior. New York: Appleton-Century-Crofts, 1976.

14 Lego, S. The one-to-one nurse patient relationship. (History and review of research on the nurse as therapist, with extensive bibliography.) Perspectives in Psychiatric Care, 18 (2), Mar/Apr 1980, 67-89.

15 Leib, A.C. and others The staff nurse as primary therapist: a pilot study. (Comparison of results of treatment by psychiatric resident and nurses.) Journal of Psychiatric Nursing and Mental Health Services, 14 (10), Oct 1976, 11-18.

16 McCann, J. Termination of the psychotherapeutic relationship. Journal of Psychiatric Nursing, 17 (10), Oct 1979, 37-39, 45-46.

17 McDonagh, M.J. and others Nurse-therapists in a state psychiatric hospital. American Journal of Nursing, 80 (1), Jan 1980, 102-104.

18 McMorrow, M.J. and others The use of the Premack principle to motivate patient activity attendance. An investigation of how a behavioral modification technique can motivate institutionalized mental patients to increase their activity attendance. (Research study.) Perspectives in Psychiatric Care, 16 (1), Jan/Feb 1978, 14-20.

19 Martin, G.L. Behavior modification to develop self control. Canadian Journal of Psychiatric Nursing, 56 (6), Nov/Dec 1975, 8-10.

20 Matheson, W.E. and others Control of food aversion using a reward model. Journal of Psychiatric Nursing and Mental Health Services, 14 (9), Sep 1976, 35-36.

21 Matheson, W.E. and others Control of screaming behavior using aversive conditioning and time-out. Journal of Psychiatric Nursing and Mental Health Services, 14 (9), Sep 1976, 27-28.

22 Niemeier, D.F. and Allison, T.S. Nurses can be effective behavior modifiers. Journal of Psychiatric Nursing and Mental Health Services, 14 (1), Jan 1976, 18-21.

23 Philp, I. Behaviour therapy in psychiatric nursing. Canadian Journal of Psychiatric Nursing, 18 (1), Jan-Feb 1977, 7, 12.

24 Randolph, G.T. Experiences in private practice. (A nurse's experiences as a psychotherapist.) Journal of Psychiatric Nursing and Mental Health Services, 13 (6), Nov/Dec 1975, 16-19.

25 Stokes, G.A. and Fitzpatrick, P.E. Teaching students psychotherapy. (University of Illinois Medical Center.) American Journal of Nursing, 77 (2), Feb 1977, 247-253.

26 Szasz, T. The myth of psychotherapy: mental healing as religion, rhetoric and repression. New York: Anchor Press/Doubleday, 1978.

c CRISIS INTERVENTION

1 Aguilera, D.C. and Messick, J.M. Crisis intervention: theory and methodology. 3rd ed. St. Louis: Mosby, 1978.

2 Ballou, M. Crisis intervention and the hospital nurse. Journal of Nursing Care, 13 (1), Jan 1980, 15-19.

3 Chen, M.E. Applying Yalom's principles to crisis work...some intriguing results. (Crisis intervention in group setting.) Journal of Psychiatric Nursing and Mental Health Services, 16 (6), Jan 1978, 15-22, 27.

4 Cooper, J.E. Crisis admission units and emergency psychiatric services. Copenhagen: WHO, 1979. (Public health in Europe; 11.)

5 Ewing, C.P. Crisis intervention as psychotherapy. New York: Oxford University Press, 1978.

6 Farewell, T. Crisis intervention. (The work of a community psychiatric team at Napsbury Hospital, St. Albans.) Nursing Mirror, 143, 2 Sep 1976, 60-61.

7 Finkelman, A.W. The nurse therapist: outpatient crisis intervention with the chronic psychiatric patient. Journal of Psychiatric Nursing and Mental Health Services, 15 (8), Aug 1977, 27-32.

8 Goldstein, D. Crisis intervention: a brief therapy model. Nursing Clinics of North America, 13 (4), Dec 1978, 657-663.

9 Grier, A.M. and Knight Aldrich, C. The growth of a crisis intervention unit under the direction of a clinical specialist in psychiatric nursing. Perspectives in Psychiatric Care, 10 (2), Apr/Jun 1972, 73-83.

10 Johnston, D. Crisis intervention skills. 1. What is the crisis? 2. Putting the skills to work. Journal of Practical Nursing, 28 (1), Jan 1978, 16-19; (2), Feb 1978, 20-23.

11 Knight, L. Emotional rescue in Tower Hamlets. (Walk-in emergency clinic at St. Clements psychiatric hospital run by nurse.) Mind Out, 41, Jul/Aug 1980, 16-17.

12 Lancaster, B.J. and Berkovsky, D. An ecological framework for crisis intervention. Journal of Psychiatric Nursing and Mental Health Services, 16 (3), Mar 1978, 17-23.

13 Mitchell, C.E. Identifying the hazard: the key to crisis intervention. American Journal of Nursing, 77 (7), Jul 1977, 1194-1196.

14 Narayan, S.M. and Joslin, D.J. Crisis theory and intervention: a critique of the medical model and proposal of a holistic nursing model. Advances in Nursing Science, 2 (4), Jul 1980, 27-39.

15 Richards, C. The crisis of mental illness in the home. (Problems of emergency compulsory admissions to psychiatric hospitals and possible alternatives.) New Society, 52, 10 Apr 1980, 60-61.

16 Scott, R.D. and Seccombe, P. Community psychiatry—setting up a service on a shoestring. (Crisis intervention service at Napsbury Hospital.) Mind Out, 17, Jul/Aug 1976, 5-7.

d FAMILY THERAPY

1 Adams, R. Naming of parts: support

groups for family therapy practice. (Include nurses and other professionals.) Social Work Services, 22, Feb 1980, 24-28.

2 Benton, D.W. Family therapy: problems encountered in defocusing the identified patient. Journal of Psychiatric Nursing, 17 (5), May 1979, 28-32.

3 Cade, B. Family therapy: an interactional approach to problems. Health Visitor, 52 (2), Feb 1979, 33-34.

4 Clement, J.A. Family therapy: the transferability of theory to practice. Journal of Psychiatric Nursing and Mental Health Services, 15 (8), Aug 1977, 33-37, 42-43.

5 Daines, B. and Holdsworth, V. Sexual problems: when two's better than one. (Therapy for a husband and wife.) Nursing Mirror, 148, 14 Jun 1979, 26-27.

6 Friedman, D. Blaming: an impasse in marital conflict—strategies for intervention. Journal of Psychiatric Nursing, 17 (4), Apr 1979, 8-13.

7 Headley, L. Adults and their parents in family therapy: a new direction in treatment. Plenum, 1977.

8 Hill, P. Conjoint family therapy. Midwife, Health Visitor and Community Nurse, 12 (11), Nov 1976, 355, 357, 358.

9 Howells, J.G. Emotion and the HV. The case for the HV as a mental health worker for the whole family. Nursing Times, 73, 28 Apr 1977, 598-599.

10 Lansky, M.R. and others Family treatment training for psychiatric nurses: a report on serial in-service workshops. Journal of Psychiatric Nursing and Mental Health Services, 16 (5), May 1978, 19-22.

11 Lantz, J.E. Family therapy: using a transactional approach. Journal of Psychiatric Nursing and Mental Health Services, 15 (4), Apr 1977, 17-23.

12 Mills, G. Family therapy involving several agencies. (Work of Child and Family Psychiatric Service in Dunstable.) Social Work Today, 10, 10 Apr 1979, 18-20.

13 Scharer, K. Nursing therapy with abusive and neglectful families. Journal of Psychiatric Nursing, 17 (9), Sep 1979, 12-21.

14 Seeger, P.A. A framework for family therapy. (A psychiatric nurse practitioner's role in solving marital problems illustrated by a case study.) Journal of Psychiatric Nursing and Mental Health Services, 14 (7), Jul 1976, 23-28.

15 Simons, H.R. and Lambley, A.M. Educating patients and staff. Conjoint therapy. (Therapy for sexual problems by a team of health professionals at Harlow House Psychiatric Day Hospital, High Wycombe.) British Journal of Occupational Therapy, 39 (10), Oct 1976, 245-246.

16 Stewart, B. Counselling. Hidden conflicts: a case study of the Fisher family. (Counselling by a psychiatric nurse.) Occupational Health, 31 (12), Dec 1979, 568-578; 32 (1), Jan 1980, 22-29; (2), Feb 1980, 76-83.

17 Walrond-Skinner, S. Family therapy: the treatment of natural systems. Routledge and

Kegan Paul, 1976. (Library of social work series.)

e GROUP THERAPY

1 Adamson, K. Silence in psychotherapy groups. (Its nature and therapeutic value.) Nursing Mirror, 146, 18 May 1978, 25-27.

2 Authier, J. and Gustafson, K. Group intervention techniques: a practical guide for psychiatric team members. Journal of Psychiatric Nursing and Mental Health Services, 14 (7), Jul 1976, 19-22.

3 Bines, J. and Masterson, P. The effect of pregnancy on patients receiving group therapy. (Case study of one patient's reaction to pregnancy in context of other members of therapy group.) Nursing Times, 74, 20 Jul 1978, 1220-1221.

4 Bowman, K. and Ware, P. Group therapy with middle-aged depressives. (Living at home.) Social Work Today, 10, 29 Aug 1978, 19-21.

5 Claxton, V. The evocative technique. (Type of group therapy.) British Journal of Occupational Therapy, 42 (5), May 1979, 111-114.

6 Fochtman, G.A. Therapeutic factors of the informal group. American Journal of Nursing, 76 (2), Feb 1976, 238-239.

7 Hager, R. Evaluation of group psychotherapy—a question of values. Journal of Psychiatric Nursing, 16 (12), Dec 1978, 26-33.

8 Holbrook, B. The quiet group. (Group therapy at Whitecroft Hospital, Isle of Wight, allowing the shy and introverted to participate in smaller groups.) Nursing Mirror, 142, 22 Apr 1976, 69-70.

9 King, P.D. Life cycle in the 'Tavistock Study Group'. (Mental health professionals participate in group therapy.) Perspectives in Psychiatric Care, 8 (4), Oct/Dec 1975, 180-184.

10 Loomis, M.E. Group process for nurses. St. Louis: Mosby, 1979.

11 McIvor, D.L. and Rosario, A. Group therapy for women going through divorce. Canadian Journal of Psychiatric Nursing, 20 (3), May/Jun 1979, 11-13.

12 Palmer, J.D. Group psychotherapy in a state mental hospital: who needs it? Journal of Psychiatric Nursing and Mental Health Services, 14 (3), Mar 1976, 19-22.

13 Whiteley, J.S. and Gordon, J. Group approaches in psychiatry. Routledge and Kegan Paul, 1979.

14 Williams, R.A. A contract for cotherapists in group psychotherapy. Journal of Psychiatric Nursing and Mental Health Services, 14 (6), Jun 1976, 11-14.

77 PSYCHIATRIC HOSPITALS

a GENERAL

1 Bickford, J.A.R. and Bickford, M.E. The

private lunatic asylums of the East Riding. Beverley: East Yorkshire Local History Society, 1976.

2 Cope, D. and Cox, S. Organization development in a psychiatric hospital: creating desirable changes. Journal of Advanced Nursing, 5 (4), Jul 1980, 371-380.

3 Department of Health and Social Security Working Group on Organisational and Management Problems of Mental Illness Hospitals. Report. DHSS, 1979. (Chairman: T.E. Nodder.) Summary in Nursing Times, 76, 31 Jan 1980, 180.

4 Eason, R.J. and Grimes, J.A. In-patient care of the mentally ill: a statistical study of future provision. Health Trends, 8 (2), May 1976, 13-18.

5 Edmonstone, J.D. Changing hospital organisation using outside consultants: evaluation of one example. (Evaluation of change in a psychiatric hospital by Trent RHA Organisation Development Unit.) Hospital and Health Services Review, 76 (1), Jan 1980, 5-8.

6 Hassall, C. and Cross, K.W. Closing a mental hospital admissions: predictions and predicaments. (Closure of Powick Hospital as part of Worcester Development Project and fate of residual population.) Hospital and Health Services Review, 75 (11), Nov 1979, 393-395.

7 Hilton, J. Point of view: how many places? (Need for long-stay beds in psychiatric hospital or alternative provision.) Journal of Community Nursing, 3 (4), Oct 1979, 17, 32.

8 Inskip, J.H. and Edwards, J.G. Mental hospital inquiries. (Suggests how they can be avoided, with advice on decision-making and reducing their impact on hospital life.) Lancet, 1, 24 Mar 1979, 658-660.

9 International Hospital Federation Psychiatry and architecture: the right to normal living conditions. World Hospitals, 12 (1), 1976, 52-82.

10 King's Fund Centre The mental hospital in the psychiatric service. (Report of conference.) Hospital and Health Services Review, 72 (12), Dec 1976, 435-436.

11 King's Fund Centre Psychiatric provision drawing on large institutions: organising and managing to develop better services. King Edward's Hospital Fund, 1978.

12 Lloyd, T. Who holds the reins? (Challenges facing management in psychiatric hospitals.) Nursing Mirror, 150, 26 Jun 1980, Supplement, x-xii, xiv.

13 Martin, I. Planning for a two-year system? (Future of the large mental hospital and the district general psychiatric unit.) New Psychiatry, 3 (3), 5 Feb 1976, 14-16.

14 Philip, A.E. and others Bed usage as an index of the work of a psychiatric hospital. (Bangour Village Hospital, West Lothian.) Health Bulletin, 34 (3), May 1976, 159-162.

15 Rodgers, S.J. Organisation and management problems of mental illness hospitals. (Nodder report.) British Medical Journal, 281, 20 Sep 1980, 820-821.

16 Rollin, H.R. Are mental hospitals really necessary? (A survey of past trends.) Public Health, 90 (2), Jan 1976, 49-52.

17 Smith, J.P. The changing role of the large psychiatric hospital. (King's Fund conference.) Nursing Mirror, 143, 4 Nov 1976, 41.

18 Towell, D. and Harries, C. editors Innovation in patient care: an action research study of change in a psychiatric hospital. Croom Helm, 1979.

19 Towell, D. Large institutions reconsidered: an approach to the management of transition. (Comment on Nodder Report.) Hospital and Health Services Review, 76 (3), Mar 1980, 87-90.

20 Watkin, B. Strategy for simplification. (Summary of Nodder Report.) Health and Social Service Journal, 90, 8 Feb 1980, 184-185.

21 Wertheimer, A. Co-ordination or chaos — the rundown of psychiatric hospitals. Royal Society of Health Journal, 95 (3), Jun 1975, 136-138, 163.

22 Whitehead, T. A plan for psychiatric hospitals. (The conversion of large hospitals into hostels and flatlets and the creation of units in general hospitals.) Health and Social Service Journal, 86, 29 May 1976, 981.

23 Young, P. Organisational and management problems of mental illness hospitals. (Summary of Nodder Report.) Nursing Times, 76, 11 Sep 1980, 1600-1602.

b DAY HOSPITALS

1 Bradley, M.E. Establishment of a day hospital (for psychiatric patients at Whiteabbey General Hospital, Co. Antrim). Nursing Times, 73, 17 Feb 1977, 246-249.

2 Brandon, D. Cheap and cheerful: Knowsley day centres. (Two day centres in Knowsley, Lancashire.) Mind Out, 43, Nov 1980, 20-21.

3 Cobb, J. Tottenham Mews day hospital — a profile. (At the Middlesex Hospital.) Nursing Focus, 1 (8), Apr 1980, 309-311.

4 Enticknap, B.C. Harlow House. (Day hospital forming part of psychiatric unit at Wycombe General Hospital.) Nursing Times, 74, 6 Jul 1978, 1121-1124.

5 Fairclough, F. Community and day hospital care. (Liverpool Psychiatric Day Hospital.) Nursing Mirror, 143, 5 Aug 1976, 67-68.

6 Harper, G. Driving force behind day care for the mentally ill. (Day centre in Derbyshire.) Health and Social Service Journal, 90, 18 Jan 1980, 88-89.

7 Higgins, P. A mobile day unit. (In Exeter health district.) Nursing Times, 76, 12 Jun 1980, 1062-1064.

8 Howat, J.G.M. and Kontny, E.L. What price the ambulance? A survey of psychiatric day patient transport. (Editorial comment, p.1242-1243.) British Medical Journal, 2, 12 Nov 1977, 1208.

9 Huggins, C. Day care on a shoestring. (Informal day centre for the mentally ill in Havering.) Health and Social Service Journal, 86, 24 Jul 1976, 1348-1349.

10 Kelly, P. Community psychiatric nursing. A psychiatric day unit. (Laurel House, Bromley AHA.) Nursing Times, 72, 4 Nov 1976, 1717.

11 Mitchell, R.G. Psychiatric day centres — a sound investment. Nursing Times, 72, 22 Apr 1976, 634.

12 Shires, J. A travelling day hospital. An experiment in rural community psychiatric care. (West Dorset.) Social Work Today, 8, 22 Mar 1977, 16-18.

13 Williamson, F. A day hospital within the diversions of a troubled community. (Psychiatric day hospital in Belfast.) International Journal of Social Psychiatry, 24 (2), Summer 1978, 95-103.

c INDIVIDUAL HOSPITALS

1 Bangour — Johnstone, T. Bangour village hospital. (Psychiatric hospital in Edinburgh with associated day hospitals.) Nursing Times, 75, 18 Jan 1979, 124-125.

2 Banstead — Cowper-Smith, F. Banstead Hospital. (Psychiatric hospital originally opened in 1877 as a pauper lunatic asylum.) Nursing Times, 73, 22/29 Dec 1977, Archive, 41-44.

3 Broadmoor — Smythe, T. MIND and Broadmoor — a disturbing correspondence. (Problems faced by MIND in representing patients at the hospital. See also editorial on p.1.) Social Work Today, 10, 21 Nov 1978, 8-10.

4 Broadmoor Allegations of staff brutality against patients in another 'secret hospital': 'everything that is alleged to have happened in Rampton has occurred in Broadmoor,' say nurses. Mind Out, 37, Nov/Dec 1979, 3-5.

5 Broadmoor — Cowper-Smith, F. Broadmoor survives slings and arrows. (Report of visit.) Nursing Times, 75, 29 Nov 1979, 2059-2062.

6 Brookwood — Surrey Area Health Authority Report of the Committee of Inquiry into standards of patient care at Brookwood Hospital. Guildford: the Authority, 1980.

7 Carstairs — Ritchie, M. Daunting challenge of care with maximum security. (Experiences of a visit to Carstairs State Mental Hospital.) Health and Social Service Journal, 86, 10 Dec 1976, 2190-2191.

8 Darlington As it seems. (Comments on the reports of enquiry at St. Augustine's and Darlington Hospitals.) Hospital and Health Services Review, 72 (9), Sep 1976, 307.

9 Darlington — Beckwith, G. Staff shortages and ward layout blamed in psychiatric unit deaths. (Inquiry at Memorial Hospital, Darlington.) Nursing Times, 72, 20 May 1976, 756.

16 Darlington Changes made at Darlington Hospital. Nursing Times, 72, 22 Jul 1976, 1105.

11 Darlington — Northern Regional Health Authority Report of the Committee of Inquiry held at Memorial Hospital Darlington between 1 Dec 1975 and 10 Jan 1976. The Health Authority, 1976. (Chairman: Harold Day.)

12 Darlington Nurse shortage blamed for patient deaths. (Darlington inquiry.) Nursing Mirror, 142, 20 May 1976, 35.

13 Darlington — Pigache, P. Unfitting Memorial. (Achievement of the inquiry into Darlington Memorial Hospital.) World Medicine, 12 (5), 1 Dec 1976, 17-20, 23, 25.

14 Ely — Ross, T. Ely Hospital 10 years on. Nursing Mirror, 148, 12 Apr 1979, 16-19.

15 Friern — Ashton, K. Off the record. (Recent adverse publicity on Friern Hospital and report of visit by author.) Nursing Times, 74, 2 Mar 1978, 346-349.

16 Friern — Halpern, S. Why this bulldozing will not clear the dumping ground. (Comment on recent reports calling for closure of Friern Hospital, Barnet.) Health and Social Service Journal, 87, 5 Aug 1977, 1128-1129.

17 Friern 'Radical appraisal' for Friern Hospital. AHA recommends district-based psychiatric service. (Summary of report by a Camden and Islington AHA working party.) Nursing Times, 73, 1 Dec 1977, 1855.

18 Friern — Young, P. Friern hospital: what is the real truth? (Report of visit and assessment of care patients receive.) Nursing Mirror, 146, 16 Mar 1978, 7-10.

19 Powick — Morris, L.N. Changing care pattern — Powick Hospital 1852-1977. (Hospital involved in Worcester development project.) Nursing Times, 73, 14 Jul 1977, 1069-1071.

20 Rampton — Department of Health and Social Security Report of the review of Rampton Hospital. HMSO, 1980. (Chairman: Sir John Boynton.) (Cmnd 8073)

21 Rampton — Ellis, S. A costly mistake? The implications of the Yorkshire TV documentary, 'The secret hospital'. (Rampton.) Nursing Times, 75, 31 May 1979, 907.

22 Rampton — Galley, J. Behind the barbed fence. (Impressions of Rampton Hospital.) Health and Social Service Journal, 86, 10 Dec 1976, 2191.

23 Rampton — Mind Out MPs suggest Rampton reforms. (Six reforms suggested by All-Party Parliamentary Mental Health Group.) Mind Out, 37, Nov/Dec 1979, 6.

24 Rampton — Morris, P. Rampton: why were Elliott's fears ignored? (Elliott report of 1973.) Nursing Mirror, 148, 7 Jun 1979, 6.

25 Rampton — Thorold, O. The future of Rampton. (Report on MIND's submission to the Rampton Review Team.) Mind Out, 37, Nov/Dec 1979, 7-8.

26 St. Augustine's — Ankers, B. Back to square one? (Comments on the emergency panel report by Kent AHA members on St. Augustine's Hospital.) Nursing Times, 73, 14 Apr 1977, 512-513.

27 St. Augustine's — Ankers, W.B. A good report, but... Critiques of policy at St. Augustine's. Nursing Times, 72, 1 Jul 1976, 997-999.

28 St. Augustine's Another dismal report. (St. Augustine's Hospital, Chartham Down, Kent.) Lancet, 1, 3 Apr 1976, 733.

29 St. Augustine's Mental nurses criticised for cruelty and neglect. (Report of inquiry into care at St. Augustine's Hospital, Chartham Down, Kent.) Nursing Mirror, 142, 8 Apr 1976, 37.

30 St. Augustine's — Newstead, K. News feature...certainly anti-therapeutic, possibly hell. (Comments on the St. Augustine's Hospital enquiry by a former principal tutor at the school of nursing.) Nursing Times, 72, 27 May 1976, 200-202.

31 St. Augustine's — Price, C. Money is not the root of the problem. (An MP's view of the lessons to be learnt from the St. Augustine's Hospital enquiry.) Nursing Times, 72, 27 May 1976, 202-203.

32 St. Augustine's — Rowden, R. St. Augustine's aftermath. Nursing Times, 72, 1 Jul 1976, 996-997.

33 St. Augustine's — South East Thames Regional Health Authority Report of Committee of Inquiry (into the care and treatment of patients at) St. Augustine's Hospital, Chartham, Canterbury. The Health Authority, 1976.

34 St. Augustine's — Swaffield, L. Policy by default. Report on conditions in the long-stay wards at St. Augustine's Hospital, near Canterbury. Nursing Times, 72, 8 Apr 1976, 520-521.

35 St. Augustine's — Thompson, S. Team work is vital. (Comments on the report of inquiry into St. Augustine's Hospital, Chartham, Canterbury, Kent.) New Psychiatry, 3 (8), 15 Apr 1976, 4.

36 St. Augustine's Yet another enquiry. (St. Augustine's Hospital, Chatham.) Hospital and Health Services Review, 72 (5), May 1976, 149-150.

37 St. Crispin — Ayres, H. A changing community: the brief history of St. Crispin Hospital, Duston, Northampton 1876-1976. Northamptonshire Area Health Authority, 1976.

38 St. Crispin — Callow, F.J. St. Crispin celebrates centenary. Nursing Mirror, 143, 25 Nov 1976, 66-68.

39 St. Crispin St. Crispin Hospital. Nursing Times, 73, 13 Jan 1977, Archive, 1-4.

40 Shenley Shenley Hospital. (Psychiatric hospital in Middlesex opened in 1934.) Nursing Times, 73, 9 Jun 1977, Archive, 21-24.

41 Warlingham — Croydon Area Health Authority Committee of Inquiry into Warlingham Park Hospital. Report. The Health Authority, 1976. (Chairman: David Sullivan.)

d THERAPEUTIC COMMUNITY

1 Adelson, P.Y. The back ward dilemma. (Need for therapeutic community in long term care.) American Journal of Nursing, 80 (3), Mar 1980, 422-425.

2 Benton, D.W. The significance of the absent member in milieu therapy. Perspectives in Psychiatric Care, 18 (1), Jan/Feb 1980, 21-25.

3 Campbell, W. The therapeutic community: a history. Nursing Times, 75, 15 Nov 1979, 1985-1987.

4 Campbell, W. The therapeutic community: problems encountered by nurses. Nursing Times, 75, 22 Nov 1979, 2038-2040.

5 Deitrich, G. Nurses in the therapeutic community (in the hospital showing advantages over traditionally run institutions.) Journal of Advanced Nursing, 1 (2), Mar 1976, 139-154.

6 DeVierno, G. Nursing administrative

process: a patient tool in the therapeutic community. Supervisor Nurse, 11 (2), Feb 1980, 41-42.

7 Hall, B.A. Mutual withdrawal: the non-participant in a therapeutic community. Perspectives in Psychiatric Care, 14 (2), Apr/Jun 1976, 75-77, 93.

8 Hanvey, C. What is a therapeutic community? (With history of their development.) Mind Out, 43, Nov 1980, 11-13.

9 Hinshelwood, R.D. and Manning, N. editors Therapeutic communities: reflections and progress. Routledge and Kegan Paul, 1979.

10 Jones, M. Nurses can change the social systems of hospitals. (Therapeutic community.) American Journal of Nursing, 78 (6), Jun 1978, 1012-1014.

11 Jones, M. Why the Henderson must stay. (History of the therapeutic community by founder of Henderson Hospital.) Mind Out, 37, Nov/Dec 1979, 20-21.

12 Kynaston, T. A special kind of help. (Role of nurses in therapeutic community at the Henderson Hospital.) Nursing Mirror, 150, 20 Mar 1980, 26-28.

13 Mills, G.L. An experience of death — the closure of a therapeutic community. (Hereward House, Fulbourn Hospital, Cambridge.) Social Work Today, 8 (4), 20 Oct 1976, 15-17.

14 Mills, V.H. Mutuality in nursing leads to vulnerability for patient and nurse in a psychotherapeutic community. (Comparison of social defence systems used in general nursing with those used in a psychotherapeutic community after a weekend duty at the Cassel Hospital, London.) Journal of Advanced Nursing, 2 (1), Jan 1977, 21-28.

15 Morris, P. Henderson hospital. (Value of therapeutic community.) Mind Out, 44, Dec 1980, 17-19.

16 Murphy, S.A. Patients' and staff's perceptions of therapy and milieu in a short-term private psychiatric hospital. International Journal of Nursing Studies, 16 (2), 1979, 159-167.

17 Rasinski, K. and others Practical implications of a theory of the 'therapeutic milieu' for psychiatric nursing practice. (Therapeutic community.) Journal of Psychiatric Nursing, 18 (5), May 1980, 16-20.

18 Robertson, P.A. The therapeutic community and the nurse: a blurring of traditional roles. Journal of Psychiatric Nursing and Mental Health Services, 14 (4), Apr 1976, 28-31.

19 Salvage, J. Communities under threat. (Threatened closure of two therapeutic communities at the Henderson Hospital and John Conolly Hospital.) Nursing Mirror, 150, 31 Jan 1980, 6.

20 Sharp, V. Social control in the therapeutic community. Farnborough: Saxon House, 1975.

21 Wolf, M.S. A review of literature on milieu therapy. Journal of Psychiatric Nursing and Mental Health Services, 15 (5), May 1977, 26-33.

e PSYCHIATRIC UNITS IN GENERAL HOSPITALS

1 Baruch, G. and Treacher, A. Treating the mentally ill. (Short-stay psychiatric units in general hospitals.) New Society, 44, 20 Apr 1978, 125-127.

2 Bowman, M.J. and Sturgeon, D.A. A clinic within a general hospital for the assessment of urgent psychiatric problems. (At University College Hospital, London.) Lancet, 2, 19 Nov 1977, 1067-1068.

3 Campbell, W. Problems of the small unit. (Problems of coping with violent, elderly and long-stay patients in small psychiatric units.) Health and Social Service Journal, 88, 24 Feb 1978, 218.

4 Coverdale, P. New patterns of contact. (Psychiatric unit at St. Luke's Hospital, Middlesbrough, which runs clinics, groups and family therapy.) Nursing Times, 76, 12 Jun 1980, 1061.

5 Fullerton, A.G. and Young, R. From mental hospital to psychiatric department. (Psychiatric care in a district general hospital in Dudley.) Health and Social Service Journal, 86, 31 Jan 1976, 210-211.

6 Hamill, J.P. and Matthei, E.H. Mental health unit serves many needs. (Design features.) Hospitals, 54 (4), 16 Feb 1980, 126, 129-130, 132, 134.

7 Hospital and Health Services Review New psychiatric unit at Whittington Hospital. Hospital and Health Services Review, 72 (9), Sep 1976, 313-314.

8 Jeevendrampillai, V. and Campbell, W. A study of new long-stay patients in a psychiatric unit. (Research study.) Nursing Times, 75, 12 Apr 1979, 633-637.

9 Keane, B. Psychiatric wards in general hospitals. Australian Nurses Journal, 8 (10), May 1979, 37-38.

10 Macilwaine, H. The nursing of female neurotic patients in psychiatric units of general hospitals. PhD thesis, University of Manchester, 1980.

11 Saunders, B. New chronic patients in a psychiatric unit. (Study of patients served by a general hospital psychiatric unit without access to a back-up hospital.) Social Work Today, 7 (2), 15 Apr 1976, 41-42.

12 Tutt, P.M. Acute psychiatry within a general hospital. (Yeovil District General Hospital.) Nursing Times, 72, 30 Sep 1976, 1529-1531.

13 Watts, C. In praise of units: the advantages of a psychiatric unit in a general hospital. Health and Social Service Journal, 87, 30 Sep 1977, 1378.

f PATIENTS' VIEWS AND WELFARE

1 Barton, R. Institutional neurosis. 3rd ed. Bristol: Wright, 1976.

2 Bayer, M. The multipurpose room: a way-out outlet for staff and clients. (Locked, soundproof room where patients and staff can give vent to feelings of anger and frustration.) Journal of Psychiatric Nursing, 18 (10), Oct 1980, 35-37.

3 Brandon, D. A day in the life of a patient at Moss Side. Mind Out, 44, Dec 1980, 19-20.

4 Breton, S. and Cockram, M.E.A. A simple programme designed to counteract some of the effects of institutionalization in long term psychiatric wards. (At Parc Hospital, Bridgend.) Journal of Advanced Nursing, 2 (5), Sep 1977, 495-501.

5 British Medical Journal Medicolegal. Mental patients and the vote. British Medical Journal, 1, 20 Mar 1976, 720.

6 Campbell, W. John Conolly...pioneer of freedom. (19th-century doctor who advocated more humanitarian treatment for the mentally ill.) Nursing Mirror, 146, 23 Mar 1978, 30-32.

7 Clare, A. One flew over the cuckoo's nest. (Film review.) Lancet, 1, 17 Apr 1976, 851.

8 Dorado, J. The right to one's own. (How a scheme of personalised clothing for psychiatric patients was developed at Runwell Hospital, Wickford, Essex.) Nursing Mirror, 150, 10 Apr 1980, 40.

9 Dunn, A. and Martin, A.J. Out of the cuckoo's nest. Could it happen here? (Comments on the film 'One flew over the cuckoo's nest'.) Nursing Times, 72, 20 May 1976, 764-766.

10 Dwyer, M. and others Effect of hospitalization on weight of psychiatric patients. (Research study on patients hospitalised for long periods and receiving psychotropic drugs.) Journal of Advanced Nursing, 3 (5), Sep 1978, 433-436.

11 Foster, C.E. Awareness group with institutionalised patients. British Journal of Occupational Therapy, 40 (8), Aug 1977, 194-195.

12 Gajos, M.J. A programme for long-stay patients. (At Broadgate Hospital, Beverley.) Nursing Times, 76, 31 Jan 1980, 204-207.

13 Goldmeier, D. and others Relatives and friends group in a psychiatric ward. (To enable them to meet the staff and discuss anxieties and problems. The experiment proved successful.) British Medical Journal, 1, 7 Apr 1979, 932-934.

14 Hirsch, S.R. and others Shortening hospital stay for psychiatric care: effect on patients and their families. British Medical Journal, 1, 17 Feb 1979, 442-446.

15 Hobson, M. This place is a madhouse. (Novel set in a psychiatric ward.) Heinemann, 1980.

16 Howell, R.G. Introducing a patient information system at a psychiatric hospital. (Hellingly Hospital.) Hospital and Health Services Review, 73 (1), Jan 1977, 10-12.

17 Inter-Departmental Working Party on Electoral Registration of Patients in Mental Hospitals (Interim report.) DHSS, 1977.

18 Jacobs, M.A. Promoting responsibility and mutual concern through a modified form of patient government. (In psychiatric wards.) Journal of Psychiatric Nursing and Mental Health Services, 15 (2), Feb 1977, 30-34.

19 Long, A. Implementation of a personalised clothing policy for long stay psychiatric patients: a study of communication. Journal of Advanced Nursing, 4 (4), Jul 1979, 415-427.

20 McKerrow, L.W. The dilemma of psychiatric hospitals: patients' rights vs. public safety. Hospital Administration in Canada, 18 (3), Mar 1976, 67-68.

21 Mark, B. From 'lunatic' to 'client': 300 years of psychiatric patienthood. Journal of Psychiatric Nursing, 18 (3), Mar 1980, 32-36.

22 Mark, B. Hospital treatment of borderline patients: toward a better understanding of problematic issues. Journal of Psychiatric Nursing, 18 (8), Aug 1980, 25-31.

23 MIND Polling power — Government responds. (Summary of MIND's observations on the DHSS consultative document on voting rights.) Mind Out, 22, May/Jun 1977, 16-17.

24 Moore, J. and Moore, G. The role of a sick unit in a psychiatric hospital. (Study at Littlemore Hospital, Oxford.) Nursing Mirror, 142, 20 May 1976, 67-69.

25 Murray, E.W. Why not night hospitals? The case for night treatment to enable psychiatric patients to hold their jobs. Nursing Mirror, 149, 30 Aug 1979, 10.

26 Nelson, P. and Chartrand, L. How we bridged the generation gap in our psych unit. (Adolescents and adults in the same psychiatric unit.) RN Magazine, 41 (2), Feb 1978, 56-57.

27 Raphael, W. Psychiatric hospitals viewed by their patients. 2nd ed. King Edward's Hospital Fund for London, 1977.

28 Royal College of Psychiatrists Confidential records under threat. (Recent report.) Nursing Times, 72, 25 Aug 1977, 1298.

29 Schrock, R.A. Psychiatry under review. 10. The rights of mental patients. Nursing Times, 76, 15 May 1980, 884-887.

30 Sheldrick, W. Patients are people. The disadvantages of hospital. (For psychiatric patients: student nurse project.) Nursing Times, 73, 9 Jun 1977, 850.

31 Thorner, N. Nurses violate their patients' rights. (Study of how nurses dealt with patient refusals of medications.) Journal of Psychiatric Nursing and Mental Health Services, 14 (1), Jan 1976, 7-12.

32 Turner-Smith, A. and Thomson, I.G. Patient's opinions. A survey of the effectiveness of a psychiatric hospital. (Based on questionnaire.) Nursing Times, 75, 19 Apr 1979, 675-679.

33 Whitehead, T. The court of protection. (For mentally ill patients incapable of managing their own affairs.) Health and Social Service Journal, 90, 28 Mar 1980, 422-423.

34 Whitehead, T. The gaslight phenomenon: the motives behind fraudulent incarceration in mental homes. (With case histories.) Nursing Mirror, 145, 29 Dec 1977, 31-32.

g SPECIAL HOSPITALS, SECURE UNITS, LOCKED WARDS

1 Bluglass, R. Plans for a secure future. (Implementing secure hospital units recommended by the Butler Committee on Mentally Abnormal Offenders.) Health and Social Service Journal, 87, 7 Jan 1977, 10.

2 Bluglass, R. Regional secure units and interim security for psychiatric patients. British Medical Journal, 1, 25 Feb 1978, 489-493.

3 Bluglass, R. Secure units or hospitals? Mind Out, 27, Mar/Apr 1978, 5-8.

4 Bluglass, R. Sin or sickness? — Stealing, vandalism and violence. A mind diseased? (Mentally abnormal offenders.) Royal Society of Health Journal, 96 (5), Oct 1976, 224-225, 229.

5 British Medical Journal Dangerous patients and prisoners. (Assessment of dangerousness by psychiatrists and nursing staff.) British Medical Journal, 2, 24 Sep 1977, 782-783.

6 Carney, M.W.P. and Nolan, P.A. Area security unit in a psychiatric hospital. (At Shenley Hospital, for disturbed patients.) British Medical Journal, 1, 7 Jan 1978, 27-28.

7 Carney, M.W.P. and Nolan, P.A. Management of the disturbed patient. (In secure unit at Shenley Hospital.) Nursing Times, 75, 1 Nov 1979, 1896-1899.

8 Castle, P. Turning critics into allies. (Problems of public resistance to setting-up of interim secure units.) Health and Social Service Journal, 89, 22 Mar 1979, 288-289.

9 Christie, L.S. Are security units really necessary? Nursing Mirror, 143, 5 Aug 1976, 69-70.

10 Clarke, J. Security systems in high-security hospitals. Nursing Mirror, 146, 22 Jun 1978, 23-26.

11 Cobb, J.P. and Gossop, M.R. Locked doors in the management of disturbed psychiatric patients. (Study at Maudsley Hospital of the effectiveness of locked wards.) Journal of Advanced Nursing, 1 (6), Nov 1976, 469-480.

12 Cohen, R. Where did the money go? (Failure of DHSS to provide secure units for mentally abnormal offenders.) Health and Social Service Journal, 87, 30 Sep 1977, 1379.

13 Confederation of Health Service Employees NHS secure treatment units: a policy statement. Banstead: COHSE, 1979.

14 Devlin, R. Towards a more secure future? (Lack of progress on regional secure units and opening of first one at St. Luke's Hospital, Middlesbrough.) Nursing Mirror, 151, 4 Dec 1980, 8.

15 Hinton, J. and others Simple behaviour rating scales for maximum security patients: development and validation. (For use by nurse custodians.) British Journal of Social and Clinical Psychology, 17 (3), Sep 1978, 255-259.

16 Journal of Medical Ethics Where are the promised secure units for the mentally ill? (Editorial.) Journal of Medical Ethics, 3 (1), Mar 1977, 2-3.

17 Kilgalen, R.K. The effective use of seclusion. (As restraint procedure for psychiatric patients.) Journal of Psychiatric Nursing and Mental Health Services, 15 (1), Jan 1977, 22-25.

18 Kilroy-Silk, R. Lead needed on the non-treatment of mentally ill. (Problem of patients languishing in special hospitals awaiting transfer to NHS psychiatric hospitals.) Health and Social Service Journal, 89, 29 Jun 1979, 788.

19 Knight, L. Secure units: fact or fiction? (Lack of progress by RHAs with map showing distribution.) Mind Out, 33, Mar/Apr 1979, 10-12.

20 Lancet Secure psychiatric units. (Lack of progress in implementing the 1961 memorandum.) Lancet, 2, 4 Sep 1976, 526-527.

21 Lancet Who's for the locked ward? Lancet, 1, 28 Feb 1976, 461.

22 MacCulloch, M.J. Some problems of placing psychiatric patients. (Sources of DHSS guidance on security for psychiatric patients and procedure for application for a Special Hospital place.) Health Trends, 9 (3), Aug 1977, 59-62.

23 Mellor, P.T. Secure units. (Letter criticising NUPE's opposition to regional secure units from nurse adviser to Rcn Society of Psychiatric Nursing.) Nursing Times, 74, 27 Apr 1978, 717-718.

24 Morris, P. The scandal of the Prestwich secure unit. (Attempts to close it by NUPE.) Nursing Mirror, 147, 12 Oct 1978, 8-9.

25 Nursing Mirror What's happened to the secure units? (Survey of provisions in each region.) Nursing Mirror, 151, 28 Aug 1980, 5.

26 Quinn, S. Management of an interim secure unit. (Lyndhurst Unit at Knowle Hospital, Hampshire.) Nursing Times, 75, 8 Feb 1979, 237-240.

27 Robertson, G. and Gibbens, T.C.N. Transfers from prisons to local psychiatric hospitals under section 72 of the 1959 Mental Health Act. (Results of survey.) British Medical Journal, 280, 24 May 1980, 1263-1266.

28 Rollin, H.R. The care of the mentally abnormal offender and the protection of the public. Journal of Medical Ethics, 2 (4), Dec 1976, 157-162.

29 Royal College of Nursing. Society of Psychiatric Nursing Seclusion and restraint in hospitals and units for the mentally disordered. Rcn, 1979.

30 Russell, D.H. and others Please lock me away... (The Villa locked ward at the Maudsley Hospital.) Nursing Mirror, 142, 8 Jan 1976, 68-70.

31 South East Thames Regional Health Authority Secure but not secured: a special assessment and supervision service for the South East Thames Region. Croydon: SETRHA, 1976.

32 Strutt, R. and others Seclusion: can it be justified? (Transcript of some of the issues raised at a debate among nurses and doctors at Netherne Hospital.) Nursing Times, 76, 11 Sep 1980, 1629-1633.

33 Walshe-Brennan, F.S. Risks in psychiatric nursing: a review of current legislation and recommendations for the assessment and treatment of mentally abnormal offenders. Nursing Mirror, 144, 14 Apr 1977, 53-54.

34 Weaver, S.M. and others Behavioural principles applied in a security ward. (Research project at St. George's Hospital, Morpeth, Northumberland.) Nursing Times, 74, 5 Jan 1978, 22-24.

35 Weaver, S.M. and others Some patterns of disturbed behaviour in a closed ward environment. (Research study by three psychologists.) Journal of Advanced Nursing, 3 (3), May 1978, 251-263.

36 Whaley, M.S. and Ramirez, L.F. The use of seclusion rooms and physical restraints in the treatment of psychiatric patients. (Research study.) Journal of Psychiatric Nursing, 18 (1), Jan 1980, 13-16.

37 Whitehead, T. Security and the locked ward. Health and Social Service Journal, 86, 28 Aug 1976, 1552.

h VIOLENCE

1 Allen, M. Striking the right balance between patient care and nurses' safety. (Violence in hospitals.) Nursing Mirror, 147, 7 Dec 1978, 9.

2 Anders, R.L. When a patient becomes violent. (Nursing care.) American Journal of Nursing, 77 (7), Jul 1977, 1144-1148.

3 Basque, L.O. and Merhige, J. Nurses' experiences with dangerous behavior: implications for training. Journal of Continuing Education in Nursing, 11 (5), Sep/Oct 1980, 47-51.

4 Block, B. Preparing students for physical restraint. Journal of Psychiatric Nursing and Mental Health Services, 14 (10), Oct 1976, 9-10.

5 Bowden, P. The psychology of violence. Nursing Mirror, 146, 15 Jun 1978, 13-16.

6 British Medical Journal Assaults on doctors. (Violence to health service staff.) British Medical Journal, 1, 13 May 1978, 1229-1230.

7 Campbell, W. and Mawson, D. Violence in a psychiatric unit. (At John Conolly Hospital, Birmingham.) Journal of Advanced Nursing, 3 (1), Jan 1978, 55-64.

8 Coffey, M.P. The violent patient. (Keynote address, Rcn conference, 1976.) Journal of Advanced Nursing, 1 (5), Sep 1976, 341-350.

9 Confederation of Health Service Employees The management of violent or potentially violent patients: report of a...working party... Banstead: COHSE, 1977. Summary in Nursing Mirror, 145, 22 Sep 1977, 3.

10 Darby, C. Inquiry demand after sister is killed. (Stabbing at Tooting Bec Hospital.) Nursing Mirror, 146, 18 May 1978, 2. See also Ashton, K. The awareness factor. (Interviews with COHSE officials regarding the incident.) Nursing Times, 74, 13 Jul 1978, 1155.

11 De Felippo, A.M. Preventing assaultive behavior on a psychiatric unit. (By means of therapeutic intervention.) Supervisor Nurse, 7 (6), Jun 1976, 62-65.

12 Department of Health Guidelines. The management of violent or potentially violent patients. The Department, 1976. (HC(76) 11 and appendix.)

13 DiFabio, S. and Ackerhalt, E.J. Teaching the use of restraint through role play. (For dealing with violent patients.) Perspectives in Psychiatric Care, 16 (5/6), Sep/Dec 1978, 218-222.

14 Donnelly, G. Violence—nurse versus patient. Nursing Mirror, 145, 17 Nov 1977, 4.

15 Frazier, S.H. Harvard psychiatrist discusses treatment of violent patients. (Report of lecture.) Journal of Psychiatric Nursing and Mental Health Services, 15 (9), Sep 1977, 39-40.

16 Hodgkinson, P.E. Psychological approaches to violence. (Attitudes and behaviour of hospital staff.) Nursing Times, 76, 7 Aug 1980, 1399-1401.

17 Holbrook, B. and others Aggression—a different approach. (Methods used in the psychiatric admission ward, Whitecroft Hospital, Newport, Isle of Wight.) Nursing Mirror, 144, 21 Apr 1977, 45-48.

18 Jacobson, Z. Therapeutic management of the assaultive patient. Supervisor Nurse, 7 (10), Oct 1976, 44-46, 51.

19 Journal of Medical Ethics Five papers and summary from London Medical Group conference on violence. Journal of Medical Ethics, 5 (3), Sep 1979, 105-132.

20 Kroner, K. Dealing with the confused patient. (Excerpt from recent Nursing Skillbook, with section on coping with violent patient.) Nursing (U.S.), 9 (11), Nov 1979, 71-78.

21 Lemmer, B. A slap in the face. (Violence in psychiatric hospitals and how nursing process can help in prevention.) Nursing Mirror, 149, 30 Aug 1979, 18-19.

22 Leopoldt, H. and others Nursing staff accidents in a psychiatric hospital. (Six-month survey revealed that most accidents were caused by aggressive acts of patients.) Nursing Times, 74, 26 Oct 1978, Occ. papers, 121-123.

23 Lewis, E. Outside the safety of the hospital. (Critical comment on the DHSS circular on violent or potentially violent hospital patients, with reference to lack of advice for ancillary staff such as ambulancemen.) Health and Social Service Journal, 88, 3 Nov 1978, 1252-1253.

24 Loucas, K. The interpretation of psychopathology. (Causes of violence in patients.) Nursing Mirror, 146, 22 Jun 1978, 20-22.

25 McPhail, N.I. Behavioural disturbances in a general hospital psychiatric unit. (Research study in Glasgow.) Health Bulletin, 36 (2), Mar 1978, 79-88.

26 Martin, A. The case for self-defence. (Legal position of staff with violent patients.) Health and Social Service Journal, 88, 16 Jun 1978, 697.

27 Matheson, W. and others Coping with the aggressive patient: an alternative to punishment. Canadian Nurse, 72 (7), Jul 1976, 18-19.

28 Modly, D.M. An adaptation of ego function assessment techniques during transactions with a schizophrenic existence. (Assessment by nurse therapist using Ego Function Profile.) Journal of Psychiatric Nursing, 17 (3), Mar 1979, 16-20.

29 Mounsey, N. Psychiatric intensive care. (Unit at Old Manor Hospital in Salisbury for difficult and violent patients.) Nursing Times, 75, 18 Oct 1979, 1811-1813.

30 Nursing Mirror Nurses' attitude to violence rings keynote in DHSS guidelines. Nursing Mirror, 142, 18 Mar 1976, 34.

31 Nursing Times COHSE rejects violence guidelines: but Rcn urges immediate action after five years' delay. Nursing Times, 72, 18 Mar 1976, 394.

32 O'Gorman, G. Means of restraint. (Letter commenting on HC(76)11 and appendix.) Nursing Times, 72 (20), 20 May 1976, 785.

33 Packham, H. Managing the violent patient. Nursing Mirror, 146, 22 Jun 1978, 17-20.

34 Perspectives in Psychiatric Care Issue on the aggressive patient. (With two articles on handling the patient and methods of restraint.) Perspectives in Psychiatric Care, 16 (5/6), Sep/Dec 1978, 202-232.

35 Phillips, M. Aggression control in the psychiatric hospital. Dimensions in Health Service, 54 (3), Mar 1977, 39-41.

36 Royal College of Psychiatrists Report on management of violent patients. RCP, 1978. Report in Nursing Times, 74, 3 Aug 1978, 1264. 'Rigid attitudes threaten mental care'.

37 Sines, D. The mentally handicapped: a group at risk. (Dealing with violent behaviour and self-inflicted injury.) Nursing, 14, Jun 1980, 597-600.

38 South East Thames RHA Management of violence. (Stills from film and details of film and accompanying booklet.) Nursing Times, 73, 17 Nov 1977, 1782-1783.

39 Surrey Area Health Authority Guidelines to staff on the management of violent or potentially violent patients. Guildford: Surrey AHA, 1979.

40 Walshe-Brennan, K.S. Teenage violence in psychiatric wards. Nursing Mirror, 143, 23 Sep 1976, 63-64.

i VOLUNTEERS

1 Harris, J. Psychiatry under review. 4. The contribution of non-professionals in psychiatric care. (Volunteers.) Nursing Times, 76, 3 Apr 1980, 602-603.

2 Lewis, M. The volunteer in action. (Volunteers at Napsbury Hospital.) Nursing Mirror, 142 (8), 26 Feb 1976, 57-59.

78 COMMUNITY PSYCHIATRIC NURSING

a UNITED KINGDOM

1 Barker, C. A community psychiatric service. (Part of the Worcester Development Project.) Nursing Times, 73, 14 Jul 1977, 1075-1079.

2 Beard, P. Community psychiatric nursing —a challenging role. (Role of the CPN and various organisational models.) Nursing Focus, 1 (8), Apr 1980, 306-308.

3 Caldwell, J. A new recruit joins the team. (Community psychiatric nurse describes her role and contacts with other members of primary care team.) Nursing Mirror, 150, 31 Jan 1980, 33.

4 Caldwell, J. Working from a health centre. (Work of CPN based in health centre in Manchester.) Nursing Times, 76, 12 Jun 1980, 1066.

5 Carr, P.J. and others Community psychiatric nursing: caring for the mentally ill and handicapped in the community. Edinburgh: Churchill Livingstone, 1980.

6 Clark, C. The CPN: here to stay. (Her role, with reference to existing schemes.) Nursing Times, 75, 8 Feb 1979, 227.

7 Clarke, M.G. Psychiatric liaison with health visitors. (Description of series of seminars at which health visitors discussed principles of case assessment and management with a psychiatrist.) Health Trends, 12 (4), Nov 1980, 98-100.

8 Community Outlook Community psychiatric nursing. (Two articles, on role of nursing officer, and Rotherham's CPN service.) Nursing Times, 74, 9 Nov 1978, Community Outlook, 356, 357-358.

9 Community Psychiatric Nurses Association Community psychiatric nurses identify their own special skills. (First annual general meeting.) Nursing Times, 73, 2 Jun 1977, 804.

10 Community Psychiatric Nurses' Association Community psychiatric nursing—a bibliography. The Association, 1979.

11 Copping, A.J. Report on psychiatric community nursing in the United Kingdom. (Squibb Scholarship.) S.A. Nursing Journal, 53 (11), Nov 1976, 27-29.

12 Corrigan, J. and Soni, S.D. Community psychiatric nursing: an appraisal of its impact on community psychiatry in Manchester, England. Journal of Advanced Nursing, 2 (4), Jul 1977, 347-354.

13 Dawe, A.M. A case for community psychiatric nurses. (Review of development of community psychiatric nursing from 1960s with statistics on cost of service based on Shenley Hospital.) Journal of Advanced Nursing, 5 (5), Sep 1980, 485-490.

14 Donnelly, G. Community nursing. A day in the life of a psychiatric community nurse. Nursing Mirror, 145, 15 Sep 1977, 38.

15 Donnelly, G. CPNs at the crossroads: the role of the community psychiatric nurses. Nursing Times, 74, 13 Jul 1978, 198-199.

16 Donnelly, G. Relationships: the social worker and psychiatric community nurse. Nursing Mirror, 145, 22 Sep 1977, 39-40.

17 Donnelly, G. Observation. The need for a new set of rules when the psychiatric community nurse makes a report on his patients. Nursing Mirror, 145, 11 Aug 1977, 24.

18 Greene, J. Discharge and be damned: the nursing response. (The work of community psychiatric nurses.) Royal Society of Health Journal, 98 (3), Jun 1978, 104-107.

19 Griffith, J.H. and Mangen, S.P. Community psychiatric nursing—a literature review. (With extensive bibliography.) International Journal of Nursing Studies, 17 (3), 1980, 197-210.

20 Griffith, J.H. and Mangen, S.P. Published literature on community psychiatric nursing: indexed bibliography. St. George's Hospital Medical School, Department of Psychiatry, 1979.

21 Harker, P. and others Attaching community psychiatric nurses to general practice. (Scheme at Littlemore Hospital, Oxford.) Journal of the Royal College of General Practitioners, 26, Sep 1976, 666-671.

22 Heales, K. Community psychiatric experience in Ipswich. (Community module training for psychiatric student nurses.) Nursing Times, 73, 10 Nov 1977, Community Outlook, 102, 105-106.

23 Hudson, B. The community psychiatric nurse and the social worker. Nursing Times, 72 (21), 27 May 1976, Community Care Supplement, xviii, xx, xxii.

24 Hunter, P. Social work and community psychiatric nursing—a review. (Of research by author and others.) International Journal of Nursing Studies, 17 (2), 1980, 131-139.

25 JOINT Board of Clinical Nursing Studies. 2. Community psychiatric nursing. Nursing Mirror, 143, 5 Aug 1976, Nursing Care Supplement, 2, i-iv.

26 Knight, L. Community care isn't dead yet. (Work of community psychiatric nursing service based at Shenley Hospital.) Mind Out, 38, Jan/Feb 1980, 17-18.

27 Laird, D.A. Report on a survey to determine the need for psychiatric nursing services within primary health care teams. Nottingham: the Author, 1978.

28 Leopoldt, H. Community psychiatric nursing. (General background and development with special reference to Littlemore Hospital, Oxford.) Nursing Times, 75, 17 May 1979, Occ. papers, 53-56; 24 May 1979, Occ. papers, 57-59.

29 Lewis, D. Bridging the gap. (The work of a community psychiatric nurse illustrated by case studies.) Nursing Times, 73, 27 Jan 1977, 132-134.

30 Littlechild, J. Community nursing care study. Father and son. Nursing Times, 72, 12 Aug 1976, 1234-1235.

31 Marais, P.A. Community psychiatric nursing. An alternative to hospitalisation (in Bromley AHA). Nursing Times, 72, 4 Nov 1976, 1708-1710.

32 Marks, B.E. Patients referred to community psychiatric nurses. (Describes referrals by GPs during experimental attachment scheme in Salford. Letter.) British Medical Journal, 2, 29 Oct 1977, 1154.

33 Millar, E.C. Nurse therapy in general practice. (Symposium paper.) Nursing Mirror, 144, 12 May 1977, 47-50.

34 Mitchell, A.R.E. The role of the district nurse in mental health education. Health Education Journal, 36 (1), 1977, 11-16.

35 Nursing Times Community psychiatric nursing. (Six articles by P.R. Coverdale, P. Higgins, M. Greenfield, P. Masters, J. Caldwell and A. McDonald.) Nursing Times, 76, 12 Jun 1980, 1061-1066.

36 Parnell, J.W. Community psychiatric nurses: a descriptive study. Queens Nursing Institute, 1978. Abridged edition, 1978.

37 Petroyiannaki, M. and Raymond, M.J. How one community psychiatric nursing service works. (Based at Sutton General Hospital.) Journal of Community Nursing, 1 (8), Feb 1978, 21.

38 Roberts, L. CPNs unite. A spring meeting is planned to launch the first national association for community psychiatric nurses. Nursing Times, 73, 3 Feb 1977, 153.

39 Roberts, L.A.M. The community psychiatric nurse. (Early development and current role.) Nursing Times, 72, 23/30 Dec 1976, 2020-2021.

40 Ryce, S.W. Psychiatric nursing—from a health centre. (Author's work as community psychiatric nurse in Livingston New Town.) Nursing Mirror, 147, 17 Aug 1978, 35-36.

41 Scottish Association for Mental Health Update no 1: community psychiatric nursing services. (Reprints from nursing journals.) Edinburgh: SAMH, 1978. (9 articles.)

42 Sencicle, L. Out of the wards. (Review of research on community psychiatric nursing and possible future directions for the service.) Nursing Mirror, 151, 21 Aug 1980, 40-42.

43 Sharpe, D. Figures tell their own story. (Effects of Croydon's community psychiatric nursing service with statistics.) Nursing Mirror, 150, 10 Jan 1980, 34-36.

44 Shaw, A. CPN attachment in a group practice. (Crawley, Sussex.) Nursing Times, 73, 24 Mar 1977, Health Centre, ix-x, xiii, xiv, xvi.

45 Sladden, S. Psychiatric nursing in the community: a study of a working situation. Edinburgh: Churchill Livingstone, 1979. (Edinburgh University, Dept. of Nursing Studies; Monograph 6.)

46 Todd, J. CPN—a lifeline keeping psychiatric patients at home. (With reference to the work done at High Royds Hospital, Ilkley.) Nursing Mirror, 147, 12 Oct 1978, 46-48.

47 Ward, D.V. Where have all the patients gone? (Community psychiatric nursing service based on Warlingham Park Hospital.) Nursing Times, 76, 28 Aug 1980, 1536-1537.

b OVERSEAS COUNTRIES

1 Birnbaum, M.A. Assessment of community nurses' adherence to community mental health ideology. (Research study with community health nurses, OH nurses and school nurses.) Journal of Psychiatric Nursing and Mental Health Services, 16 (8), Aug 1978, 13-16.

2 Chisholm, M.M. and others Psychiatric community mental health nursing case studies: 51 case histories. Flushing: Medical Examination Publishing Co., 1976.

3 Clark, C.C. Mental health aspects of community health nursing. New York: McGraw-Hill, 1978.

4 Covert, A.B. Community mental health nursing: the role of the consultant in the nursing home. (Community mental health nurse consultant with the institutionalised elderly.) Journal of Psychiatric Nursing, 17 (7), Jul 1979, 15-19.

5 Davis, A.J. and Underwood, P. Educational preparation for community mental health nursing. (Survey of the educational background of 44 nurses to see how this helped them to function in their new role.) Journal of Psychiatric and Mental Health Services, 14 (3), Mar 1976, 10-15.

6 Davis, A.J. and Underwood, P. Role, function, and decision making in community mental health. (Survey of 44 nurses' perceptions of their role and function in four urban mental health centres.) Nursing Research, 25 (4), Jul/Aug 1976, 256-258.

7 Garrison, J. and others Community mental health nursing: a social network approach. Journal of Psychiatric Nursing and Mental Health Services, 15 (1), Jan 1977, 32-36.

8 Harris, M. and Solomon, K. Roles of the community mental health nurse. Journal of Psychiatric Nursing and Mental Health Services, 15 (2), Feb 1977, 35-39.

9 Hover, D. Mental health consultation with public health nurses, using transactional analysis as a tool. Journal of Psychiatric Nursing and Mental Health Services, 14 (6), Jun 1976, 15-19.

10 Lancaster, J. Community mental health nursing: an ecological perspective. St. Louis: Mosby, 1980.

11 Morrison, K.J. and others Differential attitudes of community agencies toward mental illness: a new dilemma for the psychiatric nurse. (Research study.) Journal of Psychiatric Nursing and Mental Health Services, 15 (7), Jul 1977, 25-29.

12 Santopietro, M.C. and Rozendal, N.A. Teaching primary prevention in mental health. (Outline of a course teaching intervention with high risk members of the community to prevent psychiatric illness.) Nursing Outlook, 23 (12), Dec 1975, 774-777.

13 Sloboda, S.B. What are mental health nurses doing? (Survey by questionnaire of community health nursing roles in a metropolitan area.) Journal of Psychiatric Nursing and Mental Health Services, 14 (4), Apr 1976, 24-27.

14 Strumwasser, I. and others The plight of the nurse in community mental health centers. (Need for community psychiatric nurses in the USA to have in-service training.) International Journal of Nursing Studies, 15 (2), 1978, 67-73.

15 Vincent, P. and Price, J.R. Evaluation of a VNA mental health project. (Visiting Nurse Association of Cleveland.) Nursing Research, 26 (5), Sep/Oct 1977, 361.

79 PSYCHIATRIC DISORDERS

a GENERAL AND PSYCHIATRY

1 Bailey, C.L. Mental illness—a logical misrepresentation? Nursing Times, 75, 3 May 1979, 761-762.

2 Baruch, G. and Treacher, A. Psychiatry observed. Routledge and Kegan Paul, 1978.

3 Bracegirdle, H. Psychosis, psychiatry and antipsychiatry. (Medical versus social models of madness.) Nursing Mirror, 145, 7 Jul 1977, 15-16.

4 Bruce, M.J. Refresher course. Medical and social models in psychiatry. Nursing Times, 73, 6 Jan 1977, 24-25.

5 Clare, A.W. Ethical issues in psychiatry. Practitioner, 223, Jul 1979, 89-96.

6 Clare, A.W. Psychiatry in dissent. Nursing Mirror, 143, 7 Oct 1976, 61-62.

7 Clare, A.W. Psychiatry in dissent: controversial issues in thought and practice. Tavistock, 1976.

8 Clare, A.W. The state of psychiatry. Mind Out, 34, May/Jun 1979, 16-18.

9 Craig, A.E. and Hyatt, B.A. Chronicity in mental illness: a theory on the role of change. Perspectives in Psychiatric Care, 16 (3), May/Jun 1978, 139-144, 153-154.

10 DICTIONARY of psychiatry, edited by Harold Thakurdas and Lyn Thakurdas. Lancaster: MTP, 1979.

11 Donnelly, G. The psychiatric interview. (Basis of questions asked by doctors.) Nursing Mirror, 146, 12 Jan 1978, 21.

12 Fish, F. Outline of psychiatry for students and practitioners. Edited by Max Hamilton. 3rd ed. Bristol: Wright, 1978.

13 Iveson-Iveson, J. Disease: its cause and effect. 11. Psychosomatic disease. Nursing Mirror, 149, 22 Nov 1979, 20-21.

14 Lader, M. Psychiatry on trial. Harmondsworth: Penguin, 1977.

15 Maxwell, H. Psychosomatic medicine for nurses. 2nd ed. Macmillan, 1978.

16 Mayberry, B. Sigmund Freud—his work and contribution to psychiatry. Nursing Mirror, 147, 10 Aug 1978, 20-22.

17 Merskey, H. Psychiatric illness: diagnosis, management and treatment for general practitioners and students. 3rd ed. Baillière Tindall, 1980.

18 Nursing Times Psychiatry under review. Macmillan Journals, 1980.

19 Priest, R.G. and Steinert, J. Insanity: a study of major psychiatric disorders. Macdonald and Evans, 1977.

20 Sencicle, L. Taking the labels off: the ambiguity of nomenclature in psychiatry. Nursing Times, 74, 12 Jan 1978, 52.

21 Stafford-Clark, D. and Smith, A.C. Psychiatry for students. 5th ed. Allen and Unwin, 1978.

22 Wing, J.K. Reasoning about madness. Oxford University Press, 1978.

23 World Psychiatric Association Declaration of Hawaii. (Code of ethics adopted in 1977.) Journal of Medical Ethics, 4 (2), Jun 1978, 71-73.

b SOCIAL ASPECTS

1 Ashton, J. and Edwards, G. Marching

bands and mass hysteria. A psychological look at the 'Mansfield Sunday' syndrome. (With reference to previous outbreaks including Royal Free episode.) New Society, 53, 24 Jul 1980, 166-167.

2 **Clare, A.W.** The mind of the kidnapper. Nursing Mirror, 142, 8 Apr 1976, 47-48.

3 **Elms, R.R. and others** Cross-cultural study of initial visits to psychiatric outpatient clinics. (Interviews with patients in an Irish clinic and a U.S. clinic.) Nursing Research, 28 (2), Mar/Apr 1979, 81-84.

4 **Ineichen, B.** Mental illness. Longman, 1979. (Aspects of modern sociology: the social structure of modern Britain.)

5 **Kyriacou, C.** High anxiety. (Survey of stress in teachers and methods of overcoming it.) Times Educational Supplement, 6/6/80, 12.

6 **MacAnespie, H.** Mental illness in school teachers. (Need for assessment and help as seen by a senior school medical officer.) British Medical Journal, 2, 22 Jul 1978, 257-258.

7 **McCulloch, J.W. and Prins, H.A.** Signs of stress: the social problems of psychiatric illness. Macdonald and Evans, 1977. (Psychiatric topics for community workers.)

8 **Orford, J.** The social psychology of mental disorder. Harmondsworth: Penguin, 1976.

9 **Roberts, L.** Has psychiatry come in from the cold? Public attitudes to mental illness, and the part played by community services in changing them. Nursing Times, 72, 15 Jul 1976, 1070-1071.

10 **Segal, M.** Psychiatry and the shoplifter. (Symposium paper on social offenders.) Practitioner, 218, Jun 1977, 823-827.

11 **Thorold, O.** Is shoplifting a cry for help? (Review of research with some reference to case of Lady Isobel Barnett.) Mind Out, 43, Nov 1980, 18-20.

12 **Walshe-Brennan, K.S.** The psycho-dynamics of shoplifting. Nursing Mirror, 143 (23), 2 Dec 1976, 45-47.

c TREATMENT

DRUGS

1 **Aslam, M. and Stockley, I.H.** Drugs in psychiatry. (The major divisions of mental disease and the drugs used in their treatment.) Nursing Times, 75, 6 Sep 1979, 1539-1544.

2 **Ballinger, B.R.** Less commonly prescribed psychotropic drugs in a psychiatric hospital. (Study at Royal Liff Hospital, Aberdeen.) Health Bulletin, 34 (3), May 1976, 163-166.

3 **Davis, C.** Project lithium. (Formulation of a soluble preparation by hospital team.) Nursing Times, 74, 2 Nov 1978, 1802-1804.

4 **Fottrell, E. and others** Long stay patients with long stay drugs. (Survey of psychiatric patients at Tooting Bec Hospital.) Lancet, 1, 10 Jan 1976, 81-82.

5 **Grahame-Smith, D.G.** Drugs which alter the mind. Nursing Times, 42, 2 Dec 1976, 1881-1883.

6 **Health and Social Service Journal** Drugs and their side effects. (In mental illness.) Health and Social Service Journal, 88, 7 Jul 1978, 770-771.

7 **Hitchens, E.A.** Helping psychiatric outpatients accept drug therapy. American Journal of Nursing, 77 (3), Mar 1977, 464-466.

8 **Irons, P.D.** Psychotropic drugs and nursing intervention. New York: McGraw-Hill, 1978.

9 **Lader, M.** The mind-benders. (History of mind-altering substances from alcohol to psychotropic drugs.) 2. Tranquillisers and sleeping pills. Mind Out, 40, May/Jun 1980, 12-14; 41, Jul/Aug 1980, 19-20.

10 **Lader, M.** Tranquillisers: panacea or plague? Nursing Mirror, 149, 21 Jun 1979, 16-18.

11 **Moreton, K.** Narcosis therapy. (For range of psychiatric disorders.) Nursing Times, 74, 1 Jun 1978, 923-925.

12 **O'Brien, J.** Teaching psychiatric inpatients about their medications. (With reference to encouraging patient compliance.) Journal of Psychiatric Nursing, 17 (10), Oct 1979, 30-32.

13 **Sayle, D.** Drugs used in the treatment of mental disorder. Nursing Mirror, 142, 22 Apr 1976, 61-64.

14 **Waghorn, J.M.** Influences affecting the increasing use of psychotropic drugs—especially by women. Health Education Journal, 35 (4), 1976, 231-237.

15 **WHO Chronicle** Psychotropic drugs and mental illness. WHO Chronicle, 30 (10), Oct 1976, 420-424.

16 **Williams, P.** Recent trends in the prescribing of psychotropic drugs. Health Trends, 12 (1), Feb 1980, 6-7.

ELECTROCONVULSIVE THERAPY

17 **Bird, J.M.** Effects of the media on attitudes to electric convulsion therapy. (Survey of ECT patients in Bristol.) British Medical Journal, 2, 1 Sep 1979, 526-527.

18 **British Medical Journal** Effects of electric convulsion therapy. (Review of recent studies.) British Medical Journal, 281, 13 Dec 1980, 1588.

19 **Citizens Commission on Human Rights** A suitable treatment? (Investigation of the use of ECT.) Nursing Times, 73, 3 Mar 1977, 292-293.

20 **Deakin, H.D.** ECT therapy. (Letter on this and behavioural approaches to the treatment of depression with three references.) Nursing Times, 73, 30 Jun 1977, 1001-1002.

21 **Elithorn, A.** Identifying the patient who needs ECT treatment. Journal of Community Nursing, 1 (7), Jan 1978, 4-6.

22 **Gill, D. and Lambourn, J.** Indications for electric convulsion therapy and its use by senior psychiatrists. (Questionnaire survey in the Wessex Region.) British Medical Journal, 1, 5 May 1979, 1169-1171.

23 **Illman, J.** ECT: therapy or trauma? The history of the treatment and evidence for and against its use in the light of RCP report. Nursing Times, 73, 11 Aug 1977, 1226-1227.

24 **Johnson, R.** Turn off those bad vibrations.

(Criticism of ECT by psychiatrist who is also GP.) Health and Social Service Journal, 88, 16 Jun 1978, 700-701.

25 **Johnstone, E.C. and others** The Northwick Park electroconvulsive therapy trial. (70 patients allocated course of real or simulated ECT.) Lancet, 2, 20/27 Dec 1980, 1317-1320.

26 **Lancet** Commentary from Westminster. (Proposed inquiry into electroconvulsive therapy.) Lancet, 2, 22 Jul 1978, 220-221.

27 **Lancet** Electroconvulsive therapy. (Comment in light of recent report by Royal College of Psychiatrists.) Lancet, 2, 17 Sep 1977, 593-594.

28 **Lancet** ECT at Broadmoor. (Allegations of use of unmodified ECT.) Lancet, 1, 16 Feb 1980, 348-349; See also Commentary from Westminster, 23 Feb 1980, 433; Correspondence on unmodified ECT, 1 Mar 1980, 486; 15 Mar 1980, 599.

29 **Melville, J.** Electric therapy. (Issue of electro-convulsive therapy raised by the report of inquiry on St. Augustine's Hospital, Canterbury.) New Society, 36, 8 Apr 1976, 81; See also correspondence from a nursing assistant, 22 Apr 1976, 201-202.

30 **Minshull, D.** Out-patient ECT. (At Farm House Day Hospital, Chichester.) Nursing Mirror, 148, 22 Feb 1979, 28-29.

31 **Mulaik, J.S.** Nurses' questions about electroconvulsive therapy. (Answers to questions often asked.) Journal of Psychiatric Nursing, 17 (2), Feb 1979, 15-19.

32 **Mind Out** ECT—Royal College rules. (Summary of Royal College of Psychiastrists' guidelines on usage of ECT.) Mind Out, 23 Jul/Aug 1977, 2-3.

33 **Royal College of Psychiatrists** Memorandum on the use of electroconvulsive therapy. The College, 1977. (British Journal of Psychiatry, 1, 31 Sep, 261-272.) Summary and comments in Nursing Times, 73, 11 Aug 1977, 1220.

34 **Smith, A.C.** Talking point. The benefits of ECT. Nursing Times, 73, 17 Mar 1977, 368-369.

35 **Stern, M.** Talking point. A suitable treatment? (Collection of evidence on ECT by Citizens' Commission on Human Rights.) Nursing Times, 73, 3 Mar 1977, 292-293; Readers' views, 7 Apr 1977, 478-479.

36 **Taylor, P. and Fleminger, J.J.** ECT for schizophrenia. (Evaluation in a double blind trial.) Lancet, 1, 28 Jun 1980, 1380-1382.

37 **Thomas, S.P.** Uses and abuses of electric convulsive shock therapy. (History and review of research.) Journal of Psychiatric Nursing, 16 (11), Nov 1978, 17-23.

38 **Wells, D.** Refresher course. Electroplexy. Nursing Times, 72, 3 Jun 1976, 848-849.

RELAXATION

39 **Evans, V.** Learning to take it easy. (Leicestershire health education department's classes in relaxation techniques.) Health and Social Service Journal, 90, 11 Apr 1980, 474.

40 **Fairburn, C.G. and Fairburn, S.M.** Relaxation training in psychiatric admission units.

British Journal of Occupational Therapy, 42 (11), Nov 1979, 280-282.

41 Garrison, J. and Scott, P.A. A group self-care approach to stress management. (Procedure for teaching patients the use of relaxation as a coping skill.) Journal of Psychiatric Nursing, 17 (6), Jun 1979, 9-14.

42 Kennedy, C. and Broome, A.K. Yoga and anxiety: an account of how yoga techniques helped a patient with anxiety-based problems. (At Tynemouth Day Hospital, with patient's comments on p.1837.) Nursing Times, 75, 25 Oct 1979, 1836-1837.

43 Martin, I.C.A. Twitch and between. 1. Aspects of the relaxation technique. (Including insomnia.) 2. Further applications of the relaxation technique. (Social gatherings and examinations.) 3. The relaxation technique in the treatment of illness. (Physical and psychiatric.) Nursing Times, 74, 8 Jun 1978, 953-955; 15 Jun 1978, 1017-1018; 22 Jun 1978, 1056-1059.

44 Mellor, B. Relaxation therapy. (West Bank psychiatric unit, Wellington, Shropshire.) Nursing Times, 72, 11 Nov 1976, 1776-1777.

PSYCHOSURGERY

45 Bridges, P. and Williamson, C. Psychosurgery today. (Review of developments over last forty years.) Nursing Times, 73, 1 Sep 1977, 1363-1367.

46 Caulfield, C. The unkindest cut of all? The use of psychosurgery in the treatment of mental patients is questioned. Nursing Mirror, 147, 28 Sep 1978, 21-22.

47 Goston, L.O. Ethical considerations of psychosurgery: the unhappy legacy of the pre-frontal lobotomy. (With commentary by a surgeon on p.154-156. See also editorial on p.115-116.) Journal of Medical Ethics, 6 (3), Sep 1980, 149-154.

48 Gostin, L. and Knight, L. Psychosurgery: do the doctors know what they're doing? (With statement of MIND policy.) Mind Out, 41, Jul/Aug 1980, 12-15.

49 Patterson, D. The violence of psychosurgery. (With reference to legal case in USA over case of surgery to control violent behaviour.) New Scientist, 81, 8 Feb 1979, 374-376.

d ANOREXIA NERVOSA

1 Armstrong-Esther, C.A. Anorexia nervosa: aspects of care and treatment. (A literature review.) Journal of Advanced Nursing, 2 (2), Mar 1977, 127-135.

2 Bhanji, S. Anorexia nervosa: two schools of thought. (Medical and psychiatric.) Nursing Times, 76, 21 Feb 1980, 323-324.

3 Bhoyrub, P. The girl who would not eat: a study of anorexia nervosa. Nursing, 11, Mar 1980, 498-500.

4 Blatch, P. Nursing care study. Anorexia nervosa: an obsession with starving. (By first-year student nurse.) Nursing Mirror, 150, 24 Jan 1980, 32-35.

5 British Medical Journal Anorexia nervosa: fear of fatness or femininity? British Medical Journal, 1, 7 Jan 1978, 5.

6 Bruch, H. The golden cage: the enigma of anorexia nervosa. Open Books, 1978.

7 Butler, B. and others Anorexia nervosa: a nursing approach. (Includes case study and nursing care plan.) Canadian Nurse, 73 (6), Jun 1977, 22-24.

8 Dally, P. and others Anorexia nervosa. Heinemann, 1979.

9 Dexter, J.M. Nursing care study. Anorexia nervosa. (Treatment in a medical ward without psychotherapy.) Nursing Times, 76, 21 Feb 1980, 325-327.

10 Dunseith, B.L. Personal view. (Author's account of anorexia nervosa.) British Medical Journal, 1, 24 Jun 1978, 1694.

11 Grossniklaus, D.McC. Nursing interventions in anorexia nervosa. Perspectives in Psychiatric Care, 18 (1), Jan/Feb 1980, 11-16.

12 Hawkins, C. Diseases of the alimentary system. Anorexia and loss of weight. British Medical Journal, 2, 4 Dec 1976, 1373-1375.

13 Kauffer, R. Anorexia nervosa—the patient's view. Nursing Mirror, 146, 6 Apr 1978, 26-27.

14 Lacey, J.H. Anorexia nervosa. Nursing Times, 72, 18 Mar 1976, 407-408.

15 McNelly, P. and Hickey, P. Anorexia nervosa: a challenge to the nurse. (Nursing care including regime of management.) Nursing Mirror, 147, 7 Sep 1978, 32-34.

16 Marshall, M.H. Anorexia nervosa: dietary treatment and re-establishment of body weight in 20 cases studied on a metabolic unit. Journal of Human Nutrition, 32 (5), Oct 1978, 349-357.

17 Martin, J.E. Anorexia nervosa: a disorder of weight. (Includes occupational therapy.) British Journal of Occupational Therapy, 41 (9), Sep 1978, 304-309.

18 Melville, J. Anorexia—fear eats the soul. New Society, 53, 25 Sep 1980, 612-613.

19 Orr, R. Anorexia nervosa. A self-imposed starvation. Nursing Care, 9 (10), Oct 1976, 28-31.

20 Schlemmer, J.K. and Barnett, P.A. Management of manipulative behavior of anorexia nervosa patients. Journal of Psychiatric Nursing and Mental Health Services, 15 (11), Nov 1977, 35-37, 40-41.

e DEPRESSION

1 American Journal of Nursing Helping depressed patients in general nursing practice. Programmed instruction. American Journal of Nursing, 77 (6), Jun 1977, P.I, 1-32.

2 Authier, J. and others Clinical management of the tearfully depressed patient: communication skills for the nurse practitioner. Journal of Psychiatric Nursing, 17 (2), Feb 1979, 34-41.

3 Bastable, E. and others Standards of care for psychiatric nursing. The behavioral concepts of depression and anxiety: a working document. Vancouver: Registered Nurses' Association of British Columbia, 1977.

4 Bhanji, S. Treatment of depression by sleep deprivation. Nursing Times, 73, 14 Apr 1977, 540-541.

5 Brown, G.W. and Harris, T. Social origins of depression: a study of psychiatric disorder in women. Tavistock, 1978.

6 Brown, G.W. and others Women psychiatric disorder and social class. Working class rather than middle class women are more at risk of depressive illness. Midwife, Health Visitor and Community Nurse, 13 (2), Feb 1977, 37-45.

7 Dentith, S. Depressive illnesses: early recognition and treatment. Queen's Nursing Journal, 19 (4), Jul 1976, 103-104.

8 Frost, M. Endogenous depression complicated by carcinoma. (A case study.) Nursing Mirror, 143, 8 Jul 1976, 73-74.

9 Goble, I.W.J. Nursing care study. Endogenous depression: an illness that keeps on recurring. Nursing Mirror, 148, 15 Feb 1979, 41-43.

10 Hamadah, K. Depression. Nursing Mirror, 145, 10 Nov 1977, 13-15.

11 Hutchings, J. and Gathercole, C. Community nursing and psychology. 5. Depressed behaviour. (In a separated mother of small child.) Journal of Community Nursing, 2 (5), Nov 1978, 32-33.

12 Jacobson, A. Melancholy in the 20th Century: causes and prevention. (With models of causes and prevention and section on depression in women.) Journal of Psychiatric Nursing, 18 (7), Jul 1980, 11-21.

13 Johnson, D.A.W. and Mellor, V. The severity of depression in patients treated in general practice. Journal of the Royal College of General Practitioners, 27, Jul 1977, 419-422.

14 McMullen, D.K. Study of depressive illness among patients in a group practice (with a health visitor attached). Nursing Times, 72, 1 Apr 1976, 504-508.

15 Moreton, K. Nursing care study. Wayne—a patient with recurrent reactive depression. Nursing Times, 72, 17 Jun 1976, 945-947.

16 Mottram, E.M. The sister's role in group therapy in a general practice. (Nurse as co-leader of group for depressed patients.) Nursing Times, 76, 7 Feb 1980, 253-254.

17 Murphy, B.C. Nursing care study. Depression. Nursing Times, 72, 29 Apr 1976, 659-661.

18 Roberts, L. Community nursing care study. Marianne is not sick—yet. (Community psychiatric care of depressed 30-year-old divorcée.) Nursing Times, 74, 26 Jan 1978, 142-146.

19 Rodman, M.J. Pathways to the cure of mental depression. (Drug treatment.) RN Magazine, 40 (11), Nov 1977, 73-74, 77, 79.

20 Rowe, D. The experience of depression. Chichester: Wiley, 1978.

21 Shmagin, B.G. and Pearlmutter, D.R. The pursuit of unhappiness: the secondary gains of depression. Perspectives in Psychiatric Care, 15 (2), Apr/Jun 1977, 63-65.

22 Watts, A. Why do people get the 'blues'? 1. Assembling the jigsaw. (Discussion of causes.) 2. A biochemical explanation. 3. What the nurse can to help. Nursing Mirror, 147, 23 Nov 1978, 32-33; 30 Nov 1978, 40-41; 7 Dec 1978, 41-42.

23 White, C.L. Nurse counselling with depressed patient. (Case study by nurse psychotherapist.) American Journal of Nursing, 78 (3), Mar 1978, 436-439.

f FEAR, PHOBIAS, NEUROSIS, STRESS

1 American Journal of Nursing Stress. (Four articles, with one by Hans Selye, one on the Type A individual and two on relaxation.) American Journal of Nursing, 79 (10), Nov 1979, 1953-1964.

2 Bell, J.M. Stressful life events and coping methods in mental-illness and -wellness behaviors. Nursing Research, 26 (2), Mar-Apr 1977, 136-141.

3 Blakey, R. and Greig, K. Severe cat phobia. (Behavioural therapy and one patient's case history with patient's own account.) Nursing Times, 73, 21 Jul 1977, 1106-1116.

4 Brooker, C. Nursing care study. The behavioural management of a complex case. (Middle-aged lady with agoraphobia.) Nursing Times, 76, 28 Feb 1980, 367-369.

5 Carruthers, M. Passions that poison and deadlines that kill. (Effects of stress upon disease.) New Society, 38, 11 Nov 1976, 303-304.

6 Crichton, S. We are seeking progress. (WASP self-help group for phobias by a sufferer.) Nursing Mirror, 151, 24 Jul 1980, 40-41.

7 De Silva, D. Behaviour therapy for obsessional neurosis. (With case history.) Nursing Mirror, 146, 2 Feb 1978, 15-17.

8 Eveleigh, C. Behavioural psychotherapy to encourage self-treatment of a patient with an obsessive-compulsive neurosis. (Case study.) Nursing Times, 73, 7 Jul 1977, 1036-1038.

9 Goodwin, S. Curbing the caveman in us. (Body's response to stress and value of relaxation.) Nursing Mirror, 150, 26 Jun 1980, 22-24.

10 Hutchings, J. Community nursing and psychology. 7. . . . and frightened Miss Muffet away. (Part 1. Fear and avoidance behaviour.) Journal of Community Nursing, 2 (8), Feb 1979, 22-23.

11 Hutchings, J. Community nursing and psychology. 9. You can if you try. (Management of fears and avoidance behaviours.) Journal of Community Nursing, 2 (10), Apr 1979, 22-23.

12 Hutchings, J. It's nothing to be frightened of. (Psychological approaches to dealing with fear and avoidance behaviours.) Journal of Community Nursing, 2 (9), Mar 1979, 16-17.

13 Langendoen, S. Panic. (With details of panic routine to help patients regain control.) RN Magazine, 41 (12), Dec 1978, 45-47.

14 Little, J. Stress during the human lifecycle. (With Rahe's stress scale listing stress scores for various life events.) Health Visitor, 53 (9), Sep 1980, 373-376.

15 Macdonald Wallace, J. Stress and tension control. (Advice on relaxation.) Nursing, 10, Feb 1980, 451-454.

16 Macilwaine, H. Mobility and mental stress. (Mobility as indication of mental stress and tool to relieve it.) Nursing, 4, Jul 1979, 190, 193-194.

17 Martin, I.C.A. Clinical parable. The English malady. (Hypochondriasis.) Nursing Times, 74, 4 May 1978, 768-769; 18 May 1978, 843-844.

18 Nursing Issue on stress. Nursing, 10, Feb 1980, 418-459.

19 Parry, R. Emotions and illness. (Fear, anxiety and depression.) Nursing Mirror, 146, 20 Apr 1978, 27-30.

20 Pollitt, J. Symptoms of stress. 1. Types of stress and types of people. 2. The effects of stress. Nursing Mirror, 144, 16 Jun 1977, 13-14; 23 Jun 1977, 24-26.

21 Roberts, L.A.M. Community nursing care study. Obsessional compulsive (psycho) neurosis. Nursing Times, 73, 17 Nov 1977, 1789-1793.

22 Rouhani, G.C. Understanding anxiety. Nursing Mirror, 146, 9 Mar 1978, 25-27.

23 Rowe, J. Controlling a tense moment. (Review of research on the aetiology of stress and value of relaxation.) Nursing Mirror, 151, 10 Jul 1980, 28-29.

24 Ryland, R.K. and King, M.J. Queer turns. (Hysterical fits illustrated by three case studies.) Nursing Mirror, 143, 2 Sep 1976, 63-65.

25 Sell, K. Don't worry—there's help on the way. (Work of Phobic Trust.) Journal of Community Nursing, 3 (9), Mar 1980, 34-35.

26 Sims, A. Long-term consequences of neurosis. Nursing Mirror, 143, 23 Sep 1976, 68, 67.

27 Skidmore, D. Measuring fear. (Study of responses to 74 specific fears.) Nursing Mirror, 143, 16 Sep 1976, 68-69.

28 Stern, R.S. Nursing care supplement. Series 3. 2. Neurosis and psychosis. Nursing Mirror, 143, 14 Oct 1976, Nursing care supplement series 3, i-iv.

29 Sutherland, S. Breakdown: a personal crisis and a medical dilemma. Weidenfeld and Nicolson, 1976.

30 Tyrer, P.J. and Remington, M. Controlled comparison of day-hospital and outpatient treatment for neurotic disorders. Lancet, 1, 12 May 1979, 1014-1016.

31 Wallace, J.M. Living with stress. (Causes and treatment.) Nursing Times, 74, 16 Mar 1978, 457-458.

32 Wondrak, R. Nursing care study. Agoraphobia: another brick in the wall. (Care involving behaviour therapy and psychiatric social worker.) Nursing Mirror, 150, 17 Apr 1980, 42-44.

33 Woolstone, A.S. Stress—a call for a humane approach. Nursing Times, 74, 6 Apr 1978, 599-600.

34 Yoder, S.A. Alienation as a way of life. (Self-rejection and anxiety.) Perspectives in Psychiatric Care, 15 (2), Apr/Jun 1977, 66-71.

g PERSONALITY DISORDERS

1 Barber, R. Nursing care study. Psychopathic personality with paranoid traits. Nursing Mirror, 146, 11 May 1978, 26-27.

2 Berlyne, N. Delusions. (Symptoms of psychotic disorder.) Nursing Mirror, 144, 9 Jun 1977, 29-30.

3 Cambridge, M. Nursing care study. Psychotic depression. Nursing Times, 74, 27 Apr 1978, 711-712.

4 Carser, D. The defense mechanism of splitting: developmental origins, effects on staff, recommendations for nursing care. (Used by individuals with borderline personality.) Journal of Psychiatric Nursing, 17 (3), Mar 1979, 21-28.

5 Davis, C. Nursing care study. Personality disorder. Nursing Times, 72, 6 May 1976, 695-697.

6 Devlin, D. Nursing care study. Acute psychotic episode in a chronic paranoid personality. Nursing Times, 72, 13 May 1976, 750-751.

7 Frost, M. Nursing care study. Manic depressive psychosis. Nursing Times, 72, 15 Jan 1976, 60-61.

8 Gartside, G. Nursing care study. Manic depressive psychosis. Balancing body and mind. (By ward sister.) Nursing Mirror, 150, 27 Mar 1980, 31-32.

9 Gover, S.M. Nursing care study. A personality disorder in an adolescent with cerebral palsy. (By student psychiatric nurse.) Nursing Times, 75, 6 Dec 1979, 2111-2114.

10 Herron, W.G. The borderline problem. (Syndrome in which individuals display anger, defect in affectionate relationships, limited self-identity and depressive loneliness.) Perspectives in Psychiatric Care, 16 (4), Jul/Aug 1978, 188-190.

11 Hussey, T. Nursing care study. Manic-depressive psychosis with rapid and profound changes of mood. Nursing Times, 75, 1 Feb 1979, 193-195.

12 Hussey, T. Nursing care study. Personality disorder. Nursing Times, 74, 5 Oct 1978, 1641-1642.

13 Lynch, V.J. and Lynch, M.T. Borderline personality. Perspectives in Psychiatric Care, 15 (2), Apr/Jun 1977, 72-75, 87.

14 Neadley, A.W. Nursing care study. Paranoid depression. Nursing Times, 73, 13 Oct 1977, 1590-1592.

15 Schwartzman, S.T. The hallucinating patient and nursing intervention. Journal of Psychiatric Nursing and Mental Health Services, 13 (6), Nov/Dec 1975, 23-36.

16 Simmons, S. Nursing care study. Care for a stranger. (Psychogenic psychosis in Nigerian male patient in psychiatric hospital.) Nursing Times, 74, 16 Feb 1978, 269-272.

17 Stevens, P.F. Nursing care study. A professional patient. (A hypomaniac.) Nursing Times, 72, 4 Mar 1976, 334-335.

18 Stevenson, C. A patient with manic depressive psychosis. (Care study.) Nursing Times, 76, 3 Jul 1980, 1184-1186.

19 Storey, P. Organic psychoses. Nursing Mirror, 142, 6 May 1976, 66-68.

20 Walshe-Brennan, K.S. The psychopathic personality. Nursing Mirror, 145, 15 Dec 1977, 29-31.

21 Walshe-Brennan, K.S. Psychopathological factors in arson. Nursing Mirror, 145, 4 Aug 1977, 13-15.

h SCHIZOPHRENIA

1 American Journal of Nursing Working with schizophrenic patients. (Three articles.) American Journal of Nursing, 76 (6), Jun 1976, 941-949.

2 'Anne', pseud Self-help psychiatry. Coping with schizophrenia. Mind Out, 33, Mar/Apr 1979, 14-15.

3 Beaumont, S. Nursing care study. A new life at 61. (A chronic schizophrenic.) Nursing Times, 76, 15 May 1980, 863-865.

4 Billett, G. Nursing care study. Sam—a long-term psychiatric patient. (A schizophrenic.) Nursing Times, 75, 15 Feb 1979, 277-279.

5 Bull, A. Nursing care study. Schizophrenia. Nursing Times, 74, 16 Mar 1978, 442-444.

6 Burnside, B. and Allinson, M. Nursing care study. Rolling the dice towards success. (Behaviour therapy with a paranoid schizophrenic leading to discharge.) Nursing Mirror, 151, 10 Jul 1980, 40-41.

7 Butler, R.J. The evolution of a token economy programme for female chronic schizophrenic patients. (At High Royd Hospital in Yorkshire.) Journal of Advanced Nursing, 4 (3), May 1979, 307-318.

8 Childs-Gowell, E. A study of schizophrenics in transactional analysis treatment report of ethnographic research. (At the Cathexis Institute and community in Oakland, California.) International Journal of Nursing Studies, 14 (4), 1977, 215-221.

9 Community Outlook Care study—Margaret. Institutionalised at home. (Patient with paranoid schizophrenia treated in the token economy ward.) Nursing Times, 73, 11 Aug 1977, Community Outlook, 27-30.

10 Craig, Y. Counselling and the schizophrenias. British Journal of Guidance and Counselling, 6 (1), Jan 1978, 35-53.

11 Davis, C. Dietary pathogenesis of schizophrenia: an investigation into the effects of gluten. (Clinical trials.) Nursing Times, 74, 7 Dec 1978, 2020-2021.

12 Delamothe, K.J. Nursing care study. Schizophrenia—or not? (By third-year student on psychiatric secondment.) Nursing Times, 75, 27 Sep 1979, 1662-1665.

13 Donoghue, M. Nursing care study. Token economy treatment. (Of schizophrenic man at Shenley Hospital.) Nursing Mirror, 145, 15 Dec 1977, 34-35.

14 Fish, F.J. Schizophrenia; edited by Max Hamilton. 2nd ed. Bristol: Wright, 1976.

15 Gough, H. Nursing care study. Schizophrenia: silence filled with sound. Nursing Mirror, 151, 7 Aug 1980, 42-46.

16 Grainger, L. Nursing care study. Paranoid schizophrenia. (Care prior to discharge of middle-aged woman suffering from delusions.) Nursing Mirror, 147, 30 Nov 1978, 47-50.

17 Green, D.E. Schizophrenia: some problems for the nurse. New Zealand Nursing Journal, 73 (1), Jan 1980, 11-13, 34.

18 Grigg, W. Nursing care study. Chronic schizophrenia. Nursing Times, 75, 9 Aug 1979, 1350-1352.

19 Hardin, S.B. Comparative analysis of nonverbal interpersonal communication of schizophrenics and normals. Research in Nursing Health, 3 (2), Jun 1980, 57-68.

20 Heywood-Jones, I. The National Schizophrenia Fellowship. (Pressure and self-help group.) Nursing Times, 75, 1 Nov 1979, 1906.

21 Hopkins, S. The slow march of knowledge. (Evidence linking schizophrenia with a lack of the physiologically active substance prostaglandin PGE.) Nursing Mirror, 151, 31 Jul 1980, 37.

22 Klein, H.E. and others Transcultural nursing research with schizophrenics. (Research study of professional care of the patient in hospital; physical environment of home and hospital; and social, religious and recreational activities at home and in hospital.) International Journal of Nursing Studies, 15 (3), 1978, 135-142.

23 Lawton, K. Schizophrenia: Laura learns to make friends. Nursing Mirror, 148, 14 Jun 1979, 32-33.

24 Lemmer, B. Nursing care study. Curing a nine-year fixation: a successful self-improvement programme on a paranoid schizophrenic patient. Nursing Mirror, 147, 3 Aug 1978, 24-25.

25 McPherson, F.M. and others The restoration of one aspect of communication in chronic schizophrenic patients. (Improving use of speech by behaviour modification programme.) Health Bulletin, 37 (5), Sep 1979, 227-231.

26 Mate-Kole, C. and Wilkie, D. Scientific weaknesses among the jungle of theories. (The double bind and biological theories in the aetiology of schizophrenia.) Nursing Mirror, 147, 19 Oct 1978, 44-46.

27 Murray, E.W. Nursing care study. A kind of success. (Case study of a schizophrenic.) Nursing Mirror, 142, 29 Apr 1976, 58-59; 6 May 1976, 54-55.

28 National Schizophrenia Fellowship Coping with schizophrenia, edited by Henry R. Rollin. Burnett Books, 1980.

29 Office of Health Economics Schizophrenia: biochemical impairments, social handicaps? OHE, 1979. (Studies of current health problems, no.65.)

30 Owens, D.G.C. Dopamine and schizophrenia. (Its suggested role in causing the disorder.) Nursing Mirror, 146, 2 Feb 1978, 23-26.

31 Putnam, M. Nurse could you care more? (Current attitudes to causes and treatment of schizophrenia with recommendations for nursing care.) Nursing Times, 76, 10 Jan 1980, 56.

32 Reveley, A. The risks of inheriting schizophrenia. Mind Out, 39, Mar/Apr 1980, 16.

33 Roberts, L. and Clare, A. What is schizophrenia? New Society, 36, 20 May 1976, 410-412.

34 Roseman, T.B. Schizophrenics get sick too. (Their care during physical illness.) RN Magazine, 40 (12), Dec 1977, 39-41.

35 Sargant, W. Giving schizophrenics a better chance. (Use of ECT, drugs, modified sleep and lithium.) Nursing Mirror, 147, 24 Aug 1978, 26.

36 Sartorius, N. and Jablensky, A. Transcultural studies of schizophrenia. WHO Chronicle, 30 (12), Dec 1976, 481-485.

37 Sattin, S.M. The psychodynamics of the 'Holiday Syndrome'. The meaning and therapeutic use of holidays in group therapy with schizophrenic patients. Perspectives in Psychiatric Care, 8 (4), Oct/Dec 1975, 156-162.

38 Sawford, R. and Lee, S. Nursing care study. Restoring speech: the end of a long silence. (Operant conditioning with a mute schizophrenic.) Nursing Mirror, 148, 1 Mar 1979, 34-35.

39 Stevens, P. Nursing care study. Paranoid schizophrenia. Nursing Mirror, 142, 15 Apr 1976, 49-51.

40 Szasz, T. Schizophrenia: the sacred symbol of psychiatry. Oxford: OUP, 1979.

41 Toner, E. and Cabanban, P.A. Schizophrenia: a sense of identity. The nursing problems of caring for the chronic schizophrenic patient. Nursing Mirror, 147, 5 Oct 1978, 35-37.

42 Vaughan, C. Nursing care study. Schizophrenia. Nursing Times, 72, 11 Mar 1976, 373-375.

43 Wescott, P. One man's schizophrenic illness. (Personal experience.) British Medical Journal, 1, 14 Apr 1979, 989-990.

44 Wing, J.K. Diagnosing schizophrenia. (Medical, social and psychological models.) New Society, 44, 8 Jun 1978, 535-536.

45 Wright, I. and others The schizophrenic in the 19th, 20th and 21st centuries. (Essay entered in N.W. Thames regional nursing competition.) Nursing Times, 74, 5 Jan 1978, 36.

i SCHIZOPHRENIA: COMMUNITY AND FAMILY

1 Psychiatric Rehabilitation Association Not the same as you? The social situation of 190 schizophrenics living in the community. The Association, 1977.

2 Pyke, J. Nutrition and the chronic schizophrenic. (Research study of food intake and eating patterns of socially isolated chronic schizophrenics living in the community.) Canadian Nurse, 75 (10), Nov 1979, 40-43.

3 Pyke-Lees, P. Care of the schizophrenic at home. Midwife, Health Visitor and Community Nurse, 14 (9), Sep 1978, 300-302.

4 Scott, T. and others Beginning research. Care of the schizophrenia patient. (Survey of two groups of schizophrenia patients at Cherry Knowle Hospital, showing importance of domiciliary nursing service.) Nursing Times, 73, 19 May 1977, 740-741.

5 Stanford, J. Schizophrenia. An end to relapses. (Introduction of a community psychiatric nursing service and prescription of phenotiazone injections at Powick Hospital.) Nursing Times, 72, 18 Mar 1976, 418-420.

6 Wilson, H.S. Fairing: control of staff work in a healing community for schizophrenics. (Sociological analysis of ways nurses' work is organised.) Journal of Psychiatric Nursing and Mental Health Services, 16 (3), Mar 1978, 24-32, 37-38.

7 Wilson, H.S. Limiting intrusion—social control of outsiders in a healing community. (Study at an experimental treatment community for schizophrenics.) Nursing Research, 26 (2), Mar/Apr 1977, 103-111.

8 Wood, C. What kind of maintenance therapy for schizophrenic patients in the community? (Report of five-year trial of oral administration of drugs.) Journal of Community Nursing, 2 (4), Oct 1978, 11, 13.

j SLEEP DISORDERS

1 British Medical Journal Unquiet sleep. (Sleepwalking and night terrors in adults and children.) British Medical Journal, 2, 20/27 Dec 1980, 1660-1661.

2 Felstein, I. The sufferer who doesn't suffer. (Causes and treatment of snoring.) Nursing Mirror, 148, 12 Apr 1979, 42-43.

3 Hearne, K. Insight into 'lucid' dreams. Nursing Mirror, 150, 6 Mar 1980, 20-22.

4 Hearne, K. Terror lurking in the dark. (Research on nightmares.) Nursing Mirror, 151, 14 Aug 1980, 18-20.

5 Hediger, K.H. The place of the dream in therapy. Perspectives in Psychiatric Care, 17 (5), Sep/Oct 1979, 223-227.

6 Kogeorgos, J. and Scott, D.F. Sleep and sleep disorders. Practitioner, 224, Jul 1980, 717-721.

7 Navin, H.L. and Wilson, J.A. Caffeine consumption and sleep disturbances in acutely ill psychiatric inpatients. (Research study.) Journal of Psychiatric Nursing, 18 (3), Mar 1980, 37-42.

8 Oswald, I. No peace for the worried. (Sleep disorders and their management.) Nursing Mirror, 150, 13 Mar 1980, 34-35.

9 Parkes, J.D. The sleep patient. (Sleep disorders including narcolepsy and Kleine-Levin syndrome.) Lancet, 1, 7 May 1977, 980-993.

10 Regestein, Q.R. and Barbiasz, J.E. Sleep disorders: recognizing them in patients. Journal

of Practical Nursing, 30 (11), Nov/Dec 1980, 21-22, 62.

11 Tait, T. and others Sleep problems in mental subnormality. (Nursing care study.) Nursing Mirror, 143, 15 Jul 1976, 69-70.

12 Watts, C.A.H. The threshold to sleep. (Pre-sleep sensations and phenomena.) Nursing Mirror, 145, 29 Sep 1977, 18-19.

k SUICIDE

1 Ashton, J.R. and Donnan, S.P.B. Suicide by burning—a current epidemic. British Medical Journal, 2, 29 Sep 1979, 769-770.

2 Barraclough, B.M. and others Suicide prevention by the Samaritans. A controlled study of effectiveness. (In county boroughs with and without Samaritans.) Lancet, 2, 30 Jul 1977, 237-239.

3 Burke, A.W. Attempted suicide among Commonwealth immigrants in Birmingham. (Survey.) International Journal of Social Psychiatry, 24 (1), Spring 1978, 7-11.

4 Farmer, R.D.T. Suicide mortality in Greater London: changes during the past 25 years. British Journal of Preventive and Social Medicine, 31 (3), Sep 1977, 171-177.

5 Farmer, R.D.T. and Hirsch, S. editors The suicide syndrome. Croom Helm, 1980.

6 Fox, R. The suicide drop—why? (Statistical changes since the Second World War and preventive measures such as the formation of the Samaritans.) Royal Society of Health Journal, 95 (1), Feb 1975, 9-13, 20.

7 Hart, N.A. and Keidel, G.C. The suicidal adolescent. American Journal of Nursing, 79 (1), Jan 1979, 80, 82-84.

8 Hatton, C.L. and others Suicide: assessment and intervention. New York: Appleton-Century-Crofts, 1977.

9 Knight, L. Suicide. (Research into reasons for increase.) Mind Out, 44, Dec 1980, 14-16.

10 Kreitman, N. The coal gas story: United Kingdom suicide rates 1960-1971. British Journal of Preventive and Social Medicine, 30 (2), Jun 1976, 86-93.

11 Lancet Suicide and the Samaritans. Lancet, 2, 7 Oct 1978, 772-773.

12 Lodge, P. Look to the living—easing the pain of aftermath to suicide. (Review of insensitive procedures that follow a suicide.) Social Work Today, 11, 25 Mar 1980, 10-12.

13 Morgan, H.G. Death wishes?: the understanding and management of deliberate self-harm. Chichester: Wiley, 1979.

14 Reed, D. Anna. (The story of a woman's mental breakdown and suicide told by her husband.) Secker and Warburg, 1976.

15 Reynolds, D. Youngsters who go off the rails. (Treatment of suicide attempts by teenagers.) Nursing Mirror, 148, 8 Mar 1979, 16-18.

16 Reynolds, D.K. and Farberow, N.L. Suicide inside and out. Berkeley: University of California Press, 1977.

17 Roberts, L. Attempted suicide. Nursing Mirror, 144, 20 Jan 1977, 65-66.

18 Roberts, L. Suicide. Nursing Mirror, 144, 13 Jan 1977, 68-69.

19 Samaritans Answers to suicide: presented ...to Chad Varah on the occasion of their 25th anniversary of founding. Constable, 1978.

20 Temple, S. and Catalan, J. Group work with patients following deliberate self-poisoning or self-injury. Description of some therapeutic strategies. British Journal of Occupational Therapy, 40 (12), Dec 1977, 306-308.

21 Varah, C. editor The Samaritans in the '70s: to befriend the suicidal and despairing. 3rd ed. Constable, 1977.

l SUICIDE: NURSING CARE AND ATTITUDES

1 Bhagat, M. Attempted suicide. (Attitudes of hospital staff to these patients.) Nursing Mirror, 146, 9 Feb 1978, 26-27.

2 Bourne, G. and Lindley, P. Suicide. Nursing Mirror, 143 (3), 15 Jul 1976, Nursing care supplement, 9, i-iv.

3 Bray, D.E. Suicide. 1. Good night nurse... and good-bye... (Nursing intervention.) 2. When prevention fails. Journal of Practical Nursing, 25 (12), Dec 1975, 16-17, 32; 26 (1), Jan 1976, 19-20.

4 Cowley, S.A. We may need the bed. (Attitudes of hospital staff to self poisoned patients.) Nursing Times, 74, 9 Feb 1978, 248.

5 Cowper-Smith, F. Caring about the suicidal patient. (Report of Rcn study day on suicide.) Nursing Times, 74, 16 Nov 1978, 1880-1881.

6 DiVasto, P.V. and others A framework for the emergency evaluation of the suicidal patient. Journal of Psychiatric Nursing, 17 (6), Jun 1979, 15-20.

7 Hart, N.A.C. and Prophit, P. Adolescent suicide. (With role of nurse discussed.) Pediatric Nursing, 5 (6), Nov/Dec 1979, 12-17.

8 Hawton, K. and others Management of attempted suicide in Oxford. (With assessment by psychiatric team including nurses.) British Medical Journal, 2, 27 Oct 1979, 1040-1042.

9 Horoshak, I. How to spot and handle high-risk patients. (Suicidal patients.) RN Magazine, 40 (9), Sep 1977, 58-63.

10 Keane, B. Parasuicide is a health hazard. (With nursing assessment of potentially suicidal patients.) Australian Nurses Journal, 8 (8), Mar 1979, 41-42.

11 Large, S. Nursing care study. Reactive depression: a problem of personality. (Care of 17-year old girl who attempted suicide.) Nursing Mirror, 149, 5 Jul 1979, 44-46.

12 Martin, A. The nurse and the law. Whose life is it anyway? (Nurses' responsibility in relation to suicidal patients.) Journal of Community Nursing, 3 (6), Dec 1979, 9.

13 Miskiman, D.E. Cry wolf? A look at teenage suicide. (Including the nurse's role.)

Canadian Journal of Psychiatric Nursing, 19 (5), Sep/Oct 1978, 8-9.

14 Pyle, P.L. An attempted suicide. (Care study of psychiatric patient who attempted suicide while in hospital.) Nursing Times, 76, 10 Jul 1980, 1233-1234.

15 Schuyler, D. Counselling suicide survivors. Nursing Digest, 2 (8), Oct 1974, 66-67.

16 Spry, W.B. Prevention of suicide. (The role of the occupational health nurse in recognising and acting on symptoms.) Occupational Health, 28 (7), Jul 1976, 354-358.

17 Sumner, F.C. and Gwozoz, T.A. A nurse for suicidal patients. (Use of a clinical nurse specialist.) American Journal of Nursing, 76 (11), Nov 1976, 1792-1793.

80 PSYCHIATRIC REHABILITATION

a REHABILITATION

1 Ashton, J.R. Rehabilitation in psychiatry. Community Health, 9 (4), May 1978, 216-220.

2 Barrington, P. The self-care unit: a bridge to the community. (Experimental unit at Lakeshore Psychiatric Hospital to ease transition from hospital to community.) Canadian Nurse, 73 (2), Feb 1977, 39-41.

3 Barton, G.M. and Krone, C.H. Creation of an aftercare program. (In Michigan.) American Journal of Nursing, 78 (5), May 1978, 864-867.

4 Bayer, M. Easing mental patients' return to their communities. American Journal of Nursing, 76 (3), Mar 1976, 406-408.

5 Bell, V. Occupational therapy with young disturbed adolescents. British Journal of Occupational Therapy, 40 (5), May 1977, 116-117.

6 Bennie, E.H. and others A rehabilitation programme for long term psychiatric patients. (Levendale Hospital, South Glasgow.) Nursing Times, 72, 26 Aug 1976, 1325-1327.

7 Brennan, J.O. The Welcome Club. (To help psychiatric patients' transition from hospital to community at Walsgrave Hospital.) Nursing Times, 73, 17 Mar 1977, 393.

8 Calvert, J.M. and Long, V. Long term patients—2. What is a holiday? (Holiday for patients at Naburn Hospital, Fulford, Yorkshire.) British Journal of Occupational Therapy, 39 (8), Aug 1976, 196-197.

9 Cheadle, A.J. Long-stay patient rehabilitation. (At St. Wulstan's Hospital, Malvern.) Nursing Times, 74, 17 Aug 1978, 1382-1384.

10 Christie, H. Reality therapy. (Philosophy of method used for rehabilitation in Eden Ward, Dingleton Hospital.) Nursing Times, 42, 2 Dec 1976, 1896-1899.

11 Darby, C. Stanley Wilson: the man who made rehabilitation a reality. The nurse who established two unique rehabilitation programmes for psychiatric patients at Sheffield's

Middlewood Hospital. Nursing Mirror, 146, 12 Jan 1978, 3.

12 Fletcher, P. Work for minds on the mend. ('Restore', a pioneer scheme in Oxford to provide sheltered work.) Health and Social Service Journal, 90, 11 Jul 1980, 909-910.

13 Gittoes-Davies, A. and Montes-Palma, A.M. Occupational therapists working in the community. (Scheme at Napsbury Hospital for psychiatric patients.) British Journal of Occupational Therapy, 41 (4), Apr 1978, 119-120.

14 Hammacott, C. Patients' holidays—no gimmicks here. (Self-catering holidays for psychiatric patients.) Nursing Times, 75, 15 Feb 1979, 295-296.

15 Hawkins, D. The changing role of an occupational therapist in a child and family psychiatric clinic. British Journal of Occupational Therapy, 41 (12), Dec 1978, 405-408.

16 Hickes, P. Ending the waiting game. (Ex-patient of Broadmoor describes difficulties in rehabilitation.) Health and Social Service Journal, 89, 15 Jun 1979, 731.

17 Hulland, F. Advice and information for patients leaving hospital. (With addresses of useful organisations.) Mind Out, 36, Sep/Oct 1979, 11.

18 Hume, C.A. and Pullen, I.M. Rehabilitation in psychiatry. (Edinburgh service.) British Journal of Occupational Therapy, 42 (11), Nov 1979, 283-285.

19 Ingram, J.A. Discharge and be damned. Who cares? (The role of the family in psychiatric rehabilitation.) Royal Society of Health Journal, 98 (3), Jun 1978, 108-112.

20 Jones, K. Community projects for mental health. (The community based club using 'The Stepping Stones Club' as an example.) Social Work Today, 7 (7), 24 Jun 1976, 210-211.

21 LaDuke, D.L. and others Operation: homeward bound—a military psychiatric transition program. (Programme at Walter Reed Army Medical Center.) Journal of Psychiatric Nursing, 18 (7), Jul 1980, 22-28.

22 Laurie, F. Time for a change. (Report by student nurse on caravan holiday for long-stay psychiatric patients from Knowle Hospital.) Nursing Times, 76, 10 Apr 1980, 653-655.

23 Leamy, G. and others A breath of fresh air. (Camping holiday with elderly patients from St. Augustine's Hospital, Canterbury.) Nursing Times, 73, 3 Feb 1977, 175-176.

24 McCowen, P. and Wilder, J. Lifestyle of 100 psychiatric patients: some cost and policy implications for rehabilitation. Psychiatric Rehabilitation Association, 1975.

25 McDonald, C. How we rehabilitated 42 long-stay psychiatric patients. (A rehabilitation programme for 'graduate' patients who had grown old in a psychiatric hospital resulted in 42 discharges into residental homes.) Geriatric Medicine, 9 (6), Jun 1979, 53-54, 57.

26 MIND The next step: community care for former psychiatric patients in six towns. Mind, 1976.

27 MIND You can't have one without the

other: a report on the integration of a hospital based rehabilitation scheme and a community based resettlement project for the mentally ill in North Gwent. Cardiff: Mind, 1977.

28 Mitchell, L. Occupational therapy in the department of psychiatry, Barnet General Hospital. (Description of proposed policies.) British Journal of Occupational Therapy, 40 (8), Aug 1977, 180.

29 Murray, E.W. Rehabilitation of the mentally ill. Nursing Mirror, 145, 1 Dec 1977, 39-40.

30 Murray, J. Better prospects: rehabilitation in mental illness hospitals. A report on facilities in 84 hospitals. Mind, 1977.

31 Physiotherapy Physiotherapy and psychiatry. (Six articles including the role of the physiotherapist and setting up a physiotherapy service in a psychiatric hospital.) Physiotherapy, 66 (12), Dec 1980, 398-410.

32 Price, J. and Vincent, P. Progress evaluation: what to ask before you start. (Using follow-up service for discharged mental patients as an example.) Nursing Outlook, 24, Feb 1976, 84-86.

33 Rich, V. The Vineyard project. (Centre in Richmond to help reintegration of ex-psychiatric patients into the community.) Nursing Times, 74, 23 Mar 1978, 484-485.

34 Sackett, J. What of the future? Occupational therapy in psychiatric hospitals and the community. British Journal of Occupational Therapy, 42 (2), Feb 1979, 46-47.

35 Shafar, S. and Ruddick, N. Collaboration: a physiotherapist in the psychiatric team. Physiotherapy, 62 (3), Mar 1976, 80-82.

36 Sketty, A. Community psychiatric nursing. The Stepping Stones Club. (Psychiatric rehabilitation centre, Bromley AHA.) Nursing Times, 72 (44), 4 Nov 1976, 1713-1714, 1715.

37 Slavinsky, A.T. and others Back to the community: a dubious blessing. (Interviews with 200 chronically ill psychiatric patients following hospital discharge showing the lonely and impoverished lives which many lead.) Nursing Outlook, 24 (6), Jun 1976, 370-374.

38 Stanley, T.E. Away from it all. (Nursing officer describes how he arranged holiday in Majorca for ten long-stay psychiatric patients from St. David's Hospital, Carmarthen.) Nursing Times, 74, 13 Apr 1978, 614-615.

39 Wilder, J. An aid to community care. Psychiatric Rehabilitation Association, 1978. Revised ed. 1980.

b GROUP HOMES AND HOSTELS

1 Abrahamson, D. and others The good life at Goodmayes. (Group home scheme.) Health and Social Service Journal, 89, 25 May 1979, 633-635.

2 Aston, G. and Wheatley, M. Building up the foundation of rehabilitation. (Rehabilitation of psychiatric patients in Epsom and Ewell through group homes.) Health and Social Service Journal, 89, 18 May 1979, 606-607.

3 Bosanquet, N. Inside the social services. Services for the mentally ill. (Hostels and day centres.) Nursing Times, 73, 24 Nov 1977, 1850-1851.

4 Donnelly, G. Group survival. How careful groundwork and tactful intervention can help patients in a new community home to become a happy integrated group. (Advice to community psychiatric nurse.) Nursing Times, 74, 9 Feb 1978, 252-253.

5 Durrant, B.W. Back to the community with a hospital made family. (Scheme at Oakwood Hospital, Maidstone, of group homes for discharged psychiatric patients.) Health and Social Service Journal, 86, 4 Sep 1976, 1592-1593.

6 Goldstone, L.A. and Tooley, D.M. Aspects of hostel facilities for the mentally ill in Greater Manchester. Community Health, 8 (2), Oct 1976, 86-93.

7 Hartie, M. Community nursing care study. A social outcast. (The problems of a psychiatric patient after discharge into the community.) Nursing Times, 72, 9 Sep 1976, 1392-1394.

8 Hughes, D. How psychiatric patients manage out of hospital: community provision, living standards and financial needs. Disability Alliance/Mental Health Foundation, 1978.

9 Leopoldt, H. and McStay, P. The psychiatric group home. The Oxford Group-Home Organisation. (Alternative to hospital care for long-term mentally ill.) Nursing Times, 76, 8 May 1980, 829-832; 15 May 1980, 866-868.

10 Leopoldt, H. Sheltered accommodation for the mentally ill. Nursing Mirror, 142, 22 Jan 1976, 57-59.

11 Mungovan, R. Home from hospital. (Establishment of a Housing Council at Fulbourn Hospital, Cambridge, to assist in the resettlement of psychiatric patients in the community.) Nursing Times, 73, 28 Apr 1977, 620-621.

12 Murray, E.W. Just passing through—to independence. (Hostels for the mentally ill.) Nursing Mirror, 146, 22 Jun 1978, 39-40.

13 Roets, G.A. and Good, D.W. Group home program. (Treatment of the institutionalised of the chronic mental patient by small group homes in the community.) Journal of Psychiatric Nursing and Mental Health Services, 14 (5), May 1976, 15-17.

14 Ryan, P. and Hewett, S. A pilot study of hostels for the mentally ill. (Survey of after care paid for by three south-east London boroughs.) Social Work Today, 6 (25), 18 Mar 1976, 774-778.

15 Stephens, A. and Nattress, P. A study of day centres. Mind, 1978.

16 Thornicroft, G. Group homes—a success? (House where former psychiatric patients live together without supervision.) Nursing Times, 75, 11 Jan 1979, 84-85.

17 Toke, E. and Clews, B. The function and effectiveness of a local authority day centre in the rehabilitation of psychiatric conditions. British Journal of Psychiatric Therapy, 40 (4), Apr 1977, 75-78.

18 Wilder, J. Neighbourhood orienteering with a day centre as base. (Needs of the psychiatric patient in the community.) Health and Social Service Journal, 86, 14 Jan 1976, 64-65.

c WORK THERAPY AND EMPLOYMENT

1 Burns, D.B. Resettlement and employment of psychiatric patients. (Scheme in Dundee.) Nursing Times, 75, 10 May 1979, 799-801.

2 Jones, K. First steps on the long road that leads back to work. (Rehabilitative work centre for the mentally ill in Essex.) Health and Social Service Journal, 86, 26 Nov 1976, 2104-2105.

3 Lamont, L.O. Toil without tears. (Scheme at St. George's Hospital, Morpeth, involving work for National Trust and Forestry Commission.) Nursing Times, 75, 18 Oct 1979, 1809-1810.

4 Massey, G. Certified sane. (Author's experience of the stigma of mental illness and its effects on his career.) Nursing Mirror, 146, 8 Jun 1978, 7-8.

5 Melville, J. Mental block. (Stigma of psychiatric illness affects future employment prospects.) New Society, 42, 8 Dec 1977, 519-520.

6 Price, B. Mental illness: a case for company concern. (Discrimination by employers against ex-patients.) Personnel Management, 10 (12), Dec 1978, 39-43.

81 MENTAL HANDICAP

a GENERAL AND SERVICES

1 Association of Professions for the Mentally Handicapped Breaking the bounds and forging the links: a collection of papers given at the 2nd annual congress of APMH, Nottingham University, 14-17 April 1975. The Association, 1976.

2 Association of Professions for the Mentally Handicapped Working together: aspects of providing a multi-disciplinary service for mentally handicapped people. AMPH, 1979.

3 Berry, P. editor Language and communication in the mentally handicapped. Arnold, 1976.

4 Bosanquet, N. Inside the social services. Services for the mentally handicapped. Nursing Times, 73, 27 Oct 1977, 1686-1687.

5 Campaign for the Mentally Handicapped An enquiry into joint planning of services for mentally handicapped people. The Campaign, 1979.

6 Campaign for the Mentally Handicapped Looking at life in a hospital, hostel, home or unit. CMH, 1978. (Enquiry paper, no.7.)

7 Campaign for the Mentally Handicapped No longer a child. CMH, 1977. (CMH discussion paper, no.6.)

8 Campaign for the Mentally Handicapped Plans and provisions for mentally handicapped people: a further enquiry into the work of Regional Health Authorities, five years after the White Paper. The Campaign, 1976.

9 Campaign for the Mentally Handicapped Who's consulted? The future role of the medical specialist in mental handicap. CMH, 1978. (CMH enquiry paper, no.8.)

10 Cowie, V. De Lange syndrome: disorder with many peculiarities. Nursing Mirror, 149, 11 Oct 1979, 35-37.

11 Cowie, V. A fortunately rare pair. (Cockayne's Syndrome and Waardenburg Syndrome.) Nursing Mirror, 150, 7 Feb 1980, 36-37.

12 Cowie, V. Laurence-Moon-Biedl-Bardet syndrome: the factor that can blind a family. Nursing Mirror, 147, 14 Dec 1978, 36-37.

13 Cowper-Smith, F. Focus on Colchester— 2. (Mental handicap services.) Nursing Mirror, 142 (18), 29 Apr 1976, 55-57.

14 Craft, M. editor Tredgold's mental retardation. 12th ed. Baillière Tindall, 1979.

15 Davidson, N. Against the tide…the growing disquiet over the National Development Team on mental handicap and the way its work so far is revealing guiding principles many would challenge. Health and Social Service Journal, 88, 16 Jun 1978, 703.

16 Department of Health and Social Security Mental handicap: progress, problems and priorities. DHSS, 1980.

17 Development Team for the Mentally Handicapped First report: Jul 1976 to Dec 1977. HMSO, 1978.

18 Durrant, P. Mental handicap in Bristol—a review. (Production of booklet on services available, by Bristol Campaign for the Mentally Handicapped.) Social Work Today, 10, 10 Jul 1979, 13-15.

19 Eden, D.J. Mental handicap: an introduction. Allen and Unwin, 1976. (Unwin education books, no.26.)

20 Farrell, P.J. Who cares for the mentally handicapped? Nursing Mirror, 143, 16 Sep 1976, 63-64.

21 Fraser, W. The ultimate blueprint: policies for the mentally handicapped. Social Work Today, 7 (1), 1 Apr 1976, 4-5.

22 Griffiths, P. and Matthews, G.G. A policy group at work—lessons learnt. (Report on methods used and problems experienced by multidisciplinary and joint authority group developing policy framework for mental handicap services in Kent.) Hospital and Health Services Review, 76 (3), Mar 1980, 90-92.

23 Grunewald, K. editor The mentally handicapped: towards normal living. Hutchinson, 1978.

24 Hallas, C.H. and others The care and training of the mentally handicapped: a manual for the caring professions. 6th ed. Bristol: Wright, 1978.

25 Health and Social Service Journal The questions they leave unanswered. (Comment on National Development Team's report on care for the mentally handicapped in Wessex.) Health and Social Service Journal, 88, 17 Feb 1978, 197.

26 Hegarty, J.R. Psychological assessment of the mentally handicapped. Nursing Mirror, 143.
1. The beginnings of psychological assessment. 12 Aug, 54-56.
2. Uses and abuses of intelligence tests. 16 Sep 1976, 56-58.
3. Assessment for learning. 14 Oct 1976, 64-66.

4. The evaluation of social attainment. 18 Nov 1976, 62-64.
5. The psychologist, his tests, and the nurse. 16 Dec 1976, 59-60.

27 **Innes, G. and others** Mental subnormality in north-east Scotland: a multi-disciplinary study of total population. Scottish Home and Health Department, 1978. (Scottish health service studies, no.38.)

28 **Institute of Mental Subnormality** Language and the mentally handicapped: 3. Proceedings of the conference held at Coleshill Hall Hospital, Coleshill, Birmingham, 7 May 1975. Kidderminster: IMS, 1977.

29 **Iveson-Iveson, J.** The mentally handicapped adult. Report on a recent Anglo-American conference held at the Middlesex Polytechnic. Nursing Mirror, 145, 11 Aug 1977, 9.

30 **Joblin, M. and Parfit, J.** How to set up a resource centre on handicap. Institute for Research into Mental and Multiple Handicap, 1977.

31 **Martindale, A.** Symposium on ascertainment of national needs. 2. A case register as an information system in a development project for the mentally handicapped. (Sheffield Register.) British Journal of Mental Subnormality, 22 (2), Dec 1976, 70-76.

32 **Mittler, P.** People not patients: problems and policies in mental handicap. Methuen, 1979. (University paperbacks; 674.)

33 **National Development Group for the Mentally Handicapped** Helping mentally handicapped school leavers. The Group, 1977. (Pamphlet, no.3.)

34 **National Development Group for the Mentally Handicapped** Mental handicap: planning together. Revised ed. The Group, 1977. (Pamphlet, no.1.)

35 **National Development Group for the Mentally Handicapped** Residential short-term care for mentally handicapped people: suggestions for action. Department of Health and Social Security, 1977. (Pamphlet, no.4.)

36 **Office of Health Economics** Mental handicap: ways forward. OHE, 1978. (Studies of current health problems, no.61.)

37 **Oswin, M.** We must lift our head out of the sand. (Views on National Development Group report, by Peter Mellor, Sid Ambler and others.) Health and Social Service Journal, 88, 3 Nov 1978, 1238-1239.

38 **Pilkington, T.L.** Psychiatry and the mentally handicapped. Public Health, 90, Jul 1976, 227-230.

39 **Raynes, N.V. and others** Organisational structure and the care of the mentally retarded. Croom Helm, 1979.

40 **Scottish Home and Health Department** and **Scottish Education Department** A better life: report on services for the mentally handicapped in Scotland. Edinburgh: HMSO, 1979.

41 **Sealby, J.** Helping the profoundly and severely subnormal. Physiotherapy, 63 (8), Aug 1977, 259-262.

42 **Shearer, A.** A life of your own: mentally handicapped people. Liverpool Institute of Socio-Religious Studies, 1976. (Pastoral investigation of social trends working paper, no.2.)

43 **Tredinnick, A.** Public scandal of the seventies. (Claims that reorganisation of the health and social work services was disastrous for the mentally handicapped.) Health and Social Service Journal, 88, 3 Mar 1978, 250.

44 **Webster, R.C.** Mental handicap today. Royal Society of Health Journal, 97 (2), Apr 1977, 64-66.

45 **Wertheimer, A.** Researching into mental handicap. (Review.) Mind Out, 40, May/Jun 1980, 16-18.

46 **Yeaworth, R.C.** The agonizing decisions in mental retardation. American Journal of Nursing, 77 (5), May 1977, 864-867.

b OVERSEAS COUNTRIES

1 **Murray, R.** Providing medical care to the profoundly retarded requires initiative and innovation. Canadian Journal of Psychiatric Nursing, 18 (2), Mar/Apr 1976, 7.

2 **Townsend, D.** Actions not words. (Sweden's system of community-based care for the mentally handicapped.) Health and Social Service Journal, 89, 15 Feb 1979, 154-156.

c COMMUNITY CARE

1 **Campling, J.** Community care and mental handicap. (Work of CARE in providing villages for mentally handicapped adults.) Social Service Quarterly, 51 (4), Apr/Jun 1978, 147-149.

2 **Davidson, N.** How the real world hit a city's dream. (Report on the evaluation of the Sheffield Development Project on Services for the Mentally Handicapped.) Health and Social Service Journal, 88, 14 Apr 1978, 428-429.

3 **Davidson, N.** The not so immaculate concept of a revolution. (Impact of a changing professional climate on the Sheffield Development Project for the Mentally Handicapped.) Health and Social Service Journal, 88, 21 Apr 1978, 458-459.

4 **Evans, E.C.** Assisting retarded people into the community. Royal Society of Health Journal, 97 (2), Apr 1977, 67-69.

5 **Fotherby, M. and Froggatt, A.** Noting the patterns of unpredictability. (Based on their experience of working with mildly mentally handicapped patients the authors discuss the need to build trust and play a parental role.) Social Work Today, 11, 8 Jul 1980, 21-22.

6 **Gathercole, C.** Home is where the heart is. (Need for residential accommodation for the mentally handicapped to be as home-like as possible.) Health and Social Service Journal, 89, 7 Sep 1979, 1143.

7 **Halpern, S.** No place like home. (The Gloucester Centre in Peterborough for the mentally handicapped.) Health and Social Service Journal, 88, 1 Sep 1978, 992-994.

8 **Heley, R.W.** Continuity of care. (Beechcroft day care unit, Rotherham District General Hospital, for the severely retarded and handicapped.) Nursing Times, 72, 24 Jun 1976, 975-977.

9 **Jaehnig, W.** A family service for the mentally handicapped. Fabian Society, 1979. (Fabian tract, no.460.)

10 **Locker, D. and others** Knowledge of and attitudes towards mental handicap: their implications for community care. (Study of community reaction to a hostel for the mentally handicapped.) Community Medicine, 1 (2), May 1979, 127-136.

11 **Mathieson, S. and Blunden, R.** Nimrod is piloting a course towards a community life. (New project for the community care of mentally handicapped people in South Glamorgan.) Health and Social Service Journal, 90, 25 Jan 1980, 122-124.

12 **Meacher, M.** After one and a half million years in hospital. (Existing community services for the mentally handicapped.) Social Work Today, 7 (6), 10 Jun 1976, 162-163.

13 **Mittler, P. and Simon, G.** Building support for the mentally handicapped and their families. (Special role of community mental handicap teams alongside district handicap teams recommended by Court committee.) Health and Social Service Journal, 88, 12 May 1978, 541-542.

14 **National Development Group for the Mentally Handicapped** Day services for mentally handicapped adults. The Group, 1977. (Pamphlet, no.5.)

15 **Nellist, I.** Making sense by turning the numbers upside down: the value and problems involved in community action in helping the mentally handicapped towards normalisation. Health and Social Service Journal, 87, 7 Jan 1977, 12-13.

16 **Nursing Mirror** New concept in community hospitals. (Gloucester Centre for the Mentally Handicapped near Peterborough.) Nursing Mirror, 145, 13 Oct 1977, 9.

17 **Pushkin, R.** Community confusion over abnormality needs a remedy. (Survey of public perceptions and knowledge of mental handicap in Manchester.) Health and Social Service Journal, 86, 15 Oct 1976, 1856-1857.

18 **RIDGE Hill:** a new style of care for the mentally handicapped. (Unit in Stourbridge, Worcs, with homely atmosphere which forms base for comprehensive community service.) Nursing Mirror, 147, 28 Sep 1978, 8.

19 **Rose, V.** A family of their own. (L'Arche communities for the mentally handicapped.) Nursing Mirror, 142, 29 Apr 1976, 67-69.

20 **Royal Society of Health Journal** The mentally handicapped – is community care the best solution? (Two articles, one by a psychiatrist, the other by an officer of the National Society for Mentally Handicapped Children.) Royal Society of Health Journal, 98 (4), Aug 1978, 181-186.

21 **Tooth, T.** Philosophy of care for mental handicap services. (Plans for integrated community-based service in Coventry.) Health and Social Service Journal, 90, 1 Feb 1980, 156-157.

22 **Tyne, A.** Where there is care but no life at home. (Problems in residential care for mentally handicapped adults.) Health and Social Service Journal, 87, 21 Oct 1977, 1464-1464.

23 **Wilkin, D.** Community care of the mentally handicapped. 1. Family support. 2. The role of the services. Nursing Mirror, 146, 27 Apr 1978, 39-40; 4 May 1978, 45-46.

24 **Wing, J.K. and Olsen, R. editors** Community care for the mentally disabled. Oxford: Oxford University Press, 1979.

25 **World Health Organization. Regional Office for Europe** Care of the mentally retarded in the community: report on a conference, Santiago de Compostela, 25-29 Jun 1976. Copenhagen: WHO, 1978.

d HOSPITALS

1 **Alaszewski, A.** Problems in measuring and evaluating the quality of care in mental handicap hospitals. Health and Social Service Journal, 88, 10 Mar 1978, Centre eight papers, A9-A15.

2 **Armstrong, J. and others** Two mixed sex wards for severely and profoundly mentally handicapped adults. British Journal of Mental Subnormality, 22 (1), Jun 1976, 35-40.

3 **Birchall, G. and others** A patients' bank in a hospital for the mentally handicapped. (Darenth Park Hospital, Dartford.) Hospital and Health Services Review, 73 (8), Aug 1977, 270-274.

4 **Bosanquet, N.** The hospital handicap race. (Criticism of continuing hospital care for mentally handicapped people.) New Society, 50, 11 Oct 1979, 75-76.

5 **Davidson, N.** Why are we waiting? (Comment on recent report by National Development Group on the care of mentally handicapped people in hospital.) Health and Social Service Journal, 88, 27 Oct 1978, 1208-1209.

6 **Department of Health and Social Security** The facilities and services of mental illness and mental handicap hospitals 1975. HMSO, 1977. (Statistical research report, no.19.)

7 **Gillott, J.S. and others** The sectorisation of a large hospital for the mentally handicapped. Hospital and Health Services Review, 75 (6), Jun 1979, 189-197.

8 **Grubb, D.G.W.** The castle concept. The siege mentality of hospitals for the mentally handicapped. Nursing Mirror, 146, 12 Jan 1978, 38-39.

9 **McKay, R.** Strengthening links. (Care of mentally handicapped patients at Church Hill House Hospital and Binfield Park Hospital, both in Bracknell.) Health and Social Service Journal, 88, 8 Dec 1978, 1382-1383.

10 **Mittler, P.** Action now for a better life in hospital. (Explanation and reactions to National Development Group report on hospital care for the mentally handicapped.) Nursing Mirror, 148, 28 Jun 1979, 24-25.

11 **National Development Group for the Mentally Handicapped** Helping mentally handicapped people in hospital. Department of Health and Social Security, 1978. (Chairman: P. Mittler.)

12 **Phillips, M.** Subnormality. (Problems of falling standards in mental subnormality hospitals.) New Society, 35, 8 Jan 1976, 54.

13 **Primrose, D.A.** The development of mental deficiency hospitals in Scotland. Health Bulletin, 35 (2), Mar 1977, 63-65.

14 **Primrose, D.A.** A therapeutic environment. (The benefits of care in a mental deficiency hospital.) Health Bulletin, 35 (2), Mar 1977, 70-72.

15 **Roberts, R.W.** Talking point. The hospital's place. (Case for the extension of the hospital's role in mental handicap care.) Nursing Times, 72, 22 Apr 1976, 606.

16 **Spencer, D.A.** Morale in mental handicap hospitals. (Letter stating ten areas of concern.) British Medical Journal, 1, 7 Jan 1978, 44.

17 **Thompson, S.** An agenda for bedlam. (Health authority plans for the closure of mental subnormality hospitals.) Health and Social Service Journal, 86, 21 Aug 1976, 1519.

18 **Tudor-Davies, E.R.** Looking forward. (Views on hospital care for the mentally handicapped as seen in evidence to the Jay Committee and a National Society for Mentally Handicapped Children conference.) Nursing Times, 72, 23 Sep 1976, 1462-1463.

e INDIVIDUAL HOSPITALS

1 **Brentry Hospital**—(Originally a reformatory for inebriates, now a mental handicap hospital.) Nursing Times, 73, 12 May 1977, Archive, 17-20.

2 **Brockhall**—Nine articles on preparation for Christmas at Brockhall Hospital in Lancashire. Health and Social Service Journal, 89, 21/28 Dec 1979, 1644-1655.

3 **Darenth Park**—**Gillott, J.S. and others** The organisation and management of patient training services at Darenth Park Hospital. (Radical changes in a hospital for the mentally handicapped which could be implemented in any kind of long stay hospital.) Hospital and Health Services Review, 74 (3), Mar 1978, 77-83.

4 **Darenth Park**—**Gillott, J.S. and others** The use of management by objectives in developing services for the mentally handicapped at Darenth Park Hospital. Hospital and Health Services Review, 74 (12), Dec 1978, 425-427.

5 **Lightwood House**—The first hospital unit in the Sheffield Development Project for an integrated service for the mentally handicapped. Hospital and Health Services Review, 73 (11), Nov 1977, 394-396.

6 **Lightwood House**—**Bottomley, L.** Nursing the mentally handicapped at Lightwood House. (Hospital unit with residential and day accommodation in Sheffield.) Nursing Mirror, 146, 30 Mar 1978, 26-28.

7 **Lynbank**—**Fraser, W. and others** The first eight years of a mental handicap service. (Lynbank Hospital, Dunfermline.) Health Bulletin, 35 (2), Mar 1977, 66-70.

8 **Normansfield**—**Ashton, K.** Grasping the nettle. (Report of visit to Normansfield Hospital and future plans of hospital.) Nursing Times, 74, 7 Dec 1978, 2006-2007.

9 **Normansfield**—**Bavin, J.** After Normansfield—what next. (Suggests solutions to current problems in the mental handicap field.) Lancet, 1, 28 Apr 1979, 918-919.

10 **Normansfield**—**British Medical Journal** The Normansfield inquiry. (Extracts from the report, including the main conclusions and recommendations. See also editorial on p.1518 and comment on p.1580.) British Medical Journal, 2, 2 Dec 1978, 1560-1563.

11 **Normansfield**—**Committee of Inquiry into Normansfield Hospital** Report. HMSO, 1978. (Chairman: Michael Sherrard.) (Cmnd 7357.)

12 **Normansfield**—**Darby, C.** The challenge at the end of an unhappy affair. (Background, findings and future implications of the Normansfield Report.) Nursing Mirror, 147, 30 Nov 1978, 8-9.

13 **Normansfield**—**Davidson, N.** No room for revolt at the top. (Dilemmas facing regional teams of officers highlighted by Normansfield report.) Health and Social Service Journal, 89, 20 Apr 1979, 440-443.

14 **Normansfield**—**Dyson, R.** Normansfield: anatomy of the strike. (Examination of wider implications of the report's account of the strike.) British Medical Journal, 1, 27 Jan 1979, 283-285.

15 **Normansfield**—**Health and Social Service Journal** The shame and the blame. (Two articles on the Normansfield report including conclusions and recommendations.) Health and Social Service Journal, 88, 24 Nov 1978, 1326-1329.

16 **Normansfield**—**Hill, S.G.** Normansfield—its implications for health service administrators. (With reference to areas of responsibility.) Hospital and Health Services Review, 75 (6), Jun 1979, 208-210.

17 **Normansfield**—**Hospital and Health Services Review** Normansfield. (Comment on issues raised in the report with summary of report, 441-443.) Hospital and Health Services Review, 74 (12), Dec 1978, 423-424.

18 **Normansfield**—**James, D.** A concerted effort. (Interview with Diana James, ANO Kingston and Richmond AHA on Normansfield Hospital for the mentally handicapped. Editorial on p.475.) Nursing Times, 74, 23 Mar 1978, 482-483.

19 **Normansfield**—**Klein, R.** Normansfield: vacuum of management in the NHS. (Critique of NHS consensus management with reference to the Normansfield report.) British Medical Journal, 2, 23/30 Dec 1978, 1802-1804.

20 **Normansfield**—**Lancet** Commentary from Westminster. Normansfield inquiry. Lancet, 2, 25 Nov 1978, 1162.

21 **Normansfield**—**National Association of Health Authorities in England and Wales** Normansfield enquiry. The Association, 1979.

22 **Normansfield**—**Nursing Mirror** Normansfield inquiry gets under way. Nursing Mirror, 144, 7 Apr 1977, 36; Further reports, 145, 10 Nov 1977, 3; 17 Nov 1977, 5.

23 **POUCHLANDS Hospital.** (South Chailey, Sussex, originally a workhouse, now providing long-term care for geriatric and mentally handicapped patients.) Nursing Times, 73, 14 Jul 1977, 25-28.

24 **St. Ebba's**—**Merton, Sutton and Wandsworth Area Health Authority** Inquiry at St. Ebba's Hospital, Epsom, into the circumstances leading to the death of John James Henry

Matthews on 4 June 1975. The Health Authority, 1976.

25 St. Lawrence's—Solman, F. Joey's book starts a new community village. (Autobiography of spastic led to village community in the grounds of St. Lawrence's Hospital, Caterham.) Nursing Mirror, 146, 23 Mar 1978, 8-9.

26 St. Lawrence's—Solman, F. Mentally subnormal at home in hospital. (Care and work of action group at St. Lawrence's Hospital, Caterham.) Nursing Mirror, 146, 30 Mar 1978, 7-10.

27 St. Lawrence's—Sylvester, P.E. Adventure play for the handicapped. (Adventure playground at St. Lawrence's Hospital, Caterham, for the mentally handicapped.) Nursing Times , 73, 3 Nov 1977, 1702-1704.

f NURSING

1 Alaszewski, A.M. Suggestions for the reorganisation of nurse training and improvement of patient care in a hospital for the mentally handicapped. Journal of Advanced Nursing, 2 (5), Sep 1977, 461-477.

2 Barker, P. Jack of all trades nurse with a specialty in custodial care: the therapeutic role of the nurse in caring for the mentally handicapped in hospital. Health and Social Service Journal, 87, 15 Apr 1977, 666-667.

3 Blackwell, M.W. Care of the mentally retarded. Boston: Little, Brown and Co., 1979. (For nurses.)

4 British Journal of Mental Subnormality Symposium on structural training and nursing. 4. Self help skills in the profoundly subnormal. British Journal of Mental Subnormality, 22 (2), Dec 1976, 105-111.

5 Cooper-Smith, F. Teaching excellence in residential care of the severely handicapped. (Week's course organised by the Rcn and The Royal Hospital and Home for Incurables.) Nursing Times, 72, 23/30 Dec 1976, 2001-2004.

6 Curry, J. B. and Peppe, K.K. editors Mental retardation: nursing approaches to care. St. Louis: Mosby, 1978.

7 Fitzgerald, L.P. The role of the nurse in mental handicap. World of Irish Nursing, 7 (5), May 1978, 6-7; (6), Jun 1978, 2.

8 General Nursing Council for Scotland Syllabus for mental deficiency nursing. Edinburgh: the Council, 1980.

9 Gibson, J. and French, T. Nursing the mentally retarded. 4th ed. Faber, 1977.

10 Gladstone, R. Patients who never complain. (Defends need for nurses to care for mentally handicapped.) Nursing Mirror, 148, 7 Jun 1979, 22-23.

11 Harris, D. The Wales Court trial. (Charges of ill treatment and neglect against six mental handicap nurses who used form of behaviour modification.) Social Work Today, 10, 14 Nov 1978, 8.

12 Hay, D.N. Controversy corner. Caring for the mentally handicapped. Nursing Mirror, 142, 29 Apr 1976, 41.

13 Hosking, G. Don't disband the RNMS—improve it! Nursing Mirror, 148, 29 Mar 1979, 7.

14 Hull, D. Look and learn with 'Roy'. (Staff training programme at Lightwood House, Sheffield, hospital for the mentally handicapped.) Health and Social Service Journal, 88, 28 Jul 1978, 852-854.

15 Hulme, J. Boys will be boys. (Problems of nursing high dependency mentally subnormal males.) Nursing Times, 72, 8 Apr 1976, 550-551.

16 Malin, N. Mental handicap—the role of the auxiliary. (Research at the Department of Administration, University of Strathclyde, Glasgow.) Nursing Mirror, 143, 30 Sep 1976, 61-62.

17 Malin, N. Staff attitudes in mental handicap. Glasgow: Scottish Society for the Mentally Handicapped, 1978.

18 May, A.E. A psychologist's view of nursing the mentally handicapped. Nursing Mirror, 143, 26 Aug 1976, 56-58.

19 May, A.E. and others The consequences of vigilance in subnormality and psychiatric hospitals. (Demand for vigilance by nurses reduces their opportunity to improve organisation and physical environment. Advocates improved staff/patient ratio at certain times of the day.) British Journal of Mental Subnormality, 24 (2), Dec 1978, 109-112.

20 Moores, B. and Grant, G.W.B. The 'Avoidance' syndrome in hospitals for the mentally handicapped. (Follow-up article giving analysis of interactions received by patients in two institutions to examine the extent to which nurse staffing levels affected the pattern of patient care and staff activities.) International Journal of Nursing Studies, 14 (2), 1977, 91-95.

21 Moores, B. and Grant, G.W.B. Feelings of alienation among nursing staff in hospitals for the mentally handicapped. (A study of staff participation in 33 hospitals.) International Journal of Nursing Studies, 14 (1), 1977, 5-12.

22 Moores, B. and Grant, G.W.B. On the nature and incidence of staff-patient interactions in hospitals for the mentally handicapped. International Journal of Nursing Studies, 13 (2), 1976, 69-81.

23 Moores, B. and Grant, G.W.B. Optimists and pessimists: attitudes of nursing staff towards the development potential of mentally handicapped patients in their charge. International Journal of Nursing Studies, 14 (1), 1977, 13-18.

24 Nursing Times 'Commitment comes first', in mental handicap nursing. (Report of Mental Handicap Week conference.) Nursing Times, 73, 14 Jul 1977, 1058.

25 Nursing Times A job for professionals. (Case for hospital care of the mentally handicapped argued by nurses from Royal Earlswood Hospital, Surrey.) Nursing Times, 72 (10), 11 Mar 1976, 364.

26 Pounds, V.A. The things they say. (Personal experiences of a mental handicap nurse.) Nursing Times, 72, 17 Jun 1976, 951.

27 Taylor, S. and others Patient-nurse dependency. (Study in Leybourne Grange Hospital for the mentally handicapped.) Nursing Times, 74, 4 May 1978, 755-758.

28 Thompson, A. Applying the nursing process to the care of the mentally handicapped. Nursing Mirror, 148, 8 Mar 1979, 26-28.

29 Thurman, R.L. and Snowe, R.J. The nurse practitioner for the mentally retarded—are they compatible? (Seminar discussing the possible benefits of a co-operation between mental handicap institution and a university based paediatric nurse practitioner program.) Journal of Psychiatric Nursing and Mental Health Nursing, 14 (5), May 1976, 7-10.

30 Tierney, A.J. Behaviour modification in mental deficiency nursing. PhD thesis, Edinburgh University, 1976.

31 Williams, P. The future of mental handicap nurses. Nursing Mirror, 142, 17 Jun 1976, 67-68.

32 Williams, P. Time for nurses to lead. (Establishing the separate identity of mental handicap nurses could be a vital step in the movement towards community care of the mentally handicapped.) New Psychiatry, 3 (1), 8 Jan 1976, 10-11.

g NURSING: JAY REPORT

1 Allen, M. and Darby, C. Jay will urge mental handicap nursing should be phased out. (Report on likely proposals of Jay Committee. See also editorial 1.) Nursing Mirror, 146, 29 Jun 1978, 2.

2 Altschul, A. Jumping ahead with Jay. (Assessment of the Jay Report and its implementations.) Nursing Mirror, 148, 26 Apr 1979, 17-19.

3 Association of Nurse Administrators ANA plans for mentally handicapped. (Evidence to the Jay Committee.) Nursing Mirror, 142, 3 Jun 1976, 34.

4 Bavin, J. Jay Report critique. 1. Why the recommendations will not succeed. A view that the underlying premises of the report are open to question. Nursing Times, 75, 17 May 1979, 821-825.

5 Bavin, J. Jay report critique. 2. The Gloucestershire project. Alternatives to the recommendations of the Jay report are put forward on the basis of a scheme which has already been implemented. Nursing Times, 75, 24 May 1979, 887-890.

6 Bosanquet, N. The choice is yours. (Following Jay Report mental handicap nurses can either fight to keep RNMS or press for their own statutory training council.) Nursing Mirror, 148, 12 Apr 1979, 7-8.

7 Bosanquet, N. Parting of the way. (Why author dissented from majority report of Jay Committee.) Health and Social Service Journal, 89, 29 Mar 1979, 300-301.

8 Brown, A. Counting the cost of Jay. (Comment on the report's recommendations.) Nursing Mirror, 148, 15 Mar 1979, 4-5.

9 Campaign for the Mentally Handicapped A submission of views to the Committee of Inquiry into Mental Handicap Nursing and Care. The Campaign, 1976.

10 Committee of Enquiry into Mental Handicap Nursing and Care Progress report. DHSS, 1976. (Chairman: Pegg Jay.)

11 **Committee of Enquiry into Mental Handicap Nursing and Care.** Report. 2 vols. HMSO, 1979. (Chairman: Peggy Jay.)

12 **Confederation of Health Service Employees** COSHE takes stand on mental training. (Evidence to the Jay Committee.) Nursing Mirror, 142 (19), 6 May 1976, 34.

13 **Darby, C.** 'Full debate' assurance on the Jay proposals. (Response of Jay committee to Nursing Mirror's exclusive revelations in previous issue with letter from Peggy Jay.) Nursing Mirror, 147, 6 Jul 1978, 2.

14 **Day, K.A.** A new caring profession for the mentally handicapped? (Proposal by Briggs Committee which Jay Committee is studying.) Nursing Times, 74, 6 Apr 1978, 566.

15 **Dopson, L.** According to Jay. (Support for Jay recommendations from two nurses who work at Hawthorn Lodge, a Cheshire Home for mentally handicapped.) Nursing Times, 76, 3 Jan 1980, 8-9.

16 **Dopson, L.** Nursing Times explains. CCETSW—the council Jay prefers. (Central Council for Education and Training in Social Work.) Nursing Times, 75, 21 Jun 1979, 1033.

17 **Dugdale, R.** Beware of the Jay. (Rejection of Jay report's recommendations.) Nursing Times, 75, 22 Mar 1979, 474.

18 **General Nursing Council** Nurses caring for the mentally handicapped. (Evidence presented to the Jay Committee including an historical survey.) Nursing Times, 72, 22 Apr 1976, 619-623.

19 **General Nursing Council** Now the GNC says 'No' to Jay. (Summary of GNC comments on Jay report.) Nursing Mirror, 150, 3 Jan 1980, 4.

20 **Gorman, V.** A bright new future. (Support for Jay report's proposals.) Nursing Times, 75, 22 Mar 1979, 473-474.

21 **Greenhalgh, K.** Care-giving within boundaries. (Asks whether nursing can thrive between the boundaries of care-giving professions with reference to the Jay report.) Nursing Mirror, 148, 7 Jun 1979, 24.

22 **Hansard** Jay Committee report. Statement by Secretary of State. 8 Mar 1979, WA 814-817.

23 **Health and Social Service Journal** In the bold footsteps of Jay—the professions now reply. (Comments from a director of Social Services, clinical psychologist, sector administrator and Peter Mellor, Rcn nurse adviser.) Health and Social Service Journal, 89, 30 Mar 1979, 348-349.

24 **Health Visitors Association** Nursing the mentally handicapped. Evidence to the Jay Committee. Health Visitor, 49 (6), Jun 1976, 191-193.

25 **Hospital and Health Services Review** Jay Committee. (Statement of progress.) Hospital and Health Services Review, 72 (10), Oct 1976, 339.

26 **Hudson, B.** Who needs hospitals?—facing up to alternative models of care. (For the mentally handicapped in the light of the Jay Report.) Social Work Today, 11, 8 Jul 1980, 16-21.

27 **Institute of Health Service Administrators** Mental handicap nursing: IHSA comments. (Evidence to the Jay Committee of Inquiry into Mental Handicap Nursing.) Hospital and Health Services Review, 72 (5), May 1976, 169-171.

28 **Jay, P.** A formula for growth. (King's Fund conference on utilising Jay at which Peggy Jay was a speaker.) Nursing Times, 75, 24 May 1979, 861.

29 **Jay, P.** Peggy Jay: bête noire or Messiah? (Interview on aspects of the Jay report by A. Dunn and L. Dopson.) Nursing Times, 75, 15 Mar 1979, 434-435.

30 **Jay, P.** Ready to roll up her sleeves. (Interview with Peggy Jay by S. Lewis on implications of Jay report and reactions to it.) Health and Social Service Journal, 89, 20 Apr 1979, 445-447.

31 **Jay, P. and McCree, H.** Why we propose a new model of care. (Outline of main proposals of report by chairman and vice-chairman of Jay Committee.) Nursing Mirror, 148, 8 Mar 1979, 4-5.

32 **Joinson, P.** Why did Jay ignore us? (By community nursing officer (mental handicap).) Nursing Mirror, 149, 11 Oct 1979, 31.

33 **Lewis, S.** To live life to the full is Jay's guiding light. (Summary of Jay report and list of Jay committee's terms of reference.) Health and Social Service Journal, 89, 22 Mar 1979, 274-277.

34 **Nursing Mirror** Should the CSS replace the RNMS? (Views of 14 nurses on the Jay Report proposals.) Nursing Mirror, 148, 19 Apr 1979, 6-7.

35 **Nursing Times** The Jay recommendations. (Summary of main report and minority reports.) Nursing Times, 75, 8 Mar 1979, 392-394.

36 **Olsen, R.** Take the Jay train. (Nursing reactions to Jay report and its implementation.) New Society, 53, 11 Sep 1980, 508-509.

37 **Oswin, M.** The challenge of Jay. (Comment on the Jay report with reference to its implications for handicapped children's residential services.) Nursing Times, 75, 15 Mar 1979, 435-436.

38 **Rodgers, J.S.** Care of the mentally handicapped. The Jay Committee Report. (Comment.) Lancet, 1, 14 Apr 1979, 816-817.

39 **Royal College of Nursing** Jay: no new caring profession needed says Rcn. (Rcn evidence to Jay Committee on nursing the mentally handicapped.) Nursing Times, 72, 20 May 1976, 757; Nursing Mirror, 142, 20 May 1976, 34.

40 **Royal College of Nursing** Report of the Committee of Enquiry into Mental Handicap Nursing and Care (Jay Report): Rcn response. Rcn, 1979.

41 **Savage, D.** Facing the facts. (Interview with David Savage who opposes Jay Report, by S. Ellis.) Nursing Times, 75, 16 Apr 1979, 655.

42 **Williams, D.** Why I wouldn't sign the Jay report. Nursing Mirror, 148, 15 Mar 1979, 6-7.

h TREATMENT

1 **Armstrong, J.** Progress through persistence. (Care study of disturbed mentally handicapped woman who responded to training programme regarding behaviour, personal hygiene and incontinence. By senior nursing officer.) Nursing Times, 76, 10 Apr 1980, 656-659.

2 **Barker, P.** 'Changing image.' The reduction of self-stimulatory behaviour in four profoundly retarded males. (Study at Strathmartine Hospital, Dundee.) International Journal of Nursing Studies, 13 (3), 1976, 179-186.

3 **Barker, P. and others** 'Showing an improvement': an examination of variables central to the token economy system. (Research programme involving nursing staff on paediatric ward of a mental handicap hospital.) International Journal of Nursing Studies, 17 (1), 1980, 25-37.

4 **Barton, E.S. and others** The modification of drooling behaviour in the severely retarded spastic patient. British Journal of Mental Subnormality, 24 (2), Dec 1978, 100-108.

5 **British Journal of Mental Subnormality** Symposium on teaching methods for the severely subnormal. British Journal of Mental Subnormality, 22 (1), Jun 1976, 5-25.

6 **Bushby, S.** 'Eat your food Simon'. (Teaching a severely mentally handicapped adult how to feed himself using behaviour therapy.) Nursing Mirror, 151, 25 Sep 1980, 22-24.

7 **Bushby, S.** The reinforcers. (Training project for severely mentally handicapped patients at Leybourne Grange hospital based on behaviour therapy.) Nursing Mirror, 151, 18 Sep 1980, 18-20.

8 **Cullen, C.N.** Errorless learning with the retarded. Some procedures are described for teaching the mentally handicapped to discriminate colour, size, and weight, and for teaching them reading, writing and copying. Nursing Times, 72 (12), 25 Mar 1976, Occ. papers, 45-47.

9 **England, P.M. and others** An experiment in health education. (Using token economy therapy as part of scheme of social competence training for the mentally handicapped.) Nursing Times, 75, 30 Aug 1979, 1491-1492.

10 **Hall, S.** Behaviour therapy: a speech target for Mark. (Plan of care for high dependency mentally handicapped patient who is mute.) Nursing Mirror, 149, 20 Sep 1979, 46-48.

11 **Hegarty, J.R.** Teaching machines for the severaly retarded: a review. British Journal of Mental Subnormality, 21 (2), Dec 1975, 103-114.

12 **Hockaday, S.** Nursing care study. Kate—slow but sure progress. (Behaviour modification programme for severely subnormal woman.) Nursing Mirror, 150, 24 Apr 1980, 44-45.

13 **Jefferies, K.A.** Nursing care study. Mental subnormality. (Middle-aged mentally handicapped woman in a psychiatric hospital.) Nursing Times, 75, 25 Jan 1979, 155-157.

14 **Kirk, A.** Nursing care study. Mike—a man with tuberous sclerosis. (Long-term care of severely subnormal patient in mental handicap hospital.) Nursing Mirror, 147, 31 Aug 1978, 24-25.

15 **McCoull, K. and Gardiner, S.** Nursing care study—persistent emesis. 'Good boy, Hugh, clean mouth'. (Behaviour modification

programmes with profoundly handicapped young man.) Nursing Mirror, 149, 13 Dec 1979, 37-39.

16 May, A. Nursing care study. Hairpulling: cured by a motor cycle helmet. (Behaviour modification with mentally handicapped woman.) Nursing Mirror, 148, 7 Jun 1979, 37-38.

17 Moore, P. Behaviour modification programme (for a severely mentally retarded boy at the Bethlem Royal and Maudsley Hospital). Nursing Times, 72, 2 Sep 1976, 1356-1359.

18 Murphy, G.H. and McArdle, M. Behaviour modification with the retarded. (Treatment techniques taught in Maudsley Hospital JBCNS course.) Nursing Mirror, 146, 27 Apr 1978, 31-34.

19 Murray, A. Implementing a behaviour modification programme: (for mental subnormality patients at Ladybridge Hospital, Banff). Nursing Times, 73, 3 Feb 1977, 171-174.

20 Naylor, A. Handicap—integration or segregation? (With reference to 61-year-old lady with spastic quadriplegia and mental age of six years.) Nursing Times, 76, 25 Sep 1980, 1708-1709.

21 Nursing Times Sign language aids mentally handicapped. Nursing Times, 72, 18 Nov 1976, 1786.

22 Patrick, A.E. and Rafferty, J.A. Modifying behaviour in the institution. (Behaviour modification programme with severely mentally handicapped man.) Nursing Times, 74, 9 Nov 1978, 1840-1845.

23 Perkins, E.A. and others Helping the retarded: a systematic behavioural approach. Kidderminster: Institute of Mental Subnormality, 1976.

24 Sabulsky, D.J. Behaviourism and its application to the profoundly retarded. (How to implement behavioural programme.) Canadian Journal of Psychiatric Nursing, 20 (5), Sep/Oct 1979, 10-13.

25 Sandall, S.M. and Bailey, R.D. Makaton at the manor. (Non-verbal communications system for mentally handicapped people.) British Journal of Occupational Therapy, 43 (3), Mar 1980, 97-98.

26 Simon, G. Rewarding behaviour: toilet training programmes for the mentally handicapped. Health and Social Service Journal, 87, 25 Nov 1977, 1626.

27 Thomson, K. Tuberous sclerosis: how my daughter mirrored the facts. (Genetic disorder affecting the development of the brain and skin, with description of formation of Tuberous Sclerosis Association.) Nursing Mirror, 147, 14 Dec 1978, 30.

28 Thorpe, J.G. Time out or seclusion? (The difference between time out from positive reinforcement and seclusion, both used with the mentally handicapped.) Nursing Times, 76, 3 Apr 1980, 604.

29 Ticktum, R.J. Nursing care study. A mentally handicapped patient with manic depressive psychosis. Nursing Times, 73, 24 Feb 1977, 269-271.

30 Ulmer, R.A. On the development of a token economy mental hospital treatment program. Washington: Hemisphere Publishing Corp., 1976. (Clinical and community psychology series.)

31 Williams, C. Towards teaching communication skills: a model for use with the profoundly mentally handicapped. 2nd ed. Kidderminster: British Institute of Mental Handicap, 1980.

32 Yule, W. and Carr, J. editors Behaviour modification for the mentally handicapped. Croom Helm, 1980.

i REHABILITATION AND RECREATION

1 Baranyay, E. A lifetime of learning: a survey of further education facilities for mentally handicapped adolescents and adults. National Society for Mentally Handicapped Children, 1976.

2 British Journal of Mental Subnormality Symposium on preparing for life in the open community. British Journal of Mental Subnormality, 21 (2), Dec 1975, 61-83.

3 Brough, D. and Hooyveld, L. The role of the community O.T. in a multiprofessional psychiatric team. British Journal of Occupational Therapy, 41 (6), Jun 1978, 196-199.

4 Chisholm, I. Down on Warm Comfort Farm. (Thrift Farm near Bletchley, a training centre for the mentally handicapped.) Health and Social Service Journal, 89, 28 Sep 1979, 1242-1243.

5 Field, N. Kaboodling—don't knock it till you've tried it. (Course at St. Margaret's hospital for the mentally handicapped in Birmingham consisting of games, exercises and experiences to encourage participation and involvement.) Health and Social Service Journal, 89, 21/28 Dec 1979, 1642-1643.

6 Garioch, G. Mental health hostels—a waste of money? (For mentally handicapped adults.) Social Work Today, 9, 4 Jul 1978, 26-28.

7 Glanfield, J. Pushing out the frontiers: an adventure holiday in Devon. (For the mentally handicapped.) Social Work Today, 8, 1 Feb 1977, 16-17.

8 Health Care Evaluation Research Team The pattern of residential services for mentally handicapped people in Hampshire: implications of the current Wessex strategic policy and of implementing the recommendations made by the Development Team. Southampton: The Team, 1978.

9 Institute of Mental Subnormality Forms of rehabilitation for the mentally handicapped: proceedings of the conference, Lea Castle Hospital, 2 Jul 1975. Kidderminster: Institute of Mental Subnormality, 1977.

10 Johnson, R. Why adult training centres are failing to meet needs: the redeployment of resources to improve services for the mentally handicapped. Health and Social Service Journal, 87, 13 May 1977, 805-807.

11 Lawlor, T. and Cursley, V.F. A pocket money scheme. (Experiment at Normansfield Hospital for the mentally handicapped.) Health and Social Service Journal, 86, 29 May 1976, 983-984.

12 McKeown, R. and McKeown, C. Who can live independently at home? Assessment of mentally handicapped adults. British Journal of Occupational Therapy, 39 (4), Apr 1976, 100-101.

13 McNab, P. Community care of the mentally handicapped. 3: Educational facilities. Nursing Mirror, 146, 11 May 1978, 40-42.

14 Maxwell, J. and Parfitt, M. Village community for the mentally handicapped. (South Ockendon Hospital, Essex.) Nursing Mirror, 142, 12 Feb 1976, 68-69.

15 May, A.E. A new hostel for the mentally handicapped and its effects on social development. British Journal of Mental Subnormality, 2 (1), Jun 1976, 41-46.

16 Nea, T.F. and Doble, D.P. A programme for living. (Brunswick House, a small unit for the mentally handicapped with details of rehabilitation project.) Nursing Times, 74, 23 Mar 1978, 499-502.

17 Race, D.G. and Race, D.M. The Cherries Group Home: a beginning. HMSO, 1979.

18 Robinson, W. Aldingbourne House. Camp site for the mentally handicapped. Nursing Mirror, 143 (24), 9 Dec 1976, 58-60.

19 Spear, S. A cookery book for self-catering mentally handicapped. Journal of Human Nutrition, 34 (1), Feb 1980, 54-57.

20 Tyne, A. Residential provision for mentally handicapped adults. Social Work Today, 7 (6), 10 Jun 1976, 163-164.

j SEX

1 Craft, A. and Craft, M. Subnormality in marriage. Happiness and the quality of life among married subnormals. (Analysis of 25 couples.) Social Work Today, 7 (4), 13 May 1976, 98-101.

2 Craft, M. and Craft, A. Sex and the mentally handicapped. Routledge and Kegan Paul, 1978.

3 Lee, G.W. Sex education and the mentally retarded. National Society for Mentally Handicapped Children, 1976.

4 Lowes, L. Sex and social training: a programme for young adults. National Society for Mentally Handicapped Children, 1977.

k VOLUNTEERS

1 British Journal of Occupational Therapy Community participation in the long-stay hospital. One-to-One Day at Harperbury Hospital, Radlett, Herts. British Journal of Occupational Therapy, 39 (5), May 1976, 133-134.

2 Health and Social Service Journal The handshake that spans a gulf in the minds of men. (How Warley Hospital in Essex organised a one-to-one day to recruit volunteer help.) Health and Social Service Journal, 89, 6 Jul 1979, 826-827.

3 Health and Social Service Journal One-to-one projects. Health and Social Service Journal, 86, 17 Jul 1976, 1310-1311.

4 Limbrick, P. editor One-to-one: an experiment with community participation in long-stay hospitals. Inter-Action Advisory Service, 1976. (Inter-Action Advisory Service handbook; 51327, 52697, 58538.)

5 Nursing Times Happiness is a friend.

(Conference held by One-to-one organisation which involves the community with hospitals for the mentally handicapped.) Nursing Times, 73, 26 May 1977, 766-767.

6 Nursing Times How to organise a One-to-one project (to bring volunteers into mental

handicap hospitals). Nursing Times, 72, 25 Mar 1976, 434.

7 Nursing Times One-to-one project. (Illustrations of volunteers helping the mentally handicapped at Bromham Hospital, Bedfordshire.) Nursing Times, 72, 22 Apr 1976, 604-605.

DISEASES AND TREATMENT

82 CANCER

a GENERAL

1 **Baum, M.** Testing for cancer: the contribution that physical tests for cancer have made to accurate diagnosis and localisation. Nursing Mirror, 146, 8 Jun 1978, 21-24.

2 **British Medical Journal** Research and cancer education. (Prevention, screening and prompt diagnosis.) British Medical Journal, 1977, 1, 21 May 1977, 1302-1303.

3 **Browne, M.K.** Hodgkin's disease. Nursing Mirror, 146, 16 Feb 1978, 14.

4 **Buchanan-Davidson, D.J.** Where is that cancer? 1. Using fibroscopy for diagnosis. 2. Detection by lymphography, CAT scans, ultrasound and other techniques. Journal of Practical Nursing, 27 (11), Nov 1977, 12-15, 31; (12) Dec 1977, 22-25.

5 **Charlton, A.** Cancer and cancer education — opinions of some secondary school teachers in Northern England. (Research study.) Health Education Journal, 38 (3), 1979, 77-83.

6 **Charlton, A.** Cancer education and the young. (Preparing educational materials for use in schools.) Journal of Community Nursing, 3 (11), May 1980, 26-27.

7 **Charlton, A.** Cancer: opinions of some secondary school pupils in Northern England. International Journal of Health Education, 20 (2), 1977, 112-119.

8 **Charlton, A.** An evaluation study of two different approaches to teaching about cancer in secondary schools. International Journal of Health Education, 22 (1), 1979, 42-48.

9 **Collins, P.H.** Hodgkin's disease. Progress and problems. Journal of Practical Nursing, 26 (9), Sep 1976, 16-19, 38.

10 **Deeley, T.J.** Attitudes to cancer. SPCK, 1979.

11 **Department of Health and Social Security** Understanding cancer: a guide for the caring professions. HMSO, 1977.

12 **Elkind, A.K.** 'Can it really be cured?': what people ask nurses about cancer. International Journal of Health Education, 21 (1), 1978, 16-25.

13 **Harwood, A.** Nursing care study. Hodgkin's disease. (With patients account on p.1621-1623.) Nursing Times, 75, 20 Sep 1979, 1617-1623.

14 **Hennekens, C.H. and others** Use of permanent hair dyes and cancer among registered nurses. Lancet, 1, 30 Jun 1979, 1390-1393.

15 **Hovenden, A.L.** Hodgkin's disease. Nursing Times, 73, 29 Sep 1977, 1520-1522.

16 **Jackson, B.S. and Armenaki, D.W.** Tumor classification system. American Journal of Nursing, 76 (8), Aug 1976, 1320-1322.

17 **Lamerton, L.F.** The long search. (For a cure for cancer.) Nursing Mirror, 147, 31 Aug 1978, Supplement, viii-ix.

18 **Lewin, R.** Cancer hazards in the environment. New Scientist, 69, 22 Jan 1976, 168-169.

19 **Lowry, S.** Public cancer education. Health Education Journal, 38 (1), 1979, 23-29.

20 **Macleod, R.A.H.** Staging laparotomy in Hodgkin's disease. Nursing Mirror, 146, 16 Feb 1978, 15-17.

21 **Michielutte, R. and others** Knowledge of cancer: a cross-cultural comparison among students in the US and the UK. International Journal of Health Education, 22 (4), 1979, 242-248.

22 **Raven, R.W. editor** Outlook on cancer: (proceedings of 7th and 8th annual symposia of the Marie Curie Memorial Foundation on Cancer...) Plenum Press, 1977.

23 **Robinson, W.** The community versus cancer. Report of a one day symposium. (Women's National Cancer Control Campaign.) Nursing Mirror, 143, 7 Oct 1976, 36.

24 **Rustin, G.J.S.** Research into tumour markers. (How substances produced by tumours can now be accurately measured.) Nursing Mirror, 150, 13 Mar 1980, 41-43.

25 **Scott, R.B.** Cancer: the facts. Oxford: Oxford University Press, 1979.

26 **Smith, I.E.** Hodgkin's disease: working towards a cure for all. Nursing Mirror, 147, 7 Dec 1978, 37-39.

27 **Tiffany, R.** Oncology. Nursing Mirror, 142 (22), 27 May 1976; Nursing Care Supplement, 2, i-iv.

28 **Winters, W.D.** Viruses and cancer. (Their possible role as carcinogens.) American Journal of Nursing, 78 (2), Feb 1978, 249-253.

b NURSING

1 **Adams, A.B.** Modern management of cancer patients: a multidisciplinary approach. Hospital Progress, 58 (2), Feb 1977, 50, 52, 82.

2 **Ashton, K.** The honest art of cancer nursing. (Report of papers given at International Cancer Nursing Conference on terminal care, communication skills and community care and education.) Nursing Times, 74, 21 Sep 1978, 1551-1552; 28 Sep 1978, 1587-1588.

3 **Baldonado, A.A. and Stahl, D.A.** Cancer nursing: a holistic multidisciplinary approach. Kinipton, 1978. (Nursing outline series.)

4 **Barckley, V.** OR nurse wears cancer nurse's cap. (Role of the operating room nurse in care of the cancer patient.) AORN Journal, 23 (2), Feb 1976, 290-292, 294, 296.

5 **Barkes, P.** An American adventure. (Report of six-month exchange visit to the National Cancer Institute in Bethesda, Maryland.) Nursing Mirror, 147, 6 Jul 1978, 21-24.

6 **Barnes, J.A.** Nursing care study. Molly — terminal cancer patient. Nursing Times, 75, 21 Jun 1979, 1039-1042.

7 **Boettger, L.** Metastatic disease without a primary? (Care study of woman with metastatic adenocarcinoma in axilla who underwent surgery in search for primary growth.) Nursing Times, 75, 25 Jan 1979, 153-154.

8 **Bouchard, R. and Owens, N.F.** Nursing care of the cancer patient. 3rd ed. St. Louis: Mosby, 1976.

9 **Burkhalter, P.K. and Donley, D.L.** Dynamics of oncology nursing. New York: McGraw-Hill, 1978.

10 **Carey, R.G. and Posavac, E.J.** Holistic care in a cancer care center. (Assessment of approach at Lutheran General Hospital, Illinois, based on recognition of interdependence of the patient's physical, emotional and spiritual needs.) Nursing Research, 28 (4), Jul/Aug 1979, 213-216.

11 **Dean, C.H.** Nursing care study. Disseminated sarcoma. (Terminal care in a general ward.) Nursing Mirror, 146, 29 Jun 1978, 18-20.

12 **Dodd, M.J.** Oncology nursing case studies. New York: Medical Examination Pub.Co., 1978.

13 **Donovan, M.I. and Pierce, S.G.** Cancer care nursing. New York: Appleton-Century-Crofts, 1976.

14 **Elkind, A.K.** The nurse as health educator: the prevention and early detection of cancer. (Survey of nurses' opinions of cervical

smear test, breast self-examination and not smoking.) Journal of Advanced Nursing, 5 (4), Jul 1980, 417-426.

15 **Fisher, R.A.** The Macmillan Unit for cancer care. (A unit at Christchurch Hospital, Dorset, giving help with spiritual and social problems.) Nursing Times, 72, 15 Jan 1976, 74-75.

16 **Gray, J.C. and others** Quick cancer screen. (During nursing history-taking.) RN Magazine, 43 (1), Jan 1980, 42-50.

17 **Hennessey, S.A. and Wright, C.C.** Oncology nurse education: the first step. (Programme for community nurses.) Journal of Continuing Education in Nursing, 11 (1), Jan/Feb 1980, 24-28.

18 **Isler, C.** Delivering total care—everywhere. (Programme at a California hospital using oncology nurses to coordinate hospital and home care for cancer patients.) RN Magazine, 41 (4), Apr 1978, 59-62.

19 **Isler, C.** Emerging in cancer care. The regional ambulatory center. (Mountain States, Tumor Institute, Boise, Idaho.) RN Magazine, Feb 1977, 33-40, 42, 46.

20 **Iveson-Iveson, J.** Disease: its cause and effect—5. Neoplastic disease. (Treatment and nursing care.) Nursing Mirror, 149, 11 Oct 1979, 32-33.

21 **Joint Board of Clinical Nursing Studies** 3. Oncological nursing. Nursing Mirror, 143, 12 Aug 1976, Nursing care supplement, series 2, i-iv.

22 **Kellogg, C. and Sullivan, B.P. editors** Current perspectives in oncologic nursing. Vol.2. St. Louis: Mosby, 1978. (Mosby's current practice and perspectives in nursing series.)

23 **Koons, S.B.** The future of cancer nursing. RN Magazine, 39 (8), Aug 1976, 23, 27, 28, 32, 34.

24 **Kruglet, J.A.** Bibliography: nursing literature on cancer, 1965-1975. 1976-1978. Houston: University of Texas System Cancer Center, Research Medical Library, (n.d.) 2 vols.

25 **Lang, C.** Cancer nursing management in the Far East. (Study tour report.) Nursing Times, 72, 4 Nov 1976, 1735-1738.

26 **Law, D. and Price, B.** A developing framework for oncology nursing. (Including patient care team with research nurse and clinical nurse specialist.) Canadian Nurse, 76 (8), Sep 1980, 44-47.

27 **McClintock, E.M.** Community nursing care study. A patient with carcinomatosis nursed at home. Nursing Times, 73, 24 Mar 1977, 412-414.

28 **McKenzie, S.** The cancer care team in the community hospital. (By the oncology nursing coordinator.) Supervisor Nurse, 9 (8), Aug 1978, 17, 20-22.

29 **Moore, H.** Community nursing care study. Nine months in the life of a cancer patient. Nursing Times, 73, 13 Jan 1977, 59-60.

30 **NATIONAL Cancer Assocaition of South Africa.** International project. (Details of a study to prepare a teaching programme and manual for training cancer nurse.) S.A. Nursing Journal, 49 (1), Jan 1977, 26-27.

31 **New Zealand Nursing Journal** Cancer care overseas. Study leave to attend symposium. (Visits to Memorial Sloan Kettering Cancer Center Hospital, New York; Princess Margaret Hospital, Toronto; Royal Marsden Hospital, London, England.) New Zealand Nursing Journal, 69 (5), May 1976, 20-22.

32 **Nirenberg, A. and Rosen, G.** The day hospital: ambulatory care for the adolescent with cancer. American Journal of Nursing, 79 (3), Mar 1979, 500-504.

33 **Nursing Clinics of North America** Symposium on the nursing management of the cancer patient receiving chemotherapy. Nursing Clinics of North America, 13 (2), Jun 1978, 267-380.

34 **Nursing Mirror** Against a subtle enemy. (Supplement on aspects of research and care for cancer patients.) Nursing Mirror, 147, 31 Aug 1978, Supplement, i, iii, v, vii-viii, ix, xi, xiii.

35 **Nursing Mirror International Cancer Nursing Conference** Proceedings of the Nursing Mirror International Cancer Nursing Conference; in association with the Royal Marsden Hospital, London and Sutton. September 4th-8th, 1978. Reported in Nursing Mirror, 7 Sep 1978, 4-5; 14 Sep 1978, 4-8.

36 **Oleske, D.** Cancer prevention and nursing practice. Occupational Health Nursing, 24 (8), Aug 1976, 13-19.

37 **Parent, M.** Coping with cancer. Journal of Practical Nursing, 26 (7), Jul 1976, 34, 41.

38 **Paulen, A. and Sylvester, S.** Caring for the patient who's 'well'. (Minimal-care unit in University of Wisconsin Hospital for ambulatory cancer patients undergoing diagnostic tests and treatment.) RN Magazine, 41 (4), Apr 1978, 56-58.

39 **Peterson, B.H. and Kellogg, C.J. editors** Current practice in oncologic nursing. St. Louis: Mosby, 1976. (Mosby's current practice and perspectives in nursing series.)

40 **Rice, M.M.** JBCNS Courses, Nos. 237 and 243 in oncological nursing. Nursing Mirror, 143 (7), 12 Aug 1976, Nursing care supplement, series 2, ii-iii.

41 **Rockliff, M.** A study to investigate the nurses' opinions about the character of malignant disease and the factors (if any) that influenced these opinions. MSc thesis, Faculty of Medicine, Manchester University, Oct 1977.

42 **Rogers, J.M.** The case for a cancer nurse. (Nurse who is cancer patient describes her hospital experience and calls for post of specialist nurse to be set up.) Nursing Mirror, 151, 14 Aug 1980, 34-35.

43 **Smith, C.E.** Cancer: nursing assessment and care. New York: McGraw-Hill, 1980. (A programmed text.)

44 **Smith, E.A.** A comprehensive approach to rehabilitation of the cancer patient: a self-instructional text. New York: McGraw-Hill, 1976. (For nurses and others.)

45 **Staunton, A.** Patient care study: Carcinomatosis. Queen's Nursing Journal, 19, Aug 1976, 144.

46 **Tennell, P.** The essence of cancer nursing. Journal of Practical Nursing, 26 (7), Jul 1976, 35, 40.

47 **Tiffany, R.** Cancer education and training: nursing. Contained in: Raven, R.W. editor Outlook on cancer... Plenum Press, 1977, 109-117.

48 **Tiffany, R. editor** Cancer nursing: medical. Faber, 1978.

49 **Tiffany, R.** Cancer nursing is Nursing. (Interview with Director of Nursing at the Royal Marsden Hospital.) Nursing Mirror, 147, 31 Aug 1978, Supplement, i.

50 **Tiffany, R.** Commitment by the nurse as the foundation of cancer nursing. (With reference to the role of the clinical nurse specialist.) Journal of Advanced Nursing, 5 (4), Jul 1980, 409-416.

51 **Tiffany, R.** Nursing at the Royal Marsden. (Comment on articles by Patricia MacMillan.) Nursing Times, 76, 22 May 1980, 898.

52 **Tiffany, R. editor** Oncology for nurses and health care professionals. Allen and Unwin, 1978. Vol.1: Pathology, diagnosis and treatment. Vol.2. Care and support.

53 **United States Department of Health, Education and Welfare. Public Health Service, National Institutes of Health, Clinical Center, Nursing Department** The challenge of cancer nursing. The Department, 1976.

54 **Valencius, J.** Impact of a continuing education program in cancer nursing. 1. Results affecting patient care. 2. Results affecting the learner. Journal of Continuing Education in Nursing, 11 (2), Mar/Apr 1980, 14-18; (3), May/Jun 1980, 23-27.

55 **Wang, R. and Kelley, A.M.** Self-assessment of current knowledge of oncology nursing. New York: Medical Examination Pub.Co., 1979. (Multiple choice questions.)

56 **White, L.N. and others** Concern screening and detection manual for nurses. New York: McGraw-Hill, 1979.

57 **Wilson, M.** Nursing care study. Carcinomatosis. Nursing Times, 74, 12 Jan 1978, 56-58.

58 **Yano, B.S.** Group therapy for oncology nurses. What about us? (To give a greater understanding of the needs of the dying patient and relieve the intense psychological stress of the nurse.) Journal of Practical Nursing, 27 (3), Mar 1977, 28-29, 34, 38.

c THERAPY

1 **Andrysiak, T. and others** Marijuana for the oncology patient. (To relieve adverse side-effects of chemotherapy.) American Journal of Nursing, 79 (8), Aug 1979, 1396-1398.

2 **Baker, J.** Radiotherapy. (Symposium on gynaecological cancer.) Nursing Mirror, 143, 9 Sep 1976, 50-54.

3 **Barkes, P.** Hyperthermia in cancer treatment: some tumours don't like it hot. (Trial at National Cancer Institute, Maryland.) Nursing Mirror, 149, 2 Aug 1979, 26-28.

4 **Bingham, C.A.** The cell cycle and cancer

chemotherapy. American Journal of Nursing, 78 (7), Jul 1978, 1201-1205.

5 Breckman, B. Care of the ostomist undergoing radiotherapy and anti-tumour chemotherapy. Nursing Times, 76, 4 Sep 1980, 1568-1573.

6 Burns, N. Cancer chemotherapy: a systematic approach. Nursing, 8 (2), Feb 1978, 56-63.

7 Calman, F.M.S. Radiotherapy. (Symposium on cancer in children.) Nursing Mirror, 144, 7 Apr 1977, 56-58.

8 Carter, J. Role of the oncology nurse in regional infusion chemotherapy. AORN Journal, 25 (4), Mar 1977, 662-668.

9 Cox, S. and Wark, E. Cancer—the delivery of nursing care. 1. (Teletherapy, a type of radiotherapy.) 2. (Other forms of treatment.) Nursing Mirror, 147, 31 Aug 1978, 7-9; 7 Sep 1978, 7-11.

10 Dowd, C. Cryotherapy: cancer cells left out in the cold. (Use of liquid nitrogen for treating skin cancer.) Nursing Mirror, 149, 19 Jul 1979, 32-33.

11 Golden, S. Cancer chemotherapy and management of patient problems. Nursing Forum, 14, 1975, 278-303.

12 Gullo, S. Chemotherapy: what to do about special side-effects. (By a nurse-oncologist.) RN Magazine, 40 (4), Apr 1977, 30-32.

13 Hubbard, S. and Devita, V. Chemotherapy research nurse. (Work of a research nurse at the National Cancer Institute, Bethesda, Maryland, evaluating new drugs.) American Journal of Nursing, 76 (4), Apr 1976, 560-565.

14 Iveson-Iveson, J. IFs and buts of cancer treatment. (Interferon.) Nursing Mirror, 151, 31 Jul 1980, 34-36.

15 Law, D. Successful chemotherapy: quality care for the cancer patient. Canadian Nurse, 76 (2), Feb 1980, 19-22.

16 Leahy, I.M. and others The nurse and radiotherapy: a manual for daily care. St. Louis: Mosby, 1979.

17 Levitt, D.Z. Cancer chemotherapy: those dreaded side effects and what to do about them. RN Magazine, 43 (6), Jun 1980, 53-56; (8), Aug 1980, 57-60.

18 Lum, J.L.J. and others Nursing care of oncology patients receiving chemotherapy. (Correlation between nursing activity, patient outcome and other patient variables.) Nursing Research, 27 (6), Nov/Dec 1978, 340-346.

19 Marchant, J. Prophylactic chemotherapy following breast cancer: a personal experience. Nursing Times, 73, 7 Jul 1977, 1050.

20 Miller, S.A. Oncology nurse and chemotherapy. American Journal of Nursing, 77 (6), Jun 1977, 989-992.

21 Neidle, S. Some developments in cancer chemotherapy. Nursing Mirror, 146, 23 Mar 1978, 18-20.

22 Ostrowski, M.J. Continuous intravenous infusion of cytotoxic agents. An infusion pump

offers a fail-safe method. (Cancer chemotherapy.) Nursing Times, 75, 31 May 1979, 919-920.

23 Plant, J. Teaching hospital nurtures growth of community oncology clinics. (Primary cancer care, including drug and radiation therapy, in Boston.) Hospitals, 52 (6), 16 Mar 1978, 121-122, 126-127, 130.

24 Rapp, M.A. and others Hyperalimentation: special nutrition therapy for the cancer patient. RN Magazine, 39 (8), Aug 1976, 55-61.

25 Robbins, S.E. and Crawford, D. Nursing and the pion irradiation project. (Research to compare the effects of pion radiation and conventional X rays.) American Journal of Nursing, 76 (9), Sep 1976, 1445-1449.

26 Scott, G.M. Interferon and cancer. Journal of Community Nursing, 3 (12), Jun 1980, 4-6.

27 Scott, G.M. and Tyrrell, D.A.J. Interferon: therapeutic fact or fiction for the '80s? British Medical Journal, 280, 28 Jun 1980, 1558-1562.

28 Sikora, K. Does interferon cure cancer? British Medical Journal, 281, 27 Sep 1980, 855-858.

29 Tattersall, M.H.N. and Tobias, J.S. How strong is the case for intensive cancer chemotherapy? Lancet, 2, 13 Nov 1976, 1071-1072.

30 Tiffany, R. Cancer nursing: radiotherapy. Faber and Faber, 1979. (Cancer nursing series.)

31 Tiffany, R. Chemotherapy and the nurse. 3. Nursing care in anti-tumour drug therapy. (Royal Marsden Hospital.) Nursing Mirror, 142, 1 Apr 1976, 70-73.

32 Walter, J. Cancer and radiotherapy: a short guide for nurses and medical students. 2nd ed. Churchill Livingstone, 1977.

33 Young, P. Treatment of cancer—a progress report. (From the Cancer Research Campaign.) Nursing Mirror, 143, 25 Nov 1976, 41.

d PATIENT AND FAMILY

1 American Journal of Nursing Group approaches for cancer patients. (Three articles on use of groups for patient teaching and group therapy.) American Journal of Nursing, 79 (5), May 1979, 910-913.

2 Baker, K. Oncology support groups for out-patients. Hospital Topics, 55 (1), Jan/Feb 1977, 40-42.

3 Bond, S. Processes of communication about cancer in a radiotherapy department. PhD thesis, Edinburgh University, 1978.

4 Brewin, T.B. The cancer patient: communication and morale. British Medical Journal, 2, 24/31 Dec 1977, 1623-1627.

5 Cassileth, B.R. editor The cancer patient: social and medical aspects of care. Philadelphia: Lea and Febiger, 1979.

6 Cowper-Smith, F. Mending the broken spirit. (Cancer patients' need for information and

support.) Nursing Times, 75, 10 May 1979, 772-773.

7 Cullinan, J. Quality of life is the challenge —not quantity. (Report of Second International Cancer Nursing Conference.) Nursing Times, 76, 11 Sep 1980, 1604-1605.

8 DeWys, W.D. Changes in taste sensation and feeding behaviour in cancer patients: a review. Journal of Human Nutrition, 32 (6), Dec 1978, 447-453.

9 Downie, P.A. Cancer rehabilitation: an introduction for physiotherapists and the allied professions. Faber, 1978.

10 Few, E. 'People with cancer need a special kind of love.' (Address at symposium of the Marie Curie Memorial Foundation.) Nursing Times, 73, 26 May 1977, 762.

11 Flynn, E.D. What it means to battle cancer. (A nurse's experience.) American Journal of Nursing, 77 (2), Feb 1977, 261-262.

12 Giacquinta, B. Helping families face the crisis of cancer. American Journal of Nursing, 77 (10), Oct 1977, 1585-1588.

13 Greany, L. The Visiting Nursing Service. (Run by the Peter MacCallum Hospital to provide specialised home nursing for cancer patients.) Australian Nurses Journal, 8 (9), Apr 1979, 32-34.

14 Greer, S. Psychological consequences of cancer. Practitioner, 222, Feb 1979, 173-178.

15 Hayes, M. Waiting for diagnosis: personal experience of a nurse who was examined for breast cancer. Nursing Times, 72, 29 Jul 1976, 1175.

16 Haynes, B. Institutionalization: what happens to patients in a long term treatment center. Canadian Nurse, 76 (3), Mar 1980, 43-45.

17 Hillier, E.R. Let the patient set his own goal. (Need for staff and cancer patients to have the same aims, and methods to achieve goals by 'interventions'.) Nursing Mirror, 147, 14 Dec 1978, 40.

18 Jaffe, L. and Jaffe, A. Terminal candor and the Coda syndrome. (A married couple face a wife's imminent death from acute leukemia.) American Journal of Nursing, 76 (12), Dec 1976, 1938-1940.

19 Jennings, B.M. Blitz course for a homecoming. How the family of a critically ill woman was taught in four days to cope with the complex care they would assume at home. American Journal of Nursing, 78 (5), May 1978, 856-858.

20 Kastenbaum, B.K. and Spector, R.E. What should a nurse tell a cancer patient? (Includes statement of beliefs of Massachusetts Cancer Nurses' Group related to giving cancer patients information.) American Journal of Nursing, 78 (4), Apr 1978, 640-641.

21 Kay, E. I faced the facts—in my own time. (Patient's account of treatment for breast cancer and spine tumour who is now facing death.) Nursing Mirror, 149, 25 Oct 1979, 18-19.

22 Lamerton, R.C. Cancer patients dying at home: the last 24 hours. (Treatment, nursing care and advice to relatives.) Practitioner, 223, Dec 1979, 813-817.

23 MacInnes, C. Cancer ward. (Experiences of a cancer patient.) New Society, 36, 29 Apr 1976, 232-234.

24 McIntosh, J. Communication and awareness in a cancer ward. Croom Helm, 1977.

25 McIntosh, J. Patients' awareness and desire for information about diagnosed but undisclosed malignant disease. (Interviews with 74 patients in a Scottish teaching hospital.) Lancet, 2, 7 Aug 1976, 300-303.

26 Meares, A. Our attitude of mind in the psychological treatment of cancer. Australian Nurses Journal, 9 (7), Feb 1980, 29-30.

27 Miller, G.L. and others Assisting the psychosocial problems of cancer patients: a review of current research. International Journal of Nursing Studies, 13 (3), 1976, 161-166.

28 Naylor, V.M. Befriending the cancer patient. Liverpool: Kershaw, 1979.

29 Penson, J. Home care service for cancer patients (at the Macmillan Unit, Christchurch Hospital, Dorset.) Nursing Times, 72, 23 Sep 1976, 1492-1493.

30 Pohl, C.R. Because you care: let's talk about cancer. A rehabilitation course for families and for personnel work on an oncology unit. (At the Baptist Medical Center in Oklahoma City.) Supervisor Nurse, 9 (4), Apr 1978, 54-55.

31 Rose, M.A. Problems families face in home care. (Survey of 26 families of cancer patients.) American Journal of Nursing, 76 (3), Mar 1976, 416-418.

32 Simon, M.A.S. No one should face cancer alone — not even a nurse. (Nurse with cancer of the thyroid describes her experiences.) RN Magazine, 41 (3), Mar 1978, 79, 84, 86.

33 Stredl, D.R. Is there sex after...? (Effects of cancer of the uterus, vulva prostate and breast on sexual relations.) Journal of Practical Nursing, 26 (9), Sep 1976, 25-27, 38.

34 Strohl, R. Why your cancer patient won't eat. (Alteration of taste perception.) RN Magazine, 43 (5), May 1980, 74, 76.

35 Tiedt, E. The psychodynamic process of the oncological experience. (Emotional support of patients and relatives awaiting the outcome of cancer diagnosis.) Nursing Forum, 14 (3), 1975, 264-267.

36 Watson, P.G. Psychosocial aspects of the cancer experience. Canadian Nurse, 74 (7), Jul/Aug 1978, 45-48.

37 Winder, A.E. and Elam, J.R. Therapist for the cancer patient's family: a new role for the nurse. (Nurse therapist.) Journal of Psychiatric Nursing, 16 (10), Oct 1978, 22-27.

e SPECIFIC REGIONS

1 Beckman, J.S. For lip cancer — better results with surgery. RN Magazine, 39, Jan 1976, OR 6, 7.

2 Bibbings, J. Nursing care study. Superior vena cava obstruction. Anyone for tennis? (Malignant lymphoma of bronchus treated by radiotherapy.) Nursing Mirror, 150, 28 Feb 1980, 47-49.

3 Boxall, F.M. Theatre nursing care study. Partial cystectomy for adenocarcinoma of the bladder. (By clinical teacher.) Nursing Times, 76, 20 Mar 1980, 502-507.

4 Boyer, M.W. Treating invasive lung cancer. (Case study and tables.) American Journal of Nursing, 77 (12), Dec 1977, 1916-1923.

5 Bradley, J.E.A. Glucagonoma syndrome. (Care study of patient with tumour in the tail of the pancreas.) Nursing Times, 76, 28 Feb 1980, 370-372.

6 Carstens, G.A. Nursing care study. Osteoclastoma of cervical vertebrae. (Giant cell tumour affecting bone tissue.) Nursing Times, 73, 9 Jun 1977, 858-863.

7 Carter, R.L. How tumour cells reach bone. (Skeletal metastases.) Nursing Mirror, 147, 14 Dec 1978, 39-40.

8 Corkery, P.H. Tumours of the bone. Nursing Mirror, 146, 29 Jun 1978, 15-17.

9 Deeley, T.J. Carcinoma of the bronchus. Nursing Times, 72.
1. Incidence and aetiology. 22 Jan 1976, 98-99.
2. Symptomatology. 29 Jan 1976, 137-139.
3. Pathology. 5 Feb 1976, 185-186.
4. Treatment. 12 Feb 1976, 233-234.
5. Aftercare. 19 Feb 1976, 271-272.
6. The future. 26 Feb 1976, 314-315.

10 Falconer, W. Nursing care study. Testicular teratoma. The knitted woollen hat club... Nursing Mirror, 148, 26 Apr 1979, 41-44.

11 Fredericks, E. Cancer of the prostate and testes. Journal of Practical Nursing, 29 (3), Mar 1979, 19-23, 37, 39.

12 Gallannaugh, S.C. Tumours of bone. (Benign and malignant.) Nursing Times, 73, 27 Oct 1977, 1662-1663.

13 Garland, C. Nursing care study. Pancreatic islet cell carcinoma: an uncommon malignancy. Nursing Mirror, 149, 9 Aug 1979, 38-39.

14 Grey, A.J. Nursing care study. A new lease of life. (79-year-old man with carcinoma of the bladder who had total cystectomy and ileal conduit urinary diversion.) Nursing Times, 76, 11 Sep 1980, 1616-1620.

15 Guy, M. Nursing care study. Splenectomy. Nursing Mirror, 143, 21 Oct 1976, 59-60.

16 Hall, R.R. Carcinoma of the bladder. Nursing Times, 72, 6 May 1976, 690-692.

17 Harding, R. and Whitehouse, A. Wilms' tumour 2. Elaine: nursing care study. Nursing Mirror, 146, 1 Jun 1978, 30-32.

18 Heald, R. A staple in time saves a stoma. (Surgery in rectal cancer using stapling devices which avoid need for colostomy.) Nursing Mirror, 150, 3 Jan 1980, 30-32.

19 Hendry, W.F. Carcinoma of the kidney. (Clinical features, investigation and treatment.) Nursing Times, 73, 19 May 1977, 730-733.

20 Howat, J.M. Wilms' tumour 1. A malignant neoplasm of the immature kidney. Nursing Mirror, 146, 1 Jun 1978, 27-29.

21 Jackson, A.S. Nursing care study. A conduit for life. (Ward sister describes pre- and postoperative care of patient having cystectomy and ileal conduit for bladder carcinoma.) Nursing Times, 76, 4 Sep 1980, 1564-1567.

22 Jepsen, L. Malignant melanoma. Rare cancer, unique problems. (Treatment and nursing care.) Nursing, 7 (12), Dec 1977, 38-43.

23 Jones, E. and others Nursing care study: stay among friends for your op. (Pre- and postoperative care of elderly patient with carcinoma of the rectum in geriatric intensive care unit.) Nursing Mirror, 150, 10 Jan 1980, 42-45.

24 Lavelle, V.E. Theatre nursing care study. Cystoscopy and trans-urethral resection of a bladder tumour. NATNews, 17 (9), Sep 1980, 29-32.

25 Little, E. Nursing care study. Phaeochromocytoma. (Tumour obstructing the right kidney.) Nursing Mirror, 146, 23 Feb 1978, 21-23.

26 Maconachy, M.M. Nursing care study. The riddle of communication — 2. (Patient with carcinoma of the bronchus with metastases whose knowledge of her condition was uncertain.) Nursing Times, 75, 30 Aug 1979, 1493-1496.

27 MacDonald, D.M. Skin cancer. Nursing Times, 73, 26 May 1977, Dermatology series, 17-20.

28 MacKenzie, J. Nursing care study. Carcinomatosis from a primary bronchogenic tumour. (By Diploma in Nursing student.) Nursing Times, 75, 13 Sep 1979, 1567-1569.

29 Morrison, E. Papilloma of the bladder. Nursing Times, 72, 19 Feb 1976, 252-253.

30 Murray, B.L.S. and Wilcox, L.J. Testicular self-examination. (To detect tumours.) American Journal of Nursing, 78 (12), Dec 1978, 2074-2075.

31 Nirenberg, A. High dose methotrexate: for the patient with osteogenic sarcoma. American Journal of Nursing, 76 (11), Nov 1976, 1776-1780.

32 Pendower, J.E.H. Carcinoma of the rectum (including colostomy management). Nursing Times, 72, 19 Aug 1976, 1266-1269.

33 Poole-Wilson, P.A. Angiosarcoma of the heart. Nursing Mirror, 144, 17 Mar 1977, 55-56.

34 Raven, R.W. Carcinoma of the stomach. Nursing Times, 72, 5 Aug 1976, 1196-1197.

35 Siegler, D. The respiratory system. 7. Carcinoma of the bronchus. Nursing Mirror, 146, 26 Jan 1978, 30.

36 Stewart, S. Nursing care study. Gastroenterostomy for pyloric obstruction. Nursing Mirror, 143, 7 Oct 1976, 45-47.

37 Tanser, A.R. Types of lung cancer. Nursing Times, 73, 15 Dec 1977, 1959-1960.

38 Toy, J. Multiple myeloma. Nursing Mirror, 143, 30 Sep 1976, 50-53.

39 Trout, J.K. Nursing care study. Pituitary tumour. Nursing Times, 73, 26 May 1977, 777-779.

40 Trwoga, A. Community nursing care study. Terminal carcinoma of the lung. Nursing Times, 73, 24 Nov 1977, 1827-1828.

41 Varrow, A. and Snoad, P. Nursing care study. Carcinoma of the rectum. A staple success. (Pre- and postoperative care of patient underoing 'staple-gun' surgery.) Nursing Mirror, 150, 31 Jan 1980, 45-46.

42 Vaughan, A.B. Nursing care study. Carcinoma of the stomach. Nursing Times, 73, 1 Dec 1977, 1867-1868.

43 Venables, C.W. Carcinoma of the stomach. Nursing Times, 72, 22 Apr 1976, 613-615.

44 Washington, C.S. Surgical treatment of malignant melanoma. AORN Journal, 28 (4), Oct 1978, 734, 736, 738, 742, 744.

45 Weaver, P.C. The black cancer—malignant melanoma. Nursing Times, 72, 15 Apr 1976, 582-584.

46 Whiteford, A. Nursing care study. Whipple's pancreaticoduodenectomy. Restless nights. (Pre- and postoperative care of patient with carcinoma of the pancreas.) Nursing Mirror, 151, 17 Jul 1980, 48-50.

f BREAST CANCER

1 American Journal of Nursing Breast cancer. Confronting one's changed image. Alternative therapy. Prevention. (Eight articles on treatment, rehabilitation and prevention.) American Journal of Nursing, 77 (9), Sep 1977, 1440-1451.

2 Armstrong, K. Nursing care study. One day at a time. (Pre- and postoperative care of mastectomy patient, by SEN.) Nursing Mirror, 150, 10 Jan 1980, 20-21.

3 Baum, M. The curability of breast cancer. British Medical Journal, 1, 21 Feb 1976, 439-442.

4 Baum, M. Mastectomy: counselling removes patients' fear. (Research study in Cardiff.) Nursing Mirror, 148, 8 Mar 1979, 38.

5 Bayley, J. and others The effectiveness of registered nurses in breast self-examination. (Research study.) Australian Nurses Journal, 9 (9), Apr 1980, 42-44.

6 Bloom, J.R. and others The effect of social support on patient adjustment after breast surgery. (Research study of effect of counselling and information.) Patient Couselling and Health Education, 1 (2), Fall 1978, 50-59.

7 Brand, P.C. and Van Keep, P.A. editors Breast cancer: psychosocial aspects of early detection and treatment. Lancaster: MTP, 1978.

8 British Breast Group Screening for breast cancer. Statement by British Breast Group. British Medical Journal, 2, 15 Jul 1978, 178-180.

9 British Medical Journal Back-up for screening for breast cancer. (Leading article.) British Medical Journal, 2, 15 Jul 1978, 153.

10 Buchanan-Davidson, D. Why are some women more susceptible to breast cancer? Journal of Practical Nursing, 29 (4), Apr 1979, 15.

11 Burger, D. Breast self-examination. American Journal of Nursing, 79 (6), Jun 1979, 1088-1089.

12 Butler, A. Breast cancer. (Patients' reactions to and rehabilitation after surgery.) Canadian Nurse, 72 (6), Jun 1978, 17-22.

13 Bywaters, J.L. and Knox, E.G. The organisation of breast cancer services (in the West Midlands). Lancet, 1, 17 Apr 1976, 849-851.

14 Community Outlook A plain woman's guide to BSE. (Breast self-examination.) Nursing Times, 75, 11 Oct 1979, Community Outlook, 312-313.

15 Cox, J. Nursing care study. Breast tumour: taking the patient's point of view. (Account by mature student nurse of her feelings and action on discovering a lump in her breast.) Nursing Mirror, 148, 22 Mar 1979, 47-48.

16 Dostal, E.R. and Elder, L.E. Breast cancer: special nursing considerations. (Pre- and postoperative care and care during radiation and chemotherapy.) Journal of Practical Nursing, 29 (4), Apr 1979, 16-18, 45.

17 Downie, P.A. Post-mastectomy survey. (Breast clinic, University Hospital of South Manchester.) Nursing Mirror, 142, 25 Mar 1976, 65-66.

18 Dulcey, M.P. Addressing breast cancer's assault of female sexuality. (Physical and psychological concerns of patients.) Topics in Clinical Nursing, 1 (4), Jan 1980, 61-68.

19 Duncan, W. and Kerr, G.R. The curability of breast cancer. British Medical Journal, 2, 2 Oct 1976, 781-783.

20 Edinburgh Breast Screening Clinic Screening for breast cancer. Report from Edinburgh Breast Screening Clinic. British Medical Journal, 2, 15 Jul 1978, 175-178.

21 Elliott, R. Nursing care study. Treatment without surgery for carcinoma of the breast. Radiation treatment. Nursing Times, 76, 29 May 1980, 958-960.

22 Fitzpatrick, G. Caring for the patient with cancer of the breast. Nursing Care, 9 (1), Jan 1976, 9-18; (2), Feb 1976, 8-14; (3), Mar 1976, 16-20.

23 George, W.D. and others Hospital work load produced by breast-cancer screening programme run by trained non-medical staff. (Nurses and radiographers.) British Medical Journal, 281, 6 Sep 1980, 653-655.

24 George, W.D. and others Role of non-medical staff in screening for breast cancer. (Feasibility study using nurses and radiographers.) British Medical Journal, 280, 10 Jan 1980, 147-149.

25 George, W.D. and others Screening for breast cancer. (Study of the feasibility of mass population screening at the University Hospital of South Manchester.) British Medical Journal, 2, 9 Oct 1976, 858-860.

26 Greer, S. and others Psychological response to breast cancer: effect on outcome. (Assessment of patients' responses 3 months postoperatively and their relationship to outcome 5 years after operation.) Lancet, 2, 13 Oct 1979, 785-787.

27 Heywood Jones, I. The Mastectomy Association. Nursing Times, 75, 25 Oct 1979, 1862.

28 Hobbs, P. and others Motivation and education in breast cancer screening. (Review of recent studies.) Public Health, 91 (5), Sep 1977, 249-252.

29 Hubbard, S.M. Breast cancer: nurse's role is vital in early detection. (Risk factors, screening procedures, diagnosis and treatments.) Nursing Mirror, 147, 7 Dec 1978, 31-37.

30 Issa, M. and Yeadon, B.E. Nursing care study. Breast reconstruction. (After mastectomy. By sister in plastic surgery unit.) Nursing Times, 75, 15 Nov 1979, 1969.

31 Jenkins, H.M. Self concept and mastectomy. (Research study using Tennessee self-concept scale.) Journal of Obstetric and Gynecological Nursing, 9 (1), Jan/Feb 1980, 38-42.

32 Jones, M. Beginning research. Mastectomy. (Study of the nursing problems involved in nursing patients undergoing mastectomy.) Nursing Times, 73, 21 Apr 1977, 559-562.

33 Kaplan, I. Mastectomy complications reduced by Laser beam. Nursing Mirror, 143, 23 Sep 1976, 35.

34 Krauss, M. Nursing care study. Metastatic carcinoma of the breast. Nursing Mirror, 146, 16 Feb 1978, 20-24.

35 McDowell, P.G. and Wylie, M.E. Mastectomy and insertion of prosthesis. (Details of operation and review of psychological aspects.) Nursing Times, 76, 17 Jul 1980, 1258-1261.

36 McLoughlin, G.A. and Fox, M.C. A new mastectomy dressing. (Post-mastectomy support bandage devised by the authors, with photograph.) Nursing Times, 74, 2 Mar 1978, 377.

37 Maguire, P. and others Planning a caring programme. (Scheme in Manchester involving monitoring by nurse of social and psychological adjustment of women after mastectomy.) Nursing Mirror, 150, 17 Jan 1980, 35-37.

38 Maguire, G.P. and others Psychiatric problems in the first year after mastectomy. (Survey.) British Medical Journal, 1, 15 Apr 1978, 963-965.

39 Marchant, J. Rehabilitation of mastectomy patients: a handbook. Heinemann, 1978.

40 Marchant, J. Rehabilitation of the mastectomy patient. Nursing Times, 73, 21 Apr 1977, 564-566.

41 Mastectomy Association Practical help for mastectomy patients. (Activities and publications.) Nursing Times, 73, 19 May 1977, 753.

42 Mauldin, B. Breast reconstruction after mastectomy. AORN Journal, 31 (4), Mar 1980, 612-617.

43 Miller, S.H. and others Breast reconstruction following mastectomy. (An implantable silicone prosthesis.) AORN Journal, 25 (5), Apr 1977, 945, 948-949, 952-953, 956-957, 960.

44 Noe, B. Nursing care study. A time for reassurance. (31-year-old woman after mastectomy.) Nursing Mirror, 151, 31 Jul 1980, 40-41.

45 Nursing Pictures in nursing. Mastectomy and body image. Nursing, 16, Aug 1980, 694-695.

46 Occupational Health Reassurance on wheels. (Marks and Spencer mobile breast screening unit.) Occupational Health, 28 (3), Mar 1976, 147-150.

47 Osborne, S. Clinical nurse specialist—3. The role of the specialist in the breast unit. (At the Royal Marsden Hospital.) Nursing Times, 74, 20 Jul 1978, 1201-1202.

48 Pope, B. Reach to recovery. (Report on first European conference of self-help group for mastectomy patients.) Nursing Times, 76, 10 Jul 1980, 1203.

49 Priestman, T.J. and Baum, M. Evaluation of quality of life in patients receiving treatment for advanced breast cancer. Lancet, 1, 24 Apr 1976, 899-900.

50 Robinson, N. and Swash, I. Mastectomy: a patient's guide to coping with breast surgery. Wellingborough: Thorson, 1977.

51 Searle, C. Psychosocial aspects of mammary carcinoma. Curationis, 3 (2), Sep 1980, 12-15.

52 Seefeld, B. Breast cancer. 1. New approaches to treatment, care and counselling. 2. Prostheses and reconstructive techniques. Journal of Practical Nursing, 20 (3), Mar 1980, 27-29; (4), Apr 1980, 15-19.

53 Stevens, P. and Conkling, V. We teach breast self-examination to hospital patients. RN Magazine, 40 (1), Jan 1977, 25-31.

54 Stillman, M.J. Nursing decisions. Experiences in clinical problem solving. Series 2. Number 1. Mary E. A mastectomy patient. RN Magazine, 38 (10), Oct 1976, 31-36.

55 Stillman, M.J. Women's health beliefs about breast cancer and breast self-examination. Nursing Research, 26 (2), Mar/Apr 1977, 121-127.

56 Tait, A. and others Plan into practice. (Scheme of monitoring mastectomy patients by specialist nurse.) Nursing Mirror, 150, 24 Jan 1980, 19-21.

57 Toombs, M.E. Nursing care study. Breast cancer. (Domiciliary care following radiotherapy.) Nursing Times, 74, 16 Feb 1978, 279-280.

58 Tully, J.P. and Wagner, B. Breast cancer. Helping the mastectomy patient live life fully. (Includes preoperative teaching and nursing care during radiotherapy.) Nursing, 8 (1), Jan 1978, 18, 20-25.

59 Turnbull, E.M. Effect of basic preventive health practices and mass media on the practice of breast self-examination. (Survey measuring changes in practice following mass media coverage of Mrs Betty Ford's mastectomy.) Nursing Research, 27 (2), Mar/Apr 1978, 98-102.

60 Turner, M. Mastectomy and the health visitor's role. Health Visitor, 51 (2), Feb 1978, 44.

61 Westgate, B. Breast prostheses in the UK.

(Guide to types and suppliers.) Nursing Times, 76, 17 Jul 1980, 1262.

62 Westgate, B. Personal view. (Effects on the family after mastectomy and some breast prostheses, by a sufferer.) British Medical Journal, 280, 10 May 1980, 1184.

63 Woods, N.F. and Earp, J.A.L. Women with cured breast cancer: a study of mastectomy patients in North Carolina. (Four years after surgery.) Nursing Research, 27 (5), Sep/Oct 1978, 279-285.

g GYNAECOLOGICAL

1 Andrews, F.J. and others Cervical cancer in younger women. Lancet, 2, 7 Oct 1978, 776-778.

2 Beard, P. Nursing care study. Carcinoma of the ovary. Nursing Times, 74, 26 Jan 1978, 140-141.

3 Brindle, G. and others Cervical smears: are the right women being examined? British Medical Journal, 1, 15 May 1976, 1196-1197.

4 Brindle, G. and others Response to a mobile cervical screening unit in an industrial area of England. (Women's National Cancer Control Campaign mobile trailer visit to Salford.) Public Health, 90 (4), May 1976, 165-169.

5 Buchanan-Davidson, D.J. Cancer in women: developments in diagnosis. 1. Reproductive organs. Journal of Practical Nursing, 28 (11), Nov 1978, 21-25.

6 Cooper, W. Joining up a jigsaw. (New clues to the cause of cervical cancer.) Nursing Mirror, 149, 9 Aug 1979, 28-29.

7 Cox, S. Nursing care. (Symposium on gynaecological cancer.) Nursing Mirror, 143, 9 Sep 1976, 58-61.

8 Fitzpatrick, G. Caring for the patient with cancer of the cervix. Nursing Care, 9 (10), Oct 1976, 17-22; (11), Nov 1976, 21-25.

9 Harding, P. Colposcopy: detecting the first tumour. (Development of service at Wandle Valley Hospital.) Nursing Mirror, 148, 3 May 1979, 38-41.

10 Hildebrand, B.F. Nursing process and chemotherapy for the woman with cancer of the reproductive system. (With example of nursing care plan.) Nursing Clinics of North America, 13 (2), Jun 1978, 351-368.

11 Jackson, J. Screening in general practice: cervical cytology for higher risk women. Public Health, 93 (5), Sep 1979, 300-305.

12 Jenner, G.M. The extended role of a cervical cytology clinic. (Diagnosing minor gynaecological complaints as well as cancer.) Health Bulletin, 36 (1), Jan 1978, 19-24.

13 Jordan, J.A. Sexual activity and cervical squamous carcinoma. Nursing Mirror, 143, 7 Oct 1976, 48-49.

14 Lancet Cervical smears. When and how often? (Leading article.) Lancet, 1, 18 Jun 1977, 1297.

15 Lancet Screening for cervical cancer in young women. Lancet, 2, 11 Nov 1978, 1029-1030.

16 Nirmal, S. Cytology. (Vaginal cytology and screening for cancer.) Nursing Mirror, 145, 24 Nov 1977, 24-26.

17 Nursing Mirror A symposium on gynaecological cancer. Nursing Mirror, 143 (11), 9 Sep 1976, 45-61.

18 Spriggs, A.I. and Husain, O.A.N. Cervical smears. Policy document from the British Society for Clinical Cytology. British Medical Journal, 1, 11 Jun 1977, 1516-1518.

19 Sredl, D. Cytologic screening for cancer. Journal of Practical Nursing, 26 (4), Apr 1976, 24-26, 32.

20 Tomkinson, J.S. Carcinoma of the cervix. Nursing Times, 74, 28 Sep 1978, 1605-1607.

21 Tomkinson, J.S. Carcinoma of the vulva. Nursing Times, 72, 3 Jun 1976, 854-855.

22 Trott, P.A. Pathology and methods of screening. (Symposium on gynaecological cancer.) Nursing Mirror, 143, 9 Sep 1976, 46-48.

23 Williamson, J. Carcinoma of the body of the uterus. Nursing Times, 72, 27 May 1976, 822-823.

h HEAD, FACE AND NECK

1 Baines, A. Surgery for head and neck cancer: keeping up good appearances. (Postoperative nursing care including teaching about measures to improve cosmetic appearance.) Nursing Mirror, 149, 6 Sep 1979, 38.

2 Beveridge, S. Maxillo—facial surgery (after removal of a malignant tumour). Nursing Times, 72, 29 Jul, 1976, 1166.

3 Briggs, M. Diagnosing brain tumours. Nursing Mirror, 144, 10 Feb 1977, 65-68.

4 Carr, A.R.E. Nursing care study. A patient with cerebral tumours. Nursing Times, 73, 10 Nov 1977, 1745-1747.

5 Cook, S. Nursing decisions. Bronchogenic carcinoma: pre-op and post-op care. RN Magazine, 41 (9), Sep 1978, 83-88, 90, 92, 94, 96.

6 Daly, K.M. Oral cancer: everyday concerns. (Patient describes her experiences with advice for nurses.) American Journal of Nursing, 79 (8), Aug 1979, 1415-1417.

7 Fenner, M.L. Cancer of the tongue. Nursing Times, 74, 10 Aug 1978, 1341-1342.

8 Ford-Krauss, M. Management of patients with brain tumours. Nursing, 9, Jan 1980, 383-388.

9 Garrett, G. Left upper lobectomy for carcinoma. Nursing Times, 72 (38), 23 Sep 1976, Key clinical, 29-32.

10 Goddard, G.M. An oesophagectomy. (Nursing care study of woman patient with oesophageal carcinoma.) Nursing Mirror, 146, 18 May 1978, Nursing care supplement, i-iv.

11 Harrison, D.F.N. Nasopharyngeal carcinoma. Nursing Times, 72, 25 Nov 1976, 1835-1837.

12 Hess, J. How well I remember. (Patient's experience of a laryngectomy.) Nursing Forum, 19 (1), 1980, 94-103.

13 **Knowles, J.E.A.** Malignant disease of the mouth. Nursing Times, 72, 29 Jan 1976, 132-134.

14 **Krauss, M.** Nursing care study. A patient with an intracranial tumour. (Radiotherapy and drug treatment at the Royal Marsden Hospital, Sutton.) Nursing Times, 75, 22 Mar 1979, 481-486.

15 **Lindsay, S.** Nursing care study. Excision and repair of left cheek for fibrosarcoma. Nursing Mirror, 144, 28 Apr 1977, 48-50.

16 **Mackety, C.J.** Caring for the cancer patient who has an esophageal endoprosthesis. RN Magazine, 40 (10), Oct 1977, 51-53.

17 **Newman, M.** Nursing care study. Carcinoma of the lateral wall of the nose. Nursing Mirror, 147, 2 Nov 1978, 24-26.

18 **Smith, C.J.** Oral leukoplakia. Nursing Times, 72, 20 May 1976, 771-773.

19 **Stillman, M.J.** Nursing decisions. Series 3. Number 1. Experiences in clinical problem solving. Joseph K: A laryngectomee. (Pre- and postoperative care for patient with carcinoma of the epiglottis.) RN Magazine, 40 (11), Nov 1977, 65-72.

20 **Tierney, E.A.** Accepting disfigurement when death is the alternative. (Case study of a patient with cancer of the head and neck.) American Journal of Nursing, 75 (12), Dec 1975, 2149-2150.

21 **Wadsworth, P.V. and others** Tumours of the nose and accessory sinuses. An outline of the pre- and postoperative treatment for these uncommon tumours. Nursing Times, 75, 29 Mar 1979, 526-529.

22 **Wheeler, P.** Care of a patient with a cerebellar tumor. American Journal of Nursing, 77 (2), Feb 1977, 263-266.

i LEUKAEMIA AND CHILDHOOD CANCER

1 **Atkin, M.E.** Counselling families. (Symposium on cancer in children.) Nursing Mirror, 144, 7 Apr 1977, 62-64.

2 **Australasian Nurses Journal** Care of the child with cancer. (Three papers from a seminar for nurses.) Australasian Nurses Journal, 8 (4), Jan/Feb 1979, 12-15.

3 **Barker, S.M.** Blood cell products in the supportive care of patients with acute leukaemia. Nursing Times, 76, 24 Jan 1980, 152-154.

4 **Bremner, G.** Nursing management of childhood leukaemia. New Zealand Nursing Journal, 70 (4), Apr 1977, 12-15.

5 **Chambers, J.M.** Nursing care study. Chronic granulocytic leukaemia in blast transformation. (Radiotherapy and care in plastic isolator during acute phase of disease.) Nursing Times, 75, 8 Mar 1979, 400-403.

6 **Dennis, T.** Nursing care study. Embryonic sarcoma. A brave child loses her fight. Nursing Mirror, 149, 29 Nov 1979, 48-50.

7 **Duberley, J.D.** The adjustment of mothers to a child with leukaemia. MSc thesis, University of Manchester, Department of Nursing, Oct 1976.

8 **Fife, B.L.** Childhood cancer is a family crisis: a review. Journal of Psychiatric Nursing, 18 (10), Oct 1980, 29-34.

9 **Fochtman, D.** Leukemia in children. Pediatric Nursing, 2 (3), May/Jun 1976, 8-13.

10 **Foley, G. and McCarthy, A.M.** The child with leukemia: the disease and its treatment. American Journal of Nursing, 76 (7), Jul 1976, 1108-1110, 1112-1114.

11 **Foley, G. and McCarthy, A.M.** The child with leukemia: in a special hematology clinic. (Massachusetts General Hospital.) American Journal of Nursing, 76 (7), Jul 1976, 1115-1119.

12 **Gadsby, J.G.** Nursing care study. Acute myelomonocytic leukaemia. Nursing Times, 74, 12 Oct 1978, 1680-1683.

13 **Gleeson, C.** Nursing care study. Erythroblastic leukaemia. Parents can't accept the diagnosis. (Care of an adolescent with a fatal illness — identifying the nursing problems, the formulation and implementation of the care plan and its evaluation.) Nursing Mirror, 148, 19 Apr 1979, 34-36.

14 **Gouldstone, J.** Nursing care study. Leukaemia — to live or let die? A dilemma for the caring team. (A 20-year-old girl.) Nursing Times, 75, 31 May 1979, 914-918.

15 **Greene, T.** Current therapy for acute leukemia in childhood. Nursing Clinics of North America, 11 (1), Mar 1976, 3-19.

16 **Innes, E.M.** Leukaemia in children — progress and problems. Nursing Times, 75, 15 Mar 1979, Paediatric News, 3.

17 **Iveson-Iveson, J.** Cancer in children. (Report of one-day conference. N.B. Incorrect photographs have been used with this article.) Nursing Mirror, 146, 9 Feb 1978, 6-8.

18 **Jurk, I.** The increased responsibility of nursing staff in leukaemia management. UNA Nursing Journal, 74 (2), Mar/Apr 1976, 20-22.

19 **Karpas, A.** Leukaemia and viruses: a possible tool for prevention. (Research into cause of leukaemia.) Nursing Mirror, 148, 14 Jun 1979, 30.

20 **Kay, H.E.M.** Leukaemia in childhood. (Treatment and prognosis.) Nursing Mirror, 144, 16 Jun 1977, 15-17.

21 **Kernahan, J.** Leukaemia in childhood. Nursing Times, 72 (36), 9 Sep 1976, 1389-1391.

22 **Kikuchi, J.** An adolescent boy's adjustment to leukemia. Maternal Child Nursing Journal, 6 (1), Spring 1977, 37-49.

23 **Kikuchi, J.** Mirroring. (A clinical nurse specialist describes how leukemic children learnt about their illness by observing other children.) Canadian Nurse, 73 (3), Mar 1977, 31-33.

24 **Little, A.** Nursing care study. Childhood leukaemia. Nursing Mirror, 144, 5 May 1977, 45-47.

25 **Macfarlane, I. and Macfarlane, N.** Nursing the dying child at home. (Parents' account of care of child with leukaemia.) Nursing Times, 76, 19 Jun 1980, ABPN, 2-3.

26 **Mackay-Paterson, S. and Urbaniak, S.J.** The continuous flow cell separator. (Device to make possible the transfusion of leucocytes and platelets to leukaemia victims.) Nursing Times, 74, 30 Nov 1978, 1970-1974.

27 **Martinson, I.** The child with leukemia: parents help each other. American Journal of Nursing, 76 (7), Jul 1976, 1120-1122.

28 **Morgan, S.B.** Nursing care study. Chronic myeloid leukaemia in pregnancy. Nursing Mirror, 142 (17), 22 Apr 1976, 50-52.

29 **Nursing Mirror** Cancer in children. A guide to the pattern of care devised by the nursing staff, Royal Hospital for Sick Children, Bristol. Nursing Mirror, 146, 23 Feb 1978, 8.

30 **Nursing Mirror** Childhood cancer. (Includes leukaemia and Hodgkins Disease.) Nursing Mirror, 151, 28 Aug 1980, Supplement, i-ii, iv, viii, x-xvi, xx, xxii, xxiv-xxv, xxvi-xxxii, xxxiv.

31 **Parker, M. and Mauger, D.** Children with cancer: a handbook for families and helpers. Cassell, 1979.

32 **Peck, B.** Effects of childhood cancer on long-term survivors and their families. (Survey revealed need of families for more information, support and counselling.) British Medical Journal, 1, 19 May 1979, 1327-1329.

33 **Pochedly, C.** Nursing the child with leukaemia. (With nursing care plan.) Journal of Practical Nursing, 28 (9), Sep 1978, 16-21.

34 **Price, B.J.** Caring for the child with cancer: the nurse practitioner. (Her role in Southern Alberta Pediatric Oncology Program involving outpatient clinic and home visits.) Canadian Nurse, 75 (11), Dec 1979, 48-50.

35 **Robbins, E.** Test yourself. Leukaemia. Nursing Mirror, 143 (23), 2 Dec 1976, 64-66.

36 **SYMPOSIUM** on cancer in children. Nursing Clinics of North America, 11 (1), Mar 1976, 1-113.

37 **A SYMPOSIUM** on cancer in children. Nursing Mirror, 144, 7 Apr 1977, 47-64.

38 **Varriochio, C.G.** Nursing care during total body irradiation. (Of leukaemia patients prior to bone marrow transplantation.) American Journal of Nursing, 77 (8), Aug 1977, 1314-1317.

39 **Zimmerman, S. and others** Bone marrow transplantation. (In leukaemia. Nursing care.) American Journal of Nursing, 77 (8), Aug 1977, 1311-1315.

j OCCUPATIONAL CANCER

1 **Ackerman, A.** The death of Frank. (How co-worker's impending death affected the health of other workers and formed the basis for educational programme on cancer prevention.) Occupational Health Nursing, 25 (10), Oct 1977, 24-25.

2 **Association of Scientific, Technical and Managerial Staffs** The prevention of occupational cancer. ASTMS, 1980. (ASTMS Health and safety policy series; 3.)

3 **Bibbings, J.** Occupational health. 5. When leaving the job may be too late. (Occupational cancer and role of nurse.) Nursing Mirror, 151, 28 Aug 1980, 18-21.

4 Buchanan, W.D. Carcinogens and mutagens. (With reference to occupational cancer.) Occupational Health, 31 (9), Sep 1979, 415-421.

5 Lancet What proportion of cancers are related to occupation? Lancet, 2, 9 Dec 1978, 1238-1240.

6 Moses, M. Cancer and the workplace. American Journal of Nursing, 79 (10), Nov 1979, 1985-1988.

7 Parker, D.E. The employee and cancer chemotherapy. Occupational Health Nursing, 25 (12), Dec 1977, 22-24.

8 Phillips, M.R. The ASTMS strategy—will it work? (Review of their policy on the prevention of occupational cancer.) Occupational Health, 32 (6), Jun 1980, 309-314.

83 CARDIOVASCULAR SYSTEM

a GENERAL

1 American Journal of Nursing Programmed instruction. Patient assessment: pulses. American Journal of Nursing, 79 (1), Jan 1979, 115-132.

2 Bjeletich, J. and Hickman, R.O. The Hickman indwelling catheter. (Modification of Broviac catheter commonly used for total parenteral nutrition, used for monitoring CVP and taking blood.) American Journal of Nursing, 80 (1), Jan 1980, 62-65.

3 Bricker, P.L. The intense nursing demands of the intra-aortic balloon pump. RN Magazine, 43 (7), Jul 1980, 23-29.

4 Diethrich, E.B. editor Advances in cardiovascular nursing. (Papers presented at the 5th annual cardiovascular nursing symposium of the Arizona Heart Institute.) Bowie, Md.: Robert J. Brady, 1979.

5 Farquhar, J.W. and others Community education for cardiovascular health. (Experiment in three California towns.) Lancet, 1, 4 Jun 1977, 1192-1195.

6 Fisher, R.E. Measuring central venous pressure: how to do it accurately...and safely. Nursing (U.S.), 9 (10), Oct 1979, 74-78.

7 Gilbert, J.C. Drugs affecting the heart and blood vessels. Nursing Mirror, 143, 7 Oct 1976, 58-59.

8 GIVING cardiovascular drugs safely. Horsham: Intermed Communication, 1977. (Nursing skillbook.)

9 Graham, E. Central venous pressure. (Procedure of inserting intravenous catheter to measure CVP.) Nursing Mirror, 145, 15 Dec 1977, 22.

10 Greenwald, S.E. Assessment of blood vessel function by ultrasound. Nursing Mirror, 145, 15 Dec 1977, 23-25.

11 Hathaway, R. The Swan-Ganz catheter: a review. Nursing Clinics of North America, 13 (3), Sep 1978, 389-407.

12 Haughey, B. CVP lines: monitoring and maintaining. American Journal of Nursing, 78 (4), Apr 1978, 635-638.

13 Lalli, S.M. The complete Swan-Ganz. (Catheter to measure central venous pressure. Insertion and withdrawal procedures, dressings and maintenance.) RN Magazine, 41 (9), Sep 1978, 66-75.

14 Lamb, J. Intra-arterial monitoring: rescinding the risks. Nursing, 7 (11), Nov 1977, 65-71.

15 Mechner, F. and Brown, G.E. Patient assessment: examination of the heart and great vessels. Part 1. American Journal of Nursing, 76 (11), Nov 1976, PI 1-24.

16 Miller, K.M. Assessing peripheral perfusion. (Development of standardised scale for evaluating peripheral arterial pulse volume.) American Journal of Nursing, 78 (10), Oct 1978, 1673-1674.

17 Moore, K. and Maschak, B.J. How patient education can reduce the risks of anticoagulation. Nursing, 7 (9), Sep 1977, 24-29.

18 Moran, E. and Wilcox, P. The cardiovascular client: a teaching program. Thorofare: Slack, 1978. (For nurses.)

19 Roberts, A. Systems of life. Nursing Times 76. No.66-69. Systems and signs. The cardiovascular system. 1-4. 5 Jun 1980, (4); 3 Jul 1980, (4); 7 Aug 1980, (4); 4 Sep 1980, (4).

20 Smith, R.N. Invasive pressure monitoring. (Insertion of catheter into blood vessel, heart chamber or cerebrospinal fluid.) American Journal of Nursing, 78 (9), Sep 1978, 1514-1521.

21 Turner, P.P. The cardiovascular system. Churchill Livingstone, 1976. (Penguin Library of Nursing.)

22 Woods, S.L. Monitoring pulmonary artery pressures. (Use of the Swan-Ganz catheter.) American Journal of Nursing, 76 (11), Nov 1976, 1765-1771.

b DISEASES

1 Del Portzer, M. Geriatric cardiovascular problems. American Association of Nurse Anesthetists Journal, 44 (6), Dec 1976, 609-618.

2 Dendy, A. Nursing care study. Peripheral arterial disease: road to rehabilitation. Hospital and community care given to an elderly patient following an above-knee amputation. Nursing Mirror, 151, 21 Aug 1980, 44-45.

3 Eddy, M.E. Teaching patients with peripheral vascular disease. Nursing Clinics of North America, 12 (1), Mar 1977, 151-159.

4 Ellis, B.W. Prevention is better than cure: sepsis and central venous catheters. Nursing Times, 75, 8 Feb 1979, 248-249.

5 Fryer, J.A. Nursing care study. Right iliac artery occlusion due to atheroma. Nursing Times, 72, 5 Aug 1976, 1192-1195.

6 Harrison, M.J.G. Transient cerebral ischaemic attacks. Nursing Times, 73, 2 Jun 1977, 824-825.

7 Holland, J.M. Cardiovascular nursing: prevention, intervention and rehabilitation. Boston: Little, Brown and Co., 1977.

8 Hunt, A. Care study. A patient with a leading aortic aneurysm. (With detailed nursing care plan.) NATNews, 15 (11), Nov 1978, 36-40b.

9 Isaacson, P. Theatre nursing care study. Left femoral embolectomy. Nursing Times, 74, 5 Oct 1978, 1637-1640.

10 Jackson, B.S. Nursing decisions. Experiences in clinical problem solving. Chronic peripheral vascular disease. RN Magazine, 38, Dec 1975, 33-39.

11 Kenyon, J.R. Carotid artery stenosis and extra-cranial arterial disease. Nursing Mirror, 145, 10 Nov 1977, 23-24.

12 Laver, G.H. Nursing care study. Subacute bacterial endocarditis. Nursing Mirror, 142, 18 Mar 1976, 49-51.

13 McConnell, E.A. Fitting antiembolism stockings: how to step up your skills. Nursing, 8 (9), Sep 1978, 67-71.

14 Morris, G.K. Prevention of venous thromboembolism. A survey of methods used by orthopaedic and general surgeons. Lancet, 2, 13 Sep 1980, 572-574.

15 Nursing Clinics of North America Symposium on patients with peripheral vascular disease. Nursing Clinics of North America, 12 (1), Mar 1977, 87-168.

16 Portal, R.W. Bacterial endocarditis. Nursing Mirror, 144, 31 Mar 1977, 51-52.

17 Ream, I. Counseling patients with leg pain: a review of peripheral vascular disease. Nursing, 7 (10), Oct 1977, 54-57.

18 Riordan, S. Ultrasound in the investigation of atherosclerosis in the lower limb. (At King's College Hospital.) Nursing Mirror, 146, 30 Mar 1978, 30-31.

19 Robson, A.K. Theatre nursing care study. Aorto-femoral graft. (Insertion of bifurcation prosthesis for peripheral vascular disease.) Nursing Times, 75, 4 Jan 1979, 18-22.

20 Royal Institute of Public Health and Hygiene The problems of cardiovascular diseases. Papers presented at annual conference. Community Health, 8 (4), May 1977, 226-234.

21 Ryan, R. Thrombophlebitis: assessment and prevention. American Journal of Nursing, 76 (10), Oct 1976, 1634-1636.

22 Weir, L. Nursing care study. Lower limb ischaemia. (By first year student nurse. Includes pre- and postoperative care of amputation and terminal care.) Nursing Times, 75, 24 May 1979, 865-868.

23 Winslow, E.A. and Powell, A.H. Sick sinus syndrome. American Journal of Nursing, 76 (8), Aug 1976, 1262-1265.

c DEEP VEIN THROMBOSIS

1 Crandon, A.J. and others Postoperative deep vein thrombosis: identifying high-risk patients. (Study to assess predictive index.) British Medical Journal, 281, 2 Aug 1980, 343-344.

2 Douglas, A. Venous thrombosis and pulmonary embolism: a disease of hospitals. Nursing Mirror, 147, 26 Oct 1978, 44-46.

3 Heatley, R.V. and others Preoperative and postoperative deep vein thrombosis. Lancet, 1, 28 Feb 1976, 437-439.

4 Holford, C.P. Graded compression for preventing deep venous thrombosis (during major surgery). British Medical Journal, 2, 23 Oct 1976, 969-970.

5 Knight, M.T.N. and Dawson, R. Effect of intermittent compression of the arms on deep venous thrombosis in the legs. Lancet, 2, 11 Dec 1976, 1265-1268.

d HYPERTENSION AND HYPOTENSION

1 Aldermann, M.H. editor Hypertension: the nurse's role in ambulatory care. New York: Springer, 1977.

2 American Journal of Nursing Hypertension. (Home-study feature of five articles.) American Journal of Nursing, 80 (5), May 1980, 925-946.

3 British Medical Journal Screening for hypertension: a hospital-based home-visiting programme. (Survey in Hove with home visits by nurses.) British Medical Journal, 2, 15 Dec 1979, 1556.

4 Canadian Nurse Hypertension: pediatric hypertension—think about it. Canadian Nurse, 75 (4), Apr 1979, 32-33.

5 Conceicao, S. and others Defects in sphygmomanometers: an important source of error in blood pressure recording. British Medical Journal, 1, 10 Apr 1976, 886-888.

6 Cooper, P. Drugs for hypertension. Part 1. Midwife, Health Visitor and Community Nurse, 14 (1), Jan 1978, 22.

7 Cumming, A.M.M. Hypertension in juvenile patients. (Case presentations at International Symposium on Juvenile Hypertension in Italy in June 1979.) Nursing Times, 76, 7 Feb 1980, 245-247.

8 Daniels, L.M. and Kochar, M.S. What influences adherence to hypertension therapy. (Factors affecting patient compliance). Nursing Forum, 18 (3), 1979, 231-245.

9 Dowdall, S.A. Breathing techniques that help reduce hypertension. (Class run by nurse with ten hyperactive elderly people.) RN Magazine, 40 (10), Oct 1977, 73, 76.

10 Errico, E. Effect of cardiac monitoring on blood pressure, apical rate and respiration with and without information feedback. (Consisting of patient's receiving explanations and watching monitor.) International Journal of Nursing Studies, 14 (2), 1977, 77-90.

11 Fairchild, C. Hypertension counseling. Occupational Health Nursing, 17 (9), Sep 1979, 25-29.

12 Foster, S. and Kousch, D.C. Promoting patient adherence. (To a treatment regime for hypertension.) American Journal of Nursing, May 1978, 829-832.

13 Given, C.W. and others The association of knowledge and perception of medications with compliance and health states among hypertension patients: a prospective study. Research in Nursing Health, 1 (2), Jul 1978, 76-84.

14 Hamilton, M. The management of hypertension. Nursing Mirror, 146, 23 Mar 1978, 14-16.

15 Haslam, P. Hypertension: antihypertensives and how they work. Canadian Nurse, 75 (4), Apr 1979, 26-31.

16 Hill, M.N. Helping the hyperactive patient control sodium intake. American Journal of Nursing, 79 (5), May 1979, 906-909.

17 Hill, M.N. What can go wrong when you measure blood pressure. (Sources of error and guide to perfecting techniques.) American Journal of Nursing, 80 (5), May 1980, 942-946.

18 Hodes, C. and Rogers, P. High blood pressure and psychiatric disorder in general practice. Queen's Nursing Journal, 19 (11), Feb 1977, 302-304.

19 Horoshak, I. How RNs lower the pressure. (Hypertension screening program in New York using nurses to screen, supervise therapy and do the follow-up.) RN Magazine, 39 (1), Jan 1976, 38-41.

20 Jones, L.N. Hypertension: medical and nursing implications. Nursing Clinics of North America, 11 (2), Jun 1976, 283-295.

21 Kochar, M.S. and Daniels, L.M. Hypertension control for nurses and other health professionals. St. Louis: Mosby, 1978.

22 Lancet Measuring blood pressure. (New apparatus.) Lancet, 2, 21 Aug 1976, 409.

23 Lancour, J. How to avoid pitfalls in measuring blood pressure. American Journal of Nursing, 76 (5), May 1976, 773-775.

24 Lattimore, S. and others Is hypertension a problem in industry? (Screening and education programme for workers in a springs factory.) Occupational Health Nursing, 27 (10), Oct 1979, 19-21.

25 Logan, A.G. and others Work-site treatment of hypertension by specially trained nurses. A controlled trial. (In Toronto.) Lancet, 2, 1 Dec 1979, 1175-1178.

26 Long, M.L. and others Hypertension. What patients need to know. American Journal of Nursing, 76 (5), May 1976, 765-770.

27 McElnea, J. Hypertensive retinopathy. (Case study of nine-year-old boy by ward sister.) Nursing Times, 76, 7 Feb 1980, 244.

28 McGilloway, F. Nursing care study. Hypertension. What is to become of me? (Fictitious study of 'career' of hypertensive patient.) Nursing Mirror, 151, 11 Dec 1980, 42-43.

29 McLaughlin, F.E. and others Nurses' and physicians' performance on clinical education test: hypertension. Research in Nursing Health, 2 (2), Jun 1979, 61-72.

30 McNally, J.M. Is your number up? Ask the nurse. (A nurse conducts a high blood pressure screening program on educational administrators and support personnel in a university.) RN Magazine, 38 (12), Dec 1975, 43, 46, 48.

31 Maloney, R. Helping your hypertensive patients live longer. (Includes chart of drugs with side effects and implications for patient teaching.) Nursing, 8 (10), Oct 1978, 26-34.

32 Miller, C. and Grim, C. Personality and emotional stress measurement on hypertensive patients with essential and secondary hypertension. (Research study.) International Journal of Nursing Studies, 16 (1), 1979, 85-93.

33 Miller, C.L. and others Personality factors of the hypertensive patient. (Review of research.) International Journal of Nursing Studies, 16 (3), 1979, 235-251.

34 Milne, B. and Logan, A. Hypertension: management in industry—an expanded role for nurses. Canadian Nurse, 75 (4), Apr 1979, 21-23.

35 Mitchell, E.S. Protocol for teaching hypertensive patients. (Objects and syllabus.) American Journal of Nursing, 77 (5), May 1977, 808-809.

36 Murphy, A.J. Implications of hypertension control in the work setting. (Nurse-administered screening and follow-up programme.) Occupational Health Nursing, 25 (8), Aug 1977, 27-30.

37 North, L.W. Accuracy of sphygmomanometers. (Research study.) AORN Journal, 30 (5), Nov 1979, 996, 998, 1000, 1004.

38 O'Neill, M.F. Patients with hypertension: a study of manifest needs with self-actualization. Nursing Research, 25 (5), Sep/Oct 1976, 349-351.

39 O'Neill, M.F. A study of white males with hypertension: manifest needs and self-actualization. International Journal of Nursing Studies, 17 (2), 1980, 121-126.

40 RN Magazine Good patient compliance laid to clinic's nurses. (Care by nurse practitioners for hypertensive patients.) RN Magazine, 40 (11), Nov 1977, 9-10.

41 Roberts, A. Systems of life. No.67. Systems and signs. The cardiovascular system. 2. (Hypertension, measurement of blood pressure and factors affecting it.) Nursing Times, 76, 3 Jul 1980, (4).

42 Robinson, A.M. Detection and control of hypertension: challenge to all nurses. (Recommendations of the Task Force on Nursing in High Blood Pressure Control.) American Journal of Nursing, 72 (5), May 1976, 778-780.

43 Sackett, D.L. and others Patient compliance with antihypertensive regimens. Patient Counselling and Health Education, 1 (1), Spring 1978, 18-21.

44 Schulman, B.A. and Swain, M.A. Active patient orientation. (Study of hypertensive patients showing way to increase patients' involvement in care.) Patient Counselling and Health Education, 2 (1), First Quarter 1980, 32-37.

45 Silverberg, D.S. Seven steps to a successful hypertensive screening programme. (In Alberta, using nurses and doctors.) Canadian Nurse, 72 (10), Oct 1976, 25-26.

46 Silverberg, D.S. and others The

unsupported arm: a cause of falsely raised blood pressure readings. British Medical Journal, 2, 19 Nov 1977, 1331.

47 **Skidmore, E. and Marshall, A.** Towards a more accurate measurement of blood pressure. Nursing Times, 72, 11 Mar 1976, 376-378.

48 **Tam, G.** A comparison of two electronic sphygmomanometers with the traditional mercury type: a cost-effective study. Nursing Times, 75, 24 May 1979, 880-885.

49 **Taylor, L. and others** Divergent views of hospital staff on detecting and managing hypertension. (Survey of attitudes of doctors and qualified nurses.) British Medical Journal, 1, 17 Mar 1979, 715-716.

50 **Ward, G.W. and others** Treating and counseling the hypertensive patient. American Journal of Nursing, 78 (5), May 1978, 824-828.

51 **Wilcox, R.G.** Essential hypertension. Nursing Times, 74, 6 Apr 1978, 584-586.

52 **Wilkinson, P.R. and Raftery, E.B.** Patients' attitudes to measuring their own blood pressure. (Report of scheme with hypertensive patients at Northwick Park Hospital.) British Medical Journal, 1, 1 Apr 1978, 824.

53 **World Health** Issue on hypertension. World Health, Feb/Mar 1978, 2-35.

e VARICOSE VEINS AND ULCERS

1 **Allen, S.** A true team concept. (Teaching in varicose ulceration to health professions at the Rank Teaching Centre, Battersea Central Mission Varicose Clinic.) Nursing Mirror, 144, 3 Mar 1977, 63.

2 **Allen, S.** Varicosities and the sequelae. (Oedema, staining, eczema and ulcers.) Geriatric Medicine, 10 (7), Jul 1980, 59-62.

3 **Allen, S. and West, K.J.** Field specialists. (Two letters outlining the roles of community clinical nurse specialists in leg ulcer clinics.) Nursing Times, 74, 25 May 1978, 878.

4 **Bailey, J.L.** Leg ulcers. Nursing Times, 72, 11 Nov 1976, 1752.

5 **Bayliss, D.** Varicose ulcers: new cure for an old problem. (Trial of Synthaderm, a new plastic dressing material.) Nursing Mirror, 149, 16 Aug 1979, 34-36.

6 **Bryant, E.** Care study. One man and his leg. (Care of man with varicose ulcer by OH nurse with editorial comment on role of OH services.) Nursing Times, 76, 11 Sep 1980, Community Outlook, 271-272, 274.

7 **Burnard, K.G.** Management of varicose veins of the legs. Nursing Mirror, 144, 17 Mar 1977, 45-48.

8 **Camp, R.** Leg ulcers. (Due to increased venous pressure and other causes.) Nursing Times, 73, 25 Aug 1977, Dermatology, 25-28.

9 **Cargill, D.** How to heal leg ulcers. (Work of Stanley Allen at the Battersea Mission Varicose Clinic.) World Medicine, 15 (17), 31 May 1980, 77-78.

10 **Chant, A.D.B. and Callaghan, R.** A comparison of support bandages. (Shaped and straight Tubigrip for use during injection therapy

of varicose veins.) Nursing Times, 75, 21 Jun 1979, 1057.

11 **Community Outlook** Varicose ulcers. (Fact sheet based on visit to Dr. Stanley Allen's clinic in Battersea.) Veins at Staines. (Nurse-run clinic.) Nursing Times, 76, 14 Aug 1980, Community Outlook, 228-229, 231-232.

12 **Cysewski, A.** Nursing care study. Varicose veins and heart failure: towards a peaceful end. (Care including terminal care of elderly man.) Nursing Mirror, 148, 7 Jun 1979, 40-41.

13 **Fentem, P.H. and others** Support for varicose veins. (Comparison of support hosiery.) British Medical Journal, 1, 31 Jan 1976, 254-256.

14 **Gunn, A.D.G.** No magic cure for varicose veins and ulcers. (Review of treatment.) Journal of Community Nursing, 1 (2), Aug 1977, 4-5.

15 **Howell, R.G.** Gravitational ulcers. Nursing Times, 73, 14 Apr 1977, 516-518.

16 **Marzella, N.** A sore subject. (Review of methods of treating varicose ulcers and report of small trial by Dr. Stanley Allen's methods of Viscopaste PB7 and 4in Elastocrepe bandage.) Nursing Mirror, 151, 11 Sep 1980, Supplement, xviii, xx, xxii-xxiii, xxv-xxvi.

17 **Moore, J.** A clinic for the treatment of varicose ulcers. (Staines Health Centre.) Nursing Times, 72, 11 Nov 1976, 1756-1757.

18 **Reid, A.** Nursing care study. Varicose ulcer. Nursing Times, 72, 3 Jun 1976, 867-868.

19 **Speight, M.** Nursing care study. Healed after 41 years. (Leg ulcer treated by a district nurse.) Nursing Times, 72, 11 Nov 1976, 1754-1755.

20 **Thorne, N.** Evaluation of Debrisan in the treatment of ulceration of the lower limb. British Journal of Clinical Practitioners, 33 (9), Sep 1979, 263-265.

21 **Wilson, D.** Horses for courses at Staines. (Varicose ulcer clinic at Staines Health Centre, run by nurses.) Journal of Community Nursing, 1 (2), Aug 1977, 18-19.

22 **Zuckerman, C.** Legs to the centre. (Problems in setting up a new leg ulcers clinic.) Community View, Sep 1979, 4-5.

f CARDIAC SURGERY

1 **Bramoweth, E.** Acute aortic dissection. American Journal of Nursing, 80 (11), Nov 1980, 2010-2012.

2 **Chow, R.K.** Cardiosurgical nursing care: understandings, concepts, and principles for practice. New York: Springer, 1976.

3 **Darby, C.** Cardiac transplantation: like a miracle, like a light. (Report of visit to Stanford University Medical Center.) Nursing Mirror, 149, 5 Jul 1979, 37-39.

4 **Garrett, G.** Coronary artery bypass grafting—the nurse's role. (Procedures at Harefield Hospital, Middlesex.) Nursing Times, 73, 28 Apr 1977, 607-610.

5 **Haberman, S.** Putting a price on life. (Cost-effectiveness of heart transplants.) Health and Social Service Journal, 90, 4 Jul 1980, 877-879.

6 **Jamieson, S. and others** Cardiac transplantation: new heart, new hopes. (Description of techniques used at Stanford University Medical Center with brief history and survival rates.) Nursing Mirror, 149, 21 Jun 1979, 24-27.

7 **Linley, G.** History and techniques of heart/lung bypass. 1. Why bypass is used and how it is set up. 2. The management of the bypass. Nursing Mirror, 142, 17 Jun 1976, 52-54; 24 Jun 1976, 52-54.

8 **Lockie, E.** Heart valve transplantation (with particular reference to the homograft valve). Nursing Times, 72, 5 Aug 1976, 1190-1191.

9 **Macleod, A.** The current state of heart valve replacement. Chest, Heart and Stroke Journal, 1 (2), Summer 1976, 34-37.

10 **Terry, H.J.** Measurement of blood flow in arterial surgery. (Electromagnetic induction and ultrasonic measurement.) Nursing Times, 74, 29 Jun 1978, 1086-1089.

11 **Walker, D.R.** Surgical treatment of truncus arteriosus. Nursing Times, 72, 15 Jan 1976, 49-51.

12 **Wyatt, A.P.** Aneurysms. (Surgical techniques.) Nursing Mirror, 143, 19 Aug 1976, 52-53.

g CARDIAC SURGERY: NURSING

1 **Brewer, C.** Nursing care study. Triple coronary vein-grafts. (Revascularisation of the heart as treatment for coronary heart disease.) Nursing Times, 76, 25 Sep 1980, 1680-1693.

2 **Bryant, R.** The nursing care and management of coronary artery grafts (revised). (Update of author's previous article in Nov 1973.) Australian Nurses Journal, 8 (8), Mar 1979, 32-36.

3 **Chin, S.M.** Nursing care study. Aortic valve replacment. Nursing Times, 72, 1 Apr 1976, 489-491.

4 **Crawford, P.E. and others** Is an intermediate cardiac surgical intensive care unit really necessary? (Research study.) Heart Lung, 8 (4), Jul/Aug 1979, 685-689.

5 **Crowe, L.** Post-op care of the cineangiography patient. (Cine coronary arteriography using tracing of dye by fluoroscope and closed circuit TV.) Journal of Nursing Care, 12 (10), Oct 1979, 21.

6 **Duffield, C.S.** Theatre nursing care study. Meso-caval jump graft. (In treatment of portal hypertension.) Nursing Times, 73, 25 Aug 1977, 1314-1317.

7 **Evans, A.** Nursing management of aneurysms. (Intensive care of a patient undergoing major vascular restrictive surgery.) Nursing Mirror, 143, 19 Aug 1976, 54-55.

8 **Ford, P. and others** Historical evolution of cardiac surgical nursing. (From 1920s.) Heart Lung, 8 (5), Sep/Oct 1979, 907-912.

9 **Foster, G.A. and Hibbert, S.** Nursing care study. Transposition of the great arteries. Nursing Times, 73, 4 Aug 1977, 1193-1195.

10 **Journal of Community Nursing** Treatment trends in district nursing: heart transplants and

you. Journal of Community Nursing, 4 (6), Dec 1980, 28, 30.

11 Katz, E. Nursing care study. Femoral endarterectomy and femoro-popliteal bypass graft. (For atherosclerosis of the leg.) Nursing Times, 75, 29 Mar 1979, 530-534.

12 Lachenmyer, J. and others Cardiac transplantation: nursing—detection and teaching. (From preoperative care to discharge and long-term checks.) Nursing Mirror, 148, 28 Jun 1979, 34-36.

13 Laguea, J. and others The first 100 days of a nursing triumph. (Nursing care of heart transplant patient.) Nursing Mirror, 149, 29 Nov 1979, 19-23.

14 Luck, S. Nursing care study. A patient with right common iliac stenosis treated by aorto-iliac disobliteration. (By clinical teacher, with care plan based on Henderson's 14 components of basic nursing care.) Nursing Times, 76, 17 Apr 1980, 684-690.

15 Rakoczy, M. Waiting for cardiac surgery. (Counselling by nurse.) Canadian Nurse, 72 (10), Oct 1976, 30-31, 34-35.

16 Sadler, P.D. Nursing assessment of post-cardiotomy delirium. (Research study.) Heart Lung, 8 (4), Jul/Aug 1979, 745-750.

17 Smith, M.M. Nursing care study. Tetralogy of Fallot. (Surgery and pre- and postoperative care.) Nursing Mirror, 147, 5 Oct 1978, 25-28.

h CARDIAC SURGERY: PATIENT

1 Baum, S.S. A programme for teaching cardiac surgery patients. AORN Journal, 23 (4), Mar 1976, 591-599.

2 Brown, J.S. and others Sex differences in sick role behavior during hospitalization after open heart surgery. (Comparison of 50 male and 50 female patients.) Research in Nursing Health, 1 (1), Apr 1978, 37-48.

3 Bryant, R.B. The desirability of a pre-operative teaching programme for cardiac surgical patients. (Programme and evaluation by survey.) Australian Nurses' Journal, 6 (11), May 1977, 28-30.

4 Christopherson, L. Cardiac transplantation: need for patient counselling. Nursing Mirror, 149, 5 Jul 1979, 34-36.

5 Czerwinski, B.S. The coordinator role of the cardiovascular nurse specialist. (Discharge care for patients after coronary artery bypass surgery.) Supervisor Nurse, 9 (2), Feb 1978, 49-52.

6 Derrick, H.F. How open heart surgery feels. (Patient's account.) American Journal of Nursing, 79 (2), Feb 1979, 276-285.

7 Devlin, R. A change for life. (Interview with Paul Coffey, nurse who had heart transplant.) Nursing Mirror, 151, 3 Jul 1980, 20-22.

8 Elliott, S.M. Denial as an effective mechanism to allay anxiety following a stressful event. (Illustrated by cardiac surgery patients.) Journal of Psychiatric Nursing, 18 (10), Oct 1980, 11-15.

9 Linde, B.J. and Janz, N.M. Effect of a teaching program on knowledge and compliance of cardiac patients. (Valve replacement and coronary artery by-pass surgery.) Nursing Research, 28 (5), Sep/Oct 1979, 282-286.

10 Meyer, R.M.S. and Latz, P.A. What open heart surgery patients want to know. (Research study of patients' need for pre-discharge information and recall of teaching received.) American Journal of Nursing, 79 (9), Sep 1979, 1558-1560.

11 Swan, J.T. Coronary bypass. (Experiences of a patient undergoing open heart surgery.) American Journal of Nursing, 75 (12), Dec 1975, 2142-2145.

12 Yuille, S.R. On the other side of the sheets—a personal account of cardiac surgery. Nursing Times, 73, 28 Apr 1977, 610-611.

i CARDIAC SURGERY: CHILDREN

1 Clark, J. Kelly—an infant with heart defects. (Home nursing following surgery with completed nursing care plan.) American Journal of Nursing, 77 (11), Nov 1977, 1823-1827.

2 Cortez, A. and others The utilization of nurses in expanded roles to deliver pediatric cardiology health care. (Children's Heart program of South Texas.) Pediatric Nursing, 1 (3), May/Jun 1975, 22-29, 32.

3 D'Antonio, I.J. Mother's responses to the functioning and behaviour of cardiac children in child rearing situations. (Monograph 5.) Maternal-Child Nursing Journal, 5 (1), Winter 1976, 207-259.

4 Monro, J.L. Paediatric cardiac surgery. Physiotherapy, 63 (1), Jan 1977, 5-9.

84 CARDIAC AND CORONARY CARE

a CARDIAC DISORDERS

1 American Journal of Nursing Congenital cardiac defects. (Four articles in unit for self-study.) American Journal of Nursing, 78 (2), Feb 1978, 255-278.

2 Coulshed, N. Heart block. Nursing Times, 74, 26 Jan 1978, 149-153; 2 Feb 1978, 190-193.

3 Czerwinski, B.S. Manual of patient education for cardiopulmonary dysfunctions. St. Louis: Mosby, 1980.

4 Iveson-Iveson, J. The heart. (Anatomy and physiology.) Nursing Mirror, 148, 1 Mar 1979, 22-24.

5 Moore, P. and Garraway, M. Patients' knowledge of heart disease in general practice. Journal of the Royal College of General Practitioners, 27, Apr 1977, 221-225.

6 Robbins, E. Test yourself. Congestive cardiac failure. (Multiple choice questions.) Nursing Mirror, 143, 4 Nov 1976, 64-66.

7 Robbins, E. Test yourself. Ischaemic heart disease. Part 1. (Multiple choice questions.) Nursing Mirror, 143, 7 Oct 1976, 54-57.

8 Rose, G. and others Heart disease prevention project: a randomised controlled trial in industry. British Medical Journal, 1, 15 Mar 1980, 747-751.

9 Royal College of Physicians and **British Cardiac Society. Joint Working Party on Coronary Heart Disease** Prevention of coronary heart disease. Royal College of Physicians, 1976. (Chairman: A.G. Shaper.)

10 Thompson, D.R. Reducing the risk of sudden death from heart disease. Occupational Health, 31 (3), Mar 1979, 124-126.

11 Thornton, W.E. and Pray, B.J. Ventricular arrhythmia and thioridazine: a case report. American Journal of Nursing, 76 (2), Feb 1976, 245-246.

12 Westfall, U.E. Electrical and mechanical events in the cardiac cycle. American Journal of Nursing, 76 (2), Feb 1976, 231-235.

13 Woods, J.O. and others The prevention of coronary heart disease in general practice. (Including screening by health visitors and involvement of area health education officer and dietician.) Journal of the Royal College of General Practitioners, 30, Jan 1980, 52-57.

b CARDIAC NURSING

1 Andreoli, K.G. and others Comprehensive cardiac care: a text for nurses, physicians, and other health practitioners. 4th ed. St. Louis: Mosby, 1979.

2 Barrie-Shevlin, P. Nursing care study. The intra-aortic balloon pump in left ventricular failure. Nursing Mirror, 142, 12 Feb 1976, 48-51.

3 Benchimol, A. Noninvasive techniques in cardiology for the nurse and technician. New York: Wiley, 1978.

4 Cleeton, C.A. A nurse's guide to intra-aortic balloon assistance. (Technique used in treatment of cardiogenic shock.) Nursing Times, 74, 16 Nov 1978, 1890-1895.

5 Cogen, R. Preventing complications during cardiac catheterization. American Journal of Nursing, 76 (3), Mar 1976, 401-405.

6 Collier, P.S. and Dohoo, P.J. The intra-aortic balloon pump. (Used in cardiogenic shock.) Physiotherapy, 66 (5), May 1980, 156-157.

7 Fenton, M. Nursing care study. Ischaemic heart disease with angina pectoris. Nursing Times, 74, 27 Apr 1978, 704-705.

8 Finesilver, C. Preparation of adult patients for cardiac catheterization and coronary cine-angiography. (Research study to test the effects of information and emotional support.) International Journal of Nursing Studies, 15 (4), 1978, 211-221.

9 Finlayson, M. Catheterisation of the heart. (Nursing care during procedure based on case study.) Nursing Times, 74, 9 Nov 1978, 1835-1839.

10 Grant, J.A. Nursing care study. Endo-carditis. (Replacement of infected valve by homograft and subsequent deterioration in condition due to septicaemia.) Nursing Times, 76, 14 Feb 1980, 283-286.

11 Griffiths, M. Nursing care study. Bacterial

endocarditis. Nursing Times, 73, 10 Mar 1977, 339-341.

12 **Gronim, S.S.** Helping the client with unstable angina. American Journal of Nursing, 78 (10), Oct 1978, 1677-1680.

13 **Hayward, R.P.** Emergency care of the cardiac patient. Nursing Mirror, 144, 14 Apr 1977, 45-49.

14 **Holmwood, C.** Nursing care study. Subacute bacterial endocarditis: Louise's losing battle. Nursing Mirror, 151, 3 Jul 1980, 42-44.

15 **Jewell, S.** Nursing care study. Sub-acute bacterial endocarditis. Nursing Times, 72, 14 Oct 1976, 1593-1594.

16 **Kaiser, K.** Nursing care study. Congenital transposition of great arteries. Nursing Mirror, 147, 19 Oct 1978, 20-26.

17 **King, G. and Folger, G.M.** The nurse in the cardiac catheterization laboratory. Supervisor Nurse, 9 (9), Oct 1978, 37-38, 43-44.

18 **McIntyre, R.** Nursing care study. Ruptured aortic aneurysm. (Pre- and postoperative care of elderly man.) Nursing Mirror, 146, 4 May 1978, 32-34.

19 **Meyer, R.M.S. and Morris, D.T.** Alcoholic cardiomyopathy: a nursing approach. (Assessment during home care of nursing interventions developed to reduce the frequency of hospitalisation and improve patient's condition.) Nursing Research, 26 (6), Nov/Dec 1977, 422-427.

20 **Nursing Clinics of North America** Symposium on cardiac care. (Nine articles including cardiac pacing, resuscitation and monitoring.) Nursing Clinics of North America, 13 (3), Sep 1978, 387-530.

21 **Schreiber, L.A.** Haemodynamic monitoring in the management of cardiogenic shock in coronary care units. Curationis, 1 (2), Sep 1978, 32-35, 56.

22 **Strong, A.B.** Caring for cardiac catheterization patients. Nursing, 7 (11), Nov 1977, 60-64.

23 **Sweetwood, H.** Cardiac tamponade when dyspnea spells sudden death. RN Magazine, 43 (10), Oct 1980, 35-41.

24 **Thompson, D.** Cardiac catheterisation. (History and its uses today.) Nursing Mirror, 148, 29 Mar 1979, Supplement, i-ii, v, vii.

25 **Thompson, D.R.** Nursing care study. Supra-ventricular tachycardia. (In coronary care unit.) Nursing Mirror, 146, 5 Jan 1978, 22-23.

26 **Walker, D.R. and Sheppard, L.C.** An automated cardiac intensive care unit. Nursing Times, 72, 19 Feb 1976, 273-275.

c CARDIAC MONITORING

1 **Adler, J.** Patient assessment: abnormalities of the heartbeat. Programmed instruction. American Journal of Nursing, 77 (4), Apr 1977, PI, 1-26.

2 **Allen, F.R.** What is an E.C.G? Nursing Times, 72, 29 Jan 1976, Key Clinical, 1-4.

3 **Badura, F.K.** Nurse acceptance of a computerized arrhythmia monitoring system. (Results of surveys.) Heart Lung, 9 (6), Nov/Dec 1980, 1044-1048.

4 **Blowers, M.G. and Smith, R.J.** How to read an ECG: basic interpretation for nurses and other health workers. Revised ed. Orddell: Medical Economics Co., 1977.

5 **Bowman, G. and Priestley, B.** Refresher course. Cardiac monitoring. Nursing Times, 72, 2 Sep 1976, 1354-1355.

6 **Carlson, M.** Demystifying diagnostic procedures. Part IV: Hospital admission—EKGs. Journal of Practical Nursing, 29 (8), Aug 1979, 26-29.

7 **Etling, T. and others** Invasive monitoring of heart, circulation. AORN Journal, 23 (2), Feb 1976, 199-205.

8 **Fleming, J.S.** Interpreting the electrocardiogram. Update Books, 1979.

9 **Fontaine, G. and others** The essentials of cardiac pacing. Heinemann/Cedig, 1976. (For nurses and others.)

10 **Hammond, C.** Plain talk about cardiac monitors. RN Magazine, 42 (9), Sep 1979, 35-43.

11 **Hampton, J.R.** The E.C.G. made easy. 2nd ed. Edinburgh: Churchill Livingstone, 1980.

12 **Hurber, P.** Nurses' guide to cardiac monitoring. 3rd ed. Baillière Tindall, 1980.

13 **Miller, J. and others** Charting v computers in a postoperative cardiothoracic ITU. (Computer-assisted monitoring of patients at the Westminster Hospital.) Nursing Times, 74, 24 Aug 1978, 1423-1425.

14 **Schamroth, L.** An introduction to electrocardiography. 5th ed. Oxford: Blackwell Scientific, 1976.

15 **Schroeder, J.S. and Daily, E.K.** Techniques in bedside hemodynamic monitoring. St. Louis: Mosby, 1976.

16 **Sweetwood, H.M.** Evaluation of cardiac arrhythmias. (With illustrations of ECG tracings.) Nurse Practitioner, 3 (2), Mar/Apr 1978, 12-22.

17 **Thompson, D.R.** Introduction to ECG. Nursing Mirror, 147, 7 Sep 1978, 17-21.

d CORONARY CARE

1 **Briggs, R.S. and others** The Brighton resuscitation ambulances: a continuing experiment in prehospital care by ambulance staff. (Mobile coronary care service.) British Medical Journal, 2, 13 Nov 1976, 1161-1165.

2 **Chamberlain, D.A. and Williams, J.H.** The Brighton experiment: an appraisal of a coronary ambulance system. Health Magazine, 12 (3), Autumn 1975, 11-15.

3 **Cochrane, A.M.G. and others** Analysis of time intervals involved in admission to a coronary care unit. (From the onset of symptoms the media 'total delay' was 3 hours 30 minutes.) Journal of the Royal College of General Practitioners, 26, Sep 1976, 648-653.

4 **Colling, A. and others** Home or hospital care for coronary thrombosis? (Working paper and discussion.) British Medical Journal, 1, 13 May 1978, 1254-1259.

5 **Farnfield, M.I.** Crisis theory in the coronary care unit. Australian Nurses Journal, 7 (6), Dec/Jan 1978, 29-31.

6 **Farquhar, J.W.** Perspectives on coronary risk. Part 1. You can cut the odds on coronary risk. RN Magazine, 40 (2), Feb 1977, 23-26.

7 **Fleming, H.A.** Nurses can give heart to the sufferers. (General discussion of causes and treatment of coronary heart disease.) Journal of Community Nursing, 2 (12), Jun 1979, 10-11.

8 **Geertsen, H.R. and others** The subjective aspects of coronary care. (Measurement by questionnaire of patient satisfaction with hospital care.) Nursing Research, 25 (3), May/Jun 1976, 211-215.

9 **Graham, P.B. and Foster, S.A.** Coronary disease. Nursing Mirror, 142, 20 May 1976, Nursing care supplement, 1, i-iv.

10 **Hamilton, W.P. and Lavin, M.A.** Decision making in the coronary care unit. 2nd ed. St. Louis: Mosby, 1976.

11 **Hampton, J.R. and Nicholas, C.** Randomised trial of a mobile coronary care unit for emergency calls. (In Nottingham.) British Medical Journal, 1, 29 Apr 1978, 1118-1121.

12 **Liversuch, A.** Mobile coronary care. (Brighton coronary ambulance service.) Nursing Times, 72, 7 Oct 1976, 1559-1560.

13 **Mackintosh, A.F. and others** The Brighton resuscitation ambulances: review of 40 consecutive survivors of out-of-hospital cardiac arrest. British Medical Journal, 1, 29 Apr 1978, 1115-1118.

14 **O'Rourke, M.F. and others** Impact of the new generation coronary care unit. (Thirty bed ward at St. Vincent's Hospital, Darlinghurst, New South Wales.) British Medical Journal, 2, 9 Oct 1976, 837-839.

15 **Rawles, J.M. and Kenmure, A.C.F.** The coronary care controversy. (Home versus hospital treatment and the value of mobile coronary care.) British Medical Journal, 281, 20 Sep 1980, 783-786.

16 **Sleet, R.** The team approach to the care of patients with coronary heart disease. General Practice Team, 56, Apr/May 1976, 1-2, 4-6, 8.

17 **Sweetwood, H.** The patient in the coronary care unit. New York: Springer, 1976.

18 **West, R.** Let not your heart be troubled. (Causes of coronary heart disease.) Nursing Mirror, 146, 12 Jan 1978, 16-18.

e CORONARY CARE NURSING

1 **Bothamley, V.A.** Coronary care in the subcontinent of India. (Development of post-basic course for trained nurses.) Nursing Times, 75, 20/27 Dec 1979, 2215-2216.

2 **Daukes, M.** Coronary care district nurse. (Specialising in continuity of care for patients with hypertension, myocardial infarction and cardiac bypass surgery.) New Zealand Nursing Journal, 71 (2), Feb 1978, 13-14.

3 **Doerr, B.C. and Jones, J.W.** Effect of

family preparation on the state anxiety level of the CCU patient. (Assessment of value of booklet of information and interview.) Nursing Research, 28 (5), Sep/Oct 1979, 315-316.

4 Dunbar, J. Perspectives on coronary risk. 2. These nurse-specialists are changing the risk picture. (Work of five nurses.) RN Magazine, 40 (2), Feb 1977, 27-32.

5 Goodland, N.L. Coronary care. 3rd ed. Bristol: Wright, 1978. (For nurses.)

6 Iveson-Iveson, J. Disease: its cause and effect. 4. Degenerative diseases. (Treatment and nursing care of coronary heart disease including myocardial infarction.) Nursing Mirror, 149, 4 Oct 1979, 30-31.

7 Leslie, J. Nutrition and diet. 4. Care of the post-coronary patient. Nursing Mirror, 145, 28 Jul 1977, 21-23.

8 Mayer, G.G. and Peterson, C.W. Theoretical framework for coronary care nursing education. American Journal of Nursing, 78 (7), Jul 1978, 1208-1211.

9 Medaglia, M. A coronary care unit implements primary nursing. (At Montreal General Hospital.) Canadian Nurse, 74 (5), May 1978, 32-34.

10 Mills, M.E. and others Effect of pulse palpation on cardiac arrhythmia in coronary care patients. Nursing Research, 25 (5), Sep/Oct 1976, 378-382.

11 O'Brien, Sister H.P. and others Coronary care 1977. (Role of coronary care units and of nurses.) Cardio-Vascular Nursing, 12 (1), Jan/Feb 1977, 1-6.

12 Pinneo, R. and Briody, M. Coronary care nursing. The best is yet to be. (With history of CCUs in USA from 1962.) Heart Lung, 8 (5), Sep/Oct 1979, 876-881.

13 Walther, V.Y. Don't let CCU duty elevate your blood pressure. (Nursing procedures.) RN Magazine, 40 (9), Sep 1977, 48-51.

14 Wicks, M.K.B. and Wicks, R.J. The coronary care unit: practical psychological aspects of specialized nursing. Journal of Nursing Education, 18 (2), Feb 1979, 20-24.

f DRUG THERAPY

1 Deberry, P. and others Teaching cardiac patients to manage medications. American Journal of Nursing, 75 (12), Dec 1975, 2191-2193.

2 Hand, J. Keeping anticoagulants under control. (How they work and nursing care implementations.) RN Magazine, 42 (4), Apr 1979, 25-29.

3 Hansen, M.S. and others Relative effectiveness of nitroglycerin ointment according to site of application. (Research study of use with patients with angina pectoris and myocardial infarction.) Heart Lung, 8 (4), Jul/Aug 1979, 716-720.

4 Hansen, S. and Woods, S.L. Nitroglycerin ointment — where and how to apply it. American Journal of Nursing, 80 (6), Jun 1980, 1122-1124.

5 Manzi, C.C. Cardiac emergency! How to use drugs and C.P.R. to save lives. (Explanation

of cardiac arrest trolley equipment and effect of drugs.) Nursing, 8 (3), Mar 1978, 30-39.

g MYOCARDIAL INFARCTION

1 Baxter, P.J. Investigating heart attacks at work. Journal of the Society of Occupational Medicine, 30 (3), Jul 1980, 109-112.

2 British Medical Journal Mobilisation after myocardial infarction. British Medical Journal, 2, 10 Sep 1977, 651-652.

3 Flood, M. and DiCiancia, P. Acute myocardial infarction. Keys to assessment and intervention. (Case study.) Journal of Practical Nursing, 26 (4), Apr 1976, 16-21.

4 Gadsby, J.G. A patient with myocardial infarction. (Care study by nursing officer.) Nursing Times, 75, 8 Nov 1979, 1941-1946.

5 Gelson, A.D.N. and others Course of patients discharged early after myocardial infarction. British Medical Journal, 1, 26 Jun 1976, 1555-1558.

6 Hampton, J. Paradox at the heart of a high speed service. (Results of experimental scheme in Nottingham using 'cardiac ambulance' with special facilities for the treatment of myocardial infarction.) Health and Social Service Journal, 88, 21 Jul 1978, 819-820.

7 Hastings, M. Nursing care study. Myocardial infarction with complications. Nursing Mirror, 146, 8 Jun 1978, 25-27.

8 Hill, J.D. and others Comparison of mortality of patients with heart attacks admitted to a coronary care unit and an ordinary medical ward. British Medical Journal, 2, 9 Jul 1977, 81-83.

9 Hill, J.D. and others A randomised trial of home-versus-hospital management for patients with suspected myocardial infarction. Lancet, 1, 22 Apr 1978, 837-841.

10 Hill, S.R. Nursing care study. Myocardial infarction: six days of uphill struggle. (Patient with supraventricular tachycardia.) Nursing Mirror, 150, 26 Jun 1980, 38-39.

11 Houser, D. Ice water for MI patients? Why not? (A study of the physiological effects of ice water on post myocardial infarction patients.) American Journal of Nursing, 76 (3), Mar 1976, 432-434.

12 Joseph, S.P. Acute myocardial infarction. (Signs and symptoms.) Nursing Times, 75, 23 Aug 1979, 1453-1454.

13 Keen, L. Current nursing management of myocardial infarction as practiced at Johannesburg Hospital. S.A. Nursing Journal, 52 (12), Dec 1975, 5-6, 8-9.

14 Kennedy, R.D. Home or hospital after a heart attack: what tips the balance? (In the elderly.) Modern Geriatrics, 8 (5), May 1978, 17-18, 20.

15 Khosla, T. and others Who is at risk of a coronary? British Medical Journal, 1977, 1, 5 Feb 1977, 341-344.

16 Larter, M.H. 'M.I. wives' need you. (Study of wives' attitudes to changes in life style after a husband's myocardial infarction.) RN Magazine, 39 (8), Aug 1976, 44-48.

17 McEwen, J. Patterns of recovery following myocardial infarction. (Research study.) Health Bulletin, 37 (5), Sep 1979, 208-213.

18 MacLean, U. and Cockshutt, A. How women cope with their menfolk's heart attacks. (Survey in Edinburgh.) New Society, 49, 26 Jul 1979, 183-185.

19 Mather, H.G. and others Myocardial infarction: a comparison between home and hospital care for patients. (Survey.) British Medical Journal, 1, 17 Apr 1976, 925-929.

20 Mayou, R. and others Attitudes and advice after myocardial infarction. (Interviews with 40 patients and relatives showed a lack of understanding of medical advice.) British Medical Journal, 1, 26 Jun 1976, 1577-1579.

21 Miller, M.K. and Lazure, L.A. Four steps for better cardiac care in the E.R. (Care plan for heart attack patient in accident and emergency department.) Nursing, 8 (8), Aug 1978, 40-42.

22 Mitchell, R.G. Nursing care study. Myocardial infarction. After the storm. (Care of patient who was brain-damaged following myocardial infarction and subsequent defibrillation.) Nursing Mirror, 150, 31 Jan 1980, 43-44.

23 Monk, S.J. Nursing care study. Acute myocardial infarction. Nursing Mirror, 143, 8 Jul 1976, 59-63.

24 Pisa, Z. Saving the victims of heart attacks. Rehabilitation, 100, Jan-Mar 1977, 36-40; WHO Chronicle, 31 (1), Jan 1977, 25-28.

25 Smith, M.V. Nursing care study. Myocardial infarction. (In an 82-year old man.) Nursing Times, 74, 27 Jul 1978, 1243-1245.

26 Tanner, G. Heart failure in the MI patient. American Journal of Nursing, 77 (2), Feb 1977, 230-234.

27 Urrows, S.T. Fluid and electrolyte balance in the patient with a myocardial infarction. Nursing Clinics of North America, 15 (3), Sep 1980, 603-615.

28 Webb, K.A. A patient with myocardial infarction. (Care in a CCU, by sister.) Nursing Times, 76, 10 Jan 1980, 74-77.

h PACEMAKERS

1 Bryant, R.B. and Waddy, J.L. The pacemaker patient and his management. Australian Nurses Journal, 4 (3), Sep 1974, 29-32, 35.

2 Kerley, J.N. A case study: pacemaker implants with general anesthesia. American Association of Nurse Anesthetists Journal, 44 (4), Aug 1976, 405-407.

3 Manwaring, M. What patients need to know about pacemakers. American Journal of Nursing, 77 (5), May 1977, 825-830.

4 Myco, F. Refresher course. Heart block. The treatment of heart block and the use of the pacemaker. Nursing Times, 73, 25 Aug 1977, 1318-1319.

5 Obendorf, L. Nursing care during pacemaker implantation. AORN Journal, 26 (4), Oct 1977, 771, 774, 776.

6 O'Brien, G.J. The nursing care of patients

with cardiac pacemakers. Nursing Times, 75, 25 Jan 1979, 147-152.

7 Sowton, E. Use of cardiac pacemakers in Britain. British Medical Journal, 2, 13 Nov 1976, 1182-1184.

8 Wall, M. Cardiac pacemaker. Nursing Mirror, 143, 2 Sep 1976, 45-47.

i PSYCHOLOGICAL PROBLEMS

1 Bragg, T.L. Psychological response to myocardial infarction. Nursing Forum, 14 (4), 1975, 383-395.

2 Cassem, N.H. and Hackett, T.P. 'Ego infarction': psychological reactions to a heart attack. Journal of Practical Nursing, 29 (10), Oct 1979, 17-20, 39.

3 Castledine, G. Psychological problems (of nursing the cardiac arrest patient). Nursing Mirror, 143 (1), 1 Jul 1976, 61.

4 Connolly, J. The person, the coronary, and the nurse. (Psychological factors in coronary heart disease.) Nursing Mirror, 142, 20 May 1976, 45-46.

5 Dean, J. Patients' reactions to a coronary care unit. Nursing Mirror, 143 (5), 29 Jul 1976, 65-66.

6 Francois, M. Nursing care study. Myocardial infarction and some of the psychological factors involved. (With review of literature including reactions of wives.) Nursing Times, 76, 4 Sep 1980, 2147-2150.

7 Hill, O. The coronary care unit. (Stress associated with myocardial infarction and intensive care.) Chest, Heart and Stroke Journal, 2 (1), Spring 1977, 34-36.

8 Koon, G.T. Patients' anxiety in coronary care unit. (Research study.) Nursing Journal of Singapore, 17 (2), Nov 1977, 58-61, 64.

9 Lethbridge, B. and others The transfer process. (From CCU to medical ward. Survey of 26 patients' reactions.) Canadian Nurse, 72 (10), Oct 1976, 39-40.

10 MacFarlane, P. The stress test. (For the cardiac patient.) Canadian Nurse, 76 (4), Apr 1980, 39-40.

11 Mayou, R. and others The psychological and social effects of myocardial infarction on wives. (Results of study of 82 wives.) British Medical Journal, 1, 18 Mar 1977, 699-701.

12 Naismith, L.D. and others Psychological rehabilitation after myocardial infarction. (Research study and suggestion that this could be done by specifically trained nurse counsellor.) British Medical Journal, 1, 17 Feb 1979, 439-446.

j RESUSCITATION

1 Abdel-Hadi, O. and others Cardiac resuscitation. (With criteria which should be fulfilled before patient over 75 is resuscitated.) Geriatric Medicine, 10 (9), Sep 1980, 78.

2 Baskett, P.J.F. and others Resuscitation teaching room in a district general hospital: concept and practice. (Using models and audio visual aids to train a wide variety of staff.) British Medical Journal, 1, 6 Mar 1976, 568-570.

3 Birmingham, J.M. Cardiac arrest equipment — a CSSD service. Nursing Times, 73, 1 Dec 1977, 1869-1871.

4 Blaylock, S. Cardiopulmonary resuscitation in emergency cardiac care. (When and how to use it.) Occupational Health, 29 (12), Dec 1977, 508-514.

5 Castledine, G. Cardiac arrest. (Winning essay in a competition.) Nursing Mirror, 143, 1 Jul 1976, 58-60.

6 Castledine, G. Student nurses' reactions to cardiac arrest. (Study of 116 nurses in Central Manchester hospitals.) Nursing Times, 72, 13 May 1976, 752-753.

7 Cochrane, G.M. Saving a life after cardiac arrest. (Diagnosis and treatment.) Nursing Mirror, 147, 13 Jul 1978, 17-20.

8 Deasy, P. and Boyington, J. Emergency resuscitation in a psychiatric hospital. Design and trial of a portable resuscitation kit for all wards. (At Middlewood Hospital, Sheffield.) Nursing Times, 75, 9 Aug 1979, 1373-1374.

9 Hart, R. What to do when you're number 1: CPR review. (Advice on resuscitation with detailed photographs.) Nursing, 8 (6), Jun 1978, 48-53.

10 Hart, R. What to do when you're number 1: a review of CPR for adults. Nursing (U.S.), 9 (2), Feb 1979, 54-59.

11 LeFort, S. Cardiopulmonary resuscitation (CPR). Step-by-Step. (With 62 photographs showing resuscitation in various situations.) Canadian Nurse, 74 (2), Feb 1978, 38-47.

12 Mackintosh, A.F. and others Hospital resuscitation from ventricular fibrillation in Brighton. (Use of resuscitation equipment in A and E departments and general wards as well as CCUs by non-medical staff including nurses.) British Medical Journal, 1, 24 Feb 1979, 511-513.

13 Occupational Health Occupational first aid. No.2. Cardiopulmonary resuscitation. Occupational Health, 30 (12), Dec 1978, Supplement, (4).

14 Peatfield, R.C. and others Survival after cardiac arrest in hospital: a ten-year experience of cardiac arrests in a district general hospital. (The Central Middlesex Hospital.) Lancet, 1, 11 Jun 1977, 1223-1225.

15 Supervisor Nurse CPR policies: the art of the possible. (Three articles on ethical and policy issues of orders to resuscitate or not.) Supervisor Nurse, 10 (8), Aug 1979, 16-18, 21-22, 25-26, 29-30.

16 Thompson, D.R. Resuscitation of patients with cardiac arrest following myocardial infarction. (Analysis of patient records in a CCU and review of research.) Nursing Times, 76, 3 Jan 1980, 36-37.

k REHABILITATION

1 Anderson, I. Advances in measurement techniques in cardiac rehabilitation. Journal of the Society of Occupational Medicine, 27 (2), Apr 1977, 63-66.

2 Comoss, P.McC. and others Cardiac rehabilitation: a comprehensive nursing approach. Philadelphia: Lippincott, 1979.

3 Dehn, M.M. and others Rehabilitation of the cardiac patient. (Five articles on exercise, patient teaching and hospital liaison.) American Journal of Nursing, 80 (3), Mar 1980, 435-450.

4 Fardy, P.S. and others Cardiac rehabilitation: implications for the nurse and other health professionals. St. Louis: Mosby, 1980.

5 Fielding, R. A note on behavioural treatment in the rehabilitation of myocardial infarction patients. British Journal of the Society of Clinical Psychologists, 19 (2), Jun 1980, 157-161.

6 Fisher, M.L. Helping acutely ill patients put out the fire. (Teaching of post myocardial infarction patient to stop smoking, based on behaviour modification.) American Journal of Nursing, 79 (6), Jun 1979, 1104-1105.

7 Garcia, R.M. Rehabilitation after myocardial infarction. New York: Appleton-Century-Crofts, 1979. (Myocardial infarction; unit 2.) (Continuing education in cardiovascular nursing; 1.)

8 Gilliland, M.McG. The Coronary Club. (Voluntary group of post-coronary patients organised by nurse.) Supervisor Nurse, 10 (3), Mar 1979, 50-51.

9 Goble, R.E.A. and others Rehabilitation in heart disease. A study following patients after myocardial infarction and brady-arrhythmias treated with artificial cardiac pacemakers. British Journal of Occupational Therapy, 39 (11), Nov 1976, 281-284; Physiotherapy, 62 (11), Nov 1976, 365-368.

10 Gomph, B. Helping them back to a normal lifestyle: a practical and effective coronary teaching and rehabilitation program. Hospital Administration in Canada, 18 (4), Apr 1976, 39-43.

11 Gulko, C.S. Rehabilitation begins in the CCU. (Nursing care and patient education.) Journal of Practical Nursing, 29 (10), Oct 1979, 21-23, 42.

12 Hughes, D.T. Successful planning and implementation of a hospital-based community self-help group for patient and community cardiac education. Hospital Topics, 58 (2), Mar/Apr 1980, 25-27.

13 Jessop, P. Stepping stones: a road to coronary rehabilitation programs. (Organisation and evaluation.) Canadian Nurse, 72 (11), Nov 1976, 18-21.

14 McCoy, P. Rehabilitation after uncomplicated myocardial infarction. (Including exercises in a class and at home.) Physiotherapy, 64 (6), Jun 1978, 183-185.

15 McGann, M. Group sessions for the families of post coronary patients. Supervisor Nurse, 7 (2), Feb 1976, 17-19.

16 Milazzo, V. A study of the difference in health knowledge gained through formal and informal teaching. (Study with coronary patients showing greater effectiveness of formal teaching.) Heart Lung, 9 (6), Nov/Dec 1980, 1079-1082.

17 Morgan, D.M. Post coronary care in the community. (Work of the Ontario Heart Foundation of counselling, education and rehabilitation.) Dimensions in Health Service, 53 (9), Sep 1976, 27, 29-30.

18 Murdaugh, C.L. Effect of nurses' knowledge of teaching-learning principles on knowledge of coronary care unit patients. (Study showing effectiveness of training nurses in teaching but also problems.) Heart Lung, 9 (6), Nov/Dec 1980, 1073-1078.

19 Naimark, B. Cardiac rehabilitation: applying the benefits of exercise. Canadian Nurse, 76 (4), Apr 1980, 41-42.

20 Newby, K. Aftercare of cardiac surgery patients. (Patient teaching including group meetings.) Nursing Times, 76, 18 Sep 1980, 1658-1660.

21 Nursing Clinics of North America Symposium on teaching and rehabilitating the cardiac patient. Nursing Clinics of North America, 11 (2), Jun 1976, 211-383.

22 Owens, J.F. and others Cardiac rehabilitation: a patient education program. (Research study to measure increase in knowledge.) Nursing Research, 27 (3), May/Jun 1978, 148-150.

23 Pozen, M.W. and others A nurse rehabilitator's impact on patients with myocardial infarction. (Patient teaching and counselling.) Medical Care, 15 (10), Oct 1977, 830-837.

24 Puksta, N.S. All about sex—after a coronary. Facts, fears and concrete recommendations. American Journal of Nursing, 77 (4), Apr 1977, 602-605.

25 Stevens, P. Our patients think we've found the better way. (Team-teaching approach in cardiac rehabilitation.) RN Magazine, 40 (7), Jul 1977, 31-36.

26 Storlie, F. Learning as a life experience: the case of the cardiac patient. (General principles of teaching and learning, with special reference to patient teaching.) Supervisor Nurse, 8 (7), Jul 1977, 61-62, 65-67, 69.

27 Topics in Clinical Nursing Two articles on sex and post-myocardial infarction patients. Topics in Clinical Nursing, 1 (4), Jan 1980, 75-89.

28 Toth, A. and Toth, S. Post-coronary patients receive group therapy. (Conducted by a cardiac teaching nurse and social service director for patients and relatives at Sisters of Charity Hospital of Buffalo, NY.) Hospital Progress, 58 (8), Aug 1977, 72-75.

29 Toth, J.C. Effect of structured preparation for transfer on patient anxiety on leaving coronary care unit. Nursing Research, 29 (1), Jan/Feb 1980, 28-34.

30 Wilson-Barnett, J. Rehabilitation for coronary patients: the nurse's role. Nursing Times, 76, 10 Apr 1980, 637-638.

31 Winslow, E.H. The role of the nurse in patient education. Focus: the cardiac patient. Nursing Clinics of North America, 1 (2), Jun 1976, 213-222.

32 Woske, M. and Kratzer, J. C.T. Cardiac Teaching. Preparing the patient for a different life. Nursing, 77 7 (5), May 1977, 10-12.

85 COMMUNICABLE DISEASES

a GENERAL AND MISCELLANEOUS.

1 Antrobus, M. 1. Best of friends? (Diseases transmitted by animals.) 2. Animals should carry a health warning. Journal of Community Nursing, 3 (7), Jan 1980, 16-18, 20; (8), Feb 1980, 4-6.

2 Aronson, S.P. Communicable disease nursing. Kimpton, 1978. (Nursing outline series.)

3 Bhandari, P. Communicable diseases. 1. Ways of communication. 4. Food poisoning. 5. Brucellosis. Midwife, Health Visitor and Community Nurse, 12 (7), Jul 1976, 223-224; 13 (4), Apr 1977, 112-116; 13 (7), Jul 1977, 220, 222.

4 Brent, L. Immunology—why bother? (Its importance in medicine in the future.) Nursing Mirror, 146, 29 Jun 1978, 28-30.

5 Castle, M. and Watkins, J. Fever: understanding a sinister sign. Nursing (U.S.), 9 (2), Feb 1979, 26-33.

6 Christie, B. Diphtheria. This killing disease must never be allowed to return. Nursing Mirror, 147, 26 Oct 1978, 47-50.

7 Clayden, G. Whooping cough: a clinical overview. Journal of Community Nursing, 1 (8), Feb 1978, 4-5, 15.

8 Cook, G.C. The spread of disease—some important problems in the latter years of the twentieth century. (Communicable diseases forming major health problems.) Royal Society of Health Journal, 97 (5), Oct 1977, 218-220.

9 Cramer, K.A. and others Botulism: nursing care in an epidemic. Nursing (U.S.), 8 (11), Nov 1978, 63-69.

10 Dharan, M. The immune system. Immunoglobulin abnormalities. American Journal of Nursing, 76 (10), Oct 1976, 1626-1628.

11 Galbraith, N.S. and others Changing patterns of communicable disease in England and Wales. 1. Newly recognised diseases. (Including Legionnaire's disease.) 2. Disappearing and declining diseases. 3. Increasing infectious diseases. British Medical Journal, 281, 9 Aug 1980, 427-430; 16 Aug 1980, 489-495; 23 Aug 1980, 546-549.

12 Galbraith, N.S. and Young, S.E.J. Communicable disease control: the development of a laboratory associated national epidemiological service in England and Wales. (The Communicable Disease Surveillance Centre.) Community Medicine, 2 (2), May 1980, 135-143.

13 Glasser, R.J. How the body works against itself...autoimmune diseases. Nursing, 7 (9), Sep 1977, 38-43.

14 Green, D. Nursing care study. Toxoplasmosis. (Infection transmitted from animals causing congenital abnormality in man.) Nursing Mirror, 144, 17 Mar 1977, 53-54.

15 Harper, J.R. Whooping cough. Nursing Times, 72, 23/30 Dec 1976, 1996-1997.

16 Harris, T.J.R. Swine vesicular disease virus. Nursing Mirror, 143, 26 Aug 1976, 52-53.

17 Hawkins, C.M. The containment of exotic diseases. (Unit at Ham Green Hospital near Bristol.) Nursing Times, 74, 31 Aug 1978, Contact, 6.

18 Hendrickse, R.G. Infectious diseases. Dysentry. Nursing Mirror, 142, 8 Jan 1976, 64-66.

19 Hunneyball, I.M. The chemistry of immune reactions for trained nurses. Nursing Mirror, 144, 19 May 1977, 16-19.

20 Iveson-Iveson, J. Disease—its cause and effect: 7. Infectious disease. (Treatment and nursing care.) Nursing Mirror, 149, 25 Oct 1979, 22-23.

21 Jamieson, W.M. Bornholm disease. Nursing Mirror, 143, 25 Nov 1976, 60-62.

22 Johnson, S.A.N. Glandular fever. Nursing Mirror, 143, 18 Nov 1976, 59-60.

23 Kneale, S.J. Q fever in Cyprus. Nursing Times, 72, 15 Jan 1976, 62-63.

24 Lamb, R. Infectious diseases. Anthrax. Nursing Mirror, 142, 5 Feb 1976, 60-64.

25 Lawrence, C. Bubonic plague—extinct disease or present danger? (With historical illustrations.) Nursing Mirror, 145, 24 Nov 1977, 13-16.

26 McQuillan, W.J. Weil's disease. Nursing Mirror, 143, 23 Sep 1976, 40-41.

27 Nysather, J.O. and others The immune system: its development and functions. American Journal of Nursing, 76 (10), Oct 1976, 1614-1616.

28 Occupational Health Tampon disease puzzles experts. Occupational Health, 32 (11), Nov 1980, 590-591.

29 O'Grady, R. and Dolan, T. Whooping cough in infancy. American Journal of Nursing, 76 (1), Jan 1976, 114-117.

30 Packer, V. Diphtheria—analysis of an outbreak. (Tower Hamlets.) Health Visitor, 49 (5), May 1976, 149-150.

31 Parker, D. Introduction immunology. Nursing Times, 74.
1. What is immunity? 4 May 1978, 744-746.
2. The cells and mechanisms underlying immune reactions. 11 May 1978, 803-805.
3. Immunological diseases. 18 May 1978, 840-842.
4. Immunology in diagnosis and treatment. 25 May 1980, 875-877.

32 Pattison, J.R. Unidentified virus infections. Nursing Mirror, 144, 21 Apr 1977, 39-40.

33 Pattison, J.R. and Scading, M.M. Virus disease. Nursing Mirror, 143 (4), 22 Jul 1976, Nursing care supplement, 10, i-iv.

34 Pilsworth, R. The control and management of communicable disease: a short guide for nurses, doctors and environmental health officers. Lewis, 1980.

35 Playfair, J.H.L. Immunology at a glance. Oxford: Blackwell Scientific, 1979.

37 RN Journal Tampon-related disease can be fatal. RN Magazine, 43 (10), Oct 1980, 21.

38 Robottom, B.M. Care of the child with whooping cough. Journal of Community Nursing, 1 (8), Feb 1978, 14-15.

39 Smith, H. Infectious diseases. Opportunistic infection. (Vulnerability to infection of patients undergoing medical treatment.) Nursing Mirror, 142, 18 Mar 1976, 57-58.

40 Stronge, J.L. Screening for bacteria in Dublin schoolgirls. Nursing Times, 72, 30 Sep 1976, 1534-1536.

41 Sugden, F.G. Infectious diseases—the role of the environmental health department. Queen's Nursing Journal, 18 (12), Mar 1976, 318-319.

42 Thomson, W. Have typhoid, will travel. Nursing Mirror, 151, 17 Jul 1980, 42-43.

43 Turner, A.C. Prevention of infected persons and animals entering the country. Nursing Times, 72 (15), 15 Apr 1976, ICNA Supplement, 28-30.

44 Watson, K.C. Botulism. Nursing Mirror, 144, 30 Jun 1977, 14-16.

45 Watson, K.C. Immunology. Nursing Mirror, 148.
1. Such an important role to play. (The immune response and cells involved.) 1 Mar 1979, 26-28.
2. All about antigens and antibodies. 8 Mar 1979, 35-37.
3. Damage from immune response. 15 Mar 1979, 40-41.
4. Immunodeficiency diseases. 22 Mar 1979, 44-45.
5. Protection against infection. 29 Mar 1979, 41-42.
6. Autoimmunity and disease. 5 Apr 1979, 42-44.
7. Why many transplants fail. 12 Apr 1978, 38-40.
8. Investigations in the laboratory. 19 Apr 1978, 30-32.

46 Young, S.E.J. Clinical aspects of some infectious diseases. Queen's Nursing Journal, 18 (12), Mar 1976, 320-321.

47 Zahra, A. Communicable diseases. World Health, Nov 1980, 3-31.

b IMMUNISATION AND VACCINATION

1 Barnes, J. Immunization in infancy. (Its effects, factors affecting policy and recommended schedules.) Royal Society of Health Journal, 99 (2), Apr 1979, 82-83.

2 Bellman, M.H. Investigation into reactions to whooping cough vaccine. (National Childhood Encephalopathy Study.) Health Visitor, 49 (7), Jul 1976, 215-216.

3 Bradney, D. The vaccine damage campaign. New Scientist, 70, 20 May 1976, 404-407.

4 Brian, V. Have jabs, will travel. (Knowledge of vaccination needed by nurse in university health service with reference to overseas travel.) Nursing Mirror, 149, 8 Nov 1979, 30-31.

5 Brian, V. The persuader and dissuader. (Role of nurse in vaccination clinic in student health service.) Nursing Mirror, 149, 15 Nov 1979, 32-33.

6 Christie, A. Geography versus jabs.

(Challenge of immunisation in developing countries.) Nursing Mirror, 148, 15 Mar 1979, 24-26.

7 Clarke, S.J. Whooping cough vaccination: some reasons for non-completion. (Survey in Leicestershire.) Journal of Advanced Nursing, 5 (3), May 1980, 313-319.

8 Clode, D. Epidemic indecisions over whether or not to vaccinate. (Debate over whooping cough vaccination.) Health and Social Service Journal, 88, 13 Jan 1978, 30-31.

9 Community Outlook Special report. Whooping cough. (Controversy over vaccination.) Nursing Times, 73, 11 Aug 1977, Community Outlook, 13-17, 19-20.

10 Cranston, L. Communicable diseases and immunizations. Canadian Nurse, 72 (1), Jan 1976, 34-40.

11 Donley, D.L. The immune system. Nursing the patient who is immunosuppressed. American Journal of Nursing, 76 (10), Oct 1976, 1619-1625.

12 Dudgeon, A. Compensation for handicaps as a result of vaccination. Midwife, Health Visitor and Community Nurse, 14 (10), Oct 1978, 341, 343, 345-346.

13 Edwards, J. and Ellis, J. Accentuate the positive. (Problems of poor uptake of immunisation with reference to study of 100 mothers.) Nursing Mirror, 150, 21 Feb 1980, 42-43.

14 Ehrengut, W. Whooping cough vaccination. Comment on report from Joint Committee on Vaccination and Immunisation. Lancet, 1, 18 Feb 1978, 370-371.

15 Joint Committee on Vaccination and Immunisation Dear Sir—Vaccination—your questions answered. Nursing Times, 73, 13 Oct 1977, Community Outlook, 75, 77-78.

16 Joint Committee on Vaccination and Immunization Review of the evidence on whooping cough vaccination. HMSO, 1977. (Chairman: Sir Charles Stuart-Harris.)

17 Joint Committee on Vaccination and Immunisation Immunisation against communicable diseases. Joint committee statement on policy. Midwives Chronicle, 90, Jul 1977, 160-161.

18 Lancet Acceptance of measles vaccine. (Effectiveness and problems of obtaining high acceptance rates.) Lancet, 2, 20 Aug 1977, 387-388.

19 Lancet Vaccination against measles. Lancet, 2, 15 Jul 1976, 132-134.

20 McKinnon, J.A. The impact of the media on whooping cough immunization. Health Education Journal, 37 (3), 1979, 198-202.

21 Mallesson, P.N. and Bennett, J.C. Whooping cough admissions to a paediatric hospital over ten years. The protective value of immunisation. (Derbyshire Children's Hospital.) Lancet, 1, 27 Jan 1977, 237-239.

22 Martin, A. The nurse and the law. A shot in the long arm. (Immunisation injections.) Journal of Community Nursing, 3 (4), Oct 1979, 6, 32.

23 Miller, C.L. Reactions to vaccines.

Midwife, Health Visitor and Community Nurse, 14 (4), Apr 1978, 100, 102.

24 Miller, C.L. Ten years of measles vaccinations. (Its advantages and hazards.) Nursing Times, 74, 14 Dec 1978, 2059-2060.

25 Parliamentary Commissioner for Administration Sixth report for session 1976-77: whooping cough vaccination. HMSO, 1977.

26 Pollard, R. Relation between vaccination and notification rates for whooping cough in England and Wales. Lancet, 1, 31 May 1980, 1180-1182.

27 Roden, A.T. and Heath, W.C.C. Effects of vaccination against measles on the incidence of the disease and on the immunity of the child population in England and Wales. Health Trends, 4 (9), Nov 1977, 69-72.

28 Royal College of Nursing. Professional Nursing Department Guidelines on immunisations. Rcn, 1977.

29 Stewart, G.T. Vaccination against whooping cough. Efficacy versus risks. Lancet, 1, 29 Jan 1977, 234-237.

30 Stuart-Harris, C. Triumphs and defeats in the control of infection by immunization. Royal Society of Health Journal, 98 (3), Jun 1978, 99-103; Reprinted in Midwives Chronicle, 92, Mar 1979, 68-73.

31 Valman, H.B. The first year of life. Contraindications to immunisation. British Medical Journal, 280, 3 May 1980, 1138-1139.

32 Wilkinson, P. and others Professional attitudes towards vaccination and immunization within the Leeds Area Health Authority. (Research study with GPs, HVs and clinic doctors.) Public Health, 93 (1), Jan 1979, 11-15.

33 Wilson, J. Some complications of immunisation. The dangerous side effects attributed to pertussis vaccine. Nursing Mirror, 144, 13 Jan 1977, 39-41.

34 World Health Issue on immunization of children. World Health, Feb-Mar 1977, 4-35.

35 World Health Organization. Regional Office for Europe Immunization programmes for children: report on a working group... Copenhagen, 1-3 Sep 1976. Copenhagen: WHO, 1977.

c CHOLERA

1 Watson, E. Cholera in Kenya. Nursing Mirror, 144, 21 Apr 1977, 62-63.

d HEPATITIS

1 American Association of Nephrology Nurses and Technicians Hepatitis B as an occupational risk for neprhology nurses and technicians. AANNT, 6, 1979 Supplement edition, i-v, 47-48.

2 Banatvala, J.E. Hepatitis updated. Nursing Mirror, 143, 23 Sep 1976, 53-57.

3 Bauer, D. Preventing the spread of hepatitis B in dialysis units. American Journal of Nursing, 80 (2), Feb 1980, 260-261.

4 British Medical Journal Immunisation

against hepatitis B. British Medical Journal, 281, 13 Dec 1980, 1585-1586.

5 Burrell, C.J. and others The Chief Scientist reports...Prevalance of antibody to hepatitis B antigen among hospital personnel. (Survey at Royal Infirmary, Edinburgh.) Health Bulletin, 34 (3), May 1976, 173-174.

6 Dent, S. Nursing care study. Amoebic hepatitis. Nursing Mirror, 143, 1 Jul 1976, 53-54.

7 Galbraith, R.M. and others Variants of chronic hepatitis. Nursing Times, 72, 3 Jun 1976, 856-857.

8 Goodwin, S. Self-interest says 'keep quiet'. (Pregnant woman who is hepatitis B carrier who was refused dental care.) Nursing Mirror, 149, 6 Dec 1979, 33-34.

9 Keck, J. and Swerhun, P. Hepatitis B and occupational risk. Canadian Nurse, 76 (11), Dec 1980, 33-35.

9 Lancet Hepatitis B vaccine. Lancet, 2, 6 Dec 1980, 1229-1230.

10 Public Health Laboratory Service Hepatitis B in retreat from dialysis units in United Kingdom in 1973. (Survey of the incidence of hepatitis since 1968.) British Medical Journal, 1, 26 Jun 1976, 1579-1581.

11 Stevens, C.E. and others Hepatitis B vaccine: immune responses in haemodialysis patients. Lancet, 2, 6 Dec 1980, 1211-1213.

12 Turner, G.C. Infectious diseases. Hepatitis: two elusive viruses. Nursing Mirror, 142, 22 Jan 1976, 54-56.

13 Vella, E.E. Updating the Australia antigen. 2. Diagnosing, treating and preventing infective hepatitis. Nursing Mirror, 144, 27 Jan 1977, 64-65; 3 Feb 1977, 62-63.

14 Waterson, A.P. and Batterson, P. Viral hepatitis. NATNews, 14 (1), Jan 1977, 8-9.

15 Zuckerman, A.J. Hepatitis-B vaccine: safety criteria and non-B infection. Lancet, 1, 26 Jun 1976, 1396-1397.

16 Zuckerman, A.J. Viral hepatitis: the risk to police personnel. (From handling the contaminated syringes and needles of drug addicts.) Practitioner, 219, Sep 1977, 379-380.

e LEPROSY

1 Browne, S.G. Leprosy in Britain. Nursing Times, 73, 27 Oct 1977, 1667-1669.

2 Browne, S.G. Leprosy: new hope and continuing challenge. Revised ed. Leprosy Mission, 1977.

3 Communicable Disease Surveillance Centre Leprosy in England and Wales, 1951-79. British Medical Journal, 280, 5 Apr 1980, 1026.

4 Department of Health and Social Security and Welsh Office Memorandum on leprosy. HMSO, 1977.

5 Maitland, J. Leprosy today. A worldwide attack on leprosy has recently been launched. Nursing Times, 75, 11 Jan 1979, 68-69.

6 Noussitou, F.M. and others Leprosy in

children. Geneva: World Health Organization, 1976.

7 Nursing Mirror A symposium on leprosy. Nursing Mirror, 142, 4 Mar 1976, 47-61. Includes: Browne, S.G. The nurse's job in leprosy, 48-50; Ledger, J. Nursing care in leprosy, 51-52.

8 Sansarricq, H. Into battle against leprosy. World Health, Jul 1976, 26-29.

9 World Health Organization A guide to leprosy control. Geneva: WHO, 1980.

f MALARIA

1 Ellis, C. Keeping watch for a hidden danger. (Malaria.) Nursing Mirror, 149, 25 Oct 1979, 42-43.

2 Kouznetsov, R.L. Malaria control—benefits of past activities in tropical Africa. WHO Chronicle, 31 (93), Mar 1977, 98-101.

3 Lyster, A. Nursing care study. Malaria. Nursing Times, 72, 18 Nov 1976, 1796-1799.

4 Ree, G.H. Malaria. Nursing Times, 73, 2 Jun 1977, 826-829.

g RABIES

1 Aoki, F.Y. Rabies vaccines. Nursing Times, 72, 13 May 1976, 728-731.

2 Bhandari, P. Communicable diseases. 2. Rabies. Midwife, Health Visitor and Community Nurse, 12 (9), Sep 1976, 291-292.

3 Cohen, S.L. and others A case of rabies in man: some problems in diagnosis and management. British Medical Journal, 1, 1 May 1976, 1041-1042.

4 Department of Health and Social Security and Welsh Office Memorandum on rabies. HMSO, 1977.

5 Dunlop, J.M. 'A hair of the dog'. (Rabies.) Journal of the Royal College of General Practitioners, 28, May 1978, 293-296.

6 Dunlop, J.M. A 'missing link' in the spread of rabies. Public Health, 91 (1), Jan 1977, 11-12.

7 Gamet, A. Prevention of rabies in man. Nursing Times, 72, 13 May 1976, 727-728.

8 Gardner, S.D. Prevention of rabies in man. Health Trends, 9 (2), May 1977, 35-38.

9 Gode, G.R. and others Intensive care in rabies therapy. Clinical observations. Lancet, 2, 3 Jul 1976, 6-8.

10 Heath, R.B. Rabies. Human disease and vaccination. Royal Society of Health Journal, 96 (4), Aug 1976, 160-163.

11 Leaning, J. Post-exposure treatment for rabies. Nursing Times, 73, 17 Mar 1977, 372-378.

12 Office of Health Economics Rabies. The Office, 1976. (Studies of current health problems, no.56.)

13 Robertson, S. Nursing care study. Rabies. (University College Hospital, Intensive Care Unit.) Nursing Times, 73, 17 Mar 1977, 372-376.)

14 Threlkeld, J.M. Rabies. Government legislation and control measures. Royal Society of Health Journal, 96 (4), Aug 1976, 156-157.

15 Vella, E.C. Research into rabies. Nursing Times, 73, 17 Mar 1977, 370-371.

16 West, G. Rabies—topical questions answered. Nursing Mirror, 143, 19 Aug 1976, 39-41.

17 WHO Chronicle Rabies: controlling the spread in Europe. WHO Chronicle, 32 (3), Mar 1978, 105-108.

18 Worsley, M.A. Nursing care study. Rabies—the Manchester case. (Care of patient and vaccination of staff.) Nursing Mirror, 145, 14 Jul 1977, 14-15.

h RESPIRATORY TRACT INFECTIONS

1 British Medical Journal Legionnaires' disease. British Medical Journal, 1, 7 Jan 1978, 2-3.

2 British Medical Journal Mumps. (Leading article on its incidence and the case for and against immunisation.) British Medical Journal, 1, 11 Jun 1977, 1489-1490.

3 Carr-Locke, D.I. Psittacosis. Nursing Times, 74, 30 Mar 1978, 529-531.

4 Cullinan, J. Legionnaires' disease. (Comment on recent cases.) Nursing Times, 74, 20 Apr 1978, 653.

5 Devereux, P.M. and Goldstein, E.J.C. Legionnaires' disease: finding answers to the riddle. American Journal of Nursing, 80 (1), Jan 1980, 81-85.

6 Goodman, M. Influenza in the elderly: the case for immunisation. Geriatric Medicine, 10 (9), Sep 1980, 68, 71.

7 Hicks, C. Not to be sneezed at. (The Common Cold Research Unit at Salisbury.) Nursing Times, 75, 4 Jan 1979, 40-41.

8 Isler, C. What if Legionnaires' disease turns up in your hospital? RN Magazine, 41 (11), Nov 1978, 23-25.

9 Iveson-Iveson, J. Legionnaires' identity parade. (History and pathology.) Nursing Mirror, 151, 28 Aug 1980, 8.

10 Laver, G.H. Nursing care study. Lobar pneumonia necessitating ventilation in a poliomyelitis victim. Nursing Mirror, 142, 15 Jan 1976, 50-52.

11 Lyster, A. Legionnaires' disease. (Care study by ward sister.) Nursing Times, 76, 13 Mar 1980, 460-462.

12 Meers, P.D. Hospitals...should do the sick no harm. 9. Respiratory tract infection. Nursing Times, 76, 18 Sep 1980, (4).

13 Schilder, E.J. Legionnaires' disease: an old enemy with a new name. Canadian Nurse, 76 (3), Mar 1980, 46-47.

14 Scott, J. Legionnaires' disease: facts and fancies. Occupational Health, 32 (11), Nov 1980, 551-552.

15 Spicer, A.J. Legionnaires' disease. Practitioner, 224, Dec 1980, 1267-1269.

i RUBELLA

1 Davies, A. Is there a case to answer? (Reasons why rubella campaign is not succeeding fully.) Nursing Mirror, 150, 10 Jan 1980, 38.

2 Dudgeon, J. German measles: reducing the risk of rubella. Nursing Mirror, 149, 12 Jul 1979, 25-27.

3 Edmond, E. and others Rubella epidemic: Scotland 1978. Comments on the rubella immunisation programmes. (Weaknesses highlighted and improvements suggested.) Health Bulletin, 38 (2), Mar 1980, 54-56.

4 Goldwater, P.N. and others Maternal rubella at St. Thomas' Hospital: is there a need to change British vaccination policy? Lancet, 2, 16 Dec 1978, 1298-1300.

5 Jones, S.A.M. Health education to improve rubella immunisation in schools. (Study of London schoolgirls.) British Medical Journal, 281, 6 Sep 1980, 649-650.

6 Mair Owen, C. The educative seven. (Roles of seven types of specialist nurse in education about rubella vaccination.) Nursing Mirror, 150, 10 Apr 1980, 42-43.

7 Morrison, A. and others Rubella vaccination related to immunological status. (Method of ensuring mass immunization of 13-year-old Edinburgh schoolgirls.) Health Bulletin, 35 (4), Jul 1977, 192-196.

8 Peckham, C.S. and others Rubella vaccination of schoolgirls: factors affecting vaccine uptake. British Medical Journal, 1, 19 Mar 1977, 760-761.

9 Rose, A.J. and Mole, K.F. Rubella immunisation and contraception—a case for re-examining the policy of the Department of Health and Social Security. (The value of screening women attending for contraception advice.) Journal of the Royal College of General Practitioners, 26, Nov 1976, 817-821.

10 Stuart-Harris, C. Rubella immunization in the USA and in Great Britain. Midwives Chronicle, 93, Aug 1980, 278-279.

11 Yates, C. Rubella vaccination. (Association with congenital defects after rubella in pregnancy.) Occupational Health, 28 (3), Mar 1976, 141-146.

j SMALLPOX

1 Breman, J.G. Smallpox: no hiding place. World Health, Apr 1978, 24, 26, 28-29.

2 British Medical Journal When do we stop vaccinating against smallpox? British Medical Journal, 2, 13 Aug 1977, 413-414.

3 Magee, J. Africa wins freedom from smallpox. World Health, Oct 1979, 16, 18-19.

4 Tulloch, J.L. The last 50 years of smallpox in Africa. WHO Chronicle, 34 (11), Nov 1980, 407-412.

5 Vetter, S.D.G. Smallpox in Bangladesh—the final story. Nursing Times, 72, 1 Jul 1976, 1000-1001.

6 World Health Issue on the eradication of smallpox. World Health, May 1980, 3-39.

k TETANUS

1 Branton, P. Nursing care study. Total dysphagia due to mild tetanus. Nursing Times, 72, 23/30 Dec 1976, 1998-1999.

2 Edmondson, R.S. and Flowers, M.W. Intensive care in tetanus: management, complications and mortality in 100 cases. British Medical Journal, 1, 26 May 1979, 1401-1404.

3 Furste, W. and Aguirre, A. Preventing tetanus. American Journal of Nursing, 78 (5), May 1978, 834-837.

4 Griffith, D.L. Nursing care study. Tetanus. (Nursing care in ITU and in theatre during excision of wound and tracheostomy.) Nursing Times, 74, 29 Jun 1978, 1078-1082.

5 McLennan, A. Nursing care study. Tetanus: a dirty foul. (Care and physiotherapy following football injury.) Nursing Mirror, 151, 25 Sep 1980, 45-47.

6 Searle, C. Tetanus: the costly cure. (Nursing care study with bibliography of 36 items.) Canadian Nurse, 75 (7), Jul/Aug 1979, 18-24.

7 Smith, J.W.G. Tetanus. (Treatment and prevention.) Nursing Times, 73, 16 Jun 1977, 905-906.

8 Walley, R.V. Infectious diseases. Tetanus. Nursing Mirror, 142, 4 Mar 1976, 63-64.

l TUBERCULOSIS

1 Ansell, J.M. Community nursing study. The forgotten disease. (Tuberculosis.) Nursing Times, 73, 28 Jul 1977, 1152-1153.

2 Archer, C.R. Nursing care study. Tuberculosis—one woman's fight. (Papua, New Guinea.) Nursing Mirror, 144, 24 Mar 1977, 51-53.

3 Arokianathan, A. Tuberculosis in West Malaysia. An integrated programme involving rural health centres and the hospitals. Nursing Times, 76, 14 Feb 1980, 296-297.

4 Bentham, I.A. Tuberculosis—an old enemy stages a comeback. (Five case studies by a TB health visitor.) Nursing Mirror, 145, 8 Dec 1977, 44-46.

5 Bentham, I.A. Tuberculosis: specialty or just another disease? (With reference to role of HV.) Nursing Times, 75, 26 Jul 1979, 1273-1274.

6 British Medical Journal Isolation of patients with pulmonary tuberculosis. British Medical Journal, 280, 5 Apr 1980, 962-963.

7 Buchanan, M. X-rays in focus. Pulmonary tuberculosis. Nursing Times, 73, 17 Mar 1977, Post Basic, 9-12.

8 Bulla, A. Tuberculosis beds—too many now? (Provision and costs of hospital treatment.) WHO Chronicle, 31 (7), Jul 1977, 287-293.

9 Bulla, A. Tuberculosis patients—how many now? (Tentative overall picture of T.B. infection, morbidity and mortality.) WHO Chronicle, 31 (7), Jul 1977, 279-286.

10 Card, D. Tuberculosis: the great leap forward. (Changes in care and treatment in the early 1900s.) Nursing Mirror, 148, 25 Jan 1979, 26-27.

11 Clarke, M. and others Tuberculosis morbidity amongst immigrants: notification and hospitalization. (Survey of Asians in Leicestershire.) Community Medicine, 1 (1), Feb 1979, 23-28.

12 Cowper-Smith, F. TB: the unconquered killer. (Report of study day at the London Chest Hospital.) Nursing Times, 74, 5 Jan 1978, 9.

13 Cummings, K. Nursing care study. Miliary tuberculosis. Nursing Times, 73, 6 Oct 1977, 1550-1553.

14 Dalyell, T. Tuberculosis visitors. New Society, 70, 17 Jun 1976, 659.

15 Garrett, G.E.R. Nursing care study. Miliary tuberculosis. Nursing Mirror, 143, 2 Sep 1976, 48-50.

16 Grenville-Mathers, R. Tuberculosis in Britain today. Midwife, Health Visitor and Community Nurse, 15 (5), May 1979, 179-181.

17 Hitze, K.L. Tuberculosis: a half told story? World Health, Apr 1978, 18-22.

18 Joint Tuberculosis Committee Tuberculosis among immigrants in Britain. Memorandum from the Joint Tuberculosis Committee. British Medical Journal, 1, 22 Apr 1978, 1038-1040.

19 Khogali, M. Tuberculosis among immigrants in the United Kingdom: the role of occupational health services. Journal of Epidemiology and Community Health, 33 (2), Jun 1979, 134-137.

20 Peterson, L.D. and Green, J.H. Nurse managed tuberculosis clinic. (Miami Veterans Administration Hospital.) American Journal of Nursing, 77 (3), Mar 1977, 433-435.

21 Radha, T.G. Miliary tuberculosis. (With case history of Asian woman.) Nursing Times, 74, 17 Aug 1978, 1362-1364.

22 Redmond, I. Recent trends in pulmonary tuberculosis. (Treatment and nursing care.) Nursing Times, 75, 8 Mar 1979, 404-405.

23 Seaton, A. Diseases of the respiratory system. Tuberculosis. (Current methods of treatment.) British Medical Journal, 1, 18 Mar 1978, 701-703.

24 Siegler, D. The respiratory system. 6. Pulmonary tuberculosis. Nursing Mirror, 146, 19 Jan 1978, 31-32.

25 Spires, R. Tuberculosis today: the siege isn't over yet. RN Magazine, 43 (8), Aug 1980, 43-47.

26 Stilwell, J.A. Benefits and costs of the schools BCG vaccination programme. British Medical Journal, 1, 24 Apr 1976, 1002-1004.

27 Toman, K. Mass radiography in tuberculosis control. WHO Chronicle, 30 (2), Feb 1976, 51-57.

m SEXUALLY TRANSMITTED DISEASES

1 Adler, M.W. The terrible peril: a historical perspective on the venereal diseases. (With special reference to the Middlesex Hospital.) British Medical Journal, 281, 19 Jul 1980, 206-211.

2 Barlow, D. Sexually transmitted diseases: the facts. Oxford: Oxford University Press, 1979.

3 Caffyn-Parsons, U. Venereal diseases. (Study written during an 'A' level Human Biology Course.) Nursing Mirror, 146, 25 May 1978, Nursing care supplement, i-iv.

4 Donald, W.H. The changing pattern of sexually transmitted diseases in adolescents. Practitioner, 222, Mar 1979, 383-385.

5 Fong, R. Talking to patients in special clinics. (Reactions of staff.) Nursing Times, 73, 20 Oct 1977, 1648-1649.

6 Gould, D. The scourge of venus. (Veneral disease.) World Health, Nov 1976, 8-11.

7 Jackson, D.H. Asymptomatic sexually transmitted disease. Nursing Mirror, 143, 9 Dec 1976, 50-52.

8 Jacobs, J. On the VD trail. (Problems in tracing contacts.) New Society, 44, 25 May 1978, 425-426.

9 Kahl, I. A potential defaulter. (From special clinic for sexually transmitted diseases.) Nursing Times, 73, 15 Sep 1977, 1452-1453.

10 Kinghorn, G.R. Gonorrhea—a new strain. Nursing Times, 73, 3 Feb 1977, 150-151.

11 Marson, S. and Shaw, E. A new kind of nurse—4. The nurse and the microscope. (Development of self-instructional package for nurses in veneral disease clinic.) Nursing Mirror, 149, 30 Aug 1979, 22-23.

12 Morton, B.M. V.D.: a guide for nurses and counselors. Boston: Little, Brown and Co., 1976.

713 Schofield, E.M. The nurse in a 'special' clinic. (Dealing with patients social and psychological problems in a sexually transmitted diseases clinic by correct personal attitude, education and counselling.) Nursing Times, 72, 8 Jul 1976, 1059-1060.

14 West, J. Veneral disease contact tracing. Nursing Mirror, 142, 27 May 1976, 60-61.

n POLIOMYELITIS

1 Arnold, A. Poliomyelitis—a present threat. Nursing Mirror, 146, 18 May 1978, 16-17.

2 Bennett, M.L. Poliomyelitis. (The development of immunisation.) Nursing Mirror, 143, 25 Nov 1976, 64-65.

3 Community Outlook The summer tragedy. (Polio, with statistics of recent cases and immunisation rates.) Nursing Times, 74, 10 Aug 1978, Community Outlook, 216, 219.

4 Gunn, A.D.G. Poliomyelitis protection. Nursing Times, 73, 13 Jan 1977, 58.

5 Huckstep, R.L. Poliomyelitis: a guide for developing countries, including appliances and rehabilitation for the disabled. Edinburgh: Churchill Livingstone, 1975. (Medicine in the tropics series.)

6 Librach, I. Acute poliomyelitis: still an ever-present threat. Nursing Mirror, 149, 27 Sep 1979, 33.

7 WHO Chronicle A system of poliomyelitis surveillance. WHO Chronicle, 30 (2), Feb 1976, 72-75.

8 Wyatt, V. Polio—the triumph and the risk. (Danger of its return.) New Scientist, 75, 25 Aug 1977, 464-466.

86 DERMATOLOGY

a GENERAL

1 Amann, L.P. Psoriasis. Nursing Times, 72, 15 Jul 1976, 1081-1083.

2 Amann, L.P. Psoriasis—looking for a cure. (Present treatment and research.) Nursing Times, 75, 8 Mar 1979, 407-410.

3 Atkins, J. Care of the hair and scalp. Nursing Mirror, 144, 3 Mar 1977, 45-48.

4 Bentley-Phillips, C.B. Fungal infections of the skin. Nursing Times, 73, 28 Jul 1977, Dermatology, 21-24.

5 Bhanji, S. Psychosomatic aspects of skin disease. Nursing Times, 72, 5 Feb 1976, 180-181.

6 Bielan, B. What that rash really means. RN Magazine, 42 (2), Feb 1979, 58-63.

7 Blair, C. Browntail rash. (Caused by caterpillar of browntail moth.) Nursing Times, 75, 6 Dec 1979, 2117-2118.

8 Blair, C. and others Scabies. Nursing Times, 73, 24 Feb 1977, ICNA Supplement, 43-48.

9 Boss, J.M. Exfoliative dermatitis. Nursing Times, 74, 26 Oct 1978, 1773-1775.

10 Bounds, J.C. and Damon, J. What to do when you think there's nothing you can do. (Hidradenitis suppurativa, a chronic infection of the sweat glands.) Nursing (U.S.), 9 (10), Oct 1979, 34-38.

11 Burton, J.L. and Thompson, L. What do dermatology patients believe? (Survey of 151 outpatients attending the Dermatology Department, Bristol Royal Infirmary.) Journal of Advanced Nursing, 1 (4), Jul 1976, 293-302.

12 Cohen, S. Skin rashes in infants and children. (Programmed instruction.) American Journal of Nursing, 78 (6), Jun 1978, P.I. 1-32.

13 Derbes, V.J. Rashes: recognition and management. Nursing, 8 (3), Mar 1978, 54-59.

14 Eaves, D. Nursing care study. Pemphigus vulgaris: a reassuring touch. Nursing Mirror, 150, 21 Feb 1980, 45-46.

15 Fleming, P. Nursing care study. A patient with pre-senile dementia complicated by mycosis fungoides. (Rare skin disease of unknown causation.) Nursing Mirror, 145, 18 Aug 1977, 15-16.

16 France, D.M. Atopic eczema and its management. Health Visitor, 51 (8), Aug 1978, 294-295.

17 Galles, E.M.L. Identifying dermatological conditions in blacks. (With colour photographs.) Journal of Education in Nursing, 4 (6), Nov/Dec 1978, 56-62.

18 Gange, R.W. Bacterial and viral skin infections. Nursing Times, 73, 27 Jan 1977, Dermatology, 1-4.

19 Glasser, J. Psoriasis: trends in therapy. Nursing Care, 9 (8), Aug 1976, 12-15.

20 Hanron, J.S. Directing your care to the lupus patient's needs. RN Magazine, 38 (5), May 1975, 46-49.

21 Hawkins, K. Wet dressings: putting the damper on dermatitis. Nursing, 8 (2), Feb 1978, 64-67.

22 Huckbody, E. Advances in dermatology. (Short history of research and therapy at St. John's Hospital for Skin Diseases and the Institute of Dermatology.) Nursing Times, 73, 20 Jan 1977, 97-99.

23 Huckbody, E. Nursing procedures for skin diseases. Churchill Livingstone, 1977.

24 Hull, J. and Isaacs, B. The skin: a programmed text. Sheffield: NHS Learning Resources Unit, 1978.

25 Klaber, M. and Tulloch, M. Psoriasis: success for photochemotherapy. (Experimental treatment (also called PUVA) at the London Hospital.) Nursing Mirror, 147, 2 Nov 1978, 40-43.

26 Launer, J. Self help society for eczema sufferers and their families. (National Eczema Society.) British Medical Journal, 2, 18 Dec 1976, 1494-1495.

27 Liddell, K. Nails: clues in your claws. (Nail disorders.) Nursing Mirror, 148, 18 Jan 1979, 31-35.

28 Lloyd, P. Hazards of treatment with ultra-violet light. (To nurse and patient. Used for treatment of psoriasis.) Occupational Health, 32 (6), Jun 1980, 283-285.

29 Maher, A. Nursing care study. Mycosis fungoides. Nursing Times, 74, 18 May 1978, 830-832.

30 Marriott, P.J. Staphylococcal skin disease. Nursing Times, 72, 24 Jun 1976, 971-974.

31 Munro, D.D. and Kirby, J. Acne. Nursing Times, 72, 27 May 1976, 806-808.

32 North, C. and Weinstein, G.D. Treatment of psoriasis. American Journal of Nursing, 76 (3), Mar 1976, 410-412.

33 Nursing Times Dermatology. (A collection of articles.) Macmillan Journals, 1978.

34 Orton, P. Self-help for eczema sufferers. (National Eczema Society.) Social Service Quarterly, 50 (2), Oct/Dec 1976, 214-216.

35 Pegum, J.S. Eczema. Nursing Mirror, 144, 17 Feb 1977, 53-55.

36 Rickitt, C. Nursing care study. Toxic epidermal necrolysis. (Lyell's syndrome or scalded skin syndrome in two-year-old boy.) Nursing Times, 76, 13 Mar 1980, 455-459.

37 Roberts, A. Systems of life. No.64. Systems and signs. The skin. Nursing Times, 76, 3 Apr 1980, (4); 1 May 1980, (4).

38 Rushton, H. Dandruff—a re-appraisal. (Of possible causes.) Nursing Mirror, 145, 21 Jul 1977, 29.

39 Russell, R. Cosmetic camouflage: a new venture of the British Red Cross Society. Health Trends, 12 (1), Feb 1980, 12-13.

40 Rycroft, R.J.G. 3. Dermatitis. Nursing Mirror, 143 (17), 21 Oct 1976, Nursing care supplement, series 3, i-iv.

41 Rycroft, R.J. Eczema. Nursing Times, 73, 31 Mar 1977, Dermatology, 9-12; 28 Apr 1977, Dermatology, 13-16.

42 Senter, G.W. Scabies and other itches. Journal of Community Nursing, 3 (9), Mar 1980, 10, 12.

43 Senter, G.W. Spot cash for research shows little results. (Treatment of acne.) Journal of Community Nursing, 3 (11), May 1980, 4-6, 30.

44 Sneddon, I.B. and Church, R.E. Practical dematology. 3rd ed. Arnold, 1976.

45 Stamper, J. S.C.O.P.E.: Skin Condition of Patients Encountered. (Assessment tool with plan for action.) Journal of Gerontological Nursing, 4 (1), Jan/Feb 1978, 48-51.

46 Taaffe, A. Stevens-Johnson syndrome: a challenge to nursing care. Nursing Mirror, 143, 28 Oct 1976, 58-59.

47 Tighe, S.M. Urticaria. Nursing Times, 73, 8 Sep 1977, 1397-1399.

48 Tring, F.C. Disorders of hair growth. Nursing Times, 72, 9 Dec 1976, 1938-1939.

49 Tring, F.C. Disorders of the skin. Acne vulgaris: hair disorders/itchy skin. Nursing Times, 72, 2 Sep 1976, 1344-1350.

50 Tring, F.C. Stretch marks. Nursing Times, 72 (42), 21 Oct 1976, 1638-1639.

51 Warin, A.P. Fungus disease of the skin. Nursing Mirror, 144, 17 Feb 1977, 49-52.

52 Warin, A.P. Psoriasis. Nursing Times, 73, 24 Feb 1977, Dermatology, 5-8.

53 Wells, T.J. In geriatric patients: that 'minor' skin problem could be trouble. Here's how to make sure it won't be... (Skin hygiene.) RN Magazine, 41 (7), Jul 1978, 41-46.

54 Wilkinson, D.S. The nursing and management of skin diseases. 4th ed. Faber, 1977.

55 Woolfson, H. The psyche and the skin. (Skin disorders related to stress.) Queen's Nursing Journal, 19 (11), Feb 1977, 300-301.

b INDUSTRIAL DERMATOLOGY

1 Alberman, K. Skin care in the chemicals industry. Occupational Safety and Health, 8 (5), May 1978, 22-24.

2 Barnard, J.M. The control and prevention

of dermatitis at work. Occupational Health, 31 (1), Jan 1979, 14-18.

3 Ebert, F. Solving an occupational dermatitis puzzle. Occupational Health Nursing, 28 (8), Aug 1980, 13-16.

4 Swarbrick, P. Vitiligo as an occupational disease. (Skin condition resulting from exposure to chemical agents.) Occupational Health, 32 (9), Sep 1980, 442-448.

5 Wilkinson, D.S. The role of the dermatologist in industrial medicine. Journal of the Society of Occupational Medicine, 26 (1), Jan 1976, 3-8.

87 DIGESTIVE SYSTEM

a GENERAL

1 Allan, D. Complications of T-tube drainage of the common bile duct. Nursing Times, 73, 18 Aug 1977, 1270-1271.

2 Amies, E. The care of upper gastro-intestinal fibreoptic endoscopes. NATNews, 15 (10), Oct 1978, 34, 38.

3 Axon, A. The value of digestive endoscopy. (Includes microbiological hazards.) Health and Social Service Journal, 89, 4 May 1979, 536, 538.

4 Ayliffe, G.A.J. and Deverill, C. Decontamination of gastroscopes. Health and Social Service Journal, 89, 4 May 1979, 538, 541.

5 Belinsky, I. Fibreoptic advances. Visualizing the pancreatic and biliary ducts. American Journal of Nursing, 76 (6), Jun 1976, 936-937.

6 Bell, J. and others Just another patient with gallstones? Don't you believe it. (Pre- and postoperative care after cholecystectomy.) Nursing (U.S.), 9 (10), Oct 1979, 26-33.

7 Carr-Locke, D.L. Gastro-intestinal endoscopy. Nursing Times, 73.
1. Basic principles. 1 Sep 1977, 1348-1351.
2. Oesophago-gastro-duodenoscopy. 8 Sep 1977, 1403-1406.
3. Endoscopic retrograde cholangiopancreatography. 15 Sep 1977, 1443-1449.
4. Colonoscopy. 22 Sep 1977, 1482-1484.

8 Cheffins, P. Nursing care study. Cholecystectomy. The care of a patient before, during and after an operation for the removal of the gall bladder. NATNews, 14 (8), Nov 1977, 24-25.

9 Cherry, F.M. The Russian gun. (Used for oesophageal transection in treatment of bleeding varices.) Nursing Times, 74, 28 Sep 1978, 1601-1602.

10 Clark, A.W. Diagnosing appendicitis. (Problems and the nurse's contribution.) Nursing Mirror, 147, 31 Aug 1978, 26-27.

11 Collis, K. Aspects of geriatric care. (Care of the bowels and bladder.) Nursing Times, 72, 15 Jul 1976, Care of the elderly supplement, xiv, xvi.

12 Fitzgerald, S.J. Theatre nursing care study. Appendicectomy. Nursing Times, 73, 8 Sep 1977, 1395-1396.

13 Fowler, E. and others How to cope when

your patient has an enterocutaneous fistula. American Journal of Nursing, 80 (3), Mar 1980, 426-429.

14 Francone, C.A. 'My battle against Wilson's disease.' American Journal of Nursing, 76 (2), Feb 1976, 247-249.

15 Fryer, J.A. Theatre nursing care study. Heller's operation for a patient with oesophageal achalasia. Nursing Times, 72, 22 Apr 1976, 607-609.

16 Given, B.A. and Simmons, S.J. Gastroenterology in clinical nursing. 3rd ed. St. Louis: Mosby, 1979.

17 Griffith, D. Theatre nursing care study. Cholecystectomy and operative cholangiogram for gall stones. Nursing Times, 74, 29 Jun 1978, 1100-1104.

18 Hinchliffe, R. Nursing care study. In search of an obstruction. (Elderly patient with gall-stone ileus. By third-year student nurse.) Nursing Mirror, 149, 1 Nov 1979, 42-44.

19 Hollanders, D. Gastrointestinal endoscopy: an introduction for assistants. Baillière Tindall, 1979.

20 Johns, P.A. Theatre nursing care study. Laparotomy for intestinal obstruction and the anaesthetic nurse's role. Nursing Times, 76, 5 Jun 1980, 1002-1005.

21 Johnston, G.W. Shooting the varix. (Gun for oesophageal transection of bleeding varices.) NATNews, 16 (12), Dec 1979, 8-10.

22 Kennedy Browne, M. Peritonitis. Nursing Times, 74, 14 Sep 1978, 1531-1533.

23 Kumar, P.J. Sprue. (Tropical sprue and non-tropical sprue (coeliac disease).) Nursing Mirror, 146, 12 Jan 1978, 25-26.

24 McFarland, J. Hiatus hernia. Nursing Mirror, 144, 14 Apr 1977, 50-52.

25 NATNews Nurses and technicians training —fiberoptic endoscopes. NATNews, 13 (5), Jul 1976, 16.

26 Ramsden, E. Nursing care study. Cholecystectomy: patients have feelings too. (By student nurse.) Nursing Mirror, 150, 14 Feb 1980, 52-54.

27 Rice, H.V. Gastrointestinal nursing. Henry Kimpton Publishers, 1978. (Nursing Outline Series.)

28 Robbins, J. Refresher course. Haematemesis. Nursing Times, 72, 5 Aug 1976, 1202.

29 Roberts, A. Body fluids 13. Saliva and gastic juices. 14. Pancreatic and intestinal juices. 15. Bile. Nursing Times, 74, 22 Jun 1978, Body fluids, 49-52; 20 Jul 1978, Body fluids, 53-56; 24 Aug 1978, Body fluids, 57-60.

30 Roberts, A. Systems of life. Nos.14-18. Digestive system. 1-5. Nursing Times, 72, 5 Feb 1976, (4); 4 Mar 1976, 8 Apr 1976, 6 May 1976, 3 Jun 1976.

31 Royal College of Nursing Endoscopy nurses. (Report of Rcn conference on endoscopy and gastro-intestinal nursing.) Nursing Standard, 71, Apr 1978, 16.

32 Schiller, K.F.R. and Peachey, J. Gastrointestinal fibre-endoscopy. (Its applications and limitations and the role of the endoscopy assistant who should preferably be a nurse.) Nursing Mirror, 147, 30 Nov 1978, Supplement, i-xii.

33 Stillman, M. Experiences in clinical problem solving. Nursing decisions: nursing intervention in acute pancreatitis. RN Magazine, 41 (12), Dec 1978, 67-73.

34 Summerfield, J.Y. Theatre nursing care study. Heller's operation for achalasia of the cardia. Nursing Times, 76, 21 Aug 1980, 1470-1473.

35 Sutherland, M. Peutz-Jeghers syndrome. (Nursing care study.) Nursing Times, 75, 4 Jan 1979, 23-24.

36 Taylor, J. Nursing care study. Cholecystectomy. Nursing Times, 72, 8 Apr 1976, 530-532.

37 Turnberg, L.A. Hepatic abscess. Nursing Times, 72, 12 Feb 1976, 217-218.

38 Wales, R. Nursing care study. Cholecystectomy for cholesterolosis. (Patient is trained nurse.) Nursing Mirror, 147, 9 Nov 1978, 25-27.

39 Williams, C.B. Achalasia. (Failure of oesophageal sphincter to relax.) Nursing Mirror, 146, 27 Apr 1978, 18-20.

40 Winifred, Sister Nursing care study. Cholecystectomy. Nursing Mirror, 143, 22 Jul 1976, 45-46.

b GASTRO-INTESTINAL DISORDERS

1 Bamforth, J. Duodenal ulcers. Medical treatment. Nursing Mirror, 143, 23 Sep 1976, 60.

2 Baron, J.H. Abdominal disturbances experienced abroad. Nursing Mirror, 143, 21 Oct 1976, 61-63.

3 Bentley, R.J. Intestinal fistula. Nursing Times, 42, 2 Dec 1976, 1879-1880.

4 Cook, G.C. Dysentery—bacillary and amoebic. Nursing Mirror, 144, 24 Mar 1977, 54-57.

5 Cooper, P. Progress in therapeutics. The treatment of constipation. Midwife, Health Visitor and Community Nurse, 12 (5), May 1976, 165.

6 Currie, J.E.J. Whole gut irrigation: an assessment of this technique for geriatric patients. (To treat faecal impaction.) Nursing Times, 75, 13 Sep 1979, 1570-1571.

7 Dudley, H.A.F. 9. Abdominal pain. Nursing Mirror, 143 (24), 9 Dec 1976, Nursing care supplement, series 3, i-iv.

8 Geels, W. and others The enterocutaneous fistula: supplanting surgery with meticulous nursing care. (Postoperative care after small bowel resection.) Nursing, 8 (4), Apr 1978, 52-55.

9 Gibson, J.A. 7. The diarrhoeas. Nursing Mirror, 143 (22), 25 Nov 1976, Nursing care supplement, series 3, i-iv.

10 Goble, I.W.J. Nursing care study.

Vagotomy and pyloroplasty for duodenal ulcer. Nursing Times, 72, 15 Jul 1976, 1078-1079.

11 Green, G.F. Special care at St. Mark's. (Procedures and care at this hospital specialising in gastro-intestinal diseases.) Nursing Mirror, 146, 2 Mar 1978, 27-28.

12 Gribble, H.E. Gastroenterological nursing. Baillière Tindall, 1977. (Nurses' aids series special interest text.)

13 Gunn, A.D.G. Food poisoning. Nursing Times, 72, 3 Jun 1976, 842-844.

14 Habeeb, M.C. and Kallstrom, M.D. Bowel program for institutionalized adults. Changing dietary intake and bowel evacuation regimens for disabled adults in a long term setting improved patient and staff morale. American Journal of Nursing, 76 (4), Apr 1976, 606-608.

15 Harris, W. Bran or aperients? (To combat constipation.) Nursing Times, 76, 8 May 1980, 811-813.

16 Iveson-Iveson, J. Student's forum. Gastrointestinal tract. (With multiple choice and long answer questions.) Nursing Mirror, 150, 26 Jun 1980, 26-29.

17 Janes, L. Constipation: keeping a true perspective. Nursing Mirror, 149, 27 Sep 1979, NM Supplement, i-ii, iv-v, viii, x.

18 Jobson, G.P. Nursing care study. Perforated gastric ulcer. Nursing Times, 73, 11 Aug 1977, 1242-1245.

19 Jones, F. The management of constipation. Nursing Mirror, 142, 26 Feb 1976, 53-54.

20 Jorgensen, B. Nursing care of patients with amoebic and bacillary dysteneries. Nursing Mirror, 144, 24 Mar 1977, 58-60.

21 Law, V. and Gray, L. Disorders of the gastro-intestinal tract. Nursing Mirror, 143, 8 Jul 1976, Nursing care supplement, 8, i-iv.

22 Leeds, A.R. Constipation. Queen's Nursing Journal, 19 (2), May 1976, 40-41, 42.

23 Leslie, J. Nutrition and diet. 8. Care of the patient with gastro-intestinal disease. Nursing Mirror, 145, 22 Sep 1977, 28-30.

24 Lewin, D. Prizewinning essay. Care of the constipated patient. (Reckitt and Colman award.) Nursing Times, 72, 25 Mar 1976, 444-446.

25 Literte, J.W. Nursing care of patients with intestinal obstruction. American Journal of Nursing, 77 (6), Jun 1977, 1003-1006.

26 Loach, G.A. Laparotomy for abdominal pain of unknown origin. (Care study by student on JBCNS operating theatre course.) Nursing Times, 76, 31 Jan 1980, 196-198.

27 Long, G.D'O. Managing the patent with abdominal aortic aneurysm. Nursing, 8 (8), Aug 1978, 20-27.

28 Quinn, S.J. Nursing care study. 'Acute abdomen.' (Post traumatic pancreatitis.) Nursing Times, 72, 29 Jan 1976, 135-136.

29 Rains, A.J.H. Towards dissolving gallstones. Nursing Mirror, 143, 11 Nov 1976, 51-53.

30 Ritchie, J. The irritable bowel syndrome. Nursing Mirror, 146, 9 Mar 1978, 14-16.

31 Rowntree, T. Duodenal ulcers. Surgical treatment. Nursing Mirror, 143, 23 Sep 1976, 61-62.

32 Russo, B.A. Gastroenterology nursing continuing education review: 412 essay questions and referenced answers. Flushing: Medical Examination Publishing Co., 1976.

33 Seybert, P.L. and others The LeVeen Shunt: new hope for ascites patients. (Peritoneal-jugular shunt.) Nursing (U.S.), 9 (1), Jan 1979, 24-31.

34 Sharpley, J.A. Nursing care study. Splenectomy. Nursing Times, 73, 6 Oct 1977, Theatre Nursing, 5-6, 8.

35 Stahlgren, L.H. and Morris, N.W. Intestinal obstruction. American Journal of Nursing, 77 (6), Jun 1977, 999-1002.

36 Warmer, C.A. Nursing care study. Cimetidine therapy for a bleeding duodenal ulcer. Nursing Times, 74, 28 Sep 1978, 1597-1599.

37 Webb, K. Nursing care study. Vagotomy and pyloroplasty. (For duodenal ulcer.) Nursing Mirror, 147, 9 Nov 1978, 22-24.

38 Williams, I. and Shaffer, J.L. Gastrointestinal disorders: treatment without drugs. (With advice on diet, a sample menu and suggestions for emergency store cupboard.) Geriatric Medicine, 10 (9), Sep 1980, 20, 23-24, 27.

CROHN'S DISEASE AND ULCERATIVE COLITIS

39 Armstrong-Esther, C.A. and Williams, A. Serum immunoglobulin levels in Crohn's disease: an investigation. Nursing Times, 74, 20 Jul 1978, Occ. papers, 77-79.

40 Armstrong-Esther, C.A. and Williams, A. Serum immunoglobulin levels in ulcerative colitis: an investigation. Nursing Times, 72, 23 Sep 1976, Occ. papers, 137-139.

41 Baker, J. The nursing care of Crohn's disease. Nursing Mirror, 142, 29 Jan 1976, 52-54.

42 Byrne, P. Causing problems world wide. (Crohn's disease and ulcerative colitis.) Nursing Mirror, 151, 31 Jul 1980, 30-31.

43 Eastwood, M.A. and Ward, M. Ulcerative colitis. Nursing Times, 72, 11 Mar 1976, 371-372.

44 Foulkes, B. Nursing care study. Inflammatory disease of the bowel. (Care before and after excision of the bowel for ulcerative colitis including care of ileostomy.) Nursing Mirror, 146, 26 Jan 1978, 19-21.

45 Gazzard, B.G. and others The social toll of Crohn's disease. (Interviews and personality assessment of eighty-five outpatients.) British Medical Journal, 2, 21 Oct 1978, 1117-1119.

46 Gunn, A.D.G. Ulcerative colitis. Journal of Community Nursing, 1 (12), Jun 1978, 19-20.

47 Hill, B. Nursing care study. Acute ulcerative colitis. Facing up to fear. Nursing Mirror, 151, 31 Jul 1980, 42-43.

48 Irving, M. Ulcerative colitis. Nursing Times, 73, 22 Sep 1977, 1466-1469.

49 Joachim, G. Crohn's disease: mourning the losses. (Case study.) Canadian Nurse, 74 (8), Sep 1978, 40-43.

50 Lee, P. Patient care study: ulcerative colitis. Queen's Nursing Journal, 19 (4), Jul 1976, 97-98.

51 Lockhart-Mummery, H.E. The treatment of Crohn's disease. Nursing Mirror, 142, 29 Jan 1976, 49-51.

52 Mallett, S.J. and others Colitis. (Survey of patients' experience of its effects on their lives.) Lancet, 2, 16 Sep 1978, 619-621.

53 Marshall, J.G. The information needs of patients with Crohn's disease. (Research study by clinical librarian.) Patient Counselling and Health Education, 1 (4), Summer/Fall 1979, 142-145.

54 Mayberry, J. Crohn's disease. (With questionnaire for nurses who are sufferers to complete for research purposes.) Nursing Times, 75, 29 Nov 1979, 2070-2073.

55 Myer, S.A. The chronic threat of Crohn's disease: how to help your patients cope. RN Magazine, 41 (11), Nov 1978, 65-71.

56 Ryall, R.J. Ulcerative colitis. Nursing Times, 73, 24 Feb 1977, 266-268.

c COLON AND RECTUM

1 Crabtree, S.M. Community nursing care study. Fistula-in-ano. Nursing Times, 73, 3 Nov 1977, 1714-1715.

2 Hughes, E.M. Nursing care study. Left hepatic lobectomy following resection of pelvic colon. Nursing Times, 72, 18 Mar 1976, 403-406.

3 Thomson, J.P.S. Ano-rectal bleeding. (Diagnostic techniques.) Nursing Times, 75, 25 Jan 1979, 142-146.

4 Thomson, M. Fissure-in-ano. Nursing Times, 73, 26 May 1977, 783-784.

d LIVER DISEASES

1 Byrne, J. Liver function studies. Part 3. Tests that measure protein metabolism. Nursing, 7 (10), Oct 1977, 13-14.

2 Byrne, J. Liver function studies. Part 4. Using metabolism tests to investigate liver function. Nursing, 7 (12), Dec 1977, 15.

3 Byrne, J. Liver function studies. Part 5: using enzyme levels to assess liver function. Nursing, 8 (1), Jan 1978, 50, 52.

4 Fraser, J.A. and May, D. Liver transplant—1. Surgical aspects of orthotopic liver transplantation. Nursing Times, 75, 2 Aug 1979, 1300-1304.

5 Johnson, H. Liver transplant—2. Liver transplant operation. Nursing Times, 75, 9 Aug 1979, 1358-1361.

6 Knell, A.J. and Fawke, D. Acute liver failure. Nursing Mirror, 145, 4 Aug 1977, 16-18.

7 Law, G.M. The nursing care of patients having orthotopic liver transplants. Nursing Mirror, 147, 3 Aug 1978, Supplement, xii-xiii, xv.

8 Lok, P. Intensive care therapy for liver transplantations. Australian Nurses Journal, 8 (3), Sep 1978, 42-44.

9 Lok, P. Nursing management of liver transplant. Australian Nurses Journal, 8 (4), Oct 1978, 38-40.

10 MacDougall, B.R.D. and Williams, R. Liver transplantation. The medical aspects. Nursing Mirror, 147, 3 Aug, Supplement, iii-iv, vii, xi-xii.

11 McMaster, P. Management of liver trauma and liver transplantation. Physiotherapy, 64 (2), Feb 1978, 39-40.

12 Martin, E.J. Nursing care study. Hamartoma of the liver. (In infants.) Nursing Times, 72, 8 Jul 1976, 1043-1045.

13 Mowat, A.P. Biliary atresia. (Congenital abnormality of the liver.) Nursing Times, 72, 5 Feb 1976, 182-183.

14 Nursing Clinics of North America Symposium on diseases of the liver. Nursing Clinics of North America, 12 (2), Jun 1977, 257-356.

15 Roberts, A. and Besterman, A. Systems of life. 19-20. Liver 1-2. Nursing Times, 72, 1 Jul 1976, (4); 5 Aug 1976, (4).

16 Rodman, M.J. Drug therapy today. Controlling chronic liver disease. RN Magazine, 39 (1), Jan 1976, 79-80, 84-85; (2), Feb 1976, 75-76, 79.

17 Stubbs, J. Major surgery of the liver. Nursing Mirror, 146, 9 Mar 1978, 41.

18 Wheeler, P. and Williams, R. A better outlook. (Investigation and treatment of liver diseases including hepatitis.) Nursing Mirror, 151, 24 Jul 1980, 42-44.

19 Williams, R. and others The King's Liver Unit. (King's College Hospital.) Nursing Times, 72, 25 Nov 1976, 23/30 Dec 1976, Key Clinical, 41-48.

e PEPTIC ULCER

1 Langman, M.J.S. Medical treatment of peptic ulcer. Nursing Times, 73, 6 Jan 1977, 29-31.

f CHILDREN'S DISEASES

1 Apley, J. 'Little bellyachers'. Recurrent abdominal pain in children. Nursing Mirror, 144, 17 Feb 1977, 46-48.

2 Copeland, L. Chronic diarrhea in infancy. American Journal of Nursing, 77 (3), Mar 1977, 461-463.

3 Evans, R. Therapeutic diets for children. (Coeliac disease and cow's milk protein and lactose intolerance.) Nursing, 12, Apr 1980, 527-530.

4 Langston, G.M.D. Nursing care study. Laparotomy, removal of trichobezoar and appendicectomy. (Removal of hairball from 14-year-old girl.) Nursing Times, 76, 11 Dec 1980, 2183-2185.

5 Wherry, C.A. Treating chronic constipation in children. Nursing Times, 73, 24 Nov 1977, 1829-1831.

6 Wong, J. and Edwards, J. Nursing care study. An encopretic child. Nursing Times, 72, 5 Feb 1976, 175-176.

7 Yalden, E.M. Nursing care study. Cholecystectomy for infarction of the gall bladder. (In two-year-old child.) Nursing Times, 75, 10 May 1979, 781-782.

g STOMA CARE: GENERAL

1 Abplanalp, D.F. Obstetric considerations in stoma patients. Journal of Obstetric, Gynecologic and Neonatal Nursing, 5 (5), Sep/Oct 1976, 44-45.

2 Alexander, F.G. The role of the general practitioner in stoma care. Practitioner, 219, Jul 1977, 79-84.

3 Alexander-Williams, J. and others Magnetic continent colostomy device. (See also leading article p.1238.) British Medical Journal, 1, 14 May 1977, 1269-1270.

4 Bath, A. Nursing care study. Total colectomy and ileostomy. (Insertion of Maclet magnetic ring implant to create continent ileostomy.) Nursing Mirror, 146, 9 Mar 1978, 19-21.

5 Baum, M. and Fletcher, J.C. Porcine dressing for ileostomy retraction. American Journal of Nursing, 76 (5), May 1976, 760-761.

6 Biddulph, C. The Chairman's summary. (Symposium on stoma care.) Nursing Mirror, 142, 8 Jan 1976, 60-61.

7 Broadwell, D.C. and Sorrells, S.L. Loop transverse colostomy. American Journal of Nursing, 78 (6), Jun 1978, 1029-1031.

8 Department of Health and Social Security The provision of stoma care. DHSS, 1979.

9 Dunn, R. Comfort through thick and thin. (Hypoallergenic adhesive tape and its application to stoma care.) Health and Social Service Journal, 90, 1 Aug 1980, 1004-1005.

10 Fitzgerald, R.T.D. and others Comparative trial of skin reactions to stoma adhesives. Practitioner, 220, Apr 1978, 645-646.

11 Fussell, K. Common problems of ileostomies and colostomies. Practitioner, 216, Jun 1976, 655-664.

12 Goligher, J.C. The continent or reservoir ileostomy. Nursing Times, 73, 31 Mar 1977, 447-449.

13 Griffiths, N. Intestinal stomas. (General introduction.) Journal of Community Nursing, 2 (8), Feb 1979, 4-5.

14 Gross, L. and Bailey, Z. Enterostomal therapy: developing institutional and community programs. Wakefield, MA.: Nursing Resources, 1979.

15 Hyman, E. and others The pouch ileostomy: new nursing applications and time-tested techniques. Nursing, 7 (9), Sep 1977, 44-47.

16 Isler, C. If the ileostomy is continent, the benefits are obvious. (Continent ileostomy surgery.) RN Magazine, 40 (4), Apr 1977, 39-45.

17 Isler, C. A new ball game for colostomy patients? (Magnetic device for continent colostomy.) RN Magazine, 40 (9), Sep 1977, 52-53.

18 Keenan, K. Relief for the sensitive stoma. (Report of trial of Skin Gel.) Nursing Mirror, 147, 10 Aug 1978, 36.

19 Keenan, K. and others A trial of a new ostomy system. (Evaluation of Surgicare System 2 involving Stomahesive by stomatherapists in five units.) Nursing Times, 75, 26 Jul 1979, 1283-1285.

20 McIntyre, R. Nursing care study. Emergency colectomy for toxic megacolon. (Including postoperative care of ileostomy.) Nursing Times, 75, 22 Feb 1979, 316-319.

21 Martin-Scott, I. Skin care for ileostomists. Practitioner, 222, Feb 1979, 237-240.

22 Morgans, K.A. The attractions of magnets in stomacare. (Magnetic sealing device.) Journal of Community Nursing, 2 (12), Jun 1979, 4-5.

23 Murphy, M. Irrigation brings relief—sometimes. (Of colostomy.) Journal of Community Nursing, 2 (11), May 1979, 12, 14.

24 Murphy, M. The problem of stomal equipment disposal. Journal of Community Nursing, 4 (1), Jul 1980, 19, 22.

25 Nursing Mirror Reports of six individual workshops. (Reports presented at a symposium on stoma care.) Nursing Mirror, 142 (2), 8 Jan 1976, 56-59.

26 Phillpotts, E.A. and others The continent colostomy. (Colostomy irrigation trial at Bristol Royal Infirmary using the Hollister stoma cone method.) Nursing Mirror, 142, 20 May 1976, 53-54.

27 Plant, J. The case for stoma care. (Symposium paper.) Nursing Mirror, 142, 8 Jan 1976, 48-49.

28 Smart, M. Is it what the patient really wants? (Report of manufacturer-sponsored assessment of Stomahesive for use after urinary diversion.) Nursing Mirror, 150, 24 Jan 1980, Supplement, x, xii-xiii.

29 Starkey, R. A district stoma care service. (Brighton Health District, Sussex. Symposium paper.) Nursing Mirror, 142, 8 Jan 1976, 50-53.

30 Swailes, S. Nursing care study: be prepared. (Use of Stomahesive and condom urinal to drain faecal wound.) Journal of Community Nursing, 2 (10), Apr 1979, 16.

31 Thornton, M. Evaluation of stoma care. (Symposium paper.) Nursing Mirror, 142, 8 Jan 1976, 54-55.

32 Todd, I.P. editor Intestinal stomas. Heinemann, 1978.

33 Walker, F.C. editor Modern stoma care. Edinburgh: Churchill Livingstone, 1976.

34 Watt, R.C. Colostomy irrigation—yes or no? American Journal of Nursing, 77 (3), Mar 1977, 442-444.

h STOMA CARE: NURSE AND PATIENT

1 Auld, L.S. Pseudo-ostomy. (Nurse experiments with stoma appliances to understand her patients' feelings and problems.) American Journal of Nursing, 78 (9), Sep 1978, 1525.

2 Bailey, A.J. Beginning research. Nursing the patient with a colostomy. (Survey to compare a nursing care plan prepared by author, with care received in two hospitals.) Nursing Times, 73, 17 Mar 1977, 382-385.

3 Baum, M.E. Enterostomal therapy in the hospital. (Training and role of stoma therapists.) Supervisor Nurse, 7 (1), Jan 1976, 11-15.

4 Beadle, C. The stoma therapist and a patient with recurrent carcinoma of the colon. Nursing Times, 72, 13 May 1976, 739-741.

5 Breckman, B. Keep the customer satisfied: a personal report of consumer evaluation of urostomy bags. Journal of Community Nursing, 3 (2), Aug 1979, 4-5, 7.

6 Breckman, B.E. The nurse's dilemma in the care of patients with stoma. (Four areas where nurse's training and feelings may conflict.) Nursing Standard, 71, Apr 1978, 8-9.

7 Breckman, B.E. One means to four ends. (Special needs of four types of cancer patients with stomas.) Nursing Mirror, 150, 24 Jan 1980, Supplement, i-iii.

8 Breckman, B.E. Role of the nurse specialist in stoma care. Journal of Human Nutrition, 33 (5), Oct 1979, 383-387.

9 Breckman, B.E. Rundown on stoma problems. (Overview of stoma care including counselling of patient and family.) Journal of Community Nursing, 1 (11), May 1978, 4-6.

10 Breckman, B.E. Specialised care. 5. Care of the stoma patient. Nursing Mirror, 145, 13 Oct 1977, Nursing care supplement, i-iv.

11 Breckman, B.E. Who asks the processed patient? (Use of nursing process by stoma care nurse including getting patients' involvement.) Nursing Mirror, 149, 11 Oct 1979, 12.

12 Buchanan-Davidson, D.J. The colostomy patient. 1. Nursing concerns and considerations. 2. Caring for the patient at home. Journal of Practical Nursing, 29 (9), Sep 1979, 14-21, 36; (10), Oct 1979, 25-29, 35-36.

13 Community Outlook Opening the door: new developments in stoma care. (For adults and children.) Nursing Times, 76, 8 May 1980, Community Outlook, 131-132, 134.

14 Cronin, B. Stoma care—a personal viewpoint. Midwife, Health Visitor and Community Nurse, 12 (4), Apr 1976, 119-121.

15 Dent, D.M. What difference has the stoma therapist made to the patient with a stoma? S.A. Nursing Journal, 53 (11), Nov 1976, 20.

16 Eardley, A. Stoma care. (Research into problems experienced by patients based on interviews.) Practitioner, 222, Feb 1979, 264-266.

17 Foulkes, B. Stoma care. (Importance of meeting patients' emotional needs.) Nursing Mirror, 146, 8 Jun 1978, Supplement, i-iv.

18 Grubb, R.D. and Blake, R. Emotional trauma in ostomy patients. AORN Journal, 23 (1), Jan 1976, 52-53.

19 Gumbell, J. The ileal conduit patient. (A patient's point of view.) Nursing Mirror, 143, 26 Aug 1976, 54-55.

20 Heywood Jones, I. The Ileostomy Association. (Description of activities.) Nursing Times, 75, 22 Nov 1979, 2041. See also All in the same boat, 76, 4 Sep 1980, 1574.

21 Jackson, A.S. Nursing care study. Living with a colostomy. (Emphasises counselling of patient and relatives.) Nursing Times, 75, 11 Jan 1979, 70-75.

22 Jeter, K.F. Reality therapy: a realistic approach to enterostomy rehabilitation. (Programme of eight steps for patients to help them cope psychologically.) Nursing Forum, 17 (1), 1978, 72-83.

23 Johns, C. Nursing care study. Formation of a continent ileostomy. (Pre- and postoperative care and self management by patient at home.) Nursing Times, 74, 9 Mar 1978, 396-400.

24 Lamanske, J. Want to specialize? Consider becoming an enterostomal therapist. Nursing, 77 7 (4), Apr 1977, 18-19.

25 Lawson, A.L. The stomatherapist and the urinary diversion patient. Nursing Times, 74, 23 Nov 1978, 1938-1939.

26 Leedham, L. Living with a stoma. Marshalling resources. (Work of stoma care nurse.) Nursing Times, 75, 8 Mar 1979, Community Outlook, 76.

27 Lerner, J. and others Why pre-op stoma planning is a must: and how you can make sure it's done right. RN Magazine, 43 (8), Aug 1980, 48-51.

28 Lindensmith, S. Body image and the crisis of enterostomy. Canadian Nurse, 73 (11), Nov 1977, 24-27.

29 McKenna, S.E. A new lease of life: a positive approach to helping the stoma patient. Nursing Times, 75, 22 Feb 1979, 320-323.

30 Mahoney, J.M. Guide to ostomy nursing care. Boston: Little, Brown and Co., 1976.

31 Mahoney, J.M. What you should know about ostomies. Guidelines for giving better postop care. Nursing, 8 (5), May 1978, 74-78, 80.

32 Marzluf, M.J. Ostomies in children. Nursing Care, 10 (3), Mar 1977, 18-19, 22.

33 May, H.J. Enterostomal therapy. New York: Raven Press, 1977. (For nurses.)

34 Mayberry, J.F. and Rhodes, J. Aspects of the ileostomy appliance: a survey of the patients' difficulties. (Including skin reactions, fear of leakage and dislike of transparent bags.) Practitioner, 220, Jun 1978, 958-961.

35 Mitchell, A. Patients' views on stoma care. (Survey of ex-hospital patients of the care they received in hospital and after discharge.) Nursing Mirror, 151, 3 Jul 1980, 38-41.

36 Moser, S. Social worker's role in ileostomy. AORN Journal, 23 (1), Jan 1976, 56-59.

37 Nursing Clinics of North America Symposium on care of the ostomy patient. Nursing Clinics of North America, 11 (3), Sep 1976, 389-478.

38 Richardson, R.G. editor Stoma independence: rehabilitation of the stoma patient: proceedings of a day symposium organised by stoma care nurses... 1 Apr 1977. Queenborough: Abbott Laboratories, 1977.

39 Royal College of Nursing Nurses 'ideally placed' to counsel stoma patients. (Report of Rcn conference on the counselling of stoma care patients.) Nursing Times, 73, 22/29 Dec 1977, 1980.

40 Rush, A.M. Cancer and the ostomy patient. Nursing Clinics of North America, 11 (3), Sep 1976, 405-415.

41 Salter, M. From horror to normality. (Personal viewpoint of a district nurse ostomy patient.) Nursing Mirror, 148, 24 May 1979, 36-37.

42 Saunders, H.B. Clinical nurse consultant in stoma care. (Symposium paper.) Nursing Mirror, 142, 13 May 1976, 54-58.

43 Saunders, H.B. The nurse's role in the care of patients with a stoma. British Journal of Clinical Practice, 30 (4), Apr 1976, 81-82, 99.

44 Saunders, H.B. The stoma care course at St. Bartholomew's Hospital. (Joint Board of Clinical Nursing Studies course.) Nursing Mirror, 142, 8 Jan 1976, 62.

45 Sredl, D.R. Another look at the ostomy patient. 1. Preoperative essentials. 2. Psychological effects. 3. Complications. Journal of Practical Nursing, 27 (1), Jan 1977, 18-22, 38-39; (2), Feb 1977, 24-25, 41; (3), Mar 1977, 16-18.

46 Swaffield, L. Living with a stoma. (Four articles on finding the problems, colostomy, ileostomy, and ileal conduit.) Nursing Times, 75, 8 Mar 1979, Community Outlook, 66, 69, 70, 72, 75.

47 Tisdale, H. Helping young ostomy patients help themselves. (Teaching of stoma care through play.) Canadian Nurse, 73 (7), Jul 1977, 30-32.

48 Velangi, V. Fear fights against a stoma. (Patient's need for counselling.) Nursing Mirror, 150, 24 Jan 1980, Supplement, iv, vii-ix.

49 Vowles, K.D.J. After colostomy the problems begin. (Special problems of the elderly with colostomies.) Modern Geriatrics, 8 (1), Jan 1978, 26-27.

50 Vukovich, V.C. and Grubb, R.D. Care of the ostomy patient. 2nd ed. St. Louis: Mosby, 1977. (For nurses and others.)

51 Wentworth, A. and Cox, B. Nursing the patient with a continent ileostomy. (An ileostomy with an internal reservoir no longer requiring external appliances.) American Journal of Nursing, 76 (9), Sep 1976, 1424-1428.

52 Wood, R.Y. and Watson, P.G. People with temporary colostomies: are we meeting their needs? Canadian Nurse, 73 (11), Nov 1977, 28-30.

88 EAR, NOSE AND THROAT

a GENERAL

1 Black, L. Rhinoplasties under local anaesthesia. Nursing Times, 72, 26 Aug 1976, 1304-1305.

2 Buisseret, P. The six senses. 2. Smell and taste. 4. Hearing. Nursing Mirror, 146, 19 Jan 1978, Supplement, i-iv; 2 Feb 1978, Supplement, i-iv.

3 Burrows, A.B. Nursing care study. Elective maxillofacial surgery. (For protruding lower jaw. By sister of patient.) Nursing Times, 76, 10 Apr 1980, 633-636.

4 Coleman, B.H. Sinusitis. Nursing Mirror, 143, 16 Sep 1976, 53-55.

5 Corkery, C.M. Nursing care study. Removal of a child's tonsils and adenoids. (Preparation by parents helps child co-operate.) Nursing Times, 75, 3 May 1979, 742-743.

6 Doey, W.D. Nasal obstruction. 1. General factors, inflammatory and neoplastic causes. 2. Other causes and treatments. Nursing Times, 72, 5 Feb 1976, 177-179; 12 Feb 1976, 222-224.

7 Gladwin, B. Nursing care study. Adenotonsillectomy. Bearing up with Paddington. (Care of seven-year-old girl by student nurse.) Nursing Mirror, 150, 7 Feb 1980, 42-44.)

8 Goodall, J. Nursing care study. A patient with Wegener's granuloma. (Tumour in the nose.) Nursing Times, 74, 8 Jun 1978, 948-952.

9 Güdrün, R. Sinusitis. Nursing Times, 74, 22 Jun 1978, 1041-1044.

10 Hickish, G. All about tonsillectomy. Midwife, Health Visitor and Community Nurse, 13 (8), Aug 1977, 254-256.

11 Hope, G.A. Refresher course. Pharyngitis. Nursing Times, 72, 1/8 Jan 1976, 15-17.

12 Moore, J.C. Establishment of an outpatient ENT clinic. (Day surgery.) AORN Journal, 31 (4), Mar 1980, 620, 623, 626-627, 630.

13 Morgan, N.V. Nasopharyngeal tumours. Nursing Times, 73, 23 Jun 1977, 948-949.

14 Pracy, R. and others Ear, nose and throat surgery and nursing. Hodder and Stoughton, 1977. (Modern nursing series.)

15 Price, J.D. and others Mandibular deformity. (Nursing care study of correction of protruding lower jaw.) Nursing Times, 76, 14 Aug 1980, 1447-1452.

16 Roberts, A. Systems of life. Nos.44-46. Hearing—1-3. Nursing Times, 74, 3 Aug 1978, (4); 7 Sep 1978, (4); 5 Oct 1978, (4).

17 Roberts, A. Systems of life. No.48. Smell. (Physiology, the common cold and sinusitis.) Nursing Times, 74, 7 Dec 1978, (4).

18 Roberts, A. Systems of life. No.49. Taste. (Includes physiology and disorders of tongue.) Nursing Times, 75, 4 Jan 1979, (4).

19 Saunders, W.H. and others Nursing care in eye, ear, nose and throat disorders. 4th ed. St. Louis: Mosby, 1979.

20 Thomas, B. Nursing care study. Adenotonsillectomy. Nursing Mirror, 146, 2 Mar 1978, 18-19.

b CLEFT LIP AND PALATE

1 Daft, P. Nursing care study. Cleft lip and palate: the boy who wouldn't lie down. (Seven-year course of surgery.) Nursing Mirror, 151, 11 Sep 1980, 33-35.

2 Dencer, D. Result—a lip to be kissed with relish. (Plastic surgery for cleft lip and palate and haemangiomata.) Nursing Mirror, 151, 11 Sep 1980, 30-33.

3 Mayman, A. Nursing care study. Cleft lip and palate: three into one will go. (Five-and-a-half month old baby.) Nursing Mirror, 148, 11 Jan 1979, 31-33.

4 Nicholson, E.M. Personal notes of a laryngectomee. American Journal of Nursing, 75 (12), Dec 1975, 2157-2158.

c EAR DISEASES

1 Allan, D. Nursing care study. A patient with acoustic neuroma. (Insertion of ventriculoperitoneal shunt for tumour affecting hearing.) Nursing Times, 74, 7 Dec 1978, 2015-2108.

2 Bradbeer, T.L. Vertigo—1. In health and in disease. (Anatomy and physiology of balance mechanisms and diagnostic procedures.) 2. Causes and their treatment. Nursing Times, 73, 13 Oct 1977, 1586-1589; 20 Oct 1977, 1640-1642.

3 Brown, M. Glue ear. (Seromucinous otitis media.) Nursing Mirror, 147, 3 Aug 1978, 32-33.

4 Burgess, E.H. Earwax—and the right way to use an ear syringe. Nursing Times, 73, 6 Oct 1977, 1564-1565.

5 Carne, S. Procedures in practice. Ear syringing. British Medical Journal, 280, 9 Feb 1980, 374-376.

6 Chandra, G. and Luty, K. Acute anterior uveitis: injecting a speedier recovery. (Report of study of fifty patients treated with methylprednisolone.) Nursing Mirror, 147, 2 Nov 1978, 34.

7 Colman, B.H. Meniere's disease. Nursing Times, 72, 9 Dec 1976, 1925-1927.

8 Freeman, G. Middle ear disease. Nursing Times, 73, 13 Jan 1977, 56-57.

9 Gibson, W. and Kanagaonkar, G. Syringing the ear. Nursing Mirror, 148, 15 Feb 1979, 24-25.

10 Hornby, B. Cholesteatoma—a case history. (Pre- and postoperative nursing care of a six-year-old boy.) Australian Nurses Journal, 7 (10), May 1978, 36-37.

11 Huber, C.J. and others The BOEL tests as a screening device for otitis media in infants. (Study to evaluate the test.) Nursing Research, 27 (3), May/Jun 1978, 178-189.

12 Lancaster, V. Nursing care study. Cholesteatoma in a child. Nursing Mirror, 145, 29 Sep 1977, 13-15.

13 Mawson, S.R. Malignant otitis externa. Nursing Times, 72, 22 Jan 1976, 102.

14 **Pick, G.F.** The cochlea—normal and pathological. Nursing Mirror, 146, 9 Feb 1978, 21-23.

15 **Quattrucci, J.** Beginning research. The hygiene of stethoscopes. (Study to test whether ear pieces contribute to ear complaints experienced by nurses.) Nursing Times, 73, 10 Feb 1977, 193-195.

16 **Roberts, A.** Systems of life. No.45. Hearing—2. (Physiology and disorders of the ear.) Nursing Times, 74, 7 Sep 1978, (4).

17 **Rotter, K.** Tympanoplasty. (In treatment of chronic suppurative otitis media.) Nursing Mirror, 147, 28 Sep 1978, 28-30.

18 **Russell, G.** Theatre nursing care study. Right myringoplasty. Nursing Times, 73, 27 Oct 1977, 1664-1666.

19 **Sudworth, P.** Nursing care study. Dendritic ulcer. Nursing Mirror, 143, 12 Aug 1976, 47-49.

20 **Weir, N.** Investigation and management of vertigo in the elderly. (Symposium on care of the elderly.) Nursing Mirror, 145, 3 Nov 1977, 16-20.

21 **White, N.** OR nursing in otomicrosurgery. AORN Journal, 22 (6), Dec 1975, 889-897.

d DEAFNESS: GENERAL

1 **Anwar, M.** Communication difficulties with the elderly hard-of-hearing. (Symposium on care of the elderly.) Nursing Mirror, 145, 3 Nov 1977, 26, 29.

2 **Ballantyne, J.** Deafness. 3rd ed. Churchill Livingstone, 1977.

3 **Crammond, G.W. and Gabb, P.** Impaired hearing in the elderly. (Survey in Durham AHA.) British Medical Journal, 280, 1 Mar 1980, 612.

4 **Crine, A.** The double isolation. (Centre for the Deaf at Goodmayes Hospital, Essex.) Mind Out, 41, Jul/Aug 1980, 18.

5 **Fisch, L.** Deafness: a hearing aid alone is not enough. (Advice on communication.) Geriatric Medicine, 9 (6), Jun 1979, 28-29, 32.

6 **Gates, N.** The elderly deaf. (Day conference on community services available.) Nursing Mirror, 144, 20 Jan 1977, 67-68.

7 **Golden, P. and Ulrich, M.** Deaf patients' access to care depends on staff communication. (Use of resources and appropriate methods of communication.) Hospitals, 52 (10), 16 May 1978, 86-88, 90.

8 **Lancet** Deafness and mental illness. Lancet, 2, 16 Oct 1976, 837.

9 **Luce, R.** There's still a lot to be done: problems facing deaf people in our society. Health and Social Service Journal, 87, 4 Nov 1977, 1526.

10 **Lysons, K.** Your hearing loss and how to cope with it. David and Charles, 1978. (An RNID handbook.)

11 **McNamee, C.** Communicating. (Fifteen points of advice on communicating with the hard

of hearing.) Canadian Nurse, 74 (3), Mar 1978, 28-29.

12 **Mamaril, A.P.** Sudden deafness. American Journal of Nursing, 76 (12), Dec 1976, 1992-1994.

13 **Maquire, N.S. and Van Wagoner, R.S.** Hearing loss among hospital employees. (Survey at Foothills Hospital, Calgary.) Dimensions in Health Service, 54 (1), 1977, 16-17.

14 **Roberts, A.** Systems of life. No.47. Hearing—4. (Deafness, hearing tests and help for the deaf.) Nursing Times, 74, 16 Nov 1978, (4).

15 **Rosenblum, E.H.** Fundamentals of hearing for health professionals. Boston: Little, Brown and Co., 1979.

16 **Ross, T.** Deaf unit, Whittingham Hospital. (Description of its work, geared to the special needs of psychiatric patients.) Nursing Mirror, 145, 24 Nov 1977, 20-21.

17 **Steele, J.** Friends, Romans and countrymen. (Experiences of a deaf person.) Nursing Times, 75, 19 Apr 1979, 682-683.

18 **Ventura, F.P.** Counselling the hearing impaired geriatric patient. Patient Counselling and Health Education, 1 (1), Spring 1978, 22-25.

19 **Ward, P.R.** Treatment of elderly adults with impaired hearing: resources, outcome and efficiency. (Evaluation of effect of follow-up after fitting of hearing aids.) Journal of Epidemiology and Community Health, 34 (1), Mar 1980, 65-68.

20 **Ward, P.R.** What do they hear? Improving the communication environment for hearing impaired residents in homes for the elderly. (Pilot programme in Exeter.) Social Work Service, 22, Feb 1980, 49-53.

21 **Warren, F.** Deafness: the handicap psychiatrists ignore. (Lack of specialist psychiatric provision for the deaf, with reference to the unit at Whittingham Hospital, Preston.) Mind Out, 32, Jan/Feb 1979, 10-12.

22 **Wolf, E.M.** Communicating with deaf surgical patients. AORN Journal, 26 (1), Jul 1977, 39-47.

e DEAFNESS: CHILDREN

1 **Bickerton, M.** Detection and screening techniques. (Symposium on deafness in children.) Nursing Mirror, 143, 4 Nov 1976, 50-52.

2 **Bloom, F.** Our deaf children into the 80s. Gresham, 1978.

3 **Brooks, D.N.** Auditory screening—time for reappraisal. (Screening in school children.) Public Health, 91 (6), Nov 1977, 282-288.

4 **Dale, D.M.C.** Educating deaf and partially hearing children individually in ordinary schools. Lancet, 2, 21 Oct 1978, 884-887.

5 **Gregory, S.** The deaf child and his family. Allen and Unwin, 1976.

6 **Harris, J. and Hartley, K.** Children of deaf parents. (Family therapy by Child and Family Psychiatric Service in Dunstable.) Social Work Today, 10, 1 May 1979, 12-13.

7 **Health Visitors' Association** Survey on hearing testing: summary of findings. Health Visitor, 51 (5), May 1978, 194-195.

8 **Hickish, G.** All about children's ears. (Deafness.) Midwife, Health Visitor and Community Nurse, 13 (11), Nov 1977, 355-359.

9 **Hutchings, S.A.** Audiometric screening in schools. 1. The types of deafness and how they are detected in children. 2. A child with bilateral sensori-neural loss and secretory otitis media. (Case study.) Nursing Times, 74, 23 Nov 1978, 1947-1949; 30 Nov 1978, 1991-1994.

10 **Latham, A.D. and Haggard, M.P.** A pilot study to detect hearing impairment in the young. (Involving HVs who used a 'clues-to-hearing' leaflet for parents to help them assess child's hearing ability.) Midwife, Health Visitor and Community Nurse, 16 (9), Sep 1980, 370, 372, 374.

11 **Lesser, S.R. and Easser, R.** Psychiatric management of the deaf child. Canadian Nurse, 71 (10), Oct 1975, 23-25.

12 **Marshall, P. and Prosser, J.** Work with the deaf—a neglected area. (Social work service in Cambridgeshire for children and young people.) Social Work Today, 8, 2 Aug 1977, 13-14.

13 **National Deaf Children's Society** Deaf children and their hearing aids. The Society, 1978.

14 **National Deaf Children's Society** The deaf school-leaver. The Society, 1977.

15 **Nursing Mirror** Symposium on deafness in children. Nursing Mirror, 143, 4 Nov 1976, 48-59. Includes:
Douek, E. Diagnosis and management. 53-54.
Fisch, L. Causes of deafness in children. 48-50.
James, C. Community care. 57-59.
Wood, A.R. Educating the deaf child. 54-57.
Young, J. The National Deaf Children's Society. 59.

16 **Wright, J.** Deaf but not mute. (Case study of a deaf child who learned to communicate effectively.) American Journal of Nursing, 76 (5), May 1976, 795-799.

f DENTISTRY AND DENTAL CARE

1 **Block, P.L.** Dental health in hospitalized patients. American Journal of Nursing, 76 (7), Jul 1976, 1162-1164.

2 **Breslin, H.** Practical prevention of dental disease in schoolchildren. Public Health, 93 (4), Jul 1979, 230-234.

3 **Clewett, J.A.** A consideration of dental health education. Health Education Journal, 34 (4), 1975, 115-118.

4 **Colman, G.** Prevention of dental caries. Nursing Times, 72, 12 Aug 1976, 1238-1239.

5 **Coutts, L.** Dental health education for mothers of pre-school children. Midwife, Health Visitor and Community Nurse, 16 (8), Aug 1980, 328, 330-331.

6 **Craft, M. and Croucher, R.** Preventive dental health in adolescents: results of a controlled field trial. Royal Society of Health Journal, 99 (2), Apr 1979, 48-56.

7 **Deb, A.K.** Should geriatric patients'

dentures be marked? (Brief report of pilot study of methods.) Geriatric Medicine, 9 (5), May 1979, 79.

8 **Dexter, C.R.** Preventive dentistry and the community. Health Visitor, 49 (9), Sep 1976, 284-285.

9 **Downer, C.** Future planning of community dental care. (Manchester Business School seminar.) Hospital and Health Services Review, 72 (4), Apr 1976, 121-126.

10 **Dyer, E.D. and others** Dental health in adults. American Journal of Nursing, 76 (7), Jul 1976, 1156-1159.

11 **Farrell, J.** Sans teeth: dental care for the elderly. Journal of Community Nursing, 1 (5), Nov 1977, 4-5.

12 **Feaver, G.P.** Dental care: preventing those teething problems. The importance of dental treatment being provided in hospital for cardiothoracic patients and patients receiving radiotherapy to the mouth and cervicofacial area. Nursing Mirror, 147, 30 Nov 1978, 42.

13 **Fidler, P.E.** A comparison of treatment patterns and costs for a fluoride and non-fluoride community. Community Health, 9 (2), Nov 1977, 103-113.

14 **Royal Society of Health Journal** Fluoridation—the present case. (4 articles.) Royal Society of Health Journal, 92 (2), Apr 1977, 45-59, 63.

15 **Grenby, T.H.** Dental decay after sugary foods. Nursing Mirror, 143, 19 Aug 1976, 46-51.

16 **Hubbard-Ryland, P.A.** Dental care of the elderly. Nursing Times, 74, 16 Feb 1978, 290-291.

17 **Jackson, D.** The argument for fluoridation. Health Education Journal, 34 (4), 1975, 103-111.

18 **Jeanes, K.R. and Grant, J.R.** Children's retention of dental hygiene instruction: report of a pilot study. Nursing Research, 25 (6), Nov-Dec 1976, 452-453.

19 **Jones, P.R.** The distribution of dental care. Hospital and Health Services Review, 73 (10), Oct 1977, 351-352.

20 **Keywood, O.** The work of dental hygienists and auxiliaries. Nursing Times, 75, 8 Feb 1979, 247.

21 **King, J.** Care of children's teeth: some of the difficulties of helping handicapped children to look after their teeth. Health and Social Service Journal, 87, 30 Sep 1977, 1384.

22 **King, J.M.** Dental health: how can we achieve it? Health Visitor, 50 (9), Sep 1977, 288-289.

23 **Loach, G.A.** Total dental clearance under local anaesthetic. (Care study by nurse on JBCNS course in theatre nursing.) Nursing Times, 76, 24 Jan 1980, 155-156.

24 **May, D.** If the mountain can't come to Mohammed... (Dental Home Care Unit in South Glamorgan, for housebound patients.) Journal of Community Nursing, 1 (5), Nov 1977, 27.

25 **Morton, M.E.** Dental disease in a group of adult mentally handicapped patients. Public Health, 91 (1), Jan 1977, 23-32.

26 **Osborn, B.** Dental treatment for diabetic patients. Journal of Community Nursing, 1 (10), Apr 1978, 23.

27 **Osborn, B.** Rundown on the dental services. Journal of Community Nursing, 1 (5), Nov 1977, 18, 23.

28 **Preest, M. and Gelbier, S.** Dental health and treatment needs of a group of physically handicapped adults. Community Health, 9 (1), Aug 1977, 29-34.

29 **Royal College of Physicians. Committee on the Fluoridation of Water Supplies** Fluoride, teeth and health: a report and summary... Pitman, 1976. (Chairman: Sir Cyril Clarke.)

30 **Scully, C.** Something to bite on: dental care for mentally handicapped children. National Society for Mentally Handicapped Children, 1976.

31 **Sheiham, A.** Is there a scientific basis for six monthly dental examinations? (Review of studies.) Lancet, 2, 27 Aug 1977, 442-444.

32 **Slatterly, J.** Dental health in children. American Journal of Nursing, 76 (7), Jul 1976, 1159-1161.

33 **Smith, J.T.** Promoting childhood dental health. Pediatric Nursing, 2 (3), May/Jun 1976, 16-19.

34 **Snook, H.M.** The use of dental services by pre-school children. Health Bulletin, 34 (2), Mar 1976, 91-98.

35 **Stoner, J.E.** Planning dental services for a university population. Public Health, 93 (1), Jan 1979, 25-30.

36 **Stratford, J.M.** The health visitor and preventive dentistry. Midwife, Health Visitor and Community Nurse, 15 (4), Apr 1979, 147-149.

37 **Tee, J.H.** Dental health educational activities in the areas of England and Wales: results of a postal survey. Health Education Journal, 38 (4), 1979, 128-136.

38 **Warren, M.D. and others** Planning the provision of dental treatment for handicapped persons living at home. Public Health, 94 (1), Jan 1980, 30-39.

39 **Wildy, M. and others** Assessment of the dental knowledge of pregnant and nursing women attending four health centres. Health Education Journal, 38 (4), 1979, 123-127.

40 **Wilson, N.H.F.** The dental care of geriatric patients in hospitals. Public Health, 91 (2), Mar 1977, 97-102.

41 **Wilson, N.H.F.** A survey of the need for emergency dental services. Public Health, 90 (5), Jul 1976, 231-233.

42 **World Health Organization. Expert Committee** Planning and evaluation of public dental health services. Geneva: WHO, 1976. (Technical report series, no.589.)

g MOUTH CARE

1 **Blinkhorn, A.S.** Dentists and health visitors: an investigation into their agreement on acceptable oral hygiene regime for pre-school children. Health Education Journal, 37 (3), 1979, 193-195.

2 **British Dental Health Foundation** Home mouth care manual. The Foundation, 1976.

3 **Daeffler, R.** Oral hygiene measures for patients with cancer. 2. Cancer Nursing, 3 (6), Dec 1980, 427-432.

4 **Harris, M.D.** Tools for mouth care. (Research study in South Glamorgan based on Howarth's research.) Nursing Times, 76, 21 Feb 1980, 340-342.

5 **Hilton, D.** Oral hygiene and infection. (Care of patients' mouths at St. Columba's Hospice, Edinburgh, with care study of patient with oral carcinoma.) Nursing Times, 76, 17 Jul 1980, 1270-1272.

6 **Howarth, M.H.** Mouth care procedures for the very ill. (Abstract of MSc thesis, Manchester University, 1975. 'A study of mouth care procedure carried out by nurses for the very ill person'.) Nursing Times, 73, 10 Mar 1977, 354-355.

7 **Kirkis, E.J.** This oral care technique gets results. (Method involving mouth wash, ice chips, water and friction with sponge or applicator.) RN Magazine, 41 (10), Oct 1978, 82.

8 **Morton, C.** The mouth ulcer mystery. Health Visitor, 49 (9), Sep 1976, 287.

9 **Nally, F.F.** Infections of the mouth. Nursing Times, 73, 18 Aug 1977, 1275-1278.

10 **Schweiger, J.L. and others** Oral assessment: how to do it. American Journal of Nursing, 80 (4), Apr 1980, 654-657.

11 **Trowbridge, J.E. and Carl, W.** Oral care: of the patient having head and neck irradiation. American Journal of Nursing, 75 (12), Dec 1975, 2146-2149.

12 **Urbanska, D.K.** Care of the mouth and teeth. Nursing Mirror, 144, 1, 19 May 1977, 13-15.
2. Pregnancy. 2 Jun 1977, 29-30.
3. Infancy. 16 Jun 1977, 21-23.
4. Childhood and adolescence. 30 Jun 1977, 25-27.
5. The elderly. 14 Jul 1977, 27-39.
6. The mentally handicapped. 24-26.

13 **World Health Organization** Oral health surveys: basic methods. 2nd ed. Geneva: WHO, 1977.

14 **World Health Organization** Planning oral health services. Geneva: WHO, 1980.

15 **Young, P.** An experiment in preventive dental care. (Oral Hygiene Centre in London.) Nursing Mirror, 147, 24 Aug 1978, 7-8.

89 ENDOCRINE AND METABOLIC SYSTEMS

a ENDOCRINE SYSTEM

1 **Beardwell, C.G.** Acromegaly. Nursing Times, 73, 6 Oct 1977, 1547-1549.

2 Coupland, R.E. The adrenal glands. Nursing Times, 73, 10 Nov 1977, 1748-1751.

3 Cronin, W.E. Nursing care study. Rehabilitation of a patient with myxoedema. (Elderly lady.) Nursing Times, 74, 17 Aug 1978, 1365-1366.

4 Cumming, A.A.M. Nursing care study. Conn's syndrome. Nursing Mirror, 142, 22 Jan 1976, 50-52.

5 Felstein, I. Ten faces of a disguised disease. (How nurses assist in diagnosing myxoedema.) Nursing Mirror, 150, 7 Feb 1980, 34-35.

6 Firmin, P.B. Theatre nursing care study. Derbyshire neck. (Enlarged right lobe of the thyroid gland.) Nursing Times, 74, 16 Nov 1978, 1896-1899.

7 Hallel, J.C. Thyroid disorders. American Journal of Nursing, 77 (3), Mar 1977, 417-432.

8 Harvey, D. Children of short stature. Midwife, Health Visitor and Community Nurse, 14 (5), May 1978, 136-137, 139; (6), Jun 1978, 177-178.

9 Hipkin, L.J. Hyperparathyroidism. Nursing Times, 73, 15 Sep 1977, 1430-1432.

10 Hurwitz, L.S. Nursing implications of selected pediatric endocrine problems. Nursing Clinics of North America, 15 (3), Sep 1980, 525-534.

11 Iveson-Iveson, J. The endocrine system. (Anatomy and physiology.) Nursing Mirror, 148, 3 May 1979, 34-35.

12 Jack, S. Theatre nursing care study. Partial thyroidectomy. Nursing Times, 72, 7 Oct 1976, 1556-1558.

13 Jackson, A.S. Nursing care study. Partial thyroidectomy. Nursing Times, 74, 26 Oct 1978, 1760-1763.

14 Jeffcoate, W. A guide to the endocrine system. (Physiology and diseases.) Nursing Mirror, 144, 12 May 1977, 58-60.

15 Lancour, J. ADH and aldosterone: how to recognize their effects. Nursing, 8 (9), Sep 1978, 36-41.

16 London, D.R. Pituitary diseases. 1. The pituitary gland and its disorders. 2. Diseases of the anterior pituitary gland. 3. Hypopituitarism. Nursing Times, 72, 17 Jun 1976, 939-941; 24 Jun 1976, 966-968; 1 Jul 1976, 1012-1013.

17 McFarlane, J. Congenital adrenal hyperplasia. American Journal of Nursing, 76 (8), Aug 1976, 1290-1292.

18 McGann, M.R. Secondary hyperaldosteronism. (Nursing care study.) American Journal of Nursing, 76 (4), Apr 1976, 634-637.

19 Maisey, M.N. Thyroid disease. Nursing Mirror, 146, 4 May 1978, 15-19.

20 Newton, G.M. Nursing care study. Clitoroplasty for andrenogenital syndrome. Nursing Times, 72, 27 May 1976, 816-819.

21 Nursing Clinics of North America Symposium on endocrine disorders. (7 articles.) Nursing Clinics of North America, 15 (3), Sep 1980, 433-534.

22 Parkin, J.M. Short stature in childhood. Nursing Times, 73, 30 Jun 1977, 995-997.

23 Roberts, A. Systems of life. No.50. Hormones and homoeostasis. Nursing Times, 75, 1 Feb 1979, (4).

24 Roberts, A. Systems of life. Nos.51-53. The energy supremo—the thyroid gland. 1. The control system. 2. Searching for faults. 3. Failures of control. Nursing Times, 75, 1 Mar 1979, (4); 5 Apr 1979, (4); 3 May 1979, (4).

25 Roberts, A. Systems of life. Nos.60-62. The pituitary gland. 1. Hypopituitarism; growth and development. 3. The posterior pituitary and water homoeostasis. Nursing Times, 76, 3 Jan 1980, (4); 7 Feb 1980, (4).

26 Saunders, J. Phaeochromocytoma—surgery can bring a complete cure. (Tumour of adrenal medullary tissue.) Nursing Mirror, 147, 17 Aug 1978, 19-20.

27 Shaw, K. and Bloom, A. The nature of the endocrine system. Nursing Mirror, 144, 1, 19 May 1977, 20-22.
2. The pituitary gland. 26 May 1977, 24-26.
3. The thyroid gland. 2 Jun 1977, 26-28.
4. The adrenal gland. 9 Jun 1977, 32-35.
5. The pancreas gland. 16 Jun 1977, 26-28.
6. The parathyroid gland and calcium metabolism. 23 Jun 1977, 28-30.
7. The sex hormones. 30 Jun 1977, 32-34.
8. Gastrointestinal hormones. 7 Jul 1977, 22-24.

28 Stevens, D.W. Theatre nursing care study. Thyrotoxicosis treated by surgery. Nursing Times, 73, 31 Mar 1977, 450-451.

29 Swyer, G. Dopamine, prolactin, and bromocriptine. Nursing Mirror, 143, 16 Sep 1976, 65-66.

30 Todd, J. Achillogram test in thyroid gland disorders. Nursing Mirror, 143, 2 Dec 1976, 60-61.

31 Tunbridge, W.M.G. Acromegaly. Nursing Times, 75, 18 Jan 1979, 110-112.

b DIABETES: GENERAL

1 American Journal of Nursing Common problems in managing adult diabetes mellitus. (Seven articles by various authors on topics including diabetic ketoacidosis, patient teaching, care of the elderly and foot care.) American Journal of Nursing, 78 (5), May 1978, 871-890.

2 Blach, R.K. and Bloom, A. Diabetic eye centres for the management of diabetic eye disease. Health Trends, 4 (10), Nov 1978, 88-90.

3 Collin, J. Pancreatic transplantation (for the treatment of diabetes). Nursing Mirror, 143, 22 Jul 1976, 51-53.

4 Cook, K.A. Diabetics can be vegetarians. (With examples of diets.) Nursing (U.S.), 9 (10), Oct 1979, 70-73.

5 Cudworth, A.G. Does diabetes run in families? Nursing Mirror, 144, 31 Mar 1977, 60-61.

6 Davies, G. Diabetic retinopathy. (New treatment by photocoagulation.) Nursing Times, 74, 24 Aug 1978, 1421-1422.

7 Ellis, F.N. The diabetic in hospital. Nursing Mirror, 144, 3 Feb 1977, 52-54.

8 Fletcher, H.P. The oral antidiabetic drugs: pro and con. American Journal of Nursing, 76 (4), Apr 1976, 596-599.

9 Fox, M. Transplantation of islets of Langerhans. A new hope for diabetics. (Experimental studies in animals.) Nursing Mirror, 144, 5 May 1977, 50-52.

10 Garofano, C. Travel tips for the peripatetic diabetic. Nursing, 7 (8), Aug 1977, 44-46.

11 Greenough, A. and others Disposable syringes for insulin injection. (Survey.) British Medical Journal, 1, 2 Jun 1979, 1467-1468.

12 Guthrie, D.W. and Guthrie, R.A. DKA: breaking a vicious cycle. (Diabetic ketoacidosis.) Nursing, 8 (6), Jun 1978, 54-61.

13 Ireland, J.T. and others Diabetes today: a handbook for the clinical team. Aylesbury: HM & M, 1980.

14 Knight, M. Transplantation of Islets of Langerhans in diabetes mellitus. Nursing Mirror, 142, 20 May 1976, 55-56.

15 Koivisto, V.A. and Felig, P. Is skin preparation necessary before insulin injection? (Survey indicating that it reduces skin bacterial counts.) Lancet, 1, 20 May 1978, 1072-1073.

16 Lancet New insulin-delivery systems for diabetics. Lancet, 1, 16 Jun 1979, 1275-1277.

17 Lister, J. The syndrome of diabetes. (The two types of diabetes and contributing factors.) Nursing Mirror, 146, 27 Apr 1978, 23-24.

18 Martini, B. Diabetes: a practical approach to the problem of diet. (With the elderly.) Geriatric Medicine, 9 (7), Jul 1979, 33-34, 37-38.

19 Small, D. Special needs of the geriatric diabetic patient. Journal of Practical Nursing, 26 (11), Nov 1976, 25-27, 36.

20 Steel, J. and others How useful are patient-operated blood glucose meters? (Discussion and results of study.) Practitioner, 224, Jun 1980, 651-653.

21 Stewart, A.G. Diabetes mellitus and hypothyroidism. Nursing Mirror, 144, 3 Feb 1977, 48-51.

22 Thomas, K.P. Diabetes mellitus in elderly persons. Nursing Clinics of North America, 11 (1), Mar 1976, 157-168.

23 Walford, S. and others Self-monitoring of blood-glucose. Improvement of diabetic control. (See also leading article on p.757.) Lancet, 1, 8 Apr 1978, 732-735.

c DIABETES: NURSING AND COMMUNITY CARE

1 Blevins, D.R. editor The diabetic and nursing care. New York: McGraw-Hill, 1979.

2 Bloom, A. Diabetes explained. 3rd ed. Lancaster, MTP, 1978. (For nurses and others.)

3 Bridgman, J.F. and others Control of insulin dependant diabetes at home. (Scheme in Basildon and Thurrock district using community liaison nurse.) Practitioner, 220, Feb 1978, 193-194.

4 Cavalier, J.P. Crucial decisions in diabetic

emergencies. RN Magazine, 43 (11), Nov 1980, 32-37.

5 Doney, B.J. An audit of the care of diabetics in a group practice. Journal of the Royal College of General Practitioners, 26, Oct 1976, 734-742.

6 Farquhar, J.W. and Campbell, M.L. Care of the diabetic child in the community. (Hospital-based mobile team of experienced sisters at the Royal Edinburgh Hospital for Sick Children.) British Medical Journal, 281, 6 Dec 1980, 1534-1537.

7 Garland, C. Nursing care study. Diabetic ketosis. Nursing Mirror, 146, 25 May 1978, 26.

8 Gerber, F. Diabetes out of control! (Nursing care study.) RN Magazine, 42 (9), Sep 1979, 65-68.

9 Guthrie, D.W. and Guthrie, R.A. editors Nursing management of diabetes mellitus. St. Louis: Mosby, 1977.

10 Hayter, J. Fine points in diabetic care. American Journal of Nursing, 76 (4), Apr 1976, 594-599.

11 Hill, R.D. Community care service for diabetics in the Poole area. British Medical Journal, 1, 8 May 1976, 1137-1139.

12 Hurst, K. Nursing care study. Diabetes with complications: when illness struck three times. (Myocardial infarction and anaemia.) Nursing Mirror, 149, 19 Jul 1979, 40-43.

13 Iveson-Iveson, J. Disease: its cause and effect. 3: Disorders of metabolism—diabetes mellitus. (Treatment and nursing care.) Nursing Mirror, 149, 27 Sep 1979, 27-28.

14 Jackson, M.M. Diabetics at home. (Home stabilisation scheme in Leeds involving liaison health visitors.) Nursing Times, 75, 10 May 1979, Community Outlook, 123, 125-126.

15 Kelly, B.A. Nurses' knowledge of glycosuria testing in diabetes mellitus. Nursing Research, 28 (5), Sep/Oct 1979, 316-319.

16 Kratky, A.P. An audit of the care of diabetics in one general practice. (Basis for follow-up system involving integrated and shared care between doctor and nurse.) Journal of the Royal College of General Practitioners, 27, Sep 1977, 536-541.

17 Lancet Day care units for diabetics. Lancet, 2, 24 Jul 1976, 187.

18 Leslie, J. Nutrition and diet. Part 7. Management of the diabetic patient. Nursing Mirror, 145, 8 Sep 1977, 27-31.

19 McCarthy, J. Somogyi effect: managing blood glucose rebound. (Insulin-induced hypoglycaemia.) Nursing (U.S.), 9 (2), Feb 1979, 39-41.

20 Mahon, S. Consciousness and diabetes. (Symptoms in and care of patient during hypoglycaemic attacks.) Nursing, 8, Dec 1979, 363-364.

21 Matthes, M.L. Diabetic day care. (Hospital educational service clinic.) American Journal of Nursing, 79 (1), Jan 1979, 105-106.

22 Whitehead, A.S. Nursing care study. Neglect of diabetes leading to bilateral amputation. Nursing Times, 74, 7 Sep 1978, 1490-1493.

23 Wilkes, E. and Lawton, E.E. The diabetic, the hospital and primary care. (Medical supervision received by patients discharged from hospital and work of nurse who assisted GPs in setting up diabetic clinic.) Journal of the Royal College of General Practitioners, 30, Apr 1980, 199-206.

24 Williams, T.D. Community care of the diabetic. Nursing Mirror, 144, 3 Feb 1977, 55-56.

25 Wrench, J.G. Integration of diabetic care—a diabetic clinic in general practice. (In Livingston.) Health Bulletin, 36 (6), Nov 1978, 300-305.

26 Wrigley, P. Patient care study—diabetes mellitus. Queen's Nursing Journal, 19 (6), Sep 1976, 172-173.

27 Yudkin, J.S. and others The quality of diabetic care in a London health district. (Study of 217 patients.) Journal of Epidemiology and Community Health, 34 (4), Dec 1980, 277-286.

d DIABETES: PATIENT AND PATIENT TEACHING

1 Ayres, O. Living with diabetes. (Personal account by nurse.) Nursing, 12, Apr 1980, 532-534.

2 Bevis, S. Salisbury's progressive diabetics. (Patient education in diabetic clinic and formation of local branch of British Diabetic Association.) Nursing Times, 74, 16 Nov 1978, 1900-1901.

3 Boyles, V.A. Injection aids for blind diabetic patients. American Journal of Nursing, 77 (9), Sep 1977, 1456-1458.

4 Brock, A.M. A study to determine the effectiveness of a learning activity package for the adult with diabetes mellitus. (Pilot study in Maryland, USA.) Journal of Advanced Nursing, 3 (3), May 1978, 265-275.

5 Brock, P.A. Beginning research. Diabetic patients' understanding of their disease and its treatment. (Study of 30 patients admitted to hospital with some home interviews.) Nursing Times, 73, 21 Jul 1977, 1117-1119.

6 Fletcher, C. Personal paper. One way of coping with diabetes. British Medical Journal, 280, 26 Apr 1980, 1115-1116.

7 Fuestel, D.E. Nursing students' knowledge about diabetes mellitus. (Survey to investigate whether nurses about to graduate were able to teach patients and their families.) Nursing Research, 25 (1), Jan/Feb 1976, 4-8.

8 Garofano, C. Deliver facts to help diabetics plan parenthood. Nursing, 77 7 (4), Apr 1977, 13-16.

9 Gates, K. A candid evaluation of diabetic teaching. Dimensions in Health Service, 52 (11), Nov 1975, 13-14.

10 Isaf, J.J. and Alogna, M.T. Better use of resources equals better health for diabetics. (Setting up of Diabetes Detection and Control Centre at an Atlanta Hospital and appointment of two full-time diabetes teaching nurses.) American Journal of Nursing, 77 (11), Nov 1977, 1792-1795.

11 Iveson-Iveson, J. Teaching the teachers. Report of a recent meeting of the British Diabetic Association in conjunction with Guy's Hospital. (Methods of teaching diabetics.) Nursing Mirror, 145, 3 Nov 1977, 7.

12 Laugharne, E. and Steiner, G. Tri-hospital diabetes education centre: a cost-effective cooperation venture. (Resources shared by three hospitals.) Canadian Nurse, 73 (9), Sep 1977, 14-19.

13 Leatherdale, B.A. and others Communication with Asian diabetics. (Survey in Birmingham to assess impact of literature and signs in Asian language.) British Medical Journal, 2, 28 Oct 1978, 1197-1198.

14 Lowery, B.J. and Du Cette, J.P. Disease-related learning and disease control in diabetics as a function of locus of control. Nursing Research, 25 (5), Sep/Oct 1976, 358-362.

15 Manfredi, C. and others Developing a teaching program for diabetic patients. Journal of Continuing Education in Nursing, 8 (6), Nov/Dec 1977, 46-52.

16 Miller, B.K. and White, N.E. Diabetes assessment guide. (Questionnaire to assess patients' knowledge of their condition as guide to patient teaching.) American Journal of Nursing, 80 (7), Jul 1980, 1314-1316.

17 Morris, M.L. Why patient education? (With reference to diabetes.) Occupational Health Nursing, 27 (12), Dec 1979, 7-15.

18 Nursing Clinics of North America Symposium on diabetes: patient education and care. Nursing Clinics of North America, 12 (3), Sep 1977, 361-445.

19 Petrokas, J.C. Commonsense guidelines for controlling diabetes during illness. (Advice for diabetics at home.) Nursing, 7 (12), Dec 1977, 36-37.

20 Porter, A.L. Student participation in diabetic patient education. (Nursing module at Evanston Hospital School of Nursing.) Nursing Clinics of North America, 12 (3), Sep 1977, 407-414.

21 Porter, S.F. Diabetic education: a role for the inservice instructor. (In developing and co-ordinating a hospital/community diabetic education programme for patients.) Supervisor Nurse, 8 (5), May 1977, 49-53.

22 Reynolds, W.B. Health education for the diabetic. (Evaluation of pilot programme in industry.) Occupational Health Nursing, 26 (9), Sep 1978, 7-14.

23 West, T.E.T. A guide for patients: the care of diabetes during illness. (Reprinted from 'Balance' by the British Diabetic Association.) Nursing Mirror, 142, 22 Apr 1976, 53-54.

24 Wolfe, L. Insulin: paving the way to a new life. (Patient teaching.) Nursing, 7 (11), Nov 1977, 38-41.

25 Wotring, K.E. Problems in management: diabetes in the psychiatric patient. Journal of Psychiatric Nursing and Mental Health Services, 16 (8), Aug 1978, 26, 28.

e DIABETES: PREGNANCY

1 Brundenell, M. Diabetic pregnancy. Nursing Mirror, 142, 8 Apr 1976, 60-62.

2 Littlefield, V. and Siebert, G. The group approach to problem-solving for pregnant diabetic women. (Discussion and counselling group.) Maternal Child Nursing Journal, 3 (5), Sep/Oct 1978, 274-280.

3 Nursing Grand Rounds Panel Diabetes in pregnancy: special care for a special case. Nursing (U.S.), 10 (11), Nov 1980, 44-49.

4 Schuler, K. and others When a pregnant woman is diabetic. (Antepartal, intrapartal, postpartal care, a case study and care of the newborn.) American Journal of Nursing, 79 (3), Mar 1979, 448-460.

5 Spearing, G.J. Diabetes in pregnancy. Journal of Human Nutrition, 31 (5), Oct 1977, 329-335.

6 Stubbs, S.M. and others Management of the pregnant diabetic: home or hospital, with or without glucose meters? Lancet, 1, 24 May 1980, 1122-1124.

f DIABETES: CHILDREN AND ADOLESCENTS

1 Ames Company Rupert and his friends: a guide for the young diabetic. Slough: Ames, 1977.

2 Crosby, E.F. Childhood diabetes: the emotional adjustment of parents and child. Canadian Nurse, 73 (9), Sep 1977, 20-23.

3 Fishley, M. British Diabetic Association camps: a holiday with a difference. Nursing Mirror, 151, 14 Aug 1980, 24-25.

4 Friedland, G.M. Learning behaviors of a preadolescent with diabetes. American Journal of Nursing, 76 (1), Jan 1976, 59-61.

5 Hamilton, D.V. and others Mode of presentation of juvenile diabetes. British Medical Journal, 2, 24 Jul 1976, 211-212.

6 Iveson-Iveson, J. The diabetic child. Ways in which this condition influences a child's development. Nursing Mirror, 146, 5 Jan 1978, 5-6.

7 McDonagh, M. Nursing care study. Jean adapts to a lifelong routine. (Adolescent with acute onset diabetes mellitus. By Diploma in Nursing Student.) Nursing Mirror, 149, 22 Nov 1979, 38-40.)

8 Moens, J. Coping with diabetes insipidus. (With case study of five-year-old child.) Canadian Nursing, 75 (4), Apr 1979, 18-20.

9 Paxinos, R. and Ferguson, R. Juvenile diabetes—a team approach. (Education by multi-disciplinary team in a Melbourne hospital.) Journal of Human Nutrition, 32 (4), Aug 1978, 294-296.

10 Polowich, C. and Elliott, M.R. The juvenile diabetic: in or out of control? (Survey of problems among 11-17 year old diabetics.) Canadian Nurse, 73 (9), Sep 1977, 24-27.

11 Robinson, W. Summer camp for diabetics. (Run by British Diabetic Association.) Nursing Mirror, 145, 6 Oct 1977, 50-52.

12 Rose, V. Fun for the future. Summer camps organised by the British Diabetic Association. Nursing Times, 73, 25 Aug 1977, 1304-1305.

13 Rose, V. What teenage diabetics really think. (Talks with children at a BDA summer camp.) Journal of Community Nursing, 1 (6), Dec 1977, 11, 24.

14 Roskell, V. Beginning research. Families with diabetic children. Nursing Times, 73, 15 Dec 1977, 1948-1951.

15 Smith, T. The problems of the teenage diabetic. Journal of Community Nursing, 1 (6), Dec 1977, 12, 24.

16 Tattersall, R. Why children develop diabetes. (Physiology and pathology.) Nursing Mirror, 145, 25 Aug 1977, 28-30.

g METABOLIC SYSTEM AND ALLERGY

1 American Journal of Nursing Allergies in children. Recognition, testing and treating, teaching. (Three articles.) American Journal of Nursing, 78 (4), Apr 1978, 613-621.

2 American Journal of Nursing Metabolic acid-base disorders. Part 1. Chemistry and physiology. Programmed instruction. American Journal of Nursing, 77 (10), Oct 1977, P.I. 1-32.

3 Barbor, P. Some inborn errors of metabolism. Nursing Mirror, 147, 20 Jul 1978, 21-22.

4 Basner, N.H. Wilson's disease: a rare genetic disorder. Journal of Neurosurgical Nursing, 8 (2), Dec 1976, 144-148.

5 Benson, P. The Hunter syndrome. Nursing Mirror, 143, 18 Nov 1976, 48-49.

6 Cooksley, P.A. Nursing care study. Acute intermittent porphyria. Nursing Times, 76, 12 Jun 1980, 1041-1043.

7 Cowie, V. Inborn errors of metabolism. (Includes phenylketonuria.) Nursing Mirror, 145, 4 Aug 1977, 19-21.

8 Gracey, B. Nursing care study. Maple syrup urine disease. (Inborn error of metabolism.) Nursing Mirror, 147, 23 Nov 1978, 26-28.

9 Gunn, A.D.G. Allergen and the nurse—2. (With reference to nurse running an allergy clinic.) Journal of Community Nursing, 2 (7), Jan 1979, 4-5, 7.

10 Holzel, A. Allergy in children. Nursing Times, 72, 5 May 1977, 649-652.

11 Iveson-Iveson, J. Familial—hypercholesterolaemia. (Treatment at the MRC Lipid Metabolism Unit, Hammersmith Hospital.) Nursing Mirror, 143, 18 Nov 1976, 61.

12 Kelly, J. Nursing care study. Wilson's disease: excess copper invades the body. Nursing Mirror, 148, 22 Feb 1979, 39-41.

13 Kuzemko, J.A. A review of paediatric allergies. (Includes food allergy.) Midwife, Health Visitor and Community Nurse, 15 (10), Oct 1979, 390, 393, 395, 397.

14 McColl, K.E.L. and Fairbain, E.D.S. Acute intermittent porphyria. (For correction of error in tables see Nursing Times, 27 Sep 1979, 1688.) Nursing Times, 75, 20 Sep 1979, 1624-1628.

15 Mostafanejad, K. Nursing care study. Methylmalonic acidaemia. (Inborn error of metabolism in seven-year-old boy.) Nursing Times, 74, 20 Apr 1978, 665-666.

16 Nursing Mirror A symposium on allergies and their management. (Rhinitis, conjunctivitis and the clinical uses of sodium cromoglycate in these conditions and asthma.) Nursing Mirror, 145, 8 Sep 1977, 19-26.

17 Stordy, B.J. Food allergy—is it all true? Nursing, 12, Apr 1980, 535-537.

18 Stordy, B.J. When the body takes a stand. (The immune response with reference to allergy.) Nursing Mirror, 150, 6 Mar 1980, Supplement, i-ii, iv-v, viii-ix, xi-xii.

19 Todd, S. Allergy to food and chemicals. 1. The scope of the problem. 2. Investigation and treatment. Nursing Times, 74, 16 Mar 1978, 438-441; 23 Mar 1978, 506-510.

20 Walker-Smith, J. Forbidden fruits. (Food allergy in children.) Nursing Mirror, 151, 18 Sep 1980, 32-36.

h OBESITY

1 Department of Health and Social Security and **Medical Research Council** Research on obesity: a report of the DHSS/MRC Group. HMSO, 1976.

2 Ellis, C. Morbid obesity: a comparative study. (Report of study tour to hospitals in Vancouver, Los Angeles and San Francisco.) Nursing Times, 76, 21 Feb 1980, Occ. papers, 17-20.

3 Fletcher, R. Obesity: facing up to the fats... (Advice on slimming.) Nursing Mirror, 148, 15 Mar 1979, 34-35.

4 Garrow, J. Obesity clinic. 1. Who works there and why. 2. Treatment of refractory patients. (Northwick Park Hospital.) Nursing Times, 72, 15 Jan 1976, 78-79; 22 Jan 1976, 116-117.

5 Iveson-Iveson, J. Disease: its cause and effect. 9. Nutritional disease. (Obesity.) Nursing Mirror, 149, 8 Nov 1979, 16-17.

6 Kawasaki, G. and others Solving the very big problems of the morbidly obese. Nursing (U.S.), 10 (11), Nov 1980, 40-43.

7 Leslie, J. Nutrition and diet. 3. Management of adult obese patients. Nursing Mirror, 145, 14 Jul 1977, 21-23.

8 MacConville, C. Danger! obesity at work. (How OH nurse can help through slimming classes.) Nursing, 11, Mar 1980, 490-494.

9 MacLeod, A. Management of obesity in a subnormal patient. (Using behaviour modifications.) Nursing Times, 75, 18 Oct 1979, 1814-1815.

10 Mahan, L.K. A sensible approach to the obese patient. Nursing Clinics of North America, 14 (2), Jun 1979, 229-245.

11 Rotatori, A.F. and others A weight

reduction model for mildly retarded adults living in semi-independent care facilities. (Based on behaviour theory.) Journal of Advanced Nursing, 5 (2), Mar 1980, 179-186.

12 Tymkiw, G. Obesity: a challenge for patient teaching. Canadian Nurse, 74 (10), Nov 1978, 42-44.

13 Wineman, N.M. Obesity: locus of control, body image, weight loss, and age-at-onset. (Retrospective study.) Nursing Research, 29 (4), Jul/Aug 1980, 231-237.

14 Young, L.E. Nursing interventions with obese cardiac patients. Nursing Clinics of North America, 13 (3), Sep 1978, 449-456.

i OBESITY: CHILDREN AND ADOLESCENTS

1 Bowers, J.E. and others Obesity in children: an ecological approach. (Involving psychiatric nurse and concentrating on psychosocial problems within families.) Journal of Continuing Education in Nursing, 10 (4), Jul/Aug 1979, 40-49.

2 Copeland, R.A. Obesity in school children. Nursing Times, 75, 11 Jan 1979, Community Outlook, 18-20.

3 Crow, R.A. and Fawcett, J. Obesity in infancy. Nursing Times, 75, 11 Jan 1979, Community Outlook, 11, 15.

4 Hutchinson, M. A multidisciplinary approach to aid the overweight child. (At the Royal Belfast Hospital for Sick Children involving nurse therapist, dietician and social worker with mothers and children.) Social Work Today, 9, 27 Jun 1978, 17-18.

5 Lancet Helping obese children. (Of school age.) Lancet, 1, 3 Jun 1978, 1189-1190.

6 Robinson, A.D. An attempt to treat overweight schoolchildren. (Child obesity clinic run by dietician.) Journal of Human Nutrition, 31 (5), Oct 1977, 375-376.

7 Rotatori, A.F. and others Weight loss in retarded children—a pilot study. (Behavioural/nutritional programme directed by school nurse.) Journal of Psychiatric Nursing, 17 (10), Oct 1979, 33-34.

8 Thomas, J.E. Adolescence and weight control. (Research study to obtain information relevant to the development of an effective health education approach.) Health Education Journal, 36 (1), 1977, 19-26.

90   HAEMATOLOGY

a GENERAL AND DISORDERS

1 American Journal of Nursing Blood therapy. (Home-study feature of six articles.) American Journal of Nursing, 79 (5), May 1979, 925-948.

2 Birch, C.R. Disseminated intravascular coagulation. (Otherwise known as consumption coagulopathy or the defibrination syndrome.) Nursing Times, 74 (1), 5 Jan 1978, 15-16.

3 Blust, J. Preventing hematomas after venipuncture. (Use of pressure dressings with blood

donors.) American Journal of Nursing, 78 (10), Oct 1978, 1675-1676.

4 British Medical Journal The National Blood Transfusion Service today. British Medical Journal, 281, 9 Aug 1980, 405-406.

5 Colvin, B.T. Thalassaemia. Nursing Mirror, 145, 10 Nov 1977, 18-20.

6 Edwards, J.M. Haematology research nurse in the United States. (British nurse working at Northwestern University, Chicago.) Nursing Times, 72, 5 Feb 1976, 194-195.

7 Ellis, P.D.M. Trans-sphenoidal hypophysectomy. Nursing Mirror, 144, 21 Apr 1977, 52-54.

8 Gorman, A. Thalassaemia. Nursing Times, 76, 31 Jul 1980, 1348-1350.

9 Graham, H. A difficult match. (Autoantibodies in blood.) Nursing Mirror, 151, 4 Sep 1980, 43.

10 Habel, M. What you need to know about infusing plasma expanders. (eg Dextran.) RN Magazine, 43 (8), Aug 1980, 30-33.

11 Halward, M.A. Autotransfusion. (Procedure used at St. Joseph's Hospital, Hamilton, Ontario.) Canadian Nurse, 73 (5), May 1977, 38.

12 Hegde, U. Christmas disease. (Deficiency of a specific plasma factor in blood leading to severe bleeding.) Nursing Mirror, 143, 23 Dec 1976, 31-33.

13 Hernandez, B. Platelets: a short course. How to safely collect and transfuse them. RN Magazine, 43 (6), Jun 1980, 36-41.

14 Hollingsworth, P.K. Autotransfusion in the emergency department. (Salvaging patient's own blood and returning it.) Journal of Emergency Nursing, 3 (4), Jul/Aug 1977, 9-10.

15 Hubbard, L.J. JWs and blood transfusions. (States that Jehovah's Witnesses have no objection to the use of non-blood alternatives such as dextran and saline solution.) Nursing Mirror, 144, 16 Jun 1977, 11.

16 Iveson-Iveson, J. Anatomy and physiology. The blood. Nursing Mirror, 148, 26 Apr 1979, 35-36.

17 Iveson-Iveson, J. Anatomy and physiology. The lymphatic system. Nursing Mirror, 148, 10 May 1979, 28-29.

18 Jeffrey, H.C. Modern transfusion practice. Health Bulletin, 34 (3), May 1976, 125-140.

19 Jennings, B.M. Improving your management of DIC. (Disseminated intravascular coagulation.) Nursing (U.S.), 9 (5), May 1979, 60-67.

20 LeBourdais, E. Controlling transfusion errors. Dimensions in Health Service, 54 (8), Aug 1977, 20, 22-23.

21 Lewis, B. Attitudes and altruism. (Survey of blood donors' and the general public's attitudes to organ donorship.) Health and Social Service Journal, 90, 14 Mar 1980, 356-357.

22 Linley, G. Autotransfusion. Nursing Mirror, 142, 18 Mar 1976, 69-70.

23 Nour-Eldin, F. Current transfusion problems. Nursing Mirror, 143, 12 Aug 1976, 50-53.

24 Nursing Blood transfusions today: what you should know and should do. Nursing, 8 (2), Feb 1978, 68-70, 72.

25 O'Brian, B.S. and Woods, S. The paradox of DIC. (Disseminated intravascular coagulation.) American Journal of Nursing, 78 (11), Nov 1978, 1878-1880.

26 Parker, D. Polycythaemia. Nursing Times, 72, 9 Dec 1976, 1919-1922.

27 Reardon, N. Nursing care study. Idiopathic thrombocytopenic purpura. Nursing Times, 72, 24 Jun 1976, 980-983.

28 Roberts, A. Body fluids. The blood. Nursing Times, 73, 15 Sep 1977, Body fluids, 13-16; 20 Oct 1977, Body fluids, 17-20.

29 Roberts, A. Body fluids. The lymph. Nursing Times, 73, 17 Nov 1977, Body fluids, 21-24.

30 Roberts, A. Systems of life. 12. Lymphatic system. Nursing Times, 72, 1/8 Jan 1976, (4).

31 Roberts, A. Systems of life. 21. Haemostasis. Nursing Times, 72, 2 Sep 1976, (4).

32 Roberts, A. and Besterman, A. Systems of life. 22. Blood transfusion. Nursing Times, 72, 7 Oct 1976, (4).

33 Rossman, M. and others Pheresis therapy: patient care. (Separation of blood into its individual components, and the removal of selected components.) American Journal of Nursing, 77 (7), Jul 1977, 1135-1141.

34 Sokol, R.J. Blood transfusion. Nursing Mirror, 145, 27 Oct 1977, 13-15.

35 Thorne, R. Nursing care study. Polycythaemia vera. (Patient admitted initially to a psycho-geriatric day hospital, but whose condition was subsequently diagnosed as a blood disorder.) Nursing Mirror, 146, 15 Jun 1978, 25-26.

36 Tovey, L.A. Conquest of Rh haemolytic disease. Nursing Mirror, 143, 11 Nov 1976, 49-50.

37 Tripp, A. Hyper and hypo calcemia. American Journal of Nursing, 76 (7), Jul 1976, 1142-1145.

38 Wallace, J. and Freeman, P.A. Mouth care in patients with blood dyscrasias. (Description of care at St. Bartholomew's Hospital for patients with blood diseases.) Nursing Times, 74, 1 Jun 1978, 921-922.

39 Zucker, M.B. The functioning of blood platelets. (With illustrations and diagrams.) Scientific American, 242 (6), Jun 1980, 70-74, 83-86, 88-89.

b ANAEMIA AND SICKLE CELL DISEASE

1 Anionwu, E.N. Self help in sickle-cell anaemia. The formation in Brent of a self help group for victims of sickle-cell anaemia. World Medicine, 12 (25), 21 Sep 1977, 86, 89, 91.

2 **Anionwu, E.N.** Sickle-cell—menace in the blood. Nursing Mirror, 147, 20 Jul 1978, 16-19.

3 **Clarke-Williams, M.J.** Anaemia in the elderly. Nursing Times, 73, 3 Mar 1977, 299-301.

4 **Doswell, W.M.** Sickle cell anemia: you can do something to help. Nursing, 8 (4), Apr 1978, 65, 67-68, 70.

5 **Fawns, H.T.** Folic acid and anaemia. (Chemistry of folic acid and types of anaemia responding to folic acid therapy.) Nursing Times, 73, 19 May 1977, 737-739.

6 **Fawns, H.T.** Vitamin B12 and pernicious anaemia. Nursing Times, 72, 23 Sep 1976, 1475-1478.

7 **Gorst, D.W.** Sickle cell disease. Nursing Times, 72, 16 Sep 1976, 1436-1438.

8 **Journal of Practical Nursing** Sickle cell: the significance of screening. Journal of Practical Nursing, 27 (7), Jul 1977, 17-18.

9 **Kenny, M.W.** Sickle cell disease. Nursing Times, 76, 4 Sep 1980, 1582-1584.

10 **Linehan, M.S.** Sickle cell anaemia—the painful crisis. Journal of Education in Nursing, 4 (6), Nov/Dec 1978, 12-19.

11 **Macfarlane, J.** Sickle cell disorders. American Journal of Nursing, 77 (12), Dec 1977, 1948-1954.

12 **Meyers, A.J.** Successful bone marrow transplant for hypoplastic anaemia. (A case study.) Nursing Times, 73, 17 Feb 1977, 233-235.

13 **Robbins, R.** Pernicious anaemia. (Multiple choice questions.) Nursing Mirror, 143, 18 Nov 1976, 66-68.

c HAEMOPHILIA

1 **Cole, S. and Jones, P.** Physiotherapy in haemophilia. Physiotherapy, 62, Jul 1976, 217-221.

2 **Colvin, B.T. and others** Regional co-ordinator for haemophilia in domiciliary practice. (Nurse co-ordinates the organisation of care for haemophiliacs.) British Medical Journal, 2, 24 Sep 1977, 814-815.

3 **Drug and Therapeutics Bulletin** Home treatment for haemophilia. Drug and Therapeutics Bulletin, 16 (13), 23 Jun 1978, 49-50.

4 **Hedlin, A.** Hemostasis and the nature of its defect in hemophilia. Canadian Nurse, 76 (11), Dec 1980, 15-19.

5 **Jones, P.** Haemophilia. Physiotherapy, 62 (7), Jul 1976, 214-216.

6 **Jones, P. editor** Haemophilia home therapy. Pitman Medical, 1980.

7 **Jones, P. and others** Haemophilia. A home therapy in the United Kingdom 1975-6. (Survey of centres.) British Medical Journal, 1, 3 Jun 1978, 1447-1450.

8 **Kaufert, J.M.** Social and psychological responses to home treatment and haemophilia. (Evaluation of pilot home treatment programme at St. Thomas' Hospital and Churchill Hospital.) Journal of Epidemiology and Community Health, 34 (3), Sep 1980, 194-200.

9 **Koshy, K.T.** Haemophilia. Nursing Mirror, 142, 25 Mar 1976, 52-55.

10 **Markova, I. and Forbes, C.** Haemophilia: a study into social and psychological problems. Health Bulletin, 37 (1), Jan 1979, 24-29.

11 **Markova, I. and others** Haemophilia: a survey on social issues. (Survey of 100 patients in Glasgow area.) Health Bulletin, 35 (4), Jul 1977, 177-182.

12 **Nursing Times** New haemophilia post for nurse. Conference discusses role of nurse co-ordinator. (Regional co-ordinator in domiciliary practice at North East Thames transfusion centre.) Nursing Times, 72, 13 May 1976, 717.

13 **Rizza, C.R.** Haemophilia. Nursing Times, 73, 22 Sep 1977, 1475-1477.

14 **Royal Free Hospital. Haemophilia Centre** Haemophilia centre handbook: notes for doctors and nurses involved in the care of patients with congenital coagulation disorders. Immuno, 1980.

15 **Stuart, J. and others** Improving prospects for employment of the haemophiliac. (Results of questionnaire.) British Medical Journal, 280, 10 May 1980, 1169-1172.

16 **Swinburne, L.** A measure of acceptance: patients' attitudes to haemophilia. Lancet, 1, 14 May 1977, 1048-1049.

91 MUSCULOSKELETAL SYSTEM

a GENERAL AND DISORDERS

1 **Anwar, M.** The mechanics of walking: putting your best foot forward. (Includes gait abnormalities.) Nursing Mirror, 147, 30 Nov 1978, 36-39.

2 **Bendall, R.** Sciatica. Nursing Times, 74, 21 Sep 1978, 1555-1559.

3 **Berg, C. and Hanebuth, L.** Paget's Disease: a challenge in nursing care. (Case study of 72-year-old woman.) Journal of Gerontological Nursing, 3 (3), May/Jun 1977, 27-30.

4 **Birch, R.** A pain in the arm. (Causes of pain in the neck, shoulder joint, elbow, wrist and hand.) Nursing Mirror, 149, 15 Nov 1979, 36-38.

5 **Brooks, A.** Osteogenesis imperfecta. Nursing Mirror, 144, 12 May 1977, 61-63.

6 **Castledine, G.** Nursing assessment of the musculoskeletal system. Nursing, 3, Jun 1979, 148-149.

7 **Cowie, V.** Marfan's syndrome: recognising the 'spider' sufferers. Nursing Mirror, 148, 15 Feb 1979, 38-39.

8 **Day, B.H.** Tennis elbow. Nursing Times, 75, 2 Aug 1979, 1307-1309.

9 **Gault, P.A.** Mixed connective tissue disease. (Account of living with a chronic illness, by a nurse who has this disease.) American Journal of Nursing, 77 (11), Nov 1977, 1818-1820.

10 **Graham, K.M.** Nursing care study. Ruptured lumbar disc in the adolescent. Nursing Times, 75, 1 Feb 1979, 202-205.

11 **Hartley, B.** Systemic lupus: a patient perspective. (Based on questionnaire among 22 patients.) Canadian Nurse, 74 (2), Feb 1978, 16-20.

12 **Hill, M. and Hunter, P.M.** Nursing care study. Tempero-mandibular joint ankylosis... (In four-year-old girl. For correction of two points see Nursing Mirror, 26 Oct, 11.) Nursing Mirror, 147, 12 Oct 1978, 23-24.

13 **Hirschberg, G.G. and others** Promoting patient mobility and other ways to prevent secondary disabilities. (Muscle and joint degeneration, metabolic and circulatory disturbances.) Nursing, 77 7 (5), May 1977, 42, 44-46.

14 **Hookway, C.J.** Theatre nursing care study. Proliferative myositis. (Benign tumour in musculatory system. By nurse on JBCNS course.) Nursing Times, 75, 22 Nov 1979, 2019-2022.

15 **Hughes, G.R.V.** Systemic lupus erythematosus. Nursing Times, 73, 5 May 1977, 653-654.

16 **Janul, L.C.** Polymyositis—dermatomyositis: a perplexing disorder. American Journal of Nursing, 77 (7), Jul 1977, 1184-1186.

17 **Kocen, R.S.** The neuromuscular system. Churchill Livingstone, 1976. (Penguin Library of Nursing.)

18 **Lander, A.** Nursing care study. Periarteritis nodosa with associated renal failure. (Connective tissue disorder affecting walls of arteries and veins.) Nursing Mirror, 147, 26 Oct 1978, 26-29.

19 **Low, A.W.** The patient's view of osteoporosis. Nursing Times, 75, 4 Jan 1979, 38-39.

20 **Paterson, C.R.** Brittle bones—a plea for sensitive handling. (Osteogensis imperfecta.) Journal of Community Nursing, 2 (11), May 1979, 4-7.

21 **Paterson, C.R.** Osteogenesis imperfecta and fractures in childhood. Health Visitor, 51 (5), May 1978, 174-176.

22 **Pennington, H.E.** Nursing care study. Marfan's syndrome. (Connective tissue disorder.) Nursing Mirror, 144, 27 Jan 1977, 45-47.

23 **Pinel, C.** Metabolic bone disease in the elderly. (Types, causes and treatment of osteoporosis and osteomalacia.) Nursing Times, 72, 8 Jul 1976, 1046-1048.

24 **Roberts, A.** Synovial fluid. Nursing Times, 73, 21 Jul 1977, Body fluids, 5-8.

25 **Robinson, W.** New metabolic bone disease research unit. (Royal National Orthopaedic Hospital, Stanmore.) Nursing Mirror, 143, 14 Oct 1976, 46-49.

26 **Ross, D.S.** Case history. Haematoma of the rectus sheath. (Following lifting of heavy metal bars.) Occupational Health, 29 (12), Dec 1977, 532-535.

27 **Strong, J.A.** Paget's disease. Nursing Mirror, 142, 6 May 1976, 72-73.

28 **Swan, C.H.J.** Metabolic bone disease. Nursing Mirror, 142, 29 Apr 1976, 64-66.

29 **Taylor, J.F.** Osteomyelitis. 1. The acute

form. 2. The chronic form. Nursing Times, 72, 1 Apr 1976, 486-488; 8 Apr 1976, 535-537.

30 Torbett, M.P. and Ervin, J.C. The patient with systemic lupus erythematosus. (Treatment.) American Journal of Nursing, 77 (8), Aug 1977, 1299-1302.

31 Twomey, M.R. Arthrogryposis multiplex congenita. (Including a case study.) Nursing Times, 72 (29), 22 Jul 1976, 1117-1119.

32 Twomey, M.R. Nursing care study. Osteogenesis imperfecta. Nursing Times, 73, 27 Jan 1977, 123-126.

33 Wadsworth, T.G. and Williams, R.M. The cubital tunnel external compression syndrome. Nursing Times, 73, 1 Sep 1977, 1357-1359.

34 Walls, J. Bone densitometry (for the investigation of metabolic bone diseases). Nursing Times, 72, 3 Jun 1976, 869-870.

35 White, J.F. Teaching patients to manage systemic lupus erythematosus. Nursing, 8 (9), Sep 1978, 25, 28-34.

36 Williams, J.G.P. Strains and sprains. Nursing Times, 72, 19 Aug 1976, 1276-1278.

b BACK DISORDERS

1 Billings, R.A. and others Low back injury in sport. Rheumatology and Rehabilitation, 16 (4), Nov 1977, 236-240.

2 Chadwick, P.R. Advising patients on back care. Physiotherapy, 65 (9), Sep 1979, 277-278.

3 Cooper, S.B. A patient teaching plan for conservative treatment of low back pain. 1. Development. Orthopedic Nurse's Association Journal, 3 (10), Oct 1976, 301-306.

4 Crown, S. Psychological aspects of low back pain. Rheumatology and Rehabilitation, 17 (2), May 1978, 114-124.

5 Daniel, J.W. and others Low back pain in the steel industry: a clinical, economic and occupational analysis at a North Wales integrated steelworks of the British Steel Corporation. Journal of the Society of Occupational Medicine, 30 (2), Apr 1980, 49-56.

6 De Trense, M. Are you sitting comfortably? Will the increasing knowledge and acceptance of ergonomic principles reduce the vast amount of absenteeism caused by back pains? Occupational Health, 28 (10), Oct 1976, 470-472.

7 Fairbank, J.C.T. and others The Oswestry low back pain disability questionnaire. (For assessing patients.) Physiotherapy, 66 (8), Aug 1980, 271-273.

8 Finneson, B.E. Neurosurgical treatment of low back pain. Journal of Neurosurgical Nursing, 9 (2), Jun 1977, 54-57.

9 Grahame, H. Mind your back! (Role of ATLAS, National Organisation for Back Pain Sufferers.) Journal of Community Nursing, 3 (7), Jan 1980, 8.

10 Health Education Council Mind your back. The Council, 1976.

11 Hitch, M. Nursing assessment of a patient with low back pain. Orthopedic Nurse's Association Journal, 16 (12), Dec 1979, 484-488.

12 Muller, G.M. Disc problems and the district nurse. Queen's Nursing Journal, 19 (1), Apr 1976, 18-19, 23.

13 Nursing Mirror A symposium on low back pain. Nursing Mirror, 144, 13 Jan 1977, 45-61. Includes:
Benson, M.K.D. Surgical management. 49-53.
Coxhead, C.E. Physiotherapy in low back pain. 57-59.
O'Brien, E.A. Nursing care following back surgery. 54-56.

14 Parry, C.B.W. Minor back injuries. Nursing Times, 72, 23 Sep 1976, 1468-1471.

15 Physiotherapy Four articles and bibliography on the treatment of back pain. Physiotherapy, 66 (4), Apr 1980, 108-122.

16 Rheumatology and Rehabilitation Special World Rheumatism Year issue—Back pain. Rheumatology and Rehabilitation, 16 (1), Feb 1977, 3-69.

17 Ringer, J.H. Low back pain in industry. Occupational Health Nursing, 24 (6), Jun 1976, 11-12.

18 RN Magazine Low back pain. (Three articles including nursing care.) RN Magazine, 41 (10), Oct 1978, 71-81.

19 Society of Occupational Medicine Evidence by the Society of Occupational Medicine to the Working Group on Back Pain, Department of Health and Social Security. Journal of the Society of Occupational Medicine, 28 (1), Jan 1978, 35-36.

20 Troup, J.D.G. Chronic back pain: the management plan. Geriatric Medicine, 10 (7), Jul 1980, 33-34, 37-38.

21 Williams, T.R. Nursing care study. Low back pain. (Posterior spinal decompression and decompression of the S1 root canals.) Nursing Times, 75, 5 Apr 1979, 577-579.

c NEUROMUSCULAR DISORDERS

1 Boyle, M.A. and Cuica, R.L. Amyotrophic lateral sclerosis. (Nursing care study.) American Journal of Nursing, 76 (1), Jan 1976, 66-68.

2 Dubowitz, V. Analysis of neuromuscular disease. Physiotherapy, 63 (2), Feb 1977, 38-45.

3 Fleming, M.H. and McLaughlin, M. The family with muscular dystrophy. Journal of Practical Nursing, 26 (8), Aug 1976, 14-15, 33.

4 Fuller, D. Muscular dystrophy: a singular lack of liaison. (Care study by enrolled student district nurse.) Nursing Mirror, 150, 28 Feb 1980, 39-40.

5 Gardner-Medwin, D. Management of muscular dystrophy. Physiotherapy, 63 (2), Feb 1977, 46-51.

6 Gardner-Medwin, D. Muscular dystrophy: can it be prevented? Nursing Times, 74, 31 Aug 1978, 1441-1443.

7 Grimm, K. Nursing care study. Transient neonatal myasthenia gravis. Nursing Mirror, 147, 21 Sep 1978, 18-22.

8 Lunt, G. Getting to grips with myasthenia gravis. (Research into causes.) New Scientist, 82, 7 Jun 1979, 805-807.

9 McKeran, R.O. The muscular dystrophies. Nursing Times, 72, 30 Sep 1976, 1515-1518.

10 Marshman, G.M. and Jackman, K.V. Orthopaedic nursing in neuromuscular disorders. Nursing Clinics of North America, 14 (1), Mar 1979, 145-156.

11 Meakin, A. The nerve impulse and disordered transmission. Part 2. Myasthenia gravis. Nursing Mirror, 145, 25 Aug 1977, 34-35.

12 Muscular Dystrophy Group of Great Britain Welfare Committee The muscular dystrophy handbook. 2nd ed. The Group, 1979.

13 Pinching, A.J. Myasthenia gravis—a frustrating disability. Nursing Mirror, 147, 21 Sep 1978, 16-18.

14 Skirm, L. Myasthenia gravis: a time of quiet desperation. Journal of Practical Nursing, 25 (12), Dec 1975, 21-23, 35.

15 Walker, P.F. Welfare of the muscular dystrophy patient. Physiotherapy, 63 (2), Feb 1977, 56-58.

16 Wilson, S. Myasthenia gravis: a cure is in sight. Nursing Mirror, 148, 4 Jan 1979, 17-20.

d RHEUMATIC DISORDERS

1 Arthritis and Rheumatism Council A walking miracle: a review of surgical advances in the treatment of arthritis, particularly in total joint replacement. The Council, 1977.

2 Barnes, C.G. Rheumatoid arthritis: the team approach is the answer. (Incidence and treatment.) Nursing Mirror, 147, 30 Nov 1978, 30-35.

3 Billings, R.A. and Mole, K.F. Rheumatology in general practice—a survey in World Rheumatism Year 1977. Journal of the Royal College of General Practitioners, 27, Dec 1977, 721-725.

4 Bowden, D. Nursing care study. Illness—the last refuge of despair. (73-year-old woman who exaggerated her arthritis in order to be admitted to hospital.) Nursing Times, 76, 24 Jul 1980, 1307-1309.

5 British League Against Rheumatism Rheumatism: the price we pay. The impact of the rheumatic diseases on the individual and the country. The League, 1977.

6 Caplan, H. Temporal arthritis and polymyalgia rheumatica. Nursing Mirror, 145, 15 Dec 1977, 19-20.

7 Carr, P.A. Activity group therapy for rheumatoid arthritis. A two year experiment. Journal of Occupational Therapy, 41 (2), Feb 1978, 71-72.

8 Chamberlain, M.A. Social implications of rheumatoid arthritis in young mothers. Rheumatology and Rehabilitation Supplement, 1979, 70-73.

9 Clarke, A.K. Treating rheumatoid arthritis today. Journal of Community Nursing, 1 (1), Jul 1977, 15-16.

10 **Damerell, J.** Diagnosis bilateral osteo-arthritis of knee. Queen's Nursing Journal, 19 (1), Apr 1976, 15-16.

11 **Dieppe, P.** Microscopy in arthritis. Nursing Mirror, 144, 31 Mar 1977, 54-56.

12 **Elliott, M.** Nursing rheumatic disease. Edinburgh: Churchill Livingstone, 1979.

13 **Ferguson, K. and Bole, G.G.** Family support, health beliefs, and therapeutic compliance in patients with rheumatoid arthritis. (Research study.) Patient Counselling and Health Education, 1 (3), Winter/Spring 1979, 101-105.

14 **Figley, B.A. and others** A comprehensive approach to sexual health in rheumatic disease. Topics in Clinical Nursing, 1 (4), Jan 1980, 69-74.

15 **Haleem, M.A.** Peripheral arthropathies in the elderly. (Arthritis of the peripheral joints—hands and feet.) Nursing Times, 74, 2 Nov 1978, 1799-1801.

16 **Hamilton, A.** The problems of the arthritic patient. (Symposium paper on the sexual problems of the disabled.) Nursing Mirror, 142, 5 Feb 1976, 54-55.

17 **Hart, F.D.** History of the treatment of rheumatoid arthritis. British Medical Journal, 1, 27 Mar 1976, 763-765.

18 **Haslock, I. and others** Rheumatoid arthritis. Rheumatic disease of the shoulder. Nursing Mirror, 142, 11 Mar 1976, 51-55; 18 Mar 1976, 53-55.

19 **Hazleman, B.L.** Acute arthritis. Nursing Times, 73, 6 Oct 1977, 1554-1555; 13 Oct 1977, 1598-1600.

20 **Hernandez, L.A.** Gout. Nursing Times, 72, 10 Jun 1976, 898-900.

21 **Herr, M.** Nursing care study. Rheumatic fever. (In fourteen-year-old boy.) Nursing Times, 74, 30 Mar 1978, 526-528.

22 **Hollings, E.M. and Haworth, R.J.** Supply and use of aids and appliances: a study of 119 patients with rheumatoid arthritis. British Journal of Occupational Therapy, 41 (10), Oct 1978, 336-339.

23 **Hopkins, R. and Wright, V.** The best way to lecture in rheumatology. Different methods of teaching nurses were tested. Nursing Times, 74, 21/28 Dec 1978, 2115.

24 **Meanock, I.** Polymyalgia rheumatica. Nursing Times, 72, 16 Dec 1976, 1962-1963.

25 **Mitchell, S.H.** Nursing care study. Rheumatoid arthritis. Nursing Times, 72, 15 Apr 1976, 575-577.

26 **Nursing Times** Self help for patients with rheumatoid arthritis. (Activities of BRA (British Rheumatism and Arthritis Association).) Nursing Times, 73, 8 Dec 1977, 1918.

27 **Panayi, G.S. editor** Essential rheumatology for nurses and therapists. Baillière Tindall, 1980.

28 **Physiotherapy** Rheumatism—1. (Five articles.) Physiotherapy, 63 (12), Dec 1977, 386-399.

29 **Rhodes, H.** Community nursing care study. Rheumatoid arthritis. Nursing Times, 73, 20 Oct 1977, 1624-1626.

30 **Robbins, E.** Test yourself. Acute rheumatism and its consequences. (Multiple choice questions.) Nursing Mirror, 143, 21 Oct 1976, 68-70.

31 **Robinson, E.T. and others** Depression in rheumatoid arthritis. Journal of the Royal College of General Practitioners, 27, Jul 1977, 423-427.

32 **Savage, J.** A third hand for the arthritic. (Attachments for house and car doors to aid arthritic people.) Nursing Mirror, 148, 22 Mar 1979, 26-28.

33 **Sculco, C.D. and Sculco, T.F.** A co-ordinated team approach to one health problem. (Care of the patient with rheumatoid arthritis at the Rheumatism Foundation Hospital, Heinola, Finland.) International Nursing Review, 23 (3), May/Jun 1976, 80-83.

34 **Swinson, D.R. and Swinburn, W.R.** Rheumatology. Hodder, 1980. (Modern nursing series.)

35 **White, A. and others** Nursing care supplement. Series 3. 4. Rheumatoid arthritis. Nursing Mirror, 143, 28 Oct 1976, Nursing care supplement series 3, i-iv.

36 **World Health** Issue devoted to World Rheumatism Year. World Health, Jun 1977, 3-29.

37 **Wright, V. and Haslock, I.** Rheumatism for nurses and remedial therapists. Heinemann, 1977.

38 **Wright, V. and Hopkins, R.** Communicating with the rheumatic patient. (Research study to find out what patients, nurses and doctors mean by words relating to anatomy, symptoms, diseases and treatment.) Nursing Times, 73, 25 Aug 1977, 1308-1313.

39 **Wright, V.** Rheumatoid arthritis. Nursing Times, 73.
1. Clinical features. 17 Nov 1977, 1794-1797.
2. Nursing care of the patient at home and in hospital. 24 Nov 1977, 1832-1835.
3. Conservative management. 1 Dec 1977, 1878-1881.
4. Drug therapy. 8 Dec 1977, 1915-1918.
5. Surgical treatment. 15 Dec 1977, 1955-1958.

e SPINAL DISEASES

1 **American Journal of Nursing** The patient with scoliosis. (Four articles.) American Journal of Nursing, 79 (9), Sep 1979, 1587-1612.

2 **Braddell-Smith, S.** Patient care study. Cervical spondylosis. Queen's Nursing Journal, 18 (10), Jan 1976, 279, 281.

3 **Bucknell, E.** Nursing care study. Scoliosis: the cure that made Terri taller. (Cotrel dynamic traction and spinal operation.) Nursing Mirror, 149, 26 Jul 1979, 34-36.

4 **Clarke, A.K.** An exciting model of chronic disease. (Ankylosing spondylitis.) Journal of Community Nursing, 2 (9), Mar 1979, 4-5, 7, 32.

5 **Crank, R. and Morris, A.** Problems of nursing adolescents with idiopathic scoliosis. Nursing Times, 73, 22/29 Dec 1977, 1990-1993.

6 **Cross, V.** Physiotherapy for the ankylosing spondylitis sufferer. Journal of Community Nursing, 3 (2), Aug 1979, 20, 22, 24.

7 **Dickson, R.A. and others** School screening for scoliosis: cohort study of clinical course. British Medical Journal, 281, 26 Jul 1980, 265-267.

8 **Diekmann, E.** Understanding your scoliosis surgery: a preoperative teaching booklet for Harrington instrumentation and spinal fusion patients. Orthopedic Nurse's Association Journal, 5 (10), Oct 1978, 24-27.

9 **Fox, J.** Nursing care study. Cervical tuberculous lesion: a halo round his head. Nursing Mirror, 148, 25 Jan 1979, 29-33.

10 **Heritage, P.M.** Nursing care study. Ankylosing spondylitis. (Care before and after double osteotomy of the lumbar spine.) Nursing Mirror, 146, 2 Feb 1978, 19-21.

11 **Hogan, L. and Beland, I.** Cervical spine syndrome. American Journal of Nursing, 76 (7), Jul 1976, 1104-1107.

12 **Hudgson, P.** Syringomyelia. (Spinal cord disorder.) Nursing Times, 74, 9 Nov 1978, 1849-1852.

13 **Hunter, E. and Leonard, M.** 'Mummy, you're hurting my hand again!' (Patient's account of coping with syringomyelia.) Nursing Times, 76, 28 Aug 1980, Supplement, 3-4.

14 **Love-Mignogna, S.** Scoliosis. (Nursing care.) Nursing, 77 7 (5), May 1977, 50-55.

15 **Monro, P.** Syringomyelia: the patient who feels no pain. (Cyst in the spinal cord which destroys nerve cells and fibre pathways.) Nursing Mirror, 147, 19 Oct 1978, 38-42.

16 **Nicholls, A.** Ankylosing spondylitis. Nursing Times, 74, 26 Jan 1978, 147-148.

17 **O'Brien, J. and Van Akkerveeken, P.F.** School screening for scoliosis: results of a pilot study. (Study involving school nurses in Oswestry.) Practitioner, 219, Nov 1977, 739-742.

18 **Platts, R.G.S.** Spinal mechanics. Physiotherapy, 63 (7), Jul 1977, 224-226.

19 **Reid, U.V.** Home care after surgery for scoliosis. Canadian Nurse, 72 (11), Nov 1976, 43-47.

20 **RN Magazine** Scoliosis. (Six articles on the treatment of scoliosis.) RN Magazine, 30 (11), Nov 1976, 56-80.

21 **Robinson, H.** Community nursing. Nursing care study. Syringomyelia. (Including nursing assessment and nursing care plan.) Nursing Mirror, 145, 28 Jul 1977, 37-38; 4 Aug 1977, 34-36.

22 **Sodha, U.** Congenital scoliosis. Nursing Times, 76, 28 Aug 1980, 1524-1525.

f CHIROPODY

1 **Barrett, C.E.** Persuasive communications as related to foot health education. (Effect of health education on attitude and behaviour change.) Chiropodist, 33 (5), May 1978, 121-128.

2 **Bates, J.E.** Foot care: its relationship to

total health care. Chiropodist, 34 (2), Feb 1979, 42-44.

3 **Brocklehurst, J.C.** The opening address at the 1977 Annual Convention of the Society of Chiropodists. (On the elderly's needs for chiropody services.) Chiropodist, 32 (6), Jun 1977, 207-209.

4 **Coates, I.S.** An industrial chiropody service—a profile. (Unilever Group of Companies on Merseyside.) Chiropodist, 31 (8), Aug 1976, 199-201.

5 **Community Outlook** Feet for the future. (Campaign in City and East London AHA.) Nursing Times, 75, 9 Aug 1979, Community Outlook, 219, 221-222; Fact sheet of advice on footcare, 224-225.

6 **French, G.** Chiropody for occupational health nurses: our own two feet. Nursing Mirror, 148, 7 Jun 1979, Supplement, i, iii-iv, vii-viii.

7 **Haslock, I. and others** Disorders of the foot. Nursing Mirror, 142, 29 Apr 1976, 47-50.

8 **Karpf, A.** 'There's more to it than cutting toe-nails...' (Problems of the NHS chiropody service.) Health and Social Service Journal, 87, 1 Apr 1977, 568-569.

9 **Knight, S.E. and Lewis, J.D.** The effect of footwear on venous pressure at the ankle. (Research study using exercise sandals and ordinary shoes.) Nursing Mirror, 147, 10 Aug 1978, 22-24.

10 **Mosely, B.** Care of the feet. Nursing, 3, Jun 1979, 141-144.

11 **Neale, D.** A view from the plateau. (Review of development of chiropody services.) Chiropodist, 32 (6), Jun 1977, 191-198.

12 **Read, P.J.** Footwear, feet and form. Queen's Nursing Journal, 19 (1), Apr 1976, 12-13, 16.

13 **Rees, C.** Planning a mobile chiropody clinic. Chiropodist, 31 (4), Apr 1976, 92-94.

14 **Walton, P.** We must not drag our feet. (NHS chiropody services and lack of trained chiropodists.) Health and Social Service Journal, 89, 18 Jan 1979, 43.

92 ORTHOPAEDICS

a GENERAL AND NURSING

1 **Boardman, K.P. and Griffiths, J.C.** Effective out-patient surgery in orthopaedics. Health Trends, 9 (1), Feb 1977, 9-11.

2 **Brumbelow, S.** Editorial. (On functions of orthopaedic liaison nurse.) Orthopedic Nurse's Association Journal, 4 (3), Mar 1977, 55.

3 **Brunner, N.A.** Orthopedic nursing: a programmed approach. 3rd ed. St. Louis: Mosby, 1979. (A programmed text.)

4 **Collins, P.** Nursing care study. Treatment of Volkmann's ischaemic contracture. (In young woman who sustained supracondylar fracture of the humerus as a child.) Nursing Times, 74, 22 Jun 1978, 1038-1040.

5 **Donahoo, C.A.** Orthopedic nursing.

(Bicentennial forecast.) RN Magazine, 38 (10), Oct 1976, 19-20, 22, 26-27.

6 **Donahoo, C.A. and Dimon, J.H.** Orthooedic nursing. Boston: Little, Brown and Co., 1977.

7 **Farrell, J.** Caring for the laminectomy patient: how to strengthen your support. Nursing, 8 (5), May 1978, 65-69.

8 **Farrell, J.** Illustrated guide to orthopedic nursing. Philadelphia: Lippincott, 1977.

9 **Fox, J.A.** Orthopaedics for theatre staff. 2. The hip joint. Pathological conditions. NATNews, 17 (5), May 1980, 16-17, 19.

10 **Gregson, J.** Nursing care study. Perthes disease. (Osteochondritis of the hip. Third prize-winner in competition.) Nursing Times, 76, 18 Sep 1980, 1653-1657.

11 **Griffith, M.J.** Slipping of the capital femoral opiphysis. Nursing Mirror, 143, 30 Sep 1976, 47-49.

12 **Harrison, M.** Perthes' disease: stretching the patients' patience. Nursing Mirror, 147, 9 Nov 1978, 30-33.

13 **Hutson, L.** Nursing care study. Laminectomy. Nursing Mirror, 146, 19 Jan 1978, 18-19.

14 **Iveson-Iveson, J.** Students' forum: orthopaedics. (Including multiple choice and long answer questions.) Nursing Mirror, 150, 21 Feb 1980, 24-27.

15 **Larson, C.B. and Gould, M.** Orthopedic nursing. 9th ed. St. Louis: Mosby, 1978.

16 **Mackay, N.S.** Laminectomy 1. Relief of prolapsed intervertebral disc. (Indications for operation and pre- and postoperative care.) Nursing Mirror, 147, 6 Jul 1978, 30-32.

17 **Morris, B.** Laminectomy 2. Nursing vigilance. (Pre- and postoperative nursing care.) Nursing Mirror, 147, 6 Jul 1978, 33-34.

18 **Mourad, L.** Nursing care of adults with orthopaedic conditions. New York: Wiley Medical, 1980.

19 **Norton, T.A. and Tait, J.M.** Orthopaedic surgery. 2nd ed. Heinemann Medical, 1979. (Modern practical nursing series; 8.)

20 **Nursing Clinics of North America** Symposium on orthopedic nursing. Nursing Clinics of North America, 11 (4), 1976, 639-730.

21 **Powell, M.** Orthopaedic nursing. 7th ed. Churchill Livingstone, 1976.

22 **Preston, B.J.** Occupational health. 3. X-ray on the job. (Use in diagnosing orthopaedic disorders.) Nursing Mirror, 151, 14 Aug 1980, 21-23.

23 **Pybus, M.** Nursing care study. Hemimandibulectomy. Nursing Times, 72, 4 Mar 1976, 337-339.

24 **Quine, S.** A report of a study conducted to investigate the demand in New South Wales for the introduction of a post basic course in orthopaedic nursing. Australian Nurses Journal, 5 (10), Apr 1976, 22-23, 31.

25 **Roaf, R. and Hodkinson, L.J.** Textbook of

orthopaedic nursing. 3rd ed. Oxford: Blackwell Scientific, 1980.

26 **Robinson, W.** Advances in orthopaedics. Open day at the Royal National Orthopaedic Hospital, Stanmore. Nursing Mirror, 145, 28 Jul 1977, 7-9.

27 **Rowe, J.W. and Dyer, L.** editors Care of the orthopaedic patient. Blackwell, 1977. (For nurses.)

28 **Stone, E.M. and Pinney, E.C.** Orthopaedics for nurses. 5th ed. Baillière Tindall, 1978. (Nurses' aids series special interest text.)

29 **Stone, S.K.** Emotional reactions to alterations in body image (in orthopaedic patients). Journal of Practical Nursing, 26 (5), May 1976, 24-26.

30 **Tremlett, G.** Beginning research. Patient satisfaction in an orthopaedic ward. Nursing Times, 73, 17 Nov 1977, 1801-1804.

31 **Webb, J.T.** Notes on orthopaedic nursing. Churchill Livingstone, 1977.

32 **Yates, C.** Dislocated jaw. Nursing Times, 73, 28 Apr 1977, 604-606.

b CHILDREN

1 **Blockey, N.J.** Children's orthopaedics: practical problems. Butterworth, 1976.

2 **Dunn, B.H.** Common orthopedic problems of children. Pediatric Nursing, 1 (6), Nov/Dec 1975, 7-10.

3 **Kitching, C.** Nursing care study. Subluxation of the atlanto-occipital joint: six weeks' traction was necessary before Catrin's joint showed normal alignment. (Care of nine-year-old girl on cervical traction, by a pupil nurse.) Nursing Times, 75, 1 Mar 1979, 354-355.

4 **Mohan, J.A.** Theory to research to practice. (Implementing results of research study on preparing children for plaster cast removal, with teaching aid.) American Journal of Maternal Child Nursing, 2 (6), Nov/Dec 1977, 392-394.

c CONGENITAL MALFORMATIONS

1 **British Association of Orthopaedic Nurses** Congenital dislocation of the hip. (Winning entry of Nursing Care Study Competition describing pre- and postoperative care.) British Association of Orthopaedic Nurses, Dec 1977, 1-3.

2 **Burgess, D. and others** Orthopaedics. 2. Congenital dislocation of the hip. Nursing Mirror, 147, 14 Dec 1978, Supplement, i-iv.

3 **Day, H.J.B.** The early referral of children with congenital limb deficiencies. Health Trends, 9 (1), Feb 1977, 12-13.

4 **Davis, J. and others** Congenital dislocation of the hip. 2 parts. Nursing Times, 76, 28 Aug 1980, 1517-1518, 1519-1521.

5 **Hughes, B. and others** Orthopaedics. 3. Congenital club foot. Nursing Mirror, 147, 21 Dec 1978, Supplement, i-iv.

6 **McHugh, A.** Nursing care study.

Congenital dislocation of the hip. Nursing Mirror, 146, 6 Apr 1978, 19-21.

7 **Nichol, C.** Congenital dislocated hip. (Management and role of public health nurse.) Canadian Nurse, 73 (7), Jul 1977, 14-19.

8 **Place, M.J. and others** Effectiveness of neonatal screening for congenital dislocation of the hip. Lancet, 2, 29 Jul 1978, 249-250.

9 **Prett, C.** An advance in the treatment of leg inequality. (Nursing care study of patient treated with Wagner apparatus.) Nursing Times, 75, 4 Jan 1979, 26-29.

10 **Twomey, M.R.** Leg lengthening. (Two methods used at the Duchess of Kent Children's Orthopaedic Hospital, Hong Kong.) Nursing Times, 72, 13 May 1976, 736-738.

11 **Valman, H.B. and Finlay, H.V.L.** The first year of life. Dislocated and dislocatable hip in the newborn. British Medical Journal, 280, 10 Jan 1980, 164-166.

d AMPUTATION

1 **Baker, J.L.** Nursing care study. Traumatic sub-total amputation of the right hand. Nursing Times, 74, 23 Feb 1978, 323-325.

2 **Beattie, G.W.** On becoming an artificial arm user: a psychologist considers the effects of an accident. New Society, 48, 31 May 1979, 510-511.

3 **Coleman, A.** Rehabilitation of the elderly amputee: a review of the literature. Orthopedic Nurse's Association Journal, 6 (7), Jul 1979, 281-286.

4 **Community View** To lose a limb. (District nurse's role with amputees.) Community View, 7, Sep 1980, 3-5.

5 **Connolly, J.** Phantom and stump pain following operation. (Amputation.) Physiotherapy, 65 (1), Jan 1979, 13-14.

6 **Early, P.F.** Pictures in nursing. Limb-fitting for the amputee. Nursing, 5, Aug 1979, 238-240.

7 **English, A.W.G. and Dean, A.A.G.** The artificial limb service. Health Trends, 12 (4), Nov 1980, 77-82.

8 **Hamilton, A.** Upper limb amputees. (With details of prostheses.) Nursing, 5, Aug 1979, 232-236.

9 **Humm, W.** Rehabilitation of the lower limb amputee for nurses and therapists. 3rd ed. Baillière Tindall, 1977.

10 **MacInnes, M.S.A.** Bilateral amputation of the legs—patient care and rehabilitation. Nursing Times, 73, 7 Jul 1977, 1033-1035.

11 **Newman, E.** Specialised care. 3. The amputee. (Pre- and postoperative care.) Nursing Mirror, 145, 15 Sep 1977, Nursing care supplement, series 6, i-iv.

12 **Ritchie, J.A.** Children's adjustive and affective responses in the process of reformulating a body image following limb amputation. Maternal Child Nursing Journal, 6 (1), Spring 1977, 25-35.

13 **Wilson, J.L.** Anticipatory grief in response to threatened amputation. (In adolescent.)

Maternal Child Nursing Journal, 6 (3), Fall 1977, 177-186.

e FRACTURES

1 **Barnfield, A.M.** Nursing care study. Compound fracture of femur complicated by fat emboli. Nursing Times, 72, 18 Mar 1976, 409-412.

2 **Boucher, M.** Broken jaw guide and cookbook. (Nursing care and diet for patient with wired jaw.) American Journal of Nursing, 77 (5), May 1977, 831-833.

3 **Colbert, S. and List, S.** Fractures. Nursing, 4 Jul 1979, 174-179.

4 **Colbert, S. and others** Orthopaedics. 1. Fractures. Nursing Mirror, 147, 7 Dec 1978, Supplement, i-iv.

5 **Compton, L.** Nursing care study. A patient with a fractured facial skeleton. (Pre- and postoperative care.) Nursing Times, 75, 19 Jul 1979, 1220-1225.

6 **Crow, J.** Nursing care using a care plan. (Of two patients with fractured neck of femur. Nursing history questionnaires on p.978-982 and centre pages.) Nursing Times, 73, 30 Jun 1977, 983-994.

7 **Dunnery, E.** Fractured hip. How to position and mobilize patients—without undoing their surgery. RN Magazine, 42 (6), Jun 1979, 45-57.

8 **Fernley, H.T.** Nursing care study. A patient with severe femoral shaft fracture. Nursing Times, 74, 15 Jun 1978, 994-995.

9 **Fox, J.A.** Basic A/O techniques for theatre staff. (Internal fixation of fracture by means of screws.) NATNews, 15 (8), Aug 1978, 14-15, 17.

10 **Fox, J.A.** The hip joint and femur. (With illustrations of orthopaedic pins and prostheses used for fractures.) NATNews, 17 (4), Apr 1980, 20-24.

11 **Hogan, K.M. and Sawyer, J.R.** Fracture dislocation of the elbow. American Journal of Nursing, 76 (8), Aug 1976, 1266-1268.

12 **Isaacson, P.J.** Theatre nursing care study. Insertion of a left Kuntscher nail. (For fractured femur.) Nursing Times, 75, 5 Apr 1979, 571-576.

13 **Iveson-Iveson, J.** Nursing care supplement. 10. Fractures. Nursing Mirror, 143 (25), 16 Dec 1976, Nursing care supplement, series 3, i-iv.

14 **Johnson, D.A.** Fractured femur, compound fracture of the tibia and fibula. Nursing Times, 73, 3 Mar 1977, 305-308.

15 **Kryschyshen, P.L. and Fischer, D.A.** External fixation for complicated fractures. American Journal of Nursing, 80 (2), Feb 1980, 256-259.

16 **Lamb, K.** Effect of positioning of postoperative fractured-hip patients as related to comfort. Nursing Research, 28 (5), Sep/Oct 1979, 291-294.

17 **Lewis, M.** The nursing care of patients with fractures. Nursing, 4, Jul 1979, 180-182.

18 **Meredith, S.** Formidable: that's the only word for the external fixation device—and for

the care it demands. (With bibliography.) RN Magazine, 42 (12), Dec 1979, 18-24.

19 **Perkins, J.** Nursing care study. Fractured pelvis. (Treatment by traction.) Nursing Times, 74, 31 Aug 1978, 1444-1448.

20 **Pusey, R.** Pott's fracture. Nursing Times, 74, 3 Aug 1978, 1293-1295.

21 **Stickland, G.M.** On the wrong side of the plaster. (Experiences of a former nurse following a fracture.) Nursing Mirror, 144, 13 Jan 1977, 63-64.

22 **Stillman, M.J.** Mike J: a young man with a fractured femur. 2. Spica cast. RN Magazine, 41 (8), Aug 1978, 61-69.

23 **Sukhtian, W. and Hughes, S.** An external fixation device for the treatment of fractures. (With advertisement illustrating its use on p.14-15.) NATNews, 16 (4), Apr 1979, 13, 16.

24 **Summerfield, J.Y.** Theatre nursing care study. Bone graft to un-united fracture of neck of right femur. Nursing Times, 75, 5 Apr 1979, 580-583.

25 **Todd, R.** Fractures of the femur. Nursing Mirror, 144, 17 Mar 1977, 62-63.

26 **Woogara, R.** Nursing care study. Sub-trochanteric fracture of femur. Nursing Times, 73, 22/29 Dec 1977, 1986-1989.

27 **Williams, M.A.** Nursing activities and acute confusional states in elderly hip-fractured patients. Nursing Research, 28 (1), Jan/Feb 1979, 25-35.

f PLASTER CASTS, SPLINTS AND APPLIANCES

1 **American Journal of Nursing** Programmed instruction. Teaching a patient how to use crutches. American Journal of Nursing, 79 (6), Jun 1979, 1111-1126.

2 **Attenborough, C.G.** The Attenborough stabilised gliding prosthesis. (Symposium paper.) Nursing Mirror, 143, 14 Oct 1976, 52-56.

3 **Crout, E. and others** Boning up on a brace. (Use of Hoffman apparatus in treatment of fractures and nursing care implications.) Nursing Mirror, 149, 18 Oct 1979, 46-49.

4 **Deyerle, W.M. and Crossland, S.A.** Broken legs are to be walked on. (Two devices, the thigh lacer and the cast bracer.) American Journal of Nursing, 77 (12), Dec 1977, 1927-1930.

5 **Farrell, J.** Casts, your patients, and you. 1. A review of basic procedures. 2. A review of arm and leg cast procedures. Nursing (U.S.), 8 (10), Oct 1978, 65-69; (11), Nov 1978, 57-61.

6 **Massie, S.** Cast bracing of femoral shaft fractures. Nursing Times, 76.
1. The method and its history. 10 Apr 1980, 630-631.
2. The physics of the method. 17 Apr 1980, 700-703.
3. When to use this treatment. 24 Apr 1980, 745-747.
4. When to apply the brace. 1 May 1980, 795-796.
5. Social benefits of the cast brace. 8 May 1980, 833-834.
6. An evaluation. 15 May 1980, 882-883.

7 Meredith, S. Preparing your patient to live with his cast. RN Magazine, 42 (7), Jul 1979, 35-43.

8 Miles, S. Plastering and care of the patient in plaster. Nursing Mirror, 143, 16 Dec 1976, 45-47.

9 Physiotherapy Five articles on artificial limbs for congenital disorders and following amputation. Physiotherapy, 65 (1), Jan 1979, 3-12, 15.

10 Robinson, W. On the move: the new artificial limbfitting, rehabilitation, and outpatient department at the Royal National Orthopaedic Hospital in Stanmore. Nursing Mirror, 143, 1 Jul 1976, 39-41.

11 Sensky, T. A consumer's guide to 'bionic arms'. (Myoelectric hand compared with mechanical hand supplied at present.) British Medical Journal, 281, 12 Jul 1980, 126-127.

g TRACTION

1 Cohen, S. Nursing care of a patient in traction. (Programmed instruction.) American Journal of Nursing, 79 (10), Oct 1979, 1771-1798.

2 Jensen, J.M. and others Nursing care of the patient with Roger Anderson Well Leg traction. (With example of care plan.) Orthopedic Nurse's Association Journal, 16 (12), Dec 1979, 489-494.

3 Morgan-Jones, E. and others Orthopaedics. 4. Principles of traction. Nursing Mirror, 147, 28 Dec 1978, Supplement, i-iv.

4 Savage, J.H. Children's ward traction pulleys. (Details of construction.) Nursing Mirror, 144, 26 May 1977, 34-35.

5 Savage, J.H. Traction supports for hospital cots. (Details of construction.) Nursing Mirror, 144, 9 Jun 1977, 36-37.

h HIP, KNEE AND JOINT REPLACEMENT SURGERY

1 Armstrong, M. and Patterson, R. Arthroscopy: a new approach to knee surgery that affects patient care. RN Magazine, 41 (1), Jan 1978, 35-39.

2 Armstrong-Esther, C.A. Pictures in nursing. Joint replacement: technology with a human face. Nursing, 4, Jul 1979, 185-187.

3 Attenborough, C.G. Total knee replacement. (For arthritis, invented by author at Royal East Sussex Hospital, Hastings.) Nursing Times, 73, 29 Sep 1977, 1514-1517.

4 Boulton, C. Horizontal air flow unit: (for joint replacement surgery at Chester Royal Infirmary). Nursing Times, 72, 5 Feb 1976, 197-198.

5 Dandy, D.J. Meniscectomy. (Excision of part of medial ligament of knee.) Nursing Times, 75, 23 Aug 1979, 1437-1439.

6 Hagedorn, R.R. Summary of precautions advised following total hip replacement operations. British Journal of Occupational Therapy, 41 (9), Sep 1978, 295-296.

7 Hamerton, E. Management of total hip, femur and knee replacement. Nursing Times, 72, 29 Apr 1976, Key Clinical, 13-16.

8 Haworth, R.J. and Hopkins, J. Use of aids following total hip replacement. British Journal of Occupational Therapy, 43 (12), Dec 1980, 398-400.

9 Jackson, J.P. Internal derangement of the knee. Nursing Times, 72, 29 Apr 1976, 651-654.

10 King, I. Hip joint: a programmed text. Sheffield: NHS Learning Resources Unit, 1978.

11 King, J. Theatre nursing care study. Total hip replacment. (Charnley total hip replacement prosthesis in elderly lady with osteoarthritis.) Nursing Times, 74, 6 Jul 1978, 1126-1129.

12 Mattix, M.W. Preoperative education for the total hip patient. (Using tape slide teaching programme.) Orthopedic Nurse's Association Journal, 6 (6), Jun 1979, 251-252.

13 Meyers, M.H. and others Total hip replacement: a team effort. (With photographs and detailed advice on post-operative movement.) American Journal of Nursing, 78 (9), Sep 1978, 1485-1488.

14 Miller, A.J. and Qureshi, M.A. Arthroplasty of the knee joint. Nursing Times, 73, 16 Jun 1977, 902-904.

15 Nursing Mirror A symposium on total knee replacement. Nursing Mirror, 143, 14 Oct 1976, 51-62. Includes:
Attenborough, C.G. The Attenborough stabilised gliding prosthesis. 52-56.
Ritter, C. The nursing care of a patient with gliding stabilised knee prosthesis. 56-58.
Thomson, A. Physiotherapy in knee replacement. 59-62.

16 Paton, E.S. Knee joint replacement in Christmas disease. Nursing Times, 75, 3 May 1979, 744-746.

17 Ritter, C. The nursing care of a patient with gliding stabilised knee prosthesis. (Symposium paper.) Nursing Mirror, 143, 14 Oct 1976, 56-58.

18 Ross, D.G. A brief history of joint replacement. Orthopedic Nurse's Association Journal, 5 (6), Jun 1978, 16-17.

19 Sculco, C.D. and Sculco, T.P. Management of the patient with an infected total hip arthroplasty. American Journal of Nursing, 76 (4), Apr 1976, 584-587.

20 Spencer, S. Nursing care study. Joint replacement. (Of the hip.) Nursing Mirror, 145, 24 Nov 1977, 18-19.

21 Volz, R.G. and Jones, A.B. Upper extremity total joint replacement. (Shoulder, elbow and wrist prostheses.) AORN Journal, 28 (5), Nov 1978, 843-847.

22 Walmsley, R. Nursing care study. There's no place like home! (Lady with arthritis following hip replacement operation.) Journal of Community Nursing, 3 (9), Mar 1980, 30, 32, 35.

23 Waugh, T. Ankle replacement arthroplasty. Orthopedic Nurse's Association Journal, 6 (1), Jan 1979, 15-18.

24 Wells, M. Nurse at the receiving end of a Charnley total hip replacement. (Nurse author's account of her progress and reactions after surgery.) Nursing Mirror, 147, 10 Aug 1978, 18-19.

25 Wilcock, G.K. Benefits of total hip replacement to older patients and the community. (Evaluation of 49 people.) British Medical Journal, 2, 1 Jul 1978, 37-39.

93 NERVOUS SYSTEM—1

a NEUROLOGY AND NURSING

1 Bertwistle, H. Practical aids for coping with progressive neurological disease. (In children.) Nursing Times, 75, 11 Oct 1979, 1768.

2 Bickerstaff, E.R. Neurology. 3rd ed. Hodder and Stoughton, 1978. (Modern nursing series.)

3 Bolin, K.L. Assessing the status of neurological patients. (Assessment form with numerical scores for neurological activity.) American Journal of Nursing, 77 (9), Sep 1977, 1478-1479.

4 Buisseret, P. The six senses. 3. The peripheral sensations. (Touch, pain, heat and proprioception.) Nursing Mirror, 146, 26 Jan 1978, Supplement, i-iv.

5 Buisseret, P. The six senses. 5. The sixth sense. (The function of the cerebral cortex, memory, the emotions and atavisms.) Nursing Mirror, 146, 9 Feb 1978, Supplement, i-iv.

6 Carini, E. and Owens, G. Neurological and neurosurgical nursing; by Barbara Lang Conway. 7th ed. St. Louis: Mosby, 1978.

7 Conway, B.L. Pediatric neurologic nursing. St. Louis: Mosby, 1977.

8 Goloskov, J.W. and LeRoy, P.L. The role of the nurse in quantitative intracranial pressure determinations. Journal of Neurosurgical Nursing, 10 (1), Mar 1978, 17-19.

9 Henson, R.A. In search of the lost chord. (The neurology of music.) Nursing Mirror, 147, 21 Dec 1978, 30-33.

10 Illis, L.S. CNS regeneration and reorganisation. (Facts known about regeneration of the central nervous system and current research progress.) Nursing Mirror, 143, 16 Dec 1976, 56-58.

11 Iveson-Iveson, J. Students' forum. The brain. (With multiple choice and long answer questions.) Nursing Mirror, 150, 12 Jun 1980, 44-47.

12 Lawton, R. Autonomic nervous system: a programmed text. Sheffield: NHS Learning Resources Unit, 1978.

13 Mechner, F. Patient assessment: neurological examination. 3. Programmed instruction. American Journal of Nursing, 76 (4), Apr 1976, P.I. 1-25.

14 Mitchell, P.H. and Mauss, N.K. Relationship of patient-nurse activity to intracranial pressure variations: a pilot study. (To discover relationships between basic patient care activities and changes in ICP.) Nursing Research, 27 (1), Jan/Feb 1978, 4-10.

15 Purchese, G. Neuromedical and neurosurgical nursing. Baillière Tindall, 1977. (Nurses' aids series special interest text.)

16 **Ramirez, B.** When you're faced with a neuro patient. (Charts showing care of CVAs and intracranial pressure.) RN Magazine, 42 (1), Jan 1979, 67-76.

17 **Roberts, A.** Body fluids. Cerebrospinal fluid. Nursing Times, 73, 16 Jun 1977, Body fluids, 1-4.

18 **Roberts, A.** Systems of life. Nos.33-37. Nervous system. Nursing Times, 73-74.
3-4. Motor function 1-2. 1 Sep 1977, (4); 29 Sep 1977, (4).
5. Autonomic nervous system. 3 Nov 1977, (4).
6. Blood supply to the central nervous system. 1 Dec 1977, (4).
7. The meninges. 5 Jan 1978, (4).

19 **Roberts, A.** Systems of life. No.39. Nervous system. 9. The spine and spinal cord. Nursing Times, 74, 2 Mar 1978, (4).

20 **Savoy, J.A.** Immediate evaluation for neurological injury, simplified. American Association of Nurse Anesthetists Journal, 44 (4), Aug 1976, 390-396.

21 **Swift, N. and Mabel, R.M.** Manual of neurological nursing. Boston: Little, Brown and Co., 1978.

22 **Wehrmaker, S.L. and Wintermute, J.R.** Case studies in neurological nursing. Boston: Little, Brown and Co., 1978.

23 **Wilson, S.F.** Neuronursing. New York: Springer, 1979.

b NEUROSURGERY AND NURSING

1 **Ashton, K.** Familiar problems in a foreign place... (Report of visit to neurosurgical ward in France.) Nursing Times, 75, 30 Aug 1979, 1474.

2 **Bannister, C.M.** Extracranial-intracranial anastomosis. Keeping the lifelines open. (Microsurgery to treat atheroma in cerebral arteries.) Nursing Mirror, 151, 4 Sep 1980, 44-46.

3 **Cowper-Smith, F.** Special nurses needed for very special nursing. (Maudsley Hospital's open day for nurses to find out more about neurosurgical nursing.) Nursing Times, 75, 13 Dec 1979, 2168-2169.

4 **Howe, J.R.** Patient care in neurosurgery. Boston: Little, Brown and Co., 1977.

5 **Madeja, C. and others** The neurosurgical nurse as a departmental assistant. (Work at Cleveland Clinic, Ohio.) Journal of Neurosurgical Nursing, 7 (2), Dec 1975, 99-101.

6 **Manning, M.** Neurosurgery: the casualties of conflict. (Neurosurgery unit at the Royal Victoria Hospital, Belfast.) Nursing Mirror, 148, 28 Jun 1979, 30-32.

7 **Marshall, A.M.** The birth of an association. (American Association of Neurosurgical Nurses.) Journal of Neurosurgical Nursing, 10 (4), Dec 1978, 146-149.

8 **Miller, L.** Neurosurgical assessment: a practical approach for the critical care nurse. Journal of Neurosurgical Nursing, 11 (1), Mar 1979, 2-5.

9 **Mitchell, P.H. and Irvin, N.J.** Neurosurgical examination: nursing assessment for nursing purposes. Journal of Neurosurgical Nursing, 9 (1), Mar 1977, 23-28.

10 **Roberts, A.** Systems of life. No.38. Nervous system. 8. The skull (calvaria.) (Anatomy and nursing care of neurosurgical patients.) Nursing Times, 74, 2 Feb 1978, (4).

11 **Van Zwanenberg, D. and Adams, C.B.T.** Neurosurgical nursing care. Faber, 1979.

12 **Walleck, C.** Primary nursing: providing continuity of care to the neurosurgical patient. (Evaluation of system at University of Maryland Hospital, Baltimore.) Journal of Neurosurgical Nursing, 11 (1), Mar 1979, 21-24.

13 **White, H.** The concept of neurosurgical care in a general hospital. Journal of Neurosurgical Nursing, 7 (2), Dec 1975, 82-86.

14 **Wille, R.** Guest editorial. The nurse's role in the specialty of neurological surgery. (Address to the Society of Neurosurgical Surgeons, North Carolina, in April 1976.) Journal of Neurosurgical Nursing, 8 (2), Dec 1976, 77-79.

15 **Wille, R.L.** Neurosurgical nursing: past, present, and future. (History from prehistoric times.) Heart Lung, 8 (5), Sep/Oct 1979, 891-895.

16 **Wille, R. and others** Emergency care of the neurosurgical patient in a community hospital. (Hackensack, New Jersey.) Journal of Neurosurgical Nursing, 8 (1), Jul 1976, 11-13.

c NERVOUS SYSTEM DISORDERS

1 **Boshes, L.D.** Gilles de la Tourette's syndrome. American Journal of Nursing, 76 (10), Oct 1976, 1637-1638.

2 **Campbell, D.** Nursing care study. Guillain-Barré syndrome: light at the end of the tunnel. Nursing Mirror, 148, 8 Feb 1979, 40-43.

3 **Carse, V.** Nursing care study. Familial periodic paralysis associated with hyperkalaemia. Nursing Times, 72, 3 Jun 1976, 845-847.

4 **Carus, R.** Motor neurone disease: a demeaning illness. (Patient's account, including lack of understanding from medical profession and public.) British Medical Journal, 280, 16 Feb 1980, 455-456.

5 **COPING** with neurologic problems proficiently. Horsham, PA.: Intermed Communications, 1979. (Nursing skillbook series.)

6 **Durston, J.H.J.** Motor neurone disease. Nursing Times, 73, 1 Sep 1977, 1352-1354.

7 **Evans, B.** 'A most disgusting specimen.' (The 'elephant man', John Merrick — neurofibromatosis.) World Medicine, 15 (12), 22 Mar 1980, 85-87.

8 **Gillett, S.G. du P.** Ekbom's syndrome. (Fidgety legs due to hyper-irritability of the nervous system.) Nursing Mirror, 145, 7 Jul 1977, 13-14.

9 **Gold, P.** Nursing care study. Von Recklinghausen's disease: a family team copes with tragedy. Nursing Mirror, 148, 15 Mar 1979, 43-45.

10 **Goodwin, R.G.** Nursing care study. Sturge-Weber syndrome (naevoid amentia). Syndrome with facial haemangioma and angioma in the meninges.) Nursing Times, 73, 6 Oct 1977, 1544-1546.

11 **Hall, M.** Nursing care study. Acute exacerbation of disseminated sclerosis. Nursing Mirror, 147, 2 Nov 1978, 27-29.

12 **Hosking, G.** Topics in child neurology. Nursing Mirror 150. (Floppy infant syndrome.)
1. Born like a rag doll. 28 Feb 1980, 32-34.
3. A decrease in mobility. 6 Mar 1980, 24-26.
4. Unwelcome movements. (Ataxia.) 13 Mar 1980, 28-29.
5. Not making the miles. (Neurodegenerative disorders.) 3 Apr 1980, 32-35.

13 **Hulbert, R.** Nursing care study. Acute polyneuritis. Nursing Times, 72, 19 Feb 1976, 257-260.

14 **Kealy, S.L.** Respiratory care in Guillain-Barre Syndrome. American Journal of Nursing, 77 (1), Jan 1977, 58-60.

15 **Keiper, S.L.** Gilles de la Tourette's syndrome. As patients recall it. American Journal of Nursing, 76 (10), Oct 1976, 1639-1641.

16 **Lucid, C.** Nursing care study. Von Recklinghausen's disease. (Neurofibromatosis.) Nursing Mirror, 146, 23 Mar 1978, 28-29.

17 **McMullen, S.** Neurological disability in adolescence. Queen's Nursing Journal, 19 (5), Aug 1976, 131-132, 138.

18 **Meakin, A.** The nerve impulse and disordered transmission. 1. Related physiology. Nursing Mirror, 145, 18 Aug 1977, 17-18.

19 **Molyneux, T.F.** Personal view. (Experience of sufferer from motor-neurone disease.) British Medical Journal, 281, 26 Jul 1980, 304.

20 **Nugent, G.R.** Radiofrequency treatment of trigeminal neuralgia. Nursing Times, 74, 9 Feb 1978, 229-230.

21 **Nursing Clinics of North America** Symposium on central nervous system disorders in children. Nursing Clinics of North America, 15 (1), Mar 1980, 1-127.

22 **Nursing Mirror** Issue on spasticity — 1. Nursing Mirror, 62 (10), Oct 1976, 315-328.

23 **Perkins, C.M.** Phaechromocytoma: notable advance in management. (Rare malign tumour of the autonomic nervous system.) Nursing Mirror, 148, 8 Feb 1979, 36-38.

24 **Pinel, C.** Creutzfeldt-Jacob disease. Nursing Times, 72, 9 Sep 1976, 1396-1397.

25 **Potter, K.** My universe. (By patient with advanced motor neurone disease.) Nursing Mirror, 145, 17 Nov 1977, 28.

26 **Sanford, E.** Nursing care study. Bilateral optic neuritis. (By first-year student nurse.) Nursing Times, 76, 7 Feb 1980, 231-233.

27 **Smith, C.** Peripheral nerve lesions. 3. The lower limb. Nursing Times, 76, 4 Dec 1980, 2159-2160.

28 **Smith, M.E.** Jakob-Creutzfeld disease. Nursing Mirror, 144, 3 Mar 1977, 49-50.

29 **Twomey, Sister Mary Redempta** Neurofibromatosis. Nursing Times, 73, 4 Aug 1977, 1196-1198.

30 Wilson, J. Spastic states in childhood. Physiotherapy, 62 (11), Nov 1976, 350-353.

d BRAIN DAMAGE AND DISORDERS

1 Allwood, A.C. and Lundy, C. Cerebral artery bypass surgery. American Journal of Nursing, 80 (7), Jul 1980, 1284-1287.

2 American Journal of Nursing The brain-damaged patient: approaches to assessment, care, and rehabilitation. (Home-study feature of four articles.) American Journal of Nursing, 79 (12), Dec 1979, 2117-2138.

3 Booth, J. Nursing care study. Raised intracranial pressure and developing obstructive hydrocephalus. Nursing Mirror, 143, 28 Oct 1976, 48-51.

4 Cooksley, P.A. Nursing care study. Subfrontal meningioma. (By ward sister.) Nursing Times, 75, 11 Oct 1979, 1753-1755.

5 Cooksley, P.A. A patient with mycotic cerebral aneurysm. (Pre- and postoperative care.) Nursing Times, 75, 14 Jun 1979, 1006-1007.

6 Cowie, V. Targets are the skin and brain. (Tuberous sclerosis.) Nursing Mirror, 149, 8 Nov 1979, 32-33.

7 Cozens, S. Theatre nursing care study. Left temporal trephine for evacuation of intracerebral clot. Nursing Times, 74, 10 Aug 1978, 1319-1321.

8 Cybyk, M.E. Alzheimer's disease. (Atrophy of cerebral cortex causing pre-senile dementia.) Nursing Times, 76, 14 Feb 1980, 280-282.

9 Eardley, P.A. Nursing care study. Intracerebral hamartoma. (Tumour-like mass of cells.) Nursing Times, 74, 13 Apr 1978, 618-620.

10 Galbraith, S.L. Management of patients with subarachnoid haemorrhage. Nursing Times, 75, 25 Oct 1979, 1852-1854.

11 Gavrielides, S. Nursing care study. Meningitis. (Treatment and care in an ITU.) Nursing Times, 74, 2 Mar 1978, 367-370.

12 Hanley, J. Nursing care study. Aneurysm: suddenly, I had a violent pain... (Nurse describes her experience of surgery for aneurysm, complicated by myxoedema.) Nursing Mirror, 149, 4 Oct 1979, 40.

13 Hewitt, M. Nursing care study. Subarachnoid haemorrhage. Nursing Mirror, 144, 23 Jun 1977, 15-17.

14 Hosking, G. Topics in child neurology. 5. The CNS catches it. (Infective disorders including meningitis and encephalitis.) Nursing Mirror, 150, 20 Mar 1980, 20-23.

15 Jacobs, G.B. and others The treatment of intracranial aneurysms. Journal of Neurosurgical Nursing, 8 (2), Dec 1976, 149-154.

16 Jacobson, I. and Hutchinson, P. Brain abscess and subdural empyema. Nursing Times, 72, 21 Oct 1976, 1628-1630.

17 Jennett, B. Brain damage: predicting the quality of survival. (Development by computer

of outcome scale in Glasgow.) Nursing Mirror, 148, 1 Feb 1979, 30-31.

18 Johnston, A.F. Nursing care study. Subacute sclerosing panencephalitis. Nursing Times, 72, 26 Feb 1976, 305-308.

19 Lewin, D. and Wall, J. Primary subarachnoid haemorrhage. 1. The combined approach, by D. Lewin. 2. Nursing care, by J. Wall. Nursing Mirror, 143, 15 Jul 1976, 58-60; 22 Jul 1976, 47.

20 Loh, K.H. Nursing care study. Subarachnoid haemorrhage. Nursing Mirror, 145, 17 Nov 1977, 15-16.

21 McLennan, A. Nursing care study. A patient with meningococcal meningitis. (By a ward sister.) Nursing Times, 76, 3 Jan 1980, 29-31.

22 Newman, J. Nursing care study. Cerebral aneurysm. Nursing Times, 72, 29 Jul 1976, 1156-1161.

23 Nursing Times Royal Free disease. (Three articles on this disease, also known as myalgic encephalomyelitis.) Nursing Times, 74, 27 Apr 1978, 698-703.

24 Ozga, A. Home follow-up for the brain injured patient. (Work of rehabilitation nurse specialist.) AORN Journal, 3 (3), May/Jun 1978, 17-20.

25 Phillips, P. Nursing care study. Subarachnoid haemorrhage caused by a ruptured aneurysm. Nursing Times, 72, 19 Aug 1976, 1270-1273.

26 Pitt, N. Behaviour deviations of a brain-injured child: with some ideas to overcome them. British Journal of Occupational Therapy, 40 (1), 1977, 13-15.

27 Riley, C. Consumers viewpoint. (Experiences of disablement following a cerebral haemorrhage.) Social Work Today, 8, 25 Jan 1977, 20-21.

28 Salmon, M.A. Bacterial meningitis in infants and children. Nursing Times, 73, 8 Dec 1977, 1910-1912.

29 Salmon, M.A. The effects on growth of cerebral dysfunction. Nursing Times, 72, 28 Oct 1976, 1675-1676.

30 Sandall, S. Brain damage in adults—a personal approach to rehabilitation. (By an occupational therapist.) British Journal of Occupational Therapy, 43 (12), Dec 1980, 405-406.

31 Series, C. and Lincoln, N. Behaviour modification in physical rehabilitation. (Rivermead Rehabilitation Centre for patients with brain damage.) British Journal of Occupational Therapy, 41 (7), Jul 1978, 222-224.

32 Smellie, R. Nursing care study. Reclamation of a severely brain-damaged patient. (Care in hospital for the young chronic sick.) Nursing Times, 74, 30 Mar 1978, 532-533.

33 Whitton, T. Nursing care study. Cerebral astrocytoma. Nursing Mirror, 143, 2 Dec 1976, 59.

34 Wilkinson, O. Out of touch with reality. (Nurse describes her experience of acute organic brain syndrome.) Nursing, 9, Jan 1980, 404-406.

35 Williamson, S.M. Community nursing care study. Old before her time. (Problems following removal of cerebral cyst.) Nursing Times, 75, 11 Jan 1979, 76-77.

36 Williamson-Kirkland, T.E. and Berni, R. Neurological aspects of rehabilitation. Part 1. Brain injury. (Cerebral vascular accident, traumatic brain injury and anoxic brain damage.) AORN Journal, 5 (3), May/Jun 1980, 10-12.

e UNCONSCIOUS PATIENT

1 Adams, N.R. Prolonged coma. Your care makes all the difference. Nursing, 7 (8), Aug 1977, 21-27.

2 Darwin, J. Assessing levels of consciousness. Nursing, 15, Jul 1980, 672-673.

3 Jones, C. Glasgow coma scale. (Assessment tool to describe level of consciousness.) American Journal of Nursing, 79 (9), Sep 1979, 1551-1553.

4 Jones, D.C. and Dickerson, J.W.T. Decision making in the nutritional care of unconscious patients. (Study of 646 tube feeds showing neglect in decision making by medical and dietetic staff.) Journal of Advanced Nursing, 1 (5), Sep 1976, 359-365.

5 Loen, M. and Snyder, M. Psycho-social aspects of care of the long-term comatose patient. Journal of Neurosurgical Nursing, 11 (4), Dec 1979, 235-237.

6 Monaghan, A.M. When the patient cannot help himself. (Intensive care of the unconscious patient.) Australian Nurses Journal, 5 (6/7), Dec/Jan 1976, 22-23, 27.

7 Myco, F. and McGilloway, F.A. Care of the unconscious patient: a complementary perspective. (Parallels between world of neonate and unconscious patient and need for social aspects of care as well as physical aspects.) Journal of Advanced Nursing, 5 (3), May 1980, 273-283.

8 Nicholl, K.L. Nursing care study. Encephalitis. (Nursing care of ten-year-old girl who has been unconscious for fourteen months.) Nursing Times, 74, 22 Jun 1978, 1045-1048.

9 Nursing Altered consciousness. 2. Nursing, 9, Jan 1980, 381-416.

10 Ramirez, B. Brain integrity score simplifies patient monitoring. (Measures states of consciousness, reaction to pain and ability to move.) RN Magazine, 42 (1), Jan 1979, 74-75.

11 Rhodes, L.C. Specialised care. 6. The care of the unconscious patient. Nursing Mirror, 145, 20 Oct 1977, Nursing care supplement, series 6, i-iv.

12 Wilmot, W.M. Pictures in nursing. Turning and positioning the unconscious patient. Nursing, 9, Jan 1980, 414-416.

f CEREBRAL PALSY

1 Ansell, P. Delay in the diagnosis of cerebral palsy: an account of my daughter's first year. Health Visitor, 52 (7), Jul 1979, 269-271.

2 Crank, A. and Kelly, P. Seven points for action says cerebral palsy survey. (Survey of problems encountered by mothers of cerebral palsied children.) Health and Social Service Journal, 86, 29 Oct 1976, Rehabilitation Supplement, 12-13.

3 **Grayshon, J.R.** Nursing care study. Cerebral palsy. (Care of 21-year-old girl in a long-stay ward for mentally handicapped adults, by student nurse.) Nursing Times, 76, 6 Mar 1980, 416-419.

4 **Hare, N.** Handling cerebral palsied infants. Ways of handling cerebral palsied children, increasing their comfort and stimulation. Health and Social Service Journal, 87, 23 Sep 1977, 1362.

5 **Hitchcock, E.R.** Stereotactic surgery for cerebral palsy. (To achieve functional improvement including speech and movement.) Nursing Times, 74, 14 Dec 1978, 2064-2065.

6 **Hosking, G.** Topics in child neurology: not only...but also. (Cerebral palsy.) Nursing Mirror, 150, 21 Feb 1980, 20-22.

7 **Ratnam, S.** Nursing care study. Cerebral palsy and epilepsy. Nursing Mirror, 142, 11 Mar 1976, 49-50.

8 **Rees, J.** Nursing care study. A cerebral palsied child with mental subnormality. Nursing Times, 74, 1 Jun 1978, 908-911.

9 **Rowe, B. and Morgan, B.** Care for the handicapped adult. (A survey of the effects of cerebral palsy on a group of young adults in Newcastle.) Social Work Today, 7 (5), 27 May 1976, 134-136.

10 **Schlesinger, H.** Preparation for adult life. (Education of young men and women with cerebral palsy, with reference to the Spastics Society's Beaumont College.) British Journal of Occupational Therapy, 43 (2), Feb 1980, 54-57.

11 **Thomas, L.** Caring for the hospitalized cerebral palsy patient. Journal of Practical Nursing, 25 (12), Dec 1975, 24-25.

12 **West, J.** The Bobath Centre. (Therapeutic centre for children with cerebral palsy.) Health and Social Service Journal, 86, 12 Jun 1976, 1074-1075.

g EPILEPSY AND CONVULSIONS

1 **Arangio, A.J.** An assessment model: a systemic examination of the psychosocial needs of patients with epilepsy. Patient Counselling and Health Education, 1 (2), Fall 1978, 75-80.

2 **Beniak, J. and others** The reality of epilepsy: an up-to-date approach for patients and practitioners. Journal of Practical Nursing, 20 (3), Mar 1980, 22-26.

3 **Branson, H.K.** Understanding the epileptic and his medication. Nursing Care, 9 (7), Jul 1976, 2021.

4 **British Epilepsy Association** The nurse and epilepsy. Wokingham: the Association, 1979.

5 **Bruya, M.A. and Bolin, R.H.** Epilepsy: a controllable disease. 1. Classification and diagnosis of seizures. 2. Drug therapy and nursing care. American Journal of Nursing, 76 (3), Mar 1976, 388-397.

6 **Craig, A.G.** The epileptic worker. Occupational Health, 32 (3), Mar 1980, 137-139.

7 **Fenton, G.W.** Rehabilitation problems in people with epilepsy. Rehabilitation, 96, Jan/Mar 1976, 15-21.

8 **Gartside, G.** Nursing care study. Epilepsy: an unacceptable illness. (62-year-old epileptic patient who denied her illness and was admitted to a psychiatric unit.) Nursing Mirror, 150, 19 Jun 1980, 45-46.

9 **Grant, R.H.E.** Medical responsibilities in epilepsy. Rehabilitation, 99, Oct-Dec 1976, 37-48.

10 **Harrison, R.M.** Society at work. Epilepsy and stigma. New Society, 37, 2 Sep 1976, 497-498.

11 **Hawken, M.** If you want a real challenge, become an epilepsy nurse specialist. Nursing, 8 (9), Sep 1978, 15-17.

12 **Hawken, M. and Ozuna, J.** Practical aspects of anticonvulsant therapy. American Journal of Nursing, 79 (6), Jun 1979, 1062-1068.

13 **Hopkins, A. and Scambler, G.** How doctors deal with epilepsy. (Interview with GPs in London.) Lancet, 1, 22 Jan 1977, 183-186.

14 **Hosking, G.** Topics in child neurology 6. The eye witness fits in. (Epilepsy.) Nursing Mirror, 150, 27 Mar 1980, 22-25.

15 **Houlder, C.A.** Closure of a hospital and some people with epilepsy. (St. Faith's Hospital, Brentwood.) British Medical Journal, 1, 14 May 1977, 1266-1267.

16 **Isaacs, N.M.** The surgical treatment of epilepsy. Journal of Neurosurgical Nursing, 8 (2), Dec 1976, 155-168.

17 **Kelly, J.** Epilepsy symposium. Nursing management. Nursing Mirror, 147, 27 Jul 1978, 17-19.

18 **Laidlaw, M.V. and Laidlaw, J.** Epilepsy explained. Edinburgh: Churchill Livingstone, 1980. (Patient handbook.)

19 **Lancet** Close encounters with childhood epilepsy. (Report of survey of epileptic children and their families.) Lancet, 1, 24 Jun 1978, 1346-1347.

20 **Lopez, K.A.** Temporal lobe epilepsy: a new entity in psychiatry. Journal of Psychiatric Nursing, 18 (8), Aug 1980, 10-15.

21 **MacIntyre, I.** Epilepsy and employment. Community Health, 7 (4), Apr 1976, 195-204.

22 **Markham, G.** Epilepsy. Nursing, 8, Dec 1979, 356-359; Comment from British Epilepsy Association Nursing, 11, Mar 1980, 501.

23 **Markham, G.** Hysterical epilepsy: conflict and confusion for patient and staff. (With fit description chart.) Nursing Mirror, 148, 11 Jan 1979, 28-30.

24 **Nursing Mirror** Epilepsy symposium.
1. 147, 27 Jul 1978, 13-24. Includes:
Galbraith, A.W. Anchorman—the GP. 20-21.
Kelly, J. Nursing management. 17-19.
Reynolds, E.H. Basic concepts and diagnosis. 14-16.
Shorvon, S.D. Drug treatment. 21-24.
2. 147, 3 Aug 1978, 13-22. Includes:
Brett, E.M. Epilepsy and convulsions in children. 20-22.
Fenwick, P. Psychological changes. 13-16.
Perkins, H. Chronic idiopathic epilepsy. 16-19.

25 **Ozuna, J.** Psychosocial aspects of epilepsy. Journal of Neurosurgical Nursing, 11 (4), Dec 1979, 242-246.

26 **Pennell, E.** Helping the epileptic help himself. Nursing Care, 9 (7), Jul 1976, 16-19.

27 **Ross, E.M. and others** Epilepsy in childhood: findings from the National Child Development Study. British Medical Journal, 280, 26 Jan 1980, 207-210.

28 **Ross, E.** Epileptic children. Health and Social Service Journal, 87, 18 Nov 1977, 1600.

29 **Ross, E.** Fitting remedies: ways of managing children suffering from epilepsy. Health and Social Service Journal, 87, 4 Nov 1977, 1521.

30 **Sambrook, M.A.** The EEG in epilepsy. Nursing Times, 72, 20 May 1976, 777-780.

31 **Scott, D.** About epilepsy. 3rd ed. Duckworth, 1978.

32 **Short, E.** A patient with seizures. (Includes two case studies.) Nursing Times, 72, 29 Jul 1976, Key Clinical, 21-24.

33 **Stores, C.** The investigation and management of school children with epilepsy. (Park Hospital for Children, Oxford.) Public Health, 90 (4), May 1976, 171-177.

34 **Swift, N.** Helping patients live with seizures. Nursing, 8 (6), Jun 1978, 25-31.

35 **Walshe-Brennan, K.S.** Epileptic personality. Nursing Mirror, 142, 25 Mar 1976, 56-57.

36 **Westland, G.** Social skills training with epileptic psychiatric patients. (Course at the Maudsley Hospital.) British Journal of Occupational Therapy, 43 (1), Jan 1980, 13-16.

37 **Whitfield, W.** The epilepsies. Nursing Times, 73, 11 Aug 1977, 1251-1255.

38 **Whitlock, J. and Learner, S.** Practical aspects of O.T. with epileptic children. British Journal of Occupational Therapy, 40 (1), Jan 1977, 10-12.

39 **Whysall, D.** The role of the occupational therapist in the treatment of people with epilepsy. British Journal of Occupational Therapy, 43 (7), Jul 1980, 225-229.

h HUNTINGTON'S CHOREA

1 **Barber, R.** Nursing care study. Huntington's chorea. (Care of elderly lady in psychogeriatric ward.) Nursing Times, 74, 13 Jul 1978, 1165-1167.

2 **Davis, A.** Nursing care study. Emily—a victim of Huntington's chorea. Nursing Times, 72, 25 Mar 1976, 449-450.

3 **Evans, K. and Warren, J.** Huntington's chorea. Social Work Today, 6 (25), 18 Mar 1976, 787-788.

4 **Free, J.W. and McPhillips, C.** Huntington's disease. How to solve its unique care problems. RN Magazine, 40 (8), Aug 1977, 44-46.

5 Harper, P.S. and others Huntington's Chorea: the basis for long-term prevention. (Programme of genetic counselling in South Wales.) Lancet, 2, 18 Aug 1979, 346-349.

6 Heywood Jones, I. Association to Combat Huntington's Chorea. (Details of aims and work.) Nursing Times, 75, 8 Nov 1979, 1949.

7 Higgins, R. Huntington's chorea. Nursing Times, 72, 29 Jul 1976, 1164-1165.

8 Johnson, K.E. Nursing care study. Huntington's chorea. Nursing Mirror, 147, 23 Nov 1978, 29-31.

9 Kelly, J. Nursing care study. Huntington's chorea. A mother shunned by her family. Nursing Mirror, 148, 12 Apr 1979, 45-46.

10 Manning, M. Combating the agony of Huntington's chorea: the background to this genetically transmitted disease. Nursing Mirror, 146, 2 Mar 1978, 7-9.

11 Office of Health Economics Huntington's chorea. OHE, 1980. (Studies on current health problems.)

12 Pinel, C. Huntington's chorea. Nursing Times, 72, 25 Mar 1976, 447-448.

13 Rose, V. Huntington's chorea—the most destructive of diseases? Journal of Community Nursing, 2 (1), Jul 1978, 13, 15, 17.

14 Stevens, D.L. Huntington's chorea: a booklet for the families and friends of patients with the disease. Association to Combat Huntington's Chorea, 1976.

15 Tolliss, W. Nursing care study. Huntington's chorea. Nursing Mirror, 142, 27 May 1976, 54-55.

16 Westall, J. Research and care in Huntington's Chorea. Mind Out, 27, Mar/Apr 1978, 16-18.

i MIGRAINE AND HEADACHE

1 Bell, C.R. Headache associated with cold exposure. Occupational Health, 29 (9), Sep 1977, 393-397.

2 Bickerstaff, E.R. Cluster headaches. (Ciliary neuralgia.) Nursing Times, 73, 29 Sep 1977, 1518-1519.

3 Heathfield, K.W.G. Causes of headache. Nursing Mirror, 146, 26 Jan 1978, 13-18.

4 Marks, R.G. Intractable headache? Biofeedback could be a solution. (With reference to use in other conditions such as migraine, stress conditions and epilepsy.) RN Magazine, 42 (7), Jul 1979, 73-74, 79.

5 Migraine Trust Migraine becomes more of a headache for the researchers. (Survey into family history, symptoms, length and severity of attacks.) Nursing Mirror, 143, 1 Jul 1976, 37.

6 Nightingale, J.H. Migraine. Queen's Nursing Journal, 19 (11), Feb 1977, 298-299.

7 Nightingale, J.H. The natural history of migraine and its management in general practice. Journal of the Royal College of General Practitioners, 26, May 1976, 318-326.

8 Nursing Mirror A symposium on migraine. Nursing Mirror, 145, 11 Aug 1977, 13-24.

94 NERVOUS SYSTEM—2

a MULTIPLE SCLEROSIS

1 American Journal of Nursing Multiple sclerosis. (Home-study feature of eight articles.) American Journal of Nursing, 80 (2), Feb 1980, 273-302.

2 Bell, M.A. Adult-type relapsing multiple sclerosis presenting in childhood. (Two nursing care studies.) Nursing Times, 73, 3 Mar 1977, 294-298.

3 Birrer, C. Multiple sclerosis: a personal view. Springfield, Ill.: Charles Thomas, 1979.

4 Boyer, A. and others Nursing care. (Symposium on multiple sclerosis.) Nursing Mirror, 143, 5 Aug 1976, 52-53.

5 Burnfield, A. and Burnfield, P. Common psychological problems in multiple sclerosis. British Medical Journal, 1, 6 May 1978, 1193-1194.

6 Burnfield, A. Multiple sclerosis: a doctor's personal experience. British Medical Journal, 1, 12 Feb 1977, 435-436.

7 Catanzaro, M. Multiple sclerosis. Exploding myths that compromise patient care. (Nursing care.) RN Magazine, 40 (12), Dec 1977, 42-47.

8 Community Outlook Multiple sclerosis. (Six articles on aspects of community care.) Nursing Times, 74, 11 May 1978, Community Outlook, 130-134, 136, 138-139.

9 Connell, H.H. Social and psychological welfare. (Symposium on multiple sclerosis.) Nursing Mirror, 143, 5 Aug 1976, 56-57.

10 Cooksley, P.A. Nursing care study. A patient with multiple sclerosis. (Includes treatment for pressure sores.) Nursing Times, 75, 8 Nov 1979, 1925-1928.

11 Cross, V. Multiple sclerosis: the physiotherapist's approach. (With diagrams of exercises.) Journal of Community Nursing, 3 (8), Feb 1980, 22-23, 25-26.

12 Davies, G.M. The problems of nursing patients with advanced multiple sclerosis at home. (Research study.) Journal of Advanced Nursing, 4 (6), Nov 1979, 635-645.

13 Davies, N. Both sides of the sheets. (By male nurse with multiple sclerosis.) Nursing Mirror, 150, 12 Jun 1980, 50-52.

14 Davison, A.N. Current research. (Symposium on multiple sclerosis.) Nursing Mirror, 143, 5 Aug 1976, 50-51.

15 Davison, A. Multiple sclerosis: recent advances in research. Journal of Community Nursing, 3 (8), Feb 1980, 18, 30.

16 Dick, G. The aetiology. (Symposium on multiple sclerosis.) Nursing Mirror, 143, 5 Aug 1976, 46-47.

17 Dolan, B. Multiple sclerosis. (Including case study of nurse patient.) Journal of Neurosurgical Nursing, 11 (2), Jun 1979, 83-93.

18 Field, E.J. and Joyce, G. Multiple sclerosis: what can and cannot be done. British Medical Journal, 2, 15 Dec 1979, 1571-1572.

19 Forsythe, E. Living with multiple sclerosis. Faber, 1979.

20 Hart, L.K. Fatigue in the patient with multiple sclerosis. (Results of questionnaire.) Research in Nursing Health, 1 (4), Dec 1978, 145-157.

21 Jameson, R.M. Multiple sclerosis and the urinary tract. Practitioner, 218, Jan 1977, 91-96.

22 Johnson, G. and Johnson, R. Living with disability: a survey of social services support for multiple sclerosis patients in Scotland. Churchill Livingstone, 1978.

23 Johnson, G.S. and Johnson, R.H. Social services support for multiple sclerosis patients in West of Scotland. Lancet, 1, 1 Jan 1977, 31-34.

24 Kelly, R. Management of MS. (Symposium on multiple sclerosis.) Nursing Mirror, 143, 5 Aug 1976, 48-50.

25 Kelly, R. Multiple sclerosis. Queen's Nursing Journal, 19 (5), Aug 1976, 136-138.

26 Kelly, Y. The Bethlehem MS service. (Specialised district nursing service attached to neurological unit of Bethlehem Hospital, Melbourne.) Australian Nurses Journal, 9 (10), May 1980, 30-32.

27 Kent, H. Prisoner of the chair. How proper posture and breathing in a wheelchair can help the multiple sclerosis sufferer feel better. Nursing Mirror, 150, 12 Jun 1980, 53-54.

28 McDonnell, M. and others Problem-oriented nursing care plans. (Standard care plans for multiple sclerosis patients.) American Journal of Nursing, 80 (2), Feb 1980, 292-297.

29 McNairn, N. About multiple sclerosis. (Answers to questions commonly asked.) Canadian Nurse, 74 (7), Jul/Aug 1978, 35, 38-40.

30 Nosworthy, S.J. Physiotherapy. (Symposium on multiple sclerosis.) Nursing Mirror, 143, 5 Aug 1976, 53-55.

31 Nourse, E.M. Patient care study—multiple sclerosis. Queen's Nursing Journal, 19 (2), May 1976, 50, 61.

32 Nursing Mirror A symposium on multiple sclerosis. Nursing Mirror, 143 (6), 5 Aug 1976, 45-57.

33 Pauley, J.W. The psychological management of multiple sclerosis. Practitioner, 218, Jan 1977, 100-105.

34 Rawson, M. Cause and cure: unknown. (Multiple sclerosis.) Nursing Mirror, 150, 12 Jun 1980, 48-50.

35 Ross, J.E. The patient with multiple sclerosis at home. (Role of the district nurse.) Nursing Mirror, 145, 7 Jul 1977, 35-36.

36 Somerville, M. Community nursing. Learning to live with multiple sclerosis. Nursing Mirror, 144, 30 Jun 1977, 44-45.

37 Stevens, J. Nursing care study. When the

family rallies round... (Domiciliary care of multiple sclerosis sufferer during relapse.) Journal of Community Nursing, 1 (9), Mar 1978, 8-9.

38 Tombleson, E. Facts about multiple sclerosis. Social consequences of multiple sclerosis. New Zealand Nursing Journal, 69 (7), Jul 1976, 20-21; (8), Aug 1976, 23-24.

39 Willcocks, F. Cushioning the impact of multiple sclerosis. (Group of MS sufferers led by medical social worker.) Social Work Today, 11, 18 Mar 1980, 16-18.

40 Winter, A. The use of transcutaneous electrical stimulation (TNS) in the treatment of multiple sclerosis. Journal of Neurosurgical Nursing, 8 (2), Dec 1976, 125-131.

41 Wright, P. At home with multiple sclerosis: a patient's view. Journal of Community Nursing, 1 (10), Apr 1978, 16-17, 28.

b PARKINSON'S DISEASE

1 Beattie, A. and Caird, F.I. The occupational therapist and the patient with Parkinson's disease. (Study to establish whether assessment at home by an occupational therapist and the provision of simple aids could assist in the management of patients with Parkinson's disease.) British Medical Journal, 280, 7 Jun 1980, 1354-1355.

2 Duvoisin, R.C. Parkinson's disease: a guide for patient and family. New York: Raven, 1978.

3 Geden, C.E. Nursing care study. Rehabilitation of patient with Parkinson's disease. Nursing Times, 73, 22 Sep 1977, 1470-1471.

4 Gibberd, G. Parkinson's disease. Queen's Nursing Journal, 19 (5), Aug 1976, 126-127, 129.

5 Langan, R.J. and Cotzias, G.C. Do's and dont's for the patient on Levodopa therapy. (With Parkinson's disease.) American Journal of Nursing, 76 (6), Jun 1976, 917-918.

6 Sambrook, M.A. Parkinsonism. Nursing Times, 72, 25 Mar 1976, 454-455.

7 Stern, G. and Lees, A. The on-off effect— a side-effect of long-term levodopa treatment. (For Parkinson's disease.) Nursing Mirror, 147, 17 Aug 1978, 17-18.

8 Watson, J. Nursing care study. Parkinsonism. Nursing Mirror, 142, 25 Mar 1976, 50-51.

c SPINAL CORD INJURIES

1 American Journal of Nursing The person with a spinal cord injury. (Part of self-study series for continuing education. Physical and psychological care and two case studies.) American Journal of Nursing, 77 (8), Aug 1977, 1319-1342.

2 Barnes, A. Tetraplegia: a personal account. (With criticism of nurses' attitudes.) Nursing, 4, Jul 1979, 194-197.

3 Better, S.R. and others Complications among spinal cord injury patients following discharge. (Findings of survey.) AORN Journal, 4 (2), Mar/Apr 1979, 8-10.

4 Blackford, N. Where there's a will. (Spinal Injuries Centre at Stoke Mandeville Hospital.) Nursing Mirror, 151, 24 Jul 1980, 36-38.

5 Bromley, I. Tetraplegia and paraplegia: a guide for physiotherapists. Edinburgh: Churchill Livingstone, 1976.

6 Engstrand, J.L. A nursing challenge: effective patient education. (Review of patient teaching methods in a spinal cord injury centre.) AORN Journal, 4 (5), Sep/Oct 1979, 15-18.

7 Fine, P.R. and others The operation of a hospital based specialty home health team: activities and associated costs. (Research study of work of team of nurse, physiotherapist and vocational rehabilitation counsellor serving spinal cord injury patients.) AORN Journal, 3 (1), Jan/Feb 1978, 5-7, 9-10.

8 Foldes, M.S. and Woods, M.E. Crisis intervention: the patient with interruption of spinal cord integrity. (Case study illustrating nursing care of a paralysed patient and his family.) Journal of Neurosurgical Nursing, 7 (2), Dec 1975, 72-81.

9 Gallop, J.F. The relevance of motivation in the rehabilitation of spinal cord injuries. British Journal of Occupational Therapy, 43 (8), Aug 1980, 259-260.

10 Guttmann, L. On health deviation and rehabilitation in spinal paraplegia and tetraplegia. Community Health, 8 (4), May 1977, 186-208.

11 Hansen, A.M. Towards independence for paraplegics. (Rehabilitation.) Canadian Nurse, 72 (12), Dec 1976, 24-27, 30-31.

12 Hart, C. Care study. Sean—a world turned upside down. (Life and nursing care of paraplegic young man.) Nursing Times, 73, 10 Nov 1977, Community Outlook, 116-119.

13 Henriksen, J.D. Specialized care of the spinal cord injured patient. 3. Activities of daily living. Journal of Practical Nursing, 26 (8), Aug 1976, 17, 30.

14 Henriksen, J.D. Specialized care of the spinal cord injured patient. 5. Secondary health problems. Journal of Practical Nursing, 26 (10), Oct 1976, 21, 34.

15 Hyde, A. Fighting to save the future of the Mandeville miracle. (Report of visit to Stoke Mandeville Hospital Spinal Injuries Unit.) Health and Social Service Journal, 89, 16 Nov 1979, 1476-1478.

16 Istre, S.M. The physical aspects of counseling for persons with congenital or acquired spinal cord injury. (With reference to sexual function.) Orthopedic Nurse's Association Journal, 16 (12), Dec 1979, 468-483.

17 Jones, G. After Oswestry—what next? Rehabilitation of patients with spinal cord paralysis. Nursing, 5, Aug 1979, 214-216.

18 Kinash, R.G. Experiences and nursing needs of spinal cord-injured patients. Journal of Neurosurgical Nursing, 10 (1), Mar 1978, 29-32.

19 Larrabee, J.H. The person with a spinal cord injury. Physical care during early recovery. American Journal of Nursing, 77 (8), Aug 1977, 1320-1329.

20 Leinart, B.K. Attitudes of nurses toward spinal cord injury patients. (Study to compare attitudes of acute care nurses with those of rehabilitation nurses.) ARN Journal, 4 (1), Jan/Feb 1979, 7-9.

21 LeSieur, E. Specialized care of the spinal cord injured patient. 4. A case study. Journal of Practical Nursing, 26 (9), Sep 1976, 28-29, 39.

22 Macauley, C. Eddie: a successful quad. (Case study of quadraplegic patient following spinal cord injury.) American Journal of Nursing, 77 (8), Aug 1977, 1336-1338.

23 Mackie, J. The clinical team in action— the management of spinal injuries. Medical management. Nursing care. (Nursing Mirror Forum.) Nursing Mirror, 143, 25 Nov 1976, 47-50.

24 Mackie, J. Specialised care. 4. The paralysed patient. Nursing Mirror, 145, 22 Sep 1977, Nursing care supplement, series 6, i-iv.

25 Marshall, T. Information needs in planning spinal cord injury services. Community Medicine, 1 (4), Nov 1979, 282-285.

26 Mathews, N.C. Helping a quadriplegic veteran decide to live. (Analysis of nurse-patient interaction.) American Journal of Nursing, 76 (3), Mar 1976, 441-443.

27 Monks, J. Environment and 'debility' in spinal injury. (A survey of spinal injured patients and their relatives on the effects of social and physical environment in restricting their independence.) Nursing Times, 72, 16 Dec 1976, Occ. papers, 177-180; 23 Dec 1976, Occ. papers, 181-184.

28 Mountjoy, S. The clinical team in action— the management of spinal injuries. Community care. (Nursing Mirror Forum.) Nursing Mirror, 143, 25 Nov 1976, 57-60.

29 Nursing Times Coping with quadriplegic patient. (Personal account of difficulties of a quadriplegic patient admitted to a medical ward with a chest infection.) Nursing Times, 72, 26 Feb 1976, 303-304.

30 Pierce, D.S. and Nickel, V.H. editors The total care of spinal cord injuries. Boston: Little, Brown and Co., 1977. (For nurses and others.)

31 Roaf, R. and Hodkinson, L.J. The paralysed patient. Blackwell, 1977.

32 Rogers, M.A. Paraplegia: a handbook of practical care and advice. Faber, 1978.

33 Rottkamp, B.C. An experimental nursing study. A behavior modification approach to nursing therapeutics in body positioning of spinal cord injured patients. Nursing Research, 25 (3), May/Jun 1976, 181-186.

34 Shipp, M. The clinical team in action— the management of spinal injuries. Social implications. (Nursing Mirror Forum 76.) Nursing Mirror, 143 (22), 25 Nov 1976, 55-57.

35 Silva, A. The clinical team in action— the management of spinal injuries. Physiotherapy. (Nursing Mirror Forum 76.) Nursing Mirror, 143 (22), 25 Nov 1976, 51-52.

36 Spinal Injuries Association Nursing management in the general hospital: the first 48 hours following injury. The Association, 1980.

37 Sullivan, R.A. and others Specialized care of the spinal cord injured patient. 1. Preventing injury and promoting rehabilitation. 2. Bowel and bladder programs. Journal of Practical Nursing, 26 (6), Jun 1976, 14-17; (7), Jul 1976, 36-38.

38 Sutton, F. The clinical team in action — the management of spinal injuries. Occupational therapy. (Nursing Mirror Forum 76.) Nursing Mirror, 143, 25 Nov 1976, 53-55.

39 Williamson-Kirkland, T.E. and Berni, R. Neurological aspects of rehabilitation. Part 2. Spinal cord injury. ARN Journal, 5 (4), Jul/Aug 1980, 8-12, 17.

40 Zach, G.A. Acute therapy and rehabilitation of paraplegics. Rehabilitation, 98, Jul-Sep 1976, 13-17.

d STROKE: GENERAL AND NURSING

1 Adolphus, P. Sunnybrook stroke team — an innovative experience. (Operation of Canada's first multidisciplinary stroke unit.) Canadian Nurse, 72 (2), Feb 1976, 16-17.

2 Alexander, M.A. Nursing care study. Cerebro-vascular accident. (With chart showing positions for C.V.A. patients used by Queen Mary's Hospital, Roehampton.) Nursing Mirror, 145, 29 Dec 1977, 25-26.

3 Andrews, K. Should stroke patients be treated in hospital or at home? Chest, Heart and Stroke Journal, 1 (4), Winter 1976/11, 30-33.

4 Blower, P. and Shaukat, A. A stroke unit in a district general hospital: the Greenwich experience. British Medical Journal, 2, 15 Sep 1979, 644-646.

5 Bobath, B. Adult hemiplegia: evaluation and treatment. 2nd ed. Heinemann, 1978.

6 Brandrick, J. Nursing care study. A nursing care plan for convalescence following a cerebrovascular accident. Nursing Times, 76, 17 Jul 1980, 1253-1257.

7 Brocklehurst, J.C. Stroke patients — is admission necessary? (Survey in Manchester of reasons for admission.) Modern Geriatrics, 8 (12), Dec 1978, 56-57.

8 Carr, J. and Shepherd, R. Early care of the stroke patient: a positive approach. Heinemann Medical, 1979.

9 Carroll, S. Nursing care study. Cerebrovascular accident: teamwork aids a stroke patient. Nursing Mirror, 148, 15 Mar 1979, 47-48.

10 Cross, V. Handle with care. (Advice for community nurses and relatives on moving and positioning stroke patients.) Journal of Community Nursing, 3 (5), Nov 1979, 15, 17-18, 20.

11 Dardier, E. The early stroke patient: positioning and movement. Baillière Tindall, 1980.

12 Garraway, W.M. and others Management of acute stroke in the elderly: preliminary results of a controlled trial. (Comparison of management in a stroke unit and medical units.) British Medical Journal, 280, 12 Apr 1980, 1040-1043.

13 Garraway, W.M. and others Management of acute stroke in the elderly: follow-up of a controlled trial. (Loss after discharge of improvements achieved in stroke unit.) British Medical Journal, 281, 27 Sep 1980, 827-829.

14 Hart, G. Perceptual distortion. (After stroke.) Canadian Nurse, 76 (5), May 1980, 44-47.

15 Hodgson, S.J. Nursing care study. A patient after cerebral vascular accident. Nursing Times, 73, 14 Apr 1977, 524-526.

16 Howorth, I. and Prosser, J. Cerebrovascular accident. Nursing Mirror, 142, 3 Jun 1976, Nursing care supplement, series 3, i-iv.

17 Humm, W. Early physical treatment for the stroke patient. Nursing Times, 72, 22 Jan 1976, 103-106.

18 Isaacs, B. Five years' experience of a stroke unit. (Lightburn Hospital, Glasgow.) Health Bulletin, 35 (2), Mar 1977, 94-98.

19 Isaacs, B. The place of a stroke unit in geriatric medicine. (Lightburn Hospital, Glasgow.) Physiotherapy, 62 (5), May 1976, 152-154.

20 Jay, P.E. Help yourselves: a handbook for hemiplegics and their families. 3rd ed. Ian Henry, 1979.

21 Johnston, K. and Olsen, E. Application of Bobath principles for nursing care of the hemiplegic patient. (Weight bearing, counter-rotation and protraction.) ARN Journal, 5 (2), Mar/Apr 1980, 8-11.

22 Kennedy, B.F. The stroke unit — a physiotherapist's view. Physiotherapy, 62 (5), May 1976, 154-155.

23 Kester, R.C. Surgery for strokes resulting from extracranial arterial occlusion. Nursing Times, 74, 12 Jan 1978, 59-62.

24 Kratz, C.R. Some determinants of care of patients with stroke who were nursed in their own homes. (A study of 30 patients notified to the district nursing service in a large industrial town.) Journal of Advanced Nursing, 1 (1), Jan 1976, 89-96.

25 Moody, A. Specialised care. 1. Care of the stroke patient. Nursing Mirror, 145, 1 Sep 1977, Nursing care supplement, series 6, i-iv.

26 Muldoon, L. Hillcrest Hospital Stroke Unit. (Toronto.) Hospital Administration in Canada, 18 (6), Jun 1976, 62-64.

27 Mulley, G. Stroke: a handbook for the patient's family. Chest, Heart and Stroke Association, 1978.

28 Mulley, G. and Arie, T. Treating stroke: home or hospital? (Literature review.) British Medical Journal, 2, 11 Nov 1978, 1321-1322.

29 O'Brien, M.T. and Pallett, P.J. Total care of the stroke patient. Boston: Little, Brown and Co., 1978. (For nurses.)

30 Pallant, C. Acute nursing care in the stroke unit. (Sunnybrook Medical Centre, Toronto.) Canadian Nurse, 72 (2), Feb 1976, 18-20.

31 Parry, A. and Eales, C. Hemiplegia. Nursing Times 72.
1. The neurophysiology of normal movement. 14 Oct 1976, 1590-1592.

2. Damage to nervous pathways. 21 Oct 1976, 1640-1641.
3. Handling the early stroke patient at home and in the ward. 28 Oct 1976, 1680-1683.
4. The ambulant stroke patient at home and in the ward. 4 Nov 1976, 1726-1730.
5. The geriatric stroke patient at home and in the ward. 11 Nov 1976, 1763-1765.

32 Poole, H. Nursing care study. Cerebro-vascular accident. (Hospital care of elderly lady with glioma.) Nursing Times, 74, 24 Aug 1978, 1407-1408.

33 Rodiques, A. Nursing care study. Cerebrovascular accident. Nursing Mirror, 72, 25 Nov 1976, 1838-1840.

34 Sarno, J.E. and Sarno, M.T. Stroke: a guide for patients and their families. Rev.ed. New York: McGraw-Hill, 1979.

35 Schwartzman, S.T. Anxiety and depression in the stroke patient: a nursing challenge. Journal of Psychiatric Nursing and Mental Health Services, 14 (7), Jul 1976, 13-17.

36 Smith, G.W. Care of the patient with a stroke: a handbook for the patient's family and the nurse. 2nd ed. New York: Springer, 1976.

37 Stillman, M.J. Experiences in clinical problem solving. Stroke! Pulling your patient through the acute phase. How to care for a recovering patient. RN Magazine, 42 (10), Oct 1979, 55-60, 93, 96; (11), Nov 1979, 49-56, 94.

38 Storey, P. Depression after stroke. Chest, Heart and Stroke Journal, 1 (1), Spring 1976, 14-17.

39 Wessex Regional Library and Information Service Stroke (A bibliography.) Compiled by Robert Gann. Southampton: Wessex RLIS, 1978.

40 Wilmot, W.M. Cerebral vascular accidents and altered consciousness. Nursing, 9, Jan 1980, 390-392.

e STROKE: REHABILITATION

1 Andrews, K. and Stewart, J. Stroke recovery: he can but does he? (Less good performance of patient at home than in day hospital shows need to train chief carer and to have more home-orientated rehabilitation.) Rheumatology and Rehabilitation, 18 (1), Feb 1979, 43-48.

2 Anwar, M. Hope unfulfilled: non-neurological factors affecting stroke rehabilitation. Nursing Mirror, 146, 1 Jun 1978, 14-16.

3 Bobath, B. Treatment of adult hemiplegia. Physiotherapy, 63 (10), Oct 1977, 310-313.

4 Booker, C. Striking back at strokes. (Rehabilitation.) Journal of Community Nursing, 4 (6), Dec 1980, 4-6.

5 Brocklehurst, J.C. and others How much physical therapy for patients with stroke? (Survey of the use of physiotherapy, occupational therapy and speech therapy.) British Medical Journal, 1, 20 May 1978, 1307-1310.

6 Capildoe, R. and others Social work diagram. (Diagram showing how patients are supported by family and friends which was used as a follow-up study of patients with strokes and which could be incorporated in medical case records.) British Medical Journal, 1, 17 Jan 1976, 143-144.

7 Chest, Heart and Stroke Association Stroke clubs: a modern concept in rehabilitation. (Conference papers.) Chest, Heart and Stroke Journal, 1 (1), Spring 1976, 25-43; 2 (2), Summer 1977, 22-41.

8 Ciuca, R. and others Active range-of-motion exercises: a handbook. (For stroke patients, with detailed photographs.) Nursing, 8 (8), Aug 1978, 45-49.

9 Community Outlook How you can help. (Aids and hints for stroke patients, with list of sources of information and films on p.351.) Nursing Times, 74, 9 Nov 1978, Community Outlook, 340-341, 351.

10 Evans, C.D. How to reduce severe handicap after stroke. (Rehabilitation techniques.) Geriatric Medicine, 10 (2), Feb 1980, 77-78.

11 Graham, L. Stroke rehabilitation—a creative process. Canadian Nurse, 72 (2), Feb 1976, 22-25.

12 Hawker, M. Return to mobility: exercises for stroke patients. Chest, Heart and Stroke Association, 1978.

13 Isaacs, B. Stroke research and the physiotherapist. (Problems of research into rehabilitation after stroke.) Physiotherapy, 63 (11), Nov 1977, 366-368.

14 Johnstone, M. Restoration of motor function in the stroke patient: a physiotherapist's approach. Churchill Livingstone, 1978.

15 Johnstone, M. The stroke patient: principles of rehabilitation. Churchill Livingstone, 1976. (For nurses and others.)

16 Kester, R. Stroke group report. (Report of activities of occupational therapy stroke treatment group in Ruislip.) British Journal of Occupational Therapy, 43 (12), Dec 1980, 403-405.

17 Kratz, C.R. Care of the long-term sick in the community: particularly patients with stroke. Churchill Livingstone, 1978.

18 Lynn, P.A. and others Research in rehabilitation of stroke patients: a team approach at Bristol University and the Avon Stroke Research Unit, Frenchay Hospital. Chest, Heart and Stroke Journal, 3 (3), Autumn 1978, 25-31.

19 McLaren, M. Community nursing care study. Come on, Jiminy Cricket. (Rehabilitation of elderly lady following stroke.) Nursing Times, 73, 15 Sep 1977, 1433-1435.

20 Manuel, M. Counselling: doing it the family way. (Course at Leeds General Infirmary for stroke patients' relatives by members of the rehabilitation team.) Nursing Mirror, 149, 21 Jun 1979, 28-29, 34.

21 Mulhall, D.J. Stroke rehabilitation: counselling relatives towards a helping relationship. (Contains statistics.) Geriatric Medicine, 10 (4), Apr 1980, 39-40, 42.

22 Nursing Mirror Stroke clubs fill a need. (Report of conference.) Nursing Mirror, 142 (12), 18 Mar 1976, 35.

23 Partridge, C. and Wright, B. Helping patients to help themselves. 1. Patients with stroke. (Advice on rehabilitation in the home for district nurses.) Nursing Mirror, 146, 8 Jun 1978, 42-44.

24 Patrick, M.K. What nurses can do in stroke rehabilitation. (With diagrams showing positioning and moving of patient.) Journal of Community Nursing, 1 (11), May 1978, 4-6.

25 Poole, A.E. A stroke rehabilitation service. (Home care service in the Hove and Portslade part of the Brighton Health District.) Nursing Times, 72, 16 Dec 1976, 1977-1979.

26 Sheikh, K. and others Methods and problems of a stroke rehabilitation trial. (At Northwick Park Hospital.) British Journal of Occupational Therapy, 41 (8), Aug 1978, 262-265.

27 Smith, D.S. and others The Northwick Park Hospital stroke rehabilitation study. Rheumatology and Rehabilitation, 15 (3), Aug 1976, 163-166.

28 Smith, M.E. and others An assessment unit for measuring the outcome of stroke rehabilitation. (Royal Victoria Hospital, Edinburgh.) British Journal of Occupational Therapy, 40 (3), Mar 1977, 51-53.

29 Stickland, E. How can you help? (Detailed advice for district nurses on rehabilitation of stroke patients.) Nursing Times, 74, 9 Nov 1978, Community Outlook, 327, 329.

30 Turnbull, E.N. A male stroke patient's dressing problem. (Trouser braces to overcome problems from hemiplegia.) British Journal of Occupational Therapy, 40 (10), Oct 1977, 248-249.

31 Walton, B. Approaches to stroke management in the community. British Journal of Occupational Therapy, 41 (7), Jul 1978, 219-220.

32 Walton, M. and others How dependent are stroke patients? (Development of Nursing Dependency Index in stroke rehabilitation study in Edinburgh.) Nursing Mirror, 147, 5 Oct 1978, 56-58.

33 Wood, D.J. Rehabilitation and the DN. (Scheme using three rehabilitation district nurses who are mainly concerned with new stroke patients nursed at home.) Journal of Community Nursing, 1 (6), Dec 1977, 17.

34 Wright, W.B. and Robson, P. Crisis procedure for stroke at home. (Recommended care including role of district nurse.) Lancet, 2, 2 Aug 1980, 249-250.

f STROKE: SPEECH THERAPY

1 Carbary, L.J. Aiding the patient with aphasia. Nursing Care, 9 (1), Jan 1976, 22-24.

2 Christo, S. A nursing approach to adult aphasia. Canadian Nurse, 74 (8), Sep 1978, 34-39.

3 Codene, L. Aphasia. A nurse's guide to communicating with aphasics. Canadian Nurse, 72 (2), Feb 1976, 21.

4 Ford, M.H. Communicating with the aphasic patient. Journal of Practical Nursing, 28 (4), Apr 1978, 20-21.

5 Griffith, V.E. Observations on patients dysphasic after stroke. (Based on 14 year's experience.) British Medical Journal, 281, 13 Dec 1980, 1608-1609.

6 Griffith, V.E. and Miller, C.L. Volunteer stroke scheme for dysphasic patients with stroke. (Report of first five years of scheme started in 1973 by the Chest and Heart Association.) British Medical Journal, 281, 13 Dec 1980, 1605-1607.

7 Hopkins, A. The need for speech therapy for dysphasia following stroke. Health Trends, 7 (3), Aug 1975, 58-60.

8 Isted, C.R. Learning to speak again after a stroke. King Edward's Hospital Fund for London, 1979.

9 Law, D. Speech therapy. (For stroke victims.) Nursing Times, 74, 9 Nov 1978, Community Outlook, 333, 335.

10 Lesser, R. and Watt, M. Untrained community help in the rehabilitation of stroke sufferers with language disorder. (The Newcastle Speech-After-Stroke Project using untrained helpers to set up community clubs and home visiting.) British Medical Journal, 2, 14 Oct 1978, 1045-1048.

11 Leutenegger, R.R. Patient care and rehabilitation of communication-impaired adults. Springfield: Thomas, 1975.

12 Meikle, M. and others Comparative trial of volunteer and professional treatments of dysphasia after stroke. (Progress of two groups of patients compared.) British Medical Journal, 2, 14 Jul 1979, 87-89.

13 Piotrowski, M.M. Aphasia: providing better nursing care. Nursing Clinics of North America, 13 (3), Sep 1978, 543-554.

14 Wechsler, E.M. The problems of initiating speech therapy for the stroke patient in hospital. Chest, Heart and Stroke Journal, 2 (3), Aug 1977, 38-43.

95 OPHTHALMOLOGY

a GENERAL AND DISORDERS

1 Abramowich, F.E. A study of some ophthalmic patients' knowledge and understanding of the information given concerning their disease. MSc thesis, University of Manchester, Department of Nursing, Oct 1979.

2 Bankes, J.L.K. Modern ophthalmic precision surgery. NATNews, 11 (6), Aug 1974, 10-11.

3 Bartholomew, R.S. A survey on glaucoma in Africa. Nursing Times, 72, 8 Apr 1976, 525-526.

4 Boyd-Monk, H. Cataract surgery. (New methods and nursing care.) Nursing, 77 7 (6), Jun 1977, 56-61.

5 Boyd-Monk, H. Screening for glaucoma. (With detailed advice on use of Schiötz tonometer.) Nursing (U.S.), 9 (8), Aug 1979, 42-45.

6 Buisseret, P. The six senses. 1. Sight.

Nursing Mirror, 146, 12 Jan 1978, Supplement, i-iv.

7 **Fletcher, D.** An unexpected discovery. (Use of intraocular lens implants after cataract extraction.) Nursing Mirror, 150, 17 Apr 1980, 34-35.

8 **Gardiner, P.A.** ABC of ophthalmology. Ophthalmic services in the NHS. British Medical Journal, 1, 27 Jan 1979, 248-250.

9 **Garston, J.B.** Retinal detachment. Nursing Times, 72, 4 Mar 1976, 340-341; 11 Mar 1976, 383-385; 18 Mar 1976, 413-415.

10 **Gilkes, M.** Let there be light. (The need for preventive measures in ophthalmology by the first community ophthalmologist.) Queen's Nursing Journal, 19 (13), Apr 1977, 350, 358.

11 **Hammond, E.A. and Begley, P.K.** Screening for glaucoma: a comparison of ophthalmoscopy and tonometry. Nursing Research, 28 (6), Nov/Dec 1979, 371-372.

12 **Hunter, P.J.L.** Babies' eyes. Midwife, Health Visitor and Community Nurse, 13 (1), Jan 1977, 14-17.

13 **Ingram, R.M. and Traynar, P.M.** Five-and-a-half day ophthalmic ward. British Medical Journal, 1, 21 Feb 1976, 445-446.

14 **Kanski, J.J.** Intra-ocular infection. Nursing Times, 72, 9 Sep 1976, 1395.

15 **King, A.** Cataract surgery in village India. Nursing Times, 72, 8 Apr 1976, 527-529.

16 **Kwitko, M.L.** New lenses for old: a promising method of treating cataracts. (Intraocular lens implantation.) Canadian Nurse, 71 (11), Nov 1975, 34-38.

17 **Marsh, R.J.** Ophthalmic herpes zoster. Nursing Times, 75, 16 Aug 1979, 1405-1407.

18 **Perrin, E.D.** Laser therapy for diabetic retinopathy. American Journal of Nursing, 80 (4), Apr 1980, 664-665.

19 **Plant, R. and Crome, D.** A new ophthalmic prescription sheet. (Devised at St. Paul's Eye Hospital, Liverpool.) Nursing Times, 76, 7 Feb 1980, 238-239.

20 **Roberts, A.** Fluids of the eye. (Anatomy and pathology.) Nursing Times, 73, 18 Aug 1977, Body fluids, 9-12.

21 **Roberts, A.** Systems of life. Nos.40-42. Vision. 1-3. (3. Eyelids and their disorders.) Nursing Times, 74, 6 Apr 1978, (4); 4 May 1978, (4); 15 Jun 1978, (4).

22 **Travers, J.P.** Primary open angle glaucoma. Nursing Times, 74, 19 Jan 1978, 103-104.

23 **Treharne, J.D.** Trachoma. Nursing Times, 72, 8 Apr 1976, 523-525.

24 **Treplin, M.C.W. and Arnott, E.J.** Use of the microscope in ophthalmics: seeing eye to eye. Nursing Mirror, 147, 2 Nov 1978, 30-33.

25 **Werb, A.** Corneal grafting. Nursing Times, 73, 2 Jun 1977, 822-823.

b NURSING

1 **Boyd-Monk, H.** Helping the corneal transplant patient to see again. (Postoperative nursing care.) Nursing, 8 (2), Feb 1978, 47-50.

2 **Edwards, A.** Nursing in an eye department. New Zealand Nursing Journal, 69 (5), May 1976, 6-8.

3 **Gould, H.** How to remove contact lenses from comatose patients. American Journal of Nursing, 76 (9), Sep 1976, 1483-1485.

4 **Ingram, D.V.** Eyes and the nurse. (Work of the ophthalmic nurse in the community.) Queen's Nursing Journal, 19 (13), Apr 1977, 351-352.

5 **Kershaw, J.E.M.** The nursing care of ophthalmic patients in general wards. Nursing Times, 76, 7 Feb 1980, 234-237.

6 **Kidger, J.** Home visiting scheme for ophthalmic patients. (Postoperative visits in Sheffield.) Nursing Times, 73, 4 Aug 1977, 1212-1214.

7 **Laing, J.M.** Nursing care study. Penetrating keratoplasty. (Corneal graft.) Nursing Mirror, 146, 22 Jun 1978, 30-31.

8 **Macfadyen, J.S.** Caring for the patient with a primary retinal detachment. American Journal of Nursing, 80 (5), May 1980, 920-921.

9 **Mitchell, R.G.** Nursing care study. An accident on the golf course. (Loss of vision in one eye.) Nursing Times, 76, 19 Jun 1980, 1088-1090.

10 **Rikkhi, S.J.** Nursing care study. Glaucoma. (In 86-year-old woman.) Nursing Times, 74, 10 Aug 1978, 1325-1326.

11 **Rooke, F.C.E. and others** Ophthalmic nursing: its practice and management. Edinburgh: Churchill Livingstone, 1980.

12 **Shepherd, B.** Bilateral senile cataracts. (A case study.) NATNews, 13 (7), Sep 1976, 25, 27-29.

13 **Short, J.M.** Nursing care study. Enucleation of the eye. Nursing Times, 74, 2 Feb 1978, 184-185.

14 **Smith, J.** Focusing your care for the patient with an intraocular lens implant. RN Magazine, 41 (3), Mar 1978, 46-50.

15 **Smith, J.S.** Nursing care study. Oculomucocutaneous syndrome associated with the administration of practolol. Nursing Times, 72, 23 Sep 1976, 1472-1474.

16 **Thomson, C.E.B.** Nursing care study. Marfan's syndrome. Nursing Times, 72 (3), 22 Jan 1976, 94-97.

17 **Wilson, P.** Modern ophthalmic nursing. Arnold, 1976.

18 **Wood, C.** Nursing care study. Cataract extraction. Nursing Times, 74, 15 Jun 1978, 999-1006.

c BLINDNESS AND PARTIAL SIGHT

1 **Abel, R.A.** An investigation into some aspects of visual handicap. HMSO, 1976. (Statistical and research report series, no.14.)

2 **Chapman, E.K.** Visually handicapped children and young people. Routledge and Kegan Paul, 1978.

3 **Community Outlook** Low-vision aids. Nursing Times, 73, 13 Oct 1977, Community Outlook, 85-86.

4 **Cullinan, T.** Visually disabled people at home. (National survey showing that many elderly people are not registered as blind or partially sighted and so are not receiving appropriate help.) Health Trends, 4 (10), Nov 1978, 90-92.

5 **Cullinan, T.R. and others** Visual disability and home lighting. (Survey of elderly people suggests that better lighting would reduce the prevalence of visual disability.) Lancet, 1, 24 Mar 1979, 642-644.

6 **Cuncliffe, W.** Blindness—problems of the adolescent in rehabilitation. Rehabilitation, 96, Jan/Mar 1976, 5-7.

7 **Department of Health and Social Security** Blindness and partial sight in England 1969-1976. HMSO, 1979. (Reports on public health and medical subjects; 129.)

8 **Disabled Living Foundation** The elderly person with failing vision: a report to the DHSS, May 1979. The Foundation, 1979.

9 **Doner, F.** Blindness can be prevented. Canadian Nurse, 72 (1), Jan 1976, 27-29.

10 **Ford, M. and Heshel, T.** In touch: aids and services for blind and partially sighted people. Revised ed. British Broadcasting Corporation, 1977.

11 **Fraiberg, S.** Insights from the blind. Souvenir Press, 1977. (Human horizons series.)

12 **Gardiner, P.A.** ABC of ophthalmology. Visual difficulty in old age. British Medical Journal, 1, 13 Jan 1979, 105-106.

13 **Gardiner, P.A.** Failing vision in the elderly. (Symposium on care of the elderly.) Nursing Mirror, 145, 3 Nov 1977, 29-30.

14 **Garland, C.W.** Technical development and its part in the rehabilitation of the blind. Rehabilitation, 96, Jan/Mar 1976, 8-11.

15 **Hanson, J.** An outline of services for the blind. Queen's Nursing Journal, 19 (13), Apr 1977, 263-264.

16 **Hinds, R.** The visually handicapped child. Health Visitor, 53 (8), Aug 1980, 333-334.

17 **Kay, L. and Strelow, E.** (The blind baby controversy.) Blind babies need specially designed aids. (Reply to Tom Bower.) New Scientist, 74, 23 Jun 1977, 709-712.

18 **Klemz, A.** Blindness and partial sight: a guide for social workers and others concerned with the care and rehabilitation of the visually handicapped. Cambridge: Woodhead-Faulkner, 1977.

19 **Lovelace, B.M.** The blind child in the hospital. AORN Journal, 31 (2), Feb 1980, 256, 258, 260, 262, 264, 266, 268, 270.

20 **Neu, C.** Coping with newly diagnosed

blindness. American Journal of Nursing, 75 (12), Dec 1975, 2161-2163.

21 Pugh, R. Development in sight. (How visual handicap affects development of children.) Nursing Mirror, 151, 3 Jul 1980, 30-32.

22 Silver, J. and Thomsitt, J. Low-vision services in the United Kingdom. Health Trends, 4 (9), Nov 1977, 73-75.

23 Smith, V. and Keen, J. editors Visual handicap in children. Heinemann Medical for Spastics International Medical Publications, 1979. (Clinics in developmental medicine; 73.)

24 Spastics Society Medical Education and Information Unit Working Party on Vision in Childhood Meeting the needs of family with visually handicapped babies and young children: discussion paper. The Society, 1976.

25 Stewart, L.M. and Dawson, D.F. Blind client—sighted therapist: the interface. (Problems encountered in working with blind psychiatric patients.) Journal of Psychiatric Nursing, 17 (11), Nov 1979, 31-35.

26 Vyas, R.T. Blindness in the Third World. Nursing Journal of India, 47 (4), Apr 1976, 83-84.

27 WHO Chronicle The prevention of blindness. WHO Chronicle, 30 (10), Oct 1976, 391-397.

28 World Health Issue on blindness. World Health, Feb/Mar 1976, 3-43.

29 World Health Organization Guidelines for programmes for the prevention of blindness. Geneva: WHO, 1979.

30 World Health Organization Methods of assessment of avoidable blindness. Geneva: WHO, 1980.

d VISION DISORDERS

1 Boyd-Monk, H. Taking a closer look at contact lenses. Nursing, 8 (10), Oct 1978, 38-43.

2 British Medical Journal Screening children for visual defects. British Medical Journal, 2, 3 Sep 1977, 594-595.

3 Cameron, J.H. and Cameron, M. Visual screening of pre-school children. (Scheme in Ayrshire.) British Medical Journal, 2, 16 Dec 1978, 1693-1694.

4 Dobinson, P. The orthoptist at work. (Diagnosing and treating squints.) Nursing Times, 74, 20 Apr 1978, 680-682.

5 Dowler, P. The role of the orthoptist. Queen's Nursing Journal, 19 (13), Apr 1977, 355-357.

6 Gardiner, P.A. Visual problems in later life. Queen's Nursing Journal, 19 (13), Apr 1977, 359-360.

7 Gilkes, M.J. Eyes run on light. (Need for adequate lighting in order to see properly.) British Medical Journal, 1, 23 Jun 1979, 1681-1683.

8 Hamilton, M. Colour blindness. (Summary of a talk given by J.T. Edmunson, ophthalmic tutor, Wolverhampton Eye Infirmary.) Occupational Health, 28 (9), Sep 1976, 422-423.

9 McAllister, J. Displaced crystalline lens: this crystal ball must focus to form images. (Includes physiology of focusing.) Nursing Mirror, 147, 28 Dec 1978, 24-26.

10 MacLellan, A.V. and Harker, P. Mobile orthoptic service for primary screening of visual disorder in young children. (Oxfordshire.) British Medical Journal, 1, 14 Apr 1979, 994-995.

11 Mein, J. and Clayton, J. The profession of orthoptics. Health Services Manpower Review, 6 (1), Feb 1980, 22-25.

12 Peckham, C.S. and others Vision screening of adolescents and their use of glasses. (Data from National Child Development Study.) British Medical Journal, 1, 28 Apr 1979, 1111-1113.

13 Ridgway, A.E.A. Spontaneous displacement of the crystalline lens. Nursing Times, 73, 20 Jan 1977, 86-88.

14 Roberts, A. Systems of life. No.43. Vision—4. (Disorders of the eye, threats to sight including tropical eye diseases and blindness.) Nursing Times, 74, 6 Jul 1978, (4).

15 Rooney, M. Children with strabismus. Canadian Nurse, 74 (1), Jan 1978, 24-27.

16 Ross, D. Vision and the artist. (How visual defects may have affected some great painters.) Occupational Health, 32 (2), Feb 1980, 68-73.

17 Ruben, M. A nurse's guide to contact lenses. Nursing Mirror, 147, 31 Aug 1978, 13-15.

18 Ruben, M. The pros and cons of hard and soft contact lenses. Nursing Times, 72, 1 Jul 1976, 1018-1020.

19 Taylor, D. Aspects of strabismus in children. Nursing Times, 72, 22 Apr 1976, 610-612.

20 Voke, J. Colour vision. Nursing Times 76. Colour vision defects: their industrial and occupational significance. 7 Feb 1980, 240-243; Seeing is not always believing. 14 Feb 1980, 48-50.
Acting on impulse. (Organisation of the visual pathway.) 21 Feb 1980, 35-37.

21 Voke, J. Defective colour vision and education. (Results of a survey in England and Wales to evaluate policies of colour vision testing among school children.) Nursing Times, 74, 27 Jul 1978, 1238-1241.

22 Voke, J. Ocular entoptic phenomenon: a case of spots before the eyes. Nursing Mirror, 148, 1 Mar 1979, 30-32.

23 Woodward, E.G. Role of the ophthalmic optician in community eye care. Queen's Nursing Journal, 19 (13), Apr 1977, 260-262.

24 Yapp, J.M. Squint—an acute disease. Health Visitor, 50 (2), 1977, 37-38.

25 Zerbini, A. and Fenton, P. A modified vision screener. A school nurse redesigned the Keystone Vision Screener to make it portable. Nursing Times, 75, 24 May 1979, 672-673.

e EYE INJURIES AND OCCUPATIONAL HEALTH

1 McMillan, G.H.G. Case history. A cautionary tale. (Importance of nurse recognising possibility of presence of intraocular foreign body.) Occupational Health, 29 (8), Aug 1977, 340-341.

2 McMillan, G.H.G. Occupational eye injuries—the changing pattern. (With reference to historical incidents, eye conditions and current Eye Protection Regulations.) Journal of the Society of Occupational Medicine, 28 (2), Apr 1978, 39-43.

3 McMillan, G.H.G. Occupational eye injuries—treatment in a nurse-based service. (Based on experience in the ship repair industry.) Occupational Health, 29 (6), Jun 1977, 235-240.

4 McMillan, G.H.G. Protecting eyes in shipyards. Occupational Safety and Health, 7 (12), Dec 1977, 4-6.

5 McMillan, G.H.G. The selection of protective measures against eye injuries. Journal of the Society of Occupational Medicine, 28 (2), Apr 1978, 44-50.

6 Michell, D.R. Treatment of eye injuries. Nursing Mirror, 146, 6 Apr, 17-18.

7 Mitchell, J.A. and McConnell, E.M.J. Keeping eyes protected. Occupational Health, 31 (10), Oct 1979, 463-465.

8 Occupational Health Occupational first aid. No.1. Eyes. Occupational Health, 30 (11), Nov 1978, Supplement, (4).

9 Oshirak, P.N. The nursing role in treating occupational ocular trauma. Occupational Health Nursing, 26 (7), Jul 1978, 20-22.

10 Ross, D.S. Colour vision testing in industry—a survey. (Request for completion of questionnaire, with reference to existing research.) Occupational Health, 30 (10), Oct 1978, 479-481.

11 Ross, D.S. Safety hazard from colour vision defect. (Case history of car worker's colour vision defect and review of the literature.) Occupational Health, 29 (11), Nov 1977, 483-488.

12 Voke, J. Colour bars of an occupational kind. (Employment problems of people with defective colour vision.) Occupational Safety and Health, 9 (2), Feb 1979, 10-12.

13 Voke, J. Colour vision defects: their industrial and occupational significance. Nursing Times, 76, 7 Feb 1980, 240-243.

14 Voke, J. Colour vision defects—occupational significance and testing requirements. Journal of the Society of Occupational Medicine, 28 (2), Apr 1978, 51-56.

96 RENAL SYSTEM

a GENERAL

1 Anderton, J.L. and others, editors Living with renal failure: proceedings of a multi-disciplinary symposium... Stirling, 7-8 Jul 1977. Lancaster: MTP, 1978.

2 Andreou, A. Nursing care study. Priapism. Nursing Times, 72, 21 Oct 1976, 1631-1634.

3 British Medical Journal Selection of patients

for dialysis and transplantation. British Medical Journal, 2, 25 Nov 1978, 1449-1450.

4 **Cameron, J.S. and others** Nephrology for nurses: a modern approach to the kidney. 2nd ed. Heinemann, 1976.

5 **Evans, D.B.** Diseases of the urinary system. Management of chronic renal failure by dialysis and transplantation. British Medical Journal, 1, 18 Jun 1977, 1585-1588.

6 **Gittes, R.R.S.** Retrograde renal and ureteral brush biopsy. American Journal of Nursing, 78 (3), Mar 1978, 410-412.

7 **Greenfield, M.A.M.** Clinical nutrition in current practice. Dietary treatment of renal disease. Journal of Human Nutrition, 31 (2), Apr 1977, 127-133.

8 **Hardy, A.M.** The problems of staffing renal units. (Report of survey of 16 hospitals.) Nursing Times, 76, 17 Jan 1980, 129-130.

9 **Henari, F.Z. and others** Survival in 200 patients treated by haemodialysis and renal transplantation. (Survey at Charing Cross Hospital.) British Medical Journal, 1977, 1, 12 Feb 1977, 409-412.

10 **Herbert, B. and Winder, E.** Chronic renal failure. Nursing Mirror, 143, 1 Jul 1976, Nursing care supplement, 7, i-iv.

11 **Kagan, L.W.** Renal disease: a manual of patient care. New York: McGraw-Hill, 1979.

12 **Knapp, M.S.** Evaluating the treatment of renal failure by dialysis and transplantation. (Collection and analysis of data.) Lancet, 2, 19 Nov 1977, 1068-1070.

13 **Lancaster, L.E. editor** The patient with end stage renal disease. New York: Wiley, 1979.

14 **Mitchell, J.P.** The use and care of cystoscopes. NATNews, 17 (8), Aug 1980, 16, 28.

15 **Nicholls, A.J. and others** Integrated dialysis and renal transplantation: small is beautiful. (Aberdeen Renal Unit.) British Medical Journal, 280, 21 Jun 1980, 1516-1517.

16 **Nursing Times** X-rays in focus. The IVP in renal disease. Nursing Times, 71, 19 May 1977, Post Basic, 17-20.

17 **Office of Health Economics** Renal failure: a priority in health? OHE, 1978. (Studies of current health problems, no.62.)

18 **Parkin, D.M.** Chronic renal failure: the economics of treatment. Community Health, 9 (3), Feb 1978, 134-141.

19 **Parsons, V. and Lock, P.** Focus: current issues in medical ethics. Triage and the patient with renal failure. Journal of Medical Ethics, 6 (4), Dec 1980, 173-176.

20 **Pickering, L. and Robbins, D.** Fluid, electrolyte, and acid-base balance in the renal patient. (Including a section on complications following a kidney transplant.) Nursing Clinics of North America, 15 (3), Sep 1980, 577-592.

21 **Pincherle, G.** Services for patients with chronic renal failure in England and Wales. Health Trends, 9 (2), May 1977, 41-44.

22 **Rees, G.J.G.** Chronic renal failure. Renal bone disease. Nursing Times, 72, 17 Jun 1976, 929-931.

23 **Roberts, A.** Body fluids. 17. Peritoneal fluid. (Includes ascites and peritoneal dialysis.) Nursing Times, 74, 19 Oct 1978, Body fluids, 65-68.

24 **Roberts, A.** Systems of life. No.23. UG-1 Kidney. Nursing Times, 72, 4 Nov 1976, (4).

25 **Talf, B.** Diet therapy in renal failure. Journal of Practical Nursing, 26 (2), Feb 1976, 23-25.

26 **Ward, J.P. and Wickham, J.E.** Hypothermia in kidney surgery. Nursing Times, 72, 22 Jan 1976, 91-93.

27 **Wing, A.J.** Diseases of the urinary system. Prospects for the treatment of renal diseases. (Including haemodialysis and transplantation.) British Medical Journal, 2, 1 Oct 1977, 881-884.

28 **Wood, I.T. and others** A flexible model for planning facilities for patients with end-stage renal failure. (Study in North-west Region.) British Medical Journal, 281, 30 Aug 1980, 575-577.

b NURSING: GENERAL

1 **Baer, C.L.** The growth and development of nephrology nursing practice. Heart Lung, 8 (5), Sep/Oct 1979, 896-902.

2 **Bruce, G.L. and others** Implementation of ANA's quality assurance program for clients with end-stage renal disease. Advances in Nursing Science, 2 (2), Jan 1980, 79-95.

3 **Brundage, D.J.** Nursing management of renal problems. St. Louis: Mosby, 1976. 2nd ed. 1980.

4 **Finch, M.** Intensive care—9. Management of acute renal failure. Nursing Times, 74, 13 Apr 1978, 631.

5 **Harvey, A.** Blunt renal trauma. (Surgery and postoperative care of two patients.) Nursing Times, 75, 11 Oct 1979, 1756-1758.

6 **Hekelman, F.P. and Ostendarp, C.A. editors** Nephrology nursing: perspectives of care. New York: McGraw-Hill, 1979.

7 **Jackle, M. and Rasmussen, C.** Renal problems: a critical care nursing focus. Prentice-Hall, 1980. (A programmed text.)

8 **JOINT Board of Clinical Nursing Studies. 8.** Renal and urological nursing. Nursing Mirror, 143 (12), 16 Sep 1976, Nursing care supplement, series 2, i-iv.

9 **Mills, L.** Nursing care study. Dorothy and Rodney. Treatment of mother and son for renal failure. Nursing Times, 72, 15 Jan 1976, 52-56.

10 **National Association of Practical Nurse Education and Service** End stage kidney disease: different approaches. (Annual conference.) Journal of Practical Nursing, 26 (7), Jul 1976, 14-15.

11 **Uldall, R.** Renal nursing. 2nd ed. Blackwell, 1977.

c RENAL DIALYSIS

1 **Anger, D. and Anger, D.W.** Dialysis ambivalence: a matter of life and death. (Problems of coping with dialysis patients who would prefer to die.) American Journal of Nursing, 76 (2), Feb 1976, 276-277.

2 **British Medical Journal** Complications of vascular access devices used for repeated haemodialysis. British Medical Journal, 2, 26 Nov 1977, 1373-1374.

3 **Brown, M.** Some problems of staff stress in dialysis-transplantation units. Contained in: Anderton, J.L. and others, editors Living with renal failure... Lancaster: MTP, 1978. Section 4, part 15, 223-233.

4 **Canadian Nurse** A question of balance: the effects of chronic renal failure and long term dialysis. Part 1. Canadian Nurse, 73 (3), Mar 1977, 19-24.

5 **Davison, A.M. editor** Dialysis review. Pitman, 1978.

6 **European Dialysis and Transplant Association. Registration Committee** Dialysis dementia in Europe. (Survey.) Lancet, 2, 12 Jul 1980, 190-192.

7 **Frost, T.H. editor** Technical aspects of renal dialysis. Pitman, 1978.

8 **Gokal, R. and others** Continuous ambulatory peritoneal dialysis: one year's experience in a UK dialysis unit. (Royal Victoria Infirmary, Newcastle.) British Medical Journal, 281, 16 Aug 1980, 474-477.

9 **Gutch, C.F. and Stoner, M.H.** Review of haemodialysis for nurses and dialysis personnel. 2nd ed. St. Louis: Mosby, 1975. (Mosby's comprehensive review series.)

10 **Hooper, S.A.** The dialysis nurse's role in an interdisciplinary program. Journal of the American Association of Nephrology Nurses and Technicians, 6 (1), 1979, 20-24.

10 **Irwin, B.C.** Hemodialysis means vascular access...and the right kind of nursing care. (Care of arteriovenous shunts and fistulas.) Nursing (U.S.), 9 (10), Oct 1979, 49-53.

11 **Kerr, D.N.S.** Treatment of acute renal failure with artificial kidneys. (History from the 1950s.) British Medical Journal, 2, 28 Jul 1979, 250-252.

12 **Lavandero, R. and Davis, V.** Caring for the catheter carefully...before, during, and after peritoneal dialysis. Nursing (U.S.), 10 (11), Nov 1980, 17-23.

13 **Oag, D.** Chronic renal failure. The nurse's role in the dialysis unit. Nursing Times, 72, 17 Jun 1976, 926-928.

14 **Platzer, H.** Nursing care study. A patient suffering from chronic renal failure. (Care during haemodialysis by first year student nurse.) Nursing Times, 76, 31 Jan 1980, 191-195.

15 **Richard, C.J.** Application of heat pads to the abdomen during peritoneal dialysis in ten male subjects. (Research study.) Journal of the American Association of Nephrology Nurses and Technicians, 6 (4), 1979, 187-193.

16 **Sanderson, M.** Diet and dialysis. Nursing Times, 72, 11 Nov 1976, 1774-1775.

17 **Sausville, P.** Chronic renal failure: end stage renal disease. The nurse's role in

hemodialysis. Journal of Nursing Care, 13 (7), Jul 1980, 12-17.

18 Slaney, N. The bovine carotid artery graft and its use in the haemodialysis patient. NATNews, 14 (1), Jan 1977, 7-8.

19 Sorrels, A.J. Continuous ambulatory peritoneal dialysis. American Journal of Nursing, 79 (8), Aug 1979, 1400-1401.

20 Stenzel, K.H. and Leonard, M.O. End stage kidney disease current concepts in care. 1. Dialysis. Journal of Practical Nursing, 26 (2), Feb 1976, 16-20.

21 Taber, S.M. Rosenheim in 1977. (The case for updating the Rosenheim report which recommended procedures to prevent serum hepatitis in haemodialysis units.) Nursing Times, 73, 29 Sep 1977, 1502-1503.

22 Walls, J. Single needle dialysis. Nursing Times, 72, 30 Sep 1976, 1519-1520.

23 Winder, E. One organ medicine. (Role of nurse in multidisciplinary renal team in dialysis unit.) British Medical Journal, 2, 17 Dec 1977, 1585-1586.

24 Wing, A.J. and others Mortality and morbidity of reusing dialysers. A report by the registration committee of the European Dialysis and Transplant Association. British Medical Journal, 2, 23 Sep 1978, 853-855.

d CHILDREN

1 Chambers, T. When a child's kidneys fail. (Peritoneal dialysis in children with acute renal failure or following severe blood volume depletion in trauma or gastroenteritis.) Nursing Mirror, 149, 6 Dec 1979, 38-39.

2 Counahan, R. and others Presentation, management, complications, and outcome of acute renal failure in childhood: five years' experience. British Medical Journal, 1, 5 Mar 1977, 599-602.

3 Gilman, C.M. and others Psychosocial care of the child in renal failure. Journal of the American Association of Nephrology Nurses and Technicians, 6 (3), 1979, 143-148.

4 Lancet Dialysis and transplantation in young children. Lancet, 1, 7 Jan 1978, 26.

5 London Children's Home Dialysis Group Home haemodialysis in children. (Study to evaluate the growth and psychosocial adaption of children treated from Guy's Hospital and the Royal Free Hospital.) Lancet, 1, 29 Jan 1977, 242-246.

6 Mandleco, B. Nursing assessment of children undergoing kidney biopsy. Maternal-Child Nursing Journal, 5 (3), Fall 1976, 151-166.

7 Maternal-Child Nursing Journal Monograph 7. Orienting, resistive and adaptive responses of children undergoing hemodialysis for kidney failure. Maternal-Child Nursing Journal, 7 (4), Winter, 1978, 195-254.

8 Newton, A. Nursing care study. An infant with renal abnormality. (Retrograde pyelogram and nephrostomy in 22-month-old boy.) Nursing Times, 74, 21/28 Dec 1978, 2101-2103.

9 Pavitt, L. Chronic renal failure. Paediatric dialysis. (Home dialysis of patients from the Royal Free Hospital.) Nursing Times, 72, 17 Jun 1976, 936-938.

10 Precious, A. Nursing care study. Nephrotic syndrome in a child. Nursing Mirror, 147, 26 Oct 1978, 30-33.

11 Wheeler, D. Teaching home-dialysis for an eight-year-old boy. American Journal of Nursing, 77 (2), Feb 1977, 273-274.

12 Winder, E. Children on haemodialysis. (Includes statistics.) Nursing Times, 74, 7 Dec 1978, 2011-2014.

13 Winder, L. and Donovan, M. Nursing care study — renal failure: a father's kidney for two... (Care of adolescent patient on haemodialysis and after kidney transplant.) Nursing Mirror, 150, 3 Jan 1980, 37-39.

e PATIENT, FAMILY AND HOME DIALYSIS

1 Banks, I. Dialysis at home. (Patient's account.) Nursing Mirror, 144, 19 May 1977, 26.

2 British Association of Social Workers Social workers caring for patients with chronic renal failure. Birmingham: BASW, 1979.

3 British Medical Journal Quality of life in renal failure. (Review of studies.) British Medical Journal, 281, 12 Jul 1980, 97-98.

4 Denniston, D.J. and Burns, K.T. Home peritoneal dialysis. American Journal of Nursing, 80 (11), Nov 1980, 2022-2026.

5 Dimond, M. Social support and adaptations to chronic illness: the case of maintenance hemodialysis. (Social support was measured on three dimensions, family environment, level of spouse support and presence of a confidant.) Research in Nursing Health, 2 (3), Sep 1979, 101-108.

6 Flegle, J.M. Teaching self-dialysis to adults in a hospital. American Journal of Nursing, 77 (2), Feb 1977, 270-272.

7 Fowles, D.M. and Macdonald-Walker, E.M. Haemodialysis nursing in the community. (Project at Mossley Hill Hospital, Liverpool, employing district nurses.) Queen's Nursing Journal, 19 (7), Oct 1976, 189, 191.

8 Gabriel, R. A patient's guide to dialysis and transplantation. Lancaster: MTP, 1980.

9 Helwick, C.A. Understanding dialysis patients. (Their reactions to dialysis and their illness.) Journal of Nursing Care, 13 (4), Apr 1980, 12-14, 25.

10 Hickman, B.M. All about sex — despite dialysis. (Seminars for patients on maintenance haemodialysis.) American Journal of Nursing, 77 (4), Apr 1977, 606-607.

11 Hillman, R.L. and Walker, E.B. Minimal home (dialysis) conversions. (Adapting patients' homes to house dialysers.) Hospital and Health Services Review, 75 (9), Sep 1979, 308-311.

12 Iveson-Iveson, J. Living with renal failure. Report on a recent multidisciplinary symposium at Stirling University. (Problems faced by patients.) Nursing Mirror, 145, 13 Oct 1977, 8.

13 Knight, L. 'A very unnatural way of life' —

life on a kidney machine. (Psychological effects.) Mind Out, 34, May/Jun 1979, 9-10.

14 Laborde, J.M. Haemodialysis and renal transplantation: the family's response. (Psychosocial aspects.) Nursing Times, 76, 3 Jul 1980, 1170-1172.

15 Laborde, J.M. and Powers, M.J. Satisfaction with life for patients undergoing hemodialysis and patients suffering from osteoarthritis. Research in Nursing Health, 3 (1), Mar 1980, 19-24.

16 Livesley, W.J. Psychiatric disturbance and chronic haemodialysis. (Survey of patients attending renal unit at Royal Infirmary of Edinburgh.) British Medical Journal, 2, 4 Aug 1979, 306.

17 McGowan, M. Helping with home dialysis. (Role of primary health care team.) Community View, Dec 1979, 7-8.

18 Macniven, P.A.M. Home dialysis. (Artificial kidney unit at Withington Hospital which serves North West England.) Nursing Times, 72, 19 Aug 1976, 1286-1287.

19 Merker, J.F. and others Psychological adjustment to hemodialysis: a patient education videotape. Journal of the American Association of Nephrology Nurses and Technicians, 6 (3), 1979, 157-162.

20 O'Brien, M.E. Hemodialysis regimen compliance and social environment: a panel analysis. Nursing Research, 29 (4), Jul/Aug 1980, 250-255.

21 Platts, M.M. and others Composition of the domestic water supply and the incidence of fractures and encephalopathy in patients on home dialysis. British Medical Journal, 2, 10 Sep 1977, 657-660.

22 Voss, P. Chronic renal failure. Peter Voss talks to a doctor on home dialysis. Nursing Times, 72, 17 Jun 1976, 932-933.

23 Wash, M.G. Home dialysis: a family copes with a patient on a kidney machine. (By nurse who looked after his sister.) Nursing Times, 75, 15 Mar 1979, 449-452.

24 Watchous, S.M. and others The nurse educator and the adult dialysis patient. (Pilot study of patient teaching through programmed learning.) Nursing Forum, 19 (1), 1980, 68-84.

f TRANSPLANTATION

1 British Medical Journal Renal transplantation in the 1980s. British Medical Journal, 280, 23 Feb 1980, 503-504.

2 Campling, J. How many kidneys? (Availability of kidneys for transplantation.) New Society, 40, 7 Apr 1977, 19.

3 Carey, M.E. A child's struggle for independence following kidney transplantation. Maternal-Child Nursing Journal, 5 (1), Spring 1976, 45-54.

4 De Tornyay, R. Experiences in clinical problem solving. Pre- and post-op care of a kidney transplant patient: what you need to know. RN Magazine, 42 (4), Apr 1979, 55-63.

5 Department of Health and Social Security

Topics of our time; 2: kidney transplants and dialysis, by G. Pincherle. HMSO, 1979.

6 Fernando, O.N. and Adams, A. Renal transplantation. Nursing Times, 72, 14 Oct 1976, 1598-1600.

7 Golby, M. Twins and renal transplantation. (Account by surgeon of transplant operations on twin brothers.) Nursing Mirror, 145, 14 Jul 1977, 16-18.

8 Jones, K. Study documents effect of primary nursing on renal transplant patients. (Study to compare the effect of assigning one nurse to each patient compared with team nursing.) Hospitals, 49 (24), 16 Dec 1975, 85-86, 88-89.

9 Juliani, L. and Reamer, B. Kidney transplant: your role in aftercare. Nursing, 7 (10), Oct 1977, 46-53.

10 Kobrzycki, P. Renal transplant complications. What patients need to know to help them decide between dialysis and transplantation. American Journal of Nursing, 77 (4), Apr 1977, 641-643.

11 Lawler, M.K. An adolescent's behavioral responses to a second renal transplant. Maternal-Child Nursing Journal, 6 (1), Spring 1977, 51-63.

12 Mackenzie, C. A need to transplant new ideas into the body of ignorance. (The problems of kidney transplantation.) Health and Social Service Journal, 86, 11 Feb 1977, 240-241.

13 Masur, G. Renal transplant: your role in patient education. Journal of Practical Nursing, 30 (7), Jul 1980, 12-15, 43.

14 Moores, B. and others Public attitudes toward kidney transplantation. (Survey of 500 people interviewed by students from the University of Manchester Institute of Science and Technology.) British Medical Journal, 1, 13 Mar 1976, 629-631.

15 Morton, J.B. and Leonard, D.R.A. Cadaver nephrectomy: an operation on the donor's family. (Survey of relatives of cadaver kidney donors showing defects in system of obtaining permission.) British Medical Journal, 1, 27 Jan 1979, 239-241.

16 Nelson, B. A nursing approach to patients with long-term renal transplants. A practical application of nursing theory. (Using Orlando's definition of the nursing process.) Nursing Clinics of North America, 13 (1), Mar 1978, 157-169.

17 Riley, S.K. Nursing care study. Autotransplant of kidney for renal artery stenosis. Nursing Times, 73, 5 May 1977, 646-647.

18 Rosenberg, J.C. and others To give life to another. (Nurse's role in identifying potential kidney donors.) RN Magazine, 39 (1), Jan 1976, OR, 1, 2.

19 Sachs, B.L. Renal transplantation: a nursing perspective. Flushing: Medical Examination Publishing Co., 1977.

20 Sampson, D. RR nursing for kidney recipients. AORN Journal, 23 (2), Feb 1976, 191-198.

21 Stenzel, K.M. and Leonard, M.O. End stage kidney disease current concepts in care. 2. Transplantation. Journal of Practical Nursing, 26 (3), Mar 1976, 16-20, 39, 43.

22 Taber, S. Kidney donors: a long wait for a new kidney. The role of a transplant coordinator, a 24-hour-a-day job that could result in a dramatic increase in kidney donation. Nursing Mirror, 148, 10 May 1979, 32.

23 Taylor, J. Nursing care of twins following renal transplantation. Nursing Mirror, 145, 14 Jul 1977, 19-21.

24 Whittingham, E. Chronic renal failure. A personal view of renal transplantation. (Experiences of a doctor.) Nursing Times, 72, 17 Jun 1976, 934-936.

25 Wolf, Z.R. What patients awaiting kidney transplant want to know. American Journal of Nursing, 76 (1), Jan 1976, 92-94.

97 REPRODUCTIVE SYSTEM

a GYNAECOLOGY

1 Balfour, R.P. Operative management of vaginal prolapse. Nursing Times, 75, 7 Jun 1979, 973-974.

2 Barr, G. Laparoscopy: a multipurpose procedure. (Nurse's role in pre- and postoperative care.) Dimensions in Health Service, 53 (2), Feb 1976, 43-44.

3 Beazley, J.M. The prostaglandins. (Role in human reproduction.) Nursing Times, 72, 18 Nov 1976, 1800-1802.

4 Bevan, J. and Newton, J. Eight years' experience with a weekday gynaecological ward. (For day care or 'overnight stay' patients.) Lancet, 2, 21 Jul 1979, 137-139.

5 Chalmers, J.A. Uterine fibroids. Nursing Times, 72, 28 Oct 1976, 1672-1674.

6 Chaudhuri, G. Reproductive physiology. 1. Oxytocics. Midwife, Health Visitor and Community Nurse, 12 (9), Sep 1976, 287-288.

7 Cooper, W. Facts and fancies about menstruation. Journal of Community Nursing, 2 (7), Jan 1979, 16-18.

8 Cooper, W. The fertile years. Hutchinson, 1978.

9 Dalton, K. The curse of Eve. (Hazardous effects of menstruation.) Occupational Health, 28 (3), Mar 1976, 129-133.

10 Dalton, K. Once a month. Fontana, 1978.

11 Dalton, K. Pre-menstrual syndrome. (Interview with Dr. Katharina Dalton by L. Swaffield.) Nursing Times, 76, 6 Mar 1980, 412-413.

12 Dalton, K. The premenstrual syndrome and progesterone therapy. Heinemann, 1977.

13 Dann, T.C. Salpingitis. (Infection of the Fallopian tubes.) Nursing Mirror, 143, 16 Dec 1976, 48-50.

14 Daus, A.D. and Hafez, E.S.E. Candida albicans in women. (A study of 92 pregnant and non-pregnant patients to isolate factors affecting the incidence and severity of vaginal candidiasis.) Nursing Research, 24, Nov-Dec 1975, 430-433.

15 Dening, F.C. Psychosomatic problems in gynaecology. Report on the 5th International Congress of Psychosomatic Obstetrics and Gynaecology. Nursing Mirror, 146, 2 Feb 1978, 7-9.

16 Denniss, R.G. Vaginal bleeding. (Normal and abnormal.) Nursing Times, 73, 30 Jun 1977, 998-1000.

17 Douglas, C.P. Rupture of the uterus. Nursing Times, 73, 17 Feb 1977, 240-242.

18 Field, P.A. and Funke, J. The premenstrual syndrome: current findings, treatment and implications for nurses. Journal of Obstetric, Gynecologic and Neonatal Nursing, 5 (5), Sep/Oct 1976, 23-26.

19 Fong, R. Vaginal discharge: causes and treatment. Nursing Times, 73, 11 Aug 1977, 1256-1257.

20 Fream, W.C. Notes on gynaecological nursing. Churchill Livingstone, 1979.

21 Heywood Jones, I. The curse of Eve. (Myths and taboos surrounding menstruation.) Nursing Times, 76, 6 Mar 1980, 404-406.

22 Heywood Jones, I. The history of sanitary protection. (For use during menstruation.) Nursing Times, 76, 6 Mar 1980, 407-408.

23 Hudson, C.N. The female reproductive system. Churchill Livingstone, 1978. (Penguin library of nursing.)

24 Iveson-Iveson, J. The female reproductive system. (Anatomy and physiology.) Nursing Mirror, 148, 29 Mar 1979, 35-36.

25 Kjervik, D.K. and Martinson, I.M. editors Women in stress: a nursing perspective. New York: Appleton-Century-Crofts, 1979.

26 Langley, F.A. Premalignancy in gynaecology. Nursing Mirror, 142, 29 Jan 1976, 57-58.

27 Mylotte, M. Beaming in on women. (Use of lasers in gynaecology.) Nursing Mirror, 149, 9 Aug 1979, 26-28.

28 Phillips, A. and Rakusen, J. Our bodies ourselves: a health book by and for women. Harmondsworth: Penguin, 1978.

29 Roberts, A. Body fluids. 10. Menstrual fluid. (Physiology and disorders of menstruation.) Nursing Times, 74, 16 Mar 1978, Body fluids, 37-40.

30 Roberts, A. Systems of life. Nos.26-27. Reproduction—2-3. Nursing Times, 73, 3 Feb 1977, (4); 3 Mar 1977, (4).

31 Rockey, J. The management of menstruation in young women with congenital upper limb deficiencies. British Journal of Occupational Therapy, 43 (4), Apr 1980, 132-133.

32 Singleton, V. Division of labour. (Day care gynaecological ward, The Women's Hospital, Liverpool.) Nursing Mirror, 143, 25 Nov 1976, 69-70.

33 Steele, S.J. Amenorrhoea: what a woman fears—infertility or disease. Nursing Mirror, 147, 5 Oct 1978, 46-48.

34 Swaffield, L. Hiding the evidence: a survey of present day writing indicates that the taboos of menstruation are still with us. Nursing Times, 76, 6 Mar 1980, 414-415.

35 Taylor, D. Endometriosis — a gynaecological enigma. Nursing Mirror, 147, 31 Aug 1978, 30-32.

36 Taylor, R.W. and Watson, J.M. Premenstrual tension. (Report on current medical research at St. Thomas' Hospital.) Nursing Mirror, 145, 18 Aug 1977, 39-40.

37 Underhill, R. Gynaecological problems in children. Nursing Times, 72, 27 May 1976, 812-815.

38 Wahl, T.P. and Blythe, J.G. Chemotherapy in gynecological malignancies — and its nursing aspects. Journal of Obstetric, Gynecologic and Neonatal Nursing, 5 (5), Sep/Oct 1976, 9-14.

39 Walters, C.A. and others The association of numerous life changes with cervical dysplasia and metaplasia. Cancer Nursing, 3 (6), Dec 1980, 445-449.

b HYSTERECTOMY

1 Butts, P. Meeting the special needs of your hysterectomy patient: an important role at an important time. (Pre- and postoperative care including patient teaching.) Nursing (U.S.), 9 (11), Nov 1979, 40-47.

2 Cosper, B. and others Characteristics of posthospitalization recovery following hysterectomy. (Research study.) Journal of Obstetric, Gynecologic and Neonatal Nursing, 7 (3), May/Jun 1978, 7-11.

3 Delamothe, K.J. Nursing care study. Hysterectomy. Nursing Times, 74, 6 Apr 1978, 587-590.

4 Hamilton, A. and Kelley, P. An education program for hysterectomy patients. Supervisor Nurse, 10 (4), Apr 1979, 19-21, 25.

5 Hartgill, J. Wertheim's hysterectomy. Nursing Times, 74, 14 Dec 1978, 2061-2063.

6 Iredale, P. Nursing care study. Total abdominal hysterectomy with bilateral salpingo-oophorectomy. Nursing Times, 72, 22 Jul 1976, 1120-1122.

7 Krueger, J.C. and others Relationship between nurse counseling and sexual adjustment after hysterectomy. Nursing Research, 28 (3), May/Jun 1979, 145-150.

8 Moran, S. Vaginal hysterectomy. (Need for counselling and preoperative teaching.) RN Magazine, 42 (4), Apr 1979, 53-54.

9 Need, J. Attitudes to hysterectomy. Australasian Nursing Journal, 5 (1), Jul 1976, 27-29.

10 Phillips, C.R.N. The hysterectomy patient in the obstetrics service: a presurgery class helps meet her needs. Journal of Obstetric, Gynecologic and Neonatal Nursing, 6 (1), Jan/Feb 1977, 45-49.

11 Proops, M. Hysterectomy. (Highlighting the patient's viewpoint with the need for sympathetic advice and explanation.) Nursing Mirror, 143, 16 Sep 1976, 46-47.

12 Ritchie, M.S. Nursing care study. Total hysterectomy and bilateral salpingo-oophorectomy for endometriosis. Nursing Times, 76, 26 Jun 1980, 1133-1136.

13 Stokes, W. Nursing care study. Hysterectomy. Nursing Times, 72, 22 Jan 1976, 100-102.

14 Walker, M. Theatre nursing care study. Total hysterectomy. Nursing Times, 73, 15 Dec 1977, 1952-1954.

c MENOPAUSE

1 Anderton, K.J. Post menopausal oestrogen replacement therapy. Nursing Times, 73, 8 Dec 1977, 1923-1925.

2 Ballinger, C.B. The menopause. Mental health aspects. Royal Society of Health Journal, 96 (2), Apr 1976, 78-81.

3 Cooper, W. Don't write us off as neurotic. (Hormone replacement therapy in the menopause.) Nursing Mirror, 147, 14 Dec 1978, 21-22.

4 Cooper, W. You don't have to put up with menopause problems. (Hormone replacement therapy.) Journal of Community Nursing, 1 (12), Jun 1978, 4-6.

5 Cowper-Smith, F. Hormone replacement in menopause. Nursing Mirror, 142, 19 Feb 1976, 41.

6 Coxon, J.G. Community nursing care study. A cry for help. (Role of health visitor with menopausal woman.) Nursing Times, 74, 23 Mar 1978, 490-491.

7 Dalton, K. The menopause. Nursing Mirror, 145, 17 Nov 1977, 37-38.

8 Dosey, M.F. and Dosey, M.A. The climacteric woman. (Survey in Detroit of responses, medication and counselling during the menopause.) Patient Counseling and Health Education, 2 (1), First Quarter, 1980, 14-21.

9 Griffey, D. The menopause — a new illness? Health Visitor, 49 (5), May 1976, 150.

10 Hotchner, B. Menopause and sexuality: gearing up or down? Topics in Clinical Nursing, 1 (4), Jan 1980, 45-52.

11 Hutton, J. Oestrogens after the menopause. Midwife, Health Visitor and Community Nurse, 14 (5), May 1978, 140, 142.

12 LaRocco, S.A. and Polit, D.F. Women's knowledge about the menopause. (Study of relationship between level of knowledge and characteristics such as education and income.) Nursing Research, 29 (1), Jan/Feb 1980, 10-13.

13 Pedersen, B. and Pendleton, E. Menopause: a welcome or dreaded stage of development. (With history of attitudes and treatment.) Journal of Nurse Midwifery, 23, Fall 1978, 45-51.

14 Royal Society of Health The meaning of menopause. (Royal Society of Health meeting.) Occupational Health, 28 (3), Mar 1976, 138-140.

15 Royal Society of Health Journal The menopause. (Five articles.) Royal Society of Health Journal, 96 (2), Apr, 70-81.

16 Thomson, J. and Oswald, I. Effect of oestrogen on the sleep, mood, and anxiety of menopausal women. British Medical Journal, 2, 19 Nov 1977, 1317-1319.

17 Utian, W.H. The menopause manual: a woman's guide to the menopause. Lancaster: MTP, 1978.

d INFERTILITY

1 Alexander, N.B. and Cotanch, P.H. The endocrine basis of infertility in women. Nursing Clinics of North America, 15 (3), Sep 1980, 511-524.

2 Egerton, P.M. Subfertility: its causes and treatment. (In men and women.) Nursing Times, 74, 29 Jun 1978, 1096-1099.

3 Hall, J.E. Gonadotrophin therapy. (In infertility.) Nursing Times, 73, 25 Aug 1977, 1323-1325.

4 Houghton, P. Society at work. Childless, no choice. New Society, 40, 5 May 1977, 227-228.

5 Keywood, O. An aid to happier families. (Report of study day on artificial insemination by donor.) Nursing Mirror, 146, 18 May 1978, 30.

6 Meredith, R. and Steele, S.J. A sperm bank. (For artificial insemination by donor.) Nursing Mirror, 145, 15 Sep 1977, 20-21.

7 Mocarski, V. The nurse's role in helping infertile couples. Maternal-Child Nursing Journal, 2 (4), Jul/Aug 1977, 264-266.

8 Oyieke, J.B. Improving quality and quantity. (Male infertility.) Nursing Mirror, 150, 19 Jun 1980, 34-36.

9 Pennington, S.W. and Naik, S. Donor insemination: report of a two year study (of AID in NHS). British Medical Journal, 1, 21 May 1977, 1327-1330.

10 Snowden, R. and Mitchell, D. Anonymous AID for the childless couple. (Social implications of AID.) New Scientist, 85, 13 Mar 1980, 828-829.

11 Templeton, A. AID — What are the problems? (Artificial insemination by donor.) Midwife, Health Visitor and Community Nurse, 13 (7), Jul 1977, 208, 210-211.

12 Wiehe, V.R. Psychological reactions to infertility: implications for nursing in resolving feelings of disappointment and inadequacy. Journal of Obstetric, Gynecologic and Neonatal Nursing, 5 (4), Jul/Aug 1976, 28-32.

e MALE GENITAL SYSTEM

1 American Journal of Nursing Programmed instruction. Patient assessment: examination of the male genitalia. American Journal of Nursing, 79 (4), Apr 1979, P.I. 1-24.

2 Blandy, J.P. Benign enlargement of the prostate. Nursing Mirror, 143, 26 Aug 1976, 47-51.

3 Cranston, J.A. Nursing care study. Benign enlargement of the prostate gland. Nursing Times, 74, 11 May 1978, 789-944.

4 Green, A.N. and others Testing the effectiveness of cryosurgery for genital warts in men. Nursing Mirror, 147, 21 Sep 1978, 26-27.

5 Harden, C.L. Nursing care study. Circumcision as a day case. (In seven-year-old boy.) Nursing Times, 75, 2 Aug 1979, 1305-1306.

6 Howatt, J.M. Circumcision. Nursing Times, 72, 16 Sep 1976, 1434-1435.

7 Iveson-Iveson, J. The male reproductive system. Nursing Mirror, 148, 22 Mar 1979, 33-34.

8 Main, J.M. Prostatitis. Nursing Times, 74, 11 May 1978, 787-788.

9 Roberts, A. Systems of life. No.25. Reproduction—1. (Male reproductive system.) Nursing Times, 73, 6 Jan 1977, (4).

10 Tobiason, S.J. Benign prostatic hypertrophy. American Journal of Nursing, 79 (2), Feb 1979, 286-290.

11 Wales, R. Nursing care study. Orchidopexy for bilateral ectopic testes. (In five-year-old boy.) Nursing Mirror, 147, 16 Nov 1978, 36-38.

12 Wood, R.Y. and Rose, K. Penile implants for impotence. American Journal of Nursing, 78 (2), Feb 1978, 234-238.

f SEX

1 Anderton, K.J. Psychosexual problems in gynaecology. 1. Their nature. 2. The way they present. 3. The role of the nurse. Nursing Times, 74, 7 Sep 1978, 1499; 14 Sep 1978, 1537-1538; 21 Sep 1978, 1560.

2 Brant, H.A. The psycho-sexual problems of women. 1. (Physiology of sexual response.) 2. Female sexual dysfunctions. Midwife, Health Visitor and Community Nurse, 14 (1), Jan 1978, 12-13; (3), Mar 1978, 73, 75-76.

3 Cooper, W. The sexual spectrum. (Biological determinants of gender.) Nursing Mirror, 145, 18 Aug 1977, 25-26.

4 Daines, B. and Holdsworth, V. Sexual problems: a pattern of disharmony. (Types of problems in women.) Nursing Mirror, 148, 7 Jun 1979, 28-29.

5 Fong, R. Sexual abnormalities—1. Harmless variations. (Including homosexuality, transvestites and exhibitionism.) 2. Dangerous deviations. Nursing Times, 74, 15 Jun 1978, 1015-1016; 22 Jun 1978, 1062-1063.

6 Hill, S. The child with ambiguous genitalia. (Diagnosis and management.) American Journal of Nursing, 77 (5), May 1977, 810-814.

7 Randell, J. Transsexualism and its management. Nursing Mirror, 144, 24 Mar 1977, 45-47.

8 THE REBIRTH. An account of the treatment of a transsexual by 'John'. Nursing Mirror, 144, 24 Mar 1977, 48-49.

9 Silver, J.R. Disorders of sexual function in diseases of the nervous system. Nursing Mirror, 143, 2 Sep 1976, 58-59.

10 Simone, C.M. The transsexual patient. How you can help toward a successful surgical outcome. (Nursing care.) RN Magazine, 40 (3), Mar 1977, 37-44.

98 RESPIRATORY SYSTEM

a GENERAL AND DISEASES

1 Amborn, S.A. Clinical signs associated with the amount of tracheobronchial secretions. Nursing Research, 25, Mar-Apr 1976, 121-126.

2 Anderson, G. Cor pulmonale. (Hypertrophy of the right ventricle resulting from lung disease.) Nursing Times, 72 (43), 28 Oct 1976, 1666-1668.

3 Ashworth, P. Psychological and social aspects of respiratory care. Nursing, 7, Nov 1979, 295-299.

4 Bailey, R. Drugs and the respiratory system. Nursing, 7, Nov 1979, 315-318.

5 Boyd, D.H.A. The pneumonias. Nursing Times, 73, 11 Aug 1977, 1230-1232.

6 Capel, L.H. Refresher course. Hypostatic pneumonia. Nursing Times, 72 (13), 1 Apr 1976, 485.

7 Cardin, S. Acid-base balance in the patient with respiratory disease. Nursing Clinics of North America, 15 (3), Sep 1980, 593-601.

8 Cobell, R. An 82-year-old man with a highly malignant reticulosis. (With discussion on how patient's needs were met by hospital and community services on p.1178-1179.) Nursing Times, 75, 12 Jul 1979, 1174-1176.

9 Cohen, S. and others Blood gas and acid base concepts in respiratory care. American Journal of Nursing, 76 (6), Jun 1976, P.I. 1-30.

10 Collins, J. Blood gases, rational oxygen therapy, air flow limitations. (Causes of respiratory failure.) Physiotherapy, 62 (2), Feb 1976, 48-52.

11 Cook, F. Refresher course. Bronchoscopy. Nursing Times, 72, 4 Nov 1976, 1718-1719.

12 Coyle, N. and Arbit, E. How to protect your patients against aspiration pneumonia. (Use of Foley catheter with inflated balloon as oesophageal tube, with general advice.) Nursing, 8 (10), Oct 1978, 50-51.

13 D'Agostino, J.S. and Welch, P.L. The phrenic pacemaker. (To stimulate phrenic nerve and cause diaphragm to descend and air to be pulled into lungs.) Nursing (U.S.), 9 (5), May 1979, 41-49.

14 Doyle, J. The intracaval filter: new nursing challenge. (Device to prevent pulmonary embolism.) RN Magazine, 43 (5), May 1980, 38-42.

15 Else, D. A breath of fresh air. (Respiratory protective equipment.) Occupational Health, 31 (8), Aug 1979, 422-425.

16 Evans, C.C. Pneumonia. Nursing, 7, Nov 1979, 320, 322-323.

17 Ewertz, M. and Shpritz, D. Your best strategy when 'shock lung' strikes. RN Magazine, 43 (10), Oct 1980, 43-45.

18 Falotico, J.B. Pulmonary embolism. Don't overlook these subtle warnings. RN Magazine, 42 (2), Feb 1979, 47-52.

19 Froelich, R. Mechanisms underlying respiratory failure. (Physiology, pathology and nursing care.) Journal of Continuing Education in Nursing, 10 (4), Jul/Aug 1979, 31-39.

20 Grossbach-Landis, I. and McLane, A.M. Tracheal suctioning: a tool for evaluation and learning needs assessment. Nursing Research, 28 (4), Jul/Aug 1979, 237-242.

21 Mitchell, D.M. and others Fibreoptic bronchoscopy: ten years on. British Medical Journal, 281, 2 Aug 1980, 360-363.

22 Office of Health Economics Preventing bronchitis. OHE, 1977. (Studies of current health problems, no.59.)

23 Rau, J. and Rau, M. To breathe or be breathed: understanding IPPB. (Intermittent positive pressure breathing.) American Journal of Nursing, 77 (4), Apr 1977, 613-617.

24 Roberts, A. Body fluids, 16. Pleural and pericardial fluid. (Physiology and pleural and pericardial effusion.) Nursing Times, 74, 21 Sep 1978, Body fluids, 61-64.

25 Roberts, A. and Besterman, A. Systems of life. Nos.28-29. Respiration—1-2. Nursing Times, 73, 7 Apr 1977, (4); 5 May 1977, (4).

26 Roberts, A. Systems of life. No.72. Systems and signs. Respiration. 2. Palpation. Nursing Times, 76, 4 Dec 1980, (4).

27 Rowell, M.H. Respiratory diseases. Nursing Mirror, 142, 10 Jun 1976, Nursing care supplement, series 4, i-iv.

28 Siegler, D. The respiratory system. Nursing Mirror, 145-146.
1. Function and structure. 15 Dec 1977, 13-14.
2. Chronic bronchitis and emphysema. 22 Dec 1977, 17-18.
4. Diagnostic procedures. 5 Jan 1978, 28-29.
5. Pneumonia. 12 Jan 1978, 27-28.

29 Sinclair, D.J.M. and Ingram, C.G. Controlled trial of supervised exercise training in chronic bronchitis. (Study supervised by research nurse.) British Medical Journal, 280, 23 Feb 1980, 519-521.

30 Sweetwood, H. Acute respiratory insufficiency: how to recognize this emergency...how to treat it. Nursing, 7 (12), Dec 1977, 24, 26-31.

31 Tang, O.T. Lung function tests. Nursing Times, 72, 22 Jul 1976, 1123-1125.

32 Thompson, K.M. and others Respiratory progress chart. (Record of sputum volume and type, ventilatory function and exercise tolerance used at the St. George Hospital, Sydney.) Physiotherapy, 66 (3), Mar 1980, 88-89.

33 Tobias, M.A. Shock lung. Nursing Times, 73, 10 Mar 1977, 334-336.

34 Weatherstone, R.M. The pattern of pneumonia today. Nursing Mirror, 146, 20 Apr 1978, 22-24.

35 Welch, J. and Lennox, S.C. Treatment of spontaneous pneumothorax. Nursing Times, 75, 22 Feb 1979 , 324-326.

36 Wright, P.H. Respiratory changes

encountered in disease. Nursing Mirror, 145, 15 Dec 1977, 17-18.

b NURSING

1 **Adler, D.C.** Pulmonary nursing, 1900-1979, and future projections. (Caring for TB, poliomyelitis and pneumonia patients.) Heart Lung, 8 (5), Sep/Oct 1979, 882-890.

2 **American Journal of Nursing** Programmed instruction. How to work with chest tubes. American Journal of Nursing, 80 (4), Apr 1980, 685-712.

3 **American Journal of Nursing** Programmed instruction. Pulmonary function tests in patient care. American Journal of Nursing, 80 (6), Jun 1980, 1135-1161.

4 **Atkins, P. and McFadyen, C.** Respiratory nursing. (Two articles on using nurse specialists in community-based project to help patients maintain their independence and to teach children about lung disease.) Canadian Nurse, 74 (1), Jan 1978, 28-31.

5 **Beeharry, A.S.** Nursing care study. Spontaneous pneumothorax. (By a second-year student nurse.) Nursing Times, 75, 13 Dec 1979, 2154-2157.

6 **Bricker, P.L.** Chest tubes the crucial points you mustn't forget. RN Magazine, 43 (11), Nov 1980, 21-26.

7 **Brown, S.E.** Respiratory physiotherapy and the nurse. Nursing, 6, Sep 1979, 257-259.

8 **Chrisman, M.K. editor** Respiratory nursing continuing education review. Flushing: Medical Examination Publishing Co., 1976.

9 **Coady, T.J. and Bennett, A.** Technology in nursing. Respiratory function. Nursing Times, 74.
1. Oxygen administration. 26 Jan 1978, Scan 1-4.
2. Lung volume measurement. 23 Feb 1978, Scan 5-8.
3. Gas transfer and blood gases. 23 Mar 1978, Scan 9-12.
4. Monitoring artificial ventilation. 27 Apr 1978, Scan 13-16.
5. Respiratory failure. 25 May 1978, Scan 17-20.
6. Nebulisers and inhalation therapy. 29 Jun 1978, Scan 21-24.
7. Differential lung function studies. 27 Jul 1978, Scan 25-28.
8. Clinical aspects of inhalation therapy. 28 Sep 1978, Scan 29-32.
9. The clinical use of test results. 26 Oct 1978, Scan 33-36.
10. Challenge testing. 30 Nov 1978, Scan 37-40.
11. Research. 21/28 Dec 1978, Scan 41-44.

10 **Cobell, R.** Nursing care study. A patient with acute exacerbation of chronic bronchitis and congestive cardiac failure. (With discussion on how patient's needs were met by hospital and community services on p.1178-1179.) Nursing Times, 75, 12 Jul 1979, 1176-1178.

11 **Dubree, M. and Vogelpohl, R.** When hope dies—so might the patient. (Study of a patient with pulmonary disease who lost hope and the nursing intervention required.) American Journal of Nursing, 80 (11), Nov 1980, 2046-2049.

12 **Evans, P.M. and Massey, R.M.** Rudiments of care. 4. Helping the patient with respiration. Nursing Times, 75, 28 Jun 1979, 1106-1107.

13 **Glover, D.W. and Glover, M.Mc.** Respiratory therapy: basics for nursing and the allied health professions. St. Louis: Mosby, 1978.

14 **Harson, E.** Nursing care study. Chronic bronchitis: keeping it in the family. (Care by district nurse of elderly lady after discharge from hospital.) Nursing Mirror, 148, 3 May 1979, 44-45.

15 **Hurst, K.** Nursing care study. Cor pulmonale. A major set-back. (Patient who developed acute exacerbation of chronic bronchitis, congestive cardiac failure and polycythaemia. By charge nurse.) Nursing Mirror, 150, 7 Feb 1980, 38-40.

16 **Isacson, L.M. and Schulz, K.** Treating pulmonary edema. (With checklist of nursing care for patients receiving oxygen.) Nursing, 8 (2), Feb 1978, 42-46.

17 **Jackson, E.E.** The administration of respiratory therapy: aerosol therapy, techniques and equipment. American Association of Nurse Anesthetists Journal, 44 (4), Aug 1976, 373-389.

18 **Jarrett, J.** Nursing care study. An elderly patient with bronchopneumonia. Nursing Times, 75, 1 Nov 1979, 1884-1887.

19 **Kiely, T.** Nursing care study. Pneumonia. Chips with everything. (Five-year-old boy. With nursing care plan.) Nursing Mirror, 150, 17 Apr 1980, 40-41.

20 **Lane, C.S.** Skilled care for the pneumothorax patient. Journal of Nursing Care, 3 (2), Feb 1979, 16-17.

21 **Machner, F. and others** Patient assessment. Examination of the chest and lungs. Programmed instruction. American Journal of Nursing, 76 (9), Sep 1976, P.I. 1-23.

22 **Macleod, E. and Robinson, L.** Expanded roles in respiratory nursing. (Two Canadian nurses describe their experience as clinical nurse specialists. Two articles.) Canadian Nurse, 73 (7), Jul 1977, 35-38.

23 **Malkus, B.L.** Respiratory care at home. (Developed by the Hanover Visiting Nurse Association, Pennsylvania.) American Journal of Nursing, 76 (11), Nov 1976, 1789-1791.

24 **Meador, B.** Pneumothorax: providing emergency and long-term care. (With care during chest drainage.) Nursing (U.S.), 8 (11), Nov 1978, 43-45.

25 **Wall, M.** Nursing care study. Spontaneous pneumothorax. Nursing Times, 74, 25 May 1978, 870-872.

26 **Webber-Jones, J.E. and Davis, G.S.** Respiratory assessment guide for nurses. Burlington, Vt.: Vermont Lung Center, 1978.

27 **Wheeler, H.H.** Nursing care study. A patient with chronic bronchitis, emphysema, cor pulmonale and pulmonary embolism. Nursing Times, 76, 31 Jul 1980, 1339-1345.

c ALLERGIC DISEASES

1 **Buisseret, P.** 5. Asthma. Nursing Mirror, 143 (19), 4 Nov 1976, Nursing care supplement, series 3, i-iv.

2 **Crompton, G.K. and others** Edinburgh emergency asthma admission service: report on 10 years' experience. (1968-1978.) British Medical Journal, 2, 10 Nov 1979, 1199-1201.

3 **Ferguson, R.G. and Webb, A.** Childhood asthma: an outpatient approach to treatment. Canadian Nurse, 75 (2), Feb 1979, 36-39.

4 **Frankland, A.W.** Hay fever. Nursing Times, 73, 28 Jul 1977, 1160-1162.

5 **Harrington, V.E.** Philip: an asthmatic child. (Care study by HV with example of nursing care plan.) Nursing, 6, Sep 1979, 273-277.

6 **Hughes, D.** The seven ages of asthma. Nursing Times, 72, 7 Oct 1976, 1550-1552.

7 **Hume, K.M.** Living with asthma in adult life. Chest, Heart and Stroke Association, 1978.

8 **Kuzemko, J.A. editor** Asthma in children: natural history, assessment, treatment and recent advances. Pitman, 1976.

9 **Macleod, W.M.** Bird fanciers' lung disease. (Allergic reaction to dust from birds.) Nursing Times, 73, 17 Nov 1977, 1787-1788.

10 **Office of Health Economics** Asthma. OHE, 1976. (Studies of current health problems, no.57.)

11 **Scott, J.** Nursing care study. Tom: a boy with asthma. (Care of six-year-old boy and his distressed mother.) Nursing Mirror, 147, 13 Jul 1978, 34-36.

12 **Seaton, A.** The Cardiff Asthma Research Unit. Nursing Mirror, 143, 4 Nov 1976, 61-63.

13 **Siegler, D.** The respiratory system. 3. Bronchial asthma. Nursing Mirror, 145, 29 Dec 1977, 22-23.

14 **Speight, A.N.P.** Is childhood asthma being underdiagnosed and undertreated? (Report of survey in Newcastle-upon-Tyne.) British Medical Journal, 2, 29 Jul 1978, 331-332.

15 **Tomlin, P.** Asthma: cooperation between nurse and physiotherapist is essential if the asthmatic patient is to receive the best possible care. Nursing Times, 75, 10 May 1979, 797-798.

16 **Wieczorek, R.R. and Horner-Rosner, B.** The asthmatic child: preventing and controlling attacks. (With illustrations of postural drainage.) American Journal of Nursing, 79 (2), Feb 1979, 258-262.

d OBSTRUCTIVE LUNG DISEASE

1 **Garrett, G.E.R.** Nursing care study. Obstructive airways disease. (Care in the intensive therapy unit.) Nursing Times, 73, 23 Jun 1977, 960-962.

2 **Jacobs, M.M. and Bowers, B.** Protocol: chronic obstructive lung disease. (Nursing assessment and management.) Nurse Practitioner, 4 (6), Nov/Dec 1979, 11, 24-28.

3 **Nethercott, S.** Obstructive airway diseases in children. 5. Clearing a pathway. (Two case studies of children with Pierre-Robin syndrome showing how breathing and feeding difficulties are solved.) Nursing Mirror, 150, 24 Apr 1980, 25-27.

4 Sordelen, S.S. and Jackson, B.S. Nursing decisions. Experiences in clinical problem solving. Series 2 number 5. Dan B. A man with COPD. (Chronic obstructive pulmonary disease.) RN Magazine, 40 (3), Mar 1977, 61-67.

5 Stanley, L. You really can teach COPD patients to breathe better. (Rehabilitation programme for patients with chronic obstructive pulmonary disease.) RN Magazine, 41 (4), Apr 1978, 43-49.

e SURGERY

1 Dacko, M. Periodic deflation of the cuff is less effective. (Care of tracheostomy cuff.) American Journal of Nursing, 77 (4), Apr 1977, 590, 594.

2 Nethercott, S. Obstructive-airway diseases in children. 4. An emergency opening. (Tracheostomy for acute epiglottitis.) Nursing Mirror, 150, 17 Apr 1980, 26-28.

3 O'Donnell, B. and Gilmore, B.B. How to change tracheotomy ties—easily and safely. Nursing, 8 (3), Mar 1978, 66-69.

4 Pagana, K. Teaching your tracheostomy patients to cope at home. RN Magazine, 41 (12), Dec 1978, 63-66.

5 Rexilius, B.G. Chest drainage and suction. Philadelphia: Davis, 1977. (For nurses.)

6 Tym, G. Obstructive airway diseases in children. 1. A new breath of air. (11-month-old with subglottic stenosis who underwent tracheostomy.) Nursing Mirror, 150, 27 Mar 1980, 18-21.

7 Tym, G. Obstructive airway diseases in children. 2. The best birthday present. (Care of child following laryngotracheoplasty.) Nursing Mirror, 150, 3 Apr 1980, 36-37.

8 Tym, G. Obstructive airway diseases in children. 3. A parent needs to know. (Teaching parents to look after a tracheostomy.) Nursing Mirror, 150, 10 Apr 1980, 32-34.

9 Wines, L. Lung complications after surgery. The nurse's place in a prospective survey. Australian Nurses Journal, 5 (5), Nov 1975, 20-21.

f INTENSIVE CARE AND VENTILATION

1 Adams, N.R. The nurse's role in systematic weaning from a ventilator. Nursing (U.S.), 9 (8), Aug 1979, 34-41.

2 Carroll, S.J. Nursing care study. Patient on a ventilator: beyond the speech barrier. (Care of patient with klebsiella pneumonia.) Nursing Mirror, 148, 17 May 1979, 41-43.

3 Chusid, E.L. and others When your patient is on respiratory therapy. Nursing Digest, 4 (3), Summer 1976, 43-46.

4 Coady, T.J. and Bennett, A. Technology in nursing. Respiratory function. 4. Monitoring artificial ventilation. Nursing Times, 74, 27 Apr 1978, Scan 13-16.

5 Drain, C.B. A vigilant you can reverse respiratory distress. (Role of observation in

respiratory intensive care.) RN Magazine, 38 (12), Dec 1975, ICU 7-8, 12.

6 Feldman, S.A. and Crawley, B.E. editors Tracheostomy and artificial ventilation in the treatment of respiratory failure. 3rd ed. Arnold, 1977.

7 Fuchs, P.L. Understanding continuous mechanical ventilation. Nursing (U.S.), 9 (12), Dec 1979, 26-33.

8 Gardiner, B. Our responsibilities to the person beside the respirator. (Importance of nurse-patient communication.) New Zealand Nursing Journal, 71 (2), Feb 1978, 7-11.

9 Garrett, G. Refresher course. Care of the mechanically ventilated patient. Nursing Times, 72, 6 May 1976, 693-694.

10 Goodfield, R. and Spalding, J.M.K. A nurse's guide to artificial ventilation. Arnold, 1976.

11 Kirilloff, L.H. and Maszkiewicz, R.C. Guide to respiratory care in critically ill adults. (Suctioning procedure and tracheostomy care.) American Journal of Nursing, 79 (10), Nov 1979, 2005-2012.

12 Levi, T. Breathing equipment. 1. Oxygen therapy. 2. (Ventilators and humidifiers.) Nursing, 6, Sep 1979, 260-263; 7, Nov 1979, 336-339.

13 Michael, T.A.D. and Gordon, A.S. The oesophageal obturator airway: a new device in emergency cardiopulmonary resuscitation. British Medical Journal, 281, 6 Dec 1980, 1531-1534.

14 Milledge, J.S. Therapeutic fibreoptic bronchoscopy in intensive care. British Medical Journal, 2, 11 Dec 1976, 1427-1429.

15 Moir, J. Intensive care—6. Nursing care of patients on ventilators. Nursing Times, 74, 23 Mar 1978, 492-495.

16 Morrison, M.L. editor Respiratory intensive care nursing. 2nd ed. Boston: Little, Brown and Co., 1979.

17 Moses, R.M. and Steinberg, S. Does the MA-1 respirator make you nervous? (With reference to nursing care of patients on all types of volume ventilators.) RN Magazine, 42 (4), Apr 1979, 35-45.

18 Nursing Times Technology in nursing. Respiratory function. 4. Monitoring artificial ventilation. Nursing Times, 74, 27 Apr 1978, Scan 13-16.

19 Ostrow, L.S. Intensive respiratory care: from ICU to home. (After 3 weeks practice a wife learns to care for her husband on a respirator at home.) American Journal of Nursing, 76 (1), Jan 1976, 111-112.

20 Robinson, W. Breath of life. (Respiratory unit, South Western Hospital, Stockwell.) Nursing Mirror, 144, 17 Mar 1977, 50-52.

21 Skeates, S. Intensive care. 5. Acute respiratory failure. Nursing Times, 74, 16 Mar 1978, 445-447.

22 Sweetwood, H.M. Nursing in the intensive respiratory care unit. 2nd ed. New York: Springer, 1979.

99 URINARY SYSTEM

a GENERAL

1 Anderson, E.R. Women and cystitis. (Prevention and treatment.) Nursing, 77 7 (4), Apr 1977, 50-53.

2 Ashby, P. Refresher course. Haematuria. Nursing Times, 72, 4 Mar 1976, 336.

3 Blandy, J. Urethral stricture in the male. Nursing Mirror, 147, 10 Aug 1978, 13-16.

4 Boyarsky, S. and others Care of the patient with neurogenic bladder. Boston: Little, Brown and Co., 1979.

5 Carbary, L.J. Cystitis: a painful nuisance. Nursing Care, 8 (11), Nov 1977, 24-27.

6 Casewell, M. Urinary tract infection: bacteria danger on the ward. Nursing Mirror, 148, 17 May 1979, 37-39.

7 Cross, P.S. Ureteral reimplantation: nursing care of the child. American Journal of Nursing, 76 (11), Nov 1976, 1800-1803.

8 Dowd, J.B. Methods of urinary diversion. AORN Journal, 23 (1), Jan 1976, 37-44.

9 Fay, J. Nursing care study. Two-level congenital urinary obstruction. (Treatment of hydronephrosis and hydroureter in boy over period of seven years.) Nursing Mirror, 147, 12 Oct 1978, 20-22.

10 Fay, J. Reflux and urinary obstruction. How damage to the child can show up later on. Nursing Mirror, 147, 5 Oct 1978, 41-44.

11 Gaskell, J.D. Résumé of haematuria. Journal of Community Nursing, 1 (5), Nov 1977, 13.

12 Gibson, T. Promoting a steady flow. (Postoperative bladder drainage including bladder irrigation.) Nursing Mirror, 150, 21 Feb 1980, Supplement, xi-xii.

13 Health and Social Service Journal Clean-up. (Three short articles on hospital associated urinary tract infection and methods of prevention.) Health and Social Service Journal, 87, 21 Oct 1977, 1467-1468.

14 Hodgkinson, A. The changing pattern of urinary tract stone disease. Nuring Mirror, 142, 15 Apr 1976, 58-60.

15 Hole, R. Urinary tract infections in women. Nursing Times, 72, 12 Feb 1976, 219-221.

16 Hutchings, J. and Williams, B. Community nursing and psychology, 3: Toilet training: 1—The normal child. Journal of Community Nursing, 2 (3), Sep 1978, 22-23.

17 Iveson-Iveson, J. Students' forum. The urinary system. (Including multiple choice and long answer questions.) Nursing Mirror, 150, 28 Feb 1980, 24-26.

18 Jameson, R.M. The prevention of recurrent urinary tract infection in women. Practitioner, 216, Feb 1976, 178-181.

19 Jameson, R.M. Recurrent urinary tract infection in women. Nursing Mirror, 143, 22 Jul 1976, 55-57.

20 Kinney, A.B. and Blount, M. Effect of cranberry juice on urinary pH. (Suggested preventive or curative measure for patients with recurrent urinary tract infections.) Nursing Research, 28 (5), Sep/Oct 1979, 287-290.

21 Manchester, J. Nursing care study. Psychogenic urine retention. A graded approach. (Treatment with behaviour therapy.) Nursing Mirror, 151, 4 Sep 1980, 48-49.

22 Meers, P.D. and Stronge, J.L. Hospitals . . .should do the sick no harm. 7. Urinary tract infection. Nursing Times, 76, 24 Jul 1980, (4).

23 Mitchell, J.P. Urology for nurses. 3rd ed. Bristol: John Wright, 1980.

24 Nursing Times Four articles on urinary diversion and stoma care. Nursing Times, 74, 23 Nov 1978, 1937-1944.

25 Pattinson, A. Treatment of bladder carcinoma using hydrostatic pressure therapy. Nursing Times, 72, 19 Feb 1976, 249-251.

26 Plourde, M.C. Reflections on urinal diversions. (Nursing care of the stoma patient.) AORN Journal, 23 (1), Jan 1976, 45-51.

27 Roberts, A. Systems of life. No.24. UG 2. Ureters and bladder. Nursing Times, 42, 2 Dec 1976, (4).

28 Roberts, A. Body fluids. Urine. Nursing Times, 73, 15 Dec 1977, Body fluids, 25-28; 74, 19 Jan 1978, Body fluids, 29-32.

29 Rogers, E. Management of the neurogenic bladder and bowel. Queen's Nursing Journal, 19 (5), Aug 1976, 133-135, 138.

30 Scott, E. and others Nursing care study. One-stage urethroplasty. Nursing Mirror, 145, 1 Sep 1977, 16-18.

31 Smith, P. Prostatic and bladder neck syndromes—1. The prostatic syndrome. 2. Bladder neck obstruction. Nursing Times, 74, 8 Jun 1978, 956-960; 15 Jun 1978, 1007-1009.

32 Turner, A.G. Urinary diversion. Journal of Community Nursing, 2 (10), Apr 1979, 20-21, 28.

b NURSING

1 Bray, P.A. and Corry, M.F. Mid-stream urine collection: is preparatory cleansing essential? (Research study.) New Zealand Nursing Journal, 72 (3), Mar 1979, 13-14.

2 Chavigny, K.H. and Nunnally, D.S.M. A comparison of methods for collecting clean-catch urine specimens. Nursing Digest, 4 (4), Fall 1976, 80-83.

3 Culank, L. Detective work in the lab. (Biochemical laboratory tests on urine.) Nursing Mirror, 149, 26 Jul 1979, Supplement, xii, xiv-xv.

4 Fay, J. Colour clues to hidden danger. (Urine testing and collection of specimens for culture.) Nursing Mirror, 149, 26 Jul 1979, Supplement, iii-iv, vi-vii, x, xii.

5 Hatcher, J. Quackery, fraud and scientific method: the history of urine testing. Nursing Mirror, 142 (17), 22 Apr 1976, 65-66.

6 King, M.R. An automatic midstream urine collector. (Developed at Warley Hospital for St. Bartholomew's Hospital Medical College.) Nursing Times, 76, 5 Jun 1980, 1010-1013.

7 Moore, D.S. and Bauer, C.S. Effect of prepodyne as a perineal cleansing agent for clean catch specimens. Nursing Research, 25 (4), Jul/Aug 1976, 259-261.

8 Smith, T.C.G. Specimen testing. Nursing Mirror, 142 (19), 6 May 1976, 57-58.

9 Stronge, J. Infection control audit of a nursing procedure: collection of midstream specimens of urine. Nursing Times, 72 (15), 15 Apr 1976, ICNA Supplement, 27-28.

10 Thomas, S. Excreta. (Including urine testing.) Nursing Mirror, 148, 17 May 1979, 26-28.

11 Winter, C. and Morel, A. Nursing care of patients with urologic diseases. 4th ed. St. Louis: Mosby, 1977.

c INCONTINENCE: GENERAL

1 Age Concern (Greater London) and **Disabled Living Foundation** Improving services for the incontinent adult. Age Concern, 1979.

2 Blannin, J.P. Towards a better life. (Setting up of a nursing management clinic for incontinent patients at Ham Green Hospital, Bristol.) Nursing Mirror, 150, 20 Mar 1980, 31-33.

3 British Medical Journal Incontinence. British Medical Journal, 1, 14 Jan 1979, 61-62.

4 Browne, B. Management for continence. Mitcham: Age Concern, 1978.

5 Clay, E.C. Incontinence of urine. 1. The effects of incontinence on adults and a basis for rehabilitation. 2. (Management based on habit retraining). 3. A regime for retraining. Nursing Mirror, 146, 2 Mar 1978, 14-16; 9 Mar 1978, 36-38; 16 Mar 1978, 23-24.

6 Community Outlook Incontinence. (Three articles and information.) Nursing Times, 75, 13 Sep 1979, Community Outlook, 269-270.

7 Dufault, K. Urinary incontinence: United States and British nursing perspectives. (Review of journal articles.) Journal of Gerontological Nursing, 4 (2), Mar/Apr 1978, 28-33.

8 Hall, M.R.P. Incontinence: treatment of the uninhibited bladder. (Detrusor hyperreflexia.) Nursing Times, 75, 18 Oct 1979, 1806-1808.

9 Hood, N.A. Urinary incontinence. Health Bulletin, 34 (6), Nov 1976, 354-358.

10 Hunter, B. Beginning research. Stress incontinence. (Interviews with sufferers and relationships of stress incontinence to obstetric history.) Nursing Times, 73, 20 Oct 1977, 1636-1639.

11 Iveson-Iveson, J. Incontinence. Report of a day conference held recently by the Kent and Canterbury Hospital and the Disabled Living Foundation. Nursing Mirror, 145, 3 Nov 1977, 8-9.

12 Jay, P. At your convenience. (Ways of coping with incontinence.) Nursing Mirror, 146, 4 May 1978, 44.

13 King, M.R. A study on incontinence in a psychiatric hospital. (In women in psychogeriatric and medium and long-stay wards.) Nursing Times, 75, 5 Jul 1979, 1133-1135.

14 Knox, J.D.E. Ambulant incontinent patients in general practice. (Survey in 17 practices.) Nursing Times, 75, 27 Sep 1979, 1683.

15 Kratz, C. Management of incontinence in the home: the community nurse's view. Nursing Times, 73, 26 May 1977, 798-799.

16 Livesley, B. and Krushner, J.A. Incontinence—knowledge and caring. (Advice for community nurses on its management.) Journal of Community Nursing, 1 (3), Sep 1977, 31-32.

17 Mandelstam, D.A. Incontinence: a guide to the understanding and management of a very common complaint. Heinemann for the Disabled Living Foundation, 1977.

18 Mandelstam, D.A. Notes on incontinence. Disabled Living Foundation, 1978.

19 Mandelstam, D.A. Support for the incontinent patient. Nursing Mirror, 144, 14 Apr 1977, Supplement, xix, xxi, xxiii.

20 Mandelstam, D.A. Urinary incontinence —a new challenge. (Role of nurse in assessment and planning appropriate form of management.) Journal of Community Nursing, 3 (4), Oct 1979, 4-5.

21 Millard, P.H. The promotion of continence. (Through design of environment and patient management.) Health Trends, 1 (11), Feb 1979, 27-28.

22 Reid, E.A. The problem of incontinence. (Nursing Mirror Forum 1976.) Nursing Mirror, 142, 1 Apr 1976, 49-53.

23 Stanton, S.L. Female urinary incontinence. Lloyd-Luke, 1977.

24 Turton, P. Clean sheets: the role of a domiciliary laundry service in the care of the incontinent individual in the community. Nursing Times, 73, 8 Sep 1977, Community Outlook, 41, 43, 45-46.

25 Willington, F.L. The use of non-ionic detergents in sanitary cleansing: a report of a preliminary trial. (To compare the difference between cleansing with soap and non-ionic detergents in incontinent patients.) Journal of Advanced Nursing, 3 (4), Jul 1978, 373-382.

d INCONTINENCE: CATHETERISATION

1 Altshuler, A. and others Even children can learn to do clean self-catheterization. (Children with neurogenic bladder dysfunction master this safe, inexpensive, easy-to-learn procedure.) American Journal of Nursing, 77 (1), Jan 1977, 97-101.

2 Bellfy, L.C. You can improve your catheterized patient's care. RN Magazine, 40 (4), Apr 1977, 33-35.

3 Birley, S. Congenital abnormalities of the kidney. (Catheterisation.) Nursing Mirror, 146, 6 Apr 1978, Supplement, vii, ix, xi, xiii.

4 Champion, V.L. Clean technique for intermittent self catheterization. Nursing Research, 25 (1), Jan-Feb 1976, 13-18.

5 Clark, R. Infection control: a team approach that really works. (Reduction of urinary tract infection in patients with indwelling catheters through interdisciplinary group's programme.) Canadian Nurse, 74 (11), Dec 1978, 16-19.

6 Cule, J. Forerunners of Foley. (History of various types of catheter from 30BC to 1940s.) Nursing Mirror, 150, 21 Feb 1980, Supplement, i-ii, v-vi.

7 Dilley, J. The 'Heavitree' catheter bag holder/garment for geriatric patients. British Journal of Occupational Therapy, 40 (11), Nov 1977, 279-280.

8 Dixon, J. and Smith, P.S. Symposium on teaching methods for the severely subnormal. 3. The use of a pants alarm in daytime toilet training. British Journal of Mental Subnormality, 22 (1), Jun 1976, 20-25.

9 Fay, J. Intermittent non sterile catheterisation of children. Nursing Mirror, 146, 6 Apr 1978, Supplement, xiii, xv.

10 Ferrie, B.G. and others Long-term urethral catheter drainage. (Scheme in Glasgow based on domiciliary care by district nurses.) British Medical Journal, 2, 27 Oct 1979, 1046-1047.

11 Gaskell, J.D. Male catheter care. Queen's Nursing Journal, 18 (10), Jan 1976, 274.

12 Gurevich, I. Selection criteria for closed urinary drainage systems. Supervisor Nurse, 10 (2), Feb 1979, 39-43, 46.

13 Hartman, M. Intermittent self-catheterization: freeing your patient of the Foley. (With patient teaching aid including diagrams.) Nursing (U.S.), 8 (11), Nov 1978, 72-75.

14 Jenner, E.A. Specialised care. 8. A closed system of urinary drainage. Nursing Mirror, 145, 3 Nov 1977, Nursing care supplement, sries 6, i-iv.

15 Jorow, M. How to teach patients to catheterize themselves. RN Magazine, 38 (12), Dec 1975, 19-21.

16 Lancet Catheter-associated urinary-tract infections. Lancet, 2, 11 Nov 1978, 1033-1034.

17 Lapides, J. and others Self-catheterization in urinary tract disease. (Including a method of teaching the patient.) Journal of Practical Nursing, 26 (1), Jan 1976, 25-27.

18 Leonard, P. Catheters—a basic guide. (Fact sheet.) Nursing Times, 76, 10 Apr 1980, Community Outlook, 104-105.

19 Newman, E. 'The use of a double lumen catheter...'. (Technique of catheterizing patients with ileal urinary diversions.) American Journal of Nursing, 77 (4), Apr 1977, 588, 590.

20 O'Connor, G. Catheterization of terminally ill patients. (Procedures at St. Joseph's Hospice, Hackney.) Nursing Mirror, 146, 6 Apr 1978, Supplement, i, iii.

21 Shakeshaft, R. Closed urine drainage: an evaluation of a pre-connected system. (Trial of Bard Cath-Kit which showed that no urinary

infection occurred.) Nursing Times, 74, 7 Dec 1978, Contact, 7-8.

22 Smart, M. and Ali, N. Long-term indwelling catheters—questions nurses ask. (With section on answers to problems on p.115.) Nursing Times, 76, 10 Apr 1980, Community Outlook, 107, 109-110, 115.

23 Stronge, J.L. Infection of the urinary tract associated with catheters. Nursing Times, 72, 18 Mar 1976, 426-427.

24 Wastling, G. Long-term indwelling catheters. Nursing Times, 74, 13 Jul 1978, 1176-1177.

25 Whitfield, H.N. Non-sterile intermittent self catheterisation. Nursing Times, 72, 16 Dec 1976, 1961.

26 Whitfield, H.N. Self-catheterisation. (By patients with neuropathic bladders.) Nursing Mirror, 145, 27 Oct 1977, 38-39.

27 Withycombe, J. and others Intermittent catheterisation in the management of children with neuropathic bladder. Lancet, 2, 4 Nov 1978, 981-983.

28 Wood, R.Y. Catheterizing the patient with an ileal conduit stoma. American Journal of Nursing, 76 (10), Oct 1976, 1592-1595.

29 Woods, P.A. and Guest, E.M. Toilet training the severely retarded: the importance of evaluation. Nursing Times, 76, 1 May 1980, Occ. papers, 53-56.

e INCONTINENCE: OTHER METHODS

1 Barrett, N. Continent vesicostomy: the dry urinary diversion. American Journal of Nursing, 79 (3), Mar 1979, 462-464.

2 Beber, C.R. Freedom for the incontinent. (Evaluation of disposable brief compared with conventional methods.) American Journal of Nursing, 80 (3), Mar 1980, 482-484.

3 Bonnar, J. Silicone vaginal appliance for control of stress incontinence. (Description of device and uses.) Lancet, 2, 3 Dec 1977, 1161.

4 Bradley, C. We're still waiting for the perfect urine drainage bag! (Review of types available and problems arising.) Journal of Community Nursing, 3 (5), Nov 1979, 22-24.

5 Broughton, N. The Kylie. A ward trial of this absorbent drawsheet. Nursing Times, 75, 5 Jul 1979, 1140-1141.

6 Burton, B. Keeping the incontinent patient dry. The benefits of the Kylie absorbent bed sheet, following a study in Australia. Nursing Mirror, 148, 31 May 1979, 25-26.

7 Clay, E.C. Incontinence of urine. 4. Management by protective clothing. Nursing Mirror, 146, 23 Mar 1978, 23-25.

8 Lawson, S.D. and Cook, J.B. Condom urinals. (Preliminary study of their usefulness with patients at the Yorkshire Regional Spinal Injuries Unit.) Nursing Mirror, 145, 1 Dec 1977, 19-21.

9 Patterson, D. and Schuster, P.A. Artificial

urinary sphincter. (A new approach to the treatment of incontinence involving a patient education program at Foothills Hospital, Calgary.) Canadian Nurse, 71 (11), Nov 1975, 27-31.

10 Prinsley, D.M. and Cameron, K.P. A new nursing method for nocturnal incontinence. (Report of trial of Kylie bed sheets.) Australian Nurses Journal, 9 (1), Jul 1979, 52, 55.

11 Shepherd, A.M. and Blannin, J.P. A clinical trial of pants and pads used for urinary incontinence. (Kanga pants and pads, Mölnlycke pants and pads and Sandra pants, A and D pads.) Nursing Times, 76, 5 Jun 1980, 1015-1016.

12 Tam, G. and others A cost-effectiveness trial of incontinence pants. (Trial at Moston Hospital of Kanga and Maxi-plus pants.) Nursing Times, 74, 20 Jul 1978, 1198-1200.

13 Watson, A.C. A trial of Mölnlycke pants and diapers. (With long-stay geriatric patients.) Nursing Times, 76, 5 Jun 1980, 1017-1019.

f INCONTINENCE: CHILDREN

1 Barker, P. Nocturnal enuresis: an experimental study involving two behavioural approaches. International Journal of Nursing Studies, 16 (4), 1979, 319-327.

2 Bradshaw, J. Assistance with laundry: for parents of incontinent children. (Work of the Family Fund.) Nursing Times, 73, 9 Jun 1977, 878-879.

3 Bradshaw, J. Incontinence: a burden for families with handicapped children. Disabled Living Foundation, 1978.

4 Dische, S. The management of bed wetting. Public Health, 90 (3), Mar 1976, 131-133.

5 Drug and Therapeutics Bulletin The management of childhood enuresis. Drug and Therapeutics Bulletin, 15 (7), 1 Apr 1977, 26-28.

6 Evans, P.R. The treatment of enuresis in childhood. Nursing Mirror, 142, 25 Mar 1976, 62-63.

7 Hutchings, J. and Williams, B. Community nursing and psychology: bedwetting. Journal of Community Nursing, 1 (10), Apr 1978, 10-11.

8 Meadow, R. Diseases of the urinary system. Urinary incontinence in children. British Medical Journal, 2, 27 Aug 1977, 567-568.

9 Meadow, R. How to use buzzer alarms to cure bed wetting. (In children.) British Medical Journal, 2, 22 Oct 1977, 1073-1075.

10 Meadow, R. Problems of micturition in childhood. Nursing Mirror, 143, 16 Sep 1976, 59-61.

11 Peckham, C. Towards dry nights. (Nocturnal enuresis in children.) Health and Social Service Journal, 87, 16 Dec 1977, 1712.

12 Reilly, M. An enuresis clinic. (At St. James's Health Centre, Walthamstow.) Health Visitor, 53 (6), Jun 1980, 216, 219.

13 Shaffer, D. Nocturnal enuresis. Nursing Times, 72, 22 Apr 1976, 616-618.

g INCONTINENCE: ELDERLY

1 **Brocklehurst, J.C.** The causes and management of incontinence in the elderly. Nursing Mirror, 144, 14 Apr 1977, Supplement, xi, xiii, xv, xvii.

2 **Helps, E.P.W.** Diseases of the urinary system. Urinary incontinence in the elderly. British Medical Journal, 2, 17 Sep 1977, 754-757.

3 **Isaacs, B. and Hayward, C.** The management of urinary incontinence in departments of geriatric medicine. (Questionnaire survey.) Health Trends, 11 (2), May 1979, 42-44.

4 **King, M.R.** Treatment of incontinence. (Research study with psychogeriatric patients into effectiveness of methods of promoting continence.) Nursing Times, 76, 5 Jun 1980, 1006-1010.

5 **Lauder, M.** First, find your patient... (Advice for community nurse on discovering and helping the elderly with incontinence, with list of suppliers of aids and sources of information on p.5-6.) Journal of Community Nursing, 2 (5), Nov 1978, 4, 34.

6 **Lepine, A. and others** The incidence and management of incontinence in a home for the elderly. (Survey based on questionnaire and modified Crichton-Royal Behavioural Rating Scale.) Health and Social Service Journal, 89, 27 Apr 1979, Centre eight papers, E9-E12.

7 **Lowthian, P.** The elderly: a challenge to nursing—5. Frequent micturition and its significance. Nursing Times, 73, 17 Nov 1977, 1809-1813.

8 **McDonnell, P.** Promoting continence in psychogeriatric patients. Nursing Times, 76, 5 Jun 1980, 1014-1015.

9 **Mandelstam, D.A.** Incontinence (in the elderly). Physiotherapy, 62 (6), Jun 1976, 182-184.

10 **Mandelstam, D.A.** Incontinence: the mop-and-bucket approach is dead. (Review of eight aids.) Geriatric Medicine, 9 (4), Apr 1979, 30-34.

11 **Masterton, G. and others** The prevalence of incontinence in local authority homes for the elderly. (Research study.) Health Bulletin, 38 (2), Mar 1980, 62-70.

12 **Moore-Smith, B.** A vital balance. (Incontinence with special reference to the elderly.) Nursing Mirror, 151, 10 Jul 1980, 36-38.

13 **Schwartz, D.R.** Personal point of view—a report of seventeen elderly patients with a persistent problem of urinary incontinence. (Pilot study to discover patients' reactions to incontinence and possible care plans.) Health Bulletin, 35 (4), Jul 1977, 197-204.

14 **Smith, T.C.C.** Dignity from disaster. (Incontinence in the elderly.) Queen's Nursing Journal, 19 (3), Jun 1976, 74, 76.

15 **Willington, F.L. editor** Incontinence in the elderly. Academic Press, 1976.

AUTHOR INDEX

American Association of Industrial Nurses 26c2, 71b1, 71b2, 71b3, 71b4
American Association of Nephrology Nurses and Technicians 85d1
American Association of Occupational Health Nurses 5c2, 8c2, 71b5, 71b6, 71d1, 71f1
American Hospital Association 9b3, 66a2
American Journal of Nursing 1a1, 5b1, 5c3, 6a2, 7a1, 15a2, 15d1, 22c1, 26b2, 26b3, 28k26, 28k27, 28k28, 31d1, 34f1, 39i1, 40e1, 45d2, 52a3, 58a4, 58d2, 59b1, 68c1, 69c1, 71b7, 79e1, 79f1, 79h1, 82d1, 82f1, 83a1, 83d2, 84a1, 89b1, 89g1, 89g2, 90a1, 91e1, 92f1, 93d2, 94a1, 94c1, 97e1, 98b2, 98b3
American Nurses Association 1c1, 4a2, 5c4, 5c5, 5c6, 6a21, 12a1, 12a2, 12c1, 12c2, 12c3, 27b3, 27b4, 27b5, 27b6, 28k29, 28k30, 65b3
American Nurses' Foundation 6a3
American Society of Hospital Pharmacists 58e1
Ames, R.P. 19d1
Ames Company 89f1
Amies, E. 87a2
Amis, R.H. 70a1
Ammentorp, W. 11e6
Amoako, D. 47d8
Amonsen, S. 58d3
Amortegui, A.J. 66e1
Amos, A. 61d1
Amos, G. 31c1
Anders, R.L. 43c1, 77h2
Andersen, J. 41a1
Anderson, A. 36c1
Anderson, A.M. 52e4
Anderson, B. 31i1, 31p2
Anderson, C. 43d3
Anderson, C.J. 55c1
Anderson, C.M. 49e1
Anderson, E.M. 49f1, 58a5
Anderson, E.R. 99a1
Anderson, F. 52a4, 52a5, 52a6, 54a3
Anderson, G. 98a2
Anderson, G.C. 45e19
Anderson, I. 84k1
Anderson, J.A.D. 32g1
Anderson, J.L. 19e2
Anderson, J.M. 48c11
Anderson, M. 12k2, 12k3
Anderson, M.H. 21d1
Anderson, M.L. 15e1
Anderson, N. 27d2
Anderson, N.D. 15a3
Anderson, N.E. 21h1
Anderson, R. 29b2, 35c14
Anderson, W. 57h2
Anderson, W.A. 32e2, 70h1
Anderson, W.F. 52a7
Anderton, J.L. 96a1
Anderton, K.J. 97c1, 97f1
Andreoli, K.G. 20j1, 84b1
Andreou, A. 96a2
Andrew, R. 67d1
Andrews, A. 2 56
Andrews, A.P. 5f1
Andrews, C.T. 31i47
Andrews, F.J. 82g1
Andrews, G.A. 12k4
Andrews, G.M. 51f1
Andrews, J. 30c5
Andrews, K. 52f1, 62c4, 94d3, 94e1
Andrews, M. 10a4
Andrews, S.J. 64b1
Andrews, S.W. 42b1
Andrianos, A.F. 67c2
Andrysiak, T. 82c1
Ange, D.R.W. 96c1
Anger, D. 96c1
Angerami, E.L.S. 13d3
Angus, M. 25b1
Angus, M.D. 22b2
Anionwu, E.N. 90b1, 90b2
Ankers, B. 77c26

Ankers, W.B. 77c27
Anna, D.J. 6c3
Annandale-Steiner, D. 7d2, 9e1
Anne (pseud) 79h2
Ansell, C. 39e1
Ansell, C.J. 46a2
Ansell, J.M. 85l1
Ansell, O. 93f1
Ansett, M. 33c13
Anson, D. 30a1
Anspach, W.E. 66a9
Anstey, O. 5a4, 28d1, 28d2
Anthony, M.F. 29n2
Antrobus, M. 73e1, 85a1
Anwar, M. 34d3, 67e2, 88d1, 91a1, 94e2
Aoki, F.Y. 85g1
AORN Journal 4c1, 5d2, 5d3, 23c1, 27d1, 41e1, 51d1, 59c1, 63f1, 63g2, 64b2, 64b3, 65d1, 65d2, 65d3, 65d4, 66a3, 66d2, 66d3, 66e2, 66e3, 66e4
AORN Nursing Research Committee 65b1
Apley, J. 49a1, 51c1, 87f1
Aplin, S. 19j1
Apostoles, F.E. 75i1
Appelbaum, A.L. 6a4, 15c3
Apple, J.L. 58c1
Applegate, J. 40e2
Applegate, M. 20c5, 22b30
Appleton, P. 51e1
Applewhite, K. 58c2
Appleyard, J. 29i1
Apps, M.C.P. 17a1
Aragon, L.M. 6b1
Arakelian, M. 6c4
Arangio, A.J. 93g1
Arbit, E. 98a12
Archard, P. 38c5
Archbold, C.R. 26g2
Archbold, P.G. 54c1
Archer, A. 28b1
Archer, C.R. 85l2
Archer, R. 15b2, 67g1
Archer, S.E. 33c4, 33c5, 34c1
Archibald, E.J. 17e5
Archibald, R.M. 73e2
Ardis, M. 70h2
Arekalian, M. 52a8
Arford, P.H. 14a30
Argue, Z. 22b3
Arie, T. 52g1, 55c10, 94d28
Aries, J.M. 63a1
Arkhangelsky, G.V. 13a1
Arlidge, J.T. 70a2
Armand Smith, N.G. 72c1
Armenaki, D.W. 82a16
Armfield, J. 29h1
Armiger, B. 20j3, 27c1
Armignacco, F. 54a46
Armitage, B.E. 47d1
Armitage, M. 54a4
Armitage, P.A. 23c2
Armitage, S. 15a4, 16a3
Armour, C. 49f2
Armstrong, A.A. 44d1
Armstrong, D.M. 65d5
Armstrong, J. 29i2, 34e1, 58d7, 81d2, 81h1
Armstrong, K. 82f2
Armstrong, M. 92h1
Armstrong, M.E. 19a1, 57f2
Armstrong, P. 57h3
Armstrong, R.F. 63g3
Armstrong-Esther, C.A. 8e9, 20e4, 79d1, 87b39, 87b40, 92h2
Arndt, C. 10b2
Arndt, G. 21g10
Arndt, K. 62b1
Arne, S. 11d1
Arnold, A. 57c1, 85n1
Arnold, J. 21a1
Arnold, J.P. 54g3
Arnold, N. 3a1, 9a3, 30e2
Arnold, P.J. 32a1
Arnold, R. 64c1, 65a2

Arnott, E.J. 95a24
Arokianathan, A. 85l3
Aronson, S.P. 85a2
Arora, P. 28h37
Aroskar, M.A. 5c7, 5c8, 5c24, 20c2
Arroyave, F. 38c6
Arthritis and Rheumatism Council 91d1
Arthur, H. 38d1
Arthur, J. 44b2
Arthur, L.J.H. 51c2
Arthure, H. 39h1, 39h2, 40c2, 42e1
Artinian, B.M. 27d2
Arton, M. 57d1
Artz, C.P. 68a1
Ashby, D.J. 31d12
Ashby, P. 99a2
Ashford, N.A. 70a3
Ashikaga, T. 34c24
Ashley, A. 51e2
Ashley, J. 4a3
Ashley, J.S.A. 31c2
Ashley, M.J. 24c30
Ashton, J. 32d1, 79b1
Ashton, J.R. 29d4, 32a2, 43a2, 74c2, 79k1, 80a1
Ashton, K. 1d1, 7d3, 7d4, 8b2, 8f1, 12c4, 14a3, 15b3, 16c1, 28e75, 29j1, 30e3, 33a1, 35a2, 38c7, 39f1, 45b1, 52b1, 66a4, 67a1, 77c15, 81e8, 82b2, 93b1
Ashton, R. 39c1
Ashton, R.M. 44g2, 44g3
Ashton, W.D. 38h2
Ashworth, N.W. 73h2
Ashworth, P. 12b1, 12b2, 14a4, 16b2, 17a2, 17f2, 17f3, 98a3
Ashworth, W. 29b3, 30c6
Asken, M.J. 63e4
Aslam, M. 28b6, 34d10, 58e2, 79c1
Asperheim, M.K. 58a6
Aspinall, M.J. 12g2, 12g3, 12g4, 66a5
Aspy, V.H. 12a3
Association of British Paediatric Nurses 44a2, 44b3, 47b1, 47b2, 47b3, 48a3, 48f1
Association of Chief Administrators of Health Authorities 29f1
Association of Directors of Social Services 30b23
Association of Health Service Treasurers Research Committee 29d5
Association of Independent Hospitals and Kindred Organisations 29m1
Association of Integrated and Degree Courses in Nursing 6c5, 16b3, 20a5, 24a2
Association of Nurse Administrators 10a5, 10a6, 30a2, 81g3
Association of Operating Room Nurses 65a3, 65b2, 65b3
Association of Professions for the Mentally Handicapped 50b10, 81a1, 81a2
Association of Psychiatric Nurse Tutors (Scotland) 75g2
Association of Religious Nursing Sisters 18a1
Association of Scientific Technical and Managerial Staffs 82j2
Association of Sterile Supply Administrators 66c2
Astin, E.W. 48d1
Aston, G. 7d5, 80b2
Aston, S. 68b1
Astor, A. 75d1
Atack, S.M. 62f5
Atchison, E. 13a20
Atherley, G. 70j1
Atherley, G.R.A. 70i1
Atherley, G.R.C. 67a2, 70c1
Atkin, M.E. 82i1
Atkins, J. 86a3
Atkins, P. 98b4
Atkinson, A.B. 38h3
Atkinson, F.I. 27a1
Atkinson, J. 43a3
Atkinson, L. 62c5
Atkinson, L.D. 46b1

Rosenblum, E.H. 88d15
Rosenburgh, S.P. 59b37
Rosenkoetter, M.M. 65d40
Rosenman, H. 58c26
Rosenthal, C.J. 15a51
Rosenthal, W.P. 10b9
Rosenthall, G. 76a7, 76a8
Roskell, V. 89f14
Roskies, R. 48d19
Rosmann, J. 29n40
Ross, B.C. 73f17
Ross, C.W. 19e37
Ross, D. 70a22, 95d16
Ross, D.G. 31d2, 92h18
Ross, D.S. 70f21, 73a8, 73b10, 73d5, 73e12, 91a26, 95e10, 95e11
Ross, E.M. 45b28, 93g27, 93g28, 93g29
Ross, F. 32b30, 35c10
Ross, G.R. 22c39
Ross, H.K. 34c18
Ross, J. 50b17
Ross, J.E. 94a35
Ross, J.R.W. 57a5
Ross Laboratories 15c39
Ross, M. 10a42, 12g30
Ross, M.C. 22c39
Ross, M.S. 34c18
Ross, T. 7b17, 24a27, 28e70, 30f17, 39c32, 39d13, 39d14, 39d15, 43a17, 44d50, 45f50, 49b39, 57c22, 57f23, 57f24, 61a24, 61f23, 73h13, 74a24, 74c27, 77c14, 88d16
Rossler, L.M. 33b14
Rossman, M. 90a33
Rosswurm, M.A. 25b17
Rostron, J. 56a36, 56c15, 56c16, 56c17, 56c18, 56c19, 56c20
Rostron, P.M. 56a36, 56c19, 56c20
Rotatori, A.F. 89h11, 89i7
Rotenberg, A. 9e19, 9e20, 22a13
Roth, A. 9a26, 73i8
Roth, A.V. 9a30
Roth, B.G. 1e30
Rothenstein, L. 40a33
Rotherham, F. 38d36
Rothfeder, B. 45e21
Rothwell, H. 40b20
Rothwell, M.G. 34c19
Rotkovitch, R. 10a43, 10e35, 14a40, 24b38
Rotter, K. 88c17
Rottkamp, B.C. 5b18, 94c33
Rouch, R.E. 39h17
Rouhani, G.C. 12a34, 79f22
Rousin, S. 5c53
Rouslin, S. 44d51
Routh, J.I. 57d11, 57i10
Routledge, L. 44c41
Roux, J.P. 28f35
Rowden, R. 30e18, 77c32
Rowe, B. 15c25, 93f9
Rowe, D. 79e20
Rowe, J. 54d34, 79f23, 92a27
Rowe, R.C. 32a49
Rowe van Ort, S. 60 33
Rowe, W. 22c40
Rowell, M.H. 98a27
Rowland, B. 10b69
Rowland, H.S. 10b69
Rowland, S. 63e7
Rowlands, E.E. 75d5
Rowley, A. 32d14
Rowntree, G.R. 70h21
Rowntree, T. 87b31
Rowsell, G. 8c34
Roy, C. 6c62, 6c66, 6c67, 14b38, 20a38
Royal Association for Disability and Rehabilitation 56c21
Royal Australian Nursing Federation 28i38, 28i39
Royal College of General Practitioners 30b54, 32c23, 42d30, 51c47
Royal College of Midwives 3b23, 8g18, 8g19, 30b55, 30c54, 39c33, 39c34, 39c35, 39c36, 39c37, 39g17, 44a64, 58d26

Royal College of Midwives (Scottish Board) 30b56
Royal College of Nursing 3a21, 3a22, 3a23, 3a24, 3a25, 3a26, 4a34, 5a72, 5a73, 5c54, 5c55, 5e15, 5f29, 5h22, 5h23, 5h24, 5h25, 5h26, 5h27, 5h28, 5h29, 5h58, 5h59, 6a45, 6a46, 6a47, 6a48, 7c7, 7d58, 7d59, 7d60, 7d61, 8f32, 8g20, 9k17, 9k23, 9l11, 9l12, 12b45, 12b46, 12c83, 14a41, 16d34, 20j39, 23b10, 23b11, 26a10, 27c13, 28e39, 28e55, 28e65, 28e71, 28e74, 28e79, 28e86, 28e108, 29d70, 29d71, 29d72, 29f49, 29n41, 30b57, 30b58, 30b59, 30c35, 30c55, 30c56, 30e49, 30e50, 30e51, 32b31, 34b24, 34b25, 35a29, 42c32, 42c33, 43d17, 44a65, 44a66, 53a40, 58c27, 63h6, 63h7, 65e9, 81g40, 85b28, 87a31, 87h39
Royal College of Physicians 38h24, 70j34, 84a9, 88f29
Royal College of Physicians of Edinburgh 11b28
Royal College of Physicians of London 52a44, 73h14
Royal College of Psychiatrists 38c49, 77f28, 77h36, 79c33
Royal Commission on the National Health Service 16c17, 30b5, 30c1, 30c2, 30c61, 32b32
Royal Free Hospital 90c14
Royal Institute of Public Health and Hygiene 72a36, 83b20
Royal Society 28a24
Royal Society for the Prevention of Accidents 70j35
Royal Society of Health 20e18, 34d36, 34f25, 67c19, 97c14
Royal Society of Health Journal 29b43, 29g33, 32a50, 32h7, 38a23, 38c50, 51f20, 52a45, 54a45, 56d19, 56d20, 67c20, 73d6, 74b30, 81c20, 88f14, 97c15
Royal Society of Medicine 58c28, 58e26
Royal Victoria Hospital Belfast 69b20
Roylance, P.J. 67d4
Roys, P.J. 29a41
Royston, P. 28g18
Royston, R. 51b13
Rozendal, N.A. 78b12
Roznoy, M.S. 15e27
Rozovsky, L.E. 6a49, 16d35
Rubel, M. 12b47
Ruben, H. 67d17
Ruben, M. 95d17, 95d18
Rubenstein, R. 61d37, 73c21
Rubin, R. 27a48, 27f29, 44f30, 44f31
Rubin, S. 30d33
Rubin, S.G. 29f47
Ruch University 5a74
Ruckley, C.V. 63c9
Rudd, T.N. 52e32, 52e33, 53a41
Ruddick, N. 80a35
Ruddick-Bracken, H. 35b57, 35b58
Ruddock, R. 21f7
Rude, N.V. 27f18
Ruffing, M.A. 20b36
Ruiz, J.S. 75d9
Rule, J. 20a39
Rule, J.B. 5c56, 12c84
Rumbold, G. 35b14, 35b59
Rumfelt, J.J.M. 47b37
Rumney, S. 38a24
Rumpler, C.H. 17f22
Rumsey, J.M. 23c17
Runciman, P.J. 10j17
Runnerstrom, L. 39e26
Runswick, H. 32e49
Rush, A.M. 87h40
Rushton, A. 34e10
Rushton, E.A. 58d27
Rushton, H. 86a38
Russell, D.A. 54h32
Russell, D.H. 77g30
Russell, E.M. 54d20
Russell, G. 49e15, 88c18

Russell, H.J. 67c22
Russell, M. 26g30, 46d5
Russell, M.A.H. 38h18
Russell, M.L. 25a6
Russell, P. 49a17, 49c18
Russell, R. 86a39
Russell, S. 70b7
Russell, W. 45f51
Russo, B.A. 87b32
Russo, P.M. 19i13
Rustin, G.J.S. 82a24
Ruston, R. 56b33
Rutherford, W. 69b21
Ruthven, H. 34a21
Rutter, D.M. 16a38
Rutter, L. 61d36
Rutter, M. 51a14
Rutter, N. 45c28
Rutter, P.C. 59b38
Ryall, R.J. 87b56
Ryan, B.J. 57f25
Ryan, D. 41b11, 60 74
Ryan, J.E. 31k16, 53c12
Ryan, L.J. 75b18
Ryan, M. 28e93, 28e94, 28e95, 29l28, 30a37, 49a18
Ryan, P. 66c11, 80b14
Ryan, R. 83b21
Ryce, S.W. 74c9, 78a40
Rycroft, R.J. 86a40, 86a41
Ryden, M.B. 20c24, 22c41
Rye, D. 8b45
Ryland, R.K. 79f24

SA Nursing Journal 4d25, 28f36, 57c24, 69a35
Saarmann, S.M.V.L. 11e43
Saba, V.K. 1c16
Sabel, C. 8b46, 8f33, 29f50
Sabey, B. 67g24
Sabo, B. 63g18
Sabulsky, D.J. 81h24
Sachdev, Y. 57b12
Sachs, B.L. 96f19
Sachs, H. 34a22
Sackett, D.L. 83d43
Sackett, J. 80a34
Sackheim, G. 57d12, 57i11
Sacks, S.H. 46b51
Sadik, A.M. 7a32
Sadler, C. 45e22
Sadler, P.D. 83g16
Safier, G. 4a35, 4b18
Sager, D.P. 58d28
Sai, F.T. 42a12
Sail, L. 48a34
Sail, T. 48a34
Sainsbury, M.J.C. 15a52, 16d36
Saint-Yves, I. 6a50, 32b33, 32b34, 33b21
Sainty, A. 74a25
Salariya, E.M. 46b52
Salkind, M.R. 32b35, 32d15
Saller, D.M. 71b19, 71b20
Salmon, B. 10i8, 28i62, 31e21
Salmon, M.A. 93d28, 93d29
Salmond, G. 28i63, 34a23, 39e27
Salmond, S.W. 15c40, 61c21
Salotti, R.A. 71f12
Salter, A. 41a59
Salter, M. 87h41
Saltman, B.M. 34a24
Salvage, J. 7d62, 8e11, 9e21, 25d8, 28k80, 29d73, 29f51, 30c57, 30c58, 67a35, 72c17, 77d19
Samaras, J.T. 8c35, 11c16
Samaritans 79k19
Samborsky, V. 15c41
Sambrook, M.A. 93g30, 94b6
Sampson, C. 5c57, 22b44
Sampson, D. 96f20
Sams, C.A. 49e16
Samson, J.P. 28f37
Samuel, S.A. 21a30